Computed Tomography
and Magnetic Resonance of the Thorax

Third Edition

Computed Tomography and Magnetic Resonance of the Thorax

Third Edition

David P. Naidich, M.D.
Professor
Department of Radiology
Chief, Thoracic Imaging
New York University Medical Center/Bellevue Hospital
New York, New York

Nestor L. Müller, M.D., Ph.D.
Professor
Department of Radiology
University of British Columbia
Deputy Chief and Associate Head for Academic Affairs
Department of Radiology
Vancouver Hospital and Health Sciences Centre
Vancouver, British Columbia, Canada

Elias A. Zerhouni, M.D.
Professor and Chairman
Department of Radiology
Johns Hopkins University School of Medicine
Baltimore, Maryland

Contributing Author
Georgeann McGuinness, M.D.
Assistant Professor
Department of Radiology
New York University Medical Center/Bellevue Hospital
New York, New York

W. Richard Webb, M.D.
Professor
Department of Radiology
Chief, Thoracic Imaging
University of California, San Francisco
San Francisco, California

Glenn A. Krinsky, M.D.
Assistant Professor
Department of Radiology
New York University Medical Center
New York, New York

Stanley S. Siegelman, M.D.
Professor
Department of Radiology
Johns Hopkins University School of Medicine
Baltimore, Maryland

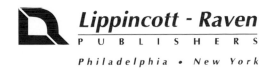
Lippincott - Raven
PUBLISHERS
Philadelphia • New York

Acquisitions Editor: Joyce-Rachel John
Developmental Editor: Brian Brown
Manufacturing Manager: Dennis Teston
Production Manager: Cassie Moore
Production Editor: Rosemary Palumbo
Cover Designer: David Levy
Indexer: Anne D. Cope
Compositor: Maryland Composition Co., Inc.
Printer: Quebecor Printing/Kingsport Press

Printed and bound in the United States of America

9 8 7 6 5 4 3 2 1

Library of Congress Cataloging-in-Publication Data

Computed tomography and magnetic resonance of the thorax/David P.
    Naidich . . . [et al.].—3rd ed.
       p. cm.
     Rev. ed. of: Computed tomography and magnetic resonance of the
thorax/David P. Naidich, Elias A. Zerhouni, Stanley S. Siegelman.
© 1991.
     Includes bibliographical references and index.
     ISBN 0-7817-1660-8
     1. Chest—Tomography. 2. Chest—Magnetic resonance imaging.
I. Naidich, David P.
     [DNLM: 1. Radiography, Thoracic. 2. Thorax—pathology.
3. Tomography, X-Ray Computed. 4. Magnetic Resonance Imaging. WF
975C7379 1999]
RC941.N27 1999
617.5′40757—dc21
DNLM/DLC
for Library of Congress   98-36942
                                 CIP

To my wife Jocelyn and my son Zachary
D.P.N.

To my wife Teresa, my children Emma,
Sonny, and Andy, and to my parents
W.R.W.

To Ruth, Alison, and Phillip
N.L.M.

To Stacie, Emma, and Reginald
G.A.K.

To Nadia, Djillali, Yasmin, and Adam
E.A.Z.

To the memory of Charles Siegelman
S.S.S.

Contents

Preface to the First Edition

Diagnostic imaging has undergone a profound and astonishingly rapid transformation over the last decade, paralleling the rapid evolution of modern computer science. The first computed tomography (CT) unit, conceived and developed by Godfrey Hounsfield, underwent initial clinical testing at the Atkinson Morley Hospital, Wimbledon, England, in 1971. This early scanner employed two sodium iodide crystals and produced an image based on an 80×80 matrix. The scan time of four and one half minutes effectively limited the machine to examination of intracranial pathology.

Within three years, Ledley developed a CT unit capable of imaging the body. In 1974 and 1975, whole body scanner prototypes were installed first at the Cleveland Clinic, then at the Malinckrodt Institute of Radiology and the Mayo Clinic. Initial reports from these institutions were enthusiastic about the role of CT in the evaluation of the pancreas, liver, and retroperitoneum, but pessimistic about the value of CT in the thorax.

Further improvements in instrumentation were necessary in order to assess the clinical role of thoracic CT. The pace of technological innovation was such that by 1977, scanners capable of scan times shorter than breath-holding had been developed. Additional improvements, including more detectors to increase resolution and finer collimation allowing a reduction in slice thickness to minimize partial volume averaging, soon became standard. As a result, initial pessimism about the role of CT in the thorax quickly gave way to considerable enthusiasm. This first became apparent as reports of the value of CT in analyzing mediastinal disease were published. Thereafter, an ever-expanding range of uses for thoracic CT has evolved and continues to evolve.

In December 1977, a CT scanner was installed at the Johns Hopkins Hospital. At that time, Drs. Naidich and Zerhouni were residents under the tutelage of Dr. Siegelman, under whose auspices the three authors of this volume enthusiastically began a series of studies concerning the utility of thoracic CT in a wide range of clinical settings. In July 1980, Dr. Naidich joined the staff at New York University Medical Center, and in January 1981, Dr. Zerhouni moved to the East Virginia Medical Center. Despite this separation, the team continued their collaborative endeavors, and in 1982 and 1983 presented instructional courses in chest CT at the annual meeting of the American Roentgen Ray Society. From these presentations, the need for a volume representing the current status of thoracic CT became apparent.

This textbook has been organized primarily around the major anatomic subunits of the thorax. These include: the mediastinum, the airways, the hila, the pulmonary parenchyma, the pleura, and the chest wall, the pericardium, and the diaphragm. Additional chapters have been added specifically on the role of CT in evaluating lobar collapse and the pulmonary nodule, as these represent discrete topics best addressed apart. This organizational scheme represents the authors' view that CT is primarily an anatomic imaging modality. Specifically excluded from consideration is the use of CT in evaluating the heart. It is only appropriate to consider cardiac CT in comparison to other cardiac imaging modalities, including angiography, echocardiography, and nuclear cardiology. It is the authors' feeling that this is outside the intended scope of the present volume as initially conceived.

Thoracic CT has become an integral part of the daily practice of radiology. With the ever-increasing number of diagnostic modalities, the task of deciding which diagnostic test is the most appropriate for a given clinical problem has become a significant part of medical practice. The authors believe that an adequate understanding of clinical issues is necessary for practicing radiologists to best help the referring physician. Consequently, throughout the text, a strong emphasis has been placed on discussing CT as it relates to clinical issues, especially as compared to other routine imaging modalities. It is to be anticipated that further technologic advances in diagnostic imaging will further complicate the role of radiologists. It is hoped that this text will prove valuable in assisting this process.

David P. Naidich
Elias A. Zerhouni
Stanley S. Siegelman

Preface to the Third Edition

It has been seven years since the second edition and 14 years since the first edition of *Computed Tomography of the Thorax* appeared in 1984. Needless to say, the recent introduction of volumetric (helical/spiral) computed tomography (CT), coupled with continued improvements in the quality of magnetic resonance (MR), especially MR angiography, have once again transformed the art of thoracic imaging. Mitigating the many challenges arising from the undertaking of a new edition of this book has been the ability of the original authors to collaborate with some extraordinary friends, both old and new.

Despite changes, the original intent of the first and second editions remains: namely, to provide within a single text a review of the current status of CT and MR for evaluating diseases of the thorax. For this purpose, the text has again been organized primarily around major anatomic units. Following an introductory chapter devoted to basic principles of thoracic CT and MR, chapters are devoted to the mediastinum, airways, focal lung disease, diffuse lung disease, the pulmonary arteries and hila, and the pleura, chest wall, and diaphragm. Additional chapters have been included to specifically address imaging lung cancer and AIDS, as these present special considerations worthy of individual attention. Deleted from the present text is pediatric and cardiac imaging. These omissions reflect the authors' desire to maintain a single accessible volume devoted primarily to clinical pulmonary imaging. In this regard, it is our feeling that adequate evaluation of the heart, in particular, requires its own text.

As before, special emphasis is placed first on scan techniques (made all the more complex by continued improvements in the quality of CT and MR scanners). A detailed evaluation of pertinent anatomy is also stressed. In the continued belief that accurate radiological interpretation requires in-depth familiarity with the clinical context in which we practice rather than simple pattern recognition, emphasis is again placed on extensive clinical correlation.

Given the daunting task of selecting from literally tens of thousands of potential images available to the authors, cases have been chosen to reflect those findings most likely to be encountered in clinical practice. Although there are enough oddities to appeal to those interested in unusual manifestations of disease, our primary intent has been to remain as practical as possible. Similarly, in this era of easily accessible computer databases, we have attempted to select only those references that are most generally useful.

It remains only to express the hope that the current edition will prove of value to all involved with the interpretation of thoracic CT and MR.

David P. Naidich

Acknowledgments

One singular pleasure in the preparation of any manuscript is the opportunity afforded to express our appreciation to the many individuals without whose support this text would never have been completed.

At New York University Medical Center we are deeply indebted to our technologists, whose willingness to be of help in obtaining and reimaging case material cannot be overstated. We thank Nelly Patino and Elba Cardona at Tisch Hospital; Debbie Harrigan, Rey Gonzalez, Fred Indiviglia, Tania Yeargin, Jennifer McNew, Carlolyn Gomez, and Debra Banini at our Faculty Practice; and John Sebellico, Ladislsav Kamenar, Carolyn Tyson, and Phil Fontana at Bellevue Hospital. We also acknowledge the assistance of Elis Nicholas and Luis Lopez, darkroom technicians extraordinaire.

We also extend our deeply felt thanks to Martha Helmers and Tony Jalandoni, whose photographic talents have contributed so much to the quality of this and previous editions of the text. We would also like to thank Phil Berman for his extraordinary skills at computer reconstructions that have added immeasurably to the appearance of this text.

It is our pleasure to also express thanks to those of our former and present residents who have given selflessly of their time and efforts to improve the quality of this work. In particular we would like to thank Edward Lubat, M.D., without whose many outstanding contributions this text would have been less complete: It is most rewarding to know that those who you have taught are able to teach you still more in return.

Finally, special mention is owed to Joyce-Rachel John at Lippincott–Raven Publishers, without whose constant moral support and creative input this work would simply never have seen the light of day.

CHAPTER 1

Principles and Techniques of Thoracic Computed Tomography and Magnetic Resonance

Since the previous edition of this textbook was published, several technologic advances and improvements have significantly influenced the diagnostic strategies now used in thoracic imaging. Foremost among these is the advent of single breath-hold volumetric computed tomography (CT) acquisition, also known as spiral or helical CT scanning (1,2). Nowhere has the impact of volumetric CT been more dramatic than in the thorax. Elimination of breath-to-breath variability and the ability to retrospectively review intermediate slices in a continuous helical data stream are two of the most fundamental advantages of volumetric CT. Furthermore, the overall shortening of total data acquisition times to less than 30 seconds allows easier attainment of uniform contrast enhancement with reliable depiction of all thoracic vascular structures (3,4). These advances, combined with newer high-heat capacity x-ray tubes and high-sensitivity solid state de-

tectors, have significantly improved patient throughput and anatomic coverage.

Perhaps as significant as the advent of helical CT are the advances in image processing, storage, and display capabilities of current computers. Larger volumetric data sets can now be manipulated in real time to achieve heretofore difficult analyses of thoracic anatomy and function. These advances in computer technology not only have made volumetric CT more practical but also have enabled new scanner designs that will, in the near future, further improve thoracic imaging.

Magnetic resonance (MR) imaging has also undergone significant changes because of the development of the high duty-cycle and more powerful gradient systems that are capable of delivering faster sequences with image acquisition times on the order of a few hundred milliseconds, and cardiac

1

gated three dimensional (3-D) acquisition schemes in single breath-hold times. The primary applications of MR in the thorax remain limited to the cardiovascular system, in which acquisition speed and the ability to use contrast agents in smaller doses than with CT is useful. The low density of lung tissue and its paramagnetic properties limit MR in the depiction of primary lung pathology. Some advances in basic research, such as the development of hyperpolarized gases that afford better visualization of air spaces, eventually may be of value but are still too experimental for clinical applications at this point in time.

In this chapter we will review and emphasize what we believe are the essential principles needed to design optimal imaging strategies in the individual patient, using current CT and MR technology.

TECHNIQUES AND STRATEGIES IN CHEST CT

With improvements in technology and greater clinical experience, the indications for thoracic CT have further expanded over the past several years. The basic imaging attributes on which the diagnostic effectiveness of CT rests are:

1. The reduction of the problem of anatomic superimposition of structures inherent to projectional imaging methods, such as plain radiography, by the use of transaxial scanning and thin imaging sections as appropriate.
2. The much greater radiographic density discrimination of CT relative to plain film methods with the preservation of sufficiently high spatial resolution.
3. The ability to generate well-registered 3-D data sets that can be used to display the entire thorax or specific structures thereof in an interactive manner with the user.

Because of these attributes, diagnostic interpretation is generally easier and less observer-dependent with CT than with other methods.

Indications for Chest CT

The chest radiograph remains the most effective study in diagnostic radiology because of the naturally high contrast of thoracic structures. CT is used as a second-line diagnostic study for problems that are unresolved by plain films. Examples of this role for CT are:

A mediastinal or hilar contour abnormality. This raises the possibility of vascular pathology such as dissection, aneurysm, congenital anomaly, normal variant, or distortion by tumor.
A pulmonary parenchymal nodule, mass, or infiltrate. In these cases, CT characterization through densitometric analysis or more precise morphologic analysis may be required. When a carcinoma is suspected, complete staging can be performed.
A diffuse abnormality on plain film. This category includes an abnormality suggestive of parenchymal or diffuse

small airway pathology in which extent and characterization of this process are needed. High resolution CT techniques are indicated in this context.
Complex cases of combined pleural and parenchymal pathology. On plain films, it is often difficult to differentiate pleural from parenchymal components. In such cases contrast-enhanced CT is indicated.
Chest wall and spinal pathology. Because of the curvature of the chest wall, no single plain film projection is adequate for full evaluation. The transaxial format of CT enables better analysis of the location and extent of such processes.
Pathology involving the cervico-thoracic or thoraco-abdominal junctional regions. Because plain films are not effective in the upper abdominal and cervical regions, CT is often indicated to clarify pathology spanning the adjacent thorax and these anatomic regions.

CT also can be used to screen patients whose chest radiographs are negative but whose clinical condition leads to a high suspicion of occult intrathoracic pathology. CT is indicated when the following conditions are suspected:

Metastatic nodules in patients with extrathoracic malignancies, especially those with a high propensity for pulmonary metastases. Certain endocrinologic or biochemical abnormalities that may be related to intrathoracic pathology, CT can be used, for example, in patients with myasthenia gravis, to rule out a thymoma; in patients with endocrine abnormalities that raise the possibility of a parathyroid adenoma following negative neck exploration; or in patients with an endocrinologically active tumor such as an ectopic pheochromocytoma or a hormonally active bronchial neoplasm.
Underlying cancer. CT is useful in patients with hemoptysis, positive sputum cytology, persistent wheezing or focal infiltrate despite therapy, or hypertrophic pulmonary osteoarthropathy.
Unknown source of infection, especially in the immunocompromised population.
CT is indicated in the evaluation of the pulmonary parenchyma in patients with abnormal pulmonary function tests but normal or near-normal chest x-rays.
Evaluation of patients with suspicion of pulmonary embolism or occult pulmonary arteriovenous malformation.
Evaluation of patients with chronic airway disease for potential lung volume reduction surgical resection.

Clearly, the expanding array of indications for CT and the boundless variations of pathologic presentations make it necessary to tailor each CT examination to the particular diagnostic task at hand. The radiologist should always review the available imaging and clinical data to determine precisely which components of the thoracic anatomy need to be depicted and to determine the best examination strategy. With modern scanners, instant reconstruction times have eased these tasks, and a firm diagnosis should be established before the patient is removed from the CT gantry. Obviously, no single technique is optimum for all indications in thoracic CT. The best approach to the effective use of thoracic CT is to develop a working knowledge of the various scanner-related and patient-related parameters that affect the diagnostic quality of the study. Once understood, these basic parameters can be combined into a strategy that embodies the principle of "maximum diagnostic value at minimum risk and cost."

Technical Parameters

CT scanners have become more complex in recent years and offer a greater array of technical parameters from which to choose. There are essentially three modes of CT imaging in current practice: conventional CT, in which contiguous slices (more than 2 mm thick) are acquired while the patient is stationary with table position incremented between acquisitions; high resolution CT (HRCT), in which very thin (less than 2 mm), typically noncontiguous slices are acquired and used for detailed analyses of lung structure; and volumetric or spiral/helical CT, in which up to 30 or more seconds of data recordings can be acquired during continuous rotation of the detector/tube assembly while the table is continuously translated at a predetermined speed. Each one of these modes offers specific advantages and disadvantages. Several technical parameters for these modes of scanning remain operator-determined and will be individually discussed.

Slice Thickness

The CT image is a two-dimensional (2-D) representation of a 3-D slice of space. Although the third dimension, or thickness, of the cross-section is not displayed, it directly affects the quality of the image in the other two dimensions. All structures within the unit volume of space represented by the slice, also known as voxel, are averaged and represented by a single CT number for the unit surface of the image, also known as pixel. Thus, the attenuation values for each pixel represent the average of the attenuation values of all structures present within the voxel. The thicker the slice, the more averaging of adjacent structures occurs. This phenomenon is known as the partial volume effect. To correct for this effect, an obvious solution is to reduce slice thickness by collimating the x-ray beam. Slice thicknesses varying from 1 to 10 mm are commonly available today. However, one should not conclude that the partial volume effect is necessarily deleterious and that the thinner the section the better the diagnostic content. Paradoxically, thick slices can have favorable attributes in thoracic CT. For example, the detection of a lesion by CT or any other modality depends essentially on the density gradient between the lesion and the surrounding normal tissue. In the lung, because normal parenchyma has a very low CT number (−800 Hounsfield Units [HU]), even a small nodule in only a portion of the slice can be detected. This is because there is enough density difference between the voxels containing the nodule and the

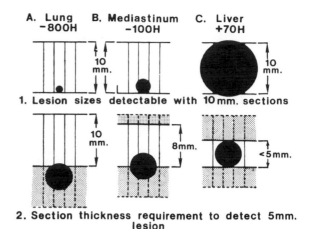

FIG. 1-1. Relationship between slice thickness, lesion size, and tissue density. **A:** (*Top*) Minimum lesion size detectable in lung (*A*), mediastinum (*B*), and liver (*C*) are illustrated for a 10-mm section thickness. With the large density gradient between aerated and pathologic lung, lesions as small as 1 mm can be easily detected. In the mediastinum with sufficient background fat, a 3-mm lesion is the smallest size detectable with a 10-mm section. In the liver, unless contrast is used, a lesion has to be 10 mm in size for detection with a 10-mm slice thickness. **B:** (*Bottom*) Slice thickness requirements to detect 5-mm lesions are illustrated for lung, mediastinum, and liver. Ten-millimeter sections are very adequate in the lung; however, 8-mm slice thicknesses are more appropriate for detecting mediastinal lymph nodes of 5 mm in diameter. In the liver it is necessary to have a slice thickness equal to the lesion size for optimal detection.

surrounding normal lung. Simple calculations show that a 1- to 2-mm lung nodule can be detected in a 10-mm thick slice. In the mediastinum, when enough contrasting fat is present, 10-mm sections allow detection of lesions as small as 3 mm (Fig. 1-1). Thus, 10-mm sections are sufficient for routine thoracic CT, requiring fewer scans and less x-ray exposure per examination than other applications.

In addition to differences in density between lesions and surrounding normal tissue, detection and recognition of lesions depend on the ability to differentiate features intrinsic to the normal background of tissue versus features of the lesion. In this regard, thick sections offer another specific advantage in the lung parenchyma. Structures such as vessels, which run obliquely to the plane of the scan, are much better appreciated using thick sections because they can be followed over a longer portion of their course, even though they fill only a small portion of each voxel (Fig. 1-2). Their branching nature can therefore be readily appreciated, and the round appearance of a small nodule is easily differentiated from vessels. On the other hand, if a thin section is used through the lungs, the vessels will be more difficult to recognize because their foreshortened cross-sections do not allow the recognition of their characteristic branching pattern. Thus, thick sections are advantageous for the detection of focal lesions in the lung parenchyma because of its high natural tissue contrast and because pulmonary vascular features are easier to recognize (Fig. 1-3). A recent alternative to thick section scanning for the recognition of small nodules is a technique known as sliding thin slab maximum intensity

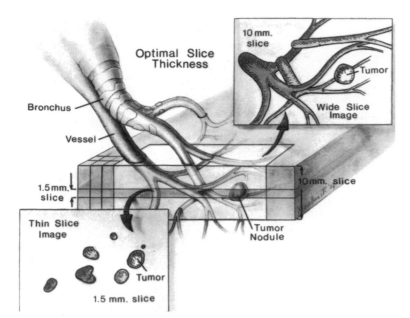

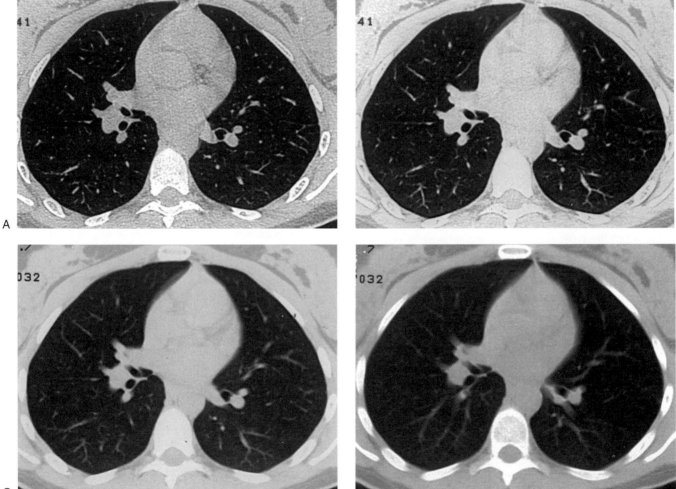

FIG. 1-2. Advantage of thick slices in lung imaging. In 10-mm thick sections, bronchovascular structures are imaged over a longer portion of their course. Thus, the branching nature of vessels and bronchi is easily recognized in thick slices (*upper right, inset*). With thinner sections, vessels and bronchi appear as round rather than tubular structures (*lower left, inset*). A tumor nodule, as illustrated, is easier to recognize against the background of branching structures in the thicker slice. See also Figure 1-3.

FIG. 1-3. Slice thickness and lung imaging. A series of four slices was obtained at the same anatomic level with 1-mm (**A**), 2-mm (**B**), 4-mm (**C**), and 8-mm (**D**) slice thicknesses. Technical parameters were kept identical except for slice thickness. Note that the branching nature of bronchial structures and vessels is progressively better appreciated as the slice thickness is increased from 1 to 8 mm. Note also the graininess of the image on the 1- and 2-mm slice thicknesses caused by higher noise levels. For routine evaluations of the pulmonary parenchyma and mediastinum, 8-mm sections offer a definite advantage since focal lesions are easily recognizable against the background of branching structures. Very thin sections should be reserved for detailed analyses of the pulmonary parenchyma. Note that even though the noise levels appear high in the chest wall and mediastinal structures on the thin-section scans, the noise level does not affect the lung parenchyma with its low radiographic density.

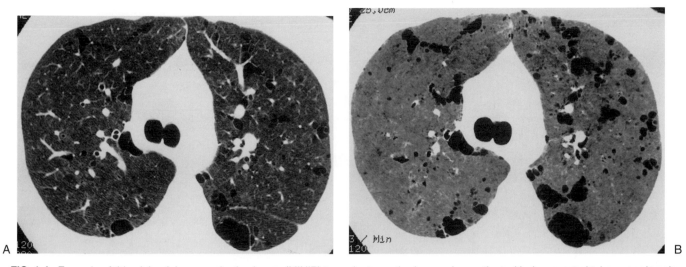

FIG. 1-4. Example of thin slab minimum projection image (MINIP) to evaluate cystic changes in a patient with documented tuberous sclerosis. **A:** Original 1-mm section. **B:** Reconstructed slab using five contiguous 1-mm sections centered at the level of the carina shows to much better advantage the true extent of cystic changes.

projection, whereby several adjacent thinner sections are added together by computer processing to form a thicker slab, and high density structures such as vessels and nodules are selectively enhanced by the processing of the original images with this algorithm. Vessels are then easily recognized by their linear branching pattern, and micronodules are better assessed than in either individual thin slices or directly acquired thick slices (5,6). Likewise, this method can be used to highlight even finer detail in parenchymal pathology (Fig. 1-4).

Conversely, partial volume effects may be detrimental in areas of the thorax in which tissue densities, such as the mediastinum and chest wall, do not demonstrate as much contrast as in the lung parenchyma.

More important, the orientation of the anatomy relative to the transaxial plane determines how much structure averaging and attendant loss of boundaries will be observed within a given slice. For example, when two structures run in a course perpendicular to the plane of scanning, they are much easier to separate than when they run obliquely. The interpreter should be keenly aware of this problem in anatomic areas in which structural boundaries are running in a course nearly parallel or at a shallow oblique angle relative to the scanned plane (Fig. 1-5). The primary areas in which this effect can be seen are the cervicothoracic junction, especially at the apex of the lungs; the aortopulmonary window; the hilar regions; the subcarinal region; and the peridiaphragmatic areas (7). In such regions, thinner sections should be used.

Thus, 7- to 10-mm thick sections, which are standard on current scanners, are generally adequate to examine the thorax. Thinner sections on the order of 3 to 5 mm are indicated when studying areas of anatomy oriented obliquely to the plane of scanning.

With very thin sections, collimation of the x-ray beam reduces the number of photons reaching the detectors. This increases noise, which is perceived as a graininess in the image. This noise will degrade resolution to a varying extent, depending on the density of the tissues examined. For example, thin-section scans demonstrate a much higher noise level in the mediastinum and chest wall regions than in the lung parenchyma, which is much less dense and requires less exposure to achieve adequate image quality (see Fig. 1-3). Thus, when the primary intent for a thin-section scan is to examine the lung parenchyma, there is only a minimal need to increase exposure factors unless graininess of the image is perceived, especially in the posterior paraspinal regions.

The most important consideration, when studying the mediastinum or chest wall, is to correct for the increased noise levels of thin slices by increasing the milliamperage or scan time. Large patients will require more exposure than small or thin patients. Unlike underexposure, which is characterized by noisy images, overexposure is difficult to perceive on CT images. As opposed to standard radiography in which the blackness of the film cannot be manipulated and overexposure is easily detected, CT images are digitized and the appearance of the image can be easily manipulated through window setting adjustments. Overexposure can, however, sometimes be recognized because it degrades image quality by generating streak artifacts near pulsatile structures like pulmonary arteries or the left heart border. Whenever streak artifacts are seen near such borders, the radiologist should make a point of verifying exposure factors and reduce them appropriately. As a guideline, adequate thoracic images can be obtained with about one-half to one-third of the exposure factors used in the abdomen (8).

Scan Time

Effective scan times have been greatly reduced over the past few years, and currently range from 0.75 to 2 seconds.

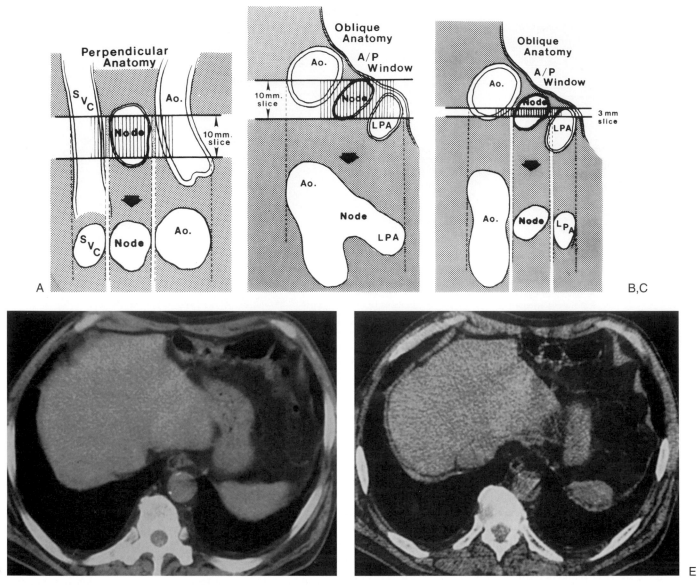

FIG. 1-5. Importance of anatomic orientation in defining optimal slice thickness. **A:** To show the importance of anatomic orientation the mediastinal region, between the superior vena cava (*SVC*) and ascending aorta (*Ao*), which are perpendicular to the axial plane, is illustrated. The node located between the aorta and the superior vena cava is easily detectable provided a minimum amount of mediastinal fat is present. Image voxels located between the node, the superior vena cava, and the aorta contain only fat and thus allow separation of the node from surrounding structures in the resultant CT image (*lower half* of **A**). **B,C:** A coronal section obtained at the level of the aortico-pulmonary window (*A/P*) is represented. Since the arch of the aorta and the left pulmonary artery (*LOA*) run an oblique course relative to the axial plane, a node located between these two structures is likely to be undetectable on a thick section scan because all pixels represent a mixture of mediastinal fat, nodal tissue, and vascular tissue, thus preventing a separation of the node from the surrounding structures on the resultant CT image. When the slice width is reduced (**C**), the node becomes visible as a distinct structure, since pixels containing only fat are now present. It is therefore important to reduce slice thickness in areas of complex anatomy oriented obliquely to the axial plane such as the hila, anteroposterior window, thoracic inlet, and peridiaphragmatic regions. Partial volume effect in thin-section scanning. As demonstrated in **A–C**, regions of oblique anatomy may require thinner section scans for delineation of structures. **D:** No separation is possible between the diaphragm and liver or the diaphragm and spleen on this 10-mm section. **E:** A 2-mm section clearly demonstrates the separation between the diaphragm and the liver and provides a better appreciation of the anatomy of the diaphragm.

Newer scanners are now produced with scan times of 0.4 to 0.5 seconds. For thoracic imaging, a short scan time is necessary to reduce the effect of respiratory motion. Furthermore, with shorter scan times, images are more often obtained within the longer and quieter diastolic period of the cardiac cycle, thereby improving visualization of cardiac structures. Whenever possible, and to the extent that short scan times are not obtained at the expense of reduced image quality, it is advisable to use the shortest scan times available on the particular scanner used. It should be remembered, however, that shorter scan times are often achieved by decreasing the number of sampling projections. A loss of resolution can therefore occur with very short scan times because the amount of data used to reconstruct the image is itself

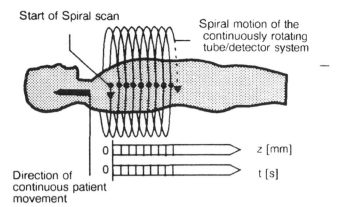

Start of Spiral scan

Spiral motion of the continuously rotating tube/detector system

z [mm]

t [s]

Direction of continuous patient movement

FIG. 1-6. Principle of spiral CT. The combination of patient translation and tube rotation provides continuous helical path for data acquisition over a large volume.

reduced. This is not correctable by using higher photon fluxes, that is, by increasing beam intensity. For studies in which high resolution is needed, it may be necessary to increase the scan time to allow for more data to be collected by the detectors.

With the short scan times currently available, scans at suspended respiration can be easily obtained in virtually every patient. Even with fast scan times, respiratory motion can degrade image quality and suspended breathing is mandatory. In most cases, scanning the thorax is performed at full lung capacity. Full inspiration promotes separation of pulmonary structures. However, the reproducibility of inspiratory breathing is less than that of breathing at resting lung volume (end-tidal volume). Thus, reproducibility when needed, as, for instance, in studying pulmonary nodules, is best achieved at resting lung breathing. The instructions to the patient in such a case are: "Breathe in, breathe out, relax, and hold your breath." Lack of breathing reproducibility can sometimes create significant problems, such as totally missing a known pulmonary nodule or inability to reconstruct 2-D and 3-D data sets without misregistration artifacts. This is one of the main reasons spiral/helical scanning is recommended whenever available (9,10).

Special Considerations for Spiral/Helical CT Scanning

When available, volumetric CT scanning using the spiral/helical acquisition method should be the dominant mode of imaging because of its inherently favorable features in thoracic CT.

The development of spiral/helical CT is due primarily to the advent of slip ring technology, which allows continuous rotation of the x-ray tube and detector assembly of the scanner combined with improvements in scanner electronics for control of table translation and more powerful computers capable of handling larger amounts of raw data (Fig. 1-6) (11). Such a combination of features allows the imaging of a large number of slices covering larger volumes of the thorax during suspended respiration, thus eliminating slice to slice

misregistration inherent to the repeated breath-holds necessary in conventional CT scanning (12,13). The main technical limit to spiral/helical CT has now become the thermal capacity of the x-ray tube. The imaging characteristics of spiral/helical scans are, however, different in crucial aspects from more conventional acquisitions. New and critical technical parameters introduced by this technique are the pitch, the data interpolation scheme, the slice sensitivity profile, and the reconstruction interval (14).

Pitch

In conventional scanning, the patient is stationary relative to the detector array while the entire set of projections needed to reconstruct a transaxial image is acquired. In spiral/helical scanning, this condition is not fulfilled and the path of the projections represents the combination of circular rotation of the detectors and simultaneous translation of the patient. Geometrically, this combination of primary rotational and translational motions results in a helicoidal pathway for the data projections. A helicoidal motion is characterized by the amount of translational motion that occurs during a full 360 degree rotation. The ratio of translation, also known as table feed, over rotation is known as the pitch of a helix. Since the width of the data acquisition is equal to the aperture of the detector, the pitch is equal to the amount of table advancement during a full rotation over the slice thickness as determined by the collimation of the detector array. For example, if we use a slice thickness of 3 mm and the patient translates by 6 mm during a full rotation of the detector-tube assembly, the pitch will be equal to 2. Because rotational scan times are different between scanners and may vary between 0.4 and 2 seconds, it is more desirable to specify scanning protocols by using the slice thickness and the pitch value rather than the translational table speed. For example, a 5-mm section scan with a pitch of 1.5 in a scanner that has a 2-second scan time means that for a full rotation, the table will advance by 7.5 mm, that is, a table speed of 3.5 mm per second. If the scan time was accelerated to 1 second, the table speed should be 7.5 mm per second. A valid and practical issue is to determine the optimum pitch value that provides maximum coverage at a similar image quality as conventional scanning within the heat capacity of the x-ray tube. As shown by Wang and Vannier, the optimum pitch for maximum coverage should be set at the value of the square root of 2, or approximately 1.4 (15). Greater pitch values can provide greater coverage at the cost of increased image noise and blurring because of a less optimum slice profile.

Data Interpolation and Slice Sensitivity Profile

Spiral/helical scanning has important consequences for data reconstruction that should be fully understood. CT images represent the mathematical reconstruction of a sufficient number of projections that measure the attenuation properties of a slice of the body using the method of filtered back projection. Ideally, in a fan beam scanner configuration, projections acquired during a complete 360-degree rotation plus two fan beam angles provide the best data set for high quality reconstruction, although reconstruction can be performed with truncated data sets representing less than 360 degrees of projection. It is assumed in such a reconstruction that all projections represent the same object. Clearly, since the patient moves during acquisition, this condition is not fulfilled in spiral/helical scanning. Appropriate steps must be taken in the reconstruction process to allow for the fact that the first measurement traverses a path that is different than the last and there is insufficient data from any one slice. The raw data projections must first be manipulated mathematically prior to reconstruction via interpolation among spatially adjacent projections to provide a near-planar data set. Linear interpolation is the dominant method used and interpolation across half scans or 180 degrees of rotation give the best results with the least amount of image blurring (14,16,17). Interpolation over greater angles results in more degradation of the slice profile. To best understand the concept of slice profile degradation, one should remember that unlike conventional CT, the slice sensitivity profile is modulated by the table motion. The slice shape is a measure of a CT scanner point-spread function in the longitudinal central axis of the scanner. In simpler terms, it describes the fidelity with which a sharp-edged point will be measured by the scanner in the longitudinal or through-plane direction. Whereas the edges of the slice sensitivity profile are more sharply defined in conventional CT, a more ill-defined slice sensitivity profile is inherent to spiral/helical scanning because objects are blurred because of their translational motion during scanning and to interpolation of projections (17–19). To minimize this effect, it is best to interpolate data from adjacent projections at the minimum feasible angle, that is, 180 degrees or half scan interpolation, since this will entail the least amount of translational distortion and blurring.

Reconstruction Interval

As can be deduced from the discussion above, it is clear that a spiral/helical slice displays data from a continuous data stream that can be computationally manipulated to represent varying amounts of projections from adjacent slices. Thus, it is possible to reconstruct slices at intervals smaller than the prescribed nominal slice thickness (20). This is a major advantage of this technique. Not only can it be used to find the best representative slice through a focalized abnormality such as a nodule (21,10), but it also helps create three-dimensional data sets with better through-plane resolution and higher quality multiplanar and volumetric displays. The overlapping reconstructed slices can improve detection of small features. However, the computational requirements can be daunting if too fine a reconstruction interval is used. Furthermore, too fine an interval may not contain additional information if the acquisition pitch is large. This is because

of the fact that fewer valid interpolations between adjacent slices of tissue can be made at higher pitch than at lower pitch since the distance traveled by any point in tissue is greater and projections are thus more separated with greater table translation speed. The more interpolations between adjacent sets of projections can be made, the more intervening slices can be reconstructed. A general rule of thumb is that three to five slices can be reconstructed at pitches less than one and about two slices for a pitch of two. Finer reconstruction intervals may not provide additional information even though the finer intervals may enhance the subjective visual effect of 3-D reconstructions.

Because of the large number of possible combinations of parameters in spiral/helical CT, it is important to remember that imaging of anatomic features is best accomplished when both the slice thickness and the table feed during slice acquisition are comparable to the size of the feature of interest. Whenever possible the slice thickness should be minimized rather than table feed as the slice sensitivity profile is better preserved with narrower collimation than with smaller table feed (20).

For example, detection of lesions or structures approximating 5 mm in size will be better accomplished with a slice thickness of 4 mm and a pitch of 1.4 than with a slice thickness of 5 mm and a pitch of 1.

In summary, spiral/helical CT scanning introduces additional variables that can be bewildering for the first-time user and requires a different approach to parameter selection than conventional CT. In addition to practical considerations related to amount of anatomic coverage as a function of patient breath-holding capacity, contrast injection requirements and the heat capacity of the x-ray tube, it is also important to choose an optimal pitch for maximum coverage while preserving image quality. Slice thickness should be near the size of the smallest feature of interest likely to be present in the image of the pathology under consideration. Two to five overlapping slice reconstructions are of value in improving anatomical depiction with more interval reconstructions indicated at lower pitch than at higher pitch, given the greater spatial proximity of the interpolated raw data projections at low pitch angles.

Recently, manufacturers have introduced scanners with multiple parallel detector arrays and faster rotational times. The multiple detectors enable acquisition of more sets of data within one slice to reduce the problems encountered with current volumetric CT techniques and reduce the need for excessive interpolation. These scanners can considerably increase the pitch beyond a factor of two. Coupled with the faster rotation of the gantry, these scanners allow coverage of much larger regions at reasonable suspended respiration times.

Field-of-View

Another important parameter in thoracic CT is the choice of an appropriate field-of-view (FOV) for image reconstruction. Although not often appreciated, the diameter of the

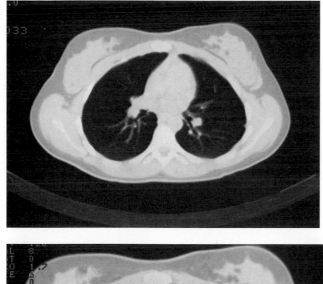

A

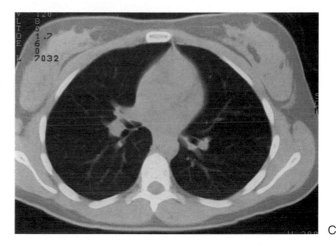

FIG. 1-7. Field-of-view. **A:** Selection of field-of-view (FOV) too large for the patient's size results in suboptimal images and a loss of anatomic detail and diagnostic information. In this example, less than half of the image matrix is used to image the patient. **B,C:** To correct for the inadequate image in **A**, simple magnification was applied (**B**) and the raw data was reconstructed with a smaller FOV (**C**). Note the difference in quality between **B** and **C**. Simple magnification does not improve spatial resolution. Structure edges are not sharp, whereas with image reconstruction with a FOV adjusted to the patient's size, better detail is seen.

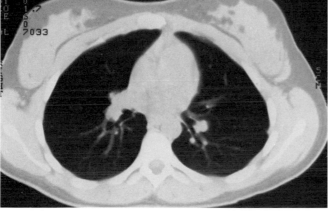

B

C

FOV has a profound effect on the image quality achieved with CT. This is because CT images are the representation of a 512 × 512 matrix of numbers. This matrix is the mathematical support of the computer calculations used to represent the space examined within the aperture of the scanner. The portion of space represented by an individual pixel depends on the size of the FOV as indicated to the computer by the operator. Because the total number of pixels in each image is limited, if we select a large area of interest, each pixel represents a proportionately larger volume of space. Resolution is then limited to the size of that pixel. For example, if we choose a 51-cm FOV, each pixel would be about 1 mm × 1 mm in size. Clearly then, it is most appropriate to adjust the diameter of the FOV to the size of the anatomic area to be examined. Ideally, pixels should be smaller than the minimum distance resolvable by a scanner. On current scanners, resolutions on the order of 0.3 to 0.4 mm can be achieved. Thus, maximum resolution is obtained only when FOVs of about 15 to 20 cm are used (15 cm divided by 512 = 0.3 mm pixels).

In practice, it is sufficient to adjust and match the diameter of the FOV to the size of the transverse diameter of the thorax. It should also be noted that simple magnification of CT images is not effective in improving details, because the pixel size is not changed with magnification (Fig. 1-7). On the other hand, retrospectively reconstructing selected areas of the object from raw data, a process known as *targeted reconstruction*, is the best way to achieve a high level of anatomic detail for high-resolution studies.

Window Settings

The full scale of CT numbers cannot be displayed in a single image because a limited number of gray shades is available for electronic display. The operator must select a portion of the CT number range to be displayed. This is done by using electronic windows and defining the width and level at which the windows will be active. Because the range of CT numbers in the thorax is the greatest of those for all body parts extending from the almost-air density of the lungs (−800 HU) to the high density of bones (−600 HU), no single window setting can properly display all the information available on a thoracic CT study. Each thoracic CT examination should be viewed with at least two and, in selected cases, three sets of window settings: one for the lung parenchyma, one for the mediastinal and chest wall structures, and, whenever needed, one for the bony structures. Although the precise window settings are often a matter of subjective preference, certain guidelines should be followed to avoid suboptimal representation of anatomic structures.

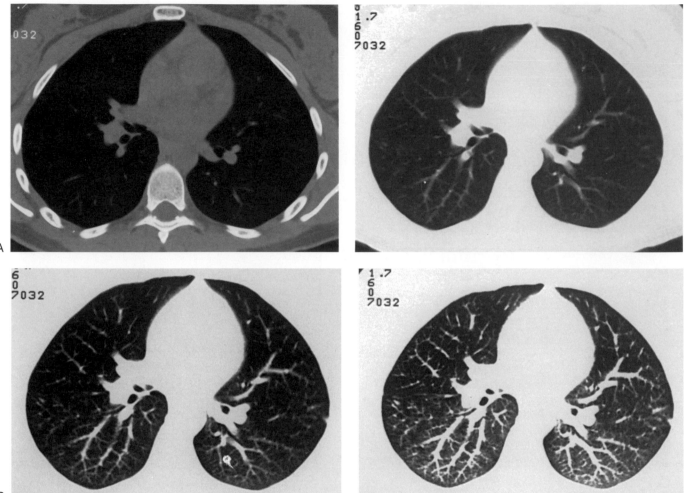

FIG. 1-8. Influence of window settings on visibility of pulmonary structures. An 8-mm thick scan in the mid-thoracic region is represented at different window settings. **A:** Small pulmonary vessels cannot be appreciated. However, at this window setting of 375 window level (*WL*) and 2,000 window width (*WW*), a good compromise is achieved between visualization of anatomic structures of the chest wall and mediastinum and those of the pulmonary parenchyma. The interface between the pulmonary parenchyma and the pleura is well delineated. Even though fine detail of the parenchymal structures is not observable, the relatively clear background helps identify focal lesions. This window setting is appropriate for routine evaluations. **B:** The effect of lowering window level and width is demonstrated. More peripheral and smaller branches of the pulmonary arteries are demonstrated. These small branches were not visible on the prior scan because their density was averaged with that of the surrounding air and was too low. However, by reducing the window width more image contrast is achievable and reducing the window level permits a better matching with the low density of these peripheral vessels. Note, however, the associated loss of visualization of the chest wall and mediastinal structures. The interface between pulmonary parenchyma and pleura is difficult to define. **C,D:** The effect of further reducing window width is illustrated. More contrast is now present between pulmonary vascular structures and lung parenchyma. Vessels appear more prominent in size and very small structures in the range of 0.5 mm can be detected with such window settings even though slice thickness is 8 mm. However, there is complete loss of detail in the mediastinum, hila, and chest wall. Note also that central vessels and bronchial walls appear falsely prominent.

It has been shown that the most accurate representation of an object is achieved when the window level is placed at a value midway between the CT number of the structure to be measured and the CT number of the surrounding tissue. For example, if a lung nodule measures 50 HU and the surrounding parenchyma measures −800 HU, the proper window level should be about −375 HU. In the lung parenchyma, as vessels become smaller from the center to the periphery of the lung, their CT density decreases proportionately because of partial volume averaging of vessel and surrounding air within the CT slice. To represent the smaller

vessels in the lung parenchyma, it is thus necessary to use proportionately lower window levels and widths (Fig. 1-8). Because of lesser partial volume effects on thin-section scans, the density of vessels is greater. Therefore, on thin-section scans, the window levels to be used for representing small vessels and parenchyma need to be higher than those used to represent the same structures on a thick-section scan (Fig. 1-9). Suggested window settings for different slice thicknesses and sizes of pulmonary structures are presented in Table 1-1.

It is also important to remember that the apparent size of

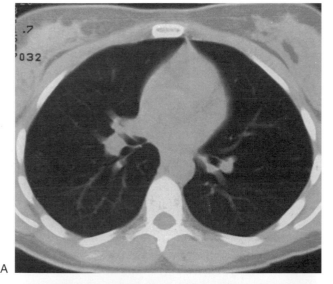

A

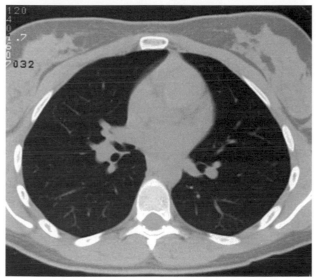

B

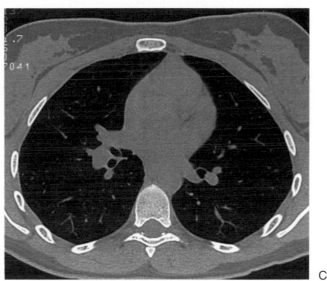

C

FIG. 1-9. Effect of slice thickness on window settings. Because partial volume effects are reduced with thinner section scans, the density of peripheral vessels are reduced with thinner section scans, the density of peripheral vessels increases on such scans. Thus, the appropriate window level will be proportionately higher on thinner section scans than with thicker section scans. Examples of a scan obtained with 8-mm (**A**), 4-mm (**B**), and 2-mm (**C**) slice thicknesses at the same anatomic level illustrate this effect. In **A**, at 675 window length (*WL*) and 2,000 window width (*WW*), a good compromise is achieved between visualization of parenchymal structures, chest wall, and mediastinal structures. To achieve the same degree of relative visualization of parenchymal, mediastinal, and chest wall structures the level of 545 WL and 2,000 WW is appropriate for a 4-mm thick scan (**B**), whereas a WL of 375 HU and a WW of 2,000 HU are needed to achieve the same degree of vascular visualization in a 2-mm thick scan (**C**).

TABLE 1-1. *Appropriate window settings as a function of slice thickness and size of pulmonary structures*[a]

Slice (mm)	Structure size (mm)						
	10	5	3	2	1	0.5	0.3
10	L −375	−587	−673	−715	−757	−780	−788
	W 2,000	2,000	2,000	1,360	688	320	192
5	L −375	−375	−545	−630	−715	−757	−775
	W 2,000	2,000	2,000	2,000	1,360	688	400
2	L −375	−375	−375	−375	−587	−694	−736
	W 2,000	2,000	2,000	2,000	2,000	1,700	1,024
1	L −375	−375	−375	−375	−375	−587	−672
	W 2,000	2,000	2,000	2,000	2,000	2,000	2,000

[a] Assumptions: Lung density is −800 HU, structure density is 50 HU. Window width is given as maximum needed to differentiate structure from surrounding lung by at least one level of gray. L, window level; W, window width.

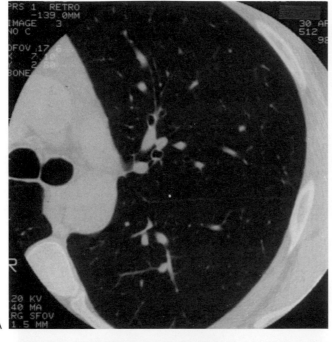

A

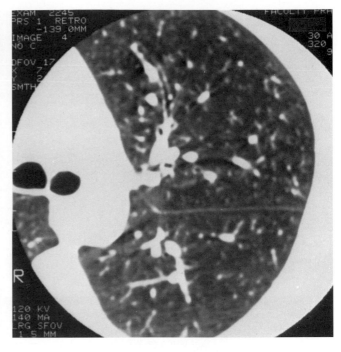

B

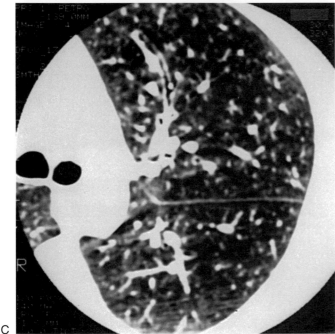

C

FIG. 1-10. Effect of window settings on apparent size of structures in the pulmonary parenchyma. **A:** At appropriate window levels and width of 375 window length (*WL*) and 2,000 window width (*WW*), accurate display of the size of pulmonary parenchymal structures is achieved. **B:** WW was narrowed to 1,000 and WL was decreased to 650. Note that the interlobar fissure is now more prominent and vessels appear larger. **C:** By further reducing WL and WW, higher contrast is achieved. However, the vascular structures, which appear very delicate in **A**, now appear abnormally prominent. Note also that the smallest structures are magnified proportionately more than larger structures. For example, note how thickened the bronchial walls appear in **C** as compared to **A**. This nonlinear preferential magnification of small structures may lead the unwary observer to over diagnosis of diffuse pathology.

structures is markedly affected by the choice of window settings, in particular by the window level. This is because of the relative blurring of edges inherent to the CT scanning process. As shown in Figure 1-10, this edge blurring will affect the apparent size of structures depending on the window settings used. More important, when an inappropriate window setting is used, the apparent size of smaller structures (e.g., blood vessels in the lung parenchyma) is much more affected than that of larger structures (e.g., the aorta). For example, a blood vessel can be magnified 300% to 400% if too low a window level is used, whereas the thoracic aorta

will be magnified 20% to 30% at most. This effect is critically important in the interpretation of diffuse parenchymal processes in which pathology can be mimicked or ignored with the use of inappropriate window settings.

Window width should be chosen so as to encompass at least the entire range of densities present within the scan. For example, in the mediastinum the range would be -100 HU for fat to -400 to -500 HU for bony structures of the sternum or spine. Thus a window width of about 500 to 600 HU is recommended. In the pulmonary parenchyma, the range extends from -800 HU for the lung parenchyma to

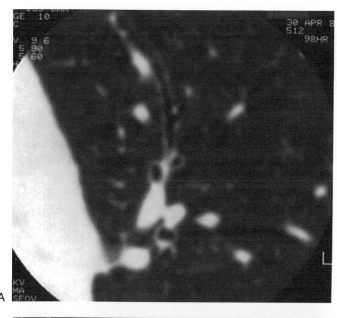

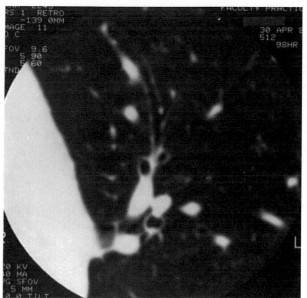

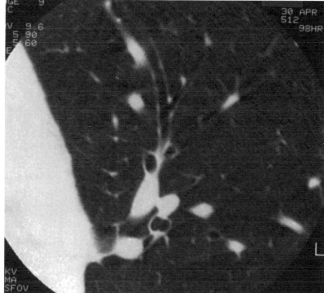

FIG. 1-11. Influence of reconstruction algorithm on image quality in high-resolution CT. High-resolution study of a left upper lobe in a normal patient with a low spatial resolution and high-contrast resolution or so-called smoothing algorithm (**A**), intermediate spatial resolution and contrast resolution (**B**), and high spatial resolution with low-contrast resolution (**C**). Note clear-cut improvement in detail in **C** compared to **B** and **A**, which exhibit blurring. Note also that the image in **C** appears noisier than either **A** or **B**. This example illustrates the trade-off between various algorithms of reconstruction. High spatial resolution software (**C**) is more appropriate for analyzing fine lung parenchymal detail.

400 to 500 HU for bone, thus a range of at least 1,300 HU and preferably 1,800 to 2,000 HU should be used. To increase conspicuity of pulmonary features, narrow window widths can be used in selected instances.

Algorithm of Reconstruction

The computer software used to reconstruct a CT image from raw data can markedly affect the characteristics of the image. For the purposes of this chapter, we will consider computer reconstruction algorithms as falling into two general classes: those designed for anatomic structures with inherently low contrast, or so-called high contrast resolution algorithms; and those designed for high-contrast anatomic structures, generally high spatial resolution algorithms (Fig. 1-11). In general, CT software designers achieve high contrast resolution by "smoothing" the image, using so-called

reconstruction filters that average the density of neighboring pixels. This is advantageous in the brain or liver because it reduces the apparent image noise, permitting the recognition of underlying lesions that are generally less dense than normal tissue by only 20 to 30 HU. However, in the thorax, this type of algorithm tends to blur the appearance of small pulmonary structures. In the lung, since natural contrast is high, it is more desirable to use high spatial resolution software, which best preserves sharp edges and detail (22,23).

A drawback of the high spatial frequency algorithms is their tendency to enhance image noise. If excessive, this "enhanced" noise may hinder the interpretation of fine details of the lung parenchyma, especially in high-resolution studies. This is particularly true in the paraspinal areas in which noise is higher because of the increased attenuation of the x-ray beam by the vertebral bodies.

High-Resolution CT

One of the primary limitations of conventional radiography in the evaluation of diffuse pulmonary parenchymal disease is the superimposition of structures caused by the 2-D projectional format of that imaging method. High-resolution computed tomography (HRCT) has become the preferred technique in the investigation of diffuse as well as focal pulmonary processes whenever detailed evaluation is required. The quality of spiral/helical CT scans is not sufficient to displace HRCT as the method of choice. Technically, HRCT simply represents the combination of 1- to 2-mm thick CT slices reconstructed with pixel sizes in the range of 300 to 400 microns, that is, FOVs of 15 to 20 cm. By using a very thin section, structural superimposition within the thickness of the scan is greatly reduced, permitting optimum evaluation of lung details. The reduction of the FOV allows optimum resolution. This technique can be performed on any modern CT scanner (24,25). As mentioned above, it is critical to use appropriate high spatial resolution reconstruction algorithms with HRCT (see Fig. 1-11). These algorithms are standard on all current scanners. HRCT can therefore be routinely implemented, provided proper technique is used.

Some technical considerations should be kept in mind. With thinly collimated sections, the signal-to-noise ratio of the image may be degraded because of the reduced number of photons reaching the detectors. Because the reconstruction software used in HRCT tends to enhance the noisiness of the image, it is important to increase exposure levels to achieve optimum image quality. However, for HRCT applications, the critical factor is the noise level within the lung parenchyma, not that in the mediastinum or chest wall. The increase in exposure can be kept to a minimum, and no increase is usually necessary in thinner patients.

As discussed above, proper window settings are critical for accurate displays of diffuse pathology. Using an inappropriate window level can make structures appear larger or smaller than they truly are. These magnification or minimization effects are much more pronounced for the fine parenchymal structures essential to the interpretation of HRCT (see Fig. 1-10). Because evaluation of the lungs with contiguous HRCT slices would be impractical and prohibitive in terms of radiation exposure, it is most appropriate to scan the lung every 10 to 20 mm when evaluating diffuse lung abnormalities with HRCT (26).

Contrast Media

Contrast agents improve subject contrast to bring it within the detection range of a particular imaging modality. Contrast agents are also used to highlight specific pathologies, which may portray different contrast agent physiology than surrounding tissues. The thorax is endowed with naturally high tissue contrast. Ribs and vessels are of markedly different density than the surrounding aerated lungs. Mediastinal structures are usually embedded in sufficient amounts of fat.

The role of contrast agents is thus more limited in thoracic CT than in other body regions. In most cases, sufficient information is available without contrast enhancement. Knowledge of mediastinal and hilar anatomy is generally sufficient to determine whether a particular structure is pathologic. Contrast enhancement, however, may be necessary when mediastinal fat is lacking, when a vascular abnormality is suspected, when patients have complex pleuroparenchymal disease, or when staging for lung cancer is required. With the advent of volumetric CT, the use of contrast has increased in thoracic imaging as better and rapid enhancement during the vascular phase of contrast distribution can be more reliably accomplished. CT angiography techniques to assess pulmonary embolism and primary vascular pathology have also gained wider acceptance and increased the need for contrast enhancement.

Physiologic Considerations and Contrast Injection Techniques

Defining sensible strategies of contrast agent administration requires a brief review of the physiology of intravenous contrast distribution in the body. First and foremost, intravenous contrast media used in CT distribute freely and rapidly from the vascular compartment into the extravascular, extracellular compartment and vice versa. The only tissue of exception is the brain, in which the vascular compartment is not permeable to contrast agents when the blood-brain barrier is intact. Rapid passage of contrast from the intravascular space into the extracellular, extravascular space occurs within seconds. Within one or two minutes after intravenous injection, equilibrium is reached. Because the extravascular space is several times larger than the vascular compartment, the majority of iodine molecules will be distributed in the extravascular space of tissues. In addition, renal excretion actively decreases the concentration of the contrast agent. Therefore, with contrast-enhanced CT, the differentiation and characterization of a lesion depends upon all of the following factors: (a) the timing of the scan relative to the amount and speed of contrast delivery; (b) the vascularity of the lesion during injection and for a few seconds thereafter, while most contrast molecules are still in the vascular space; (c) the relative size of the extravascular space of the lesion compared to normal tissue, which determines the density difference between lesion and tissue for scans obtained beyond the early vascular phase of injection; (d) the permeability of the vascular space both for exit and reentry of contrast molecules, since it determines the rate of contrast agent exchange between intra- and extravascular compartments; and (e) renal excretion. Because of these factors and given the fact that little tissue is present in the lung, most enhancement in the thorax is primarily caused by vascular structures and rapid dilution is the rule. Hence, it is paramount that the data acquisition time window fit the physiologic time window during which vessels are most opacified. The shortening of total scan time makes continuous volumetric CT more suited

TABLE 1-2. *Average thoracic transit times[a]*

	Bolus in (sec)	Bolus out (sec)
Superior vena cava	3.7 ± 1.5	9.0 ± 2.5
Pulmonary arteries	6.5 ± 2.5	10.0 ± 3.0
Ascending aorta	10.5 ± 3.0	17.8 ± 3.5
Descending aorta and neck vessels	12.3 ± 3.8	19.4 ± 3.8
Jugular vein	17.8 ± 5.0	27.0 ± 5.0
Inferior vena cava	16.0 ± 5.5	ND

[a] Two second intravenous bolus of 10 cc total volume 1 antecubital vein. Data were obtained by measuring transit times with a gamma camera set at one image per sec from start of an injection of 20 mCi of technetium-99m methylene diphosphonate. The data of 35 consecutive patients of ages varying between 19 and 72 years were averaged. These average times should be taken into consideration when setting up dynamic scan programs or when obtaining individual scans of particular areas. Scans should start at the time of bolus arrival in the structures investigated. ND, not done.

than conventional incremental CT for this purpose (27,28). The proper timing of the bolus of contrast can be optimized by using preparatory scan techniques that monitor the density of a given slice to signal the arrival of the contrast bolus. Also important is the need to achieve near complete mixing of blood and contrast to avoid pseudo-filling defects that may mimic pathology. Streaming of unopacified blood into vessels early after injection can sometimes occur (29). A better understanding of these physiologic points, along with the availability of automated injectors and nonionic or more dilute ionic solutions that are better tolerated by patients, has popularized strategies combining an extended intravenous bolus injection of contrast at high delivery rates of 3 to 5 cc per second with rapid spiral/helical scanning. This technique is extremely effective in evaluating vascular structures, especially in the mediastinal, hilar, and perihilar regions. When evaluating pleuroparenchymal abnormalities, information relative to the postvascular phase is also important. In such cases, the start of scanning may be delayed by 20 to 30 seconds to permit the distribution of some contrast agent to the extravascular space. This is helpful in differentiating inflammatory pleural processes from parenchymal infiltrates.

A working knowledge of the transit times of the intravenous bolus in the various vascular structures of the chest greatly helps in the timing of bolus injections and scans. To define this range of transit times, we have studied a series of patients to determine the average times of bolus arrival in the major vascular structures (Table 1-2). In hemodynamically normal individuals, antecubital vein to right heart transit is about 3 seconds, 6 seconds to pulmonary arteries, 9 seconds to left heart, and 12 to 15 seconds to major arteries.

One important concept to grasp for proper contrast delivery is that cardiac function strongly influences contrast delivery. For example, in normal hearts, the right ventricular ejec-

tion fraction is about 60%, which means that total ventricular contrast content, about 100 cc, can be ejected in 4 to 5 heartbeats, assuming good mixing. In a patient with ventricular failure, however, ejection fraction is lower and correspondingly more heartbeats are needed to eject the contrast bolus. Thus, cardiac rhythm as well as cardiac function can drastically affect contrast mixing and delivery. Tachycardia or bradycardia can significantly affect the transit times mentioned above. A rule of thumb that we have found useful in practice is that it is better to use heartbeats rather than seconds to time the scanning window. In a normal individual, 3 seconds after the beginning of injection a total of 8 to 10 heartbeats are needed to fully opacify the right heart chambers and the lungs and an additional 8 to 10 heartbeats are necessary to opacify the left heart chamber and proximal aorta (for a total of 16 to 20 heartbeats). In an individual with mild to moderate decreased cardiac function, the number of heartbeats is increased to 12 to 16 heartbeats for right and left heart transit (for a total of approximately 24 to 32 heartbeats). Once the injection is started, it is advisable to maintain the bolus for the entire scanning time.

Another important consideration in contrast enhancement is to use agents with a lower concentration of iodine to avoid streak artifacts in the superior vena cava related to marked differences in density between the concentrated agent and surrounding structures. With CT numbers greater than 200 to 250 HU, the abrupt change in density between the edge of the vein and mediastinum creates discontinuity in the raw projection data, leading to streak artifacts. Although agents with concentrations of about 150 mg iodine per mL will avoid this effect, higher concentrations of 240 to 300 mg iodine per mL are generally needed when good opacification of heart chambers or major aortic vessels is sought. Total bolus volume varies between 150 to 300 cc, depending upon the specific application. In our experience, nonionic contrast agents have been associated with a lower incidence of minor reactions, such as nausea and vomiting, when used with rapid, high-volume bolus injection techniques and are preferred, although the use of ionic contrast at lower concentration has also been reported. (More detailed descriptions of strategies for contrast enhancement pertaining to specific clinical indications will be presented in later chapters.)

Patient Factors

Studies of the lung parenchyma are best performed at full inspiration to promote separation of vascular structures. Scans obtained at lesser degrees of inspiration may demonstrate areas of increased densities in the dependent regions of the lung parenchyma. On conventional CT scans, these areas of dependent densities appear featureless, but on HRCT a pseudoreticular and often misleading appearance can be seen (Fig. 1-12). Classically, dependent densities have been attributed to fluid accumulation caused by gravitational effects. It has been shown that these dependent densities are caused by areas of microatelectasis (30). The best

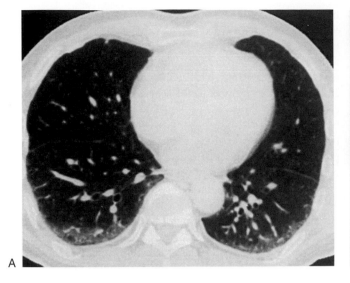

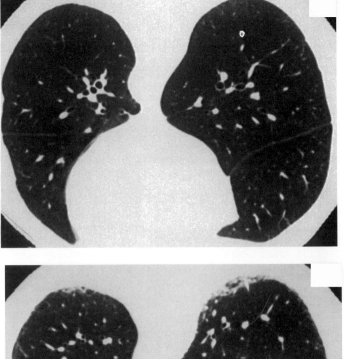

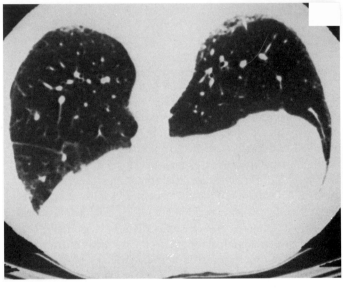

FIG. 1-12. Importance of patient positioning. **A:** Supine scan demonstrates increased dependent densities in the lower lobes. The possibility of interstitial lung disease cannot be excluded. **B:** A scan of the same region taken in prone position with full inspiratory effort demonstrates disappearance of the dependent densities, thus proving their physiologic nature. **C:** Patient with similar appearance in the dependent regions of the lungs. However, when scanned in the prone position the parenchymal changes persist despite good inspiratory effort. Patient in **C** had asbestosis. Areas of atelectasis and fluid accumulation are frequently seen in normal individuals in the dependent regions of the lungs. These areas can mimic interstitial pathology. Scans at full inspiration and in a nondependent position are helpful in differentiating physiologic from nonphysiologic causes of dependent densities.

explanation for this process is that the pressure gradient needed to expand air spaces is lower in the nondependent regions of the lungs than in the dependent regions, which are subject to the weight of the lung above them. Thus, in the recumbent position, air space expansion does not occur homogeneously. Rather, it progresses from nondependent to dependent regions during inspiration. With incomplete inspiration, partially collapsed air spaces are likely to be present in the dependent regions of the lungs. Dependent densities may simulate or obscure underlying pathology. The best way to correct for this problem is to obtain a deep inspiration scan. If the abnormality does not disappear, it is necessary to place the patient in a prone position and rescan the area after vigorous coughing and deep inspiration maneuvers have been attempted (see Fig. 1-12). Another often unrecognized patient-related artifact is the presence of atelectatic regions of lung caused by processes compressing the lung focally, such as pleural plaques, pleural masses, chest wall masses, and large osteophytes (Fig. 1-13).

Patient Positioning

Patients are usually scanned in the supine position. To prevent streak artifacts generated by skeletal structures of the upper extremity, patients should be scanned with arms elevated above the head. In patients with pleural or parenchymal fluid collections, scanning in positions other than supine is useful. The effect of gravity may help to differentiate loculated from free effusion and pulmonary edema from other causes of infiltrates. Displacement of fluids by the use of lateral decubitus or prone positioning can also help sometimes in defining any underlying pathology (Fig. 1-14).

CT PLANNING AND GUIDANCE OF PERCUTANEOUS NEEDLE BIOPSIES

CT is increasingly used to guide needle biopsy procedures in the thorax.

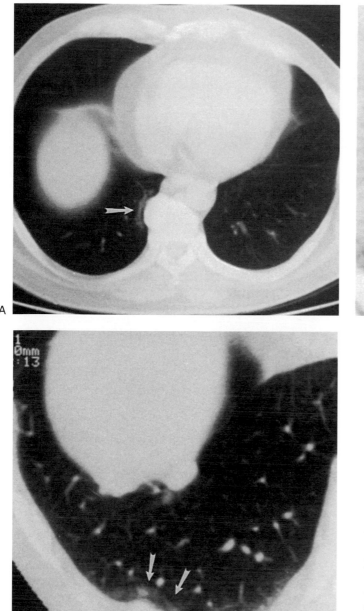

FIG. 1-13. Effect of focal pressure on lung parenchyma. Abnormal density of the lung parenchyma is often seen near processes that compress the lung. These changes are nonspecific and presumably represent areas of focal atelectasis. **A:** A focal lung compression caused by a large osteophyte. Linear area of atelectasis is seen in the subpleural region adjacent to the osteophyte (*arrow*). **B:** Example of focal subpleural atelectasis. The patient with a large callous from prior rib fracture (*arrows*). **C:** Example of same phenomenon near pleural plaque from asbestos exposure (*arrows*). Note absence of similar parenchymal changes in the regions immediately adjacent to the process that compresses the lung. These changes should not be interpreted as pathologic.

Biopsy of Pulmonary Lesions

In our experience, biplane fluoroscopic guidance is still the method of choice for pulmonary masses. Fluoroscopy has the unique advantage of visualizing the tip of the needle in real time. Observing the motion and the relationship of the needle tip to the lesion during the biopsy is the best way to ensure effective sampling. CT cannot provide such assurance. However, when lesions are poorly visualized under fluoroscopic guidance or when the lesion is seen in only one plane, CT can be used to provide in-depth information. CT can also be used to enable fluoroscopic guidance in a single plane, or to help decide whether CT should be

the guiding modality. Using CT with thin sections, if necessary, can define the optimum path for needle penetration. It is important to define the relationship of lesions to surrounding pulmonary emphysema because the risk of pneumothorax is greatly increased if the needle traverses areas of emphysema. In addition, the risk of pneumothorax increases as the number of pleural leaflets crossed by the needle increases. Needle paths crossing fissures should be avoided whenever possible.

Certain technical factors should be kept in mind when performing CT-guided needle biopsy. First, the CT slice has a given thickness, and the needle position cannot be defined

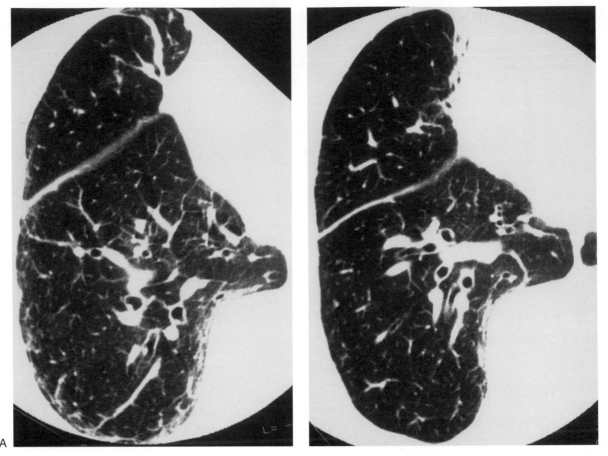

A   B

FIG. 1-14. A: Target reconstruction of 1-mm section through the right lower lobe shows diffuse reticular changes raising the possibility of pulmonary fibrosis. **B:** Section obtained at same level as **A** with the patient in a decubitus position shows marked change in appearance consistent with shifting interstitial edema.

with an accuracy greater than the slice thickness. To increase the accuracy of needle placement, we strongly recommend the use of external visual landmarks. These landmarks can help to maintain a plane of penetration exactly parallel to the scanned plane and at an appropriate angle. An error of a few angular degrees at the entry point can translate into an error of several centimeters at the lesion level. It is important to verify and document the needle tip penetration of a lesion before sampling, and a CT scan should be obtained for that purpose.

Biopsy of Mediastinal, Pleural, and Chest Wall Lesions

Unlike lung lesions, mediastinal, pleural, and chest wall lesions are almost always sampled under CT guidance (31). Uncomplicated pleural lesions are more appropriately sampled or drained under ultrasound guidance, but complex pleural or chest wall lesions are best managed with CT guidance. To avoid the risk of hemorrhage, precise identification of chest wall vascular structures is necessary. This is especially true for the subclavian and internal mammary vessels when an anterior approach is planned. Generally, anterior mediastinal lesions are best approached at the level of the

second to the fourth intercostal space anteriorly and laterally to the internal mammary vessels. To avoid errors of localization, markers should always be placed on the surface of the thorax at the time of scanning. The most practical markers are made of radiopaque angiographic catheters cut at progressive lengths and taped perpendicular to the plane of scanning on the skin surface. With such an arrangement, the number of catheters visualized precisely indicates the level of the scan on the patient's thorax.

Hilar and posterior mediastinal lesions are best sampled via a posterolateral approach. Likewise, lesions located in the superior mediastinum are also best approached posteriorly because the anterior approach runs the risk of damaging subclavian vessels. Pleural and chest wall lesions are ideally suited for CT guidance because they are difficult to visualize under fluoroscopic control (because of the curvature of the chest wall). In addition, the superficial location of pleural and chest wall lesions allows precise and easy placement of percutaneous needles (32,33).

The most important technical point to remember is that the optimum route for sampling chest wall or pleural lesions is not necessarily the direct perpendicular approach, but rather an obliquely oriented course along the main axis of

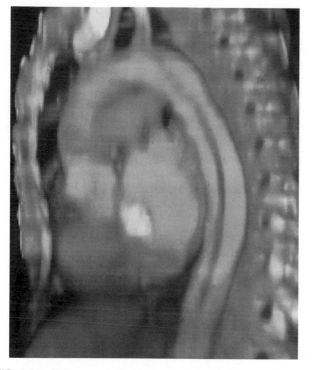

FIG. 1-15. Oblique sagittal reformation of the volumetric dataset in a patient with type B dissection. Note visualization of major aortic vessels and intimal flap. (Courtesy of Elliot K. Fishman, M.D., Baltimore, MD.)

the lesion. An oblique approach allows sampling of more of the pathology without the risk of penetrating the lung. This is particularly important in rib lesions and for chest wall and pleural lesions located near the diaphragm. A coaxial technique, using a needle with a larger bore to guide repeated sampling passes with a thinner needle, is useful in reducing procedure time.

DATA PROCESSING AND DISPLAY METHODS

Dramatic increases in computer speed, data handling, storage, and display capabilities, along with the development of properly registered large volumetric data sets, render feasible the application of advanced image processing and display techniques in thoracic CT. Volumetric display methods are most effective when image resolution is isotropic, which means that image pixels would have the same dimensions in the image plane as well as through the image plane. Obviously this is not achievable with CT in which voxels are considerably smaller within the imaging plane than through the imaging plane because of noise considerations and detector physics. However, with volumetric CT and overlapping slice reconstruction it is possible to minimize this problem.

Once a high quality data set is acquired in a volumetric fashion, several classes of image processing and display techniques can be used. For displaying the anatomy, there are two general methods to view CT data: multiplanar reformation, and 3-D rendering techniques.

Multiplanar Reformation

Multiplanar reformation is a 2-D display created through any arbitrary plane intersecting the CT volume. Typically, sagittal and coronal reformations are displayed side-by-side and, in some software packages, sagittal and coronal views extracted from the same 3-D volume of data can be shown on a single image (34). Likewise, arbitrary reformation of oblique planes can be interactively prescribed on most current display systems (Fig. 1-15). For structures that do not conform to either sagittal or coronal or oblique planes, curved planar reformation is possible. However, when displaying structures such as tortuous vessels or airways, arbitrary curved reformation along the main axis of the structure can lead to considerable anatomic distortion. If not performed properly, stenoses can be simulated in such vessels or airways.

Volumetric Rendering

Because of the limitation of multiplanar reformation, graphics software developers have sought to directly visualize the entire volume of data (34,35,36). Obviously, this approach requires that a strategy be developed to avoid confusing superimposition of structures. Because the data can be viewed from multiple angles, such superimposition problems can be partially overcome.

Two main strategies exist for creating 3-D rendering of volumetric image data. These are shaded surface displays and true volumetric rendering.

Shaded Surface Displays

Shaded surface displays require the prior identification of the surface of a particular anatomic structure of interest so as to separate it from the 3-D data set and have the remainder of the anatomy removed from the displayed set (Fig. 1-16).

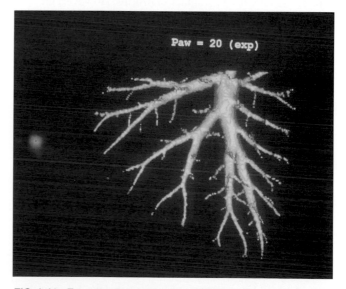

FIG. 1-16. Example of shaded surface display of bronchial tree. Note poor visualization of more peripheral branches with gaps in the data.

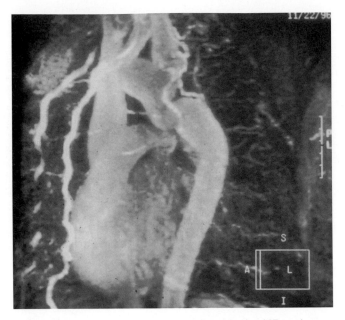

FIG. 1-17. Example of maximum intensity projection MR angiogram of the aorta in a patient with aortic coarctation. Note visualization of collateral vessels in upper thorax and prominent internal mammary arteries. Image acquired with gadolinium-enhanced single breath-hold fast three dimensional T1-weighted acquisition.

This method requires a strong density difference at the interface between the structure of interest and the surrounding tissues (37). This is why this method is most appropriate for bony structures and contrast-enhanced vascular structures or along the interface between airways and soft tissues in the mediastinum.

Once the surface is identified, the computer creates a mesh-like representation of the structure, which can then be shaded to provide color and depth cues. Because the amount of data is greatly reduced in shaded surface displays, impressive color-coded depiction of the anatomy can be easily achieved on standard computer platforms. However, the perceived size of the structure is dependent upon the exact threshold density chosen. This is of particular concern in smaller anatomic structures in the bronchial or arterial trees in which partial volume effects create gaps in the displayed surface. Therefore, shaded surface displays are most appropriate for larger anatomic structures such as the aorta and great vessels or the spine.

Volume Rendering

Because of the limitation of shaded surface displays, investigators have explored methods that would depict the entire volume of data. In volume rendering, the processing strategy is based on the use of linear projections of virtual rays through the data set to create a projectional image of the pixels of interest. The most commonly known volume rendering technique is maximum intensity projection, which is used to display structures of interest that are brighter than adjacent structures (38,39). This is of particular usefulness

in CT angiography and MR angiography (Fig. 1-17). Each pixel in the output image corresponds to the maximum pixel value encountered along the path of the ray. As the mathematical rays that analyze the data set are rotated around the entire volume of data, images representing the maximum pixel value along each projection are displayed. This technique eliminates structures that do not exhibit maximum intensity along the ray and thus "extracts" out of the image volume the relevant structures that display maximum intensity. Unlike shaded surface displays, this technique preserves relative density information since it is not surface dependent. More or less dense vessels can be appreciated and calcification, stents, or coils within vessels can be identified. Smaller structures can be visualized more easily with maximum intensity projection than with shaded surface displays and these structures are better defined. In the chest, this method suffers, however, from the large number of overlapping vessels and dense ribs. This is why it is necessary to edit, from the data set, the bony structures for better results in vascular display. In addition, because of overlapping and anatomically adjacent vascular mediastinal structures, it can be difficult to identify smaller branches in such regions. Nonetheless, maximum intensity projection methods have gained wide acceptance because of their ease of use and general applicability. Furthermore, the large density difference between lung parenchyma and vascular structures allows easy application of these algorithms.

An alternative rendering technique, the minimum intensity projection (MINIP), also has utility in the thorax. This method identifies the voxel with the minimum intensity along the projectional ray and can be useful for visualizing the airways as well as areas of emphysematous destruction because of their lower attenuation than surrounding mediastinal or pulmonary parenchyma (6,40). However, the density difference between pulmonary and airway density is small and partial volume effects in smaller airway branches diminish the usefulness of this method beyond segmental anatomy.

More computationally intensive forms of volume rendering are now increasingly used in clinical practice because of the availability and lower costs of advanced graphics computers (36). By attributing colors and opacity values to all pixels encountered around a ray, it is possible to display semitransparent data sets containing all of the anatomic structures of interest (Fig. 1-18). This method allows different tissues to be visualized either through spatial gradients used to simulate gray scale and lighting effects or different colors or opacities pegged to the expected range of CT attenuations of specific tissues. Such comprehensive volume rendering schemes require specialized workstations for their clinical application. Such advanced workstations, however, offer the possibility of additional processing steps of potential clinical value. For example, instead of creating views from points external to the data set, views can be created from viewing perspectives inside the data set. Typically, these rendering techniques try to simulate the point of view of the human eye, such as giving depth cues to create the

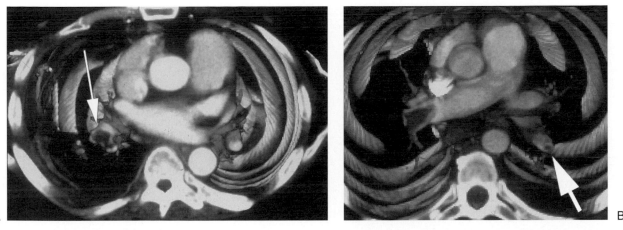

FIG. 1-18. Three dimensional volume rendering of a patient with pulmonary embolus (*arrows*) demonstrated by contrast-enhanced spiral CT. **A:** Note thrombus in right pulmonary artery. **B:** Note small thrombus in left pulmonary artery. (Courtesy of Elliot K. Fishman, M.D., Baltimore, MD.)

impression of perspective within hollow organs. These methods, termed virtual bronchoscopy or virtual angioscopy offer considerable promise in visualizing endobronchial and endovascular pathology (Fig. 1-19). These techniques, however, require intense computation. In our experience and that of others, it is generally necessary to implement software that automatically identifies the center line of either airways or vessels for optimal navigation within the structure of interest when performing virtual perspective imaging. In combination with other modes of rendering, this method may be of great use in surgical planning and surgical follow-up.

Alternative Axial Display Methods

Because of the large number of hard copy films that can be generated with volumetric CT data or volumetric MR

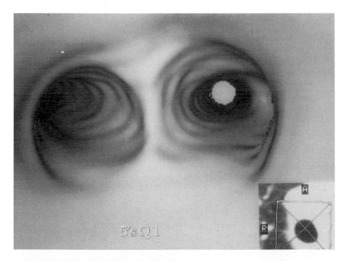

FIG. 1-19. Example of perspective rendering in virtual bronchoscopy. Note depth cues provided by lighting and shading effects. The internal morphology of the airways is demonstrated at the level of the carina. These images are displayed to simulate the appearance of the airways as seen with flexible bronchoscopy, with right-sided airways shown to the right side of the image. Note that this software simultaneously displays the corresponding axial image in the upper right corner of the image.

data, other strategies for displaying a large number of views have become necessary. For example, rapid sequential display of adjacent axial slices have been found useful because of the ability of the human brain to integrate rapidly changing scenes. Integration of anatomic data from adjacent slices that are rapidly and sequentially displayed allows the user to immediately recognize connected structures such as airways or vessels and identify nonconnected structures such as nodules (41). The implementation of such schemes on standard display stations is now common and will play an increasingly important role in the future. An alternative to rapid sequential display of adjacent images is the creation of preprocessed data slabs to both reduce the necessary hard copies and allow the identification of anatomic connectivity of given structures, such as arteriovenous malformations. This technique, known as sliding thin slab maximum intensity projection, can both reduce the number of necessary hard copies and increase lesion conspicuity (see Fig. 1-4) (39).

IMAGE SEGMENTATION METHODS

Most computer display methods in use today are based on one or more passive properties of tissues that are exploited to better depict a particular structure. Although these structures are visually extracted, they are not truly separated or segmented out from the surrounding data set. Segmentation methods are a class of algorithms that seek to automatically identify a particular structure in the image and extract all of its voxels from the data set for specific measurements and analysis. The simplest problem of this class in thoracic CT is the extraction of lung parenchyma for specific measurements of its density exclusive of vascular branches. Other applications are the specific identification of venous, arterial, and airway trees. These goals can be accomplished by three separate approaches: active contours, seed region growing algorithms, and mathematical morphologic methods.

Active contour methods have been developed to overcome

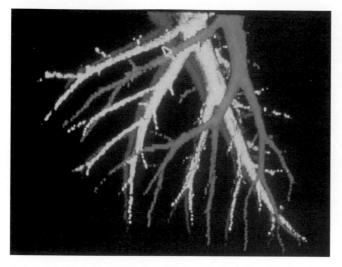

FIG. 1-20. Example of segmentation and extraction of pulmonary veins (*dark gray*), arteries (*light gray*), and airways (*white*). Paw = 5, Pv = 5.

the weakness of thresholding algorithms whereby certain pixels that belong to a given structure are mistakenly removed because partial volume effects can change the measured density of the pixel. Active contours overcome these local imperfections in the data set by computing the expected positions of neighboring pixels along any given contour. If a gap or additional spurious pixels are found, the algorithm can automatically estimate the appropriate contour by defining what the optimum contour path would be. Active contours have been used to identify endocardial and epicardial borders in the heart as well as pulmonary boundaries.

To specifically identify pulmonary tree structures in 3-D, a seed region growing algorithm can be used whereby an initial seed point is defined on the first slice within the lumen of either the main airways or pulmonary arteries or veins (Fig. 1-20). All pixels contiguous to the seed within the representative CT density range for the airway lumen are added to the seed pixel (42). The algorithm terminates when the transition area between wall and lumen is no longer measurable. The advantage of this method is that each pixel belonging to the tree structure is individually identified. From this data set, cross-sectional measurements truly perpendicular to any airway or any vessel can be accomplished. In addition, the central axis of the tree can be captured to define the branch topology and geometric features and content of each tree. This method allows the central axis to be used for fly-through virtual bronchoscopy or angioscopy as well as a point of reference to compare airways and vessels at different physiologic states (Fig. 1-21).

The third method is automated segmentation using mathematical morphology, which is based on the use of geometric structures of different shapes and size to process images (Fig. 1-22) (43). By defining the expected structural elements of a given anatomic feature, the algorithm can identify even small branches that are missed by conventional thresholding methods (44). In addition to enabling the specific extraction of anatomic features, these methods also permit intelligent recognition of features of interest at different states of inflation or after intervention and can compare changes between states (45,46). A clinical application that has been demonstrated is the ability to automatically remove vascular structures from CT data sets to enhance recognition of pulmonary metastases (Fig. 1-23) (47).

In summary, advanced image computing is gaining a strong foothold in the clinical armamentarium of thoracic imaging. Besides passive display techniques, more intelligent algorithms are now being developed for specific recognition of not only anatomic features but also other patterns

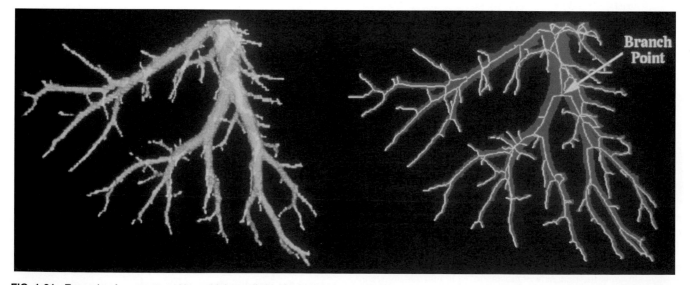

FIG. 1-21. Example of a segmented bronchial tree (**left**) obtained using a seed growing region algorithm with computation and depiction of the central axis (**right**) and branch points of airways demonstrated.

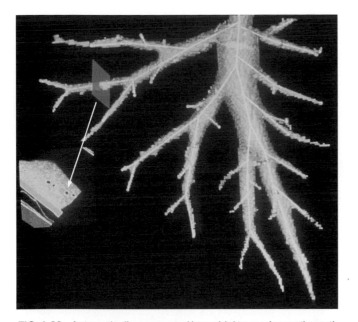

FIG. 1-22. Automatically segmented bronchial tree using mathematical morphology algorithm and automated identification of the center line performed on an advanced computer. The software displays simultaneously the original CT image at the location of the selected airway segment (*arrow*).

TECHNIQUES AND STRATEGIES IN THORACIC MR IMAGING

Because of technical limitations, magnetic resonance imaging (MRI) has not been used as extensively in the investigation of thoracic pathology as CT. There are several drawbacks to the use of MR in the thorax. Motion artifacts generated by cardiac and respiratory movements are difficult to control. Only 10% to 20% of lung parenchyma represents tissue and circulating blood; consequently, expanded lung has insufficient protons capable of generating an MR signal. Furthermore, the parenchyma is difficult to image by MR because of magnetic susceptibility effects related to the numerous air-tissue interfaces inherent to the structure of lung. Because the magnetic field is made heterogeneous by the different magnetic susceptibilities of air and tissue, the T2 relaxation time of lung tissue is short, which reduces the available signal. These characteristics mean that unless the lung becomes abnormal as a consequence of edema, consolidation, or fibrosis, it is difficult to image by MR. For example, MR is very useful in patients with an opacified hemithorax in which better tissue signal and absence of motion result in excellent images (Fig. 1-24). On the other hand, certain characteristics of MR enhance its usefulness for thoracic imaging as a second line modality to resolve problems not fully addressed with CT. These characteristics include the ability to demonstrate flow without the use of contrast agents, the multiplanar capability of the modality, and its high tissue differentiation.

The technologic advances implemented over the last few years have permitted the routine acquisition of nearly artifact-free images of the thorax at scan times of less than 1 second per image with full 3-D acquisitions within a single breath-hold. These images permit exquisite demonstration of all cardiovascular structures. With the advent of newer pulse sequences for MR angiography, MR imaging is an attractive modality for primary cardiovascular pathology.

and physiologic parameters. By enabling extraction of imaging information within and between data sets of the same patients, better diagnosis and monitoring of multiple disease entities can be foreseen. For example, such methods will be crucial, we believe, to the development of CT angiography for the detection of pulmonary embolus by allowing computers to identify areas of high suspicion for the radiologist's review. This form of computer-aided diagnosis has already found applications in breast imaging. Likewise, such methods could be of use in the screening of lung cancer in the future.

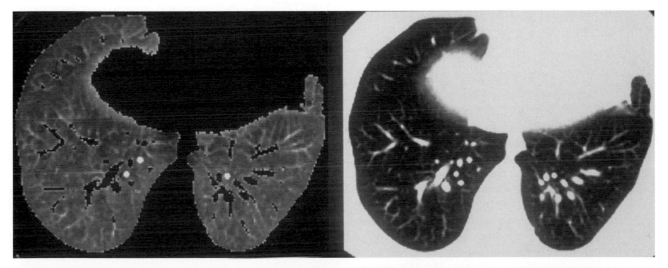

FIG. 1-23. Automatic segmentation and removal of vascular structures for enhanced detection of pulmonary nodules. On the left is the computer-processed image showing three separate metastatic nodules that could not be identified on the original image on the right (see also Fig. 4-4).

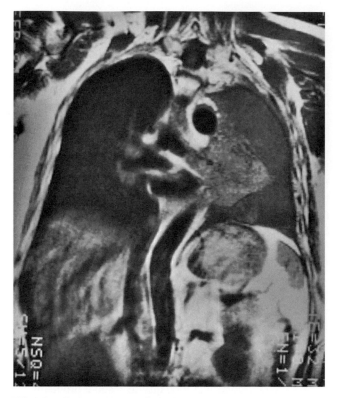

FIG. 1-24. Patient with opacified left hemithorax on chest radiograph. Coronal MR shows excellent delineation of pathology in the left lung. The left lung is collapsed. There is obstruction of the left mainstem bronchus by tumor. Associated left pleural effusion is present with shift of the mediastinum to the left side. Note the sharp demonstration of the left hemidiaphragm as compared to that of the right hemidiaphragm. MR is well suited to evaluate the opacified or partially opacified hemithorax because respiratory artifacts are nil in such cases and tissue differentiation afforded by MR permits a reliable and rapid diagnosis.

Because of its multi-planar imaging capability and the excellent depiction of musculoskeletal structures, MR is well-suited to evaluate processes located near the apex of the lung, near the spine, in the chest wall, processes suspected of involving mediastinal vessels and peridiaphragmatic regions.

Indications

MR has very limited indications in evaluating pulmonary parenchymal pathology except in cases of extensive combined pleural and parenchymal disease. The high tissue differentiation capability of MR provides an easy way to differentiate in a single examination pleural collections from areas of consolidation and associated mediastinal and chest wall involvement. It can also identify cystic lesions that may appear solid on CT such as bronchogenic cysts. MR can help differentiate residual fibrosis from residual or recurrent tumor. This can be of value for patients with lymphoma when long term monitoring is indicated (48). MR obviates the need for contrast injection in most cases and is thus

particularly useful in patients with impaired renal function. MR is also indicated for evaluating chest wall lesions (49,50). Likewise, invasion of the mediastinal structures and heart by tumors is optimally defined with MR because of its multi-planar and vascular visualization capabilities (51). This can be helpful in patients with equivocal CT findings of invasion of a critical structure (52).

MR is an effective modality in evaluating thoracic aortic dissection and aneurysms as well as in evaluating the postoperative aorta. Congenital anomalies of the aorta and major vessels are easily examined by MR. It provides exquisite demonstration of the pulmonary arteries and is accurate in the detection of central pulmonary emboli. A further indication for MR is the evaluation of the neck and upper mediastinal veins in patients with indwelling venous catheters for chemotherapy, parenteral nutrition, and long-term antibiotic therapy, and for the differentiation of masses from vascular structures (Fig. 1-25).

Clinical indications of MR for cardiac applications include the investigation of congenital heart disease, suspected intracardiac masses, pericardial disease, evaluation of the mechanical function and perfusion of the myocardium. The above indications reflect the current status of MR applications in thoracic imaging according to our experience. More recently MR has been shown capable to visualize pulmonary perfusion using contrast agents (53) and ventilation using pure oxygen gas (54). Hyperpolarized gases such as xenon (55) or helium (56) also show promise in greatly improving visualization of the pulmonary parenchyma by MR.

Safety Considerations

There are no documented, lasting, harmful effects from MR. In high field strength magnets, radio frequency (RF) power deposition has the potential to raise body core temperature, especially in children. MRI is absolutely contraindicated in patients with cardiac pacemakers. Even at very low field strengths, the operation of a pacemaker can be modified by the magnetic field. In addition, pacing leads can act as antennas and receive the RF pulses from the imaging sequence, thus pacing the heart at a very high rate. Even with inactive pacemakers, examining patients with pacing leads in place is not recommended. Multiple instances of first and second degree burns of the thorax caused by the proximity of looped electrocardiogram (ECG) wires, have been reported. It is thus very important to avoid contact of looped ECG wires with the patient's skin. Because the magnetic field induces a torque force on ferromagnetic intracranial aneurysm clips, patients with such clips should not be studied. However, nonferromagnetic clips or prosthetic materials are not dangerous. All heart valves can be imaged except for the older Starr-Edwards type, which are ferromagnetic. MR is also contraindicated in the presence of metal objects within the eye or near the spinal cord, cochlear implants, and neurostimulators connected to the patient. Metallic vascular

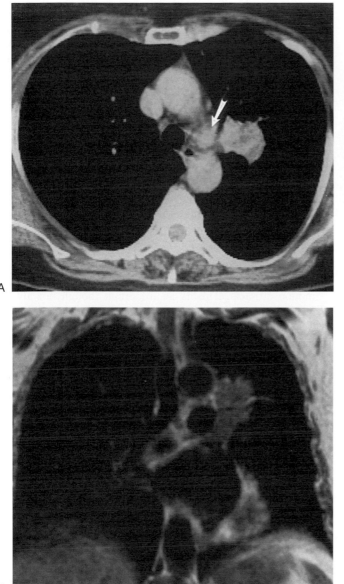

A

B

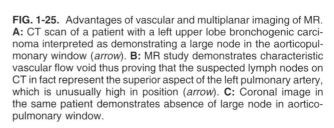

C

FIG. 1-25. Advantages of vascular and multiplanar imaging of MR. **A:** CT scan of a patient with a left upper lobe bronchogenic carcinoma interpreted as demonstrating a large node in the aorticopulmonary window (*arrow*). **B:** MR study demonstrates characteristic vascular flow void thus proving that the suspected lymph nodes on CT in fact represent the superior aspect of the left pulmonary artery, which is unusually high in position (*arrow*). **C:** Coronal image in the same patient demonstrates absence of large node in aorticopulmonary window.

stents for coronary and more peripheral vessels present some risks of dislodgement and MR is not indicated for at least 2 weeks after stent placement (57).

Technical Parameters

The thorax is probably the most difficult area of the body to examine with MR. MR is an imaging method characterized by a low signal level arising from tissues. Thus, any loss of signal or inappropriate increase in noise will degrade the image. Consequently, one should always seek to ensure an optimal signal-to-noise ratio (SNR). Another source of problems is sensitivity to motion artifacts. This problem however has been greatly reduced by the advent of new gradient systems and pulse sequences that can routinely image the entire chest in a one or two breath-holds (58,59).

Adequate Prescan Tuning

The MR signal is first generated by an RF excitation pulse and is received afterward by an antenna called a receiver coil. Because the MRI system is not absolutely stable, the resonance frequency may drift. In addition, the presence of the patient's body within the magnet changes the magnetic field slightly in a manner that varies from patient to patient. Consequently, the exact resonance frequency varies slightly for each patient. In addition, RF penetration is different from patient to patient and the RF pulse strength needed to maximize the signal will be different for each patient. It is therefore essential to perform a prescan procedure to define the exact resonance frequency and the appropriate level of RF exposure for each patient, each region of the body, and before each image sequence. Most newer scanners now offer efficient automated prescan routines.

Signal-to-Noise Considerations

Several important steps are needed to ensure an adequate SNR for a thoracic MR examination. Optimizing SNR without increasing examination time is also an important factor. It is not yet possible with MR to obtain the same spatial resolution as with CT. To maintain an adequate SNR, voxels in MRI have to be made larger than with CT. The most effective strategies to improve SNR relate to geometric factors such as slice thickness, pixel size, diameter of the FOV, and size of the receiving coil. In MR, very thin slice thicknesses are not achievable for large body parts, and slices less than 3 mm in thickness should be avoided. However, with newer 3-D acquisition pulse sequences and the use of phased array surface coils designed specifically for thoracic imaging, SNR is improved and slices as thin as 1.5 mm are now available. A frequent bias of radiologists trained in other cross sectional imaging methods is to use the finest matrix available. This lowers the SNR since each voxel is the smallest possible. In addition, scan times in MRI are directly proportional to the number of pixels in the phase-encoding direction. Generally, the spatial resolution of MR for large body parts is less than that achieved by CT. For smaller body parts or children the resolution of MR, however, is superior to that of CT. To maintain SNR, the user can select a number of image matrices, usually 256 frequency encoding steps by 256, 192, or 128 phase encoding steps. In our experience a 256 × 192 matrix is generally adequate. A 256 × 256 matrix is reserved for cases in which maximum resolution is important. Finer matrices of 512 pixels, which are now available on modern scanners, are rarely necessary in the chest.

One of the most powerful ways to affect SNR is to modify the FOV. Ideally, FOV should be equal to the size of the region of interest. However, one should remember that when the FOV is reduced, the size of the pixel is reduced in both the X and Y directions. Therefore, in MR a reduction of the FOV by a factor of two reduces pixel size by four, thus decreasing SNR by four. As a general rule, one should avoid using an FOV of less than half the diameter of the receiving coil. On the other hand, a slight increase in FOV can be very effective in improving image quality.

The best way to improve SNR in MR is to use receiving coils placed in close proximity to the body part being examined. Even more effective has been the introduction of multicoil phased arrays, which greatly enhance the reception of the MR signal (60).

Because the MR signal decays rapidly it is imperative to use very short echo-time (TE) whenever possible. Since the T2 of tissues is relatively short (about 30 to 70 milliseconds), a reduction in the TE time of a few milliseconds makes a potentially large difference. Short echo times also reduce motion artifacts. This is an important though not always available option. With current scanners TEs on the order of 3 to 4 milliseconds are routinely achievable.

Averaging signal from the same pixels by increasing the number of RF excitations can also improve SNR. For example, by doubling the number of excitations, SNR improves by the square root of two. This however increases scanning time and is a time inefficient way to improve image quality.

Prevention and Correction of Motion Artifacts

There are three major sources of motion artifacts in thoracic MR: the beating heart, blood traveling through vessels, and respiratory excursions of the anterior chest wall. A series of correcting steps need to be taken to achieve optimal image quality.

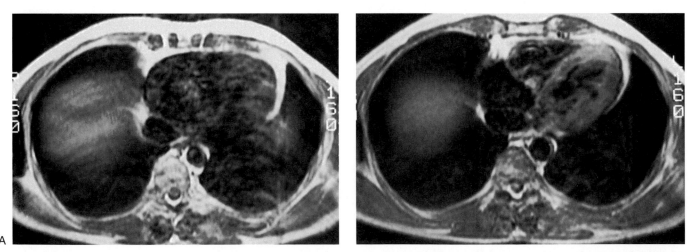

A

B

FIG. 1-26. Cranio-caudal versus caudo-cranial scanning with electrocardiogram (ECG) gating. **A:** ECG-gated image of the heart obtained with a cranio-caudal prescription in which first scan is obtained near the thoracic inlet and last scan is obtained in the cardiac region. Note absence of detail and major artifacts over the heart region. **B:** Same patient, same ECG-gating except that the scans were prescribed in a caudo-cranial direction with the early scans being obtained in the cardiac region. Intracardiac detail is now available with much decreased motion and flow artifacts. In ECG-gated thoracic scanning, scans in which maximum image quality is desired should be prescribed first to correspond with the systolic phase.

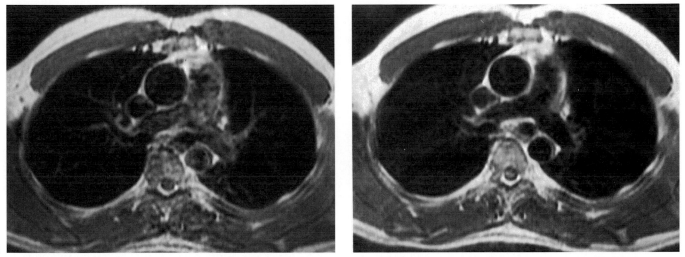

FIG. 1-27. Flow-related artifacts. **A:** Image obtained during diastolic phase shows presence of signal in most vessels caused by nearly stationary flow during diastole. Note visualization of pulmonary vessels. **B:** Same scan level obtained during systolic phase. Better flow void effect is observed because of the higher velocity of blood during systole. Note also that pulmonary vessels are not visualized on this scan.

Cardiac Gating

In thoracic MRI, we strongly recommend the systematic use of cardiac gating. By synchronizing the acquisition of the images to the heart cycle, the cardiac walls can be imaged in reproducible positions. ECG gating entails only a 10% to 15% increase in scan time but significantly improves image quality. An important technical consideration that is often overlooked is the fact that ECG gating is most reliable in the early phase of the cardiac cycle between the QRS and the T-wave of the ECG tracing (systole). The later part of the cardiac cycle is the most variable. It is, therefore, better to scan the thorax in a caudal to cranial direction, rather than from the thoracic inlet to the abdomen as usually performed in CT (Fig. 1-26). This ensures that the scans obtained over the heart are acquired during the early and most reproducible portion of the cardiac cycle, thus improving image quality.

Elimination of Artifacts Related to Blood Motion

Blood traveling in a pulsatile fashion through the major mediastinal vessels can generate variable degrees of signal, provoking ghost artifacts in the phase direction of the image. The most effective method to reduce this problem is to decrease the signal arising from blood by reducing the magnetization of incoming blood. This is accomplished by applying RF pulses adjacent to the imaged region (Fig. 1-27). The other approach is to use very fast gated sequences, thus eliminating blood motion effects during image acquisition (59).

Respiratory Motion Artifacts

Respiratory gating is never used because the cycle time of respiration is too long, necessitating excessively lengthy examination times. However, respiratory compensation techniques that change the order of acquisition of the phase encoding steps of the image can be quite effective. These techniques match the motion of the anterior chest wall to the acquisition and reconstruction of the image, significantly reducing respiratory artifacts. This method, known as respiratory-ordered phase encoding, is quite effective if the anterior chest wall motion of the patient is properly recorded. Thus, special attention should be given to the placement of the sensing device, usually a pneumatic belt or nasal thermistor.

Pulse Sequences

The thorax is best examined with pulse sequences that are less motion sensitive. In addition, mediastinal fat is an ideal contrasting tissue. Thus, sequences with long relaxation time (TR) and long TE, which decrease the contrast between fat and surrounding tissues and are extremely motion sensitive, should be reserved for purposes of tissue characterization.

T1-weighted sequences with shorter TR and TE are extremely effective in the thorax and form the backbone of the thoracic MR study. Since all studies are gated, the TR is equal to the RR interval. The TE should be short in the range of 5 to 15 milliseconds. For spin echo images, it is not necessarily productive to use TE shorter than 15 milliseconds because it tends to increase blood signal, thereby generating ghost artifacts. With a normal heart rate of 60 to 80 beats per minute, ECG gating produces pulse sequences with a TR of 700 to 1,000 milliseconds. Thus, simultaneous acquisition in a multi-slice mode of 14 to 20 images can easily be achieved. With the introduction of better hardware and software, more efficient pulse sequences have now been implemented. The most effective scheme is to use segmented K-space sequences in which multiple lines of data are acquired after each excitation (58). These methods can accelerate image acquisition time by a factor of ten or more. All scanners now offer varying versions of this general scheme allowing single images to be acquired in less than one second and full volumes in 15 to 20 seconds. These sequences can also be repeated multiple times for dynamic studies and if gated can acquire cine images of the cardiovascular system in a total of 16 to 20 seconds. Both gradient-echo and spin-echo sequences have been implemented with these rapid sequences.

In practice, it is most advantageous to first perform a coronal segmented K-space, T1-weighted series of images with a 10-mm slice thickness, 3 to 5 mm gap, 256 × 192 matrix, 1 Nex, 42 to 48 cm FOV covering the entire thorax. This series of images requires a single breath-hold of approximately 15 seconds. Based on this first sequence, a series of cardiac gated T1-weighted axial scans can then be prescribed. As mentioned earlier, it is important to acquire scans in the cardiac region early in the RR interval. Slice thickness should be 7 to 10 mm with a 256 × 192 matrix, TE 15 or 20 using respiratory compensation and presaturation above and below the imaging volume. The FOV should be adjusted to the patient's size.

Role of T2-Weighted Sequences

In our experience, the coronal and transaxial rapid T1-weighted sequences are the most effective. If no pathology is found on these sequences, it is unlikely that a T2-weighted sequence would reveal additional information. T2-weighted sequences are often necessary to characterize pathology already detected or suspected on the T1-weighted scans. With the advent of segmented K-space fast spin echo sequences

it is now practical to acquire good T2-weighted quality images of the thorax (61).

MR ANGIOGRAPHIC TECHNIQUES

Much progress has been accomplished in the development of MR angiographic techniques. After much research and development it has become evident that fast gradient echo sequences with or without cinematic acquisition offer the best approach to visualize intra luminal blood. More recently the introduction of contrast enhanced 3-D single breath-hold angiography using gadolinium-based contrast agents has enabled excellent depiction of mediastinal and pulmonary vessels (Fig. 1-28). These techniques are known as *white blood angiography* because of the high signal of blood. Other sequences rely on the elimination of signal from flowing blood and are known as *black blood angiography*. White blood angiography is best at characterizing luminal flow, and black blood angiography is best at directly demonstrating the vascular walls.

TISSUE CHARACTERIZATION BY MR IMAGING

The differences in signal intensity patterns of human tissues are based essentially on differences in proton density and T1 and T2 relaxation times. Tissue differentiation and contrast in images also depends on the particular pulse sequence used. One of the most difficult tasks for the diagnostic radiologist analyzing MR images is to develop an understanding of the meaning of signal intensity changes. Unlike CT, in which image contrast is essentially determined by atomic attenuation of x-rays, the tissue characteristics that determine MR relaxation times are more complex. In this section we will present the most important concepts underlying the interpretation of signal differences in MR images.

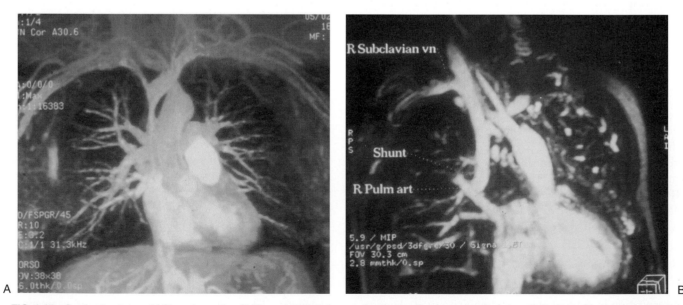

FIG. 1-28. Contrast-enhanced MR angiography. **A:** Normal patient. Image shows excellent vascular depiction. **B:** Patient with tetralogy of Fallot, status post-Glenn shunt. Study demonstrates patency of shunt between superior vena cava and the right pulmonary artery.

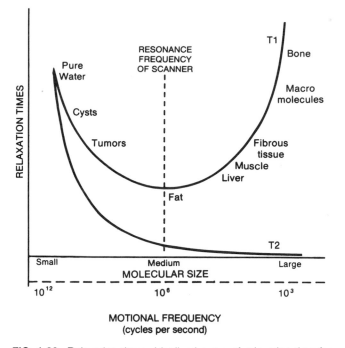

FIG. 1-29. Relaxation times. Idealized curve of relaxation time for various tissues is represented as a function of molecular size. For molecules such as fat, which have a motional frequency close to the resonance frequency of clinical scanners, T1 relaxation is most efficient and the T1 time is shortest. For smaller molecules such as pure water or larger molecules such as macromolecules, the T1 times will be much longer because they are not matched to the resonance frequency of the scanner. T2 times relate mostly to degree of freedom between molecules. For pure water, in which molecules are freely mobile, the T2 time is long. For macromolecules or bone in which atoms are restricted in motion, the T2 times are short. These factors are the main determinant of relaxation times.

Role of Molecular Motion on Relaxation Times

Relaxation times are essentially determined by the size, motional characteristics, and degrees of motional freedom of the various molecules making up tissues.

T1 Relaxation

The first step in generating an MR image is to excite hydrogen nuclei with an RF pulse. After excitation, the nuclei progressively return to rest by giving off energy to the surrounding molecules. This is known as the spin lattice, or T1 relaxation process. When the exchange of energy between the proton and the molecule on which it is located is efficient, the T1 time is short. When this exchange of energy is inefficient, the T1 time is long. The most important factor in determining efficiency of T1 relaxation is whether the resonance frequency of the MR scanner is close to the frequency of motion of the surrounding molecules.

Indeed, all molecules move or "tumble" at a given frequency. This motional frequency basically depends on the size of the molecule. For example, large tissue molecules, such as proteins or DNA, have a very slow tumbling frequency of about 1,000 cycles per second. On the other hand, water molecules, which are very small, have a much higher

frequency of motion in the range of 100 billion to 1 trillion cycles per second. Between these extremes are tissue molecules of various sizes and varying frequencies of motion.

When molecules move at a rate equal to or near the resonance frequency of the magnet, energy exchanges between the resonating protons and their carrier molecules are enhanced. In human tissues, fat molecules or triglycerides have molecular motional frequencies close to the resonance frequencies of clinical scanners. Thus, fat exhibits the shortest T1 relaxation time, ranging from 250 to 400 millisecond. For molecules larger or smaller than fat with respectively lower or higher frequencies of motion, relaxation times are less efficient than for fatty molecules (Fig. 1-29). This explains why water molecules have a much longer T1 than fat. It also explains why large macromolecules, such as those found in fibrous tissue, exhibit long T1 times. This is simply because their motional frequencies are not matched to the resonance frequencies of current clinical scanners. This also explains why T1 times of tissues are different for magnets of different field strengths. In general, as the resonance frequency increases with higher field strength, T1 relaxation becomes less efficient and T1 times increase. As a rule of thumb, there is an increase of about 500 millisecond for each tesla of increase in magnetic field strength.

Influence of Degree of Molecular Freedom on T2 Relaxation

T2 relaxation depends primarily on interactions between nuclei. In a general way, T2 depends on the degree of freedom between molecules in a particular tissue. For example, water molecules move freely and very little restrictions or interactions exist. Hence, the T2 relaxation of pure water is long. In larger molecules, spin interactions are so restricted that rapid dephasing of the magnetic vectors of nuclei is observed after RF excitation, leading to a short T2 time. One can then simplify the understanding of relaxation times by relating them to molecular size, which is itself related to molecular motion for T1, and relative freedom between molecules for T2. This concept is summarized in (Fig. 1-30). For tissues that have very short T2 times, the MR signal decays very fast and cannot be recorded within the TE time. As a consequence, macromolecules, proteins, cell membranes, and all tissues in which molecules are restricted in motion are not usually visible by MR. In essence, only mobile water and fat molecules generate signal in clinical MR. However, this does not mean that MR is simply a water/fat imaging technique. Water molecules do interact with surrounding proteins and macromolecules that make up the structure of live tissues. Thus, the motional frequency and degrees of freedom of water can be affected by the nearby molecules, thereby changing the relaxation time of water.

Influence of Macromolecular/Water Interactions on Relaxation Times

Water molecules that come close to the larger MR invisible molecules may be slowed in their motional frequency

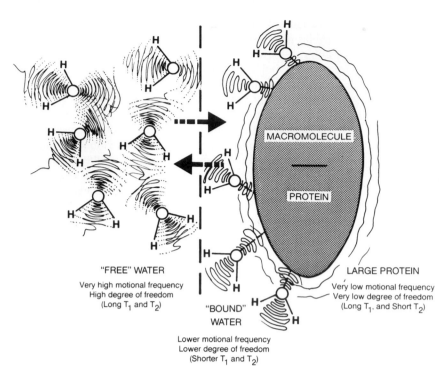

FIG. 1-30. Macromolecular/water interactions. The main determinant of relaxation times in tissues is the interaction of water with large macromolecules that are not normally visible in MR. When water is free, long T1 and T2 times are observed because of the high motional frequency and the high degree of freedom observed in free water. However, when water molecules come close to larger biologic molecules such as proteins, its motional frequency and degree of freedom are reduced, thus the T1 and T2 relaxation times are proportionately reduced. The degree of slowing down of water by the various biologic molecules is what ultimately determines in great part the appearance of tissues on MR images.

by temporary bindings near the surface of such molecules. Therefore, relaxation times of water are modulated by the presence of the various macromolecules of tissues. Even though large tissue molecules are not directly visible by MR, their effect on the water molecules surrounding them can actually be seen as a change in the relaxation time of water. This is the mechanism by which tissue contrast and tissue characterization are achieved in MR.

At the tissue level, MR signal reflects the averaged contribution of the histologic constituents of normal and patho-logic processes. Components of tissues with high free-water content (edema, inflammation, necrosis, glandular fluids, cysts, retained secretions, hemorrhage, and actively growing malignant cells) contribute to high signal intensity on T2-weighted images and to low signal intensity on T1-weighted images. Tissue components rich in structured collagen, elastic fibers, and large proteins exhibit a low signal on T2-weighted scans and a low to intermediate signal on T1-weighted images (Fig. 1-31). Clearly, the MR signal of any given tissue is the complex sum of the signals of its basic

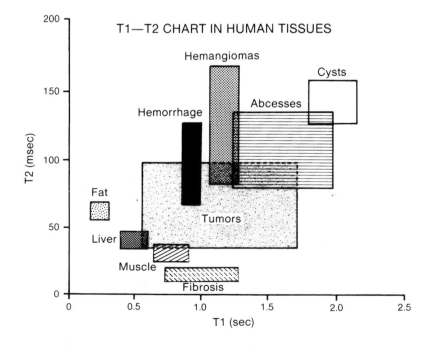

FIG. 1-31. T1/T2 chart of normal and pathologic tissues in humans. This chart summarizes current data on the range of T1 and T2 times observed in various pathologies. Note that fibrosis and tumors overlap in their T1 time but not in their T2 time, thus providing the potential for differentiation.

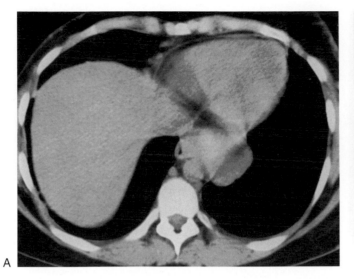
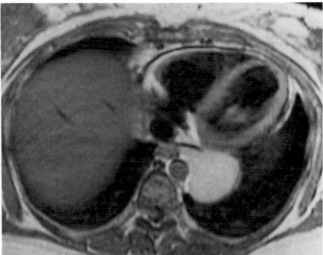
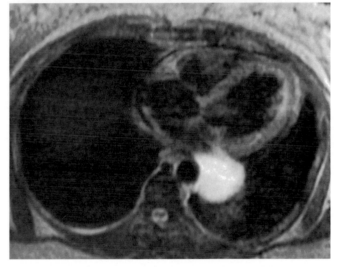

FIG. 1-32. Tissue characterization by MR. **A:** CT scan of a patient demonstrated a mass of soft-tissue density near the gastro-esophageal junction. **B:** Proton density weighted scan, relaxation time (TR) 2,700 and echo time (TE) 20, and **C:** T2-weighted scan, TR 2,700/TE 80 demonstrated a high signal intensity characteristic of fluid. At surgery a duplication cyst with a high protein content was found. Such cysts can appear very dense with CT. However, with MR, their cystic nature can easily be determined.

constituents. Because identical pathologic processes may differ in the relative amount of their constituents, they may exhibit different MR signal characteristics. Conversely, dissimilar pathologic processes may generate the same signal if the sum effect of their basic elements (necrosis, edema, connective tissue) is identical. Clearly, the MR signal of any given tissue cannot be very specific and overlap is observed across tissues. However, if the histologic composition of a tissue changes over time, MR signal is likely to change as well. This ability to track histologic modification is unique to MR and has been proposed as a mechanism for monitoring various processes such as fibrosis or tumor recurrence (48).

Influence of Paramagnetic Agents

Paramagnetic substances are capable of shortening relaxation times by interfering with the homogeneity of the local field and by their interaction with water molecules in close proximity. Indeed, when a paramagnetic substance is present, the main effect by which it reduces T1 times is by locally varying the magnetic field and increasing the range of reso-

nance frequencies of protons at the local level. This permits more effective matching between the motional frequencies of a greater range of tissue molecules and those of the hydrogen nuclei they carry thus accelerating primarily T1 relaxation times.

Tissues or pathologies with paramagnetic properties, such as subacute hemorrhage or tissues containing melanin exhibit a relatively higher signal on T1-weighted images with no effect on the T2-weighted scans. When a superparamagnetic substance such as ferrite is present in tissues it can create strong magnetic field heterogeneity, which shortens T2 times as well. This is also true when tissues are made of components with markedly different magnetic susceptibility properties, such as air spaces and interstitium of lung. Consequently, T2 is reduced and the signal intensity of these tissues is decreased on both T1- and T2-weighted scans.

Implications for Tissue Differentiation

As demonstrated in Figure 1-30, experience with clinical MR shows significant overlap between various types of pa-

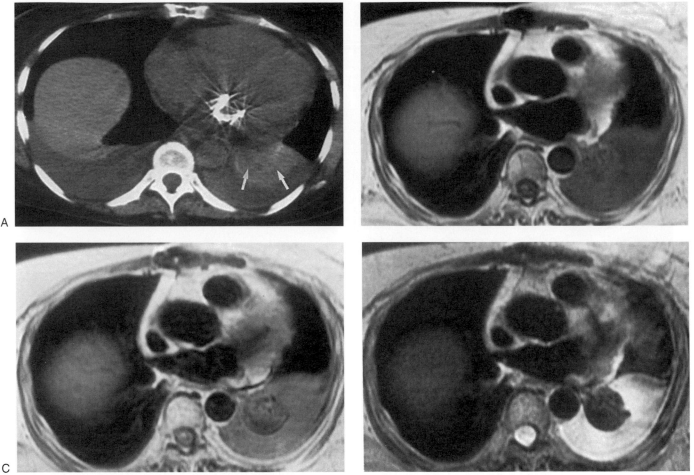

FIG. 1-33. Tissue differentiation on MR. Nonobstructive atelectasis. **A:** CT scan in a patient with large bilateral pleural effusions demonstrates compressed left lower lobe (*arrows*). **B:** On T1-weighted scan obtained several days later, effusion is again noted and compressed lung is seen with a signal intensity similar to that of the surrounding effusion. Note small areas of low signal intensity in the compressed lung represent flow void effect in small pulmonary vessels and not air bronchograms. **C:** Proton density weighted image. Compressed lung parenchyma is now slightly less intense than surrounding pleural effusion. **D:** T2-weighted scan. Compressed lung demonstrates very low signal intensity whereas pleural effusion demonstrates high signal intensity. The low signal intensity of the compressed lung is probably caused by residual air not appreciable on CT scan or T1- or T2-weighted scans. (From ref. 45, with permission.)

thologies. Since differentiation of MR signal depends on the interaction of water and surrounding molecules, limited characterization can be expected. The major differentiating tissue in the thorax is mediastinal and chest wall fat, which has a high signal intensity on T1-weighted scans because of its short T1 time. Vessels, airways, and pathologic lesions are easily contrasted against the fat background. MR is useful, however, in differentiating cysts from solid masses (Fig. 1-32) (63,64). With CT, it is common to observe high density cysts indistinguishable from solid masses. With MR, these cysts tend to have longer T2 relaxation times than solid masses and are therefore of very high intensity on T2-weighted scans, permitting differentiation. MR has been disappointing in distinguishing inflammatory from neoplastic lymphadenopathy (65). In vivo and in vitro studies both demonstrate a significant overlap between bronchogenic carcinoma, nodal metastasis, lymphoma, and granulomatous

diseases. Even though T1 and T2 relaxation times have been shown to be longer for nodes involved with bronchogenic carcinoma than for nodes involved with sarcoidosis, the clinical value of these differences is negated by considerable overlap.

MR is capable of differentiating fibrosis from tumors by virtue of the marked differences in T2 relaxation time of these two processes (66–69). Therefore, when a question of tumor versus fibrosis is raised, MR will demonstrate a low signal intensity for the fibrotic components of the tumor and a high signal intensity for the neoplastic tissue. This is helpful in differentiating residual or recurrent lymphomatous masses from residual fibrosis (48).

MR is valuable in the diagnosis and follow-up of hemorrhage and hematoma (70,71). Subacute hemorrhagic lesions characteristically show high signal intensity on T1-weighted images. This is because of a shortened T1 relaxation time,

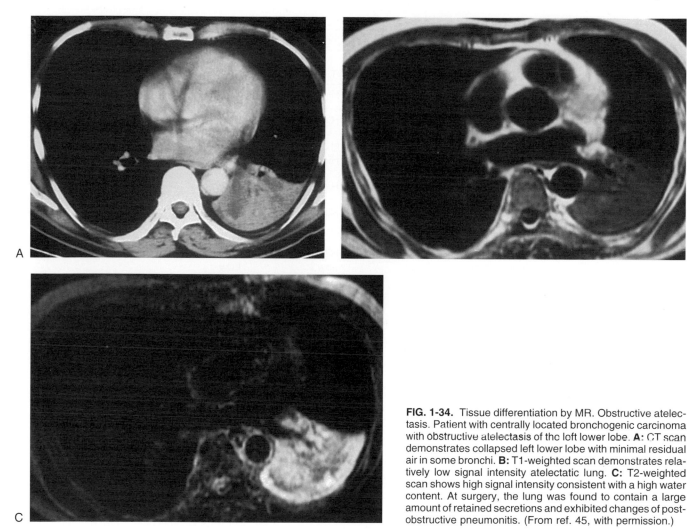

FIG. 1-34. Tissue differentiation by MR. Obstructive atelectasis. Patient with centrally located bronchogenic carcinoma with obstructive atelectasis of the left lower lobe. **A:** CT scan demonstrates collapsed left lower lobe with minimal residual air in some bronchi. **B:** T1-weighted scan demonstrates relatively low signal intensity atelectatic lung. **C:** T2-weighted scan shows high signal intensity consistent with a high water content. At surgery, the lung was found to contain a large amount of retained secretions and exhibited changes of postobstructive pneumonitis. (From ref. 45, with permission.)

resulting from the paramagnetic effects of desaturated hemoglobin and methemoglobin, which occurs as a result of the oxidation of ferrous iron to a high-spin ferric state. Except for hemorrhagic, fatty, cystic, and possibly fibrotic lesions, MR offers little in the differentiation of other malignant or benign processes.

Likewise, MR is limited in the differentiation of pulmonary parenchymal processes. The tissues involved in pulmonary consolidation exhibit substantial overlap in signal characteristics. However, alveolar proteinosis is notable for its short T1 value. Pulmonary hemorrhage may also demonstrate a short T1 behavior at some point in its evolution. Some studies suggest that active severe interstitial lung disease is associated with high signal intensity on T2-weighted scans, probably caused by alveolitis with edema. Experimental studies on rats show that MR signal intensities are elevated in alveolitis and early fibrosis, and T1 and T2 values are significantly decreased in chronic,

more advanced fibrotic lung disease. It would appear that T1 and T2 values in the lung parenchyma correlate with changes in water content of the diseased lung. Obstructive atelectasis can be distinguished from nonobstructive atelectasis on T2-weighted images. Nonobstructive atelectasis characteristically demonstrates a very low signal intensity on T2-weighted scans (Fig. 1-33), whereas obstructive atelectasis demonstrates high signal intensity (Fig. 1-34). These may be indistinguishable from each other on either CT scans or T1- and proton density-weighted images. We presume that with obstructive atelectasis, accumulation of secretions and disappearance of residual air increase the T2 time of the collapsed lung. In nonobstructive atelectasis, collateral ventilation and clearance of secretions are still active. Presumably, the magnetic susceptibility effects of microscopic residual air lead to a low T2 relaxation time. The behavior of several tissues of interest is summarized in Table 1-3.

TABLE 1-3. *Patterns of tissue signal*

	Pulse sequence				
	T1-weighted	Proton density	T2-weighted	Gradient echo	
Cyst	Low	Medium	High	Variable	Homogeneous sharp border round
Abscess	Low-medium	Medium	High	Variable	Heterogeneous ill-defined border
Seroma	Low	Medium	High	Variable	Same as cyst
Lipoma	High	High	High	Medium	Sometimes brighter than normal fat
Neurofibroma	Medium	Medium	High	Medium	Often with central area of low signal on T2
High protein content collection (bronchogenic cyst)	Medium-high	Medium	High	Variable	Initially homogeneous
Obstructive atelectasis	Low-medium	Medium	High	Variable	
Nonobstructive atelectasis	Low-medium	Medium	Low	Low	
Bronchogenic carcinoma	Low-medium	Medium	Medium-high	Medium-low	Mixed patterns are most common
Pulmonary secretions	Low	Medium	High	Variable	
Alveolar proteinosis (before lavage)	Medium-low	Low	Medium-low	Low	
Hemorrhagic collections					
Acute	Low	Medium	High	Medium-high	Homogeneous
Subacute	Medium-high	Medium	High	Low	Heterogeneous fluid-fluid level
Chronic	Low	Medium	Medium-high	Low-medium	Homogeneous with dark rim
Blood clot					
Acute	Medium	Medium	Medium-high	Medium	
Chronic	Medium	Medium-low	Medium-low	Low-very low	Gradient echo signal void is larger than clot (magnetic susceptibility)
Arteriovenous malformation	Very low	Low	Medium-low	High	Appearance depends on flow rate

REFERENCES

1. Kalender W, Vock P. Single breathhold spiral volumetric CT by continuous patient translation and rotation. *Radiology* 1989;176:181–183.
2. Kalender WA, Vock P, Polacin A, Soucek M. Spiral-CT: a new technique for volumetric scans. I. Basic principles and methodology. *Rontgenpraxis* 1990;43:323–330.
3. Remy J, Remy-Jardin M, Giraud F, Wannebroucq J. Spiral volumetric scanning and its applications in thoracic pathology (see comments). *Rev Mal Respir* 1994;11:13–27.
4. Remy-Jardin M, Remy J, Deschildre F, et al. Diagnosis of pulmonary embolism with spiral CT: comparison with pulmonary angiography and scintigraphy. *Radiology* 1996;200:699–706.
5. Remy-Jardin M, Remy J, Artaud D, Deschildre F, Duhamel A. Diffuse infiltrative lung disease: clinical value of sliding-thin-slab maximum intensity projection CT scans in the detection of mild micronodular patterns (see comments). *Radiology* 1996;200:333–339.
6. Bhalla M, Naidich DP, McGuiness G, et al. Diffuse lung disease: assessment with helical CT—Preliminary observations of the role of maximum and minimum intensity projection images. *Radiology* 1996;200:341–347.
7. Brink JA, Heiken JP, Semenkovich J, et al. Abnormalities of the diaphragm and adjacent structures: findings on multiplanar spiral CT scans. *AJR Am J Roentgenol* 1994;163:307–310.

8. Naidich DP, Marshall CH, Gribbin C, Arams RS, McCauley DI. Low dose CT of the lungs: preliminary observations. *Radiology* 1990;175:729–731.
9. Collie DA, Wright AR, Williams JR, et al. Comparison of spiral-acquisition computed tomography and conventional computed tomography in the assessment of pulmonary metastatic disease. *Br J Radiol* 1994;67:436–444.
10. Costello P, Anderson W, Blume D. Pulmonary nodule: evaluation with spiral volumetric CT. *Radiology* 1991;179:875–876.
11. Heiken JP, Brink JA, Vannier MW. Spiral (helical) CT. *Radiology* 1993;189:647–656.
12. Remy-Jardin M, Remy J, Giraud F, Marquette CH. Pulmonary nodules: detection with thick-section spiral CT versus conventional CT. *Radiology* 1993;187:513–520.
13. Kalender WA, Seissler W, Klotz E, Vock P. Spiral volumetric CT with single breathhold technique, continuous transport, and continuous scanner rotation. *Radiology* 1990;176:181–190.
14. Kalender WA, Polacin A. Physical performance characteristics of spiral CT scanning. *Medical Physics* 1991;18:910–915.
15. Wang G, Vannier M. Maximum volume coverage in spiral CT scanning. *Acad Radiol* 1996;3:423–428.
16. Polacin A, Kalender WA, Marchal G. Evaluation of section sensitivity profiles and image noise in spiral CT. *Radiology* 1992;185:29–35.
17. Polacin A, Kalender WA, Brink J, Vannier MA. Measurement of slice sensitivity profiles in spiral CT. *Medical Physics* 1994;21:133–140.

18. Wang G, Vannier M. Longitudinal resolution in volumetric x-ray computerized tomography: analytical comparison between conventional and helical computerized tomography. *Medical Physics* 1994;21: 429–433.

19. Kalender WA, Polacin A, Suss C. A comparison of conventional and spiral CT: an experimental study on the detection of spherical lesions. *J Comput Assist Tomogr* 1994;18:167–176.

20. Brink J. Technical aspects of helical (spiral) CT. *Radiol Clin North Am* 1995;33:834–851.

21. Buckley JA, Scott WW Jr, Siegelman SS, et al. Pulmonary nodules: effect of increased data sampling on detection with spiral CT and confidence in diagnosis. *Radiology* 1995;196:395–400.

22. Mayo JR, Webb WR, Gould R, et al. High resolution CT of the lungs: an optimal approach. *Radiology* 1987;163:507–510.

23. Zwirewich CV, Terriff B, Müller NL. High spatial frequency (bone) algorithm improves quality of standard CT of the thorax. *AJR Am J Roentgenol* 1989;153:1169–1173.

24. Gamsu G. Computed tomography and high-resolution computed tomography of pneumoconioses. *J Occupational Med* 1991;33:794–796.

25. Grenier P, Brauner M, Lenoir S, Cluzel P. High-resolution CT for specific diagnosis of diffuse chronic infiltrative lung disease. *J Belge de Radiologie* 1993;76:1–6.

26. Mayo JR, Jackson SA, Müller NL. High-resolution CT of the chest: radiation dose. *AJR Am J Roentgenol* 1993;160:479–481.

27. Costello P, Dupuy DE, Ecker CP, Tello R. Spiral CT of the thorax with reduced volume of contrast material: a comparative study. *Radiology* 1992;183:663–666.

28. Costello P. Thoracic helical CT. *Radiographics* 1994;14:913–918.

29. Storto ML, Ciccotosto C, Patea RL, Spinazzi A, Bonomo L. Spiral CT of the mediastinum: optimization of contrast medium use. *Eur J Radiol* 1994;18(Suppl 1):S83–S87.

30. Tokics L, Hedenstierna G, Strandberg A, Brismar B, Lundquist H. Lung collapse and gas exchange during general anesthesia: Effects of spontaneous breathing, muscle paralysis and positive end expiratory pressure. *Anesthesiology* 1987;66:157–167.

31. Klein JS, Zarka MA. Transthoracic needle biopsy: an overview. *J Thoracic Imaging* 1997;12:232–249.

32. Protopapas Z, Westcott JL. Transthoracic needle biopsy of mediastinal lymph nodes for staging lung and other cancers. *Radiology* 1996;199: 489–496.

33. Protopapas Z, Westcott JL. Transthoracic hilar and mediastinal biopsy. *J Thoracic Imaging* 1997;12:250–258.

34. Jurik AG, Albrechtsen J. Spiral CT with three-dimensional and multiplanar reconstruction in the diagnosis of anterior chest wall joint and bone disorders. *Acta Radiologica* 1994;35:468–472.

35. Drebin RA, Hanrahan P. Volume rendering. *Comput Graphics* 1988; 22:65–74.

36. Fishman EK, Magid D, Ney DR, et al. Three-dimensional imaging. *Radiology* 1991;181:321–337.

37. Levoy M. Displays of surface from volume data. *IEEE Comput Graph Appl* 1988;8:29–37.

38. Napel S, Marks MP, Rubin GD, et al. CT angiography with spiral CT and maximum intensity projection. *Radiology* 1992;185:607–610.

39. Napel S, Rubin GD, Jeffrey RB Jr. STS-MIP: a new reconstruction technique for CT of the chest. *J Comput Assist Tomogr* 1993;17: 832–838.

40. Remy-Jardin M, Remy J, Gosselin B, et al. Sliding thin slab, minimum intensity projection technique in the diagnosis of emphysema: histopathologic-CT correlation. *Radiology* 1996;200:665–671.

41. Seltzer SE, Judy PF, Adams DF, et al. Spiral CT of the chest: comparison of cine and film based viewing. *Radiology* 1995;197:73–78.

42. Wood SA, Zerhouni EA, Hoford JD, Hoffman EA, Mitzner W. Measurement of three dimensional lung tree structures by using computed tomography. *J Appl Physiol* 1995;79:1687–1697.

43. Pisupati C, Wolff L, Zerhouni EA. Tracking 3-D pulmonary tree structures. Proceedings of the IEEE workshop on mathematical methods in biomedical image analysis, 1996.

44. Pisupati C, Zerhouni EA, Mitzner W. Segmentation of 3D pulmonary trees using mathematical morphology [thesis]. Baltimore: Johns Hopkins University Press, 1996.

45. Herold CJ, Brown RH, Mitzner W, et al. Assessment of pulmonary reactivity with high-resolution CT. *Radiology* 1991;181:369–374.

46. Brown RH, Zerhouni E. New techniques and developments in physiologic imaging of airways. *Radiol Clin North Am* 1998;36:211–230.

47. Croisille P, Souto M, Cova M, et al. Pulmonary nodules: improved detection with vascular segmentation and extraction with spiral CT. *Radiology* 1995;197:397–401.

48. Rahmouni A, Tempany C, Jones R, et al. Lymphoma: Monitoring tumor size and signal intensity with MR imaging. *Radiology* 1993;188: 445–451.

49. Kuhlman JE, Bouchardy L, Fishman EK, Zerhouni EA. CT and MR imaging evaluation of chest wall disorders. *Radiographics* 1994;14: 571–595.

50. Fortier M, Mayo JR, Swensen SJ, Munk PL, Vellet DA, Müller NL. MR imaging of chest wall lesions. *Radiographics* 1994;14:597–606.

51. Webb WR. The role of magnetic resonance imaging in the assessment of patients with lung cancer: a comparison with computed tomography. *J Thoracic Imaging* 1989;4:65–75.

52. Grover FL. The role of CT and MRI in staging of the mediastinum. *Chest* 1994;106(Suppl):391S–396S.

53. Gefter WB, Hatabu H, Holland GA, Gupta KB, Henschke CI, Palevsky HI. Pulmonary thromboembolism: recent developments in diagnosis with CT and MR imaging. *Radiology* 1995;197:561–574.

54. Edelman RR, Hatabu H, Tadamura E, Li W, Prasad PV. Noninvasive assessment of regional ventilation on the human lung using oxygen-enhanced magnetic resonance imaging. *Nature Medicine* 1996;2: 1236–1239.

55. Mugler JP 3rd, Driehuys B, Brookeman JR, et al. MR imaging and spectroscopy using hyperpolarized 129Xe gas: preliminary human results. *Magn Reson Med* 1997;37:809–815.

56. Kauczor HU, Ebert M, Kreitner KF, et al. Imaging of the lungs using 3He MRI: preliminary clinical experience in 18 patients with and without lung disease. *J Magn Reson Imaging* 1997;7:538–543.

57. Hartnell GG, Spence L, Hughes LA, et al. Safety of MR imaging in patients who have retained metallic materials after cardiac surgery (see comments). *AJR Am J Roentgenol* 1997;168:1157–1159.

58. Edelman RR, Wallner B, Singer A, Atkinson DJ, Saini S. Segmented turboFLASH: method for breath-hold MR imaging of the liver with flexible contrast. *Radiology* 1990;177:515–521.

59. Foo TK, MacFall JR, Hayes CE, Sostman HD, Slayman BE. Pulmonary vasculature: single breath-hold MR imaging with phased-array coils. *Radiology* 1992;183:473–477.

60. Hatabu H, Gefter WB, Listerud J, et al. Pulmonary MR angiography utilizing phased-array surface coils. *J Comput Assist Tomogr* 1992;16: 410–417.

61. Haddad JL, Rofsky NM, Ambrosino MM, Naidich DP, Weinreb JC. T2-weighted MR imaging of the chest: comparison of electrocardiograph-triggered conventional and turbo spin-echo and nontriggered turbo spin-echo sequences. *J Magn Reson Imaging* 1995;5:325–329.

62. Schmidt HC, Tscholakoff D, Hricak H, Higgins CB. MR image contrast and relaxation times of solid tumors in the chest, abdomen, and pelvis. *J Comput Assist Tomogr* 1985;9:738–748.

63. Webb WR, Gamsu G, Stark DD, et al. Evaluation of magnetic resonance sequences in imaging mediastinal tumors. *AJR Am J Roentgenol* 1984;143:723–727.

64. Barakos JA, Brown JJ, Brescia RJ, Higgins CB. High signal intensity lesions of the chest in MR imaging. *J Comput Assist Tomogr* 1989; 13:797–802.

65. Webb WR. Magnetic resonance imaging of the hila and mediastinum. *Cardiovasc Intervent Radiol* 1986;8:306–313.

66. Glazer HS, Lee JKT, Levitt RL, et al. Radiation fibrosis: differentiation from recurrent tumor by MR imaging. *Radiology* 1985;156:721–726.

67. Rahmouni AD, Zerhouni EA. Role of MRI in the management of thoracic lymphoma. *Contemp Issues CT* 1990;11:23–33.

68. Nyman R, Rehn S, Glimelius B, et al. Magnetic resonance imaging for assessment of treatment effects in mediastinal Hodgkin's disease. *Acta Radiol Diagn* 1987;28:145–151.

69. Rholl KS, Levitt RG, Glazer HS. Magnetic resonance imaging of fibrosing mediastinitis. *AJR Am J Roentgenol* 1985;145:255–259.

70. Oliver TB, Murchison JT, Reid JH. Serial MRI in the management of intramural haemorrhage of the thoracic aorta. *Br J Radiol* 1997;70: 1288–1290.

71. Swensen SJ, Keller PL, Berquist TH, et al. Magnetic resonance imaging of hemorrhage *AJR Am J Roentgenol* 1985;145:921–927.

CHAPTER 2

Mediastinum

Computed tomography (CT) is indispensable in the radiographic assessment of the mediastinum. Although conventional radiographs can show recognizable abnormalities in many patients with mediastinal pathology, radiographs are limited in their sensitivity and ability to delineate the extent of mediastinal abnormalities and the relationship of masses to specific mediastinal structures.

Because of its excellent density resolution and tomographic format, CT is able to identify normal mediastinal structures, opacified vessels and vascular abnormalities, and is often able to characterize masses based on their attenuation, and precisely localize them as to site of origin and extent. Furthermore, the transaxial plane of CT is well-suited to the investigation of a number of mediastinal structures, such as the trachea, esophagus, aorta, and superior vena cava, which are oriented perpendicular to the plane of scan and are thus imaged in cross-section. Confusing radiographic appearances caused by superimposition of structures are readily resolved using CT, and the traditional plain radiographic "blind spots" such as the thoracic inlet, the intrapericardial vessels, and the diaphragmatic crura are much easier to evaluate (1–3).

The indications for mediastinal CT can be divided into two broad categories. First, CT is commonly used to define and characterize a mediastinal abnormality suspected or diagnosed on plain chest radiographs. When a mediastinal contour abnormality is visible on plain films, CT should generally be the next imaging procedure performed. Secondly, CT is often used to evaluate the mediastinum in patients who have normal chest radiographs yet a clinical reason to suspect mediastinal disease. For example, CT has been shown to be of significant value in the detection and assessment of mediastinal masses or lymph node abnormalities in patients with neoplasm or granulomatous disease, and in detecting a pathologic process in patients with conditions such as myasthenia gravis or surgically-resistant hyperparathyroidism, which can be associated with a mediastinal mass (thymoma and ectopic parathyroid adenoma, respectively) (1–4).

The clinical indications for mediastinal magnetic resonance imaging (MRI) are somewhat more limited (5–7). In certain situations, MRI provides diagnostic information superior to that available from CT, and MRI can be used as the primary imaging modality. Primary uses of MRI include: (a) the diagnosis of mediastinal abnormalities that are suspected to be vascular; (b) the evaluation of posterior mediastinal or paravertebral masses, and neurogenic tumors; and (c) distinguishing mass and fibrous tissue in a patient with

TABLE 2-1. *Protocol for routine thoracic/mediastinal survey[a]*

Collimation:	7–8 mm	
Pitch:	1.0–2.0. Variable pitch > 1 is recommended as needed to insure data acquisition in a single breathhold period.	
Reconstruction Interval:	7 mm q 6 mm; 8 mm q 7 mm, respectively	
Superior extent:	Above clavicles	
Inferior extent:	Below the posterior costophrenic sulci to include the adrenal glands	
IV contrast:	Concentration:	LOCM 300–320 mg I/mL, or: HOCM 282 mg I/mL (60% solution)
Low volume technique	Rate:	2 mL sec
	Scan Delay:	20 sec
	Total Volume:	60 mL
Standard volume technique	Rate:	2–3 mL sec
	Scan Delay:	15–20 sec
	Total Volume:	120 mL
Comments:	1. Precontrast images should be obtained in those cases in which there is radiographic evidence of a focal mediastinal abnormality as this may be invaluable in assessing mediastinal cysts, or aneurysms, for example.	
	2. Optimal contrast enhancement may be obtained either by use of an initial 20-cc test dose injected at the same rate as subsequently used (2–3 mL/sec) with test images obtained at 5 sec intervals up to 25 sec; or using automated scan monitoring of vascular enhancement, if available.	
	3. In select cases, 5-mm sections reconstructed q 4 mm's may be preferred, for example in patients with masses in the region of the APW.	
	4. For patients for whom a combined chest and abdomen protocol is required, images through the upper abdomen may be acquired during the portal venous phase by allowing a 15-sec interval between the 2 acquisitions. Studies for which earlier images through the liver are required should be performed separately.	

[a] Adapted from ref. 18.
LOCM, low osmolarity contrast media; HOCM, high osmolarity contrast media; APW, aorticopulmonary window.

treated lymphoma or carcinoma in whom tumor recurrence may be present. These primary uses of MRI generally relate to its ability (a) to image vessels, (b) to distinguish different tissues, (c) to image in nontransaxial planes, or (d) to obviate iodinated contrast material. In many other instances, however, MRI is best reserved as a secondary or problem-solving tool, in patients who have equivocal or confusing CT findings, or in whom specific anatomic information is required, which is less clearly demonstrated using CT. In such cases, a limited number of MR images can be helpful.

It is important to understand, however, that if MRI provides diagnostic information that is merely equivalent to that of CT, then CT is usually the most appropriate clinical study (5). CT is less expensive, more available, usually takes less time, is easier for debilitated patients to tolerate, often provides more ancillary information, and has an established role in the clinical diagnosis of a number of entities. However, it is a mistake to think of CT and MRI as necessarily competitive. Rather, CT and MRI can be complementary in many instances—each has its own particular strengths that may be advantageous in specific circumstances.

CT TECHNIQUES

The advent of spiral/helical CT has fundamentally revised our approach to scanning the mediastinum and will therefore be the focus of the following discussion. The ability to acquire a volumetric data set in a single breath-hold period eliminates misregistration between adjacent slices at the same time minimizing respiratory and, to a lesser degree, cardiac motion artifacts. As important, rapid acquisition of scan data insures optimal utilization of intravenous contrast material not only insuring that all mediastinal vessels will

be opacified on all sections, but allowing more accurate assessment of abnormal vasculature as occurs in many mediastinal lesions (Table 2-1, Fig. 2-1). Helical scanning also allows both the prospective and/or retrospective acquisition of additional scans anywhere within the scan volume, providing for overlapping reconstructions without the need for additional radiation exposure. This feature also enables a variety of high-quality retrospective reconstructions, including multiplanar reconstructions to be easily acquired (8–10).

As discussed in Chapter 1, performing a helical examination requires a number of technical choices. In addition to standard options such as kVp, mAs, field-of-view, and reconstruction algorithm, these include: collimation; pitch (P); reconstruction interval (RI), selected either prospectively and retrospectively; and breath-hold period. In addition, important choices regarding contrast administration must be made, including type of contrast agent, rate and method of infusion, as well as optimal scan delay. These decisions are further complicated by the frequent need to integrate chest imaging with neck and/or abdominal examinations.

In general, the choice of parameters for performing spiral CT of the thorax usually requires that a compromise be made between optimal collimation and breath-hold capability. Ideally, the entire thorax should be scanned in a single breath-hold period. If this is not possible, sequential acquisitions may be acquired, optimally keeping all scan parameters constant, especially the field-of-view: this is necessary for those cases, in particular for which retrospective reconstructions may be required. Although scans may be obtained during quiet respiration, whenever possible examinations should be performed following a deep inspiratory effort. In select cases this may be facilitated either by repeated deep inspirations prior to scan acquisition and/or the use of oxygen during the examination.

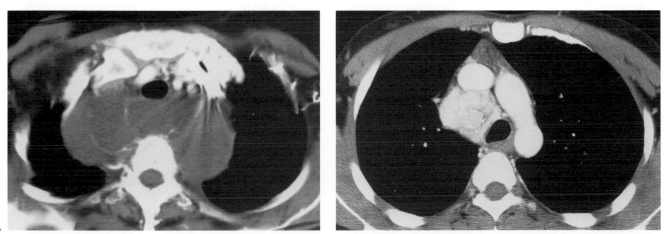

A   B

FIG. 2-1. Vascular mediastinal lesions: value of contrast-enhanced helical CT. **A:** Section through the superior mediastinum following a bolus of 120-cc. 60% contrast media injected at a rate of 2 cc/second. Although this bulky mediastinal mass was initially interpreted as probably cystic because of homogeneous low density, the presence of discrete vessels traversing the mass is an important clue to the highly vascular nature of this lesion. At surgery, biopsy led to considerable hemorrhage requiring transfusion of several units of blood. Surgically proved mediastinal chordoma. **B:** Contrast-enhanced CT section in a different patient than **A** at the level of the aortic arch shows the presence of a lobulated mass in the right paratracheal space showing marked, uniform enhancement, indicative of considerable vascularity. Biopsy proved Castleman's disease.

A slice thickness of 7 to 8 mm is sufficient for assessing most mediastinal abnormalities. However, thinner slices are sometimes required for (a) small lesions, (b) areas where anatomic structures are not oriented perpendicular to the scan plane (such as in the aorticopulmonary window), (c) when mediastinal fat is lacking, or (d) if hilar structures and bronchi also need to be assessed. In these situations, 5-mm collimation can be helpful.

Although adequate images can often be obtained without the use of intravenous contrast media, especially if the primary indication for CT is to determine the presence or absence of a mediastinal mass, in our experience, whenever possible the use of contrast administration should be encouraged (11). Contrast infusion can be indispensable in identifying and differentiating between vascular and nonvascular structures. Contrast media should be used routinely if clinical or radiographic findings suggest the possibility of (a) a vascular abnormality (Fig. 2-2), (b) a hilar mass or hilar lymph node enlargement (as in patients with lung cancer) (Fig. 2-3), or (c) a mediastinal mass which may be invading or compressing vessels (as in the presence of superior vena cava syndrome) (see Fig. 2-3). Also, the enhancement characteristics of some mediastinal lesions can be helpful in diagnosis or differential diagnosis. For example, in patients with active tuberculosis, enlarged mediastinal lymph nodes often show a low attenuation center and an enhancing rim on con-

trast enhanced CT, findings that can strongly suggest the diagnosis (Fig. 2-4) (12–14). Similarly, contrast enhancement may be an invaluable aid in assessing the presence and extent of tumor necrosis as occurs in some patients with lymphomas or germ-cell tumors, for example (see Fig. 2-4) (15,16). Use of contrast enhancement also allows differentiation of highly vascularized nodes and tumors from patients with avascular masses or cysts (see Fig. 2-1). This may be of great importance in determining the need for further histologic evaluation. In the latter case, it should be emphasized that adequate evaluation of mediastinal cysts may necessitate the acquisition of both pre and postcontrast enhanced scans as these lesions frequently have high density because of the presence of blood, debris, or even calcification (17).

If contrast is required, it is best administered in the form of a bolus, preferably utilizing a power injector. Protocols using both low and high osmolarity contrast material have been advocated (17). As reported by Costello et al., a complete helical CT examination of the thorax may be performed with as little as 60 mL of high (300 mg I/mL) osmolarity contrast material, potentially offering significant cost savings (9). In distinction, as emphasized by Schneider et al., among others, it is also possible to perform high quality studies using low osmolarity contrast media (150 mg I/mL) by diluting a 50-mL vial of 300-mg I/mL contrast material with 50 mL of saline, for example. This has the advantage of

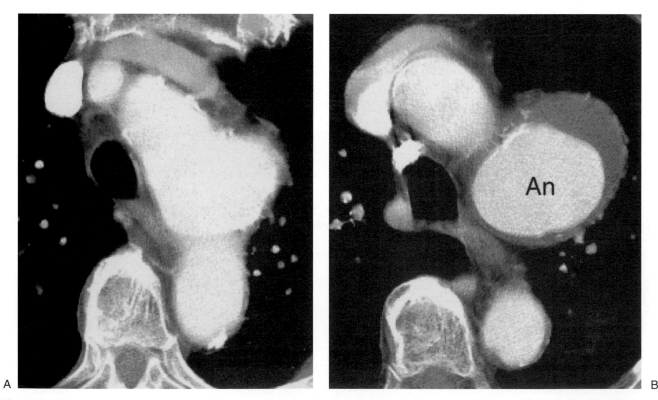

A   B

FIG. 2-2. Vascular disease: value of contrast-enhanced helical CT. **A,B:** 7-mm helical CT sections following bolus administration of 120-cc 60% iodinated contrast media at a rate of 2 cc/second in a patient with a left mediastinal mass visible on chest radiographs shows a focal saccular aneurysm of the aortic arch. Note that in **B** the contrast-opacified lumen of the aneurysm (*An*) can be clearly distinguished from clot lining its wall. In this case vascular opacification is excellent with this rate of contrast injection.

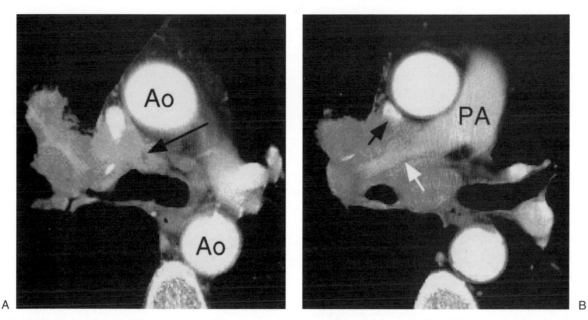

FIG. 2-3. Superior vena caval obstruction: bronchogenic carcinoma. **A:** Contrast-enhanced 7-mm. helical CT section in a patient with radiographic evidence of a right hilar mass obtained following a bolus of 120 cc of 60% iodinated contrast media injected at a rate of 2 cc/second confirm the presence of tumor invading the mediastinum (*arrow*) anterior to the right main bronchus and carina. The aorta (*Ao*) and superior vena cava are densely opacified at this rate of contrast infusion. **B:** At a lower level, tumor surrounds and narrows the right pulmonary artery (*white arrow*) and compresses the superior vena cava (*black arrow*). *PA*, main pulmonary artery.

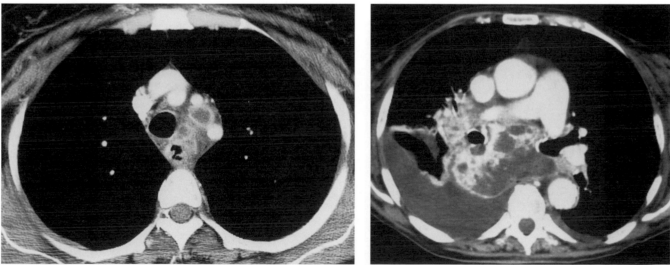

FIG. 2-4. Mediastinal lymphadenopathy: characterization with contrast enhancement. **A:** Contrast-enhanced CT section at the level of the great vessels shows several low density lymph nodes in the left paratracheal space with distinct rim enhancement. This pattern is strongly suggestive of tuberculous lymphadenitis, subsequently verified in this HIV− patient by transbronchial needle aspiration (Compare with Fig. 2-1). **B:** Contrast enhanced CT section in a different patient than in **A**, shows the presence of massively enlarged and necrotic subcarinal and right axillary lymph nodes in this patient with documented non-Hodgkin's lymphoma.

minimizing streak artifacts, especially those that arise from mediastinal venous structures, and allowing more rapid and safer infusion of contrast media, which may be advantageous in patients being evaluated for suspected pulmonary emboli. In our experience, the rate of contrast injection, rather than the volume injected, is most important in diagnosis. The total volume of contrast used, and its rate of injection, will usually be determined by the type of scanner (conventional or helical) employed, the scan protocol, and the area of the mediastinum to be scanned. It should be noted that regardless of technique, although it is common to see small bubbles of air in the most anterior part of the left brachiocephalic vein or main pulmonary artery after contrast infusion, clinically significant venous air embolism is an unusual complication of intravenous contrast injection (Fig. 2-5) (25,26).

Acknowledging that continued rapid improvements in scanner design, including subsecond gantry rotation and multiple detectors, among others, will likely radically alter routine scan protocols, at present we recommend the protocol for routine mediastinal evaluation that is presented in Table 2-1.

In cases in which there is suspected superior vena caval obstruction, vocal cord paralysis, or other abnormalities involving both the neck and chest, a combined study may be performed by first obtaining 3- to 5-mm sections parallel to the cords from the base of the tongue to the base of the neck during quiet respiration reconstructed every 2 to 4 mm, respectively, with a pitch of 1 to 2. Although the rate of contrast administration remains the same, the total volume

should be at a minimum between 120 to 150 mL, whereas the scan delay should be decreased to 15 seconds (18). Following a 15 second interscan delay, sections are then obtained through the chest as shown in Table 2-1.

MR IMAGING TECHNIQUES

In our experience, MRI is best utilized to evaluate vascular structures in patients who cannot tolerate radiographic contrast agents or as a problem-solving modality when CT has proven inconclusive (5–7). Each case is individualized according to the information needed, and no standard algorithm is universally applicable. As a rule, following acquisition of initial coronal scout images, cardiac-gated, T1-weighted axial sections are obtained through regions of interest, and are most valuable in demonstrating mediastinal structures and delineating the presence of a mediastinal mass. With gating, the effective repetition time (TR) is determined by the heart rate. Coronal and sagittal images are generally best reserved for specific indications, such as analyzing the chest wall, the aorticopulmonary window, or subcarinal space (5–7).

T1-weighted images obtained following contrast administration or T2-weighted images are usually required only in those cases for which tissue characterization is deemed necessary. T2-weighted images may be acquired either utilizing a prolonged TR (2,000 ms) without cardiac gating, or preferably utilizing cardiac gating (especially if the region of interest is near the heart or hila) with images obtained every second or third cardiac cycle. Gradient-refocused sequences with breath holding also may be of value to reduce scan time and optimize visualization of vascular pathology. With this technique, flowing blood results in an intense signal whereas soft-tissue contrast is reduced.

Although, as noted above, evaluation of mediastinal masses with MRI has traditionally relied on acquisition of conventional spin-echo (SE) T1- and T2-weighted images with electrocardiographic (ECG) triggering supplemented with cine gradient-echo images as needed, image quality is heavily dependent on a good ECG signal. As a consequence, examinations are often suboptimal or even nondiagnostic in patients with abnormal cardiac rhythms. Even with optimal triggering, examination times are lengthy, which predisposes to degradation from patient motion. Finally, respiratory motion may also degrade image quality.

Technologic advances, which include the widespread use of echo-train fast spin-echo pulse (ETFSE) sequences, specialized phased-array multicoils and magnets with high performance gradient systems now provide for a comprehensive evaluation of the mediastinum with short acquisition times. Because of these advances, many sequences can be performed during a comfortable breath hold, thus eliminating respiratory artifacts.

A typical imaging protocol for evaluation of a mediastinal mass now includes ECG-triggered ETFSE T1- and T2-

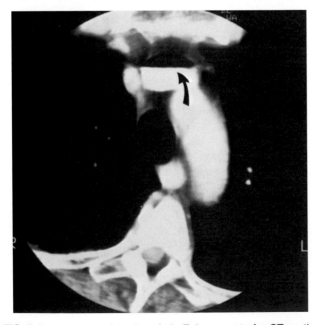

FIG. 2-5. Intravenous injection of air. Enlargement of a CT section obtained at the level of the aortic arch following the bolus injection of intravenous contrast media administered through a power injector. Note that an air-fluid level is present in the left brachiocephalic vein (*arrow*), the consequence of air within the injector. Despite the seemingly large volume of air, this patient remained asymptomatic.

weighted images (Fig. 2-6). These can be acquired with breath holding if the TR is sufficiently shortened at the expense of less slice coverage. Alternatively a ETFSE short T1 inversion recovery sequences could be used instead of T2-weighted images. In patients with abnormal cardiac rhythms and those who cannot breath hold or are otherwise uncooperative, a diagnostic quality examination can still be performed with single shot ETFSE sequences with half Fourier reconstruction (HASTE). Because each slice is acquired in under 1 second, these sequences are impervious to respiratory motion.

Finally, a comprehensive vascular evaluation can be performed with breath hold three-dimensional (3D) gadolinium-enhanced MRI. The ultrashort TR and TE inherent to these pulse sequences allows for imaging the great vessels with a temporal resolution of as little as 10 seconds. This allows clear distinction between arteries and veins. In addition the 3D technique is amenable to high quality multiplanar reformations and can be postprocessed with maximum-intensity-projection (MIP) algorithms. These MIP images resemble conventional angiographic images. Gadolinium-enhanced 3D MRI represents a significant advance from the traditional time-of-flight techniques because saturation effects and pulsatility artifacts are minimized.

THE NORMAL MEDIASTINUM: REGIONAL ANATOMY

The accurate interpretation of images of the mediastinum, whether obtained using CT or MRI, requires a detailed knowledge of normal cross-sectional anatomy. Transverse imaging is fundamental to most imaging studies. In addition, sagittal and coronal images can be valuable in selected cases and may be obtained using MRI or by reformation of spiral CT data; some knowledge of mediastinal anatomy in these planes is also essential.

The Transverse Plane

Cross-sectional anatomy is best learned using CT. In most respects, the anatomy of mediastinal structures shown using MRI is identical to that shown on CT, although the gray-scale representation of various tissues is different with the two techniques.

The anatomy of the mediastinal great vessels and airways is discussed in detail in subsequent chapters, but it also will be reviewed briefly in this section, as a knowledge of this anatomy is important in understanding the mediastinum as a whole. The aorta and its branches, the great veins, the pulmonary arteries, and the trachea and main bronchi serve as reliable guides to localizing other important mediastinal structures. Furthermore, the relationship between vessels and other mediastinal structures is important to know if the potential effects of masses on vascular structures is to be assessed.

As an aid to understanding regional mediastinal anatomy, the mediastinum can be conceptualized as divided into several compartments, respectively, from superior to inferior, (a) the superior or supraaortic mediastinum, (b) the region of the aortic arch, subaortic mediastinum, and aorticopulmonary window, and (c) the subcarinal space and azygoesophageal recess.

The Superior or Supraaortic Mediastinum

At or near the thoracic inlet (Figs. 2-7 and 2-8A), the mediastinum is relatively narrow from anterior to posterior. The trachea appears central in the supraaortic mediastinum. The esophagus lies posterior to the trachea at this level, but depending on the position of the trachea relative to the spine, the esophagus can be displaced to right or left. It is usually collapsed, and appears as a flattened structure of soft-tissue attenuation, but small amounts of air or air and fluid may sometimes be seen in its lumen (see Figs. 2-7 and 2-8A).

Above the level of the aortic arch, the large arterial branches of the aorta (i.e., the innominate artery, the left common carotid artery, and the left subclavian artery) and the brachiocephalic veins are the most apparent normal structures, other than the trachea and esophagus (see Figs. 2-7, 2-8A; Fig. 2-9A). At or near the thoracic inlet, the brachiocephalic veins are the most anterior and lateral vascular branches visible, lying immediately behind the clavicular heads. Although they vary in size, their positions are relatively constant. The great arterial branches lie posterior to the veins, and adjacent to the anterior and lateral walls of the trachea. These can be reliably identified by their consistent positions.

Below the thoracic inlet, the left brachiocephalic vein crosses the mediastinum from left to right, anterior to the arterial branches of the aorta (see Fig. 2-8B–D). The two brachiocephalic veins have very different configurations. The right brachiocephalic vein has a nearly vertical course throughout its length; the left brachiocephalic vein is longer, and, courses horizontally as it crosses the mediastinum. The horizontal segment of the left brachiocephalic vein is a convenient anatomic landmark, being the line of demarcation between the anterior mediastinum (the prevascular space) that is anterior to it, and the middle mediastinum posterior to it. The precise cepalo-caudal location of this vein is quite variable; although it is most frequently visible at the level of the great vessels, the horizontal portion of the left brachiocephalic vein also can be seen at the level of the aortic arch (see Fig. 2-9B). Because of the central location of the left brachiocephalic vein in the supraaortic mediastinum, when a mass is supected in this region, intravenous contrast medium can be injected using a left-sided arm vein. This maximizes visualization of the full length of the left brachiocephalic vein.

The innominate artery is located in close proximity to the anterior tracheal wall, near its midline or slightly to the right

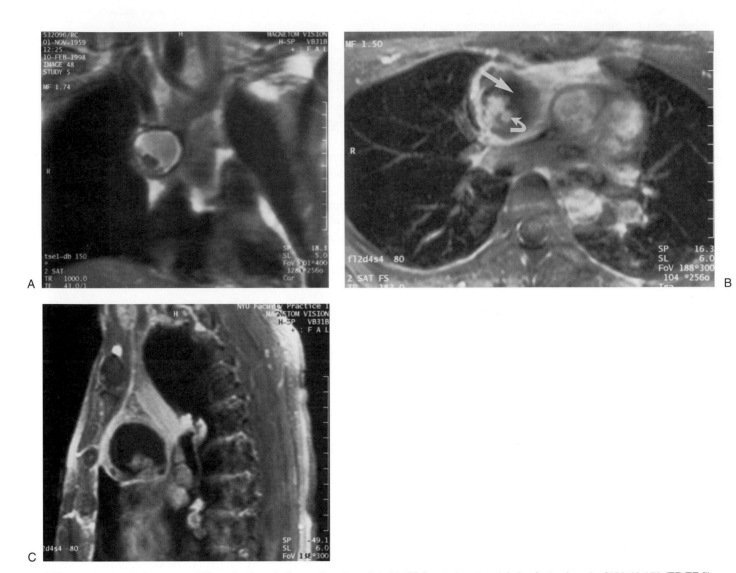

FIG. 2-6. Mediastinal teratoma: MR evaluation. **A:** Coronal nonbreath hold, ECG gated proton density, fast spin-echo [100/43/150 (TR/TE/flip angle)] image performed in phased-array coil demonstrates complex cystic anterior mediastinal mass. T1 weighting could not be achieved in this case because of the patient's relatively slow heart rate (60 beats/minute). **B,C:** Axial and sagittal breath hold, nonECG-triggered, fat-suppressed T1-weighted gradient-echo [183/4/80 (TR/TE/Flip angle)] images, respectively, performed in the body phased-array coil, after the administration of gadolinium, demonstrate an irregular, thick-walled cystic anterior mediastinal mass with both fluid-like (*arrow* in **B**) and nodular components (*curved arrow* in **B**). **D–G:** Three coronal source images from mixed arterial and venous phase (second acquisition from gadolinium-enhanced three-dimensional MRA) demonstrate minimal peripheral enhancement of the mass (*arrows* in **I** and **J**). The fourth image (a selective venogram) was obtained by subtracting the first (arterial phase) acquisition from a delayed, predominantly venous phase acquisition. **H–K:** Coronal maximum-intensity projection and three axial reformatted images from arterial phase gadolinium-enhanced three-dimensional MRA (3.8/1.3/25 [TR/TE/Flip angle]) performed in the body phased-array coil with 20 mL of contrast in conjunction with a timing examination, demonstrates an aberrant right subclavian artery (*arrows* in **H** and **K**). Note that with this sequence the mediastinal mass is all but invisible.

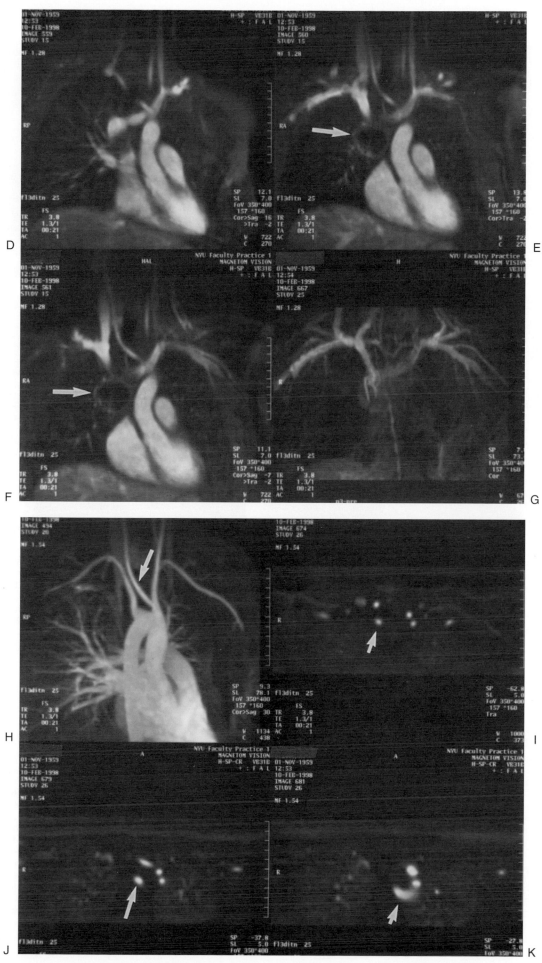

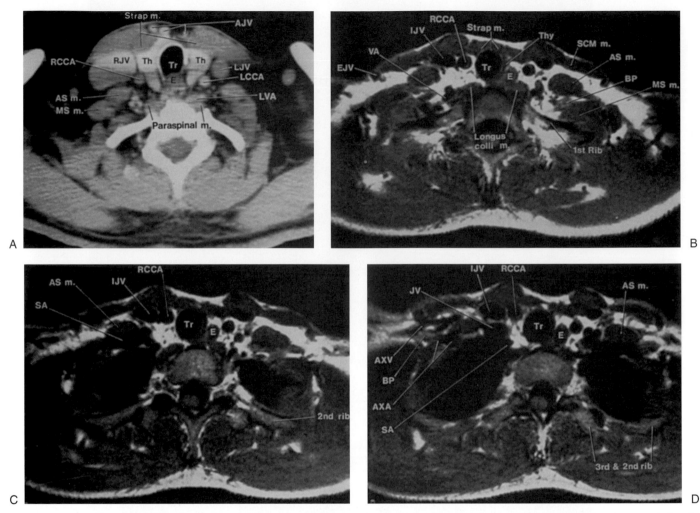

FIG. 2-7. Thoracic inlet, CT/MRI evaluation. **A:** CT section through the lower neck, just above the thoracic inlet. Note the close proximity of the thyroid gland to the trachea. **B–D:** Sequential MR images from above-downward through the thoracic inlet. The anatomy of the thoracic inlet is especially well-visualized with MRI. Note the relationship between the anterior scalene muscle and the subclavian artery that lies immediately posteriorly. The brachial plexus usually can be identified just above the subclavian artery as it passes behind the anterior scalene. *AJV*, anterior jugular veins; *ASm*, anterior scalene muscle; *AXA*, axillary artery; *AXV*, axillary vein; *BP*, brachial plexus; *E*, esophagus; *EJV*, external jugular vein; *IJV*, internal jugular vein; *JV*, jugular vein; *LCCA*, left common carotid artery; *LJV*, left jugular vein; *LVA*, left vertebral artery; *MSm*, middle scalene muscle; *RCCA*, right common carotid artery; *RJV*, right jugular vein; *SA*, subclavian artery; *SCMm*, sternocleidomastoid muscle; *Th, Thy*, thyroid; *Tr*, trachea; *VA*, vertebral artery.

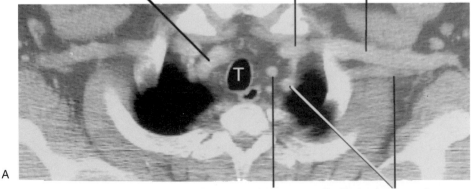

FIG. 2-8. Normal CT Anatomy. Supraaortic mediastinum. **A:** At the thoracic inlet, the trachea (*T*) is clearly seen, with the air filled esophagus posterior and to the left of it. The right and left brachiocephalic veins are located anteriorly and laterally, being seen behind the clavicular heads. The great arterial branches (innominate, left carotid, and left subclavian arteries) lie posterior to the veins, anterior and lateral to the trachea. The innominate artery appears elliptical in shape because of its orientation in the plane of scan.

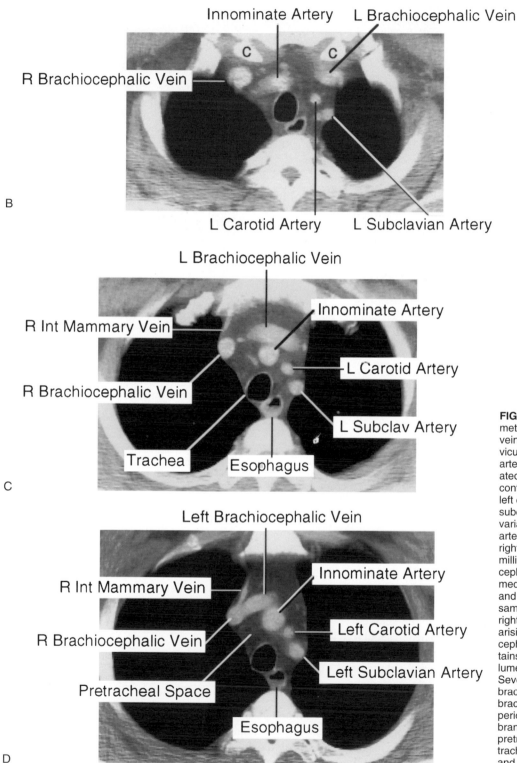

B

C

D

FIG. 2-8. *Continued.* **B:** Seven milli-meters below (**A**), the brachiocephalic veins are visible posterior to the cla-vicular heads (*C*). The left subclavian artery is most posterior, and is situ-ated lateral to the left tracheal wall, contacting the mediastinal pleura. The left carotid artery is anterior to the left subclavian artery, and is somewhat variable in position. The innominate artery is usually anterior and to the right of the tracheal midline. **C:** Seven millimeters below (**B**), the left brachio-cephalic vein is visible in the anterior mediastinum. The subclavian, carotid, and innominate arteries maintain the same relative positions as in **B**. The right internal mammary vein is visible arising from the anterior right brachio-cephalic vein. The esophagus con-tains a small amount of fluid in its lumen, with an air-fluid level visible. Seven millimeters below **C**, the left brachiocephalic vein joins the right brachiocephalic vein, forming the su-perior vena cava. The major aortic branches are again clearly seen. The pretracheal space is anterior to the trachea and posterior to the arteries and veins.

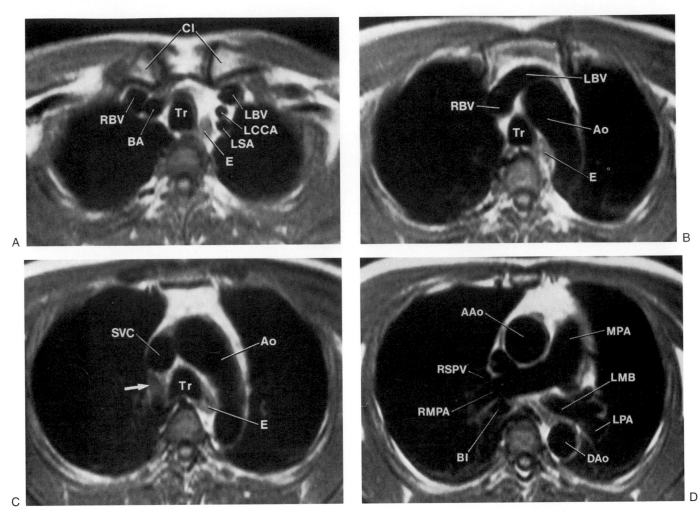

FIG. 2-9. Cross-sectional MRI anatomy. **A–D:** Cardiac-gated MR images through the mediastinum from above-downward. *Tr,* trachea; *LBV,* left brachiocephalic vein; *LCCA,* left common carotid artery; *LSA,* left subclavian artery; *E,* esophagus; *RBV,* right brachiocephalic vein; *BA,* brachiocephalic artery; *Cl,* clavicles; *Ao,* aorta; *SVC,* superior vena cava; *MPA,* main pulmonary artery; *LMB,* left main-stem bronchus; *LPA,* left interlobar pulmonary artery; *DAo,* descending aorta; *BI,* bronchus intermedius; *AAo,* ascending aorta; *RSPV,* right superior pulmonary vein; *RMPA,* right main pulmonary artery. Note that signal is present within the azygos vein, posterior to the *SVC* (*arrow* in **C**), presumably secondary to slow flow.

of midline in most normal patients; it is the most variable of all the great arteries (see Figs. 2-8A–D, 2-9A). The left common carotid artery lies to the left and slightly posterolateral to the innominate artery; generally it has the smallest diameter of the three major arterial branches. The left subclavian artery is a relatively posterior structure throughout most of its course, lying to the left of, and frequently directly lateral to the trachea. The lateral border of the left subclavian artery typically indents the mediastinal surface of the left upper lobe.

Other than the great vessels, trachea, normal lymph nodes, and esophagus, little is usually seen in the supraaortic mediastinum. Small vascular branches, particularly the internal mammary veins, can sometimes be seen in this part of the mediastinum (see Fig. 2-8A–D). In some patients, the thyroid gland may extend into superior mediastinum, and the right and left thyroid lobes may be visible on each side of

the trachea (see Fig. 2-7). This appearance is not abnormal, and does not imply thyroid enlargement. On CT, the thyroid can be distinguished from other tissues or masses; because of its iodine content, its attenuation is greater than that of soft tissue.

The Aortic Arch, Subaortic Mediastinum, and Aorticopulmonary Window

Although the supraaortic region largely contains arterial and venous branches of the aorta and vena cava, this compartment contains the undivided mediastinal great vessels, including the aorta, superior vena cava, and pulmonary arteries. This compartment also contains a number of important lymph node groups.

The aortic arch has a characteristic but somewhat variable appearance. The anterior aspect of the arch is located anterior and to the right of the trachea, with the arch passing to the left and posteriorly (see Figs. 2-9B,C; 2-10A,B). The posterior arch usually lies anterior and lateral to the spine. The aortic arch tapers slightly along its length, from anterior to posterior. The position of the anterior and posterior aspects of the arch can vary in the presence of atherosclerosis and aortic tortuosity; typically the anterior arch is located more anteriorly and to the right in patients with a tortuous aorta, although the posterior aorta lies more laterally and posteriorly, in a position to the left of the spine. At this level, the superior vena cava is visible anterior and to the right of the trachea, usually being elliptical in shape (see Figs. 2-9C, 2-10A,B). The esophagus appears the same as at higher levels, being posterior to the trachea but variable in position. Often it lies somewhat to the left of the midline of the trachea.

The aortic arch on the left, the right brachiocephalic vein or superior vena cava and mediastinal pleura on the right, and the trachea posteriorly serve to define the pretracheal or anterior paratracheal space (see Fig. 2-10A,B) (27,28). This fat filled space contains middle mediastinal lymph nodes in the pretracheal or anterior paratracheal chain. Other mediastinal node groups are closely related to this group both spatially and in regard to lymphatic drainage. It is not uncommon to see a few normal sized lymph nodes in this compartment.

Anterior to the great vessels (aorta and superior vena cava) at this level is another triangular space called the prevascular space. This compartment, which is anterior mediastinal, primarily contains lymph nodes, the thymus, and fat (see Figs. 2-9C, 2-10A,B). The apex of this triangular space represents the anterior junction line, which can sometimes be seen on chest radiographs. At higher levels in the mediastinum (see Figs. 2-8C,D), the prevascular space is anterior to the great arterial branches of the aorta and the brachiocephalic veins.

In young patients, usually in their teens or early twenties, CT shows the thymus to be of soft-tissue attenuation (19–25). The thymus has two lobes, the right and the left, but the left thymic lobe often predominates. On CT, the thymus often appears bilobed or arrowhead shaped, with each of the two thymic lobes contacting the mediastinal pleura. Each lobe usually measures one to two cm in thickness (measured perpendicular to the pleura), but this is variable. In patients in whom the left thymic lobe predominates, the thymus appears to be predominantly left sided, paralleling the aortic arch. In adulthood, the thymus gradually involutes, and soft-tissue attenuation elements are replaced by fat (19–21, 23). Thus, in patients older than 30, the prevascular space appears to be primarily fat filled, with thin strands of wispy tissue passing through the fat. Most of this, including the fat, actually represents the thymus. At higher levels, the thymus is sometimes visible anterior to the brachiocephalic arteries and veins, within the prevascular space.

At a level slightly below the aortic arch, the ascending aorta and descending aorta are visible as separate structures (Fig. 2-11A, B). Characteristically, the descending aorta is slightly smaller (mean diameter 2.6 cm) than the ascending aorta (mean diameter 3.5 cm) (26).

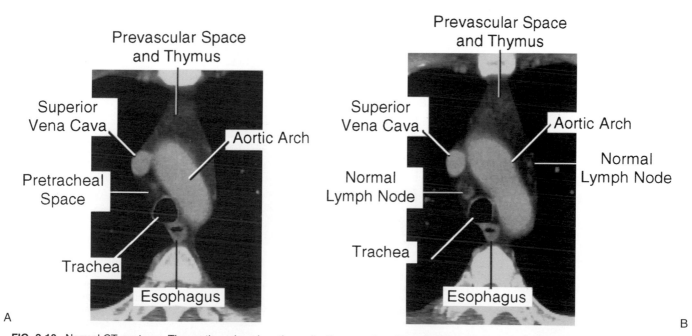

FIG. 2-10. Normal CT anatomy. The aortic arch, subaortic mediastinum, and aorticopulmonary window. **A:** Aortic arch level (same patient as in Fig. 2–8). The superior vena cava contacts the right mediastinal pleura, and along with the aortic arch delineates the anterior aspect of the pretracheal space. The prevascular space is anterior to the great vessels, and contains the thymus, which is largely replaced by fat in this patient. **B:** The location of the pretracheal node bearing space and prevascular space, containing the thymic remnant, are indicated. A normal pretracheal node is visible.

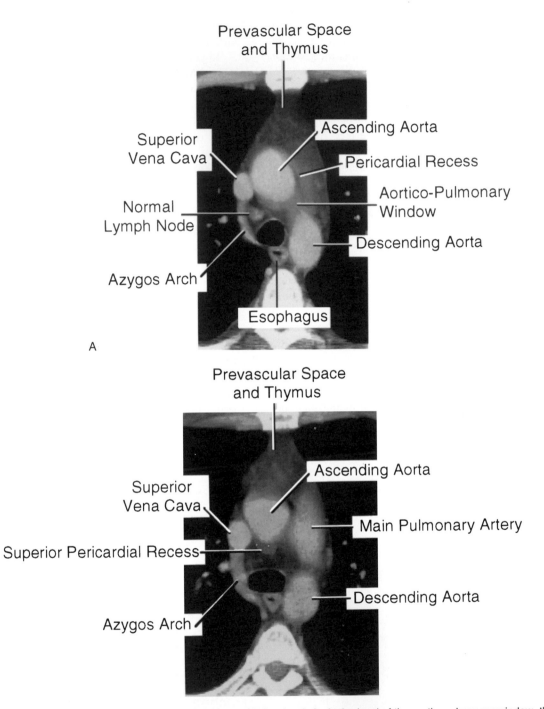

Prevascular Space
and Thymus

Ascending Aorta

Superior
Vena Cava

Pericardial Recess

Aortico-Pulmonary
Window

Normal
Lymph Node

Descending Aorta

Azygos Arch

Esophagus

A

Prevascular Space
and Thymus

Ascending Aorta

Superior
Vena Cava

Main Pulmonary Artery

Superior Pericardial Recess

Descending Aorta

Azygos Arch

B

FIG. 2-11. Normal CT anatomy. Azygos arch and aorticopulmonary window level. **A:** At the level of the aorticopulmonary window, the azygos arch (same patient as in Figs. 2–8 and 2–10) is visible arising from the posterior aspect of the superior vena cava, contacting the right mediastinal pleura, and forming the lateral margin of the pretracheal space. Fat visible under the aortic arch is in the aorticopulmonary window. **B:** At the tracheal carina, the trachea assumes an oval shape. The azygos arch remains visible. The upper aspect of the main pulmonary artery, which marginates the caudal aspect of the aorticopulmonary window, should not be confused with a mass lesion. The superior pericardial recess is visible posterior to the ascending aorta.

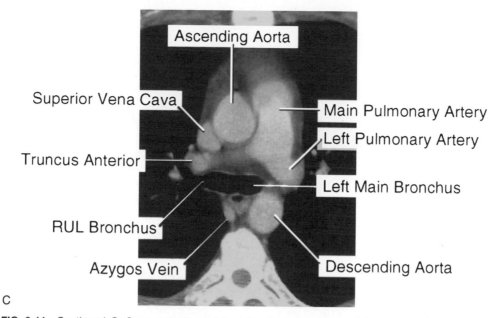

FIG. 2-11. *Continued.* **C:** Scan at the level of the left pulmonary artery and right upper lobe bronchus.

At or near this level, the trachea bifurcates into the right and left main bronchi (see Fig. 2-11B,C). Near the carina, the trachea commonly assumes a somewhat triangular shape (27,28). The carina itself is usually visible on CT. On the right side, the arch of the azygos vein enters the posterior wall of the superior vena cava, passes over the right main bronchus, and continues posteriorly along the mediastinum, to lie to the right and anterior of the spine (29). Below the level of the azygos arch, the azygos vein is consistently seen in this position. The azygos arch is often visible on one or two adjacent slices, and sometimes appears nodular (30). However, its characteristic location is usually sufficient to allow its correct identification. When the azygos arch is visible, it marginates the right border of the pretracheal space.

On the left side of the mediastinum, caudal to the aortic arch, but cephalad to the main pulmonary artery, is the region termed the aortopulmonary window (APW) (31). The APW contains fat, lymph nodes, the left recurrent laryngeal nerve, and the ligamentum arteriosum; the latter two are usually invisible. These lymph nodes freely communicate with those in the pretracheal space, and, in fact, a distinction between nodes in the medial APW from those in the left pretracheal space is rather arbitrary and generally unnecessary. In some patients, the APW is not well seen, with the main pulmonary artery lying immediately below the aortic arch. In such patients, it is usually difficult to distinguish APW lymph nodes from volume averaging of the adjacent aorta and pulmonary artery, unless thin collimation is used.

At or slightly below the aorticopulmonary window, the level the ascending aorta is first clearly seen in cross section (i.e., it is round or nearly round), a portion of the pericardial space, usually containing a small amount of pericardial fluid extends cephalad, into the pretracheal space, immediately behind the ascending aorta. This part of the pericardium is called the superior pericardial recess (see Fig. 2-11B) (32,33). Although it can sometimes be confused with a lymph node, its typical location, immediately behind and contacting the aortic wall, oval or crescentic shape, and its relatively low (water) attenuation, allow it to be distinguished from a significant abnormality. Another part of the pericardial recess can sometimes be seen anterior to the ascending aorta and pulmonary artery (see Fig. 2-11A).

Subcarinal Space and Azygoesophageal Recess

Below the level of the tracheal carina and azygos arch, the medial aspect of the right lung contacts the posterior aspect of the middle mediastinum, in close association to the azygos vein and esophagus (Fig. 2-12A,B). This part of the mediastinum, called the azygoesophageal recess, is important because of adjacent subcarinal lymph nodes, and its close relationship to the esophagus and main bronchi. The contour of the azygoesophageal recess is concave laterally in the large majority of normal subjects, and a convexity in this region should be regarded as suspicious of mass, and the scan examined closely for a pathologic process. However, a convexity in this region may also be produced by a prominent normal esophagus or azygos vein, and is particularly common in patients with a narrow mediastinum and in children (34).

In many subjects, the azygoesophageal recess is somewhat posterior to the node bearing subcarinal space, which lies between the main bronchi (35). Normal nodes are commonly visible in this space, being larger than normal nodes in other parts of the mediastinum, and up to 1.2 cm in short-axis diameter (36,37). The esophagus usually is seen immediately

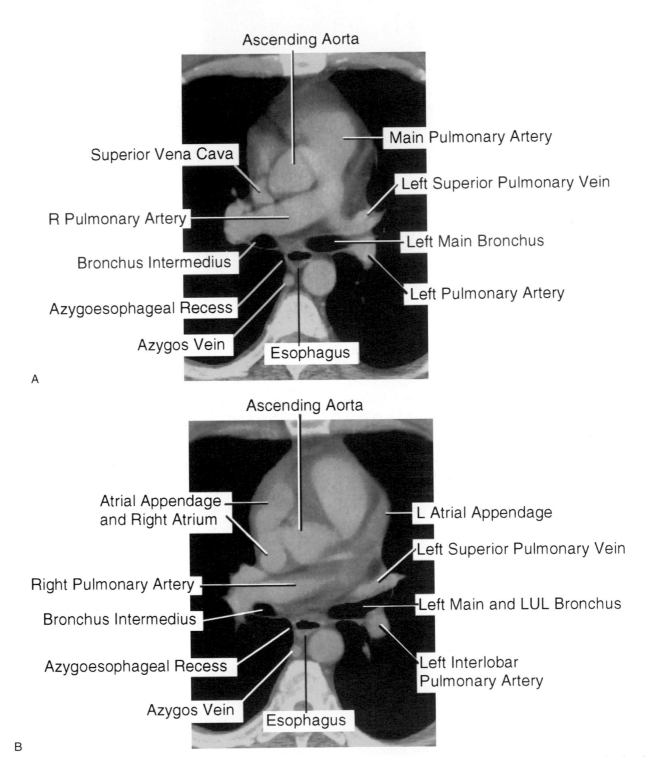

FIG. 2-12. Normal CT anatomy. Main pulmonary arteries, subcarinal space, and azygoesophageal recess. **A:** Slightly below the tracheal carina (same patient as in Figs. 2–8, 2–10, and 2–11), the right pulmonary artery is visible crossing the mediastinum, filling the pretracheal and precarinal space. A small amount of fat is visible in the subcarinal space, slightly anterior to the esophagus, azygos vein, and azygoesophageal recess. **B:** Scan at the level of the azygoesophageal recess. The recess appears concave laterally, with the mediastinal pleura closely related to the azygos vein and esophagus.

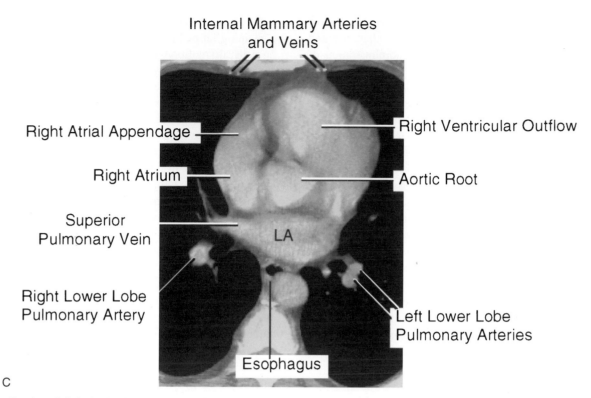

Internal Mammary Arteries and Veins

Right Atrial Appendage

Right Atrium

Superior Pulmonary Vein

Right Lower Lobe Pulmonary Artery

Right Ventricular Outflow

Aortic Root

LA

Left Lower Lobe Pulmonary Arteries

Esophagus

C

FIG. 2-12. *Continued.* **C:**At the level of the base of the heart, the azygoesophageal recess lies posterolateral to the left atrium (*LA*) and lateral to the esophagus.

behind the subcarinal space, and distinguishing nodes and esophagus may be difficult, unless the esophagus contains air or contrast material, or its course is traced on adjacent scans. At levels below the subcarinal space, the appearance of the azygoesophageal recess is relatively constant, although it narrows anteroposteriorly in the retrocardiac region (Fig. 2-12C).

Also, at or near this level, the main pulmonary artery divides into its right and left branches. The left pulmonary artery is somewhat higher than the right, usually being seen 1 cm above it, and appears as the continuation of the main pulmonary artery, directed posterolaterally and to the left (see Figs. 2-11C, 2-12A,B). The right pulmonary artery arises at an angle of nearly 90 degrees to the main and left pulmonary arteries, and crosses the mediastinum from left to right, anterior to the carina or main bronchi (see Fig. 2-9D). The right pulmonary artery limits the most caudal extent of the pretracheal space.

The azygos vein parallels the esophagus along the right side of the mediastinum, and laterally contacts the medial pleural reflections of the right lower lobe, defining the medial and posterior border of the azygo-esophageal recess (see Figs. 2-11C; 2-12A,B) (29). On the left side, the hemiazygos vein parallels the descending aorta, lying posterior to it; it is not always visible. The hemiazygos vein generally drains into the azygos vein via communicating branches that cross

the midline, behind the aorta, in the vicinity of the T-8 vertebral body. The communicating vein or veins are sometimes seen on CT in normals (38,39).

Sagittal and Coronal Planes

Although cross-sectional imaging of the mediastinum (see Figs. 2-7 and 2-9) is generally adequate to visualize most pathologic processes, sagittal and coronal imaging using MRI (Figs. 2-13 and 2-14) or reformatted spiral CT can sometimes add to our understanding of the origin and extent of disease. Utilization of multi-planar images, however, requires a detailed knowledge of normal relationships between mediastinal structures in both standard coronal and sagittal planes (see Figs. 2-13 and 2-14). Once familiar, these images can be augmented by use of select parasagittal planes that maximize visualization of select regions, such as the aortico-pulmonary window.

DIAGNOSIS OF MEDIASTINAL MASS

The differential diagnosis of a mediastinal mass on CT is usually based on several findings, including its location, identification of the structure from which it is arising; whether it is single, multifocal (involving several different areas or lymph node groups), or diffuse; its size and shape, its attenuation (fatty, fluid, soft-tissue, or a combination of these); the presence of calcification and its character and amount; and its opacification following administration of contrast agents.

The mediastinum is divided anatomically into superior, anterior, middle, and posterior compartments, and localizing a mediastinal mass to one of these divisions can facilitate their differential diagnosis on conventional radiographs. On CT, however, it is more appropriate to base the differential diagnosis of a mediastinal mass on a direct observation of the tissue or structure from which the mass is arising (e.g., lymph nodes, veins and arteries, thymus, thyroid, parathyroid, trachea, esophagus, vertebral column) rather than its location in the anterior, middle, or posterior mediastinum. If this is not possible, then localizing the mass to specific regions of the mediastinum (e.g., prevascular space, pretracheal space, subcarinal space, aorticopulmonary window, anterior cardiophrenic angle, paraspinal region) can be valuable in differential diagnosis (Table 2-2). However, it is also important to keep in mind, that although many pathologic processes have a typical location or locations, most can be seen in any part of the mediastinum.

The attenuation of mediastinal masses is also of primary importance in their differential diagnosis (40–42). Masses can be categorized as (a) fat attenuation, (b) low attenuation, having density greater than fat, but less than muscle, (c) high attenuation, with a density greater than that of muscle, and (d) enhancing, showing a significant increase in attenuation following the injection of contrast.

Fat attenuation masses, composed primarily of or partially containing fat or lipid rich tissues, include lipomatosis and fat pads; thymolipoma; teratoma; lymphangioma and hemangioma; lipoma or liposarcoma; fatty hernias; and rarely, lymph node enlargement in Whipple's disease or extramedullary hematompoeisis (42–47).

Low attenuation masses are usually cystic or fluid filled, or contain some lipid. These include a variety of congenital or acquired cysts (bronchogenic, esophageal duplication, neurenteric, pericardial, and thymic); necrotic neoplasms, including necrotic lymphoma, cystic thymoma, germ-cell tumors, and necrotic lymph node metastases; lymphangioma and hemangioma; neurogenic tumors; thoracic meningocele; fluid collections such as mediastinal abscess, mediastinitis, hematoma, seroma, or pseudocyst; cystic goiter; a dilated, fluid-filled esophagus; and fluid localized in the superior pericardial recess (12,41,48).

High attenuation masses generally contain calcium, have a high iodine content, or are related to the presence of fresh blood. They include calcified lymph nodes secondary to granulomatous infection, sarcoidosis, inhalational diseases such as silicosis, *Pneumocystis carinii* infection; lymph node calcification caused by metastatic tumor such as adenocarcinoma or sarcoma; lymphoma with calcification usually after treatment; partially calcified primary neoplasms including germ-cell tumors, thymoma, and neurogenic tumors; calcified goiter; calcified vascular lesions; calcium within a cyst; goiter with high-iodine content; and mediastinal hematoma (40).

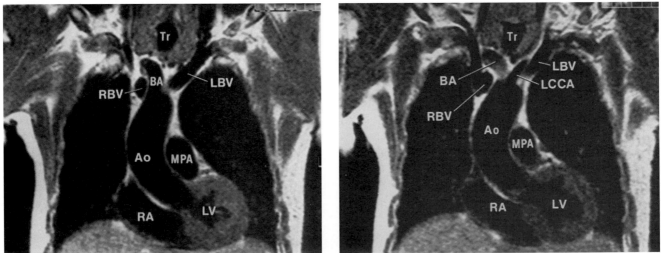

FIG. 2-13. Mediastinal anatomy, coronal MR images. **A–H:** Sequential coronal MR images from anterior to posterior. Identification of individual structures is easiest when comparison is made to the sections immediately adjacent, limiting potential problems of interpretation caused by partial volume averaging. *Ao*, aorta; *RA*, right atrium; *LV*, left ventricle; *MPA*, main pulmonary artery; *BA*, brachiocephalic artery; *RBV*, right brachiocephalic vein; *LBV*, left brachiocephalic vein; *Tr*, trachea; *LCCA*, left common carotid artery; *SVC*, superior vena cava; *RSPV*, right superior pulmonary vein; *RIPA*, right inferior pulmonary artery; *RSA*, right subclavian artery; *LSA*, left subclavian artery; *TA*, truncus anterior; *RMPA*, right main pulmonary artery; *LMPA*, left main pulmonary artery; *LSPV*, left superior pulmonary vein; *APW*, aorticopulmonary window; *RULB*, right upper lobe bronchus; *LMB*, left main-stem bronchus; *RMB*, right main-stem bronchus; *LA*, left atrium; *RMPA*, right main pulmonary artery; *LULB*, left upper lobe bronchus; *A-PSB*, apical-posterior segmental bronchus; *DAo*, descending aorta. Note that the thyroid gland is easily identified adjacent to the trachea in **A** and **B.**

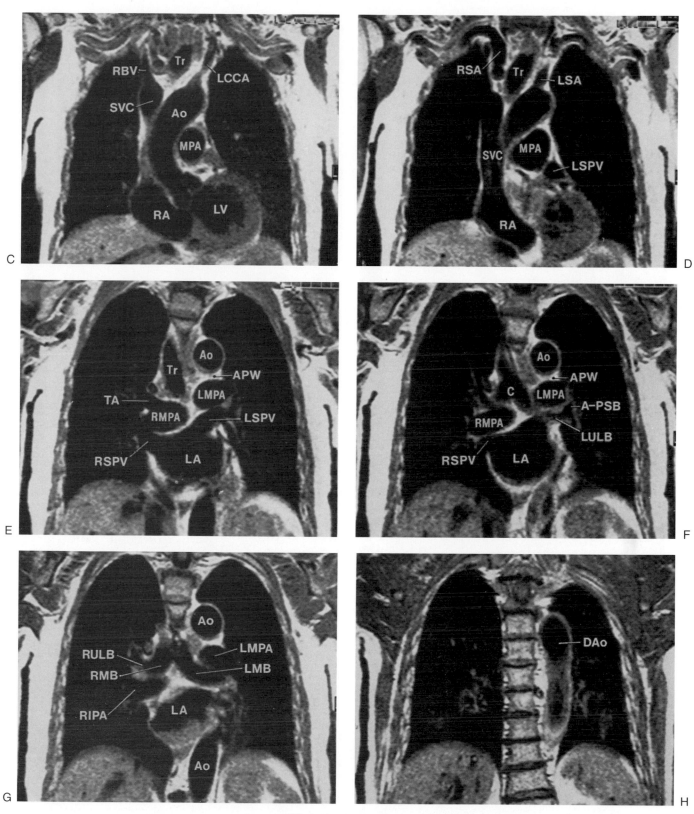

FIG. 2-13. *Continued.*

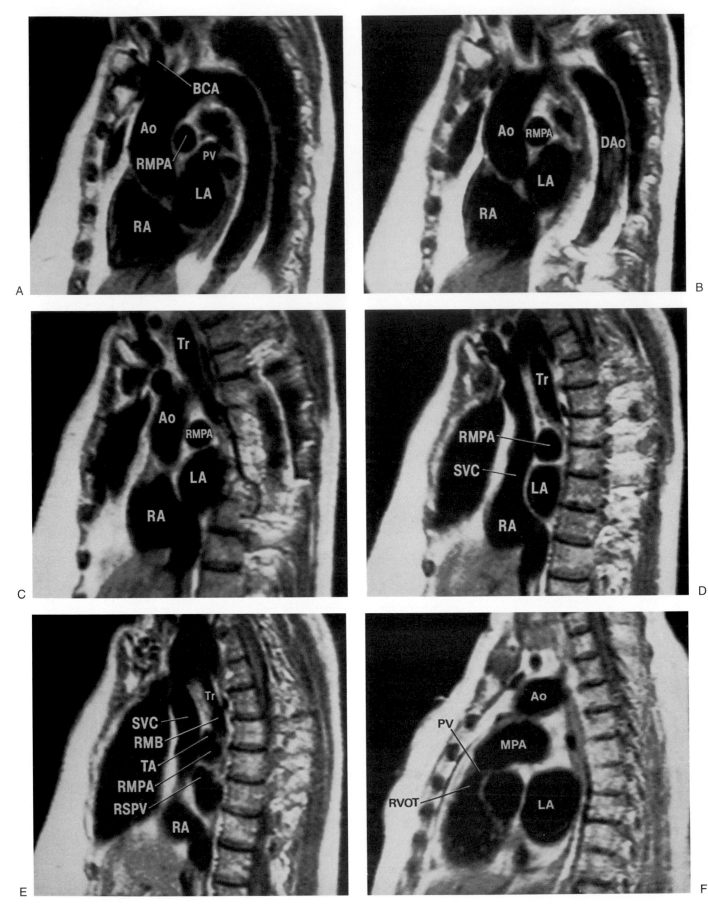

TABLE 2-2. *Differential diagnosis of mediastinal masses based on common sites of origin*

Prevascular space
- Thymic masses
  - hyperplasia
  - thymoma
  - thymic carcioma
  - thymic carcinoid tumor
  - thymolipoma
  - thymic cyst
  - thymic lymphoma and metastases
- Germ-Cell Tumors
  - teratoma
  - seminoma
  - nonsemiomatous germ-cell tumors
- Thyroid Abnormalities
- Parathyroid Tumor
- Lymph Node Masses (particularly Hodgkin lymphoma)
- Vascular Abnormalities (aorta and great vessels)
- Mesenchymal Abnormalities (e.g., lipomatosis, lipoma)
- Foregut Cyst
- Lymphangioma and Hemangioma

Cardiophrenic angle
- Lymph Node Masses (particularly lymphoma and metastases)
- Perciardial Cyst
- Morgagni Hernia
- Thymic masses
- Germ-Cell Tumors

Pretracheal space
- Lymph Node Masses
  - lung carcinoma
  - sarcoidosis
  - lymphoma (particularly Hodgkin disease)
  - metastases
  - infections (e.g., TB)
- Foregut Cyst
- Tracheal Tumor
- Mesenchymal Masses (e.g., lipomatosis, lipoma)
- Thyroid Abnormalities
- Vascular Abnormalities (aorta and great vessels)
- Lymphangioma and Hemangioma

Aorticopulmonary window
- Lymph Node Masses
  - lung carcinoma
  - sarcoidosis
  - lymphoma
  - metastases
  - infections (e.g., TB)
- Mesenchymal Masses (e.g., lipomatosis, lipoma)
- Vascular Abnormalities (aorta or pulmonary artery)
- Chemodectoma
- Foregut Cyst

Subcarinal space, azygoesophageal recess
- Lymph Node Masses
  - lung carcinoma
  - sarcoidosis
  - lymphoma
  - metastases
  - infections (e.g., TB)
- Foregut Cyst
- Dilated Azygos Vein
- Esophageal Masses
- Varices
- Hernia

Paravertebral region
- Neurogenic Tumor
  - nerve-sheath tumors
  - sympathetic ganglia tumors
  - paraganglioma
- Foregut Cyst
- Meningocele
- Extrameduallary Hematopoeisis
- Pseudocyst
- Thoracic Spine Abnormalities
- Hernias
- Esophageal Masses
- Varices
- Mesenchymal Masses (e.g., lipomatosis, lipoma)
- Lymph Node Masses
  - lymphoma (particularly non-Hodgkin)
  - metastases
- Dilated Azygos or Hemiazygos Vein
- Hernia
- Lymphangioma and Hemangioma
- Thymic Mass or Germ-Cell Tumor

Enhancing masses are highly vascular (49), and include substernal thyroid and parathyroid glands (50,51); carcinoid tumors; lymphangiomas and hemangiomas which may contain vascular elements (52,53); paraganglioma (54,55); Castleman's disease (15,56); and a variety of partially necrotic inflammatory and neoplastic lesions in which some rim enhancement is visible (12,13).

MASSES PRIMARILY INVOLVING THE PREVASCULAR SPACE

Mediastinal masses result in alterations of normal mediastinal contours, and displacement or compression of mediastinal structures; recognizing these findings can be valuable in diagnosis and in suggesting the site of origin of the mass.

Masses in the prevascular space, when large, tend to dis-

FIG. 2-14. Mediastinal anatomy, parasagittal MR images. **A–E:** Sequential parasagittal images through the mediastinum, from the level of the aortic arch to the right hilum, respectively. Familiarity with this particular plane is especially important as it intersects both the ascending and descending aorta, thus allowing visualization of the entire aorta in a single plane (see **A**). *Ao,* ascending aorta; *BCA,* brachiocephalic artery; *RA,* right atrium; *LA,* left atrium; *RMPA,* right main pulmonary artery; *PV,* left superior pulmonary vein; *DAo,* descending aorta; *Tr,* trachea; *SVC,* superior vena cava; *RSPV,* right superior pulmonary vein; *TA,* truncus anterior; *RMB,* right main-stem bronchus. **F:** True sagittal MR image through the main pulmonary artery (MPA). Note that in this plane, the relationship between the MPA and the right ventricular outflow tract is especially well seen. As shown in this example, occasionally a section at this level allows visualization of the pulmonic valves.

place the aorta and great arterial branches posteriorly, but distinct compression or narrowing of these relatively thick walled structures is unusual. Within the supraaortic mediastinum, displacement, compression, or obstruction of the brachiocephalic veins is common. Posterior displacement or compression of the superior vena cava is typical only with large or right sided masses. On the left, compression of the main pulmonary artery can be seen. Recognizing abnormalities of mediastinal contours are not particularly helpful in diagnosing masses in this region. The anterior junction line is rather variable in thickness, and cannot be relied upon as abnormal unless grossly thickened. The mediastinal pleural relections bordering the prevascular space are often convex laterally, although a marked convexity may suggest mass. The differential diagnosis of masses arising in this area include thymoma and other thymic tumors, cysts, lymphoma and other lymph node masses, germinal-cell tumors, thyroid masses, parathyroid masses, fatty masses, and lymphangioma (hygroma) (57).

CT is advantageous in the diagnosis of masses in the prevascular mediastinum (48,58). In a study of 128 patients, the correct first choice diagnosis was made in 48% of cases, based on CT, although this was possible in only 36% of cases based on plain radiographs (58). Those masses most accurately diagnosed were cystic in nature, contained fat, or had characteristic enhancement patterns, including benign germ-cell tumors, thymolipoma, omental hernia, and tuberculous lymphadenopathy.

THE THYMUS AND THYMIC MASSES

Normal Thymus

The thymus has two lobes that are fused superiorly near the thyroid gland and smoothly molded to the anterior aspect of the great vessels at lower levels. It occupies the thyropericardic space of the anterior mediastinum and extends inferiorly to the base of the heart. The thymus is very rarely found in an ectopic location, usually the neck (59).

On conventional radiographs, the thymus appears largest in the neonate and young infant. In fact, the thymus weighs an average of 22 ± 13 g at birth and increases progressively to reach a maximum weight at puberty of approximately 34 g (60). Beginning at puberty, the thymus begins to involute, and this process continues for a period of 5 to 15 years. During thymic involution, atrophied thymic follicles are progressively replaced by fat, and the relative proportion of fat to thymic tissue increases progressively, until after age 60. At this age, remaining thymic tissue is negligible (61,62). For example, in an autopsy series of 20 patients over 60 years of age, no thymus could be recognized with gross examination and only 11 had any thymic tissue visible histologically (61).

CT allows imaging of the thymus with much greater clarity than is possible using plain radiographs or conventional tomography. The CT appearance of the normal thymus has been well described in both adults and children (19,21–23,25). In interpreting CT, one must be aware, of

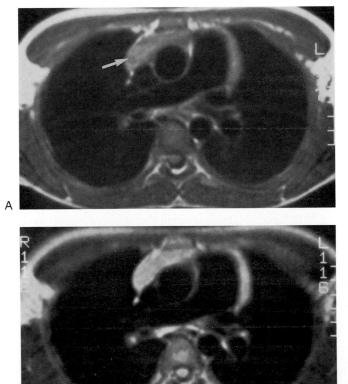

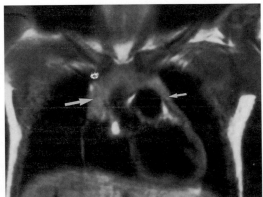

FIG. 2-15. Normal thymus in a 12-year-old boy. **A:** T1-weighted transaxial image (TR/TE = 750/20 msec) of the mediastinum shows the homogeneous intensity thymus (*arrow*) anterior to the great vessels. The right mediastinal pleura is convex laterally. In this patient, the right thymic lobe predominates. **B:** T2-weighted transaxial image (TR/TE = 2250/70 msec) shows an increase in intensity of the thymus, as compared with mediastinal fat. **C:** T1-weighted transaxial image (TR/TE = 750/20 msec) in the coronal plane shows the thymus occupying most of the superior mediastinum, extending inferiorly to the level of the right atrium. The right thymic lobe is largest (*large arrow*), but the left thymic lobe (*small arrow*) is also visible.

A

B

C

the significant changes that occur in thymic morphology with age, and the significant variation in the normal size and weight of the thymus seen in younger individuals, particularly those under the age of 25.

Appearance in Children

In children, the normal thymus occupies the retrosternal space, draping itself over the great vessels and cardiac margins (22). Its left lobe usually extends laterally, adjacent to the arch of the aorta, and posteriorly to the level of the descending aorta, but distinct lobes are not generally seen (63). Cephalad, the thymus extends an average of 1.7 cm superior to the innominate vein, and can be seen as high as the thyroid gland, where it may simulate lymph node enlargement (64). Its inferior extent is variable. In infancy, it is commonly seen at the level of the pulmonary arteries or below, but its inferior extent decreases with age.

In infants and younger children, the thymus appears quadrilateral in shape in the axial plane, but assumes a more triangular shape as the child grows. Its margins are sharp, smooth, and convex in infants, and often become straight in older children (19,22,65). On CT, the thymus is of soft-tissue

attenuation, slightly more dense than vessels, but approximately the same attenuation as muscle. The mean attenuation of the thymus has been found to be 36 Hounsfield units (HU) (65).

It is often possible to distinguish between thymus and vessels even without contrast enhancement, but contrast is required to optimally delineate the thymus, which shows homogeneous enhancement of 20 to 30 HU after bolus contrast injection. MRI clearly distinguishes the thymus from mediastinal vascular structures (Fig. 2-15) (20,24). On T1-weighted images, the signal intensity of the thymus is slightly greater than that of muscle; on T2 images, it becomes brighter than both the surrounding fat and muscle.

Thymic size can be quantitated using its length (measured in the cephalo-caudal dimension), width (measured in the transverse dimension), and thickness, measured perpendicular to its length and anteroposterior dimension (Fig. 2-16). Although thymic size increases with age in young subjects, its width shows little change. On CT, the average thickness of the thymus decreases with age, from an average of 1.4 cm in children aged 5 years or less, to an average of 1.0 cm in children aged 10 to 19 years (25).

In children, CT (22,25) and MRI (20,24) provide some-

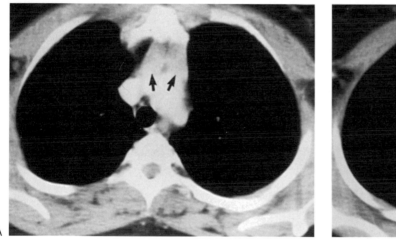

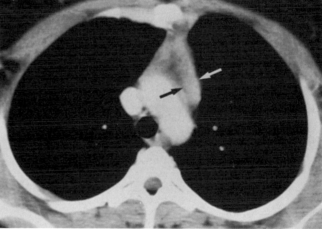

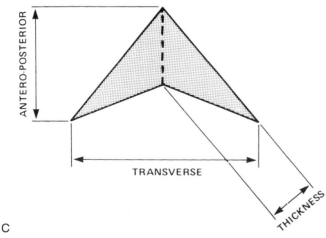

FIG. 2-16. Normal thymus, CT assessment. **A,B:** Sequential contrast-enhanced CT scans at the levels of the great vessels and aortic arch, respectively, show normal bilobed appearance of the thymus in a teenager (*arrows* in **A**). Measurements of the thymus thickness are generally most useful, as indicated by the *arrows* in **B**. **C:** Schematic diagram of the thymus. (From ref. 21, with permission.)

what different normal values for thymic size, a finding that likely reflects the fact that MRI scans are obtained during quiet breathing, whereas CT, especially in older children, is commonly performed at full inspiration (20). As compared to CT, MRI in children usually shows a slightly greater thymic width, but a marked decrease in the ratio of the size of the thymus relative to both the transverse and cephalo-caudal dimensions of the thorax. On MRI, the thymus appears to have a slightly greater thickness than noted on CT, with an average thickness of 1.8 cm for the right lobe and 2.1 cm for the left lobe. Occasionally the signal intensity characteristics of normal thymic tissue may be of value in identifying unusual configurations of the thymus, especially in children in whom posterior mediastinal extension between the superior vena cava and trachea is not uncommon (66).

Appearance in Adults

From puberty to the age of about 25 years, the thymus is recognizable as a distinct triangular or bilobed structure, usually outlined by mediastinal fat. Typically its borders are flat or concave laterally, but on occasion the thymus may show convex margins, a finding more typical in children (see Figs. 2-15 and 2-16). Its CT attenuation usually decreases to less than that of muscle because of fatty replacement. Over the age of 25 years, the thymus is no longer recognizable as a soft-tissue structure, because of progressive fatty involution. Islands or whisps of soft-tissue density within a background of more abundant fat are typically noted on CT. The rapidity and degree of thymic involution are variable in different subjects, and occasionally the thymus may still be recognized as a discrete structure up to the age of 40. With complete thymic involution, the anterior mediastinum appears to be entirely filled with fat. It should be realized however, that most of the anterior mediastinal fat is contained within the fibrous skeleton of the thymus and may have a CT density slightly higher than that of subcutaneous fat.

Normal measurements for the thymus, as shown on CT in adults have been reported (see Fig. 2-16) (19,21). Although values for the length (measured in the cephalo-caudal dimension), and width (measured in the transverse dimension) of the thymus have been defined, the most helpful value for thymic size is "thickness," measured perpendicular to the length. Under age 20, a thickness of 1.8 cm is considered the maximum allowable normal value, with 1.3 cm being the maximum normal value in older subjects. The accuracy of these dimensions has been confirmed by Francis et al. (21) and Nicolaou et al. (67). Francis showed that although thymic thickness is a sensitive indicator of thymic abnormality, thymic shape was just as reliable in separating normal from abnormal thymus, especially when the thymus was multi-lobulated (21). In fact, qualitative assessment of thymic shape alone should prove sufficient for diagnosing mass lesions of the thymus. Nicolaou et al., found a sensitivity of 100% for diagnosing thymic hyperplasia or thymoma based on a thymic thickness of greater than 1.3 cm or a focal soft-tissue density greater than 7 mm (67).

On MRI, the normal thymus (20,24,68) characteristically appears homogeneous and of intermediate signal intensity on T1-weighted images, being less intense than surrounding mediastinal fat, but greater intensity than muscle (see Fig. 2-15; Fig. 2-17). However, because of progressive thymic involution, its appearance is dependent on the age of the patient. In patients over 30 years of age, differentiation between the thymus and adjacent mediastinal fat may be difficult because of thymic involution and replacement by fat (see Figs. 2-10 and 2-11). The T2 relaxation times of the thymus are similar to fat at all ages, making visualization of the thymus more difficult than on T1-weighted images (20,68). On MRI, thymic thickness can appear considerably greater than that seen on CT, with a mean value of up to 20 mm (20).

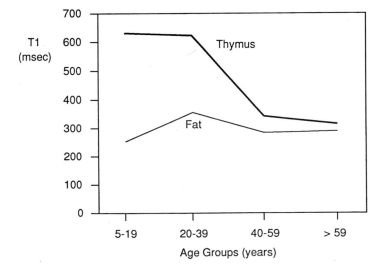

FIG. 2-17. Relative T1 values of thymus and fat in different age groups. The T1 of thymus decreases in older patients because of fatty replacement. The T1 of fat remains constant relative to age.

Thymic Enlargement

The thymus can weigh as much as 45 to 50 grams in normal individuals, and it is difficult to diagnose mild degrees of thymic enlargement. However, when the thymus results in a mediastinal mass readily detectable on plain chest radiographs in older children or young adults, it can be considered to be enlarged. Hyperthyroidism may be responsible for thymic enlargement (60). Less common associations with thymic enlargement are acromegaly, Addison's disease, and recovery from burns or chemotherapy (69).

Thymic Hyperplasia

Thymic germinal or lymphoid follicular hyperplasia (LFH) is a term used by pathologists to describe the presence of hyperplastic lymphoid germinal centers in the thymic medulla, associated with a lymphocytic and plasma cell infiltrate (60). The presence of LFH is commonly associated with myasthenia gravis, although lymphoid follicles can also be present in the medulla of the normal thymus, particularly in young subjects.

On CT, 30% to 50% of patients with LFH can have a normal appearing thymus. In many of the remaining patients, the thymus appears abnormally enlarged, but generally has a normal shape. In some patients with LFH, the thymus appears nodular or mass-like or inhomogeneous in attenuation. In a recent study of 22 patients with myasthenia gravis and LFH (67), 10 (45%) had a normal appearing thymus on CT, 7 (32%) had an enlarged thymus, and 5 (23%) had a focal thymic mass. Focal thymic masses ranged from 1.7 to 5 cm in diameter.

Although thymic enlargement can be identified on CT in some patients with LFH, the usefulness of CT in detecting this abnormality is limited (67,70,71). In one large study correlating CT with pathologic findings, thymus glands showing LFH typically appeared larger than those of age-matched controls. However, based on diffuse enlargement of the gland, CT proved only 71% sensitive for diagnosing lymphoid hyperplasia (71). In the study by Nicolaou et al. (67), only 55% of patients with LFH showed an abnormal thymus on CT. Furthermore, Castleman and Norris (72) have shown that in patients with myasthenia gravis, the weight of thymus glands showing LFH does not differ significantly from that of normal controls. Up to 50% of the thymus glands called normal on CT may prove to contain LFH after surgical removal (73).

On MRI, patients with thymic hyperplasia or thymic rebound may show enlargement of the thymus, but its signal intensity is the same as for normal thymus (68).

Thymic Rebound

The thymus involutes during periods of stress, sustaining a decrease in volume that variably depends on the age of the patient and the severity and duration of the stress. This phenomenon is most marked in children, but it has also been observed in young adults. Following involution, the thymus will generally reacquire its premorbid size within several months of the stressful episode. It may also exhibit "rebound," or growth to a size significantly larger than its original size (Figs. 2-18 and 2-19). For example, Gelfand et al. (69) found enlargement of the thymus, as determined using plain chest radiographs, in five children aged 5 to 12 who were recovering from burns. Also, largely using chest roentgenography, Cohen et al. illustrated rebound thymic growth in seven children aged 3 to 11 who had received chemotherapy for 5 months to 3 years for Wilms' tumor, malignant lymphoma, osteosarcoma, malignant teratoma, or acute lymphatic leukemia (74). In three cases, a prominent thymus was observed during the course of chemotherapy; in the remaining four patients the changes were detected 1 to 9 months after cessation of therapy.

Since CT is more sensitive than are plain chest radiographs for detecting thymic enlargement, thymic rebound is detected with greater frequency when patients are monitored with CT. Using CT, Choyke et al. (75) made serial observations of the mediastinum in a group of patients aged 2 to 35, who were receiving chemotherapy for various malignancies, including Hodgkin's disease (n = 6), osteosarcoma (n = 5), testicular neoplasms (n = 4), Wilms' tumor (n = 3), and rhabdomyosarcoma (n = 2). In this study (75), thymic volume decreased an average of 43% in response to chemotherapy. On follow-up studies, however, the thymus recovered its pretreatment volume in most cases and, in 25% of patients, thymic rebound occurred, with the volume of the thymus exceeding the baseline volume by 50%. Thymic rebound as visualized by CT has also been reported after treatment of Cushing's syndrome (76).

In most patients with extrathoracic malignancies, thymic rebound is unlikely to cause concern or diagnostic confusion. As a practical matter, thymic rebound is most problematic when it is observed in patients with malignant lymphoma, who have been treated using chemotherapy. When an enlarged thymus is seen in such patients, it can be difficult to distinguish thymic rebound from recurrent lymphoma. In our experience, however, when a patient with lymphoma shows thymic enlargement as an isolated finding after treatment (see Fig. 2-19), with no adenopathy being visible, it is reasonable to follow the patient with the presumption that thymic rebound is responsible.

In a study by Kissin et al. (77) of adults receiving chemotherapy, there was a suggestion that thymic rebound may be a favorable prognostic factor, in that 13 of 14 patients with thymic enlargement after chemotherapy were free of disease after a mean follow-up of 45 months (77).

Diagnosis of Thymic Masses

The left thymic lobe is normally larger than the right and the thymus is almost always slightly asymmetric. However, if enlargement of the thymus is grossly asymmetric or if

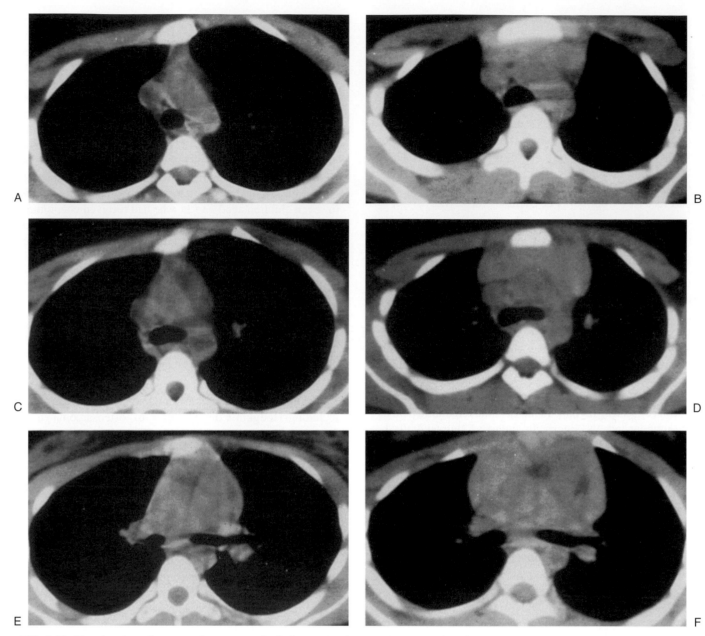

FIG. 2-18. Thymic rebound, osteogenic sarcoma. **A–C:** Sequential CT sections through the mediastinum in a 10-year-old girl with osteogenic sarcoma treated with chemotherapy show marked thymic involution. **D–F:** Sequential CT sections at the same levels as shown in **A–C**, 4 months later. Note marked thymic rebound with enlargement of both the right and left lobes.

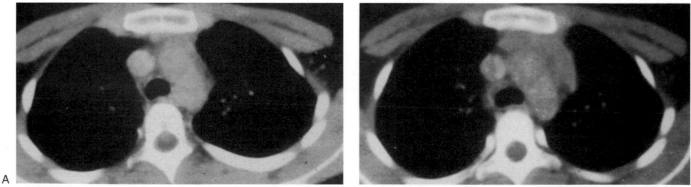

FIG. 2-19. Thymic rebound, lymphoma. **A:** 10-year-old girl with thymic involution following chemotherapy for malignant lymphoma. **B:** Follow-up CT obtained 8 months later shows enlargement of both lobes of the thymus without adenopathy.

TABLE 2-3. *Differentiation of thymoma and normal thymus: CT criteria*

Thymoma
1. Patient over 30
2. Mass spherical or lobulated with rounded margins
3. Attenuation of mass equals or exceeds muscle of chest wall
4. Lesion surrounded by fat
5. Calcification present
6. Unilateral or midline

Normal Thymus
1. Patient under 20
2. "Mass" elongated with length > width, as is typical for a normal thymic lobe
3. "Mass" diffusely infiltrated by fat, seen much better with lower window setting
4. Paucity of thymic fat—i.e., lesion represents thymus with delayed involution
5. No calcification
6. Bilateral soft-tissue prominence seen in usual location of right and left thymic lobes

the thymus has a lobular contour, a thymic mass should be suspected. Using these criteria, CT has proven extremely accurate in diagnosing thymoma and other thymic neoplasms (Table 2-3). In a study reported by Chen et al., CT proved 91% sensitive and 97% specific in establishing the presence of a mass within the thymus (71). Of 34 patients with a CT diagnosis of a mass or neoplasm, all but one proved surgically to have a thymoma (n = 31), thymic cyst (n = 1), or Hodgkin's disease (n = 1). Similar results have been reported by others (78). It must be kept in mind, however, that thymic hyperplasia can also result in a focal thymic mass, up to 5 cm in diameter (67). The role of MRI in diagnosing thymic masses is more limited (48). One important exception is in the diagnosis of vascular invasion, especially in patients for whom intravenous contrast cannot be administered (79). In these cases, MRI exquisitely delineates the extent of vascular involvement, including identification of intracardiac disease extension.

Thymic masses and tumors include thymoma, thymic carcinoma, thymic carcinoid tumors, thymic cyst, thymolipoma, and lymphoma (80). Overall, they account for approximately 20% of primary mediastinal tumors (81,82).

Thymoma

The most common primary thymic tumor is thymoma (83). It accounts for about 15% of primary mediastinal masses (83). The term thymoma should be used only to describe neoplasms originating from the thymic epithelium (84). Thymomas are rare before age 20, and are most common in patients aged 50 to 60 years. From 30 to 54% of patients with a thymoma develop myasthenia gravis. Other syndromes associated with thymoma include red cell aplasia, and hypogammaglobulinemia.

Traditionally thymomas have been classified as predominantly epithelial, predominantly lymphocytic, and mixed lymphoepithelial, regardless of cytologic abnormalities identified within the neoplastic epithelial cells (84,85). Recently, an alternate classification of thymoma has been suggested by Marino and Müller-Hermelink that categorizes thymomas as either cortical, medullary, or mixed, based on both morphology and histogenesis (86). This classification may have significant predictive value (87). As reported by Ricci et al., (88) in a study of 74 cases of thymoma, those tumors classified as medullary were benign, arose late in life, and were not associated with mortality. In distinction, cortical thymomas usually presented earlier in life and were associated with a 50% mortality at 5 years despite aggressive therapy.

Histologic appearances do not allow a reliable differentiation between benign and malignant thymoma; malignancy can only be established by documenting the presence of tumor growth into or through the tumor capsule. Thus, thymomas are most appropriately referred to as invasive or noninvasive.

Approximately 30% of thymomas are invasive. Characteristically, invasive thymomas infiltrate adjacent structures or result in pleural or pericardial implants; thymoma rarely metastasizes outside the thorax. This neoplasm grows (a) to invade local mediastinal structures, including the superior vena cava, great vessels, and even the airways; (b) to invade the adjacent lungs or chest wall; or (c) to spread by contiguity along pleural reflections, usually on one side of the chest cavity only, potentially seeding even the diaphragmatic surfaces with consequent direct extension into the abdomen (Fig. 2-20) (84,85,89–93).

Thymomas can be staged at the time of surgery, based on the presence and extent of invasion (83). Stage 1 indicates that the capsule is intact; stage 2, that pericapsular growth has resulted in invasion of mediastinal fat; and stage 3, that invasion of surrounding organs has occurred or pleural implants are present at a distance from the primary tumor. Resection is indicated in all three stages, with supplemental radiotherapy in stage 2 and radiotherapy plus chemotherapy in stage 3 (94–96). Five-year survival for thymoma is between 53 and 87% (83).

The CT appearance of thymomas has been well described (21,67,71,78,97–102). Approximately 80% of thymomas occur at the base of the heart (83). Commonly, they are subtle or invisible on chest radiographs (103). On CT, thymomas appear as homogeneous soft-tissue density masses, which are usually sharply demarcated, and oval, round, or lobulated in shape, project to one side of the mediastinum, and do not conform to the normal shape of the thymus (Fig. 2-21) (83). Most often the tumor grows asymmetrically to one side of the anterior mediastinum and prevascular space (Figs. 2-21–2-23). Because extopic thymic tissue in the neck is found in up to 21% of subjects, thymoma can occur in the neck or at the thoracic inlet, thus mimicking a thyroid mass (104). Rarely, thymomas may appear cystic, with discrete nodular

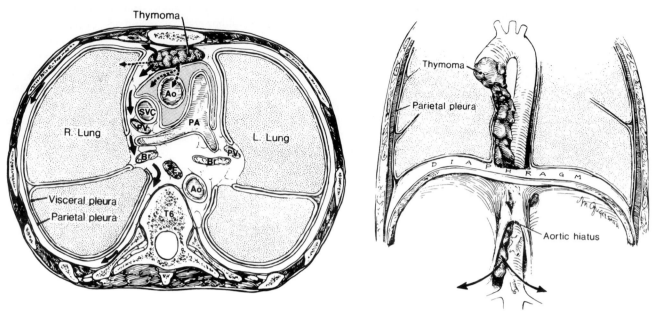

FIG. 2-20. Invasive thymoma: CT evaluation. **A,B:** The pattern of spread of invasive thymomas is graphically represented. In cross-section, the tumor can directly invade surrounding structures (*broken arrows*) or insinuate itself between the chest wall or mediastinum and the parietal pleura (*solid arrows*). Once the paraaortic—paraspinal area is reached, inferior extension through the aortic or esophageal hiatus can occur. With CT, such extension can be seen reliably and the study should always be extended to the upper abdomen. *Ao*, aorta; *PA*, pulmonary artery; *PV*, pulmonary vein; *Br*, bronchus; *E*, esophagus; *SVC*, superior vena cava. (From ref. 89, with permission.)

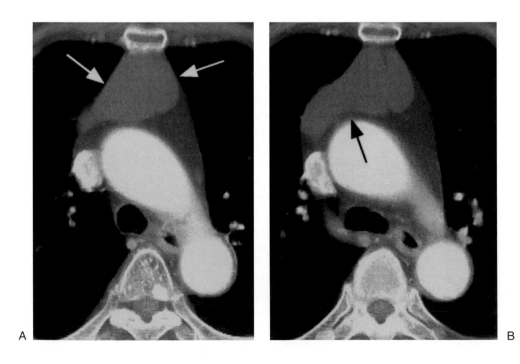

FIG. 2-21. Noninvasive thymoma. **A:** A large homogeneous mass (*arrows* in **A** and **B**) is visible in the prevascular space on a contrast-enhanced helical CT scan. **B:** It is separated from the ascending aorta by a well defined fat plane, suggesting that it is noninvasive.

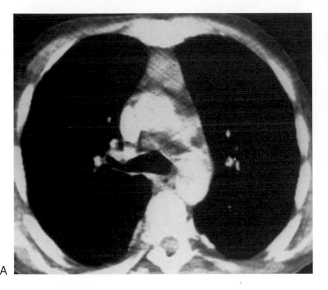

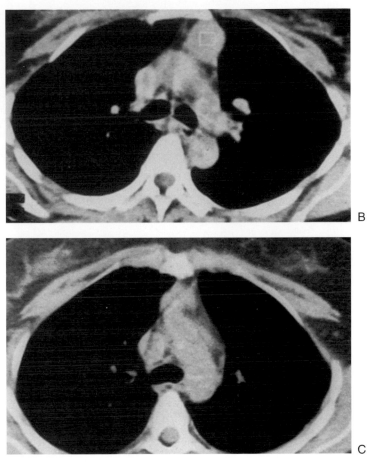

FIG. 2-22. Noninvasive thymomas in patients with myasthenia gravis. **A:** A 70-year-old man. There is an obvious solid, spherical mass in the anterior mediastinum surrounded by anterior mediastinal fat. **B:** A 45-year-old woman. A solid, spherical mass can be identified bulging into the fat in the anterior mediastinum. The attenuation value within the mass is similar to that of the chest wall muscles. **C:** A 39-year-old woman. The diagnosis of thymoma in this case is slightly more difficult because of a relative paucity of mediastinal fat. Key features are the spherical appearance of the lesion and the age of the patient.

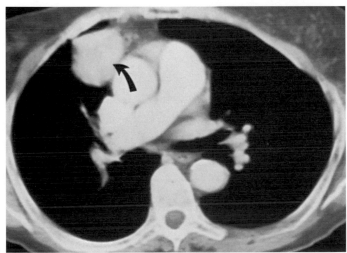

FIG. 2-23. Noninvasive thymoma, CT and MR findings. **A:** CT section at the level of the right main pulmonary artery following a bolus of intravenous contrast media. A well-defined rounded mass of soft-tissue attenuation is present on the right side (*arrow*). *(continues)*

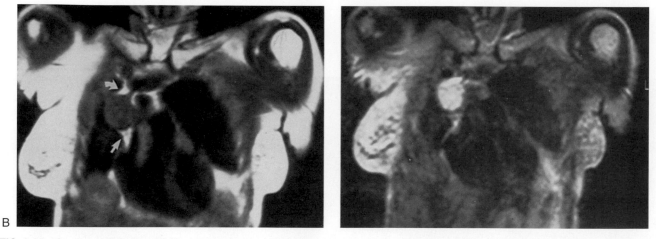

B C

FIG. 2-23. *Continued.* **B,C:** T1- and T2-weighted coronal images through the mass, respectively. On the T1-weighted image, fat clearly margin-ates both the superior and inferior borders of the mass (*arrows* in **B**), indicative of a mediastinal origin. The margins of the mass are sharply marginated. On the T2-weighted image (**C**), there is marked increase in the relative signal of the lesion.

components (Fig. 2-24). Except in patients with cystic masses, tumors usually enhances homogeneously after con-trast medium injection, and not uncommonly may contain calcium (Fig. 2-25).

The spectrum of CT findings in patients with invasive thymomas is illustrated in Figure 2-26. With CT, caution should be used to avoid over diagnosing invasion. As with other tumors, direct contact with and absence of cleavage planes between the tumor and mediastinal structures are not strictly reliable criteria for predicting invasion. On the other hand, clear delineation of fat planes surrounding a thymoma on CT should be interpreted as indicating an absence of extensive local invasion (see Fig. 2-21), especially when the

study is performed with thin collimation following a bolus of intravenous contrast medium (78). Pleural implants, when present, are often unilateral, and unlike other tumors result-ing in pleural metastases, are usually unassociated with pleural effusion. Thus, CT can show focal, well-defined pleural masses, unobscured by pleural fluid.

Invasive thymomas growing along pleural surfaces can reach the posterior mediastinum and extend downward along the aorta to involve the crus of the diaphragm and the retro-peritoneum (see Fig. 2-20) (83). These areas are "hidden" on conventional studies, but CT excels at demonstrating these sites of involvement (see Fig. 2-26) (89,90). A full CT examination of the thorax extended to include the upper

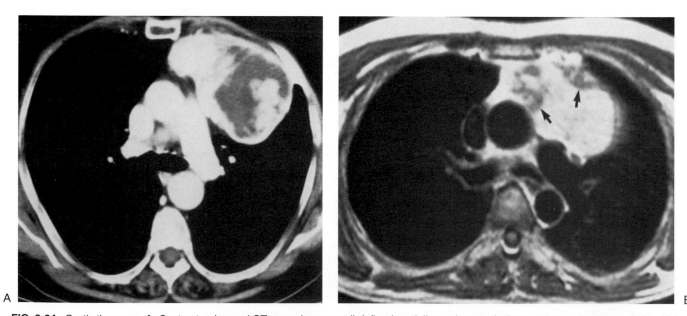

A B

FIG. 2-24. Cystic thymoma. **A:** Contrast-enhanced CT scan shows a well-defined partially cystic mass in the anterior mediastinum within which distinct soft-tissue nodules can be seen. Biopsy proved cystic thymoma. **B:** MR image in a patient different than in **A** shows a heterogeneous high-signal intensity mass in the anterior mediastinum within which discrete nodules of intermediate signal intensity can be identified (*arrows*). Although most thymomas are solid, occasional thymomas prove to be at least partially cystic. High-signal intensity within the mass proved to be secondary to complex cystic fluid and not fat. Cystic thymoma was surgically documented.

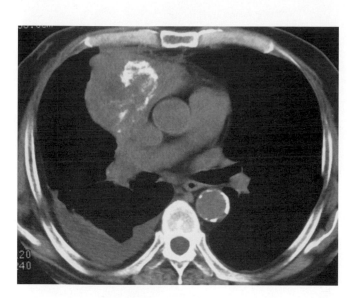

FIG. 2-25. Thymoma with calcification. A bulky mass in the prevascular space contains dense areas of calcification. The presence of pleural effusion on the side of the tumor suggests that the tumor is invasive.

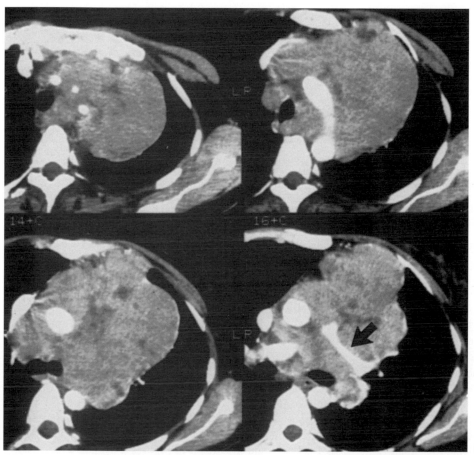

FIG. 2-26. The spectrum of invasive thymoma, CT findings. **A–D:** Sequential contrast-enhanced CT sections through the mediastinum show a bulky, nonhomogeneous soft-tissue mass deeply invading the mediastinum with encasement of all the great vessels as well as the left main pulmonary artery (*arrow* in **D**). *(continues)*

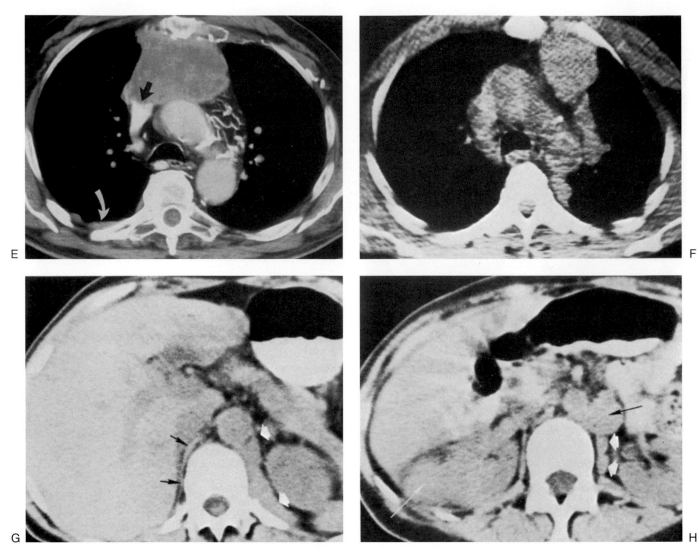

FIG. 2-26. *Continued.* **E:** Contrast-enhanced CT section through the carina in another patient shows a lobulated, slightly heterogeneous soft-tissue mass that is invading the adjacent superior vena cava (*arrow*). Markedly enlarged collateral vessels can be identified in the region of the aorticopulmonary window draining into the hemiazygos and azygos veins. Pleural implants, not appreciated on the accompanying chest radiograph (not shown), are apparent on the right side (*curved arrow*). **F–H:** CT sections at the level of the aortic arch and the hemidiaphragms, respectively, in another patient with documented invasive thymoma. The tumor has an irregular, lobulated contour. Poor definition of the interface between the tumor and the chest wall caused by invasion is noted. Invasive thymomas grow by contiguous spread, and a tongue of tumor tissue extends along the pleuromediastinal surface on the left side to reach the paraaortic region. From there it can extend inferiorly to reach the diaphragm (*white arrows* in **G**) [to be compared with the normal contralateral crus (*black arrows* in **G**)]. Further contiguous extension may lead to tumor growth into the retroperitoneum (*arrows* in **H**).

abdomen should be performed in these patients. Metastases are apt to be silent since only a minority of patients with invasive thymomas present with symptoms from intrathoracic spread. CT provides invaluable guidance for the radiotherapist and chemotherapist to adjust their treatment plans.

Because of the large size of the normal thymus in patients less than 25 years old, diagnosing thymoma in this age group can be difficult. However, thymomas are extremely rare in this age group, and, unless very obvious, we would avoid diagnosing thymoma in a patient less than 25 (73,97,101,102,105). Over the age of 40, the diagnosis of thymoma on CT usually poses no problem, as the normal thymus is largely replaced by fat. In patients ranging from

25 to 40 years, the thymus may be well seen, and, unless a definite mass is visible, as is often the case in the presence of thymoma, a definite diagnosis cannot be made. It should be noted that invasive thymomas, our main concern, are slow growing tumors, having little potential for distant metastases, and, if in doubt, a follow-up CT examination can be safely recommended. The clinical information and CT features that are most helpful in distinguishing between a thymoma and a prominent but normal thymus are summarized in Table 2-2 and illustrated in Figures 2-16 and 2-21.

On MRI, thymomas typically have a low signal intensity on T1-weighted images, which increases with T2 weighting (see Fig. 2-24; Figs. 2-27–2-30) (48,68); they may appear

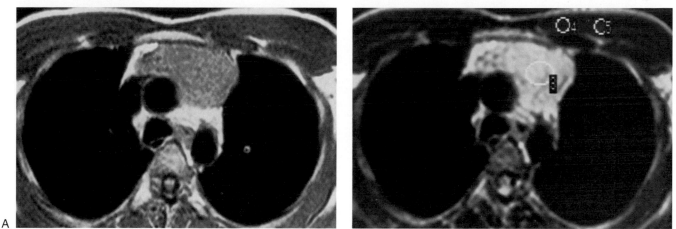

FIG. 2-27. Thymoma, MRI assessment. **A:** T1-weighted MR image at the level of the carina shows a homogeneous soft-tissue mass of intermediate signal intensity within the anterior mediastinum. **B:** T2-weighted MR image at the same level as shown in **A**. There is considerable signal enhancement within the mass that is now more difficult to differentiate from adjacent mediastinal fat. This appearance is entirely nonspecific. Biopsy proved thymoma.

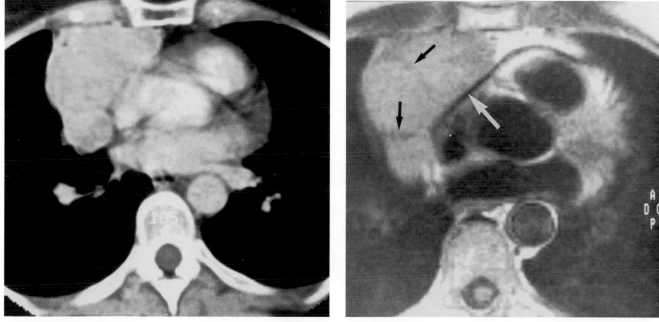

FIG. 2-28. Noninvasive thymoma. **A:** Contrast enhanced CT at the level of the aortic root shows a large thymic mass within which there is a suggestion of lobulation. **B:** T1-weighted axial MRI at the same level as in **A** shows the thymic mass is clearly distinguished from the normal fluid filled pericardium (*white arrow*). There no evidence of pericardial invasion or effusion or vascular invasion. Relatively low intensity septations (*black arrows*) delineate lobules of tumor.

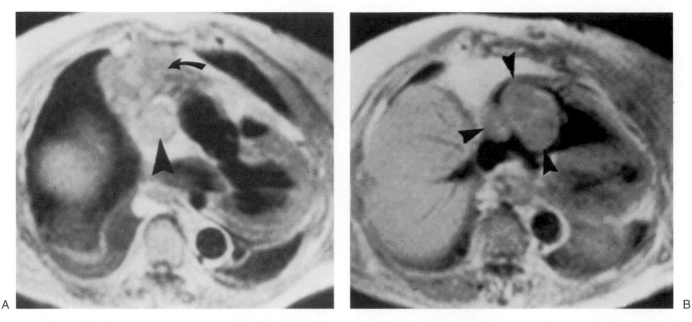

A

B

FIG. 2-29. Invasive thymoma, MRI evaluation. **A,B:** Sequential MR images through the heart show a poorly marginated mass of intermediate signal intensity within the anterior mediastinum (*curved arrow* in **A**) that is directly invading the superior mediastinum (*arrowhead* in **A**). The mass extends into the right atrium and can be seen crossing the tricuspid valve plane to enter the right ventricle (*arrowheads* in **B**). A moderately sized right pleural fluid collection is present as well. Invasive thymoma was surgically documented.

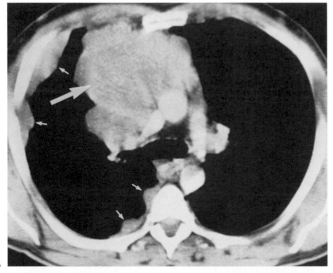

A

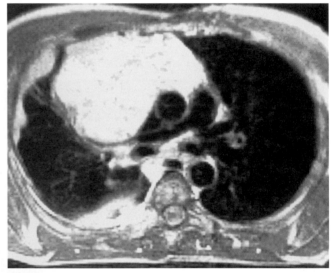

B

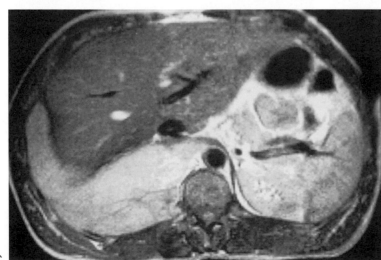

C

FIG. 2-30. Invasive thymoma. **A:** Contrast enhanced CT shows a large, lobulated thymoma (*large arrow*). There is marked displacement of the mediastinal vessels. Right pleural masses (*small arrows*) represent pleural metastases occurring because of invasion of the pleural space. **B:** TR/TE 1500/30 MRI clearly shows the relationship of the mass to great vessels. The pleural masses are visible as in **A**. **C:** MRI at a lower level shows large lobulated right pleural metastases These are typical of pleural metastases from thymoma.

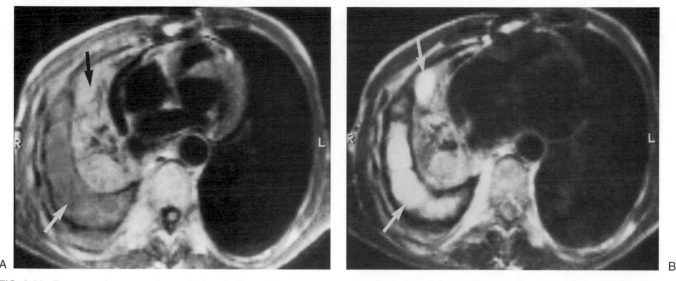

FIG. 2-31. Recurrent thymoma after radiation. **A:** T1-weighted image. Collapsed and fibrotic lung (*black arrow*) secondary to radiation fibrosis is visible medially. Tumor within the right pleural space (*white arrow*) is of similar intensity with this imaging sequence. **B:** With T2 weighting, high intensity areas (*arrows*) within the fibrotic lung and pleural space represent recurrent tumor. This was confirmed at biopsy.

homogeneous in intensity, inhomogeneous with or without cystic components (see Fig. 2-24), or may show nodules or lobules of tumor separated by relatively low intensity septations (see Fig. 2-28) (106). In a study comparing the MRI appearances of invasive and noninvasive thymomas with pathologic findings (107), it was found that nearly all thymomas appeared inhomogeneous on T2-weighted scans, because of the presence of cystic areas or areas of hemorrhage. In addition, half of the invasive thymomas showed a multinodular appearance on T2-weighted images, with tumor nodules separated by lower intensity fibrous septa. In their study, this appearance was not seen in patients with noninvasive thymoma. However, although this appearance may be regarded as suggestive of invasive thymoma, it must be considered nonspecific, as it can also be seen with noninvasive tumors (see Fig. 2-28).

MRI has proven valuable in identifying the presence or absence of vascular invasion in patients with thymoma, especially in patients for whom intravenous contrast cannot be administered. In these cases, MRI exquisitely delineates the extent of vascular involvement, including identification of intracardiac disease extension (see Fig. 2-29). Extension to other sites (see Fig. 2-30) and recurrent tumor after resection or radiation (Fig. 2-31) may also be shown using MRI.

Imaging in Myasthenia Gravis

Myasthenia gravis is commonly associated with thymic pathology. Sixty-five percent of patients with myasthenia gravis have thymic hyperplasia, thymoma is present in from 10% to 28% of patients with myasthenia gravis, and the remainder have a normal or involuted thymus.

Although there is no convincing evidence to suggest that thymectomy improves the outcome of myasthenia patients who are well controlled medically, it is generally agreed that thymectomy is indicated, regardless of thymic status, when medical therapy fails. In this setting, effective surgical treatment necessitates complete removal of all thymic tissue. Because surgical-anatomic studies have shown that both gross and microscopic thymic tissue is widely distributed throughout the mediastinum, it has been suggested that en bloc transcervical-transsternal "maximal" thymectomy be performed (108). Myasthenia patients most likely to benefit from thymectomy, in terms of disease control, are young females with a disease of short duration. Older patients and patients with long standing myasthenia rarely benefit from thymectomy.

The role of CT in patients with myasthenia remains somewhat unclear, at least partially because the role of surgery in patients with myasthenia gravis, in relation to thymic histology, is not clearly defined. Although the presence of thymic enlargement or a focal mass on CT reliably indicates the presence of FTH or thymoma (67), these findings do not have a strong correlation with surgical outcome. In one study (67) of 45 patients with myasthenia gravis having thymectomy, 17 of 19 patients showing thymic enlargement or focal thymic mass on CT improved following thymectomy, although improvement was seen in 80% of those having a normal thymus on CT. The presence of an abnormality on CT is not necessary in choosing patients for thymectomy, as a normal CT does not exclude FTH, and poor clinical response determines the need for thymic resection regardless of the presence or absence of thymic hyperplasia.

On the other hand, because thymoma is invasive in about 30% of cases, thymectomy is indicated in all patients who have thymoma, regardless of the effect of surgery on the course of the disease. The role of the radiologist in patients

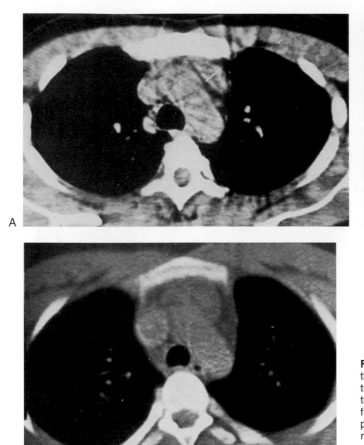

A

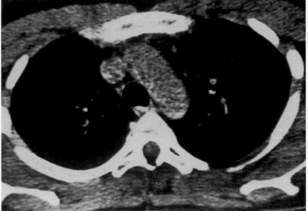

B

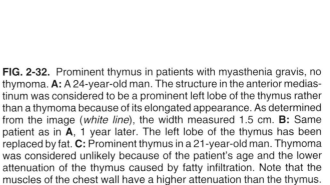

FIG. 2-32. Prominent thymus in patients with myasthenia gravis, no thymoma. **A:** A 24-year-old man. The structure in the anterior mediastinum was considered to be a prominent left lobe of the thymus rather than a thymoma because of its elongated appearance. As determined from the image (*white line*), the width measured 1.5 cm. **B:** Same patient as in **A**, 1 year later. The left lobe of the thymus has been replaced by fat. **C:** Prominent thymus in a 21-year-old man. Thymoma was considered unlikely because of the patient's age and the lower attenuation of the thymus caused by fatty infiltration. Note that the muscles of the chest wall have a higher attenuation than the thymus.

C

with myasthenia, most appropriately, is to diagnose patients in whom thymoma is likely, because of the presence of a focal thymic mass, and to distinguish them from patients who show thymic enlargement indicative of hyperplasia (FLH) (Figs. 2-32 and 2-33); such patients require surgery regardless of their likelihood of responding to thymectomy, based on their age and the duration of their symptoms.

The MRI appearance of the thymus in patients with myasthenia gravis has been described but its utility in diagnosing thymic abnormalities in this setting appears limited.

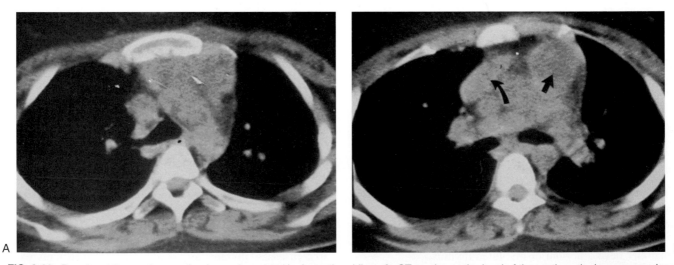

A

B

FIG. 2-33. Prominent thymus in myasthenia gravis caused by hyperthyroidism. **A:** CT section at the level of the aortic arch shows a prominent thymus in a 28-year-old woman. The appearance initially suggests a possible thymoma. **B:** CT section just below that shown in **A** demonstrates prominence of both the right (*arrow*) and left (*curved arrow*) lobes of the thymus. Enlargement of both lobes would be distinctly unusual in thymoma. In this case, the enlarged thymus was attributable to concurrent hyperthyroidism.

In a study of 16 patients with myasthenia gravis, imaged with both CT and MRI, who subsequently underwent thymectomy, MRI provided little if any distinctive information as compared with CT. Specifically, no distinctive MRI features could be identified in patients with thymomas apart from the presence of a mass (109). In seven patients with a histologic diagnosis of thymic hyperplasia, both CT and MRI displayed normal thymic morphology in five patients, and an enlarged and a small thymus in one case each, respectively. Unfortunately, MRI signal intensities were of no value in differentiating thymic hyperplasia from normal thymus.

Thymic Carcinoma

Thymic carcinoma, like thymoma, arises from thymic epithelial cells (80,110,111), but it is much less common. Thymic carcinoma accounts for about 20% of thymic epithelial tumors. Unlike thymoma, thymic carcinoma can be diagnosed as malignant on the basis of histologic criteria. The tumor is aggressive and more likely to result in distant metastases than invasive thymoma; although distant metastases are present in only about 5% of patients with invasive thymoma, they are present at diagnosis in 50% to 65% of patients with thymic carcinoma (111). Frequent sites of metastasis include the lungs (58), liver, brain, and bone (111). It has a poor prognosis.

Symptoms are usually attributable to the mediastinal mass, and superior vena cava syndrome may be present. Although paraneoplastic syndromes such as myasthenia gravis, pure red cell aplasia, and hypogammaglobulinemia are common with thymoma, they are rare with thymic carcinoma (111). Thymic carcinoma cannot be distinguished from thymoma on CT unless enlarged lymph nodes are visible in the mediastinum or distant metastases are evident

(58,80,112). A large mass with or without areas of low attenuation is typical (58,110). Thymic carcinoma is less likely than thymoma to result in pleural implants (112).

On MRI, thymic carcinoma appears higher in signal intensity than muscle on T1-weighted MR images, with an increase in signal on T2-weighted images. Heterogeneous signal may reflect the presence of necrosis, cystic regions within the tumor, or hemorrhage. It has been suggested by Endo et al. (106) that thymoma has a greater tendency to show a multinodular appearance on MRI than thymic carcinoma. Of the 15 cases of thymoma they reported (106), 79% showed lobulation, with areas of tumor separated by thick fibrous septa of lower intensity; this appearance was not seen in their 5 cases of thymic carcinoma.

Thymic Carcinoid Tumors

Thymic carcinoid tumors are believed to arise from thymic cells of neural crest origin (APUD, or cells that demonstrate amine precursor uptake and decarboxylase activity); they are usually malignant, with a tendency for local recurrence following resection (113). Although this lesion does not differ significantly from thymoma in its radiographic or CT appearance (48,80), the diagnosis can be suspected on clinical grounds. Approximately 40% of patients have Cushing's syndrome as a result of tumor secretion of adrenocorticotrophic hormone (ACTH) (114), and nearly 20% have been associated with multiple endocrine neoplasia (MEN) syndromes I and II. In some patients, a mediastinal mass may not be visible on CT despite the presence of endocrine abnormalities (113). This tumor is somewhat more aggressive than thymoma, being malignant in most cases, and superior vena cava obstruction is much more common with thymic carcinoid than with thymoma (Fig. 2-34). MRI findings are nonspecific and identical to those of thymoma (48).

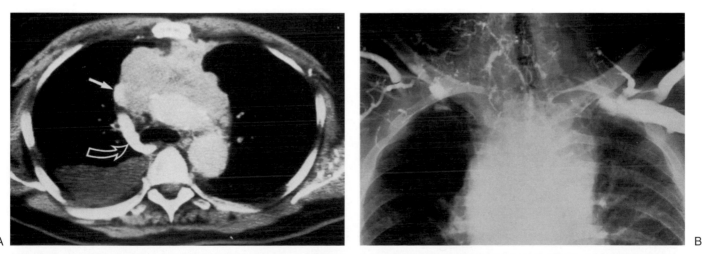

A   B

FIG. 2-34. Thymic carcinoid tumor with superior vena caval obstruction. **A:** Contrast-enhanced CT section at the level of the carina shows a bulky, somewhat heterogeneous soft-tissue mass within the prevascular space obliterating the left brachiocephalic vein and invading the superior vena cava (*arrow*). There is dense opacification of the azygos vein (*curved arrow*) serving as a collateral. **B:** Coned-down view from simultaneous bilateral antecubital fossa venous injections shows complete obstruction of the brachiocephalic veins bilaterally. At surgery this proved to be a primary thymic carcinoid tumor.

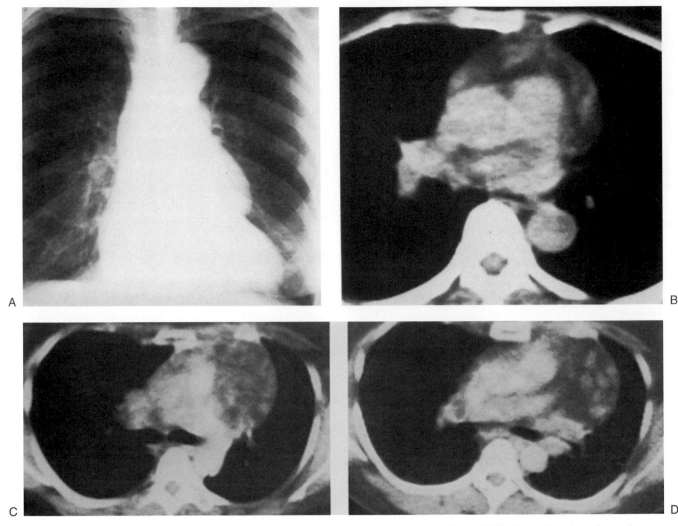

FIG. 2-35. Thymolipomas. **A,B:** A 71-year-old asymptomatic woman. Posteroanterior chest radiograph **(A)**. A smooth mass deforms the contour of the left heart border. CT at level of mass **(B)**. The mass is mostly fatty, but areas of soft-tissue density are identified within it. It is therefore unlikely to represent a simple lipoma. However, its sharp borders, the lack of compression of the nearby vessels, and its location point to benign lesion. Thymolipoma is a benign fatty tumor of the thymus that is usually of no clinical consequence. No surgery was performed. **C,D:** Another example of thymolipoma in a 51-year-old woman. Note again the inhomogeneous appearance of the mass **(C)**. Note in **D** the round areas of increased density that were found to represent lymph nodes on pathologic examination. No thymic tissue was identified.

Thymolipoma

Thymolipoma is a rare, benign, well-encapsulated thymic tumor, consisting primarily of fat but also containing variable amounts of thymic tissue; it can arise within the thymus or be connected to the thymus by a pedicle (115). It can be seen at any age, but is most common in children and young adults. In a recent review of 27 cases, 81% presented in the first four decades (115). In a majority of cases, thymolipoma is unaccompanied by symptoms or detected incidentally on chest radiographs. They are often large, ranging up to 36 cm in diameter (mean 18 cm) at the time of diagnosis, and may project into both hemithoraces (115). Because of its fatty content and pliability, it tends to drape over the heart, extending inferiorly into the cardiophrenic angles, and can simulate cardiac enlargement. Radiographically they have

also been mistaken for pleural or pericardial tumors, basal atelectasis, and even pulmonary sequestration (116). There is no known association with myasthenia gravis.

On CT, thymolipoma usually appears to contain a significant amount of fat, but three patterns have been reported (115). Most common is a combination of fat and whisps of soft tissue (Fig. 2-35); in 8 of 11 patients having CT, roughly equal amounts of fat and soft tissue were visible, with the soft tissue appearing as linear whorls intermixed with fat (seven cases) or as rounded opacities embedded within the fat (one case). The second pattern, seen in two cases was that of predominant fat attenuation, with tiny internal foci of soft tissue. The final pattern was seen in a single case in which a mass appeared to be primary of soft-tissue attenuation. In all cases, CT showed a connection between the mass and the thymic bed, which was narrow in seven cases and broad in four. When fat is visible on CT, a preoperative diagnosis can often be made. As would be expected from their fat content, MRI shows areas of high signal intensity on T1-weighted SE images, similar to the intensity of subcutaneous fat, with areas of intermediate signal intensity reflecting the presence of soft tissue (68,115,117). Despite attaining a large size, thymolipomas do not invade surrounding structures (118). However, some compression of mediastinal structures is visible in half of cases (115).

Thymic Cysts

Thymic cysts can be either congenital or acquired, but congenital thymic cysts are quite rare. Acquired thymic cysts have been reported following radiation therapy for Hodgkin's disease (119,120), in association with thymic tumors (121–123), and following thoracotomy (124). Their attenuation is usually that of water, but can be higher or lower depending on the presence of hemorrhage or lipid deposits.

One should be conservative in making the diagnosis of thymic cyst, as cystic regions can be seen in a variety of thymic tumors, including thymoma and lymphoma. CT can suggest the diagnosis if (a) the cyst appears thin walled; (b) it is unassociated with a mass lesion; and (c) it contains fluid with a density close to that of water or remains unopacified following contrast infusion. Calcification of the cyst wall can also be seen. MRI characteristics are similar to those of other cystic lesions (68).

Thymic Involvement in Lymphoma and Metastases

Hodgkin's disease has a prediliction for involvement of the thymus in conjunction with involvement of mediastinal lymph nodes (Fig. 2-36) (125). In a study of adults with newly diagnosed Hodgkin's disease involving the thorax, thymic enlargement was seen in 30% and in all, mediastinal lymph nodes were also enlarged (see Fig. 2-36 and Fig. 2-37). In a study of 60 pediatric patients with Hodgkin's disease, 17 (28%) had thymic enlargment; this represented 49% of patients with a mediastinal abnormality (126). In this study, 73% also showed mediastinal lymph node enlargment. Thymic enlargement was seen in 38% patients with intrathoracic recurrence (125). Thus, Hodgkin's disease, particularly the nodular sclerosing type, should be considered in the differential diagnosis of a thymic mass, but lymph node enlargement is typically present, at least in adults, and should suggest the correct diagnosis. Non-Hodgkin lymphoma much less commonly involves the thymus.

Thymic involvement in Hodgkin's disease and in lymphoma is usually indistinguishable from thymoma or other causes of anterior mediastinal mass. The enlarged thymus often retains its normal shape, and it may appear arrowhead shaped with convex borders (83%) or bilobed (17%) (125), but lobulation or a nodular appearance are also common (127). In adults, the thickness of the thymus measured 1.5 to 5 cm (125); in children, thickness of the larger thymic lobe ranged from 2.5 to 8.6 cm (126). The thymus usually appears homogeneous, but an inhomogeneous nodular inter-

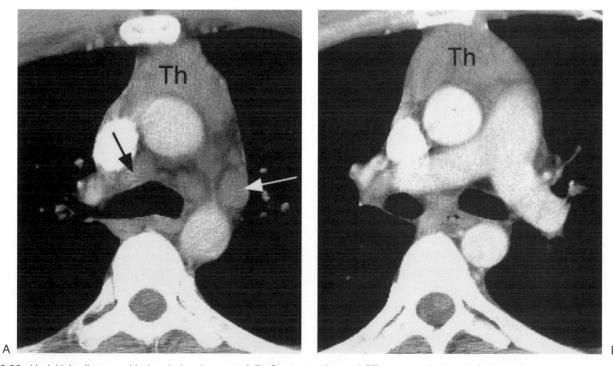

FIG. 2-36. Hodgkin's disease with thymic involvement. **A,B:** Contrast-enhanced CT scans at the level of the aorticopulmonary window and main pulmonary artery, respectively, show thymic enlargement (*Th*) and enlarged lymph nodes in the pretracheal space (*black arrow* in **A**) and aorticopulmonary window (*white arrow* in **A**). Lymph node enlargement in conjunction with thymic enlargement is typical of lymphoma involving the thymus.

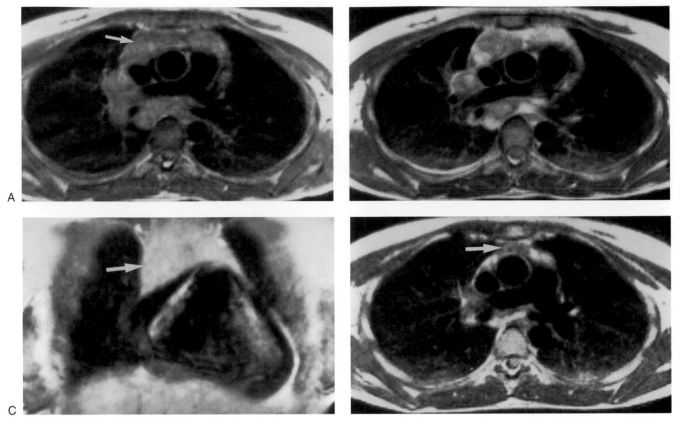

FIG. 2-37. Hodgkin lymphoma with thymic involvement: MR findings. **A:** T1-weighted transaxial image shows a large thymic mass (*arrow*), associated with right hilar and subcarinal lymphadenopathy. **B:** With T2 weighting the mass appears inhomogeneous, a finding common with lymphomas. **C:** T1-weighted coronal image shows the thymic mediastinal mass (*arrow*), associated with a large pericardial effusion. **D:** After radiation, a T2-weighted image at the same level as (**C**) shows the thymic mass (*arrow*) to be significantly reduced in size, as are the hilar lymph nodes.

nal architecture can be seen in adults (126,127). Cystic areas of necrosis may be visible at CT; this has been reported in 21% to 23% of adult patients (125,127), but is less common in children (126). Except in occasional cases, calcification does not occur in the absence of radiation (126).

On MRI, thymic lymphoma shows low intensity on T1-weighted images, with a variable change on T2-weighted images (68). In one study (24), two of seven patients with thymic lymphoma had a homogeneous appearing thymus, whereas in the remaining five, areas of increased or decreased intensity were visible on T2-weighted images (Fig. 2-38). The low intensity areas may represent fibrosis, whereas the high intensity areas could reflect hemorrhage or cystic degeneration. Although the MRI characteristics of lymphoma are not characteristic, the combination of a thymic mass with mass or lymph node enlargement in other areas of the mediastinum is very suggestive of the diagnosis.

Lung and breast carcinomas can also involve the thymus (128): in the case of lung cancer this is typically the result of direct extension, although hematogenous metastases may also occur. Involvement of mediastinal lymph nodes is also typically present. CT and MRI appearances of thymic metastases are nonspecific.

GERM-CELL TUMORS

Primary germ-cell tumors account for about 10% to 15% of primary mediastinal masses (as well as 10% to 15% of all anterior mediastinal masses) and are histologically identical to their gonadal counterparts (129). Presumably they arise from primitive germ cells that have arrested their embryologic migration in the mediastinum, frequently within the thymus (81,130). They are most common in the anterior mediastinum; only about 5% originate in the posterior mediastinum (81,82). Most germ-cell tumors present during the second to fourth decades of life. Germ-cell tumors include benign and malignant teratoma, seminomas, embryonal carcinoma, endodermal sinus (yolk sac) tumor, choriocarcinoma, and mixed types (48,131,132).

Overall, more than 80% of germ-cell tumors are benign (82), with the large majority of these being benign teratomas. Although the sex distribution of benign germ-cell tumors is about equal, there is a strong preponderance of males among patients with malignant germ-cell tumors (81,82). A striking male predominance has been noted recently in a series of three reports from the Armed Forces Institute of Pathology (133–135). Of 322 patients with primary mediastinal germ-cell tumors in this study, 320 were men including all 120

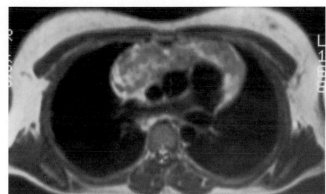

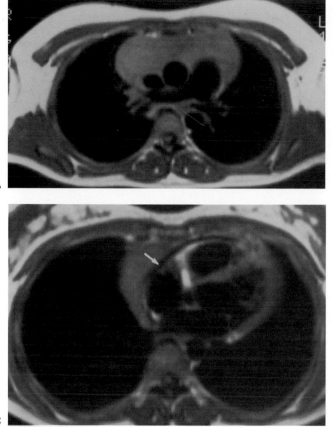

FIG. 2-38. Thymic lymphoma. **A:** A T1-weighted image (800/20) shows thymic enlargement appearing homogeneous in intensity. **B:** With T2-weighting (2400/70), the mass appears inhomogeneous. **C:** At a lower level, the relationship of the mass to the fluid filled pericardium (*arrow*) is visible on a coronal image obtained with T1 weighting.

patients with mediastinal seminomas, and all 64 cases with yolk sac tumors, embryonal carcinomas, and nonteratomatous germ-cell tumors of the mediastinum, respectively.

Among patients with malignant tumors, seminoma is most common, representing between 30% and 40% of cases (129), with embryonal carcinoma and malignant teratoma each responsible for about 10%, and choriocarcinoma and endodermal sinus tumor responsible for about 5% each; the remainder of malignancies, approximately 40% of cases represent mixed tumors (82,136).

Benign tumors are often asymptomatic, whereas malignant tumors are more likely to cause symptoms (81). Confirmation that these lesions are primary to the mediastinum requires that there be no evidence of a testicular or retroperitoneal tumor. Although of some value in diagnosis, the primary role of CT in evaluating patients with malignant germ-cell tumors is defining disease extent, and monitoring response to therapy.

Teratoma

Teratomas contain elements of all germinal layers. They are classified as mature, immature, and malignant (129). Mature teratomas account for the vast majority of cases and represent between 60% and 70% of all mediastinal germ-cell tumors (129). They are composed of well-differentiated benign tissue, with ectodermal elements such as skin and hair predominating. Dermoid cysts are said to contain elements of only the ectodermal layer of germ cells, specifically skin and its appendages, but small rests of endodermal and mesodermal cell are often present; they are benign, as are mature teratomas. Immature teratomas contain less well developed tissues more typical of those present during fetal development; in infancy or early childhood, these tumors often have a benign course, while in adults they usually behave in an aggressive and malignant fashion (81). Malignant teratomas contain frankly malignant tissues and have a very poor prognosis; they are seen almost entirely in men.

Teratomas are usually found in the prevascular space, although it is important to realize that these lesions may occur in other locations in up to 20% of cases, including both the middle and posterior mediastinum as well as in multiple compartments (137–139). Regardless of their histology, CT often shows a combination of fluid-filled cysts, fat, soft tissue, and areas of calcification (Figs. 2-39–2-41) (132,139,140). This pleomorphic appearance is an important clue to the diagnosis and often makes it possible to distinguish these lesions from thymoma and lymphoma (48,58). Calcification is seen in from 20% to 80% of cases (see Figs. 2-40 and 2-41), being focal, rim-like, or rarely representing teeth or bone (81). Fat is visible on CT in half of cases (see Figs. 2-39 and 2-40), a finding that is highly suggestive of

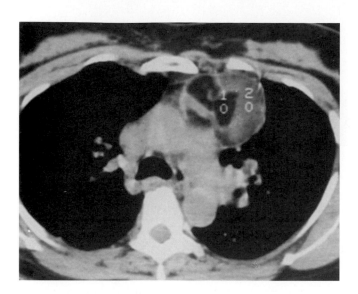

FIG. 2-39. Teratoma. CT section through the carina shows a well-encapsulated mass anterior to the left pulmonary artery, within which fat elements are clearly discernible. This was confirmed by measurements obtained within the region of interest demarcated by cursor number 1. The remainder of the lesion was composed of soft-tissue elements.

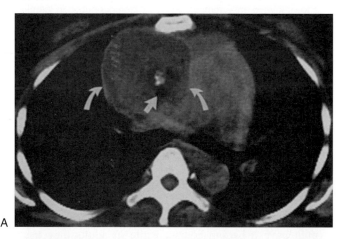

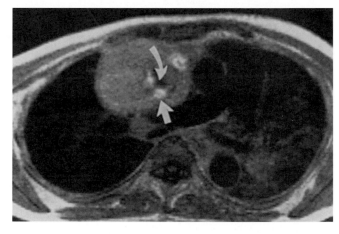

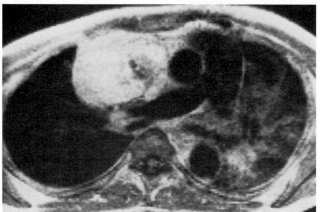

FIG. 2-40. Teratoma. **A:** Noncontrast-enhanced CT section just below the carina shows a well-encapsulated mass anterior to the right main pulmonary artery (*curved arrows*). The mass is strikingly heterogeneous with fluid, fat (*arrow*), and calcific elements clearly discernible. **B, C:** T1- and T2-weighted MR images obtained at the same level as shown in A, respectively. On the T1-weighted image, regions of high-signal intensity correspond precisely to the fatty elements seen in A (*arrow* in **B**), whereas regions corresponding to calcium demonstrate signal void (*curved arrow* in **B**). Intermediate signal is present within the remainder of the mass, in this case presumably secondary to complex fluid within the tumor. Note that there is considerable signal enhancement within these regions on the T2-weighted image, consistent with the presence of fluid within the tumor. (Case courtesy of Jeffrey Weinreb, M.D., New York, NY.)

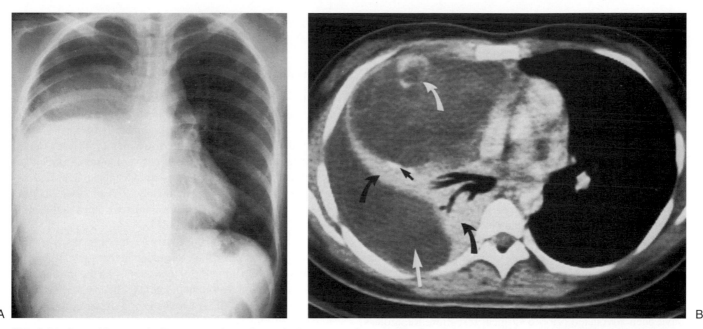

A   B

FIG. 2-41. Dermoid tumor. **A:** Posteroanterior radiograph shows extensive opacification of the mid- and lower right hemithorax in a teenage girl whose chief complaint was moderate dyspnea. The chest radiograph is nonspecific. **B:** Contrast-enhanced CT section through the midthorax shows a complex, cystic mass within which discrete septations can be recognized (*curved white arrow*), causing compression and posterior displacement of the adjacent lung (*curved black arrows*) as well as mediastinal shift to the left. Faint curvilinear calcifications can be identified posteriorly (*straight black arrow*). Although a pleural etiology was initially considered, the finding of multiple septations within this mass occurring in a young girl suggested the proper diagnosis. At surgery, the mass was found to extend posterior to the lung as well, accounting for the area of fluid density seen posteriorly (*straight white arrow*), otherwise mimicking the appearance of loculated pleural fluid.

this diagnosis. A fat-fluid level within the mass is particularly diagnostic (141–143).

Recently, Moeller et al., reported findings in a total of 66 cases of mediastinal mature teratoma (139). Although soft-tissue attenuation was identified in virtually all cases, fluid was present in 88%, fat in 76%, and calcium in 53%. Interestingly, all these elements were present in the same lesion in 39% whereas the combination of soft tissue, fluid and fat was seen in 24%. Importantly, nonspecific cystic lesions without fat or calcium were seen in a total of 15% of cases.

Mature teratomas are predisposed to rupture, occurring in some series in as many as a third of cases (144). This phenomenon has been attributed to the presence of digestive enzymes secreted by pancreatic or intestinal mucosa within these tumors leading to rupture into adjacent structures including bronchi, pleura, lung, and even the pericardium. Rarely, a fat-fluid level may be identifiable within a pleural effusion caused by rupture of the primary tumor into the pleural space (145). The fluids within the cystic parts of the tumors also vary in their CT density and may reach soft-tissue density (see Fig. 2-40). Teratomas are typically encapsulated and well-demarcated; rim enhancement can be seen.

Malignant teratomas typically appear nodular or poorly defined, and the tumor molds and compresses surrounding structures (Fig. 2-42), whereas benign teratomas are well defined and smooth. Malignant teratomas are more likely to appear solid, and less often contain fat (40%) than benign lesions (81), but they can be cystic as well. Following con-

trast infusion, malignant teratoma can show a thick enhancing capsule (81,131).

MRI can show various appearances, depending on the composition of the tumor (see Figs. 2-6 and 2-40) (48,68). They commonly contain fat, which is intense on T1-

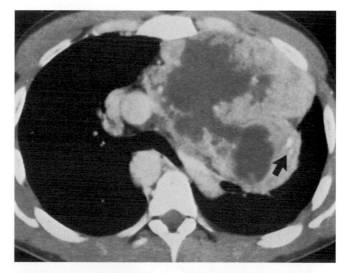

FIG. 2-42. Malignant teratoma. Contrast-enhanced CT scan through the carina shows a large, poorly demarcated tumor within the anterior mediastinum causing compression and displacement of adjacent mediastinal structures. The tumor is markedly heterogeneous with areas of low density, presumably caused by extensive tissue necrosis, as well as some punctate areas of calcification (*arrow*). These findings suggest a malignant etiology (see Figs. 2-42–2-45).

weighted images and cystic areas, which are low in intensity on T1-weighted images, but increase with T2-weighting.

Seminoma

Seminoma occurs almost entirely in white men, with a mean age at presentation of 29 years (146). They represent 40% of malignant germ-cell tumors of single histology (129). Approximately 10% with pure seminoma have evidence of elevated beta-human chorionic gonadotrpin (HCG) levels, but never elevated alpha-fetoprotein (AFP) levels. Typically, primary mediastinal seminomas present as large, smooth or lobulated, homogeneous soft-tissue masses, although small areas of low attenuation can be seen (Fig. 2-43) (48,81,131,132,147). Obliteration of fat planes is common, and pleural or pericardial effusion may be present, although direct invasion of adjacent structures has been reported to be rare (129,131). Seminomas are very sensitive to both radiation and chemotherapy: as a consequence, both have been advocated prior to surgical resection. Regardless

of approach, long term survival may be anticipated in up to 80% of cases (129).

Nonseminomatous Germ-Cell Tumors

Although other germ-cell tumors are much less common, their CT appearances have been well described (81,131,132,148–150). Nonseminomatous tumors, namely embryonal carcinoma, endodermal sinus (yolk sac) tumor, choriocarcinoma and mixed types, are often grouped together because of their rarity, similar appearance, and aggressive behavior. In approximately 20% of cases, there is an association between nonseminomatous germ-cell tumors and Klinefelter's syndrome (129).

It is worth emphasizing that over the past decade there has been a remarkable transformation in therapy of nonseminomatous malignant germ-cell tumors. With the introduction of cisplatin-based chemotherapeutic regimens the likelihood of cure has risen from 10% to 80% (151). Currently, surgery is reserved only for those patients with radiologic evidence

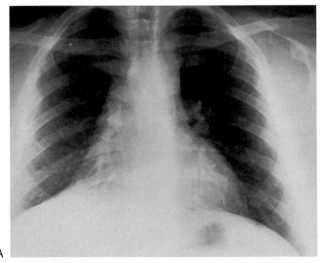

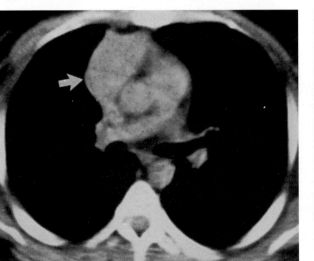

FIG. 2-43. Seminoma. **A:** Posteroanterior chest radiograph in a 35-year-old man shows poor definition of the right heart border and elevation of the right hemidiaphragm, findings initially thought to be secondary to middle lobe volume loss. **B, C:** Contrast-enhanced CT sections through the mid- and lower thorax, respectively, show a homogeneous soft-tissue mass to be present in the anterior mediastinum (*arrows* in **B** and **C**), marginating the right heart border. This appearance is entirely nonspecific. At surgery, this proved to be a seminoma.

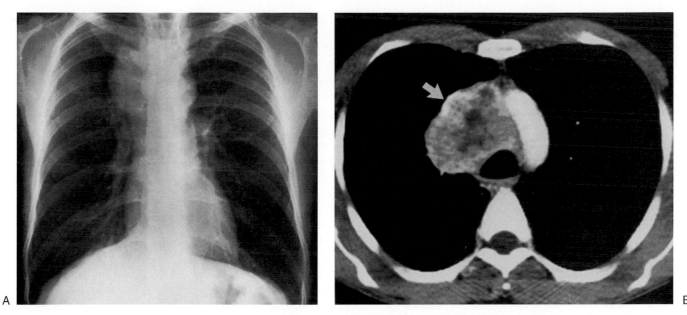

A   B

FIG. 2-44. Nonseminomatous germ cell tumor. **A:** Posteroanterior chest radiograph shows a mediastinal mass deforming the right pleuromediastinal interface. **B:** Contrast-enhanced CT section at the level of the aortic arch shows an irregular, heterogeneous tumor mass that is partially obstructing the superior vena cava (*arrow*). Although most germ-cell tumors arise in the prevascular or anterior mediastinal compartment, these tumors may originate anywhere within the thorax. Surgery confirmed a nonseminomatous malignant germ-cell tumor.

of persistent masses. In this regard, an unusual phenomenon associated with the treatment of malignant teratomas has been reported: the so-called mediastinal growing teratoma syndrome (151). This refers to the finding of an enlarging germ-cell tumor despite complete eradication of malignant cells and normalization of serum tumor markers following successful chemotherapy. Surgery may be required if growth is sufficient to impinge on adjacent mediastinal organs, despite eradication of malignant cells.

On CT, these tumors usually show heterogeneous opacity, including ill-defined areas of low attenuation secondary to necrosis and hemorrhage or cystic areas (81,131,148) (Fig. 2-44). They often appear infiltrative, with obliteration of fat planes, and may be spiculated. Calcification may be seen. MRI findings also reflect the inhomogeneous nature of these lesions (Fig. 2-45).

THYROID GLAND

Usually, diseases of the thyroid gland are first evaluated with either radionuclide scintigraphy (152), or ultrasonography, with needle aspiration biopsy as indicated. The role of CT has generally been restricted to morphologic evaluation, especially when it is suspected that thyroid abnormalities involve the mediastinum. Intrathoracic extension of thyroid tissue is common, in some series representing nearly 10% of mediastinal masses resected at thoracotomy (153). Usually representing direct contiguous growth of a goiter into the mediastinum, such lesions are almost always connected to the thyroid gland, even though on radionuclide studies the mass may appear to be separated from the thyroid (50,154). Truly ectopic mediastinal thyroid tissue is extremely rare.

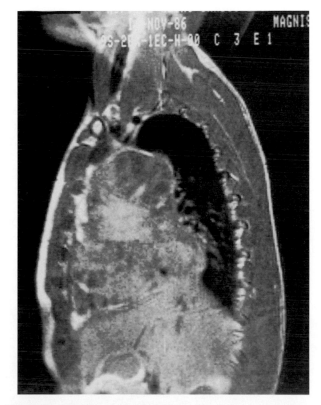

FIG. 2-45. MR of nonseminomatous germ-cell tumor: Embryonal carcinoma. T1-weighted sagittal image (TR 600 msec; TE 28 msec) shows a large inhomogeneous mass with areas of both high and low signal intensity. Low intensity regions are likely cystic, whereas high-intensity regions may represent hemorrhage.

Mediastinal involvement by thyroid masses is most often anterior (50). In 80% of cases, an enlarged thyroid extends into the thyropericardiac space anterior to the recurrent laryngeal nerve and the subclavian and innominate vessels. Posterior mediastinal goiters constitute approximately 10% to 25% of cases (50,154). Presumably arising from the posterolateral portion of the gland, posterior goiters descend behind the brachiocephalic vessels and are most commonly found on the right side, in close proximity to the trachea, bounded inferiorly by the arch of the azygos vein (154). Less often, thyroid tissue may extend either between the esophagus and trachea or even come to lie posterior to the esophagus (154).

CT Evaluation of Thyroid Disease

The CT appearances of both normal and abnormal thyroid gland have been extensively reviewed (50,153,155–165). The appearance of normal thyroid tissue is characteristic. On precontrast scans, thyroid tissue is high in attenuation, relative to adjacent soft tissues, because of its high iodine content; thus, it is easily identified (Fig. 2-46) (153,158). Attenuation values of thyroid tissue range from 57 ± 11 H in patients with chronic thyroiditis to 112 ± 10 H in normals, although in hypothyroid patients, thyroid attenuation is only slightly greater than soft tissue. Thyroid tissue typically en-

hances 25 HU or more following intravenous administration of contrast (158).

Recognizing that a mediastinal mass originates from the thyroid gland is contingent on the following observations: (a) demonstration of a communication with the cervical portion of the thyroid gland when contiguous sections are extended to include the neck; (b) high attenuation of at least of portion of the mass; (c) marked enhancement after contrast media injection, sometimes to the point of simulating a vascular lesion; and (d) prolonged contrast enhancement (153) presumably caused by the thyroid actively trapping iodine contained in the contrast medium.

Mediastinal thyroid masses commonly appear inhomogeneous and cystic on CT (Figs. 2-47–2-49). Although the appearance of low density cystic areas shown on CT correlate with areas of decreased isotope uptake on radionuclide studies, this appearance is nonspecific. Similar limitations in histologic specificity have been noted when CT is compared to high-resolution sonography (161–165). Curvilinear, punctate, or ringlike calcifications can also be seen (see Fig. 2-49); fat has not been reported in thyroid lesions and its presence can help in distinguishing a teratoma or dermoid cyst from a thyroid lesion (166). CT is of greatest value in defining the morphologic extent of a thyroid mass (see Figs. 2-47–2-49; Fig. 2-50). Marked irregularity of the gland contour, loss of distinct mediastinal fascial planes, and/or the

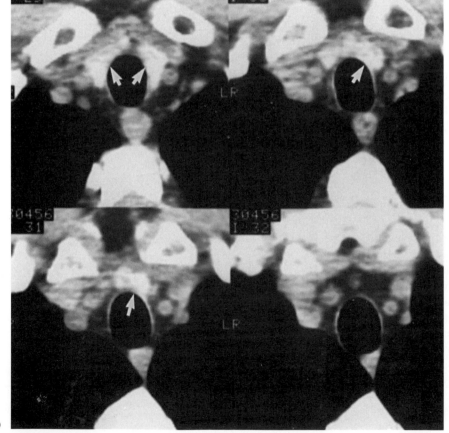

A,B

C,D

FIG. 2-46. Normal thyroid tissue. **A–D:** Enlargements of sequential nonenhanced CT sections through the superior mediastinum show characteristic appearance of both thyroid lobes, recognizable by their increased density relative to adjacent soft tissues caused by high iodine content (*arrows* in **A–C**). Note that the thyroid gland is closely applied to the anterolateral aspect of the trachea at all levels.

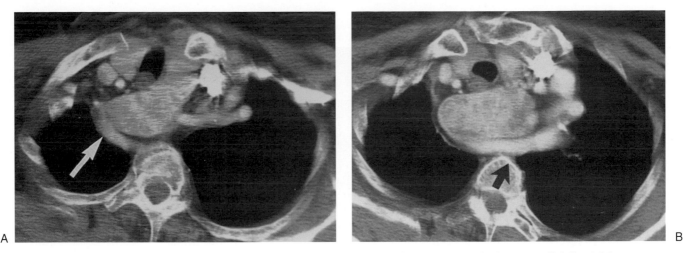

FIG. 2-47. Posterior mediastinal goiter. **A,B:** Sequential CT sections at the level of the great vessels shows a well-defined, inhomogeneous mass posterior to the trachea and esophagus that are displaced anteriorly. Note that in this case, thyroid tissue is limited posteriorly by an aberrant left subclavian artery (*arrows*).

presence of cervical or mediastinal adenopathy should signal potential malignancy (see Fig. 2-50).

CT plays an especially important role in the preoperative assessment of substernal goiters (50). It has been shown that the surgical approach to these lesions depends on precise anatomic localization. Intrathoracic goiters should be removed for symptomatic relief as well as to reduce the risk consequent to acute hemorrhage or inflammation. Although anterior substernal goiters (see Fig. 2-48) usually can be removed through a routine cervical incision, posterior mediastinal goiters require a selective approach. In these cases,

a decision as to the need for a thoracotomy or a combined cervicothoracic incision generally depends on the size of the lesion or whether or not the mass is mainly intrathoracic without a significant cervical component (154).

MR Evaluation of Thyroid Disease

The potential of MRI for evaluating the thyroid gland has long been appreciated (167,168). MRI has been shown to be a sensitive means for morphologically delineating the extent of thyroid enlargement. This includes the presence of

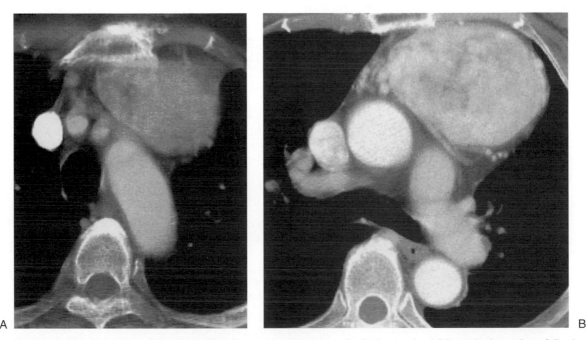

FIG. 2-48. Anterior mediastinal goiter. **A,B:** Large, inhomogeneous anterior mediastinal mass is visible on both sections following contrast enhancement with areas of low attenuation consistent with the appearance with the presence of colloid cysts. At higher levels, the mass was contiguous with the inferior aspect of the thyroid gland (not shown).

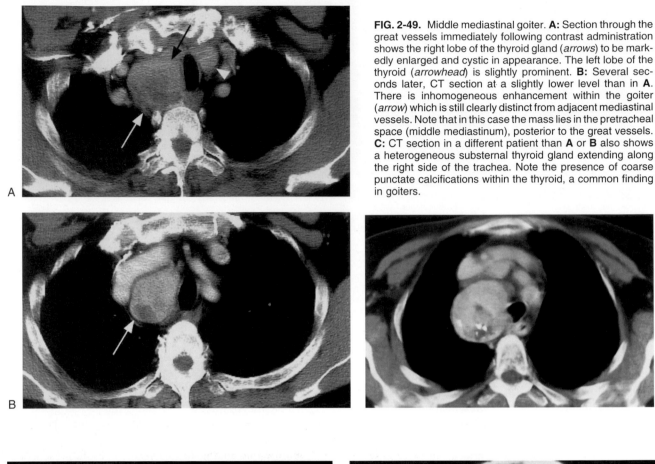

FIG. 2-49. Middle mediastinal goiter. **A:** Section through the great vessels immediately following contrast administration shows the right lobe of the thyroid gland (*arrows*) to be markedly enlarged and cystic in appearance. The left lobe of the thyroid (*arrowhead*) is slightly prominent. **B:** Several seconds later, CT section at a slightly lower level than in **A**. There is inhomogeneous enhancement within the goiter (*arrow*) which is still clearly distinct from adjacent mediastinal vessels. Note that in this case the mass lies in the pretracheal space (middle mediastinum), posterior to the great vessels. **C:** CT section in a different patient than **A** or **B** also shows a heterogeneous substernal thyroid gland extending along the right side of the trachea. Note the presence of coarse punctate calcifications within the thyroid, a common finding in goiters.

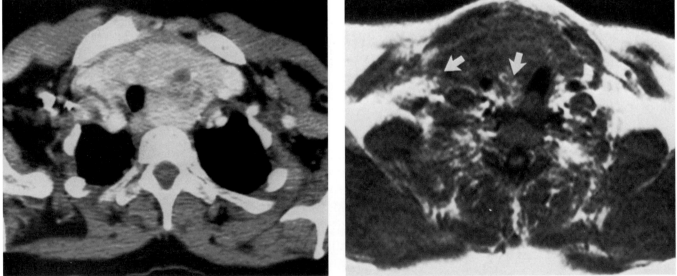

FIG. 2-50. Thyroid cancer. **A:** Contrast-enhanced CT section at the level of the thoracic inlet. Thyroid tissue is easily identifiable because of marked contrast enhancement that is characteristic following intravenous administration of contrast. Within the thyroid, areas of low tissue attenuation and foci of calcification can be identified. Although the thyroid is markedly enlarged, causing the trachea to deviate to the right, the outlines of the thyroid are still identifiable. Biopsy proved follicular carcinoma of the thyroid. **B:** T1-weighted MRI section in a patient different than in **A**. The thyroid is markedly enlarged and is poorly marginated causing loss of visualization of normally discrete fascial planes (*arrows*). Note that with T1 weighting the thyroid appears relatively homogeneous. Biopsy proved follicular carcinoma of the thyroid.

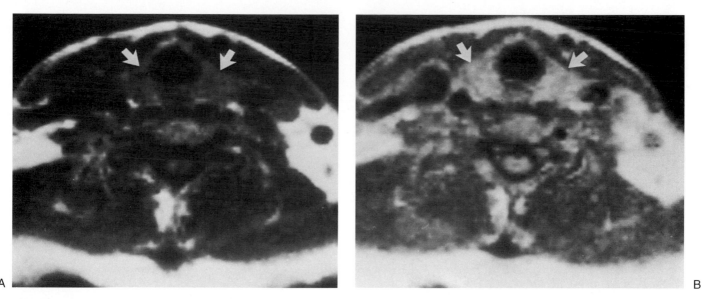

A

B

FIG. 2-51. Normal thyroid glands: MR assessment. **A, B:** T1- and T2-weighted MR images through a normal thyroid gland. On T1-weighted images the signal intensity in the normal gland is equal to or slightly greater than is seen in adjacent muscles (*arrows* in **A**). This appearance may also be seen in patients with thyroid malignancies (compare with Fig. 2–99). Note that the signal intensity within the thyroid is significantly greater with T2 weighting (*arrows* in **B**).

associated abnormalities such as cervical and/or mediastinal adenopathy, displacement of mediastinal organs such as the esophagus, trachea, and great vessels, and loss of normal cervical and intrathoracic fascial planes (169–179). Unfortunately, MRI has proven of only limited value as a means for tissue characterization.

Characteristically, on T1-weighted images, the signal intensity of the normal thyroid is equal to or slightly greater than that seen in the adjacent sternocleiodomastoid muscle; on T2-weighted scans, the signal intensity of the thyroid gland is significantly greater (Fig. 2-51) (174,175,178). Most focal pathologic processes, including adenomas, cysts, and cancer, are easily identified on T2-weighted sequences because of their markedly prolonged T2 values (Fig. 2-52). Functioning thyroid nodules, however, are an exception; these have been reported to be isointense with normal thyroid tissue on both T1- and T2-weighted scans (177).

Multi-nodular goiters are relatively hypointense as compared to normal thyroid tissue on T1-weighted images, except when there are foci of either hemorrhage or cysts, in which case focal areas of high signal intensity may be visualized. On T2-weighted images, multi-nodular goiters are typically heterogeneous, with high-signal intensity noted throughout most of the gland (see Fig. 2-52) (172–174,176–178). Although it has been suggested that benign adenomas can be differentiated from follicular carcinomas based on the presence of an intact pseudocapsule surrounding adenomas, this finding has been insufficiently documented (178,179). In most series, MRI has proven no more specific histologically than CT (168,172,174–177).

In patients with Graves' disease, Noma et al. have noted typical morphologic features, including the presence of nu-merous coarse, band-like structures traversing the thyroid gland and dilated vascular structures within the thyroid parenchyma (178). Also, in patients with Graves' disease, MRI has the capability to provide physiologic insight into the functional status of the thyroid gland (180). Typically, patients with Graves' disease have moderate to marked increased signal intensity on studies performed with both short and long TRs. Significantly, in these patients, there is a linear relationship between the thyroid-muscle signal intensity contrast ratio and both the serum thyroxine (T4) level and the 24-hour radioactive iodine uptake. Furthermore, these changes have been shown to normalize following therapy (180). The significance of these findings awaits further clinical investigation.

Descriptions of the thyroid gland in patients with Hashimoto's thyroiditis have also been published. Although this disorder is characterized by diffuse enlargement, no distinct pattern has been identified with MRI (178).

A potential role for MRI in the evaluation of patients following surgery has also been proposed (177,181). In one series of 24 patients with primary thyroid carcinoma evaluated postoperatively with MRI, MRI correctly diagnosed or excluded disease in 20 patients. However, MRI provided a false positive diagnosis in one case, and a false negative diagnosis in three cases (181).

PARATHYROID ADENOMA

Ninety percent of parathyroid glands are located near the thyroid gland. Their precise localization and number are variable. The upper pair are typically located dorsal to the

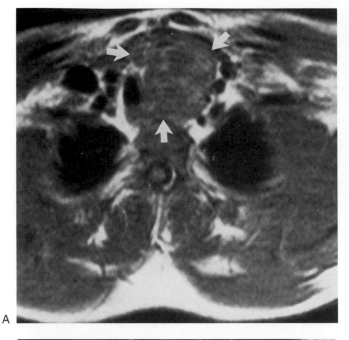

A

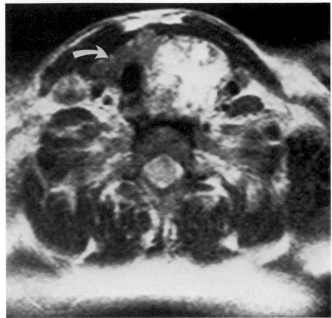

B

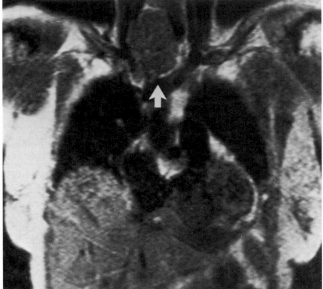

C

FIG. 2-52. Substernal goiter: MR evaluation. **A:** T1-weighted MR image through the thoracic inlet shows typical appearance of a multinodular substernal goiter. Note that the substernal thyroid is easily identified, separate from adjacent mediastinal fat and vessels, displacing the trachea to the right (*arrows* in **A**). **B:** T2-weighted MR image obtained at a slightly higher level than is shown in **A**. There is considerable increase in signal intensity within the goiter, which appears markedly heterogeneous. On T2-weighted images, multinodular goiters are typically heterogeneous, with high-signal intensity identifiable throughout the gland. Note that a portion of residual normal thyroid can be identified anterior to the trachea (*curved arrow*). **C:** Coronal T1-weighted image in another patient with a substernal goiter shows to best advantage the true extent of the thyroid. Note that inferiorly, the gland is bounded by the left brachiocephalic vein (*arrow*). Multiplanar imaging is a distinct advantage of MRI, especially in presurgical assessment.

superior poles of the thyroid gland, whereas the lower pair lie just below the lower thyroid poles, in the region of the minor neurovascular bundle. The lower pair of glands is most variable in location. Most parathyroid adenomas are found in the lower group of parathyroid glands.

Approximately 10% of parathyroid glands are ectopic. In one study, 62% of the ectopic glands were located in the anterior mediastinum, 30% were embedded within thyroid tissue, and 8% were found in the posterior-superior mediastinum, in the region of the tracheoesophageal groove (182). In a study of ectopic parathyroid tumors in the mediastinum, 81% were in the anterior mediastinum and 19% were in the posterior mediastinum (183); in another study, extopic mediastinal glands were most often within the thymus or

in the paraesophageal regions (184). Anterior mediastinal parathyroid glands are thought to result from islands of parathyroid tissue that are carried into the anterior mediastinum by the descending thymus during embryologic development. Anterior mediastinal parathyroid adenomas are intimately connected with the thymus.

Primary hyperparathyroidism results from a solitary adenoma in approximately 85% of cases. Other causes include diffuse hyperplasia (10%), multiple adenomas (5%), and rarely, carcinoma (1%) (175). Various studies are available for detecting parathyroid disease. These include high-resolution ultrasonography, radionuclide imaging using thallium or sestamibi, high-resolution contrast-enhanced CT, MRI, and selective venous catheterization.

CT Evaluation of Parathyroid Disease

The CT appearance of parathyroid adenomas has been well described (185–200). Normal glands cannot be identified on CT. Parathyroid adenomas and hyperplastic glands are usually small, but vary in size from 0.3 to 3 cm; rarely are they large enough to be detected on plain radiographs. When visible on CT, they usually appear homogeneous in density. Adenomas having their vascular supply compromised at surgery may appear cystic (195,196,200). Rarely, parathyroid adenomas appear calcified (197). No CT criteria reliably differentiate an adenoma from hyperplasia or carcinoma. In the anterior mediastinum they may be indistinguishable from small thymic remnants, small thymomas, or small lymph nodes, and are usually found in the expected location of the thymus (Fig. 2-53). An important potential source of error is to mistake a parathyroid adenoma for a thyroid adenoma (162,200). An association between thyroid and parathyroid disease is well known; as many as 30% of patients with parathyroid disease prove to have simultaneous thyroid abnormalities. In a review of 65 patients in whom parathyroid surgery was performed for primary hyperparathyroidism, Stark et al. (162) found that 40% of these patients had nonpalpable thyroid nodules detected either by CT or high-resolution sonography.

The ability of CT to detect parathyroid abnormalities is clearly related to scan technique. Utilizing contiguous 5-mm sections from the hyoid bone to the carina, prospectively reconstructed with small fields of view, a 512 matrix, and maximum contrast enhancement using 50 g of iodine injected through a power injector, Cates et al. documented that CT correctly identified parathyroid adenomas preoperatively in 81% of patients (200), although somewhat lower sensitivities have been reported by others (201). The accuracy of CT compares favorably with reported sensitivities of both high-resolution ultrasonography and thallium radionuclide imaging (198,199,202). However, CT obtained with substandard technique has a much lower accuracy (189). It should be emphasized that in patients with primary hyperparathyroidism, surgical neck exploration with resection of parathyroid tissues is curative in about 90% to 95% of cases (203,204). As a consequence, in most institutions, no imaging is done prior to surgery. However, the persistence of hyperparathyroidism following surgical resection of the cervical glands suggests the presence of an ectopic parathyroid adenoma or hyperfunctioning gland. Almost 50% of these patients will have mediastinal parathyroid glands; two-thirds of these glands will be located in the superior mediastinum, particularly in the posterior aspect near the tracheoesophageal groove (193), and one-third will be in the lower anterior mediastinum, often in relation to the thymus, although a wide variety of locations can be seen (184). Parathyroid adenomas in the aorticopulmonary window are rare, but their appearance has recently been described (51). In a review of 285 consecutive patients treated surgically for hyperparathyroidism, mediastinal parathyroid tumors were present in 22%, and were present in 38% of the patients requiring reoperation for persistent or recurrent hyperparathyroidism (183). Preoperative localization has also been advocated for patients at a high risk for surgery (201).

Reports comparing the accuracy of CT to competing modalities in postoperative patients vary significantly (189). Miller et al. (202) compared sonography, thallium scintigraphy, CT, and MR imaging in 53 postoperative patients, and found that no technique detected more than 50% of abnormal glands. Similar results have been reported by others, including false-positive rates of nearly 20%. However, in a recent study (51), CT obtained with 5-mm collimation during the infusion of contrast material was positive in eight (89%) of nine patients with a parathyroid adenoma in the aorticopulmonary window, whereas MRI was positive in 63%, arteriography was positive in 56%, and sestamibi radionuclide images were positive in all six patients in whom they were obtained. Also, higher accuracy rates have recently been reported for MR imaging and sestamibi scintigraphy (201,205,206).

MR Evaluation of Parathyroid Disease

The appearance of abnormal parathyroid glands on MRI has been well documented (169,170,172,173,175,184,202, 207–213). Similar to thyroid adenomas, most parathyroid adenomas appear intense on T2-weighted images (Fig. 2-54), increasing significantly in intensity as compared to T1-weighted images. Similar findings have been documented for parathyroid hyperplasia and carcinomas. In a small but significant percentage of cases, parathyroid adenomas fail to show increased signal intensity with T2 weighting. As shown by Auffermann et al., in a study of 30 patients with recurrent hyperparathyroidism, 13% of the abnormal glands failed to display high intensity on T2-weighted images (212).

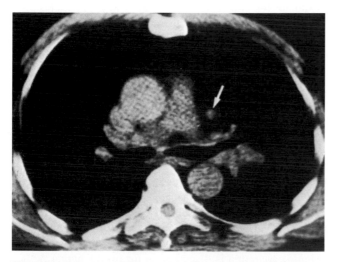

FIG. 2-53. Ectopic parathyroid adenoma. A 45-year-old patient with hyperparathyroidism not responding to surgical therapy. The CT scan reveals a small, 0.5-cm density in the anterior mediastinum (*arrow*). At surgery, a small parathyroid adenoma was found. Mediastinal parathyroid adenomas are found in the usual location of the thymus. They are difficult to distinguish from small nodes or residual thymic tissue.

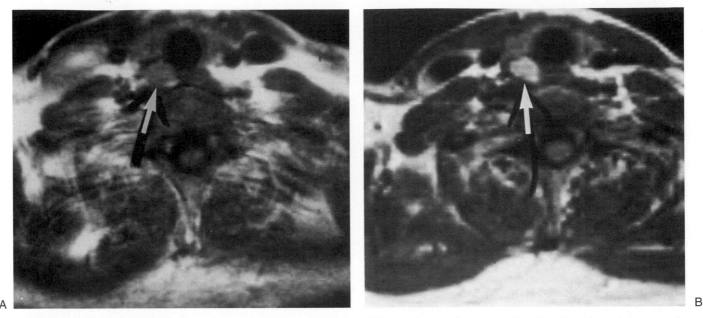

FIG. 2-54. Parathyroid adenoma: MR evaluation. **A,B:** T1- and T2-weighted images through the lower poles of the thyroid gland show a well-defined mass in the region of the tracheoesophageal groove (*arrows*). Note the marked signal enhancement within the mass on T2-weighted images. These findings are characteristic of parathyroid adenomas. Unfortunately, this same appearance can be seen in patients with thyroid adenomas, differentiation of which can be problematic, especially as a significant percentage of patients with hyperparathyroidism have concomitant thyroid disease.

Enhancement following gadolinium infusion is typical, and fat suppression images can be valuable in demonstrating parathyroid adenomas.

Reports of the accuracy of MRI, although variable, largely show that this modality is superior to other noninvasive techniques for detecting parathyroid pathology, with the exception of sestamibi radionuclide imaging (170,172,173,175, 201,202,205–212). Spritzer et al., using both T1- and T2-weighted scans to evaluate 23 patients with suspected parathyroid adenomas reported an overall sensitivity of 78% and a specificity of 95%, with a resulting overall accuracy of 90% (210). Kneeland et al., evaluating 22 patients with hyperparathyroidism, reported a 74% and 88% sensitivity and specificity of MR imaging, respectively (208).

In postoperative patients and those with mediastinal parathyroid glands, MRI has proven more sensitive than thallium/technitium scintigraphy or sonography (184). In a study of 25 patients with mediastinal lesions (184), MRI had a sensitivity of 88%, whereas thallium/technitium scintigraphy and sonography had sensitivities of 58% and 12% respectively. However, in interpreting these results, it should be kept in mind that (a) false positive MRI studies are not uncommon, because of lymph node enlargement or thyroid nodules, and (b) the sensitivity of sestamibi radionuclide imaging is higher than that of thallium (51,205,206). It has recently been suggested that a complementary role for MRI and sestamibi imaging is appropriate (201). In 25 patients with hyperparathyroidism, 17 of whom were postoperative, MRI and sestamibi imaging had sensitivities of 84% and 79% respectively, with specificities of 75% and 94%; when both studies were interpreted in conjunction, their sensitivity was 89% with a specificity of 95% (201).

Given the limited accuracy rates of the various noninvasive imaging modalities in patients with hyperparathyroidism, each case must be individualized in order to select the most appropriate study. To some extent, availability, cost, and familiarity with these procedures will determine their usage. In our experience, MRI has come to replace CT in the investigation of patients with recurrent hyperparathyroidism following surgery, and sestamibi radionuclide imaging is assuming an increased role. CT is reserved for those patients with suspected recurrent parathyroid carcinoma, especially to evaluate the lungs and the liver to rule out metastatic disease (214). Another specialized use of CT is to evaluate patients for whom angiographic ablation of mediastinal parathyroid adenomas has been performed (Fig. 2-55) (215).

MEDIASTINAL LYMPH NODES AND LYMPH NODE MASSES

Mediastinal lymph node abnormalities can be seen in any mediastinal compartment, although they most commonly involve middle mediastinal regions such as the pretracheal space, aorticopulmonary window, and subcarinal space. Their detection and diagnosis is important in the evaluation of a number of thoracic diseases, including bronchogenic carcinoma, lymphoma, and granulomatous diseases. The assessment of mediastinal lymph nodes in patients with bronchogenic carcinoma is discussed in detail in Chapter 5.

Lymph Node Groups

Mediastinal lymph nodes are generally classified by location, and most descriptive systems are based on Rouviere's

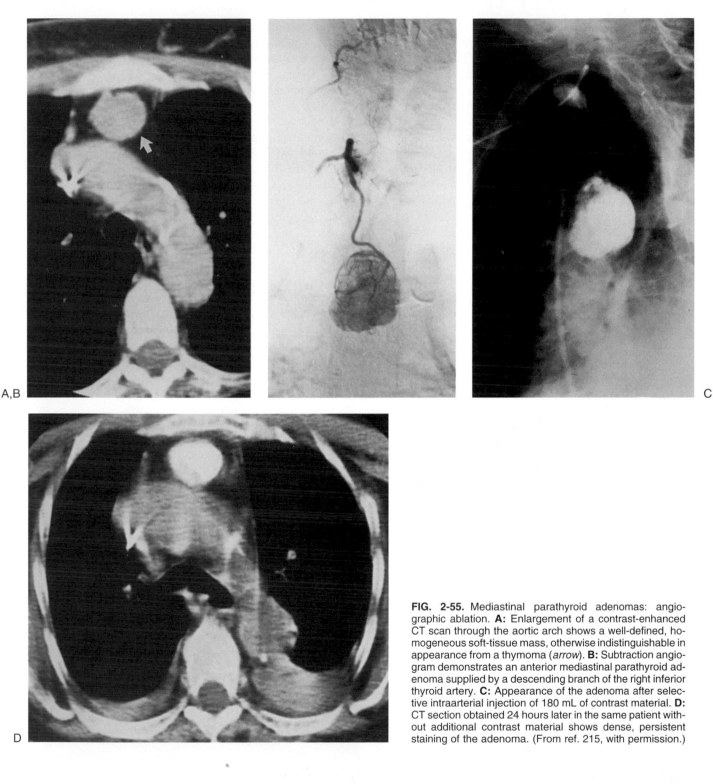

FIG. 2-55. Mediastinal parathyroid adenomas: angiographic ablation. **A:** Enlargement of a contrast-enhanced CT scan through the aortic arch shows a well-defined, homogeneous soft-tissue mass, otherwise indistinguishable in appearance from a thymoma (*arrow*). **B:** Subtraction angiogram demonstrates an anterior mediastinal parathyroid adenoma supplied by a descending branch of the right inferior thyroid artery. **C:** Appearance of the adenoma after selective intraarterial injection of 180 mL of contrast material. **D:** CT section obtained 24 hours later in the same patient without additional contrast material shows dense, persistent staining of the adenoma. (From ref. 215, with permission.)

classification of lymph node groups (216). Patterns of lymphatic drainage are also considered in defining groups of related lymph nodes, an approach that can be helpful in understanding the involvement of particular nodes in patients with diseases involving various sites in the chest (217).

Thoracic lymph nodes are usually grouped into parietal and visceral, depending on their location and drainage. The parietal lymph nodes primarily drain structures of the chest wall and are classified as internal mammary, diaphragmatic, or paracardiac, and intercostal. Visceral node groups include intrapulmonary, bronchopulmonary, tracheobronchial, paratracheal, paraesophageal, and anterior mediastinal.

Intrathoracic lymph nodes are described as belonging to specific node groups, although they freely communicate with each other via numerous lymphatic vessels. Different methods of classification of intrathoracic lymph nodes have been used by different authors, although most divide lymph nodes into parietal and visceral groups, based on their location and structures they drain. Parietal node groups are related to the chest wall and lie outside the parietal pleura. Visceral node groups are located within the mediastinum or are related to the lung hila, and drain mediastinal structures and the lungs.

The following classification is based on a modification of well recognized anatomic descriptions of lymphatic anatomy (216,218), although some terms have been modified to be consistent with current usage, and anatomic descriptions emphasize the localization of lymph nodes on imaging studies, rather than considering nodes as parietal or visceral. Anterior, tracheobronchial, and posterior nodes will be considered.

Anterior Lymph Nodes

Internal mammary lymph nodes are located in a retrosternal position, at the anterior ends of the intercostal spaces, near the internal mammary artery and veins; they are considered to be part of the parietal lymph node group. They drain the anterior chest wall, anterior diaphragm, medial breasts, and freely communicate with prevascular lymph nodes and paracardiac or diaphragmatic lymph nodes (219,220). They are most often enlarged as a result of lymphoma or metastatic breast cancer (Fig. 2-56) (221,222).

Prevascular lymph nodes lie anterior to the aorta and in relation to the great vessels (Fig. 2-57). These nodes drain most anterior mediastinal structures including the pericardium, thymus, thyroid, pleura, and the anterior hila. They represent visceral nodes. They communicate with the internal mammary chain of nodes anteriorly and paratracheal and aorticopulmonary lymph nodes posteriorly. They may be involved in a variety of diseases, notably lymphoma and granulomatous diseases, but their involvement in lung cancer is relatively uncommon.

Paracardiac or cardiophrenic angle lymph nodes (223–225) lie anterior to or lateral to the heart and pericardium, on the surface of the diaphragm (see Fig. 2-56; Fig. 2-58). They communicate with the lower internal mammary chain, and drain the lower intercostal spaces, pericardium, diaphragm, and liver. As with internal mammary nodes, paracardiac nodes are most commonly enlarged in patients with lymphoma and metastatic carcinoma, particularly breast cancer (219,220,226,227). Paracardiac lymph nodes correspond to the anterior (prepericardiac) and middle (juxtaphrenic) subgroups of the diaphragmatic parietal lymph node group (216,218). Prepericardiac nodes are located posterior to the xyphoid process and slightly lateral to it. Juxtaphrenic lymph nodes are situated adjacent to the pericardium, where the phrenic nerves meet the diaphragm. From a clinical standpoint, there is little reason to distinguish between them.

Tracheobronchial Lymph Nodes

Tracheobronchial lymph nodes generally serve to drain the lungs. Lung diseases (e.g., lung cancer, sarcoidosis, tuberculosis, fungal infections) that secondarily involve lymph nodes, typically involve these lymph nodes. Tracheobronchial lymph nodes are subdivided into a number of important node groups, which are all closely related. Paratracheal nodes lie anterior to, and on either side of, the trachea, thus occupying the pretracheal (or anterior paratracheal) space (see Fig. 2-36A; Fig. 2-59) (228,229). Retrotracheal nodes may also be seen. The most inferior node in this region is the so-called "azygos node," medial to the azygos arch. These nodes form the final pathway for lymphatic drainage from most of both lungs, excepting the left upper lobe (217).

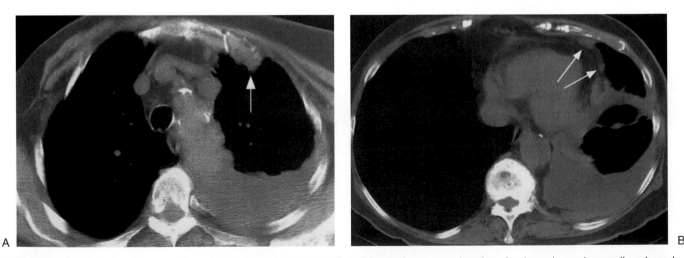

FIG. 2-56. Lymph node enlargement in metastatic breast carcinoma. **A:** Left internal mammary lymph nodes (*arrow*) are abnormally enlarged. Left pleural effusion is also present. **B:** Near the level of the diaphragm, paracardiac lymph node enlargement is also seen (*arrows*). Paracardiac and internal mammary lymph nodes are often involved in conjunction in breast cancer and lymphoma.

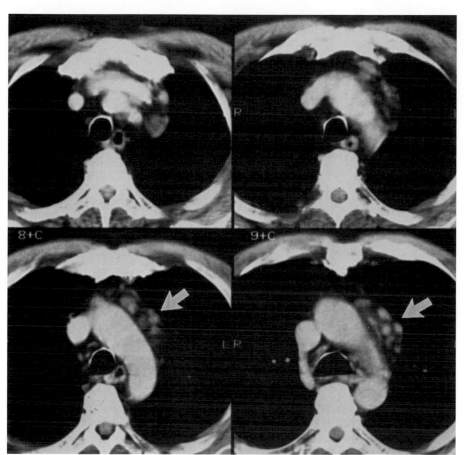

A,B

C,D

FIG. 2-57. Mediastinal lymphadenopathy, Hodgkin's disease. **A-D:** Contrast-enhanced CT sections at the level of the great vessels, aortic arch, and aorticopulmonary window, respectively. Clusters of enlarged prevascular lymph nodes are easily identifiable (*arrows* in **C** and **D**), whereas few if any enlarged nodes can be identified in the pre- or paratracheal spaces. This pattern of lymph node enlargement would be uncharacteristic of most granulomatous diseases and should suggest possible malignancy. Following therapy, these nodes regressed.

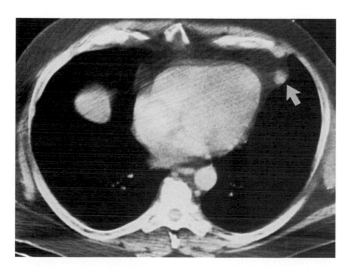

FIG. 2-58. Paracardiac lymphadenopathy, non-Hodgkin's lymphoma. Contrast-enhanced CT section through the lung bases shows a single, isolated, left paracardiac node (*arrow*).

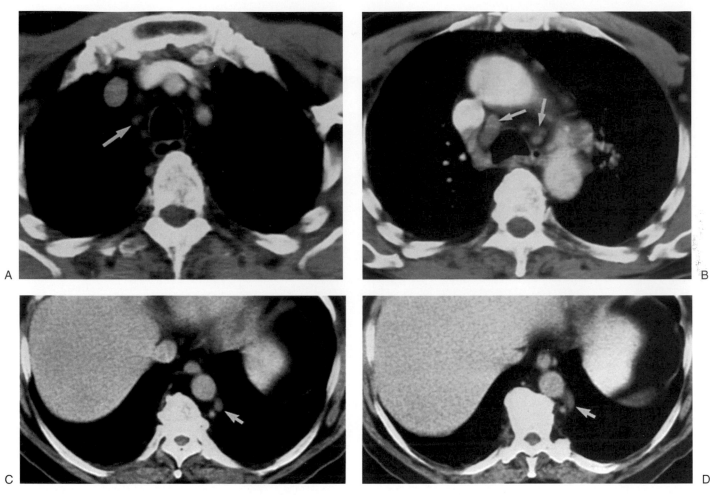

FIG. 2-59. Mediastinal lymphadenopathy, Hodgkin's disease. **A–D:** Contrast-enhanced CT sections at the level of the great vessels, the aorticopulmonary window, and the lung bases, respectively. Mediastinal lymph nodes appear as round, oval, or triangular soft-tissue densities against the lower density background of mediastinal fat (*arrows* in **A–D**). Paratracheal and pretracheal lymph node enlargement is visible in **A** and **B**. Aorticopulmonary lymph node enlargement is visible in **B**. Posterior paravertebral lymph node enlargement is visible in **C** and **D**.

Because of this, they are commonly abnormal regardless of the location of the lung disease.

Aorticopulmonary nodes are grouped by Rouviere with prevascular nodes, but because they serve the same function on the left as paratracheal nodes on the right, and freely communicate with paratracheal nodes, it is most appropriate to group them together. They lie in the aorticopulmonary window, lateral to the left main bronchus and between the aorta and pulmonary artery (see Fig. 2-36A). The left upper lobe drains via this node group.

Peribronchial nodes surround the main bronchi on each side, and lie between the main bronchi in the subcarinal space. These drain the lungs. Bronchopulmonary nodes are located distal to the main bronchi and are usually considered to be hilar.

Subcarinal nodes represent peribronchial nodes lying between the main bronchi in the subcarinal space (35,230). These nodes drain the inferior hila and lower lobes on both the right and left, and communicate in turn with the right paratracheal chain.

Posterior Lymph Nodes

Paraesophageal and inferior pulmonary ligament nodes are associated with the esophagus and descending aorta, and lie medial to the inferior pulmonary ligament. They represent visceral nodes, and drain the medial lower lobes, esophagus, pericardium, and posterior diaphragm. On the right, they are impossible to distinguish from subcarinal nodes, unless they are near the diaphragm. Retrocrural lymph nodes lie posterior to the diaphragmatic crura. They communicate with lumbar nodes and posterior mediastinal lymph nodes, and drain the diaphragm and liver, and represent the posterior group of diaphragmatic parietal lymph nodes.

Intercostal and paravertebral lymph nodes are found in the posterior intercostal spaces and adjacent to thoracic vertebral bodes (see Fig. 2-59C,D). These drain the posterior pleura, chest wall, and spine, and communicate with other posterior mediastinal lymph nodes. They are part of the parietal group.

The American Thoracic Society Lymph Node Stations

The American Thoracic Society (ATS) has developed a numerical system of lymph node localization for use in the staging of lung cancer that has recently been modified (231,232) (see Chapter 5 for an in-depth discussion). In the ATS system, nodes are classified as belonging to one of a number of 14 "node stations," for which mediastinoscopic, surgical, and CT criteria have been established. However, this system is not generally used for the clinical description of lymph node abnormalities in diseases other than lung cancer. Nonetheless, familiarity with this classification is encouraged (see Fig. 5-11 and Table 5-3).

Normal Lymph Nodes

In autopsy series, the average number of mediastinal lymph nodes is 64 (233). Almost 80% of mediastinal lymph nodes are located in relation to the trachea and main bronchi and serve to drain the lungs.

On CT, lymph nodes are generally visible as (a) discrete and surrounded by mediastinal fat, (b) round, elliptical, or triangular in shape, and (c) of soft-tissue attenuation (see Fig. 2-36A, 2-57–2-59). The node hilum can sometimes be seen to contain a small quantity of fat; this is most apparent when scans are obtained with thin collimation (see Fig. 2-10B).

Lymph nodes can usually be distinguished from vessels by their location. However, our ability to recognize and correctly identify lymph nodes is directly related to the amount of mediastinal fat surrounding them; in patients having little mediastinal fat, lymph nodes can be difficult to distinguish from vessels without contrast infusion. In many parts of the mediastinum, lymph nodes often occur in clusters of a few nodes of similar size.

A number of pitfalls in diagnosing lymphadenopathy have been described. Structures that can be mistaken for enlarged lymph nodes include both normal and anomalous vascular structures, such as an aberrant right subclavian artery or high-riding left pulmonary artery (234,235), and prominent pericardial recesses, especially the superior recess of the pericardium (see Fig. 2-11B) (32). It should be emphasized that viewing contiguous scans often can be helpful in differentiating lymph nodes from vessels; mediastinal vessels are usually visible on several adjacent scans, whereas lymph nodes are not, unless they are quite large. In difficult cases, the use of bolus intravenous contrast material injection will prove diagnostic.

Internal mammary nodes, paracardiac nodes, and paravertebral nodes are not commonly seen on CT in normals, but in other areas of the mediastinum, normal lymph nodes are often visible. The size of normal nodes varies with their location, and a few general rules apply. Subcarinal nodes can be quite large in normal patients. Pretracheal nodes are also commonly visible, but these nodes are typically smaller than normal subcarinal nodes. Nodes in the supraaortic mediastinum are usually smaller than lower pretracheal nodes, and left paratracheal nodes are usually smaller than right paratracheal nodes.

Numerous reports have addressed the issue of what constitutes the normal size, number, and appearance of mediastinal lymph nodes (36,37,228,236–238). The short axis or least diameter (i.e., the smallest node diameter seen in cross section) of a lymph node should generally be used when measuring its size (Fig. 2-60). This measurement more closely reflects actual node diameter when nodes are obliquely oriented relative to the scan plane and shows less variation

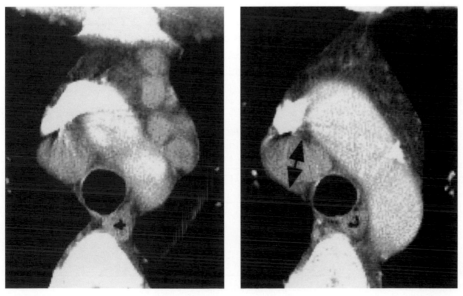

FIG. 2-60. Short-axis lymph node diameter in a patient with metastatic lung carcinoma. **A:** Pretracheal and prevascular lymph node enlargement is present. **B:** The short-axis or least diameter of the enlarged pretracheal lymph node is indicated by the *arrows*. This measurement is generally used for assessing lymph node size. In this case, the short-axis lymph node diameter is 2 cm.

A

B

among normal subjects than does the long axis or greatest diameter.

As determined both in vivo and by autopsy evaluation, the most useful upper limit of normal for mediastinal lymph nodes is 1.0 cm, as measured in its short axis (37,226,236), except in the subcarinal region. In studies by Glazer et al. (36) and Genereux and Howie (238), 95% or more of lymph nodes in normal subjects measured 1.0 cm or less in the lower paratracheal (4R), right paratracheal (10R), and aorticopulmonary window (5) regions.

However, there are significant variations in normal node size, depending on the precise location of the node. As shown by Glazer et al., in an evaluation of 56 normal patients (36), the largest lymph nodes visible using CT are subcarinal (least diameter 6.2 mm, SD 2.2 mm) and lower right tracheobronchial (least diameter 5.9 mm, SD 2.1 mm) (corresponding to ATS nodal stations 4R and 10R, respectively), whereas upper paratracheal nodes (2R) are smaller than lower paratracheal nodes (4R), and right-sided nodes in general are smaller than those on the left side (see Table 5-4). Kiyono et al. (37) reported very similar findings in an evaluation of 40 adult cadavers (see Table 5-5). In their series, mean short transverse nodal diameters ranged from 2.4 to 5.6 mm, with substantial variations noted depending on nodal station, subcarinal nodes again being largest. Based on these findings, these authors (37) recommended using short axis measurements of 12 mm as upper limits of normal for subcarinal lymph nodes, 10 mm for right tracheobronchial and low paratracheal lymph nodes, and 8 mm for all other nodal groups. Receiver operating characteristic curve analysis of node size performed by Glazer et al., (36) suggest that the optimum size for upper limits of normal for mediastinal lymph nodes in patients suspected of malignancy are 1.0 cm, except in the subcarinal region.

Diagnosis of Lymph Node Abnormalities

CT is restricted to providing the following information regarding mediastinal lymph nodes: (a) precise measurements of lymph node diameter, (b) delineation of lymph node morphology, and (c) characterization of lymph node density and the internal characteristics, both before and after intravenous contrast enhancement. Using CT, lymph nodes can be characterized as homogeneous in density, calcified, low-density and necrotic, or enhancing after contrast infusion. CT can also be valuable in localizing abnormal lymph nodes, and determining their extent and relationship to mediastinal structures such as the superior vena cava, pulmonary arteries, airways, and the esophagus. In combination, these findings frequently limit the range of differential diagnoses; they also can allow a determination of the best approach, when necessary, to establish a histologic diagnosis.

Lymph Node Enlargement

Enlargement of lymph nodes is the most common CT finding in a number of neoplastic and inflammatory diseases

(see Figs. 2-36A, 2-56–2-59, 2-60). As indicated above, a short-axis node diameter exceeding 1 cm is generally thought to indicate abnormal node enlargement, except in the subcarinal space. However, it is important to understand that a simple assessment of lymph node size has a limited accuracy in determining whether mediastinal nodes are normal or abnormal. Early in the course of a number of diseases, significant nodal pathology may be present in the absence of lymph node enlargement, and normal sized lymph nodes do not rule out a pathologic process. For example, as many as 40% of patients with lymph node metastases from bronchogenic carcinoma show no evidence of lymph node enlargment on CT (239–245). Furthermore, it must also be recognized that mediastinal lymph nodes can be enlarged in the absence of significant disease, usually as a result of hyperplasia. In patients with bronchogenic carcinoma, approximately 30% of patients without evidence of lymph node metastases at surgery show some evidence of lymph node enlargement on CT.

In general, the diameter of an enlarged lymph node correlates with its likelihood of harboring significant or active disease, and the larger the node, the more likely it indicates a significant abnormality. This has best been studied in patients with bronchogenic carcinoma; in this setting the likelihood that a mediastinal node is involved by tumor is directly proportional to its size, and no node diameter is clearly able to separate normal from abnormal nodes (Table 2-4) (244,245).

The significance given to the presence of a minimally enlarged lymph node must be tempered by a knowledge of the patient's clinical situation. For example, if the patient is known to have lung cancer, then an enlarged lymph node has a significant likelihood of being involved by tumor. However, the same node in a patient without lung cancer is much less likely to be of clinical significance. In the absence of a known disease, an enlarged node must be regarded as likely to be hyperplastic or postinflammatory.

Lymph nodes having a short axis of 2 cm or more, often reflect the presence of neoplasm, such as metastatic tumor or lymphoma, sarcoidosis or infection, and should always be treated as potentially significant. Although mediastinal

TABLE 2-4. *Relationship of least node diameter to likelihood of involvement by tumor in 143 patients with lung cancer[a]*

Number of nodes	Least node diameter (cm)	Percent malignant
336	<1	13
57	1.0–1.9	25
13	2.0–2.9	62
6	3.0–3.9	67
2	4.0 or more	100

[a] Modified from ref. 245.

lymph nodes can become enlarged in a variety of noninfectious and nongranulomatous inflammatory diseases, they are usually smaller than 2 cm (246–248).

It should also be recognized that although the least node diameter is most frequently used to assess node diameter and lymph node enlargement, it has been shown in several studies that using the long axis or greatest node diameter can also be used, with very similar accuracy rates. In patients with bronchogenic carcinoma, using a least node diameter of 10 mm, and a greatest node diameter of 15 mm had identical sensitivities and specificities for diagnosis of tumor involvement of nodes. Generally speaking, however, using greatest node diameter should be avoided if a node appears much longer than it is wide (i.e., its greatest node diameter is much longer than its least diameter).

Lymph Node Morphology

In patients with lymph node abnormalities, three patterns of involvement can be seen on CT. This pattern may be of some value in differential diagnosis. These patterns are:

1. Discrete enlarged nodes. Nodes are enlarged, as determined by measurement of least node diameter, and individual nodes are surrounded by fat and appear distinct (see Figs. 2-36A, 2-56–2-59, 2-60). Although adjacent nodes may contact each other, with focal obscuration of their margins, they remain well defined. This pattern can be seen in association with all causes of mediastinal lymph node enlargment.
2. Coalescence of enlarged nodes. With progression of

disease, a pathologic process involving several contiguous nodes may also involve surrounding mediastinal fat, and several adjacent nodes may fuse to form a single larger mass. Poor definition of node margins, or poor definition of the margins of the coalescent node mass can indicate extension of the disease process through the node capsule (see Fig. 2-3; Fig. 2-61A,B), or an associated fibrotic or inflammatory reaction. This appearance is most typical of infection, granulomatous disease, and neoplasm.
3. Diffuse mediastinal involvement. Mediastinal connective tissue and fat are diffusely infiltrated, with no recognizable nodes or node masses. Typically, mediastinal fat appears to be replaced by soft-tissue density (Fig. 2-61C). This diagnosis may be difficult to make unless the attenuation of mediastinal soft tissues is compared to the attenuation of subcutaneous fat on the same scan—they should be similar. This pattern suggests lymphoma, undifferentiated carcinoma, generalized infection, or granulomatous mediastinitis.

Lymph Node Attenuation

CT can also be used to define the density of lymph nodes, both before and after the injection of intravenous contrast media. Although enlarged nodes most often have a nonspecific appearance, being of soft-tissue attenuation, nodes can be calcified or low in density and necrotic in appearance, or can opacify following the administration of a bolus of intravenous contrast media (Table 2-5).

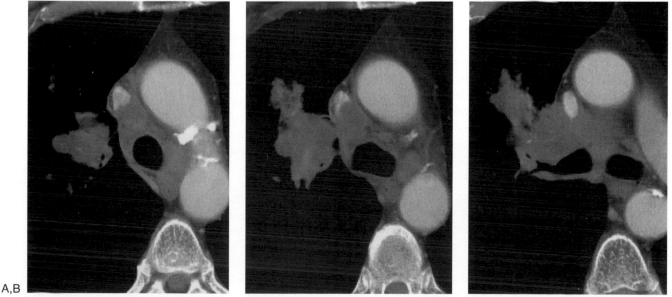

FIG. 2-61. Mediastinal lymph node metastases with extranodal involvement and mediastinal infiltration in small-cell lung carcinoma. **A:** A right hilar mass is present. Pretracheal lymph nodes are enlarged, but their margins are poorly defined. **B:** At the level of the carina, several contiguous enlarged pretracheal and aorticopulmonary lymph nodes are visible, but their margins are poorly defined. Note that the posterior wall of the superior vena cava is irregular, suggestive of direct invasion and likely impending obstruction. **C:** At the level of the right upper lobe bronchus, the precarinal mediastinal fat is infiltrated by tumor. Individual lymph nodes are not visible.

TABLE 2-5. *Mediastinal lymph node attenuation*

Calcified lymph nodes
  Common:
    Infectious granulomatous diseases
      Tuberculosis
      Fungal infections (histoplasmosis)
    Sarcoidosis
    Silicosis
    Hodgkin's disease (following treatment)
  Rare:
    Pneumocystis carinii pneumonia
    Metastases (mucinous adenocarcinoma)
    Amyloidosis
    Scleroderma
    Castleman's disease
Low-density/necrotic lymph nodes
  Common:
    Infectious granulomatous diseases
      Tuberculosis
      Fungal infections (histoplasmosis)
    Metastases
      lung cancer
      seminoma
    Lymphoma
  Rare:
    Whipple's disease
    Sarcoidosis
Enhancing lymph nodes
  Common:
    Metastases
    Castleman's disease
  Rare:
    Sarcoidosis
    Angioimmunoblastic lymphadenopathy

Calcified Lymph Nodes

Calcification of lymph nodes is most frequently seen in patients with granulomatous diseases, including tuberculosis, histoplasmosis and other fungal infections, and sarcoidosis (Figs. 2-62 and 2-63), but can also be seen in other diseases (249–252). Calcification can be dense, involving the node in a homogeneous fashion, stippled, "egg-shell" in appearance, or faint and cloud-like. The abnormal nodes are often enlarged, but can also be of normal size. Multiple calcified lymph nodes are often visible, usually in contiguity, and hilar lymph node calcifications are often associated.

Dense calcification involving all or most of an abnormal node is typical of previous granulomatous infection. Eggshell calcification is defined by the presence of calcium in the node periphery, which is often ring-like, but central calcification can be present as well. Egg-shell calcification is most often seen in patients with either silicosis or coal workers' pneumoconiosis, sarcoidosis, and tuberculosis, but it also occurs in patients with Hodgkin's disease, usually following radiation, and has occasionally been described in patients with blastomycosis, histoplasmosis, amyloidosis, scleroderma, and Castleman's disease (253–255).

Rarely, node calcification is seen in untreated lymphoma (250,252) or as a result of metastatic carcinoma, typically adenocarcinoma, and most frequently from the colon (see Fig. 2-62C and 2-63). Lymph node calcification has also been reported with metastatic bronchoalveolar carcinoma, in relation to psammoma bodies (251). Usually calcification of tumors is stippled or faint and cloud-like. Calcification may also be seen in patients with metastatic osteogenic sarcoma, as well as in patients with primary intrathoracic extraosseous osteogenic sarcomas (256). Calcified hilar and mediastinal lymph nodes have been observed in acquired immune deficiency syndrome (AIDS) patients with *Pneumocystis carinii* infection, especially in patients receiving prophylaxis with aerosolized pentamidine (see Fig. 2-62D), possibly as a result of a necrotizing vasculitis with resultant tissue infarction and dystrophic calcification (257).

Although calcified lymph nodes generally indicate the presence of old disease, it should be kept in mind that densely calcified nodes can remain functional, and can become involved by other processes, such as metastatic neoplasm.

Low-Attenuation or Necrotic Lymph Nodes

After administration of intravenous contrast media, low-attenuation lymph nodes, with or without an enhancing rim, have been described as characteristic of a number of different pathologic entities (see Fig. 2-4; Fig. 2-64) (41). Typically, low-density nodes reflect the presence of necrosis, and are commonly seen in patients with tuberculous, fungal infections, and neoplasms, such as metastatic carcinoma (see Fig. 2-4B; Figs. 2-65 and 2-66) and lymphoma (12,13,258,259).

Necrotic lymph nodes are common in patients with active tuberculosis. In a study by Im et al. (12), the CT scans of 23 patients with tuberculous lymphadenitis were reviewed. On CT, right paratracheal and tracheobronchial node enlargement predominated. After injection of intravenous contrast medium, nodes larger than 2 cm in diameter invariably showed central areas of low attenuation with peripheral rim enhancement (see Fig. 2-4A, 2-64A), and the enhancing walls were usually irregular in thickness. Smaller lymph nodes showed varying degrees of enhancement. In our experience, this appearance is particularly common in patients with infection associated with the acquired immune deficiency syndrome (AIDS).

In patients with seminoma, low density areas usually result from extensive tissue necrosis, although low density may also correlate with the presence of numerous small epithelial-lined cystic spaces (see Figs. 2-64 and 2-66) (260,261). Low-density nodes occur in patients with metastatic lung cancer (see Fig. 2-65), when the primary tumor also appears necrotic, and in metastatic ovarian, thyroid, and gastric neoplasia. Low-attenuation or necrotic lymph nodes are common in patients with lymphoma, both before and after treatment. An incidence of 10% to 21% has been reported (262,263). They have also been described in patients

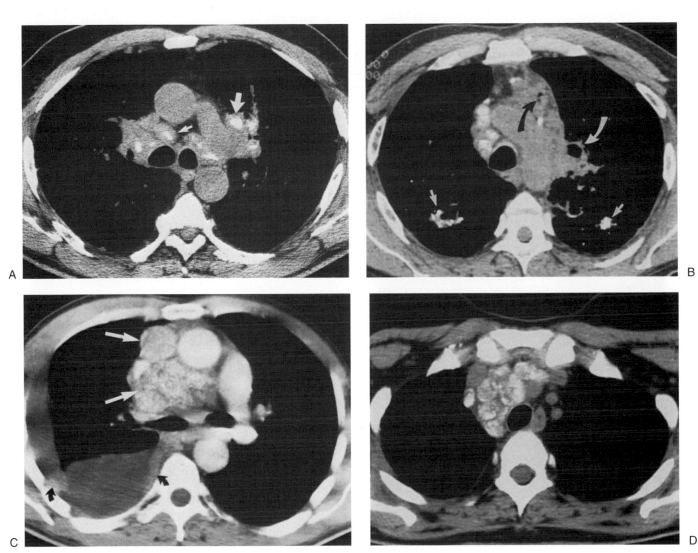

FIG. 2-62. Calcified lymph nodes, CT assessment. **A:** Nonenhanced CT section through the carina shows scattered calcified hilar and pretracheal lymph nodes in a patient with transbronchial, biopsy-documented sarcoidosis. Although these nodes frequently have been described as containing egg-shell calcifications, central or bull's eye calcifications can be identified within enlarged nodes (*arrows*) as frequently. **B:** Nonenhanced CT section through the aortic arch in a patient with documented silicosis. Calcified paratracheal nodes are easily identified, in this case associated with dense foci of parenchymal calcifications in the posterior segments of both upper lobes caused by early progressive massive fibrosis (*arrows*). In addition, air can be seen in both enlarged left hilar and prevascular nodes (*curved arrows*). This unusual appearance is secondary to superimposed tuberculosis (silicotuberculosis). Air within these nodes is presumably secondary to necrosis of peribronchial nodes, with resultant fistulization to adjacent airways. **C:** Contrast-enhanced CT section just below the carina. Amorphous calcifications can be identified within markedly enlarged pretracheal and prevascular lymph nodes (*arrows*). A large, partially loculated pleural fluid collection is present on the right within which foci of soft-tissue density can be identified (*curved arrows*). This patient has known mucin-producing colon carcinoma, metastatic to both the pleura and mediastinal nodes. Diagnosis was confirmed by mediastinoscopy. **D:** Nonenhanced CT section through the great vessels shows diffuse calcifications throughout pre- and paratracheal nodes. This patient had AIDS and was being treated prophylactically with aerosolized pentamidine. Mediastinoscopy revealed these nodes to be filled with *Pneumocystis carinii* organisms, a finding increasingly being observed in patients treated with aerosolized pentamidine.

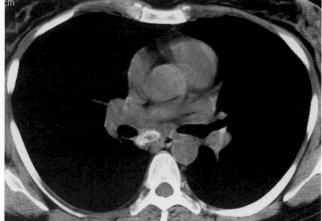

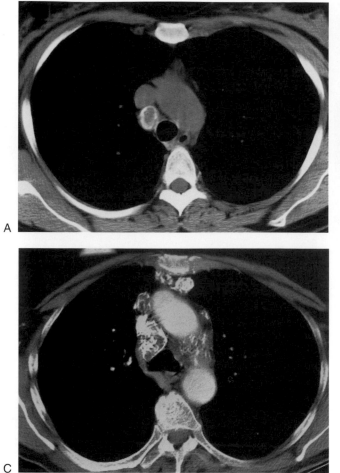

FIG. 2-63. Eggshell lymph node calcification. **A,B:** CT sections through the right paratracheal and subcarinal spaces, respectively show enlarged nodes with peripheral curvilinear calcifications, consistent with history of treatment for known metastatic mucinous adenocarcinoma. **C:** CT section at the level of the aorticopulmonary window in a different patient than in **A** and **B** again show characteristic egg-shell calcifications within nodes, in this case in a patient undergoing therapy for known metastatic gallbladder carcinoma.

with a variety of other entities, including sarcoidosis and Whipple's disease (264).

Lymph Node Enhancement

Lymph nodes can be defined as enhancing, and thus highly vascularized, when they substantially increase in attenuation following a bolus of intravenous contrast media. The distribution of intravenous contrast medium within tumors and/or nodes is a reflection of several factors, including blood flow, the total quantity and concentration of contrast medium injected, the distribution between the vascular and extravascular spaces, and renal function. The differential diagnosis of enhancing mediastinal nodes is limited, and includes Castleman's disease (15,56,265) and angioimmunoblastic lymphadenopathy, as well as vascular metastases, in particular, from renal cell carcinoma, papillary thyroid carcinoma, and small-cell lung carcinoma (see Fig. 2-1B; Fig. 2-67) (49). We have also observed considerable contrast enhancement within enlarged mediastinal and hilar nodes in some patients with sarcoidosis. Also, as indicated above,

nodes in patients with tuberculous lymphadenopathy can show significant enhancement.

Differentiation between enhancing lymph nodes and enhancing mediastinal masses may be problematic. Enhancing masses include substernal thyroid and parathyroid glands, carcinoid tumors, lymphangiomas, hemangiomas, and paragangliomas (54), both intracardiac and mediastinal (52,53,266).

Location of Enlarged Mediastinal Lymph Nodes

The differential diagnosis of lymph node enlargement at least partially depends on whether nodes are predominantly middle mediastinal (including paratracheal, subcarinal, and aorticopulmonary window nodes), and/or hilar, prevascular, internal mammary, paracardiac, or posterior mediastinal.

Approximately 30% of patients with lung cancer have mediastinal node metastases at the time of diagnosis. Lung cancer most often involves middle mediastinal node groups (see Figs. 2-61 and 2-65) (217,241,243–245). Left upper lobe cancers typically metastasize to aorticopulmonary win-

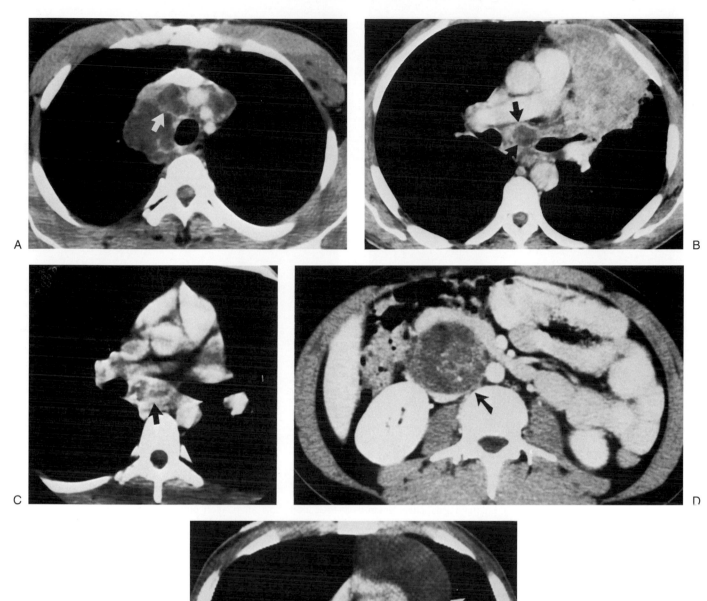

FIG. 2-64. Low-density masses/necrotic lymph nodes, CT assessment. **A:** Contrast-enhanced CT section through the great vessels. Massively enlarged low-density paratracheal and prevascular lymph nodes are present, many of which have a distinct vascular capsule (*arrow*). This appearance is especially suggestive of granulomatous infections such as tuberculous or cryptococcal infection, particularly in patients with AIDS. Tuberculous adenopathy in this case was established by mediastinoscopy. **B:** Contrast-enhanced CT section in a patient with malignant obstruction of the left upper lobe bronchus with associated left upper lobe atelectasis. An enlarged, low-density, necrotic subcarinal lymph node is present (*arrows*), surrounded by a vascular capsule. We have seen this type of necrotic lymph node in association with lung carcinomas of all histologic types. Transbronchial biopsy documented squamous cell carcinoma. **C, D:** Contrast-enhanced CT sections through the subcarinal space and the midabdomen, respectively, in a patient with known seminoma. Note the characteristic appearance of low-density, necrotic subcarinal (*arrow* in **C**) and retroperitoneal lymph nodes. A hypervascular rim can be identified around the subcarinal nodes. **E:** Contrast-enhanced CT scan through the heart shows a large, seemingly homogeneous low-density mass anteriorly (*arrow*) in a patient with documented non-Hodgkin's lymphoma. The appearance superficially resembles cystic lesions such as a pericardial or thymic cyst.

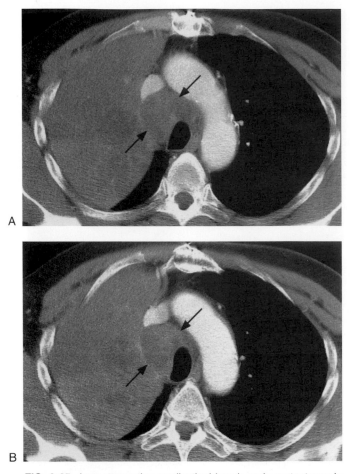

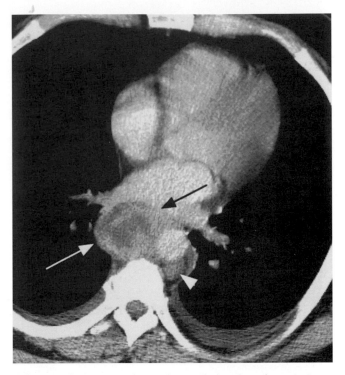

FIG. 2-65. Low-attenuation mediastinal lymph node metastases in lung cancer. **A,B:** On a contrast-enhanced CT, right upper lobe consolidation reflects bronchial obstruction. Enlarged pretracheal lymph nodes (*arrows* in **A** and **B**) are low in attenuation because of necrosis. In patients with lung cancer, necrotic lymph nodes are often associated with a necrotic primary tumor.

FIG. 2-66. Low attenuation and necrotic lymph node metastases from testicular seminoma. Lymph nodes metastases (*arrows*) in the azygoesophageal recess, posterior to the left atrium, are inhomogeneously low in attenuation.

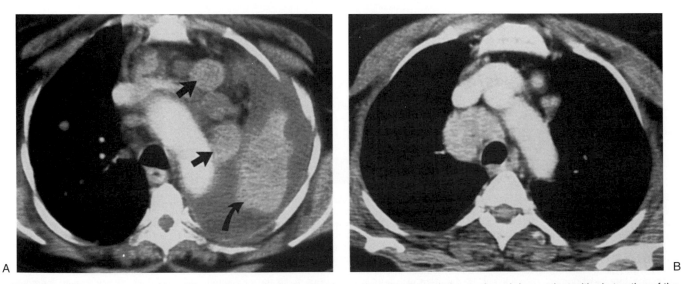

FIG. 2-67. Enhancing lymph nodes, CT assessment. **A:** Contrast-enhanced section through the aortic arch in a patient with obstruction of the left upper lobe bronchus caused by nonsmall cell carcinoma. Note that there is considerable enhancement within several enlarged prevascular lymph nodes (*arrows*). A large pleural effusion is present on the left side within which a portion of the collapsed left upper lobe can be identified, also caused by contrast enhancement of the still-vascularized parenchyma (*curved arrow*). **B:** Contrast-enhanced CT section through the aorta shows markedly enlarged, enhancing pre- and paratracheal and prevascular lymph nodes in a patient with documented sarcoidosis.

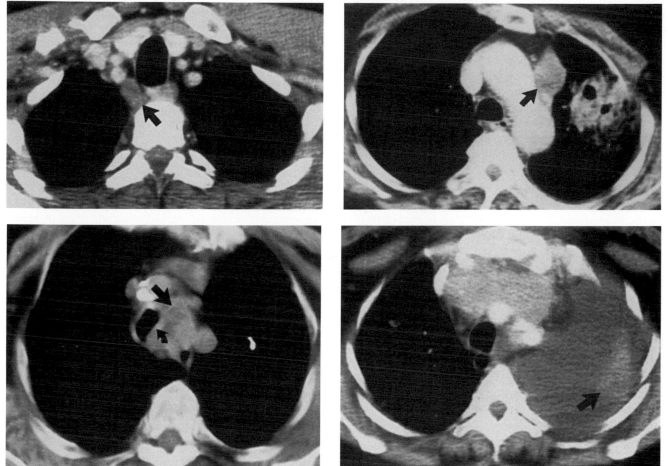

FIG. 2-68. Mediastinal adenopathy, lung cancer staging. **A:** Contrast-enhanced CT section through the superior mediastinum in a patient with known nonsmall cell lung cancer. An enlarged, 1.3 cm high right paratracheal lymph node can be identified just posterior to the right subclavian artery (*arrow*), corresponding to ATS nodal station 2R. Statistically, an enlarged node in this location is far more apt to be malignant than a similar sized lower paratracheal node. Surgery documented a metastatic lymphadenopathy. **B:** Contrast-enhanced CT section at the level of the aortic arch shows a markedly enlarged preaortic lymph node (*arrow*) in a patient with left upper lobe nonsmall cell carcinoma. Note that in this case there is an absence of pre- or paratracheal adenopathy (confirmed at other levels as well). This constellation of findings typifies the usual pattern of local lymph node metastases in patients with left upper lobe tumors. As clearly demonstrated by CT, in this case accurate staging is best accomplished by left parasternal mediastinotomy. **C:** Noncontrast-enhanced CT section at the level of the distal trachea in a patient with known nonsmall cell lung cancer associated with left vocal cord paralysis. An inhomogeneous soft-tissue mass is present (*arrow*) narrowing and displacing the trachea to the right (*curved arrow*). In this case CT not only provides the cause of the vocal cord paralysis, but additionally allows definitive noninvasive staging. **D:** Contrast-enhanced CT scan through the great vessels in a patient with an opacified left hemithorax. A large pleural fluid collection is present on the left, within which the tip of the collapsed left upper lobe can be visualized (*arrow*). Note that there is a poorly marginated soft-tissue mass extensively infiltrating throughout the mediastinum, resulting from extranodal spread of disease. This appearance in itself allows definitive CT staging, although in this case the presence of pleural fluid and contralateral metastases rendered this finding less significant.

dow nodes or anterior mediastinal lymph nodes (see Fig. 2-67; Fig. 2-68), whereas tumors involving the lower lobes on either side tend to metastasize to the subcarinal and right paratracheal chains (217). Right upper lobe tumors typically involve paratracheal nodes (see Fig. 2-65). In patients with lung cancer, the presence of enlarged lymph nodes only in an atypical location suggests that the node enlargement is unrelated to metastasis.

Sixty to ninety percent of patients with sarcoidosis develop lymphadenopathy at some time in the course of their disease. Typically enlarged nodes involve both hila, often associated with either right paratracheal node enlargment or nodes in the aorticopulmonary window. Isolated enlarged nodes, or mediastinal adenopathy in the absence of hilar

adenopathy, is distinctly unusual (267–269). Anterior or posterior lymph node enlargement can be seen on CT, but is unusual in the absence of middle mediastinal lymphadenopathy.

It is estimated in some series that more than 85% of patients with Hodgkin's disease eventually develop intrathoracic abnormalities, typically involving the superior mediastinal (prevascular, pretracheal, and aorticopulmonary) lymph nodes (see Figs. 2-36, 2-57, 2-59) (270–272). In fact, it has been suggested that the absence of involvement of these mediastinal nodes in patients with intrathoracic adenopathy should prompt one to question the diagnosis of Hodgkin's lymphoma.

Similarly, the finding of enlarged paracardiac nodes has

diagnostic significance, as these generally prove malignant (see Figs. 2-56 and 2-58). As shown by Vock and Hodler (227), in their study of 21 cases of cardiophrenic angle adenopathy, all proved to be caused by malignancy, including 12 patients with malignant lymphomas, 7 with metastatic carcinomas, and 2 with metastatic malignant mesotheliomas. Similar findings have been reported by Sussman et al. (226), who found that of 45 patients with paracardiac adenopathy, only 2 were found to have benign lymphadenopathy; the remaining patients had either lymphomas (40%), carcinomas, or sarcomas.

The ability to localize enlarged nodes is especially important in the preoperative assessment of patients with lung cancer. As indicated above, node location is predictive of the likelihood of malignancy. More importantly, accurate localization is usually of critical importance in determining the most efficacious method for definitive staging. Enlarged nodes in close association to the trachea suggest that bronchoscopy with transbronchial needle biopsy may be diagnostic. Nodes in the pretracheal space, anterior subcarinal region, and anterior to the right main bronchus are accessible to routine suprasternal mediastinoscopy, whereas nodes anterior to the left main bronchus, posterior subcarinal space, aorticopulmonary window, and anterior mediastinum are not. Left anterior mediastinal nodes and aorticopulmonary window nodes are accessible to left parasternal mediastinotomy (see Figs. 2-63A, 2-67 and 2-68).

In patients with lung cancer, CT may also be valuable in assessing node morphology. CT may allow differentiation between intra and extranodal disease in those cases where tumor transgresses the nodes capsule (see Figs. 2-60 and 2-61). CT also may provide invaluable information concerning the effects of enlarged mediastinal nodes on adjacent structures. For example, in patients presenting with signs of recurrent laryngeal nerve paralysis or airway compression, the demonstration of appropriate anatomic abnormalities frequently obviates more invasive diagnostic procedures (273).

MR Evaluation of Mediastinal Lymph Nodes

MRI is comparable to CT in identifying mediastinal and hilar lymph nodes, even though its spatial resolution is inferior to CT (see Figs. 2-5, 2-37; Fig. 2-69) (243,274–278). This probably reflects the greater contrast resolution of MRI, which makes identification of mediastinal lymph nodes especially easy when they are embedded in mediastinal fat or adjacent to mediastinal or hilar blood vessels. Although there are some differences in the MRI characteristics of benign and malignant lymph nodes (279–281), their differentiation in individual cases is not possible. Furthermore, MRI is unable to detect calcification, rendering identification of granulomatous nodes exceedingly difficult. Although MRI has been used to diagnose fibrosing mediastinitis, recognition of this entity with MRI is dependent on identifying secondary consequences such as vascular displacement and occlusion (282,283). Low signal intensity has been noted in calcified nodes on T2-weighted images in patients with fibrosing mediastinitis; however, this appearance is nonspecific (283). As will be discussed in greater detail later, a role for MRI in assessing residual or recurrent tumor has been documented for patients with lymphoma following therapy.

In some specific regions of the mediastinum, MRI can be advantageous in demonstrating mediastinal nodes, because of its ability to image in nontransaxial planes, although this advantage is uncommonly of clinical utility (230,284,285). Specifically, nodes in the aorticopulmonary window are better shown on MRI obtained in the coronal plane because volume averaging with pulmonary artery or aortic arch are

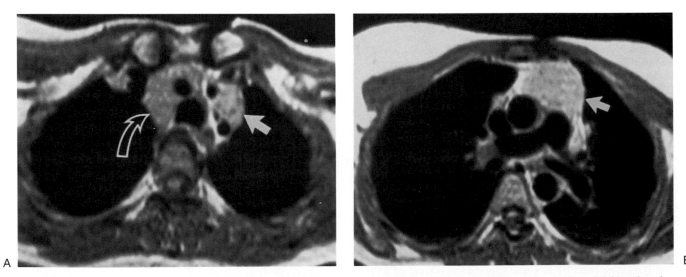

FIG. 2-69. Mediastinal lymphadenopathy, MR assessment. **A,B:** T1-weighted axial MR images through the great vessels and right main pulmonary artery, respectively. Enlarged, confluent, prevascular (*arrow* in **A**, **B**) and paratracheal (*curved arrow* in **A**) lymph nodes are easily identifiable as areas of intermediate signal intensity embedded in fat. Non-Hodgkin's lymphoma.

TABLE 2-6. *Ann Arbor staging classification for lymphoma*[a]

Stage	Definition
I	Involvement of a single lymph node region (I) or a single extralymphatic organ or site (I$_E$)
II	Involvement of two or more lymph node regions on the same side of the diaphragm (II) or localized involvement of an extralymphatic organ or site and of one or more lymph node regions of the same side of the diaphragm (II$_E$)
III	Involvement of lymph node regions on both sides of the diaphragm (III), which may also be accompanied by involvement of the spleen (III$_S$) or by localized involvement of an extralymphatic organ or site (III$_E$) or both (III$_{SE}$)
IV	Diffuse or disseminated involvement of one or more extralymphatic organs or tissues, with or without associated lymph node involvement
	The absence or presence of fever, night sweats, and/or unexplained loss of 10% or more of body weight in 6 months is denoted by the suffix A or B, respectively

[a] From refs. 271 and 286, with permission.

avoided. Similarly, subcarinal nodes can be better shown on MRI in the sagittal plane, than on CT.

Lymphoma

Lymphoma accounts for about 4% of newly diagnosed malignancies in the United States (286). Lymphomas are primary neoplasms of the lymphoreticular system and are classified in two main types: Hodgkin's disease (HD) and non-Hodgkin lymphoma (NHL). Although Hodgkin's disease is the less common of the two types, representing about 25% to 30% of cases, it is more common as a cause of mediastinal involvement (286).

Hodgkin's Disease

Hodgkin's disease occurs at all ages, but its peak incidence is in the third and eighth decades; it accounts for about 0.5% to 1% of all newly diagnosed malignancies in the U.S. (271,287). It is more prevalent in males with a male:female ratio of from 1.38 to 1.94 (271). The Ann Arbor Staging Classification is used to describe the anatomic extent of disease at the time of diagnosis, and correlates well with prognosis (Table 2-6). Radiation is used for stages I and II, with a combination of radiation and chemotherapy or chemotherapy alone being employed in stages III and IV (287). There is a 75% to 80% cure rate for adult HD and in children, the cure rate is about 95% (272).

HD has a predilection for thoracic involvement, and up to 85% of patients with HD present with mediastinal adenopathy (see Fig. 2-36, 2-37, 2-57–2-59) (126,223,271). HD most often involves prevascular and paratracheal lymph nodes (126). In one study, these node groups were abnormal in 170 (84%) of 203 patients with HD; this represented 98% of the 173 patients with intrathoracic disease (270) (Table 2-7); if these nodes appear normal on CT, intrathoracic adenopathy is unlikely to represent HD (271). Multiple node groups are commonly involved in patients with HD (Fig. 2-70). Other sites of lymph node enlargement include hilar nodes (28% to 44% of all cases), subcarinal nodes (22% to 44%), cardiophrenic angle (paracardiac) lymph nodes (8% to 10%) (219,220), internal mammary nodes (5% to 37%), and posterior mediastinal nodes (5% to 12%) (270,288). Enlargement of a single node group can be seen in some patients with HD, most commonly in the prevascular mediastinum. This often indicates the presence of nodular sclerosing histology that accounts for 50% to 80% of adult HD (271). Direct extension of lymphoma from the mediastinum to the lung or the chest wall is common with large mediastinal masses (289).

CT is advantageous in showing mediastinal lymph node

TABLE 2-7. *Plain radiograph and CT abnormalities in patients with Hodgkin's disease*[a]

	Radiograph abnormal (%)	CT abnormal (%)	Change in treatment based on CT findings (%)
Superior mediastinal nodes	77	84	0.5
Hilar nodes	21	38	1
Subcarinal nodes	7	22	3.5
Internal mammary nodes	1	5	0
Posterior mediastinal nodes	2	5	1
Paracardiac nodes	1	8	1.5
Lung parenchyma	8	8	0
Pleura	10	13	0
Pericarium	2	6	1
Chest wall	1	6	2.5
All Sites	78	87	9.4

[a] From ref. 270, with permission.

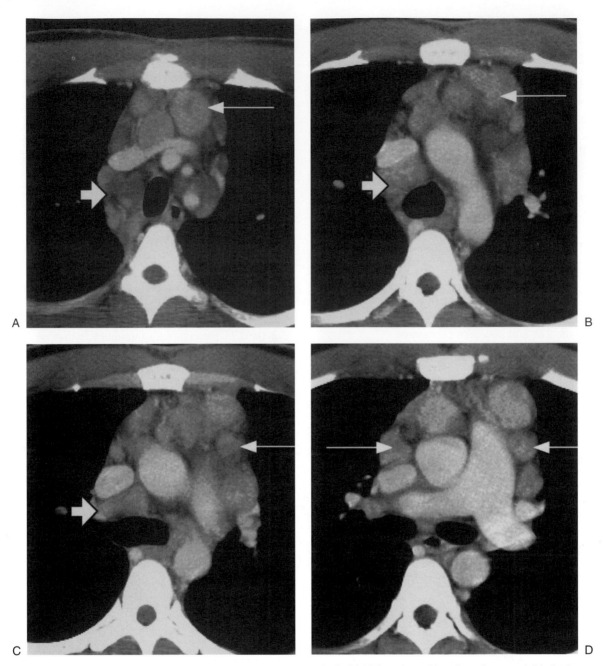

FIG. 2-70. Mediastinal lymph node enlargement in Hodgkin's lymphoma. **A–D:** Multiple enlarged lymph nodes are visible in the prevascular space (*small arrows*) and pretracheal space (*large arrows*). Some nodes appear to be low in attenuation whereas others are enhanced.

abnormalities in patients with lymphoma. For example, para-cardiac lymph node enlargment was seen on CT in 14 (6.6%) of 274 patients with HD or NHL, but in only 3 of these, was the abnormality visible on plain radiographs (224). In a study by Castellino et al. (270), of 203 patients, findings shown only on CT changed treatment in more than 9% of patients (see Table 2-7). In another study, however, it was uncommon for CT to show evidence of mediastinal adenopathy if the chest radiograph was normal, but if the radiograph was ab-normal, CT detected additional sites of adenopathy in many cases (288). In this study, CT was most helpful in diagnosing

subcarinal, internal mammary, and aorticopulmonary win-dow node enlargement not visible on radiographs. In a sig-nificant percentage of patients, the additional node involve-ment shown by CT changed therapy (272,288).

In patients with HD, enlarged lymph nodes can be variable in appearance. Nodes are of homogeneous soft-tissue attenu-ation in the majority of cases (126). Multiple enlarged lymph nodes are often seen, and they can be well-defined and dis-crete, matted, or associated with diffuse mediastinal infiltra-tion. It is not uncommon for lymph node masses to show areas of low attenuation or necrosis following contrast enhancement; cystic and necrotic appearing nodes have been reported in 10% to 21% of cases (see Fig. 2-70) (262,263). Rarely, nodes show fine flecks of calcification in untreated patients (252).

The significance of low-density nodes in patients presenting with newly diagnosed lymphoma has been studied by Hopper et al. (263). A review of 76 patients with newly diagnosed HD found that 16 patients (21%) had low-density nodes at presentation. However, no difference was found between those patients with and without necrotic nodes with respect to stage, disease distribution, cell type, disease extent, the presence of bulk disease, or most importantly, prognosis (263).

HD also has a predilection for involvement of the thymus in association with mediastinal lymph node enlargement (125,126). In a study of 50 patients with newly diagnosed disease and evidence of thoracic involvement, the thymus was enlarged in 15 (30%); in all, mediastinal lymph nodes were also enlarged. In other studies (126,127), thymic enlargement visible on CT has been reported in 17 (40%) of 43 adult patients and 17 (28%) of 60 pediatric patients. In a review of 50 episodes of recurrence of HD, 18 patients had an intrathoracic relapse, and thymic enlargement was present in 7 (38%) of the 18; in all but one patient who had a thymic cyst, mediastinal lymph nodes were also involved (125).

HD is believed by most to be unifocal in origin and typically spreads by contiguity to involve adjacent lymph node groups (271,290). It is unusual for HD to skip lymph node groups, and if areas contiguous with the mediastinum, such as the lower neck or upper abdomen, are not involved by HD, it is not generally necessary to scan regions, such as the pelvis, which are more distant from the involved nodes. However, in patients with mediastinal HD, scanning should always be extended to include the upper abdomen. Intraabdominal periaortic adenopathy can be found in 25% of patients with HD, and the spleen and liver are involved in 37% and 8% respectively (291).

It is important to note that there is no strong correlation between liver or spleen size and their involvement by lymphoma. Fewer than 30% of HD patients with hepatic involvement at autopsy have detectable hepatomegaly at clinical examination. Thus, CT or MRI demonstration of liver enlargement is of no diagnostic value. Likewise, spleen size evaluation is of limited value; solitary or multiple splenic lesions are the most reliable evidence of splenic involvement with either CT or MRI. In one series, almost two-thirds of HD nodules involving the spleen were less than 1 cm in diameter, rendering their detection difficult on both CT and MRI, although marked splenomegaly is almost always related to tumor involvement (271,292).

Non-Hodgkin's Lymphoma

The term non-Hodgkin's lymphoma (NHL) refers to a diverse group of diseases, varying in radiologic findings, clinical presentation, course, and prognosis (286, 293–296). In comparison to Hodgkin's disease, these tumors are less common as causes of thoracic disease, and occur in an older group (median 55 years) (286). Non-Hodgkin lymphoma is more common than HD in children (4).

Thoracic involvement is about half as common with NHL (40% to 50%) as with HD (85%) (223,286,293). In a study of 181 newly diagnosed patients with NHL, only 82 (45%) had intrathoracic disease (293). As with HD, the most common thoracic abnormality in patients with NHL is mediastinal lymph node involvement, although the pattern of lymph node disease is somewhat different. Involvement of one node group is much more common in patients with NHL; in one study, 40% of patients with NHL and thoracic involvement had involvement of only one node group, whereas this was seen in only 15% of patients with HD (223). Enlargment of anterior mediastinal, internal mammary, paratracheal, and hilar nodes is much less common with NHL than with HD. Nonetheless, superior mediastinal node involvement remains the most frequent abnormality seen. In one study (293), 34% of patients had superior mediastinal (prevascular and pretracheal) node involvement, and this represented 74% of the patients with an intrathoracic abnormality. Subcarinal lymph node enlargement was present in 13% of cases, hilar nodes in 9%, and cardiophrenic nodes in 7%. Involvement of posterior mediastinal nodal groups is much more common with NHL; this was seen in 10% of cases (223,293,297) (see Fig. 2-48). Rarely, calcification of node masses can be seen (250). Extranodal involvement is much more common with NHL (286). Extranodal sites of involvement include lung (13%), pleura (20%), pericardial space (8%), and chest wall (5%) (293).

CT can show evidence of intrathoracic disease when it is unrecognizable on plain radiographs and may be helpful in diagnosis (293,294). In a recent study, both CT and chest radiographic findings were positive in 65 (36%) of 181 patients with NHL, whereas CT findings were positive and chest radiographs were negative in 17 (9%) (293). In the 65 patients with abnormal CT and chest radiographs, CT showed more extensive intrathoracic disease in 49 (75%), and this resulted in an increase in stage in 16. In another study (294), chest CT showed intrathoracic disease in 28% of patients with NHL thought to have normal chest films, and 45% of patients with equivocal plain radiographic findings.

An understanding of the use of CT in patients with NHL requires some knowledge of how it is treated. NHL is usually treated using chemotherapy in patients with intermediate or high grade lymphomas regardless of their anatomic stage and in the majority of patients with low grade lymphoma (293,295). The use of primary radiotherapy is usually limited to a small subgroup of patients with early stage (I or II) low grade lymphoma; only 20% to 25% of patients with low grade lymphoma are stage I or II at diagnosis (295). Although NHL is staged using the same system as HD; staging of NHL is much less important. With HD, the anatomic extent of the tumor strongly predicts outcome; with NHL, the histopathologic classification is more predictive (286).

Although the precise role of chest CT in patients with NHL remains to be defined, it is commonly obtained in clinical practice (286,293). The use of chest CT has been called into question by Castellino et al. (293); in their study, although CT often showed more extensive thoracic disease than did plain radiographs, in none of their cases did this information alter treatment. Nonetheless, some reasonable recommendations for CT can probably be made, based on a consideration of tumor histology, clinical stage, and plain radiographic findings (294). In patients with intermediate or high grade NHL or stage III or IV disease, chest CT does not seem to have a distinct role to play, as patients are treated using chemotherapy (293,294). In fact, it should be pointed out that the lack of utility for staging NHL found for CT by Castellino et al. (293), is at least partially explained by the preponderance of intermediate and high grade NHL in their study. On the other hand, in patients thought to have stage I or II low grade NHL, CT seems appropriate for determining whether intrathoracic disease is present and, if localized, in helping to plan radiation (294).

In contrast to patient with HD, the abdomen, pelvis, and neck must be scanned in all patients with NHL, as noncontiguous spread is common; NHL is assumed to be multi-focal in origin (295). Abdominal involvement is more common than in patients with HD, and a variety of findings may be present (298); intraabdominal periaortic adenopathy is found in 49% of patients with NHL (291), the spleen is involved in 41%, and the liver in 14%. It is important to note that there is no strong correlation between liver size and liver involvement; only 57% of patients with NHL and hepatomegaly demonstrate liver lymphoma at histologic examination. In one study (299), CT of the abdomen and pelvis resulted in an upgrading of the clinical stage in 33% of patients with NHL and detected unsuspected active disease in 43% of patients thought to be in remission. This resulted in clinically important upstaging in 15% of all cases.

The incidence of NHL, particularly of the intermediate and high grades, is significantly higher in immunodeficient patients, being associated with congenital immunodeficiency syndromes, HIV infection, and immunosuppressive therapy (286,295). These tumors differ somewhat from those occurring spontaneously in immunocompetent patients, usually being polyclonal rather than monoclonal and usually involving extranodal sites (e.g., central nervous system, lung, gastrointestinal tract).

Primary mediastinal large-B-cell lymphoma has recently been described as a distinct subtype of NHL (300). Although the mediastinum is abnormal in a minority of patients with NHL, it is the primary site of involvement in this disease. In a study of 43 patients (300), an anterior mediastinal mass was the predominant finding in 42 (98%) of 43 patients studied using chest radiographs and 24 (96%) of 25 patients having CT. These tumors are thought to arise from thymic medullary B cells, explaining their common location in the prevascular space. Both clinically and radiographically, this entity is difficult to distinguish from HD. Affected patients are usually younger than other patients with NHL, with a median age of 35 years (300).

On CT, large, lobulated anterior mediastinal masses were visible, averaging 10 cm in diameter; lymph node enlargement in the subcarinal space and posterior mediastinum were much less common. Low attenuation areas of necrosis within the mass were seen in 44%, with calcification in two cases. Pleural and pericardial effusions were present in about one-third. Superior vena cava obstruction and chest wall invasion were uncommon (300). CT is valuable in determining tumor extent, as radiation is usually used; the presence of pleural effusion predicts a poor outcome.

Diagnosis of Residual Tumor After Treatment

With the development of effective treatments for lymphoma, there is a need for accurate monitoring of tumor response. Imaging studies are frequently obtained to judge the completeness of tumor response to treatment, and periodic surveillance imaging is used to determine the presence or absence of relapse (271,287). Many patients with recurrence will eventually be cured. Chest radiographs are usually used for monitoring patients in the months and years following treatment. CT is usually obtained 2 to 4 months following treatment to assess the completeness of response and to provide a baseline for subsequent studies in patients who develop radiographic abnormalities (271,287).

Reduction of tumor bulk is universally present in patients with adequately treated tumor, and this finding is commonly used when assessing the efficacy of treatment. Reduction in tumor size is satisfactorily monitored using CT. Patients showing complete resolution of the lymphoma on CT are generally considered to have had a satisfactory response.

However, monitoring the decrease in tumor size is not always an accurate measure of treatment success, as the rate of decrease in tumor size is different in different patients and varies with the size of the initial mass, its site, histology, and the type of treatment (301,302); tumors containing a significant fibrous component, such as nodular sclerosing HD, will generally show less decrease in size than tumors made up primarily of cellular elements, and residual mediastinal masses are common after treatment, even in patients who have achieved a cure.

Residual mediastinal masses following treatment often reflect so-called "sterilized" lymphoma—residual fibrous tissue components of the tumor itself, or posttreatment fibrosis (303). Pathologic studies of residual mediastinal masses in patients with treated Hodgkin's disease have shown them to be nearly acellular, hyalinized fibrous tissue (301,304,305). Prior to CT, residual masses were thought to be present in a minority of patients. However, more recent studies indicate that residual masses can be seen in as many as 88% of pa-

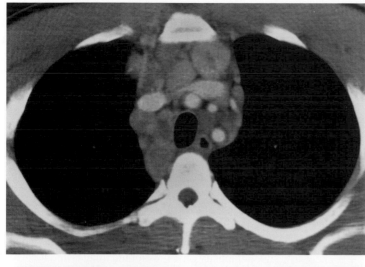

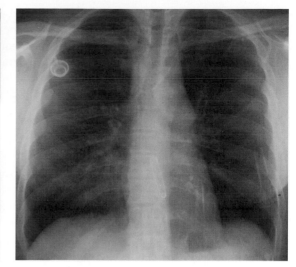

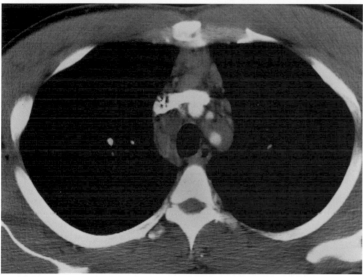

FIG. 2-71. Residual masses after treatment for Hodgkin's lymphoma: CT appearance. **A:** Pretreatment CT shows extensive mediastinal lymph node enlargement typical of Hodgkin's disease. **B:** Posttreatment radiograph shows persistent widening of the superior mediastinum. **C:** Posttreatment CT, obtained at the same time of the radiograph in **B** shows residual lymph node enlargement. Such residual masses are very common in patients with Hodgkin's disease, and if stable, do not imply recurrence.

tients with HD (Fig. 2-71) and 40% of patients with NHL (306–308). In patients with thymic enlargement resulting from HD, most show a return to normal thymic size following treatment. However, the thymus remained enlarged following treatment in 9 (38%) of 24 adult patients (127) and three (27%) of 11 pediatric patients (126). Although it is acknowledged that in patients with HD, these masses are usually benign and of no consequence, close monitoring of residual masses is recommended. In some patients, masses remaining after treatment continue to decrease in size or resolve over a period ranging from 3 to 11 months (301,309).

Recurrent HD does not commonly involve previously irradiated intrathoracic lymph nodes. However, so called "in-field recurrence" does occur. In one study (301), one of 20 intrathoracic relapses were in the treatment field, and in another (310), 13 of 60 patients with stage I or II mediastinal disease had an intrathoracic relapse, and six of these were in previously treated mediastinal nodes. All of six patients with a mediastinal recurrence had large masses (greater than one-third of the chest diameter) before treatment. Large

masses, and masses in the anterior mediastinum are generally considered to carry an increased risk of recurrence (271,301,306,310–312).

In one study, intrathoracic relapse was more than twice as frequent in HD patients who had residual masses after treatment (301). Other studies, however, have not confirmed this finding, perhaps because of differing patient populations and different findings used to diagnose mediastinal mass (306,309). On the other hand, both residual mediastinal masses and recurrence, are more common in HD patients who have a large mass initially. Also, in a series of NHL patients restaged surgically following initial therapy of NHL, residual masses were present in 20%, and persistent disease and relapses occurred mainly in areas of previous involvement (308).

In patients with recurrent tumor, CT can show an increase in size of one or more masses. CT attenuation is identical for both active and inactive residual masses in patients treated for lymphoma, and is of limited value in making this diagnosis. Recently, promising results in distinguishing active tumor from residual masses have been reported with gallium-67 imaging, which presumably monitors tumor cell viability (313,314). Ongoing research indicates that monitoring tumor metabolism with positron emission tomography may also be helpful. MRI can also provide important information in distinguishing active tumor from residual benign masses, as reviewed below (302,315–317).

MR Evaluation of Lymphoma and Residual Tumor

As discussed in Chapter 1, the basis for the MRI signal intensity differences exhibited by different tissues is fundamentally different from that resulting in density differences in CT (279,318). In simplified terms, relaxation times are primarily dependent on the proportion of water and proteins as well as the type of proteins within a given tissue. Lymphoma cells contain a large amount of water, with a relatively low proportion of proteins and thus appear intense on T2-weighted images. Conversely, fibrous tissue contains much less water and a high proportion of highly polymerized proteins and shows low intensity with T2-weighting (318).

Histologically lymphomas contain variable proportions of cells and connective tissue. For example, in nodular sclerosing HD, large amounts of fibrous tissue are typically interspersed with malignant cells (Fig. 2-72). Conversely, in diffuse NHL, tumors may be composed almost entirely of malignant cells without significant collagen. Based on these histologic differences, lymphomas can have varying MRI appearances, appearing homogeneous or heterogeneous on T2-weighed images.

In patients with a homogeneous pattern (Fig. 2-73), lesions demonstrate homogeneous high signal intensity similar to that of fat on T2-weighted images. This appearance can be seen with Hodgkin's or non-Hodgkin's lymphoma. Typically, patients with a heterogeneous pattern show mixed signal intensity on T2-weighted images, with interspersed areas of high and low signal intensity. This pattern is often seen in untreated nodular sclerosing HD, with the low-signal intensity areas on T2-weighted images related to regions of fibrosis in the tumor (Fig. 2-74), and high intensity regions representing tumor tissue or cystic regions. Furthermore, it has recently been suggested that MRI signal characteristics may be of value in differentiating low-grade from high-grade lymphomas (319). The likelihood of recurrence has been found to be higher if the signal intensity of the initial mass is high on T2-weighted MR images (302).

Several studies have demonstrated that residual inactive masses from ''sterilized'' lymphoma are composed primarily of fibrous tissue. It is therefore reasonable to suspect that some changes in the MRI signal intensity pattern may be expected during the posttreatment evolution of lymphoma. This hypothesis has been the basis of research into the potential utilization of MRI to monitor lymphoma patients showing residual masses after treatment (320). As demonstrated in Figure 2-72, differences in the histologic composition of lymphoma are paralleled by differences in their signal intensity pattern.

By systematically studying a series of patients with treated lymphoma, four characteristic MRI signal patterns have been defined on the basis of T1-weighted and T2-weighted images (316,321):

1. Homogeneous, hyperintense (active) pattern. This is characteristic of untreated lymphoma (see Fig. 2-73). The lesion demonstrates a homogeneous low signal intensity similar to that of muscle on T1-weighted images, and a high signal intensity similar to that of fat on T2-weighted images. This pattern is never seen in inactive residual lymphomatous masses.

2. Heterogeneous active pattern with mixed hypo- and hyperintensity. This pattern is characterized by homogeneous low signal intensity on T1-weighted images and heterogeneous signal intensity on T2-weighted images, with areas of both high and low signal intensity. This pattern can be seen in untreated nodular sclerosing HD, with the low-signal intensity areas on T2-weighted images presumably related to regions of fibrosis in the tumor (see Fig. 2-74). Also, it is commonly seen during the posttreatment response phase of most lymphomas, with the high signal intensity regions presumably representing residual active lymphomatous masses, areas of necrosis, or inflammation. The low signal areas likely represent fibrotic tissue (see Fig. 2-72). This pattern is seen in about 20% of patients with residual masses after treatment.

3. Heterogeneous inactive pattern with mixed areas of low and high signal intensity on both T1- and T2-weighted images. Areas of high intensity on the T1-weighted images should correspond to those seen with T2-weighting. This pattern is seen in lesions containing mixed fat (high-intensity regions) and fibrous tissue (low intensity regions), and is seen after treatment in patients with sterilized tumors.

4. Homogeneous, hypointense (inactive) pattern. This appearance is characteristic of inactive residual fibrotic masses in patients having successful therapy for lymphoma. These lesions are characterized by homogeneously low signal intensity on both T1-weighted and T2-weighted images. Approximately 80% of masses show a homogeneous hypointense pattern within 6 to 8 weeks of initiation of therapy.

One caveat must be kept in mind. In patients with inactive treated lymphoma, mediastinal fat, interspersed with residual fibrous tissue, can mimic this heterogeneous pattern on T2-weighted images. Indeed, as mediastinal lymphomas regress after treatment, mediastinal fat often appears to be mixed with the residual mass or masses. Since fat has a high signal intensity on T2-weighted images, heterogeneous intensity can result. However, on T1-weighted images these masses also appear heterogeneous, because of the high signal intensity of fat.

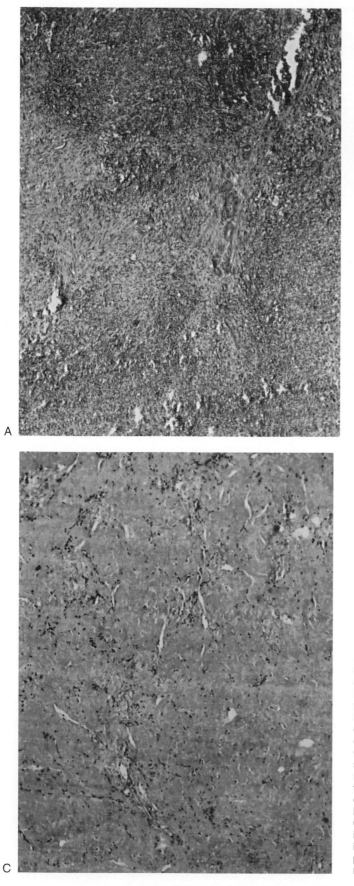

A

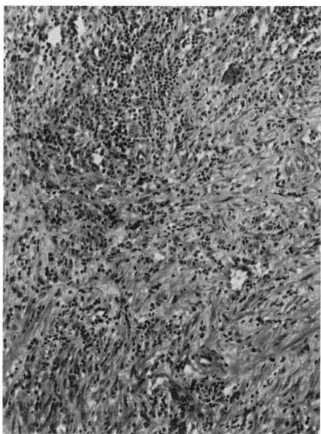

B

C

FIG. 2-72. Histologic changes before and after therapy of nodular sclerosing Hodgkin's lymphoma. **A:** Islands of highly cellular tissue are interspersed among more fibrotic, relatively hypocellular areas. Low-power photomicrograph of nodular sclerosing Hodgkin's lymphoma demonstrates typical biphasic histology with areas of predominant sclerosis with paucity of malignant cells and areas of malignant cell infiltrations. **B:** Higher magnification of **A** shows predominance of malignant cells with interspersed connective tissue components. **C:** After therapy, repeat surgical biopsy of residual mass demonstrates cell necrosis with marked hypocellularity and extensive sclerosis, presumably representing the residual fibrous component of the tumor. MR imaging of the lesion at the time of biopsy illustrated in **A** demonstrated a slightly heterogeneous pattern with predominantly high signal intensity on T2-weighted images. At time of biopsy in **C**, homogeneously low signal intensity was noted on T2-weighted images. Thus, MR appears to track, to some degree, the changes in relative proportion of cellular and fibrotic components within lymphomas because relaxation times of fibrosis and malignant cells are markedly different.

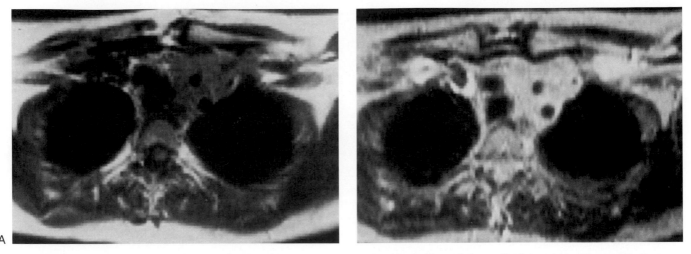

FIG. 2-73. Mediastinal lymphoma, MR assessment pretreatment. **A:** T1-weighted image through the mediastinum shows a mass of homogeneously low-signal intensity. **B:** T2-weighted image at the same level as **A** shows homogeneously high-signal intensity.

It is important to emphasize that both T1-weighted and T2-weighted images are necessary in evaluating patients with lymphoma. Active residual areas of lymphoma, necrosis, or inflammation can only be diagnosed if high signal intensity is seen on T2-weighted images, but low signal intensity is seen on T1-weighted images in the same region. Another solution to this problem would be the use pulse sequences with selective fat suppression.

In patients with lymphoma, complete regression of the tumor mass will often be observed following treatment; in such patients there is no need for MRI (315). However, in those patients having a residual mass after one or two cycles of chemotherapy, MRI should be used to assess the potential activity of the remaining lesion. A divergence of lesion size change and MRI signal intensity is common in the first 6 months after treatment. This was seen in 44 (47%) of 93 cases in one study (316). Generally in this situation, signal intensity changes were more reliable than size in assessing tumor status.

In particular, the T2-weighted intensity of a residual mass shown on MRI has a significant relationship to the likelihood of residual or recurrent tumor. Typically, the intensity of HD on T2-weighted images significantly decreases following treatment (302). In a study by Nyman et al. (302), a prompt and persistent decrease in intensity occurred after treatment in all but three cases. In two of these three, the persisting high intensity may have reflected necrosis of the mass, cysts within the treated tumor, or volume averaging with fat, but in one, an increase in intensity, accompanied by an increase in size of the mass, indicated recurrence.

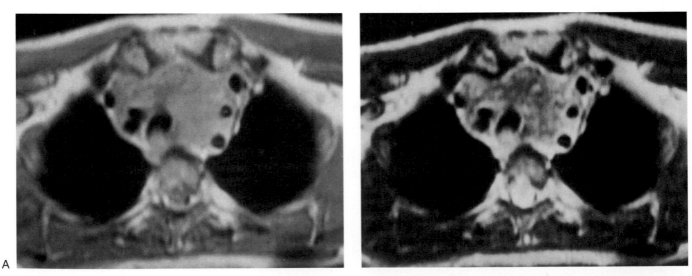

FIG. 2-74. A 48-year-old patient with newly diagnosed Hodgkin's disease. **A:** Proton density image shows mass in superior mediastinum. **B:** T2-weighted image demonstrates a heterogeneous pattern with mixed areas of high and low signal intensity. This is typical of nodular sclerosing Hodgkin's disease, with its biphasic histology comprising fibrotic areas interspersed with more cellular areas.

Also, Zerhouni and others (320), found that inactive (treated) lymphomas were significantly lower in intensity on T2-weighted images (mass/fat intensity ratio 0.3) than active lymphomas (mass/fat intensity ratio 0.9). The average mass/fat intensity ratio on the T2- weighted sequence in Nyman's study was approximately 0.8 prior to treatment, and slightly less than 0.4 after treatment. Thus, a high relative intensity with T2 weighting, although not specific for persistent or recurrent tumor, might indicate the need for biopsy or close follow-up of a residual mediastinal mass. Change in intensity from low to high during follow-up should be regarded as very significant.

In a study of 93 intervals between MRI examinations in 34 patients with treated lymphoma (316), using the four signal intensity patterns described above, seven incorrect diagnoses of tumor recurrence were made. Four were in the first 4 months after treatment, caused by the presence of necrosis or inflammation in the tumor or increased intensity in adjacent lung; two were caused by misinterpretation of a heterogeneous inactive pattern as abnormal; and an additional patient showed a heterogeneous active pattern 6 months after treatment caused by the presence of chronic inflammation.

In our experience, monitoring the MRI signal intensity of residual masses can provide a qualitative measure of tumor response, and can benefit patient management in several ways.

First, in patients showing a decrease in mass size and a homogeneous decrease in T2-weighted signal intensity, a favorable response can be expected. Of course, it must be recognized that microscopic residual tumor cannot be detected by MRI, given the low spatial resolution and the variability of signal intensities intrinsic to the method. In all such cases, continued surveillance is warranted until there is complete resolution of the residual mass. Residual masses may resolve in 12 to 18 months or persist without change in size. Reappearance of foci of high signal intensity in such masses are strong indicators of early recurrence and are usually noted before clinical symptoms.

Secondly, decrease in size of the mass with a persistent homogeneous hyperintense or heterogeneous hyperintense pattern suggests partial response. However, inflammation and necrosis may result in a similar appearance, mimicking active tumor, in the early posttherapy phase (317). In a series of 115 patients we have studied over 3 years, all instances of a false positive MRI diagnosis of residual mass caused by necrosis or inflammation of the tumoral mass, occurred within 4 months of the initiation of therapy. One should be cautious in not over interpreting these patterns as definite evidence of lack of response within the first few months following therapy.

In some patients a marked size reduction occurs, but a small residual mass or masses show heterogeneous or homogeneous high-signal intensity (Fig. 2-75). In such patients, although the size decrease would suggest tumor response (322–324), the high signal intensity shown on MRI justifies close monitoring for recurrence. In a series of 34

patients prospectively followed by serial MRI studies over 30 months, this combination of findings occurred in 23% of cases (306).

MRI signal intensity increases during follow-up of residual masses previously considered inactive. In this group of patients, "islands" of high signal intensity can be seen to reappear in low intensity residual masses. This appearance indicates recurrence. In our experience, about 20% of patients will demonstrate this MRI finding, and it can precede clinical symptoms by 8 to 12 weeks, allowing earlier detection than otherwise possible (316,321).

Certain caveats, however, should be emphasized in regard to interpretation of MRI in patients with treated lymphoma. As mentioned above, cautious interpretation should be the rule within the first 4 to 6 months following the initiation of therapy. T1- and T2-weighted images should always be interpreted in combination, or fat suppression techniques should be used, to exclude the possibility of fibro-fatty masses mimicking the appearance of recurrent tumor (316). Motion artifacts in the phase direction of the image or flow artifacts may, on occasion, render interpretation difficult. Good technique with cardiac gating and presaturation of incoming blood is usually sufficient to resolve this problem.

Another important caveat is that MRI signal intensity analysis is not necessarily valid in assessing lung abnormalities in these patients (316,318). In our experience, high signal intensity can often be seen in areas of pulmonary radiation fibrosis, in the absence of any residual tumor. Clearly, bronchial secretions accumulating in areas of previously irradiated lung can increase signal intensity on T2-weighted images. In areas of irradiated lung, the ciliated respiratory epithelium is usually damaged and mucociliary clearance of secretions from the lung is reduced. Secretions accumulate in damaged areas of lung, and in bronchi dilated because of surrounding lung fibrosis. MRI signal intensity analysis should be limited to purely mediastinal and hilar masses and exclusive of their intrapulmonary manifestations.

In summary, current experience with patients having lymphoma and other neoplasms such as rectal carcinoma, cervical carcinoma, and musculoskeletal tumors indicate that MRI signal patterns reflect, to some extent, histologic features of the tumors. The ability of MRI to assess disease activity is unique: however, since MRI is more expensive and provides anatomic information identical to that of CT, we believe that it is most appropriate to examine patients with suspected mediastinal lymphoma first using CT.

Since in many uncomplicated cases complete regression of masses will be observed, there is no need for MRI in these instances (315). For those patients in whom a residual mass is observed after one or two cycles of chemotherapy, however, MRI should be used to assess whether the signal pattern is consistent with active disease. In the majority of cases, a rapid decrease in the T2-weighted signal intensity of lymphomatous masses is the rule in the posttreatment period, with 80% of masses assuming a homogeneous hypo-

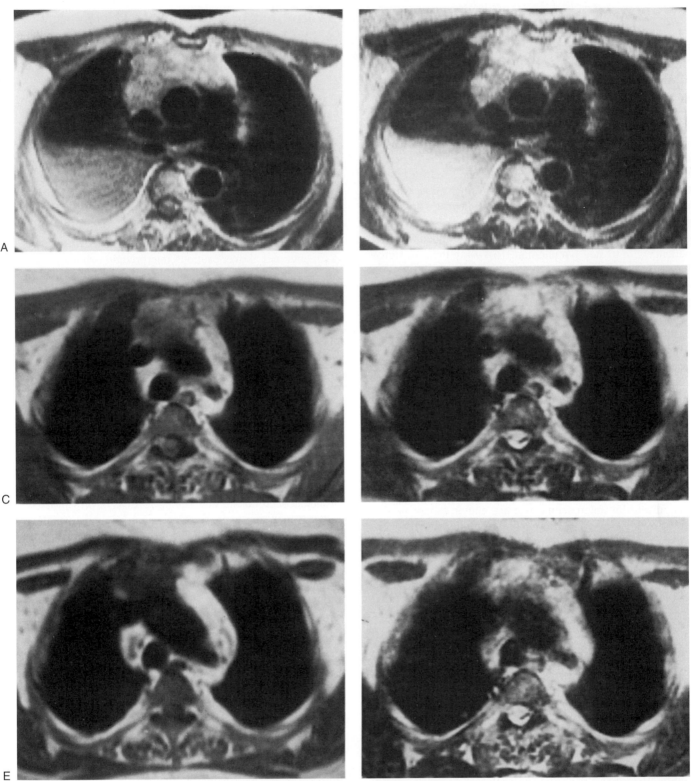

FIG. 2-75. A 27-year-old patient with Hodgkin's lymphoma in the anterior mediastinum. **A, B:** Proton density and T2-weighted images, respectively, obtained in a patient prior to the initiation of therapy demonstrate a large mass in the anterior mediastinum with large right pleural effusion. The mass appears mostly hyperintense with a signal intensity almost equal to that of surrounding fat. Slight heterogeneity is noted within regions of the mass. **C, D:** T1- and T2-weighted images, respectively, 2 months after therapy initiation. A marked decrease in the bulk of the tumor is noted. However, a small amount of residual mass is seen immediately anterior to the arch of the aorta. Note the heterogeneous, predominantly high signal intensity seen on the T2-weighted image and the correspondingly low signal intensity on the T1-weighted scan. **E, F:** Scans obtained 5 months after start of therapy. Again there is a persistent residual mass anterior to the aorta, essentially unchanged in size from the previous examination. Note the heterogeneous high signal intensity pattern on the T2-weighted image. Even though the initial mass has regressed markedly, the lack of change in size between months 2 and 5 and the persistently "active" MR signal pattern strongly suggest residual active disease. The patient was asymptomatic at this point.

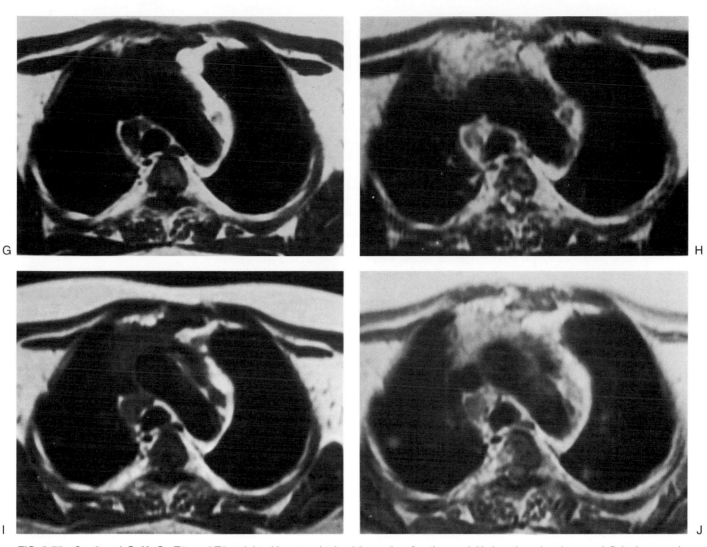

FIG. 2-75. *Continued.* **G, H:** On T1- and T2-weighted images obtained 9 months after therapy initiation, there has been a definite increase in the mass size compared to the previous examination. Note again the low homogeneous signal intensity on the T1-weighted image compared to the heterogeneous, mostly high signal intensity seen on the T2-weighted image. Additionally, an enlarged right paratracheal lymph node can now be identified. On the basis of these findings, therapy was reinitiated. **I, J:** Twelve months following the initial diagnosis, the mass has decreased somewhat in size since the previous examination. However, a pattern of high signal intensity on T2-weighted images persists, suggesting a lack of response. Note also the appearance of pulmonary lesions. The patient expired 2 months following the last study. This case represents a typical example of the dissociation between the evolution of size and that of the MR signal intensity pattern, thus demonstrating the unique information MR can provide in this category of patients.

intense pattern within 6 to 8 weeks of the initiation of therapy. If, however, an active pattern (homogeneous and/or heterogeneous hyperintense) is observed, especially beyond 4 to 6 months after therapy, a diagnosis of remission should be questioned.

Thus, even though false positive diagnoses do occur in the first 4 months of therapy, a lack of rapid response may be a significant indicator of therapy ineffectiveness. At this time, available data are insufficient to confirm this point, and assessment of signal intensities has not been reliably quantified to permit objective comparisons of disease activity status.

As demonstrated by Nyman et al., residual masses may slowly disappear over a 12- to 18-month period (317). MRI

can be used at regular intervals during that period, to ensure continued resolution of the abnormality. Indeed, in 20% of patients, MRI will reveal that the residual mass still contains areas of high signal intensity suspicious for active disease (see Fig. 2-75). In other cases, even though the pattern of the residual mass is one of inactive mass (homogeneous hypointense), it is very likely that microscopic residual tumor cannot be detected by MRI given the low spatial resolution and the variability of signal intensities intrinsic to the method. In all such cases, continued surveillance is warranted until complete resolution. Reappearance of foci of high signal intensity in such masses are strong indicators of early recurrence and are usually noted before clinical symptoms.

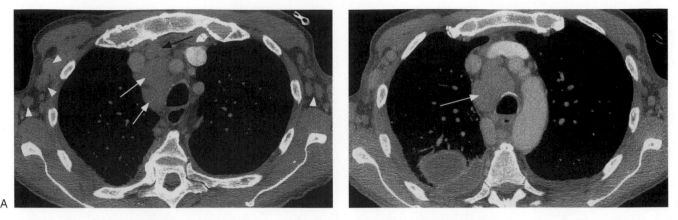

FIG. 2-76. Chronic lymphocytic leukemia with mediastinal and axillary lymph node enlargement. **A:** Contrast-enhanced CT at the aortic arch level shows large pretracheal and retrotracheal lymph nodes (*arrows*). Axillary lymph node enlargement (*arrowheads*) is also visible. **B:** At a lower level, large pretracheal lymph nodes (*arrow*) are visible. A right pleural effusion is also present.

Leukemia

Mediastinal lymph nodes can be involved in patients with leukemia, particularly lymphocytic leukemia. In one study, involvement of thoracic lymph nodes was present at autopsy in 50% and 67% of patients respectively with acute and chronic lymphocytic leukemia (Fig. 2-76) and 35% and 36% of patients with acute and chronic myelogenous leukemia (Figs. 2-77, 2-78), although lymph node enlargement was present in only 41% of these; on chest radiographs, enlarged mediastinal lymph nodes were visible in 17% (325). Mediastinal lymph node enlargement is more common than hilar node enlargement (325).

Approximately 15% of children with acute lymphoblastic leukemia have so-called ''lymphoma syndrome,'' with mediastinal mass present in more than 50% of cases; differentiation of NHL with marrow involvement from leukemia with lymphoma syndrome is difficult (4).

In patients with acute or chronic myeologeneous leukemia, masses of malignant myeloid precursor cells may be found in an extramedullary location; these masses are termed granulocytic sarcoma (326). They most commonly are present at the time of first diagnosis of leukemia. In about 50% of cases, masses involve the mediastinum (see Figs. 2-77 and 2-78), either as a focal mass or generalized widening. Lymph node enlargement or mediastinal infiltration can be seen. Any portion of the mediastinum can be affected (326).

Castleman's Disease

Castleman's disease (327) (also referred to by a number of other terms, including angiofollicular mediastinal lymph node hyperplasia, angiomatous lymphoid hamartoma, and giant mediastinal lymph node hyperplasia) is a disease of unknown etiology (265,328). Histologically, two forms of the disease have been described, the hyaline-vascular type, and the plasma cell type (328). From a clinical standpoint, Castleman's disease is also classified as localized or multicentric (15).

The hyaline-vascular type of Castleman's disease occurs in up to 90% of cases, and is characterized histologically by lymph nodes having hypervascular hyaline germinal centers marked by extensive capillary proliferation. Patients with the hyaline-vascular type are usually children or young adults, are usually asymptomatic, and their disease behaves in a benign fashion, with cure following complete surgical resection (15,329). Up to 70% of patients have an asymptomatic, localized mediastinal mass on radiographs and CT.

Unlike the hyaline-vascular type of Castleman's disease, the plasma-cell variety often presents as a multicentric process, associated with generalized lymphadenopathy and hepatosplenomegaly; most cases of multicentric Castleman's disease are of the plasma-cell variant, with some cases having mixed histology. Clinically, multicentric disease occurs in an older population than localized Castleman's disease, with most patients being in their fifth or sixth decade (329). It often results in a systemic illness, associated with anemia, infections, malignancies such as lymphoma or Kaposi's sarcoma, fever, hypergammaglobulinemia, and the POEMS syndrome (polyneuropathy, organomegaly, endocrinopathy, monoclonal protein abnormality, and skin abnormalities) (265). When associated with localized node involvement, such systemic findings usually disappear following total resection; however, the multicentric form of the disease is difficult to treat and usually progressive, even with the use of steroids and chemotherapeutic agents.

On contrast-enhanced CT, Castleman's disease localized to the mediastinum typically shows dense contrast enhancement (16,49,56,330); any mediastinal compartment can be involved, as can abdominal lymph nodes (see Fig. 2-1B; Fig. 2-79) (331). Central, dense, or flocculent lymph node calcifications can occasionally be seen (16,265,332). In a report of CT findings in six patients with multicentric Castleman's disease, all had retroperitoneal lymphadenopathy and splenomegaly; axillary, inguinal, mesenteric, peripancreatic, and mediastinal lymphadenopathy were also seen (16,333). Patients with multicentric Castleman's disease

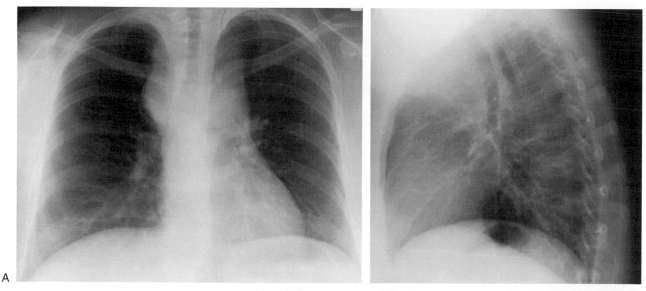

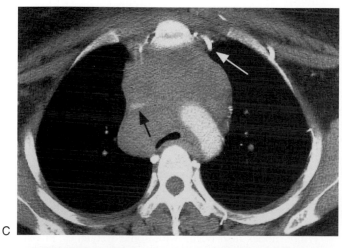

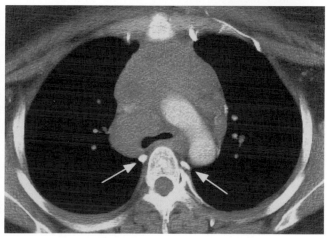

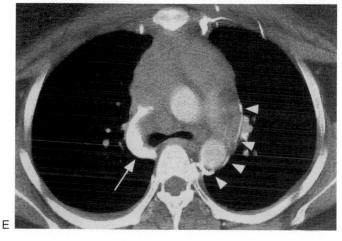

FIG. 2-77. Chronic myeologeneous leukemia with extramedullary involvement of mediastinal lymph nodes (granulocytic sarcoma). **A,B:** Posteroanterior and lateral chest radiographs show a superior and anterior mediastinal mass. **C:** CT at the level of the aortic arch shows enlarged pretracheal and prevascular lymph nodes with evidence of superior vena cava obstruction (*black arrow*). Numerous enhance veins in the chest wall including the internal mammary vein (*white arrow*) serve as collateral pathways. **D:** At a lower level, enhancement of the azygos and hemiazygos veins (*arrows*) reflects their function as collaterals. **E:** The azygos arch (*arrow*) and left superior intercostal vein (*arrowheads*) are densely opacified and represent significant collaterals.

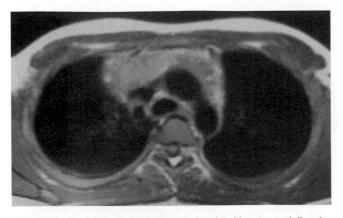

FIG. 2-78. Chronic myeologeneous leukemia with extramedullary involvement of mediastinal lymph nodes (granulocytic sarcoma): MRI appearance. T1-weighted image shows a large lobulated mass involving the anterior mediastinum. This appearance is nonspecific.

evaluated using dynamic contrast-enhanced CT have shown early, dense, uniform enhancement of enlarged mediastinal lymph nodes (15). Further imaging findings reported in patients with multicentric disease include skin thickening, pleural and pericardial effusions, and ascites (15,329,333).

Similar findings have more recently been identified in patients with AIDS, including hypervascular follicular hy-

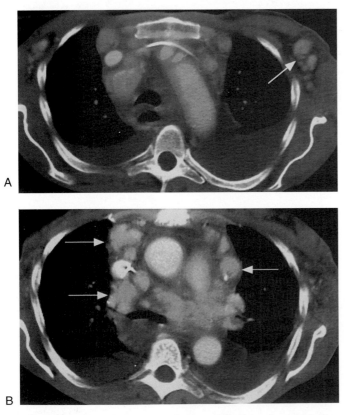

FIG. 2-79. Diffuse Castleman's disease. **A,B:** Extensive, enhancing mediastinal lymphadenopathy (*arrows* in **B**) in a patient with the diffuse form of Castleman's disease. The enhancement is typical. Enlarged axillary (*arrow* in **A**), abdominal, and inguinal lymph nodes were also visible. Bilateral pleural effusions are also present.

perplasia, indistinguishable from the plasma-cell type of Castleman's disease. Hypervascular follicular hyperplasia has also been seen in association with Kaposi's sarcoma (KS). Similar features have also been described in patients with angioimmunoblastic lymphadenopathy (AIL). This is especially significant given the propensity of AIL to evolve into malignancy.

Other Lymphoproliferative Disorders

In addition to those diseases listed above, a variety of uncommon lymphoproliferative diseases affecting the lung can be associated with hilar or mediastinal lymph node enlargement (328,334). These include posttransplantation lymphoproliferative disorders, angioimmunoblastic lymphadenopathy, lymphoid interstitial pneumonitis, and lymphomatoid granulomatosis (328,334,335). Among these, lymph node enlargement is most common with angioimmunoblastic lymphadenopathy, a disease most common in patients over 50 years of age, characterized by enlarged, hypervascular lymph nodes, constitutional symptoms, and infections (328,334).

Metastatic Tumor

Metastases to mediastinal lymph nodes from extrathoracic malignancies are uncommon. In a review of 1,071 cases of extrathoracic neoplasms, only 25 (2.3%) had evidence of hilar or mediastinal adenopathy (336). The extrathoracic tumors most likely to metastasize to the mediastinum are carcinomas of the head and neck, genitourinary tract, breast, and malignant melanoma.

Most mestastatic tumors cause lymph node enlargement without distinguishing characteristics. Hypervascularity is the exception, most often secondary to metastatic leiomyosarcoma, neurofibrosarcoma, and melanoma. Enhancing lymph nodes also occur with some frequency in patients with primary lung cancer, metastatic to mediastinal nodes. Calcification may also occur, especially in patient with metastatic mucinous adenocarcinomas (see Figs. 2-62C and 2-63).

The location of enlarged nodes is sometimes suggestive of the primary tumor site. Lymph node enlargment involving posterior mediastinal and paravertebral lymph nodes suggests an abdominal location for the primary tumor, and superior mediastinal lymph node involvement suggest a head and neck tumor. Internal mammary lymph node metastases are most likely caused by breast carcinoma (221). In a review of 219 women with breast cancer (221) who had CT, 20.5% had internal mammary lymph node enlargement. Of these, 71% had unilateral involvement, and multiple intercostal spaces were involved in 57%; the upper intercostal spaces were most frequently involved. Average node diameter was 1.95 cm (range 0.6 to 6.0 cm). Paracardiac lymph node enlargement can occur as a result of metastasis from abdominal or thoracic tumors in approximately equal numbers. In two studies (226,227) reviewing the causes of paracardiac lymph node enlargement, although a variety of metastatic tumors were responsible, the most common were colon carcinoma, lung carcinoma, ovarian carcinoma, and breast carcinoma.

Sarcoidosis

Mediastinal lymph node enlargement is very common with sarcoidosis, occurring in 60% to 90% of patients at some stage in their disease. About half of these will also show findings of lung disease on plain radiographs. In a study by Kirks et al. (268), lymph node enlargement was seen in association with lung disease in 41% of 150 patients, and in 43% it appeared as an isolated abnormality on chest radiographs. However, it must be recognized that a greater percentage of patients with lymph node enlargement caused by sarcoidosis will show abnormalities on high-resolution CT (337).

Typically, node enlargement involves the hilar as well as mediastinal node groups, and masses appear bilateral and symmetrical in the large majority of patients (268,338); this combination usually allows the differentiation of sarcoidosis from lymphoma. The presence of hilar lymph node enlargement is so typical of sarcoidosis that the absence of this finding in a patient with mediastinal lymphadenopathy should lead one to question the diagnosis. In order of decreasing frequency, paratracheal, aorticopulmonary, subcarinal, and prevascular lymph nodes are also commonly involved (Fig. 2-80); internal mammary, paravertebral, and retrocrural lymph node enlargement can also be seen, but are much less common (269). In CT studies of patients with sarcoidosis, lymph node enlargement has been reported in more than 80% (267,269,337), with the great majority showing both hilar and mediastinal lymph node enlargement.

In many patients with sarcoidosis, chest radiographic and clinical findings are sufficient for diagnosis and clinical management, but approximately 25% of cases are associated with atypical findings and CT is obtained for further evalua-

tion (267,339). Even in these patients, however, CT can often show typical lymph node abnormalities. In a group of 25 patients with sarcoidosis having CT because plain radiographs suggested malignancy or other disease, or were not diagnostic of sarcoidosis (267), 84% had right paratracheal (56%) or bilateral (28%) paratracheal lymph node enlargement, and 60% had subcarinal node enlargment. Anterior mediastinal lymph node enlargement was present in 56%; although anterior lymphadenopathy has been regarded as unusual based on plain radiographic studies, it is very common on CT. Although 81% of patients had hilar lymph node enlargement, it was bilateral in only 56% and unilateral in 25%; this atypical distribution likely reflects the groups studied.

In patients with sarcoidosis, lymph nodes can be several cm in diameter, but sarcoid is not generally associated with large localized masses as is lymphoma. Lymph nodes can calcify densely or show a stippled or egg-shell appearance (see Fig. 2-62A), and rarely enhance (see Fig. 2-67B) or appear necrotic on contrast enhanced scans (339).

A variety of patterns of pulmonary involvement from small nodules to large ill-defined masses or pulmonary fibrosis can also be seen in patients with sarcoidosis. However, it should be kept in mind that not all patients with active sarcoidosis show lymph node enlargement on CT. It is common to see typical features of sarcoid lung involvement on high-resolution CT without lymph node enlargement being visible.

Infections

A variety of infectious agents can cause mediastinal lymph node enlargement during the acute phase of disease. These include tuberculosis, a number of fungal infections including histoplasmosis and coccidioidomycosis, bacterial infections, and viral infections (see Fig. 2-67A). Typically, there will be symptoms and signs of acute infection, and chest radiographs will show evidence of lung disease, al-

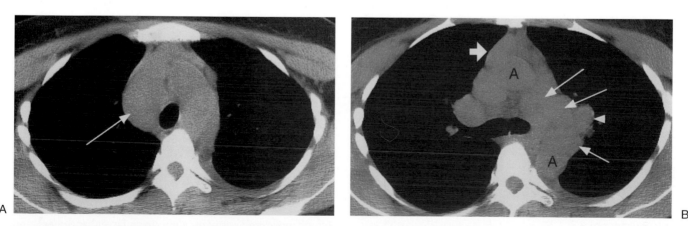

FIG. 2-80. Mediastinal lymphadenopathy in sarcoidosis. **A:** Unenhanced CT at the level of the aortic arch reveals marked enlargement of pretracheal lymph nodes (*arrow*). **B:** Aorticopulmonary window lymph node enlargement (*arrows*), left hilar lymph node enlargement (*arrowhead*), and prevascular lymph node enlargement (*short arrow*) are also seen. *A*, aorta.

though this is not always the case. In patients with prior granulomatous infections, lymph node calcification is common (249), with such nodes appearing normal in size or enlarged.

Tuberculosis

Hilar and mediastinal lymph node enlargement is commonly seen on CT in patients with active tuberculosis (TB) (259), although it is more frequently seen in children than adults (12). In a study by Im et al. (13), mediastinal lymph node enlargement was seen on CT in 9 of 29 patients with newly diagnosed disease, and in 2 of 12 patients with reactivation.

Lymph node enlargement is usually seen on the side of lung disease, but involvement of contralateral nodes can sometimes be present. Although Lee et al. (259) indicate that lymphadenopathy without lung disease is unusual in tuberculosis patients, except in the presence of AIDS, in a study by Im et al. (12), only 61% of patients with tuberculous lymphadenopathy had evidence of pulmonary tuberculosis on chest radiographs. Right sided adenopathy usually predominates (12,259); right paratracheal lymph node enlargement was seen in 87% of the cases reported by Im et al., whereas right tracheobronchial nodes were abnormal in 65% (Table 2-8). However, it should be noted that in the study by Im et al., right sided pulmonary tuberculosis was twice as common as disease on the left.

In a study by Im et al. (12) of 23 patients with active TB, nodes larger than 2 cm in diameter invariably showed central areas of low attenuation on contrast-enhanced CT, with peripheral rim enhancement. It should be noted, however, that these areas of low attenuation are not of water density, but range from about 40 to 60 H; they are visible only on contrast enhanced scans. Although smaller nodes did not typically show low attenuation, only one of the 23 patients had nodes less than 2 cm in diameter. In a small percentage of cases, areas of low attenuation can be seen extending outside nodes, with obliteration of mediastinal fat, representing tuberculous mediastinitis (340) or a cold abscess (12). In patients with large areas of low attenuation seen on CT, constitutional

symptoms were frequent. Rim-enhancing lymph nodes have also been reported in nearly 85% of AIDS patients and 67% of HIV(−) patients with culture or histologically verified tuberculosis (14).

CT more accurately defines the presence and extent of lymph node enlargement than does routine chest radiography in patients with tuberculosis. In particular, the finding of low-attenuation necrotic lymph nodes, with rim enhancement following contrast infusion, strongly suggests a diagnosis of mycobacterial infection, both in immunocompetent patients and in patients who are HIV-positive (12,14,341,342) (see Figs. 2-4A and 2-64). Although a similar appearance may be seen in patients with fungal infections, especially cryptococcosis and histoplasmosis, this appearance is less frequent in patients with lymphadenopathy resulting from metastatic neoplasm, Kaposi's sarcoma, or lymphoma, and in our experience almost always indicates the presence of a treatable infection (343). In some cases CT can serve as a guide for determining the best sites for node biopsy, and can help determine whether mediastinoscopy or parasternal mediastinotomy is most appropriate.

Three patterns of lymph node enlargement have been reported on MRI in patients with tuberculosis (344), correlating with clinical symptoms and pathologic findings, and paralleling the expected CT findings in such patients (12). In 14 (61%) of 23 cases, nodes were inhomogeneous with marked peripheral enhancement after injection of contrast material (344). Areas of enhancement were on intermediate in intensity on T1-weighted images and hypointense on T2-weighted images, corresponding pathologically to peripheral granulation tissue within nodes. Unenhanced areas were hypointense on T1-weighted images and hyperintense on T2-weighted images, corresponding to areas of central caseation or liquefaction. Almost all patients with this pattern had clinical symptoms of active TB.

In six (26%) patients with the second pattern of node involvement, nodes were relatively homogeneous and hyperintense to muscle on both T1- and T2-weighted images and enhanced homogeneously after contrast infusion (344). This pattern correlated with the presence of granulomas without necrosis or with minimal necrosis; symptoms were minimal or absent in these patients. In the remaining three patients (13%), nodes were homogeneously and hypointense on both T1- and T2-weighted images and did not enhance after contrast infusion. Such nodes were fibrocalcific and patients had no symptoms.

Histoplasmosis

Infection with Histoplasma capsulatum is a well-recognized cause of hilar and mediastinal lymph node enlargement. In reported patients with acute or subacute histoplasmosis, CT has shown paratracheal, subcarinal, and hilar lymph node enlargement with irregular enhancement and necrotic regions as in patients with tuberculosis (345). Masses ranged up to several centimeters in diameter. Rim

TABLE 2-8. *Lymph node enlargement in 23 patients with tuberculosis*

Site	ATS designation	Percent abnormal
Right paratracheal	2R	83
Left paratracheal	2L	4
Right paratracheal	4R	87
Left paratracheal	4L	9
Right tracheobronchial	10R	65
Subcarinal	7	52
Aorticopulmonary	5	35
Right hilar	11R	30
Left hilar	11L	9

enhancement or enhancing septa within the mass have been described.

Fibrosing Mediastinitis

In some patients with granulomatous disease involving mediastinal lymph nodes, extension of the disease process to involve surrounding mediastinal tissues results in extensive fibrosis (346). This is termed fibrosing or granulomatous mediastinitis. Symptomatic encasement and/or compression of a number of mediastinal structures, particularly vessels, and the trachea or esophagus, can result (347). The most common causes are histoplasmosis, tuberculosis, and sarcoidosis, but fibrosing mediastinitis can also be related to autoimmune disease, drugs, retroperitoneal fibrosis, or may be idiopathic (348–350). In patients with histoplasmosis, it has been suggested that fibrosis may result from seepage of fungal antigen from adjacent lymph nodes. Extension of the infectious process into the mediastinum, as can be seen in tuberculosis (12), may also be associated.

Typically, enlarged lymph nodes in patients with granulo-matous disease, such as histoplasmosis, tuberculosis, and sarcoidosis are sharply defined. Fibrosing mediastinitis is manifested on CT by replacement of low-density mediastinal fat by higher density fibrous tissue, often associated with calcification (Fig. 2-81). In the presence of fibrosing medi-astinitis, discrete enlarged lymph nodes cannot be identified.

Manifestations on CT include hilar and mediastinal masses, stippled or diffuse calcification, and compression and/or encasement of the trachea, main bronchi, or mediasti-nal vessels (348). Those structures most often involved are those that have the thinnest walls (e.g., superior vena cava), or the longest mediastinal course (e.g., trachea and left main bronchus and right pulmonary artery). In a study of patients with fibrosing mediastinitis, the most common complica-tions were narrowing or obstruction of the superior vena cava (39%), bronchi (33%), pulmonary artery (18%), and esophagus (9%) (351). Rarely, these findings primarily af-fect the posterior mediastinum, with esophageal encasement and dysphagia predominating (350). CT may play a very important role in these patients by suggesting the proper diagnosis and identifying compression of vascular and non-

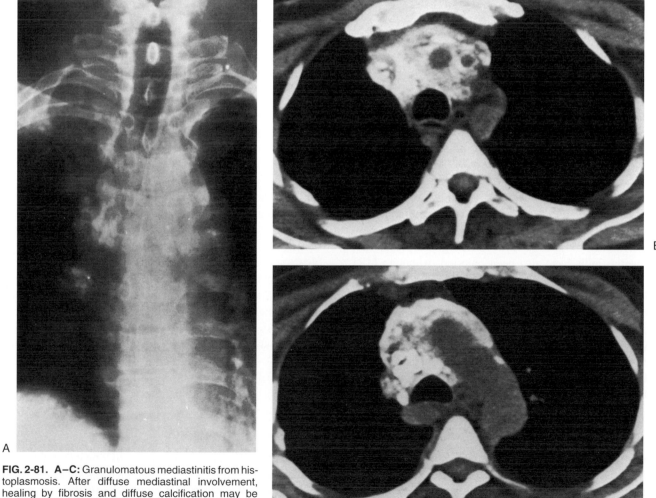

FIG. 2-81. A–C: Granulomatous mediastinitis from his-toplasmosis. After diffuse mediastinal involvement, healing by fibrosis and diffuse calcification may be seen. The superior vena cava appears obstructed.

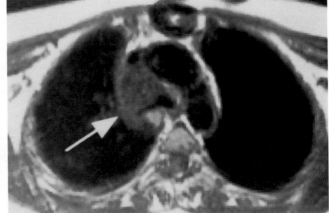

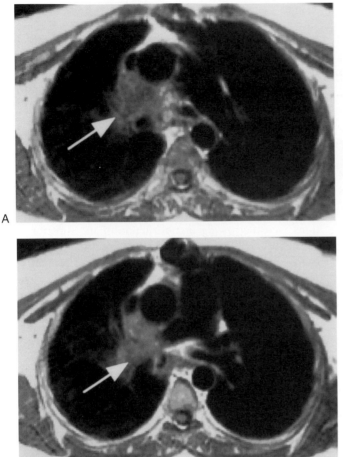

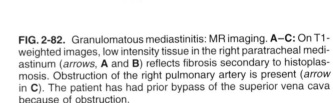

FIG. 2-82. Granulomatous mediastinitis: MR imaging. **A–C:** On T1-weighted images, low intensity tissue in the right paratracheal mediastinum (*arrows*, **A** and **B**) reflects fibrosis secondary to histoplasmosis. Obstruction of the right pulmonary artery is present (*arrow* in **C**). The patient has had prior bypass of the superior vena cava because of obstruction.

vascular structures. It may obviate more invasive and potentially dangerous procedures (348). It has also been shown that in patients with a localized pattern of fibrosis with calcification, histoplasmosis is the likely cause and steroid treatment is of little benefit, whereas those having more diffuse fibrosis without calcification likely have idiopathic disease and steroids may be of value (351).

MRI findings in patients with fibrosing and granulomatous mediastinitis have also been reported. Although MRI and CT are equivalent in defining the extent of adenopathy or fibrosis, CT is superior in demonstrating node calcification, a finding that is often important in making the diagnosis. MRI, however, was particularly valuable in assessing vascular patency without the need for intravenous contrast media (Fig. 2-82). On T2-weighted images, fibrosing mediastinitis is noted to be of relatively low signal intensity, likely the result of fibrosis and calcification.

FATTY LESIONS

Fat is specifically recognized on CT by its low CT numbers, which vary from −40 to −130 HU (2). Fat is normally present in the mediastinum and its amount may increase with age. In patients older than 25, most of the fat visible in the

anterior mediastinum is contained within the fibrous skeleton of the involuted thymus.

Normal fat is unencapsulated and equally distributed throughout the connective tissue matrix of the mediastinum. The contours of the mediastinum are not generally affected by normal amounts of fat. However, accumulations of fat in the anterior cardiophrenic angles, or epicardiac fat pads, can be assymetric and can suggest the presence of a mass on chest radiographs (352).

Abnormalities of fat distribution can be diffuse, as in mediastinal lipomatosis, or focal, as in the presence of lipomas or fat-containing transdiaphragmatic hernias. In our experience, most fatty masses are seen in the peridiaphragmatic areas and they most often represent herniation of abdominal fat (Figs. 2-83–2-85). In the large majority of cases, discovery of the fatty nature of a mass indicates its benignancy, but mediastinal liposarcomas rarely occur.

Mediastinal Lipomatosis

Lipomatosis is a benign condition in which overabundant amounts of histologically normal, unencapsulated fat accumulate in the mediastinum. Lipomatosis may be associated with Cushing's syndrome, steroid treatment, or obesity, but

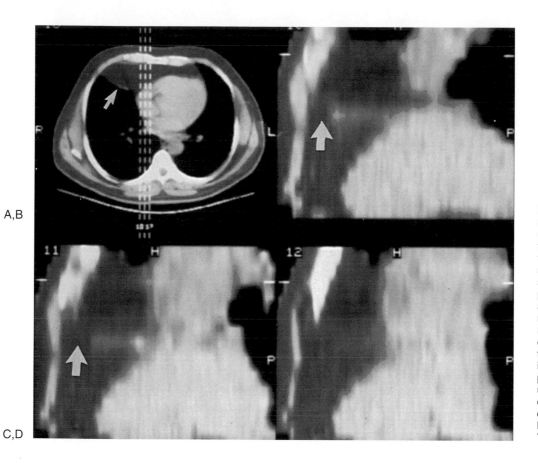

A,B

C,D

FIG. 2-83. Morgagni hernia. **A:** CT section at the level of the cardiophrenic angle. This study was performed to further evaluate a patient with a prominent paracardiac density of uncertain etiology (not shown). Excessive homogeneous paracardiac fat is present (*arrow*), accounting for the radiographic abnormality. **B–D:** Sequential sagittal reconstructions at the levels indicated by the dotted lines in **A**. Note that the paracardiac fat in this case is continuous with fat below the diaphragm which appears discontinuous (*arrows* in **B** and **C**). Surgically confirmed Morgagni's hernia. (Case courtesy of Deborah Reede, M.D., Long Island College Hospital, New York, NY.)

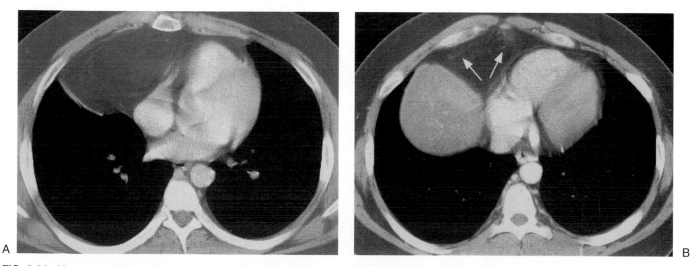

A

B

FIG. 2-84. Morgagni hernia. **A,B:** Sequential sections through the lower thorax and upper portion of the right diaphragm, respectively, show the presence of omental fat anteriorly, recognizable by the finding of visible mesenteric vessels (*arrows* in **B**) within the fat. Note that there is some compression on the adjacent right side of the heart, most pronounced in **A**.

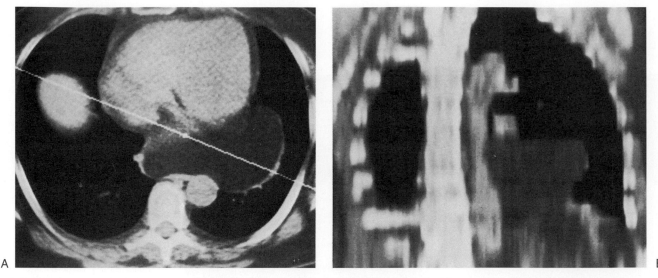

FIG. 2-85. Large paraesophageal omental hernia in a 39-year-old woman with dysphagia. **A:** CT scan at level of an apparent soft-tissue mass identified in the lower thorax overlying the left heart border on corresponding chest radiograph. Note the presence of a large, homogeneous fatty mass in the posterior mediastinum within which faint linear densities can be identified compatible with omental vessels. **B:** Oblique reconstruction through axis of line seen in **A** confirms the true intra-abdominal origin of the mass, found at surgery to represent omental fat extending into the mediastinum via a large esophageal hiatus. Peridiaphragmatic fatty masses are much more likely to represent hernias containing fat than lipomas.

these factors are absent in up to one-half of cases (353). It is unassociated with symptoms. Lipomatosis is relatively common, and is often detected incidentally in patients having chest CT.

The excess fat deposition is most prominent in the upper mediastinum, resulting in smooth mediastinal widening as shown on chest radiographs, and convex or bulging mediastinal pleural surfaces on CT (Fig. 2-86). Tracheal compression or displacement is uniformly absent (45,354,355). Less commonly, fat also accumulates in the cardiophrenic angles

and paraspinal areas (Figs. 2-87 and 2-88) (356–358). In patients with lipomatosis, the fat should appear homogeneously low in attenuation, sharply outlining mediastinal vessels and lymph nodes. If the fat appears inhomogeneous or the margins of mediastinal structures are ill-defined, superimposed processes such as mediastinitis, hemorrhage, tumor infiltration, fibrosis, or postsurgical changes should be considered. The appearance of smooth mediastinal widening on plain radiographic is characteristic of mediastinal lipomatosis, and in patients with a suitable clinical history, usu-

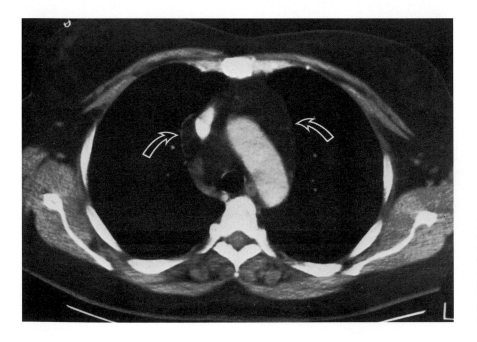

FIG. 2-86. Mediastinal lipomatosis. Contrast-enhanced CT image at the level of the aortic arch shows abundant fat throughout the mediastinum causing distortion of the normal pleuromediastinal interfaces (*arrows*). Note that the fat is similar in density to subcutaneous fat, and is exceedingly homogeneous. This patient had no history of either steroid therapy or Cushing's syndrome.

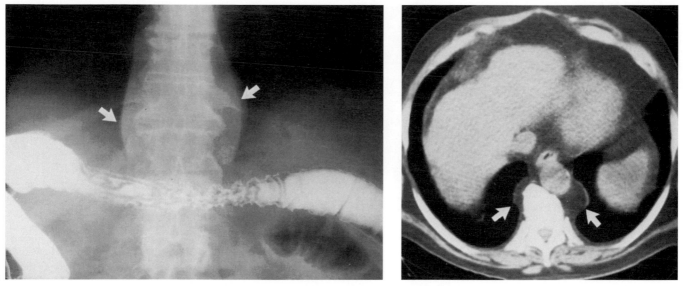

FIG. 2-87. Mediastinal lipomatosis. **A:** Coned-down anteroposterior radiograph of the lower thoracic spine in a patient undergoing a barium enema. The paraspinal interfaces are abnormally convex bilaterally (*arrows*), the appearance of which is nonspecific. **B:** CT section at the level of the distal esophagus unequivocally confirms that the abnormality seen in **A** is caused by excessive fat in the posterior mediastinum (*arrows*). Note again the homogeneous nature of the fat, confirming this as lipomatosis.

ally requires no further evaluation; however, if confirmation of this condition is desired, CT is diagnostic.

A rare condition, termed multiple symmetrical lipomatosis may mimic the appearance of simple lipomatosis on CT; however, this entity often results in compression of mediastinal structures, the trachea in particular, and does not involve the anterior mediastinum, cardiophrenic angles, or paraspinal regions. In addition, periscapular lipomatous masses are almost always present (44).

Lipoma and Liposarcoma

Mediastinal lipoma is uncommon, constituting approximately 2% of all mediastinal tumors (359,360). As with other mesenchymal tumors, lipomas can occur in any part in the mediastinum but are most common in the prevascular space. Lipomas are soft and pliable and do not result in symptomatic compression of adjacent structures unless they are very large. They may or may not be encapsulated. Although they variably contain fibrous septa, lipomas appear

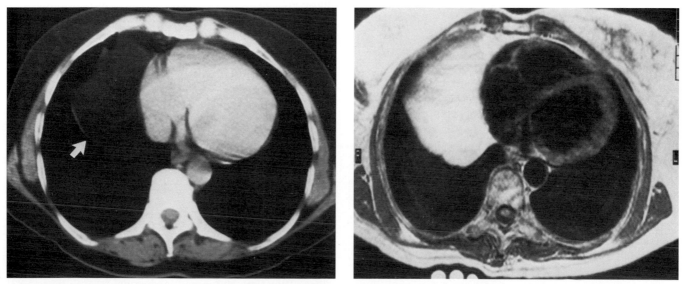

FIG. 2-88. Cardiophrenic lipomatosis. **A:** Contrast-enhanced CT image through the heart demonstrates a large accumulation of fat adjacent to the right heart border (*arrow*). Note the similarity in appearance between paracardiac and subcutaneous fat. **B:** T1-weighted MR image at the same level as shown in **A**. On T1-weighted sequences fat appears bright (compare with the signal intensity of adjacent subcutaneous fat).

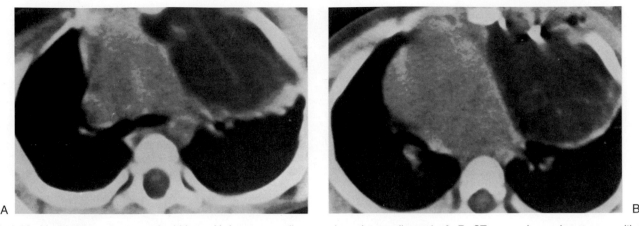

A   B

FIG. 2-89. Lipoblastoma. An 8-month-old boy with large mass discovered on chest radiograph. **A, B:** CT scans show a large mass with low CT numbers compatible with a fatty tumor. The suggestion of chest wall invasion anteriorly in **B**, the patient's age, and the minimal inhomogeneity would be unusual for a simple lipoma. Surgery was therefore recommended. A lipoblastoma, a rare benign tumor of childhood made of immature adipose tissue with rapid growth and local recurrence potential, was removed.

to have homogeneously low CT numbers. Their boundaries are typically smooth and sharply defined, and adjacent mediastinal structures appear well-defined and sharply marginated.

Mediastinal liposarcoma and lipoblastoma are rare malignant tumors, composed largely of fat. Histologic differentiation between a lipoma and well-differentiated liposarcoma depends on the presence of mitotic activity, cellular atypia, fibrosis, neovascularization, and tumor infiltration. CT findings suggesting liposarcoma or lipoblastoma include (a) inhomogeneous attenuation, with evidence of significant amounts of soft-tissue within the fatty mass, (b) poor definition of adjacent mediastinal structures, (c) evidence of infiltration or invasion of mediastinal structures (Fig. 2-89; see Fig. 2-38) (361–364). However, as documented by DeSantos et al. (365), the diagnosis of a liposarcoma is often difficult using CT. In their series of 17 liposarcomas, a preoperative diagnosis was made in only four cases (22%).

Other Fatty Masses

Other rare, fatty lesions have been reported to involve the mediastinum. Thymolipoma usually appears on CT as a large fatty mass, in the anterior mediastinum, containing wisps or strands of fibrous tissue (43) (see Fig. 2-35). Fat is also commonly identifiable as a component of mediastinal germ-cell tumors (see Fig. 2-40). In the posterior mediastinum, spinal lipomas rarely may present as primary mediastinal masses (366). Other fat-containing masses that have been identified by CT in the posterior mediastinum include angiolipomas (367,368) and even fatty transformation of thoracic extramedullary hematopoiesis following splenectomy (47). Fatty hernias are described below. Angiolipoma is a very rare benign mediastinal tumor composed of mature fat and blood vessels, which appears encapsulated on CT and contains both fat and soft tissue; it can mimic the appearance of liposarcoma (368).

Hernias Containing Fat

There are several direct connections between the abdomen and mediastinum that permit passage of intraabdominal fat into the thorax.

Omental fat is freely mobile, and can herniate through the foramen of Morgagni to create the appearance of a cardiophrenic angle mass, almost always located on the right side (see Figs. 2-83 and 2-84) (46,369). The transverse colon may accompany the omentum in patients with a Morgagni hernia. Fine linear densities can sometimes be seen within herniated omental fat and probably represent omental vessels (see Fig. 2-84). When seen within a fatty mass, these linear densities should suggest fat herniation rather than a lipoma.

Fat herniation through the foramen of Bochdalek occurs most often on the left side since the liver limits the frequency of its occurrence on the right (370,371). Although they are most often located in the posterolateral diaphragm, they can occur anywhere along the posterior costodiaphragmatic margin. Bochdalek hernias in adults usually contain retroperitoneal fat, although kidney can occasionally be present. CT has shown that small Bochdalek hernias may occur in as many as 5% of normals. Characteristically, a thinning or defect in the diaphragm is visible on CT, marginating the collection of fat.

Herniation of perigastric fat through the phrenicoesophageal membrane surrounding and fixating the esophagus to the diaphragm is the first step in the pathogenesis of hiatus hernias (372). The herniated fat can extend along the aorta and widen the paraspinal line or it can appear as a retrocardiac mass (see Fig. 2-85). Although multiplanar reconstructions are sometimes helpful for demonstrating the connections of the fatty hernia with abdominal fat (see Figs. 2-83 and 2-85), because of its multi-planar imaging capabilities, MRI may be better suited to the evaluation of such lesions (373).

MR Evaluation of Fatty Lesions

The MR appearance of fatty tissue has been well described (48,117,374,375). Typically, fat has a high signal intensity on both T1- and T2-weighted sequences, appearing identical to subcutaneous fat (see Figs. 2-41 and 2-88). Similar findings have been described, however, in patients with hematomas or hemorrhagic tumors. In an analysis of 17 patients with 18 lipomatous tumors, Dooms et al. reported that of 16 benign lesions, including 12 lipomas, the fatty components of the tumors were equally well visualized with both CT and MRI (375). As reported by London et al. in an evaluation of 15 patients with liposarcomas, MRI correctly identified the presence of fat in all eight cases in which it was present pathologically (374). Unfortunately, MRI has proven no more accurate than CT in differentiating liposarcomas from benign lipomas.

MEDIASTINAL CYSTS

Most mediastinal cysts are of congenital origin and include foregut-duplication cysts (i.e., bronchogenic, duplication, and neurenteric cysts), and pleuropericardial cysts (376). Thymic cyst, described above, may be congenital or acquired. Cysts account for about 9% of primary mediastinal masses in adults; foregut-duplication cysts account for 11% of mediastinal masses in children (4).

Bronchogenic Cysts

Bronchogenic cysts are most common, representing approximately 60% of foregut duplication cysts. They probably result from defective growth of the lung bud during fetal development (41,377). Bronchogenic cysts are lined by pseudostratified ciliated columnar epithelium, typical of the respiratory system, and frequently associated with smooth muscle, mucous glands, or cartilage in the cyst wall. Bronchogenic cysts contain fluid, which ranges in color from clear to milky white to brown; the fluid can contain variable amounts of protein and can be either serous in nature, hemorrhagic, or highly viscous and gelatenous. Cyst fluid can rarely contain milk of calcium.

On CT, bronchogenic cysts usually appear rounded or elliptical in shape, smooth in contour, and are sharply marginated. The wall of a bronchogenic cyst appears thin or is imperceptible (Fig. 2-90). Rarely, calcification of the cyst wall is present. Because of the variable composition of fluid contained within bronchogenic cysts, their attenuation on CT is highly variable (see Fig. 2-90) (4,378–384). Half of bronchogenic cysts are of water attenuation. In the other half, the CT density can vary from near that of water to higher than muscle. When dense, bronchogenic cysts may be difficult to distinguish from solid lesions. An important clue to the diagnosis can be their lack of enhancement on scans obtained following intravenous contrast enhancement. Mediastinal bronchogenic cysts rarely contain air or become infected, although this is common in patients with pulmonary cysts.

Bronchogenic cysts can be seen in any part of the mediastinum, but most are located in the middle or posterior mediastinum, near the carina (52%) (see Fig. 2-90), in the paratracheal region (19%) (Fig. 2-91), adjacent to the esophagus (14%), or in a retrocardiac location (9%) (385). A subcarinal location is most common on CT. They rarely occur in the

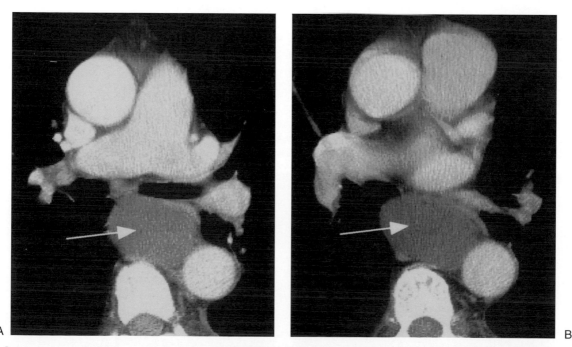

A   B

FIG. 2-90. Subcarinal bronchogenic cyst. **A,B:** A low attenuation bronchogenic cyst is visible (*arrows*) on a contrast-enhanced CT. Its wall is imperceptible.

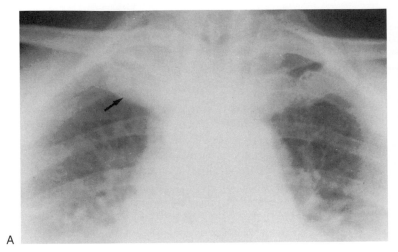

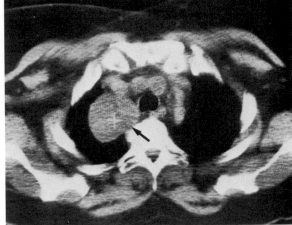

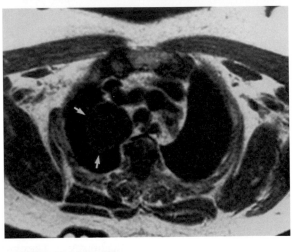

FIG. 2-91. Bronchogenic cyst: CT/MRI correlation. **A:** Coned-down view from a posteroanterior radiograph of the chest shows a mass (*arrow*) of uncertain etiology, initially felt to possibly be bronchogenic carcinoma. **B:** Nonenhanced CT section through the superior mediastinum shows a well-demarcated mass (*arrow*) with a density measuring within the range of soft tissue. This patient could not receive intravenous contrast media because of an allergy history. **C:** T1-weighted MR image at the same level as in **B** shows the mass to be of very low signal intensity (*arrows*). The mass is clearly distinct from the adjacent vessels and mediastinal fat. **D–G:** Single-level, multi-echo sequence obtained at the same levels as shown in **B** and **C**, using TEs of 30, 60, 90, and 120 msec, respectively. This technique allows acquisition of heavily T2-weighted images. Note that the signal intensity of the lesion steadily increases relative to all other tissues, including fat. This combination of findings is diagnostic of a cystic mass, in this location almost certainly a bronchogenic cyst. TE, echo time. (From ref. 404, with permission.)

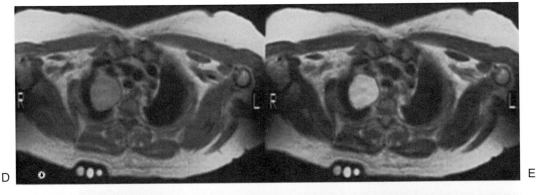

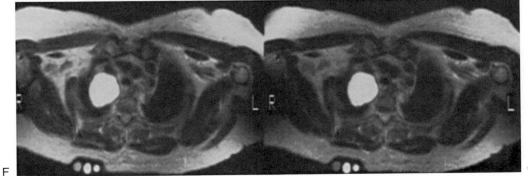

anterior mediastinum or the inferior aspect of the posterior mediastinum. Large bronchogenic cysts may be associated with symptoms because of compression of adjacent structures, such as the trachea and carina, mediastinal vessels, and the left atrium (386,387).

Small, asymptomatic cysts can be followed (388). However, enlargement over years is typical, and rapid enlargement can indicate hemorrhage or infection and be associated with pain. Because of their tendency to enlarge, surgical management has been traditional (389). Recently, percutaneous and transbronchial needle aspiration has been used for the diagnosis and treatment of bronchogenic cysts and other benign mediastinal fluid collections, including esophageal duplication cysts and mediastinal pseudocysts (388–393). In select cases, these procedures may obviate the need for more invasive procedures such as mediastinoscopy or thoracotomy.

Esophageal Duplication Cysts

Esophageal duplication cysts are lined by gastrointestinal tract mucosa and are often connected to the esophagus. Sixty percent are found in the lower posterior mediastinum, adjacent to the esophagus, and are sometimes found within its wall (Fig. 2-92) (41,392,394). Their appearance on CT is indistinguishable from that of bronchogenic cysts, except for their location (394,395). Rarely, these cysts may calcify (396).

Neurenteric Cysts

These rare lesions are connected to the meninges through a midline defect in one or more vertebral bodies, and are composed of both neural and gastrointestinal elements (41). A connection with the esophagus is often present. The appearance of neurenteric cyst on CT is the same as that of

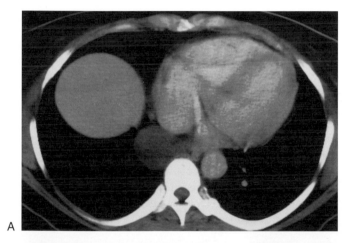

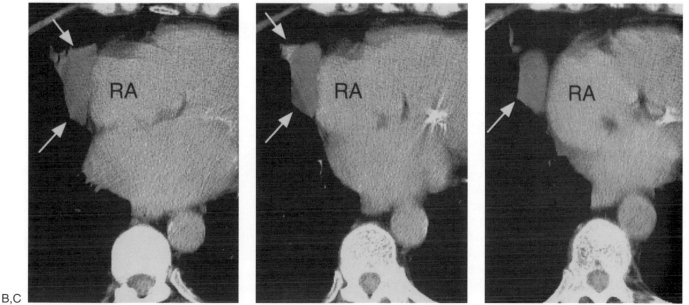

FIG. 2-92. Miscellaneous mediastinal cysts. **A:** Esophageal duplication cyst. Contrast enhanced CT section through the lower chest shows a well-defined fluid containing mass adjacent to the esophagus, findings characteristic of esophageal duplication cysts. **B–D:** Pericardial cyst. A well-defined low attenuation pericardial cyst (*arrows*) is visible in the right cardiophrenic angle on an unenhanced scan with attenuation clearly lower than the adjacent right atrium (*RA*). The key to the correct diagnosis of a pericardial cyst versus enlarged paracardiac nodes In this case is demonstration of water density within this lesion. Alternatively, images may be obtained both prior to and following administration of contrast to further confirm the avascular or cystic nature of this lesion. This approach is of particular value as mediastinal cysts frequently measure greater than water density prior to enhancement caused by the presence of prior hemhorrage, or elevated protein or debris within.

other duplication cysts, but the presence of the vertebral abnormality points to the diagnosis; vertebral anomalies are present in about half of cases (41). The cysts rarely contain air, because of communication with the viscera. They frequently cause pain and are generally diagnosed at a young age.

Pericardial Cysts

Pericardial cyst represents a defect in the embryogenesis of the coelomic cavity. Their walls are composed of connective tissue and a single layer of mesothelial cells. Most patients are asymptomatic. Approximately 90% of pericardial cysts contact the diaphragm, with 65% occurring the right cardiophrenic angle (Fig. 2-92B) and 25% in the left cardiophrenic angle; 10% are seen at higher levels. They can be seen as high as the pericardial recesses at the level of the proximal aorta and pulmonary arteries (397,398). Their appearance is usually diagnostic of their cystic nature. They are sharply marginated and have low CT numbers, although pericardial cysts with high CT numbers have been reported (see Fig. 2-92B) (399,400). Pleuropericardial cysts are not always round; they may assume different shapes when studied at different times (401). In some cases, cysts can extend into the major fissure. When small, they can sometimes be confused with enlarged cardiophrenic angle lymph nodes.

Differential Diagnosis of Cystic Masses

Differentiation of an uncomplicated congenital cyst from other cystic encapsulated lesions, such as abscess, chronic hematoma, cystic lymphangioma or hemangioma, cystic teratoma, or other cystic tumor relies on the clinical presentation, findings on correlative radiographic studies, and the location and appearance on CT of the cyst (41).

Cystic masses of the anterior mediastinum rarely represent a congenital cyst, but are more likely related to the presence of a cystic tumor or a thymic cyst. Mediastinal parathyroid cyst is a rare occurrence (196). Abscess, hematoma, and cystic tumors commonly demonstrate thick walls, with septa sometimes visible within the cystic space, and mixed-density fluids. Anterior meningocele may closely resemble a congenital cyst, but careful examination of adjacent sections should demonstrate the intraspinal connection of the mass through the neural foramen. Occasionally, loculated fluid in the superior pericardial recess can simulate a cystic mediastinal mass (402).

The potential of MRI to identify cystic or fluid-filled masses is well established (403). MRI has been used successfully to diagnose a wide range of lesions, including bronchogenic cysts, pericardial cysts, thymic cysts, colloid cysts within goiters, cystic hygromas, and even mediastinal pseudocysts (169,170,404–408). MRI is especially valuable in assessing complex cysts that do not appear fluid-filled on CT (379–383), especially when intravenous contrast cannot be administered (see Fig. 2-91) (404).

High-signal intensity is characteristically seen within cystic lesions on T2-weighted sequences regardless of the nature of the cyst contents, but variable patterns of signal intensity have been noted on T1-weighted sequences, presumably because of variable cyst contents and the presence of protein and/or hemorrhage or mucoid material (409). This variable appearance can be of some value in distinguishing the type of cyst or its contents. In patients with pericardial cysts containing serous fluid, the cysts always appeared less intense than muscle on T1-weighted images, while in patients with thymic cysts, the signal intensity ratio (SIR) of cyst to muscle ranged from 0.48 to 1.65 (409). However, in patients with bronchogenic cysts or cystic teratomas, the SIR were considerably higher, reflecting the complex nature of the cyst contents in these lesions; in all patients with these lesions, cysts appeared more intense than muscle and the SIR ranged from about 1.4 to more than 3 (409). A fluid-fluid level within a bronchogenic cyst has been reported on T1-weighted MRI (410).

VASCULAR TUMORS

Lymphangioma and Cystic Hygroma

Lymphangiomas are rare benign lesions of lymphatic origin and represent 0.7% to 4.5% of mediastinal tumors; most are present at birth and are detected in the first 2 years of life (411,412). Lymphangiomas are most common in the neck (75%) and axilla (20%). Although 10% of cervical lymphangiomas extend into the mediastinum, less than 5% of lymphangiomas are limited to the mediastinum itself (Fig. 2-93) (412). Patients may be asymptomatic, but compression of mediastinal structures can result in chest pain, cough, or dyspnea. Because of a tendency for local growth, surgery is recommended. Lymphangioma can be seen in adults, with or without a history of incomplete resection as a child. In

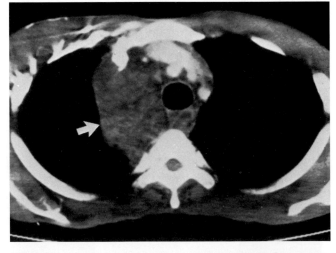

FIG. 2-93. Low attenuation mediastinal lymphangioma. Contrast-enhanced CT scan shows a heterogeneous, low-density, right paratracheal mass. Lymphangioma limited to the mediastinum is unusual.

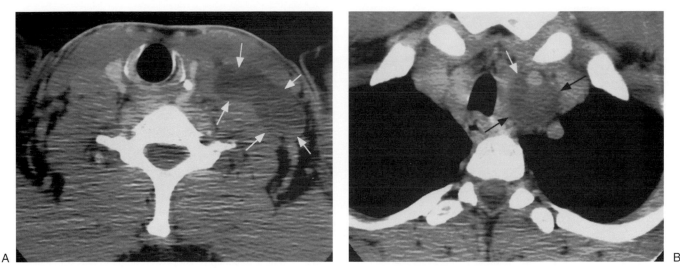

FIG. 2-94. Cystic hygroma. **A,B:** Sections through the lower neck and superior mediastinum, respectively, show a low attenuation mass (*arrows*) visible in the neck (**A**) and upper mediastinum (**B**). In **B**, the mass appears to envelop the left carotid artery.

adults, it is common for lymphangioma to be localized to the mediastinum.

Lymphangiomas are classified as capillary, cavernous, or cystic (hygroma), depending on the size of the lymph channels they contain. Cystic lymphangiomas are most common, and were seen in 63% of adult patients in one study (411); they may be either unilocular or multilocular, and contain either serous or chylous fluid (413); thin septations within the mass can sometimes be seen (413). In adults, lymphangiomas are most common in the anterior (28% to 37%) or superior (16% to 36%) mediastinum, but are also seen in the middle (20% to 26%) and posterior (16% to 28%) mediastinum. They can be quite large, ranging up to 30 cm in diameter (411,414).

On CT, their attenuation is usually homogeneous, and near to that of water (see Fig. 2-93; Figs. 2-94, 2-95), but they can be of higher attenuation, or variably composed of a combination of fluid, solid tissue, and fat; calcification is rare (411,413,415). Although they are usually well-circumscribed and localized, they may appear to envelop mediastinal structures (see Fig. 2-94) (413). Lymphangioma may be associated with vascular malformations that are easily identifiable following the administration of intravenous contrast (53,416,417). Simple lymphangiomas and hemangiomas composed of capillary-sized, thin-walled channels may appear as solid masses (see Fig. 2-85) (411). On MRI, heterogeneous signal is typical, with increased signal on T2-weighted images reflecting their fluid content (see Fig. 2-95).

Hemangioma

Hemangiomas are rare benign vascular tumors, accounting for less than 0.5% of mediastinal masses (52,418). They are composed of large interconnecting vascular channels with regions of thrombosis and varying amounts of interposed stroma, such as fat and fibrous tissue. Tumors are categorized according to the size and nature of their vascular spaces as capillary, cavernous, or venous; cavernous hemangiomas make up about 75% of cases (52). They are well defined and rarely are invasive (52).

Mediastinal hemangiomas are most common in young patients, and about 75% present before the age of 35 (52,266). One-third to one-half of cases are asymptomatic, but some patients present with symptoms of compression of mediastinal structures. Occasional cases are associated with peripheral hemangiomas or Osler-Weber-Rendu syndrome (52).

Hemangiomas most commonly arise in the anterior and posterior mediastinum. Of 14 cases studied by McAdams et al. (52), six (43%) were posterior, five (36%) were anterior, one was middle mediastinal, and two were multicompartmental. Extension into the neck may occur. In a review of 77 cases (266), 68% were primarily located in the anterior mediastinum, whereas 22% were posterior, and in 7%, extension into the neck was present. Masses may appear well marginated on CT (71%), inseparable from adjacent mediastinal structures (21%), or diffusely infiltrative (7%) (52). Apparent infiltration may or may not predict unresectability.

On CT, tumors are often heterogeneous in attenuation on unenhanced scans, and fat may occasionally be seen within them. Heterogenous enhancement is typical following contrast infusion, but is not always present (52). Enhancement may be dense, multifocal or diffuse, and central or peripheral. Opacified vascular channels can be seen within the mass, with rapid enhancement similar to that of normal mediastinal vessels. Phleboliths, though to be pathognomic, are visible up to 10% of cases on plain radiographs (266). On CT, punctate calcifications are visible in 21% and phleboliths are visible in 7% (52).

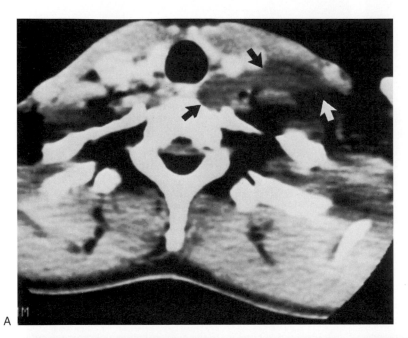

FIG. 2-95. Cystic hygroma. **A:** Contrast-enhanced CT section through the lower neck shows a well-defined cystic mass lying behind the carotid sheath; adjacent to the trachea, esophagus, and cervical spine; and extending laterally to lie behind the sternocleidomastoid muscle (*arrows*). This lesion also was visualized with CT extending inferiorly into the thoracic inlet and mediastinum (not shown). **B–E:** T2-weighted MR images through the lower neck and superior mediastinum in the same patient confirm the presence of an elongated cystic mass extending from the neck into the posterior mediastinum (*arrows*). Surgery confirmed cystic hygroma.

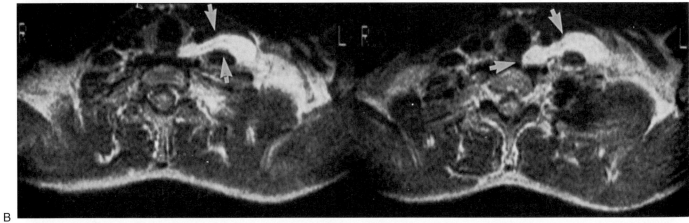

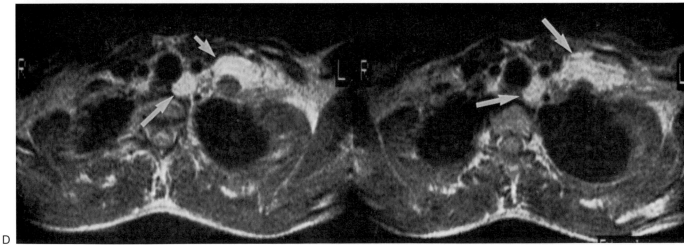

THE ESOPHAGUS

When sufficient mediastinal fat is present, the esophagus can be adequately visualized with CT. At successive levels in the mediastinum, the esophagus is in intimate contact anteriorly with the posterior or posterolateral trachea, the left mainstem bronchus, and the left atrium. The esophagus lies between the aorta on the left and the azygos vein on the right. Intraluminal air or a small amount of fluid are common and normal findings with CT (see Fig. 2-8). Evaluation of esophageal disease is limited if the esophagus is incompletely distended (419). In those cases for which assessment of the esophagus is the primary indication for the study, as for example evaluation of patient with known or suspected esophageal surgery, both pre and post surgery, or in patients with suspected esophageal perforation, 500 mL of oral contrast material may be administered approximately 30 minutes prior to the examination in order to distend the stomach and proximal small bowel, with another 250 mL given just prior to placing the patient supine. With the patient in the gantry, a final swallow of oral contrast may then be timed to coincide with helical acquisition. This has the advantage of insuring that the entire length of the esophagus is opacified during scan acquisition (Fig. 2-96).

In our experience, CT has several distinct indications in patients with suspected esophageal disease. It is indicated (a) to evaluate and stage patients with esophageal carcinoma and to provide a means for assessing response to therapy and resultant complications, (b) to evaluate and characterize esophageal contour abnormalities detected at esophagography, and their relationship to intrinsic or extrinsic masses, and (c) to evaluate patients with suspected esophageal perforation and to assess the extent of pleural and mediastinal fluid collections. CT plays no substantial role in the evaluation of most benign esophageal diseases, including benign strictures, inflammatory disease of any etiology, and disorders of esophageal motility.

Esophageal Carcinoma

Esophageal carcinoma represents approximately 10% of all cancers of the gastrointestinal tract. Excluding adenocarcinomas of gastric origin with secondary esophageal involvement, most esophageal tumors are squamous cell carcinomas, although it is worth noting that the incidence of distal esophageal adenocarcinomas has been reported in some institutions to be increasing dramatically representing nearly 20% of cases of primary esophageal tumors (420). Esophageal carcinomas usually present in an advanced stage, with 5-year survival rates varying between 3% and 20% (421). This poor prognosis results from rapid submucosal extension of the tumor and early transmural invasion, facilitated by the lack of an esophageal serosa. This leads to early spread to regional and distal lymphatics as well as the liver, adrenals, and lung in particular.

The CT manifestations of esophageal carcinoma include

(a) narrowing of the esophageal lumen or dilatation caused by obstruction; (b) thickening of the esophageal wall, either symmetric or asymmetric; (c) loss of periesophageal fat planes, with or without evidence of invasion of surrounding organs; and (d) periesophageal adenopathy (Figs. 2-97–2-100) (422). Wall thickening must be distinguished from idiopathic muscular hypertrophy of the esophagus (423).

Accurate presurgical assessment of disease extent has proven difficult (424). Esophageal carcinoma has traditionally been staged according to the primary tumor, nodal involvement, and distal metastases (TNM) classification of the American Joint Committee on Cancer (AJCC) (Table 2-9) (425).

Moss et al. have proposed an alternative classification based on CT findings, which has been further modified by Reinig et al. to include stage 1: intraluminal lesions or those that cause localized wall thickening of between 3 and 5 mm; stage 2: wall thickening greater than 10 mm, either localized or circumferential; stage 3: wall thickening associated with evidence of contiguous spread or tumor into adjacent mediastinal structures including the airways, aorta, or pericardium; and stage 4: any locally definable disease associated with distal metastases (426,427).

The role of CT in preoperative staging of esophageal carcinoma has proven controversial (426,428–441). Most reports suggest that CT is 80% to 95% accurate. Thompson et al., in a series of 76 patients (12 with carcinomas of the gastroesophageal junction and 64 with esophageal carcinomas), reported that CT correctly identified 61 of 64 patients with esophageal carcinoma, 49 of whom had surgical confirmation (432). Of these 49 patients, 42 (86%) were correctly staged using the Moss et al. classification. CT was also 88% accurate in evaluating the regional extent of disease, correctly identifying 40 of 44 patients with mediastinal invasion and 11 of 15 patients without invasion, for a sensitivity of 90% and a specificity of 79%. CT correctly identified 15 of 19 patients with distal metastases and 28 of 39 patients without metastatic disease for an overall accuracy of 88%.

More recently, the relationship between CT findings and prognosis in esophageal carcinoma has been investigated. In a retrospective study of 89 patients, Halvorsen et al. found significant correlation between decreased survival and CT findings of tracheal, aortic, or pericardial invasion (439). Evidence of mediastinal invasion and enlarged upper abdominal lymph nodes was ominous with mean survival in this group of only 90 days. These findings are consistent with data linking various parameters to 5- and 10-year survival in patients with esophageal carcinoma in a large series of patients in Japan (442).

Significantly different results have been reported by Quint et al. (434), however, who evaluated 33 patients with esophageal cancers who subsequently underwent transhiatal esophagectomies. Using a modification of the TNM system, only 13 cases (33%) were staged accurately using CT. Thirteen of 33 cases were understaged as a result of inaccurate assessment of tumor invasion through the esophageal wall

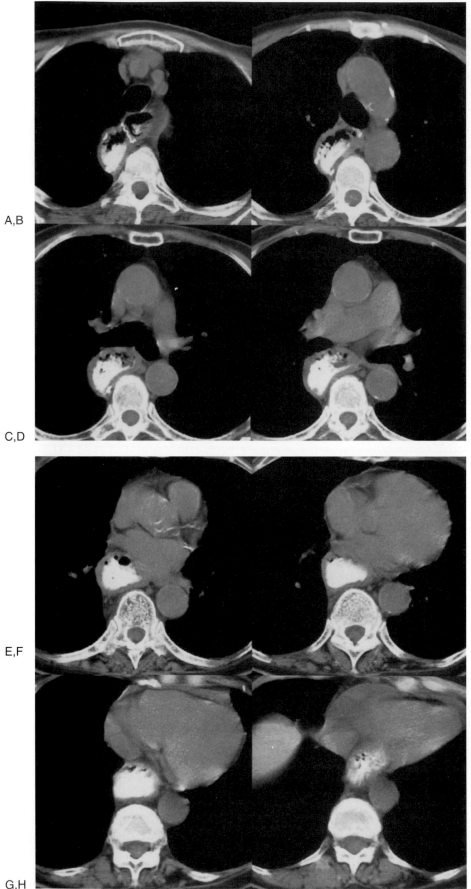

FIG. 2-96. Esophagogastrectomy: CT evaluation. **A–H:** Sequential CT sections through the thorax in a patient status postesophagogastrectomy. During administration of oral contrast 7-mm sections were obtained with a pitch of 2. There is uniform distension of the intrathoracic portion of the stomach allowing precise evaluation of the anastomosis in **A**. Note the incidental presence of a small pericardial effusion in **H**.

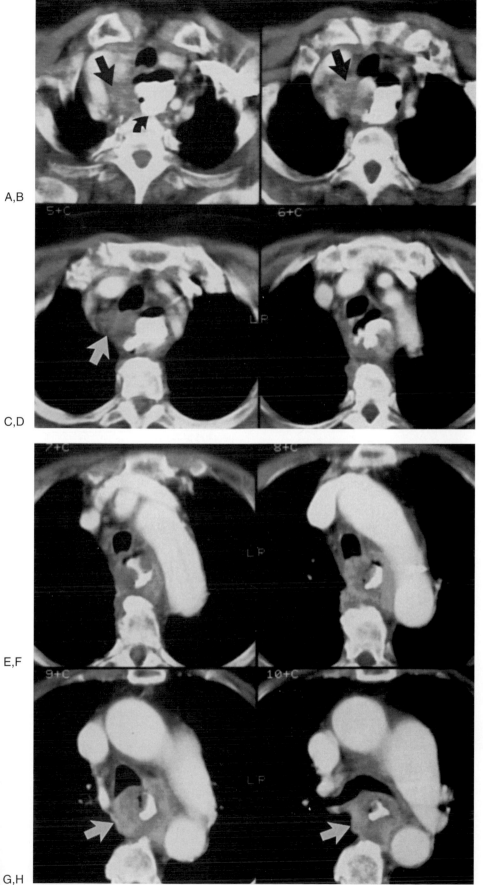

FIG. 2-97. Squamous cell carcinoma of the midesophagus. **A–H:** Enlargements of sequential contrast-enhanced CT sections through the mediastinum from above-downward following the oral administration of 2 tablespoons of 3% barium paste. An irregular mass is present, most easily identified as irregular thickening of the esophageal wall posterior to the distal trachea and left mainstem bronchus (*arrows* in **G** and **H**) extending at least 5 cm in length. Note that at the level of the tumor, the esophageal lumen is markedly irregular; superiorly, the esophagus is dilated because of partial obstruction (*curved arrow* in **A**). In addition, mediastinal adenopathy is apparent superiorly (*straight arrows* in **A**, **B**, and **C**). Note that the distal trachea and left mainstem bronchi are bowed forward. Although this appearance suggests direct extension of tumor into the airways, in our experience this finding is nonspecific. By CT criteria, this is at least a stage 3 lesion.

A,B

C,D

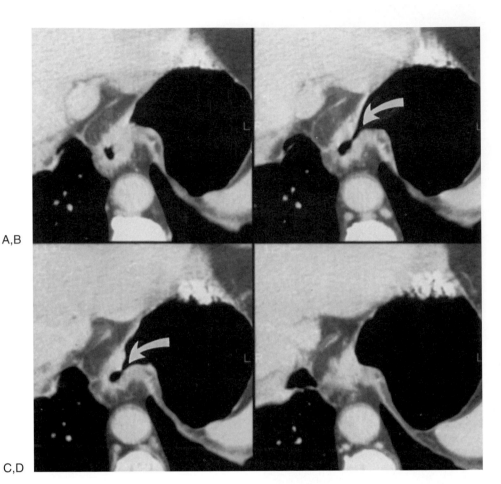

FIG. 2-98. Adenocarcinoma of the gastro-esophageal junction. **A–D:** Enlargements of sequential CT sections through the esophageal hiatus with the patient in a left lateral decubitus position to facilitate getting air into the distal esophagus. There is marked, irregular thickening of the distal esophageal wall (*arrows* in **B** and **C**). The immediate surrounding fat is intact. At surgery this proved to be a gastric adenocarcinoma with extension into the distal esophagus.

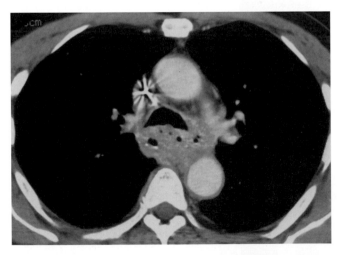

FIG. 2-99. Esophageal carcinoma: mediastinal extension. Section at the level of the carina shows posterior mediastinal mass with poorly defined borders and indistinct foci of air. Note that the mass extends to the posterior aspect of the left main pulmonary artery. Biopsy proved esophageal carcinoma with perforation and mediastinal invasion.

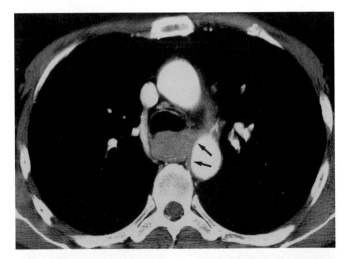

FIG. 2-100. Esophageal carcinoma: mediastinal extension. Contrast enhanced CT section through the carina shows a bulky posterior mediastinal soft-tissue mass confirmed as esophageal carcinoma at biopsy. Note that posteriorly to the left the mass extends to contact most of the medial wall of the aorta (*arrows*). Evaluation of aortic invasion is limited by CT as even this degree of contact does not necessarily preclude resection. In this case, palliative therapy only was administered because of documented metastatic disease.

TABLE 2-9. *Primary tumor, nodal involvement, and distal metastases (TNM) staging of esophageal carcinoma*

Tis = carcinoma *in situ*
T1 = tumor invasion lamina propria or submucosa
T2 = tumor invasion muscularis propria
T3 = tumor invasion adventitia
T4 = tumor invasion mediastinal structures
N0 = regional nodes uninvolved
N1 = regional nodes involved
M0 = no distant metastases
M1 = distant metastases (including nodes outside the medistinum)
Stage 0 = Tis, N0, M0
Stage 1 = T1, N0, M0
Stage 2A = T2/3, N0, M0
Stage 2B = T1/2, N1, M0
Stage 3 = T3, N1, M0 or T4, N0/1, M0
Stage 4 = T1–4, N0/1, M1

with contiguous mediastinal invasion; seven cases were overstaged because of false-positive CT diagnoses of enlarged celiac nodes. It should be noted that in this series, a significant percentage of patients proved to have adenocarcinomas of the gastroesophageal junction with secondary invasion of the esophagus. As shown by Freeny et al., the reliability of CT in staging this subset of esophageal tumors is poor (435). The addition of a substantial number of adenocarcinomas, therefore, is likely to have an adverse effect on determining the efficacy of CT. This is especially important when assessing the accuracy of CT in determining unresectability such as invasion of the trachea and mainstem bronchi and the aorta, findings far more typical of squamous cell carcinomas involving the mid-thoracic esophagus (437).

More recently, Maerz et al. reviewed CT findings in 37 patients with esophageal or proximal gastric carcinomas in whom surgical correlation was obtained (443). The sensitivity of CT for detecting direct mediastinal invasion and/or nodal or hepatic metastases proved less than 60%. Although CT specificity was greater than 90%, the negative predictive value of CT for nodal metastasis was less than 40% leading

these authors to conclude that although CT is of value in patients with extensive disease, it is less valuable for assessing patients with less bulky disease (443).

In our experience, CT assessment of resectability, especially in individual cases, is frequently problematic (see Figs. 2-97–2-100; Fig. 2-101). CT has been reported to be an accurate means for detecting invasion of the carina and the mainstem bronchi (434,439,440). However, tumors may lie adjacent to the carina or mainstem bronchi, and even compress these airways, and still be resectable (428). Usually, periesophageal invasion is easily identified in patients with bulky tumors (see Figs. 2-98–2-101). Unfortunately, definitive assessment of mediastinal invasion may be difficult in cachectic patients in whom a paucity of mediastinal fat makes visualization of the entire length of the esophagus difficult (427,429,435). Similarly, identification with CT of aortic invasion may be difficult (see Fig. 2-100) (429,432,434,436). It has been suggested that aortic invasion may be predicted on the basis of whether or not the area of contact between the aorta and adjacent tumor is less than 45, between 60 and 75, or greater than 90 (436). Although these findings may have statistical significance, they are difficult to apply in individual cases, especially if the CT interpretation results in denying a patient a chance for curative surgery. CT is controversial, as well, in its ability to identify distant metastases. The finding of enlarged mediastinal and more particularly celiac nodes is in itself nonspecific (see Fig. 2-101) (432,434,436). Unlike mediastinal adenopathy, CT is of proven value in detecting liver and lung metastases, as well as direct extension of tumor into the pleura, lung, or adjacent vertebral bodies (444,445). Rarely, CT may detect unusual complications of esophageal carcinoma, including the presence of perforation (see Fig. 2-99) even between the esophagus and the spinal canal (444,446).

If the role of CT in presurgical evaluation is controversial, there is little dispute concerning the value of CT in postsurgical follow-up (see Fig. 2-96) (447,448). As documented by Heiken et al., CT may be especially useful in detecting early postoperative complications, including anastomotic leaks

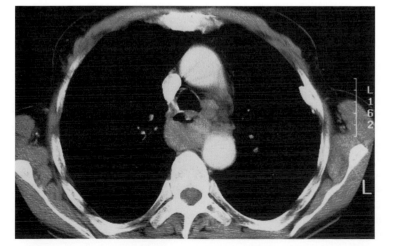

FIG. 2-101. Esophageal carcinoma: nodal metastases. Contrast enhanced CT section shows bulky posterior mediastinal mass consistent with esophageal carcinoma. Note the presence of enlarged left paratracheal nodes. Although with tumors this large the likelihood of nodal metastases is great, enlarged nodes are nonspecific and may reflect hyperplastic changes only.

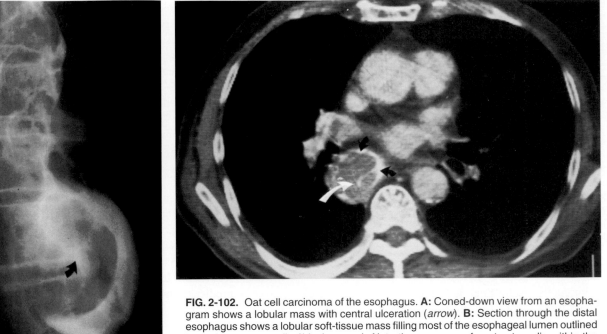

FIG. 2-102. Oat cell carcinoma of the esophagus. **A:** Coned-down view from an esophagram shows a lobular mass with central ulceration (*arrow*). **B:** Section through the distal esophagus shows a lobular soft-tissue mass filling most of the esophageal lumen outlined by oral contrast media (*black arrows*). Note the presence of contrast media within the mass because of central ulceration (*white arrow*). Biopsy proved oat cell carcinoma. (From Naidich DP. Esophagus. In: Megibow AJ, Balthazar EJ, eds. *Computed tomography of the gastrointestinal tract.* St. Louis: CV Mosby, 1986:33–98, with permission.)

with or without associated mediastinitis, parenchymal consolidation, empyema, and subphrenic abscesses (447). Equally important, CT is an accurate means for detecting early tumor recurrence. Gross et al. have reported detecting locally recurrent disease with CT in 7 of 21 patients following transhiatal esophagectomies, whereas corresponding barium studies proved positive in only four cases (448). Other unusual postoperative findings have been reported, including identifying recurrent tumor within thoracotomy incisions, as well as postoperative esophageal mucoceles (449,450).

CT has proven of little value in patients with unusual esophageal tumors, although these are occasionally encountered (Fig. 2-102).

Differentiation of Intrinsic and Extrinsic Esophageal Lesions

CT plays a major role in identifying extramural abnormalities that secondarily affect the esophagus. There are many causes of extrinsic esophageal compression. In the upper mediastinum CT is especially helpful in diagnosing vascular abnormalities. Detection of aortic aneurysms obviates the need for aortography. Aneurysmal dilatation of other arteries causing compression of the esophagus also may occasionally be identified. Rarely, these may rupture into the esophagus with resultant exsanguination (Fig. 2-103) (451). In addition, CT is useful in diagnosing a variety of vascular anomalies that cause compression or displacement of the esophagus, including aberrant right and left subclavian arteries, double

aortic arch anomalies, and pulmonary vascular slings (452,453). CT is also helpful in diagnosing substernal thyroid glands, especially when they extend posterior to the esophagus (see Fig. 2-47) (158–160). Throughout the length of the mediastinum the esophagus may be displaced by enlarged lymph nodes. In select cases, CT may allow a presumptive diagnosis. In particular, secondary involvement of the esophagus caused by low-density tuberculous lymph nodes with resultant esophago-mediastinal fistulas has been described (Fig. 2-104) (454,455). The esophagus may become secondarily involved by paraesophageal neoplasms that either obstruct the esophagus mechanically, or even invade the esophageal wall (456,457).

Esophageal Varices

CT is able to detect both esophageal and paraesophageal varices (Fig. 2-105) (458–460). Although endoscopy and esophagography are able to detect esophageal varices, paraesophageal varices have previously required angiography for definite diagnosis (458). Typically these appear as either nonspecific right- or left-sided mediastinal soft-tissue masses on chest radiographs, necessitating differentiation from enlarged periesophageal lymph nodes or other posterior mediastinal masses. Using CT during the administration of a bolus of intravenous contrast, paraesophageal varices are easily identified with CT (459). In fact, with a sufficient contrast, varices within the wall of the esophagus itself can often be seen. CT may be of value in patients following endoscopic sclerotherapy (461,462). In an assessment of

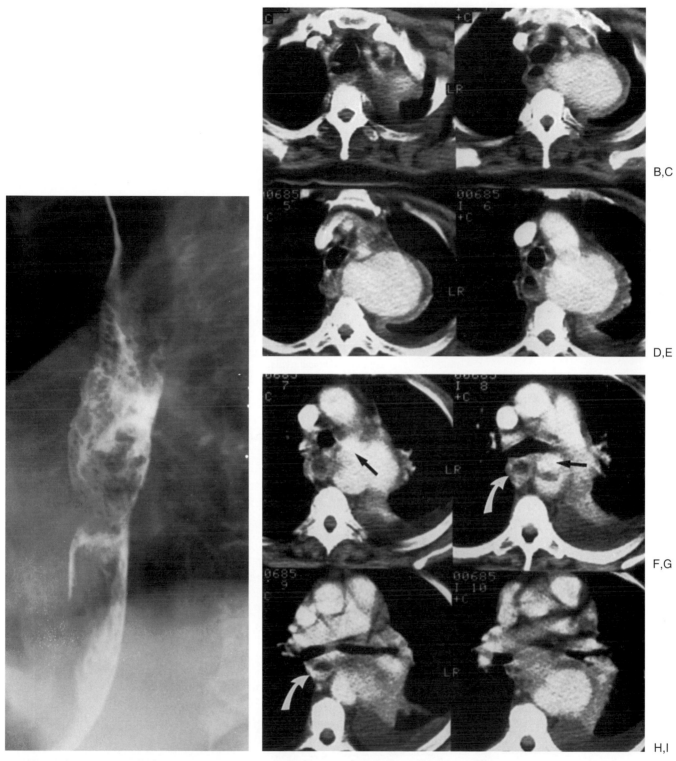

FIG. 2-103. Ruptured aortic aneurysm, CT evaluation. **A:** A coned-down view from an esophagram obtained in a patient who presented with hematemesis. A large filling defect is conspicuous within the esophageal lumen. **B–I:** Sequential contrast-enhanced CT sections from above-downward show a large aortic aneurysm involving the proximal portion of the descending aorta. At the level of the distal trachea and carina, disruption in the wall of the aneurysm can be identified (*arrows* in **F** and **G**) with resultant mediastinal hematoma and associated left pleural effusion. A blood-fluid level can also be seen within the esophageal lumen (*curved arrow* in **H**). *(continues)*

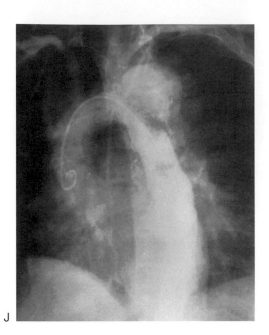

FIG. 2-103. *Continued.* **J:** Corresponding aortogram showing a large aneurysm of the aorta without apparent leak. This patient died shortly thereafter despite attempts at surgical repair.

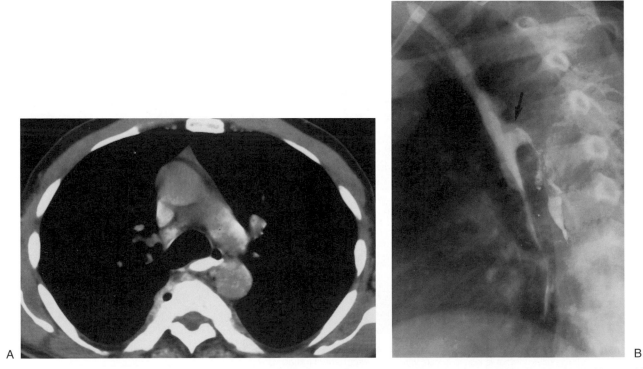

FIG. 2-104. Tuberculous esophageal fistula. **A:** CT section at the level of the carina shows oral contrast within the esophageal lumen. Note the presence of a small pocket of paraspinal air on the right. This finding is suspicious for a possible esophageal fistula. **B:** Coned down lateral view from subsequent esophagram confirms the presence of an esophageal fistula extending posteriorly (*arrow*). Patient subsequently verified to be sputum positive.

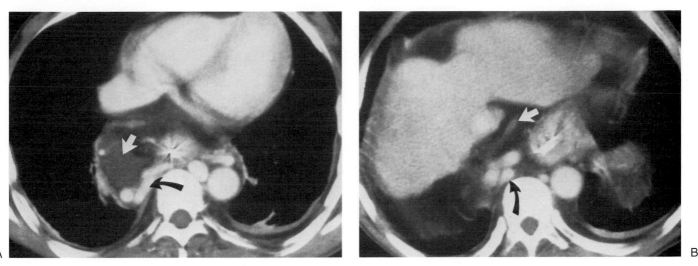

FIG. 2-105. Sliding hiatal hernia: esophageal varices. **A,B:** Sequential CT sections through the distal esophagus and esophageal hiatus, respectively, show a large sliding hiatal hernia. Note elevated medial margins of the right crus (*arrow* in **B**). In addition to the stomach, a portion of the peritoneal cavity has also herniated, within which a small quantity of ascites can be identified within the hernial sac (*arrow* in **A**). Posteriorly, numerous dilated vascular structures can also be identified (*curved arrows* in **A** and **B**), because of paraesophageal varices.

nine patients evaluated by CT following otherwise uncomplicated esophageal sclerotherapy, Mauro et al. noted the following CT findings: (a) esophageal wall thickening within which areas of low density could be identified; (b) obliteration of mediastinal fat planes, often associated with a focal fluid collection; (c) thickening of the diaphragmatic crura; and (d) associated pleural effusions and subsegmental atelectasis (462). Similar findings have been reported by Saks et al. (463).

Hiatal Hernia

Thorough familiarity with the normal cross-sectional appearance of the gastroesophageal region is a necessary pre-

requisite for accurate identification of hiatal hernias (Fig. 2-106). The esophageal hiatus is formed by the decussation of muscle fibers originating from the diaphragm around the lower esophagus. The esophagus is fixed at the level of the hiatus by the phrenicoesophageal ligament, which is not routinely visible on CT scans. The esophageal hiatus is an elliptical opening just to the left of the midline, corresponding superiorly to the level of the tenth thoracic vertebral body. The margins of the hiatus are formed by the arms of the diaphragmatic crura, which are easily identified in cross-section. Variation in the normal appearance of the crura is common, especially nodular thickening that is particularly common and may be mistaken for either abnormally enlarged lymph nodes or rarely, crural invasion by adjacent

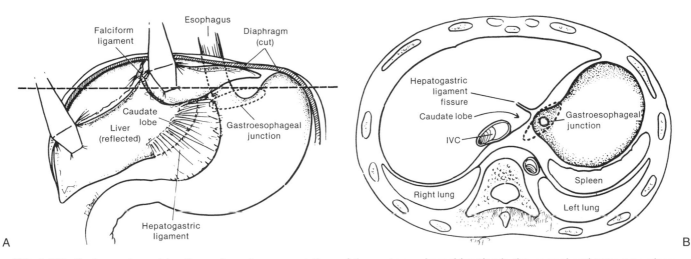

FIG. 2-106. Gastroesophageal junction: schematic representations of the gastroesophageal junction in the coronal and transverse planes, respectively. **A:** Note the relationship between the gastrohepatic ligament, the caudate lobe of the liver, and the medial wall of the gastroesophageal junction. **B:** A cross-section of the gastroesophageal region, corresponding to the level of the *dotted line* in **A**. Note that laterally the gastrohepatic ligament can be identified as a line separating the caudate lobe posteriorly from the lateral segment of the left lobe anteriorly. (From ref. 475, with permission.)

tumor (464,465). As the esophagus passes through the upper margin of the hiatus, it assumes an oblique orientation, coursing in a posterior-to-anterior and right-to-left direction. The gastroesophageal junction itself lies just below the diaphragm. As it courses through the upper abdomen the distal esophagus is enveloped by the most cranial portion of the gastrohepatic ligament, which originates from a deep cleft in the liver, separating the left lobe from the caudate. This landmark serves as a convenient reference point for identifying the esophagogastric junction (466). On cross-section the abdominal or submerged portion of the esophagus frequently appears cone-shaped with its base at the junction with the gastric fundus (467). This segment is only rarely distended by either air or barium, and hence is easily mistaken as abnormal (468). This problem may be solved by scanning patients in the left lateral decubitus position following ingestion of at least 200 mL of standard oral contrast material (469).

In a patient with sliding hiatal hernia, the most common abnormalities identified are dehiscence of the diaphragmatic crura and stretching of the phrenicoesophageal ligament, which ceases to exist for all practical purposes in most adults. These findings manifest as widening of the esophageal hiatus on cross-section, identifiable whenever the medial margins of the diaphragmatic crura are not tightly opposed (Fig. 2-107) (372). Actual measurements of the standard width of the esophageal hiatus, defined as the distance between the medial margins of the crura, have been reported. This distance has a mean measurement of 10.7 mm (SD 2.4 mm) with a maximum width of 15 mm (428). Sliding hiatal her-

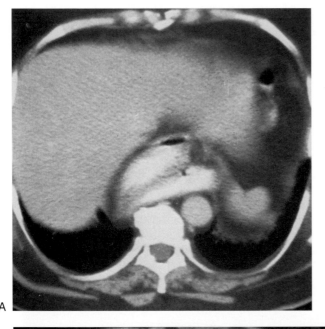

A

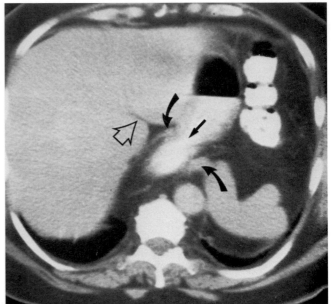

B

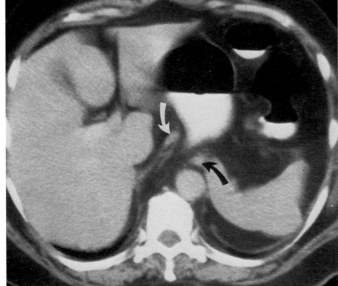

C

FIG. 2-107. Hiatal hernia. **A–C:** Sequential CT sections from above-downward following the administration of oral contrast in a patient with a moderate-sized sliding hiatal hernia. Note that the medial margins of the crura are widely separated (*curved arrows* in **B** and **C**). A portion of the contrast-filled stomach as well as peritoneal fat (*straight arrow* in **B**) can be identified between the widened margins of the crura. A few linear densities can be identified within the fat, presumably representing peritoneal vessels. The *open arrow* in **B** points to the fissure of the gastrohepatic ligament.

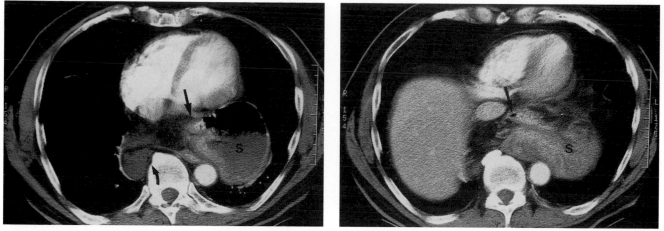

FIG. 2-108. Paraesophageal hernia. **A,B.** Contrast enhanced CT sections in a surgically documented paraesphageal hernia show that a considerable portion of the stomach (*S*) lies anterior to and alongside the distal esophagus (*arrows*) that is normal in caliber. Note the presence of fluid within a portion of herniated peritoneum to the right of the spine (*curved arrow* in **A**).

nias are frequently associated with an apparent increase in mediastinal fat surrounding the distal esophagus, secondary to herniation of omentum through the phrenicoesophageal ligament. In the presence of massive ascites, it may be possible to actually identify fluid within herniated peritoneum anterior to the contrast-filled stomach (470).

Identification of sliding hiatal hernias rarely presents much difficulty when seen on CT (464,466,467,471). Paraesophageal herniation is easily differentiated because in these cases although the stomach is herniated, the esophagogastric junction remains in a normal position (Fig. 2-108). Occasionally tumors arise in hernias; this appearance may also be mimicked by incomplete filling of the herniated stomach (472). Accurate differentiation usually requires esophagography.

MEDIASTINITIS AND MEDIASTINAL ABSCESS

Acute mediastinal infections are uncommon and usually related to surgery, esophageal perforation, or spread of infection from adjacent regions (473–475). Infections may be classified as diffuse mediastinitis or mediastinal abscess, depending on their extent. Diffuse mediastinitis has a relatively poor prognosis.

CT findings in mediastinitis include diffuse or streaky infiltration of mediastinal fat (greater than 25 H), mediastinal widening, localized fluid collections, pleural or pericardial effusion, lymph node enlargement, and compression of mediastinal structures (Figs. 2-109 and 2-110). Gas bubbles in the mediastinum, with or without associated fluid collections, are seen in up to half of cases, and are an important finding (473,474). In patients with an abscess, a localized fluid-filled space is visible, often containing air (41).

Since many cases of mediastinitis occur after median sternotomy, it is important to consider the normal postoperative appearance of the mediastinum in such patients. In subjects having CT after an uncomplicated sternotomy, findings can closely mimic the appearance of mediastinitis, and abnormal findings can persist for up to 3 weeks (473,476,477). In a study by Kay et al. (476), more than 75% of patients having median sternotomy showed retrosternal fluid collections, air, hematoma, or a combination of these in the early postoperative period. In a study assessing the accuracy of CT in diagnosing mediastinitis after sternotomy (477), a diagnosis based on the presence of mediastinal fluid or air collections had a sensitivity of 100%. In the first 14 days after surgery, these findings had a specificity of only 33%, but after 14 days, their specificity was 100% (see Fig. 2-110).

CT has also proven particularly valuable in diagnosing esophageal perforation (see Fig. 2-104; Figs. 2-111, 2-112). This is a potentially lethal condition frequently complicated by the rapid onset of severe mediastinitis, empyema, and sepsis. In addition to its association with esophageal carci-

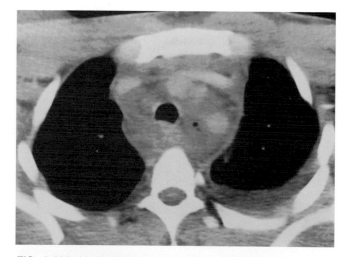

FIG. 2-109. Mediastinitis secondary to retropharyngeal abscess. Mediastinal soft tissues are of water density because of edema, and small gas bubbles are visible.

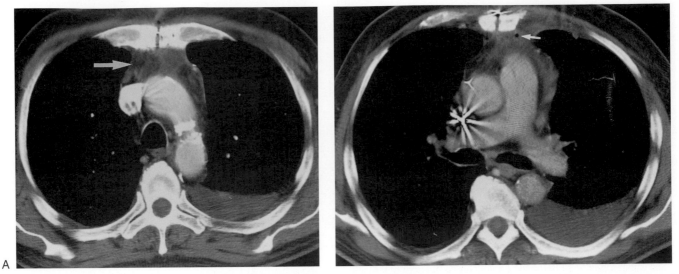

FIG. 2-110. Mediastinitis 4 weeks after median sternotomy. **A:** Mediastinal fat is increased in attenuation and a focal fluid collection in the right mediastinum (*large arrow*) represents an abscess. A small amount of gas is visible in relation to the sternotomy incision. **B:** At a lower level, a small gas bubbles (*arrow*) are visible in the mediastinum and in relation to the sternotomy. This appearance is distinctly abnormal this long after surgery.

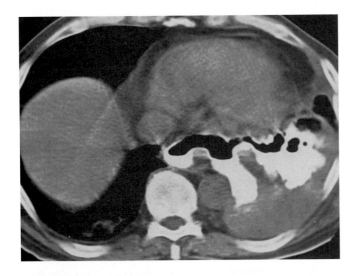

FIG. 2-111. Esophageal perforation: Boerhaave's syndrome. CT section through the distal esophagus following administration of oral contrast media. There is perforation of the esophagus with free extravasation of contrast into the mediastinum, associated with a moderate-sized left pleural fluid collection. (Case courtesy of Robert Meisell, M.D., Booth Memorial Hospital, New York, NY.)

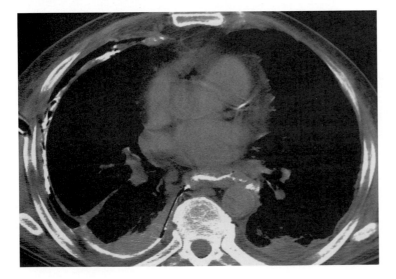

FIG. 2-112. Esophageal perforation-esophageal-pleural-cutaneous fistula. Helical CT section at the level of the distal esophagus following oral contrast administration shows the presence of an esophageal-pleural-cutaneous fistula in a patient with a history of trauma following placement of a right sided pleural tube. In this case, administration of oral contrast confirms the continuity of these spaces.

noma, perforation may occur spontaneously (Boerhaave's syndrome), or may be posttraumatic or iatrogenic, complicating endoscopy, esophageal dilatation, attempted intubation, or surgery (478). As documented by Han et al., routine radiographs may be normal in up to 12% of patients with perforations (428). Although the definitive diagnosis is generally made by esophagraphy, CT may provide valuable information concerning the extent of associated mediastinal, pleural, and parenchymal disease (479–481). Furthermore, in select cases, CT can be used to determine which patients require immediate surgical intervention and which patients can be managed conservatively; the presence of mediastinal fluid collections suggests the need for intervention. Although uncommon, the CT appearance of acquired tracheoesophageal fistulas has been reported (482). In patients having esophageal surgery, a localized fluid collection without air bubbles, may represent seroma (483). Aspiration (484) may be necessary for differentiation from abscess (41).

PARASPINAL ABNORMALITIES

A wide variety of pathologic processes may involve the paraspinal regions (485). Most frequently, masses affecting these regions are neural in origin, including neurogenic tumors, neurenteric cyst, and anterior or lateral thoracic meningocele, or are related to the spine. Infections involving the spine may lead to the development of paraspinal abscesses, most commonly in patients with tuberculosis (Fig. 2-113). In addition, lymphoma and other causes of lymph node en-

largement may result in abnormalities in this region; paraspinal lymph nodes freely communicate with lymph nodes in the upper abdomen, and contiguous involvement is common. Since the mediastinum communicates with the retroperitoneal space via the esophageal hiatus, aortic hiatus, and other defects in the diaphragm, diseases can spread between the abdomen and thorax by direct extension; inflammatory masses such as pancreatic pseudocysts can involve the paraspinal mediastinal regions. Rare entities such as extramedullary hematopoesis, primary myelolipomas of the mediastinum, benign hemangioendotheliomas, aggressive fibromatosis, and even fibrosing mediastinitis have been reported in the paravertebral regions (350,367,486,487).

Neurogenic Tumors

Neurogenic tumors account for about 9% of primary mediastinal masses in adults (488), although they are more prevalent in children, representing 29% of mediastinal tumors (488). A high proportion of posterior mediastinal masses are of neurogenic origin, particularly in children (4). Tumors may arise from peripheral nerves and nerve sheath (neurofibroma, schwannoma, malignant peripheral nerve-sheath tumors) or sympathetic ganglia (ganglioneuroma, ganglioneuroblastoma, neuroblastoma). In two reviews of thoracic neurogenic tumors in 160 and 134 patients (488,489), the most common lesions were schwannoma (31% to 32%), ganglioneuroma (25% to 26%), neuroblastoma (15% to 21%), ganglioneuroblastomas (7% to 14%),

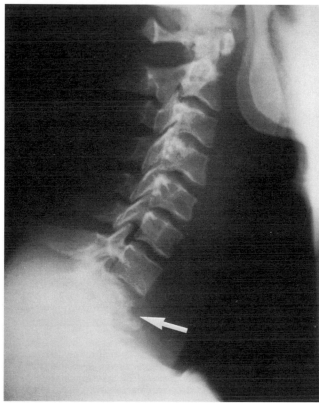

A

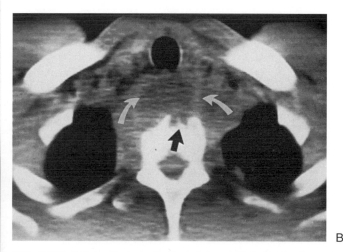

B

FIG. 2-113. Tuberculous mediastinal abscess. **A:** Lateral radiograph of the cervical spine shows destruction of the T1 vertebral body (*arrow*). **B:** Contrast-enhanced CT section confirms lytic destruction of T1 (*arrow*) associated with a large, poorly marginated posterior mediastinal fluid collection (*curved arrows*). Surgery confirmed tuberculous abscess.

and neurofibroma (5% to 10%), but the incidence varies with the patient's age. Nearly 85% of tumors in children are of ganglionic origin, whereas in adults, more than 75% are nerve sheath tumors (488). Specifically, schwannoma and neurofibroma are more common in adults whereas ganglioneuroblastoma, and neuroblastoma are more common in children. The mean ages at diagnosis for neurogenic tumors in the study by Reed et al. (489), was 5.8 years for neuroblastoma, 8.4 years for ganglioneuroblastoma, 19.6 years for ganglioneuroma, 29.7 years for neurofibroma, and 38 years for schwannoma. Similar results were reported by Ribet and Cardot (488). In their study, 23 of 28 neuroblastomas occurred before the age of 1. Patients with ganglioneuroblastomas were slightly older, but all were diagnosed before the age of 10.

Peripheral Nerve Sheath Tumors

Nerve sheath tumors included neurilemoma (schwannoma), neurofibroma, and neurogenic sarcoma. Schwanno-

mas are composed of spindle cells densely packed together (Antoni A pattern) or organized more loosely in association with a myxoid stroma (Antoni B pattern); areas of infarction are common. Neurofibromas are also variable in appearance, consisting of spindle cell, a loose myxoid matrix, neurofibrils, and collagen.

The CT findings in patients with peripheral nerve sheath tumors have been well described (490–498). They typically appear as well-marginated, smooth, rounded, or elliptical masses in the paravertebral regions or along the courses of the vagus, phrenic, recurrent laryngeal, or intercostal nerves. Enlargement of neural foramina with or without extension into the spinal canal may be associated with paravertebral tumors.

Although peripheral nerve or nerve sheath tumors can be of soft-tissue attenuation, low attenuation is characteristic, and is seen in up to 73% of cases (Fig. 2-114) (490,491,493,497). Low density areas within nerve sheath tumors can be caused by the presence of (a) lipid-rich Schwann cells; (b) adipocytes; (c) perineural adipose tissue

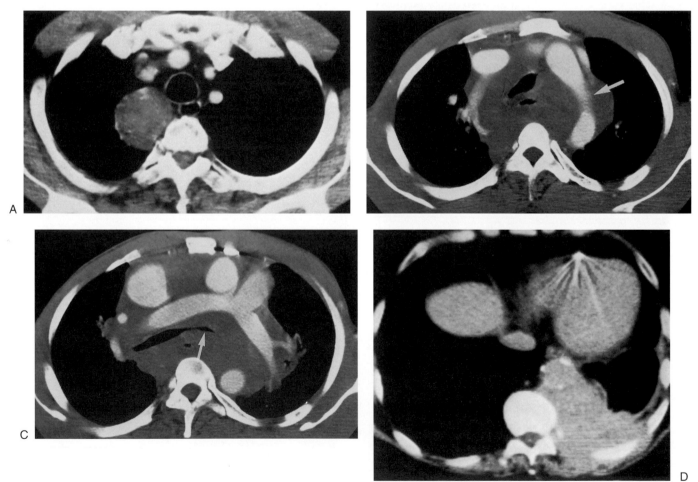

FIG. 2-114. Neurogenic tumors. **A:** Contrast-enhanced CT scan shows a well-defined, slightly heterogeneous posterior paravertebral mass. The appearance and location are typical. Biopsy proved neurofibroma. **B,C:** Contrast-enhanced CT sections in a different patient with neurofibromatosis. The mediastinum is infiltrated by a relatively homogenous soft-tissue mass, resulting in marked displacement of mediastinal vessels including the azygos vein and aortic arch (*arrow* in **B**) as well as marked narrowing of the right and especially left mainstem bronchi (*arrow* in **C**). (Case courtesy Israel Gary, Montefiore Medical Center, New York, NY.) **D:** Malignant neurofibrosarcoma. The tumor has infiltrated the chest wall.

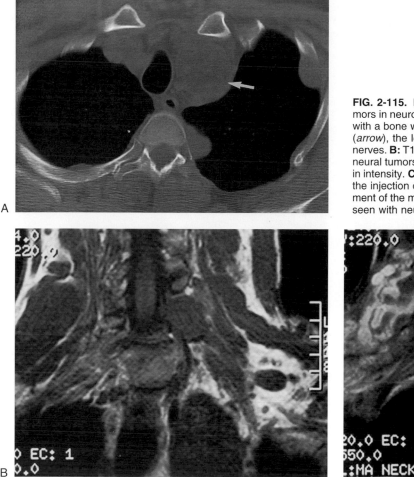

A

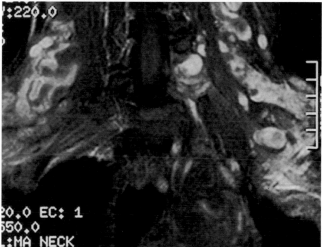

FIG. 2-115. Extensive mediastinal and intercostal neurogenic tumors in neurofibromatosis. CT and MR correlation. **A:** CT obtained with a bone window setting shows masses in the left mediastinum (*arrow*), the left paravertebral region, and in relation to intercostal nerves. **B:** T1-weighted MRI (TR/TE = 600/8 msec) shows multiple neural tumors in the neck and left mediastinum. These appear low in intensity. **C:** T1-weighted MRI (TR/TE = 550/20 msec) following the injection of contrast material shows inhomogeneous enhancement of the multiple tumors. Inhomogeneous enhancement can be seen with neurofibroma or schwannoma.

B

C

entrapped by plexiform neurofibromas; (d) cystic spaces caused by the coalescence of interstitial fluid in schwannomas with Antoni B tissue; and (e) cystic degeneration secondary to infarction (491,499). Variable enhancement of the tumor may be seen following contrast infusion; peripheral enhancement is common.

Neurofibromas may be associated with von Recklinghausen's disease, which can result in vertebral abnormalities including kyphoscoliosis, scalloped vertebrae, and lateral meningocele (500). In one study (489) more than one-third of patients with neurofibromas had neurofibromatosis.

Malignant nerve sheath tumors, termed malignant schwannoma, are relatively uncommon, but represent up to 15% of nerve sheath tumors (488,501). The CT diagnosis of malignancy can be difficult. Although benign tumors tend to be small, sharply marginated and fairly homogeneous in attenuation, and malignant nerve sheath tumors tend to be large, infiltrating, irregular, and inhomogeneous, these findings are not sufficiently reliable to obviate histologic evaluation (496,497,501). In a study of eight cases of malignant schwannoma arising in the thorax (501), tumors averaged nine cm in diameter (range 6 to 13 cm) and six showed areas of low attenuation caused by necrosis, but only three had an

irregular edge and five had a smooth margin. Both benign and malignant lesions may be symptomatic, rendering clinical differentiation of limited utility. Calcification and some degree of contrast opacification may be present with either benign or malignant tumors. Lung metastases may be present (501).

On MRI (497,502–504), neurogenic tumors typically have slightly greater signal intensity than muscle on T1-weighted images, and markedly increased signal intensity on T2-weighted images, although often in an inhomogeneous fashion (Figs. 2-115 and 2-116) (502,505). An inhomogeneous appearance on T2-weighted MRI is common. In half of cases in one study (505), schwannomas had a high intensity center and a relatively low intensity outer wall; this appearance correlated with the presence of central cystic degeneration. Neurofibromas, on the other hand, showed the central region to be less intense than the periphery on T2-weighted images, with central contrast enhancement; this correlated with the presence of tumor tissue centrally and peripheral myxoid degeneration.

Plexiform neurofibroma represents an extensive fusiform or infiltrating mass along the course of the sympathetic chains, mediastinal, or intercostal nerves (see Figs.

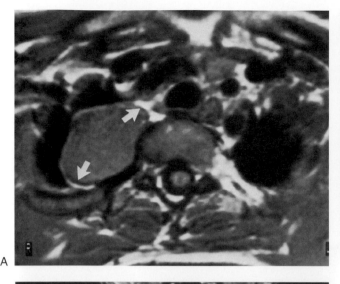

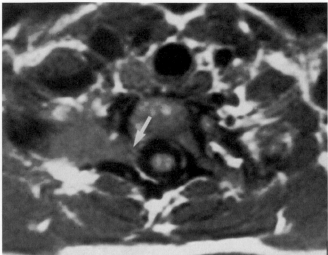

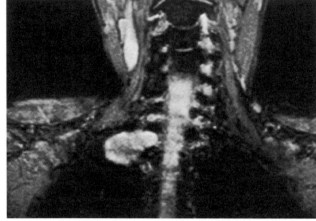

FIG. 2-116. Neurogenic tumor: MR evaluation. **A,B:** Sequential MR images through the lung apex from above-downward show a sharply defined, homogeneous mass in the right paravertebral space. A thin mantle of fat surrounds the lesion (*arrows* in **A**), confirming that this lesion arises extrapleurally. Note that the lesion clearly extends into the T1–2 foramen (*arrow* in **B**). **C:** Coronal MR image confirms extension of the lesion through the intervertebral foramen. This lesion has remained stable for 2 years, compatible with the clinical and morphologic diagnosis of a neurofibroma. (Case courtesy of Andrew Litt, M.D., New York University Medical Center, New York.)

2-114B,C and 2-115) (493). It is considered pathognomonic of von Recklinghausen's disease. As with localized nerve sheath tumors, plexiform neurofibromas appear low in attenuation as compared to muscle, with CT values ranging from 15 to 20 H on unenhanced scans. They are often multiple and lobulated, have ill-defined margins, and tend to surround mediastinal vessels with loss of normally visible fat planes (493). They can closely mimic the appearance of extensive mediastinal lymph node enlargement. Calcification and contrast enhancement can be seen.

Tumors Originating from Sympathetic Ganglia

Included in this group are ganglioneuroma, ganglioneuroblastoma, and neuroblastoma. Ganglioneuroma, a benign tumor made up of Schwann cells, collagen, and ganglion cells, is a common tumor in teenagers and young adults. It cannot be distinguished from schwannoma or neurofibroma on the basis of its appearance, although a somewhat different whorled MRI appearance has been described (505). In children, 80% of posterior mediastinal masses are derived from sympathetic ganglia (4).

Approximately 15% of neuroblastomas arise in the mediastinum (Fig. 2-117), and almost all are located posteriorly. Mediastinal neuroblastoma is seen almost exclusively in young children, under the age of five years (488,489). It is malignant and may present with a wide variety of signs and symptoms including chest pain, fever, malaise, anemia, Horner's syndrome, and extremity weakness.

On CT, neuroblastomas appear as soft-tissue attenuation masses, but up to 40% contain speckled or curvilinear calcifications. They are most common in the paravertebral regions and may extend superiorly and inferiorly for several centimeters. Neuroblastoma often shows inhomogeneous enhancement following contrast injection. CT and MRI may be used to help determine the presence and extent of mediastinal or vertebral column invasion. Invasion of the extradural spinal canal is frequent, even in the absence of neurologic signs and symptoms (506). On T2-weighted images, neuroblastoma appears intense (see Fig. 2-117). MRI has the advantage of allowing tumor and surrounding soft tissues to be distinguished more readily than on CT, and is more accurate in the recognition of bone marrow involvement. Neuroblastoma may extend from a primary site in the abdomen into

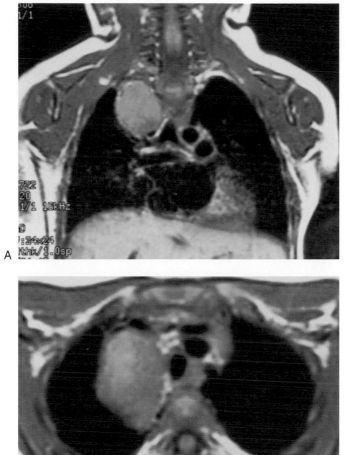

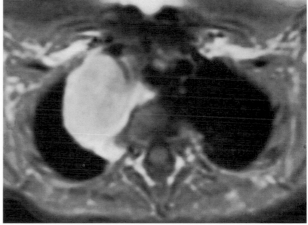

FIG. 2-117. Mediastinal neuroblastoma in a 9-month-old child. **A:** T1-weighted coronal MRI (TR/TE = 722/20 msec) shows a large right mediastinal mass. **B:** T1-weighted transaxial MRI (TR/TE = 689/20 msec) shows the mass to be relatively low in intensity. **C:** T1-weighted transaxial MRI (TR/TE = 714/20 msec) following the injection of contrast agent shows significant enhancement of the mass.

the thorax. Most commonly, this occurs by direct invasion through the retrocrural space and into the lower paravertebral regions, often on both sides. In the rare instance of adult neuroblastoma, differentiation from lymphoma may be difficult (498).

Ganglioneuroblastoma is found in somewhat older children than neuroblastoma, and is less common. Ganglioneuroblastomas are regarded by some as partially matured malignant neuroblastomas (488), and are somewhat intermediate in histology between neuroblastoma and ganglioneuroma. Their imaging characteristics are indistinguishable from neuroblastoma. They can present as either a large, smooth spherical mass or as a small, elongated sausage-shaped mass. Some of the large ones are of low, homogenous density and show little, if any, contrast enhancement.

MR Evaluation of Neurogenic Tumors

Compared with other imaging modalities including CT, MR has several distinct advantages for imaging neurogenic tumors. In addition to identifying the tumor, MR is especially helpful in assessing intraspinal extension, as well as the presence of associated spinal cord pathology (see Figs. 2-115–2-117). The ability to obtain multiplanar images is particularly helpful as many of these tumors demonstrate longitudinal extension into structures along the axis of the spine. Recently, MRI findings have been shown to accurately reflect underlying pathologic findings in patients with neurogenic tumors (505). For these reasons, MRI has largely replaced CT as an initial imaging modality in the evaluation of patients with suspected neurogenic tumors. Unfortunately, MRI is no more specific than CT in differentiating benign from malignant lesions. As documented by Levine et al., in these cases, gallium scintigraphy appears to be a promising screening technique, as radiogallium uptake appears to occur only in malignant lesions (497).

Paraganglioma

Paraganglioma (chemodectoma) is a rare tumor originating from neuroectodermal cells located in relation to the autonomic nervous system, especially in the region of the aorticopulmonary window and the posterior mediastinum (Fig. 2-118) (54); they have also been identified within the

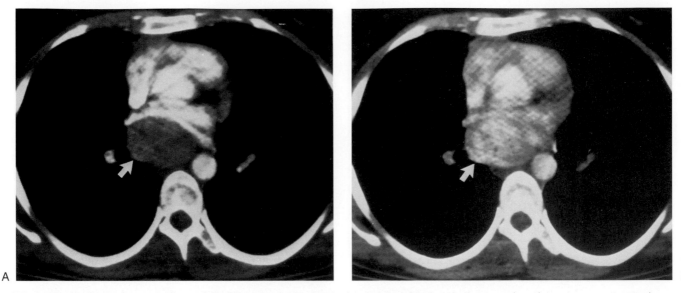

FIG. 2-118. Mediastinal paraganglioma. **A,B:** CT scans obtained at the level of the left atrium, both pre- and postintravenous contrast enhancement, respectively. A large, homogeneous, low density mass can be identified causing marked compression of the left atrium (*arrows* in **A** and **B**). Note that following intravenous contrast administration there has been marked contrast enhancement within the mass. Without benefit of the precontrast image, this mass could easily be overlooked as representing a normal left atrium. (Case courtesy of Barry Gross, M.D., Detroit, MI.)

atria. In the study of thoracic neurogenic tumors reported by Reed et al. (489), only 4% were paragangliomas. On unenhanced CT, paraganglionoma has no characteristic features. However, scanning during bolus contrast infusion shows dense enhancement, and marked hypervascularity is seen on angiography (54). Patients are often asymptomatic and detected incidentally, although compression of mediastinal structures may result in symptoms. Approximately 10% of these lesions are malignant or invasive. Paravertebral paragangliomas are more easily resectable than aorticopulmonary tumors and have a better prognosis. Local recurrence is common following surgery in patients with aorticopulmonary paraganglioma.

About half of patients with paravertebral paraganglionoma have symptoms of catecholamine secretion by the tumor or associated tumors in other locations, but catecholamine secretion is rare in patients with aorticopulmonary tumors. Identification of hormonally active lesions has been greatly aided recently by use of 131-I metaiodobenzylguanidine (131-I-MIBG) scintigraphy which localizes to catecholamine-producing tumors, including neuroblastoma and carcinoid tumor (55,507,508).

Anterior or Lateral Thoracic Meningocele

This entity represents anomalous herniation of the spinal meninges through an intervertebral foramen or a defect in the vertebral body. It results in a soft-tissue mass visible on chest radiographs. In many patients, this abnormality is associated with neurofibromatosis; most are detected in adults (509).

Meningoceles are described as lateral or anterior, depending on their relationship to the spine. They are slightly more common on the right (509). On CT they appear low in attenuation, as they contain cerebrospinal fluid (Figs. 2-119 and 2-120). Findings that suggest the diagnosis include rib or vertebral anomalies at the same level or an association with scoliosis. The mass is often visible at the apex of the scoliotic curve (509). MRI is diagnostic, as is filling of the meningocele with contrast at CT myelography (see Figs. 2-119, 2-120). As with meningocele, neurenteric cysts are fre-

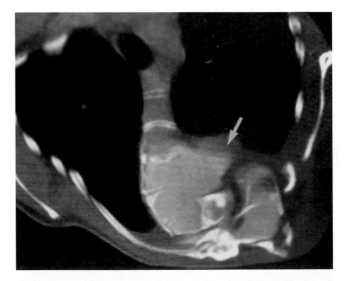

FIG. 2-119. Anterior thoracic meningocele associated with neurofibromatosis: CT myeolography. Vertebral defects and scoliosis are evident. The meningocele (*arrow*) is opacified.

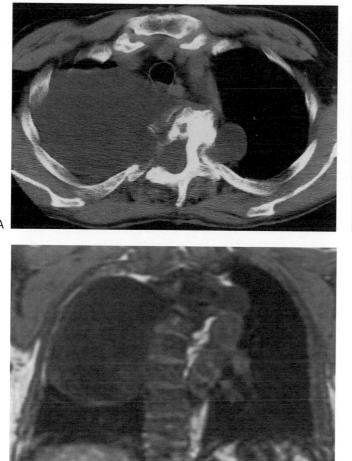

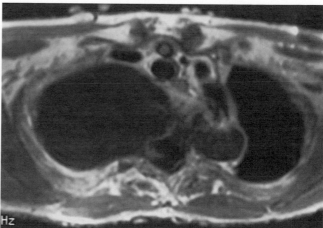

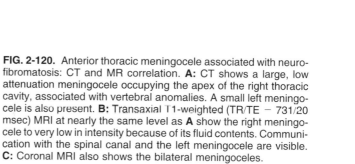

FIG. 2-120. Anterior thoracic meningocele associated with neurofibromatosis: CT and MR correlation. **A:** CT shows a large, low attenuation meningocele occupying the apex of the right thoracic cavity, associated with vertebral anomalies. A small left meningocele is also present. **B:** Transaxial T1-weighted (TR/TE − 731/20 msec) MRI at nearly the same level as **A** show the right meningocele to very low in intensity because of its fluid contents. Communication with the spinal canal and the left meningocele are visible. **C:** Coronal MRI also shows the bilateral meningoceles.

quently associated with vertebral anomalies or scoliosis. They rarely fill with myelographic contrast.

Extramedullary Hematopoiesis

Extramedullary hematopoiesis can result in paravertebral masses in patients with severe hemolytic anemia caused by excessive destruction of blood cells. It can be seen in the presence of thalassemia, hereditary spherocytosis, and sickle-cell anemia (42,510,511). These masses are of unknown origin but may arise from herniations of vertebral or rib marrow through small cortical defects, or may arise from lymph nodes or elements of the reticuloendothelial system.

Lobulated paravertebral masses, usually multiple and bilateral and caudad to the sixth thoracic vertebra, are typically seen. They appear well marginated and of homogeneous soft-tissue attenuation (30–65 H) (510) or may show areas of fat attenuation (− 50 H) that may increase after treatment (42,47,512). The diagnosis can be suggested by the presence of chronic anemia and radiographic or CT findings in the skeleton suggesting a bone marrow abnormality. Coursening of the trabecular pattern, rib expansion, and periosteal new bone may be seen (510). Although not always present, splenomegaly is common (Figs. 2-121 and 2-122).

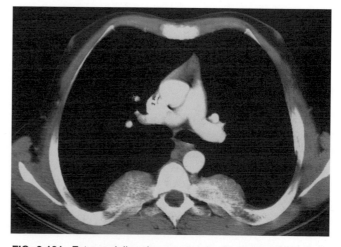

FIG. 2-121. Extramedullary hematopoesis. Contrast enhanced CT section through the mid thorax shows marked expansion of the medial aspects of the ribs bilaterally with evidence of bony trabecullae extending through the cortex to form paraspinal masses. This patient had long standing thalassemia.

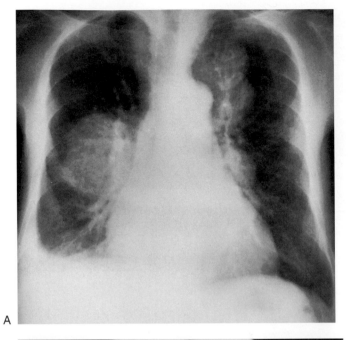

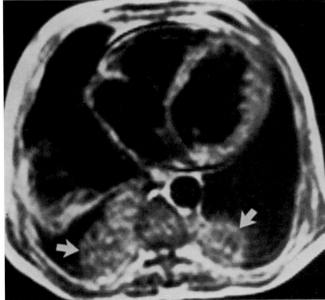

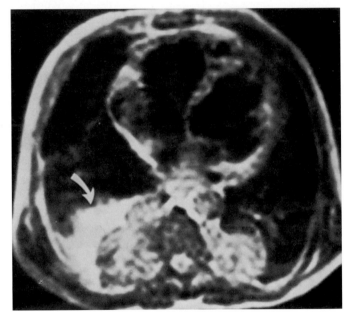

FIG. 2-122. Extramedullary hematopoiesis: MR evaluation. **A:** Posteroanterior chest radiograph shows massive, bilateral, paravertebral masses. **B,C:** T1- and T2-weighted MR images show typical appearance of bilateral, heterogeneous paravertebral masses (*arrows* in **B**). Note that there is a considerable increase in signal intensity within these lesions on the T2-weighted scan, although nowhere as near as much as in the associated right pleural fluid effusion (*curved arrow* in **B**). This patient had longstanding thalassemia.

Mediastinal Pseudocyst

Pancreatic pseudocyst represents an encapsulated collection of pancreatic secretions, blood, and necrotic material (513). Mediastinal extension of a pancreatic pseudocyst is rare (393), but can occur via the aortic hiatus, esophageal hiatus, or through a defect in the diaphragm. Symptoms are generally those of pancreatitis. CT shows a cystic and low attenuation mass in the posterior mediastinum or adjacent thoracic cavity, associated with compression or displacement of the esophagus or splaying of the diaphragmatic crura (393,394). Mediastinal pseudocysts are commonly located under and posterior to the heart, anterior to the aorta and esophagus, and medial to the inferior vena cava. The fluid can be of water density or higher, depending on the presence of blood or infection. The presence of an abdominal component is common, but not invariably present (408). CT may also be helpful in percutaneous catheter drainage of a mediastinal pseudocyst (393). Reported MRI findings are compatible with the cystic nature of this lesion (408).

REFERENCES

1. Baron RL, Levitt RG, Sagel SS, Stanley RJ. Computed tomography in the evaluation of mediastinal widening. *Radiology* 1981;138: 107–113.
2. Webb WR. Advances in computed tomography of the thorax. *Radiol Clin North Am* 1983;21:723–739.

3. Sones PJ, Torres WE, Colvin RS, et al. Effectiveness of CT in evaluating intrathoracic masses. *AJR Am J Roentgenol* 1982;139:469–475.
4. Merten DF. Diagnostic imaging of mediastinal masses is children. *AJR* 1992;158:825–832.
5. Webb WR, Sostman HD. MR imaging of thoracic diseases: clinical uses. *Radiology* 1992;182:621–630.
6. Gefter W. Chest applications of magnetic resonance imaging: an update. *Radiol Clin North Am* 1988;26:573–588.
7. Weinreb JC, Naidich DP. Thoracic magnetic resonance imaging. *Clin Chest Med* 1991;12:33–54.
8. Kalender WA. Technical foundations of spiral CT. *Seminars Ultrasound, CT and MRI* 1994;15:81–89.
9. Costello P, Dupuy DE, Ecker CP, Tello R. Spiral CT of the thorax with reduced volume of contrast material: a comparative study. *Radiology* 1992;185:663–666.
10. Heiken JP, Brink JA, Vannier MW. Spiral (helical) CT. *Radiology* 1993;189:647–656.
11. Cascade PN, Gross BH, Kazerooni EA, et al. Variability in the detection of enlarged mediastinal lymph nodes in staging lung cancer: a comparison of contrast-enhanced and unenhanced CT. *AJR* 1998;170:927–931.
12. Im JG, Song KS, Kang HS, et al. Mediastinal tuberculous lymphadenitis: CT manifestations. *Radiology* 1987;164:115–119.
13. Im JG, Itoh H, Shim YS, et al. Pulmonary tuberculosis: CT findings early active disease and sequential change with antituberculous therapy. *Radiology* 1993;186:653–660.
14. Pastores SM, Naidich DP, Aranda CP, McGuinness G, Rom WN. Intrathoracic adenopathy associated with pulmonary tuberculosis in patients with human immunodeficiency virus infection. *Chest* 1993;103:1433–1437.
15. Kirsch CFE, Webb EM, Webb WR. Multicentric Castleman's disease and POEMS syndrome: CT findings. *J Thoracic Imaging* 1997;12:75–77.
16. Moon WK, Im JG, Kim JS, et al. Mediastinal Castleman's disease: CT findings. *J Comput Assist Tomogr* 1994;18:43–46.
17. Schneider P. Contrast techniques for spiral CT of the thorax. In: Remy-Jardin M, ed. *Spiral CT of the thorax*. Frankfurt: Springer-Verlag, 1997:57–99.
18. Silverman P, ed. *Helical/spiral computed tomography. A practical approach to clinical protocols*. Philadelphia: Lippincott-Raven, 1998.
19. Baron RL, Lee JK, Sagel SS, Peterson RR. Computed tomography of the normal thymus. *Radiology* 1982;142:121–125.
20. de Geer G, Webb WR, Gamsu G. Normal thymus: Assessment with MR and CT. *Radiology* 1986;158:313–317.
21. Francis IR, Glazer GM, Bookstein FL, Gross BH. The thymus: reexamination of age-related changes in size and shape. *AJR Am J Roentgenol* 1985;145:249–254.
22. Heiberg E, Wolverson MK, Sundaram M, Nouri S. Normal thymus: CT characteristics in subjects under age 20. *AJR Am J Roentgenol* 1982;138:491–494.
23. Moore AV, Korobkin M, Olanow W, et al. Age-related changes in the thymus gland: CT-pathologic correlation. *AJR Am J Roentgenol* 1983;141:241–246.
24. Siegel MJ, Glazer HS, Weiner JI, Molina PL. Normal and abnormal thymus in childhood: MR imaging. *Radiology* 1989;172:367–371.
25. St. Amour TE, Siegel M, Glazer HS, Nadel SN. CT appearances of the normal and abnormal thymus in childhood. *J Comput Assist Tomogr* 1987;11:645–650.
26. Aronberg DJ, Glazer HS, Madsen K, Sagel SS. Normal thoracic aortic diameters by computed tomography. *J Comput Assist Tomogr* 1984;8:247–250.
27. Gamsu G, Webb WR. Computed tomography of the trachea: normal and abnormal. *AJR Am J Roentgenol* 1982;139:321–326.
28. Gamsu G, Webb WR. Computed tomography of the trachea and mainstem bronchi. *Semin Roentgenol* 1983;18:51–60.
29. Smathers RL, Buschi AJ, Pope TL, Brenbridge AN, Williamson BR. The azygos arch: normal and pathologic CT appearance. *AJR Am J Roentgenol* 1982;139:477–483.
30. Rockoff SD, Druy EM. Tortuous azygos arch simulating a pulmonary lesion. *AJR Am J Roentgenol* 1982;138:577–579.
31. Jolles PR, Shin MS, Jones WP. Aortopulmonary window lesions: detection with chest radiography. *Radiology* 1986;159:647–651.
32. Aronberg DJ, Peterson RR, Glazer HS, Sagel SS. The superior sinus of the pericardium: CT appearance. *Radiology* 1984;153:489–492.
33. McMurdo KK, Webb WR, von SG, Gamsu G. Magnetic resonance imaging of the superior pericardial recesses. *AJR Am J Roentgenol* 1985;145:985–988.
34. Fitzgerald SW, Donaldson JS. Azygoesophageal recess: normal CT appearance in children. *AJR Am J Roentgenol* 1991;158:1101–1104.
35. Müller NL, Webb WR, Gamsu G. Subcarinal lymph node enlargement: Radiographic findings and CT correlation. *AJR Am J Roentgenol* 1985;145:15–19.
36. Glazer GM, Gross BH, Quint LE, et al. Normal mediastinal lymph nodes: number and size according to American Thoracic Society mapping. *AJR Am J Roentgenol* 1985;144:261–265.
37. Kiyono K, Sone S, Sakai F, et al. The number and size of normal mediastinal lymph nodes: a postmortem study. *AJR Am J Roentgenol* 1988;150:771–776.
38. Takasugi JE, Godwin JD. CT appearance of the retroaortic anastomoses of the azygos system. *AJR Am J Roentgenol* 1990;154:41–44.
39. Smathers RL, Lee JKT, Heiken JP. Clinical image: anomalous preaortic interazygous vein. *J Comput Assist Tomogr* 1983;7:732–733.
40. Glazer HS, Molina PL, Siege MJ, Sagel SS. Pictorial essay. High-attenuation mediastinal masses on unenhanced CT. *AJR Am J Roentgenol* 1991;156:45–50.
41. Glazer HS, Siege MJ, Sagel SS. Pictorial essay. Low-attenuation mediastinal masses on CT. *AJR Am J Roentgenol* 1989;152:1173–1177.
42. Glazer HS, Wick MR, Anderson DJ, et al. CT of fatty thoracic masses. *AJR Am J Roentgenol* 1992;159:1181–1187.
43. Mendez G, Isikoff MB, Isikiff SK, Sinner WN. Fatty tumors of the thorax demonstrated by CT. *AJR Am J Roentgenol* 1979;133:207–212.
44. Enzi G, Biondetti PR, Fiore D, Mazzoleni FD. Computed tomography of deep fat masses in multiple symmetrical lipomastosis. *Radiology* 1982;144:122–124.
45. Lee WJ, Fatal G. Mediastinal lipomatosis in simple obesity. *Chest* 1976;70:308–309.
46. Rohlfing BM, Korobkin N, Hall AD. Computed tomography of intra-thoracic omental herniation and other mediastinal fatty masses. *J Comput Assist Tomogr* 1977;1:181–183.
47. Martin J, Palacio A, Petit J, Martin C. Fatty transformation of extra-meduallary hematopoiesis following splenectomy: CT features. *J Comput Assist Tomogr* 1990;14:477–478.
48. Brown LR, Aughenbaugh GL. Masses of the anterior mediastinum: CT and MR imaging. *AJR Am J Roentgenol* 1991;157:1171–1180.
49. Spizarny DL, Rebner M, Gross BH. CT of enhancing mediastinal masses. *J Comput Assist Tomogr* 1987;11:990–993.
50. Katlic MR, Wang C, Grillo HC. Substernal goiter. *Ann Thorac Surg* 1985;39:391–399.
51. Doppman JL, Skarulis MC, Chen CC, et al. Parathyroid adenomas in the aortopulmonary window. *Radiology* 1996;201:456–462.
52. McAdams HP, Rosado-de-Christenson ML, Moran CA. Mediastinal hemangioma: radiographic and CT features in 4 patients. *Radiology* 1994;193:399–402.
53. Joseph AE, Donaldson JS, Reynolds M. Neck and thorax venous aneurysm: association with cystic hygroma. *Radiology* 1989;170:109–112.
54. Drucker EA, McLoud TC, Dedrick CG, et al. Mediastinal paraganglioma: radiologic evaluation of an unusual vascular tumor. *AJR Am J Roentgenol* 1987;148:521–522.
55. Sheps SG, Brown ML. Localization of mediastinal paragangliomas (pheochromocytoma). *Chest* 1985;87:807–809.
56. Onik G, Goodman PC. CT of Castleman disease. *AJR Am J Roentgenol* 1983;140:691–692.
57. Mullen B, Richardson JD. Primary anterior mediastinal tumors in children and adults. *Ann Thorac Surg* 1986;42:338–345.
58. Ahn JM, Lee KS, Goo JM, et al. Predicting the histology of anterior mediastinal masses: comparison of chest radiography and CT. *J Thoracic Imaging* 1996;11:265–271.
59. Martin KW, McAliste WH. Case report. Intratracheal thymus: a rare cause of airway obstruction. *AJR Am J Roentgenol* 1987;149:1217,1218.
60. Goldstein G, Mackey IR. *The human thymus*. St. Louis: Warren H. Green, 1969.
61. Perlo VP, Arnason B, Castleman B. The thymus gland in elderly patients with myasthenia gravis. *Neurology* 1975;25:294–295.
62. Dixon AK, Hilton CJ, Williams GT. Computed tomography and histologic correlation of the thymic remnant. *Clin Radiol* 1981;32:255–257.
63. Day DL, Gedgaudas E. The thymus. *Radiol Clin North Am* 1984;22:519–538.
64. Cory DA, Cohen MD, Smith JA. Thymus in the superior mediastinum simulating adenopathy: appearance on CT. *Radiology* 1987;162:457–459.

65. Salonen OLM, Kivisaari ML, Somer JK. Computed tomography of the thymus of children under 10 years. *Pediatr Radiol* 1984;14:373–375.

66. Rollins NK, Currarino G. Case report. MR imaging of posterior mediastinal thymus. *J Comput Assist Tomogr* 1988;12:518–520.

67. Nicolaou S, Müller NL, Li DKB, Oger JJF. Thymus in myasthenia gravis: comparison of CT and pathologic findings and clinical outcome after thymectomy. *Radiology* 1996;20:471–474.

68. Molina PL, Siegel MJ, Glazer HS. Thymic masses on MR imaging. *AJR Am J Roentgenol* 1990;155:495–500.

69. Gelfand DW, Goldman AS, Law EJ, et al. Thymic hyperplasia in children recovering from thermal burns. *J Trauma* 1972;12:813–817.

70. Goldberg RE, Haaga JR, Yulish BS. Case report. Serial CT scans in thymic hyperplasia. *J Comput Assist Tomogr* 1987;11:539–540.

71. Chen J, Weisbrod GL, Herman SJ. Computed tomography and pathologic correlations of thymic lesions. *J Thorac Imaging* 1988;3:61–65.

72. Castleman B, Norris EH. The pathology of the thymus in myasthenia gravis. *Medicine* 1949;28:27–58.

73. Brown LR, Muhm JR, Sheedy PF, et al. The value of computed tomography in myasthenia gravis. *AJR Am J Roentgenol* 1983;140:31–35.

74. Cohen M, Hill CA, Cangir A, Sullivan MP. Thymic rebound after treatment of childhood tumors. *AJR Am J Roentgenol* 1980;135:151–156.

75. Choyke PL, Zeman RK, Gootenberg JE, Greenberg JN, Hoffer F, Frank JA. Thymic atrophy and regrowth in response to chemotherapy: CT evaluation. *AJR Am J Roentgenol* 1987;149:269–272.

76. Doppman JL, Oldfield EH, Chrousos GP. Rebound thymic hyperplasia after treatment of Cushing's syndrome. *AJR Am J Roentgenol* 1986;147:1145–1147.

77. Kissin CM, Husband JE, Nicholas D, Eversman W. Benign thymic enlargement in adults after chemotherapy: CT demonstration. *Radiology* 1987;163:67–70.

78. Keen SJ, Libshitz HI. Thymic lesions. Experience with computed tomography in 24 patients. *Cancer* 1987;59:1520–1523.

79. Weinreb JC, Mootz A, Cohen JM. MRI evaluation of mediastinal and thoracic inlet venous obstruction. *AJR Am J Roentgenol* 1986;146:679–684.

80. Freundlich IM, McGavran MH. Abnormalities of the thymus. *J Thorac Imaging* 1996;11:58–65.

81. Hoffman OA, Gillespie DJ, Aughenbaugh GL, Brown LR. Primary mediastinal neoplasms (other than thymoma). *Mayo Clin Proc* 1993;68:880–891.

82. Wychulis AR, Payne WS, Clagett OT, Wollner LB. Surgical treatment of mediastinal tumors: a 40-year experience. *J Thorac Cardiovasc Surg* 1971;62:379–391.

83. Morgenthaler TI, Brown LR, Colby TV, Harper CM, Coles DT. Thymoma. *Mayo Clin Proc* 1993;68:1110–1123.

84. LeGolvan DP, Abell MR. Thymomas. *Cancer* 1977;39:2142–2157.

85. Bergh N, Gatzinsky P, Larson S, Ludin P, Ridell B. Tumors of the thymus and thymic region: 1. clinicopathological studies on thymomas. *Ann Thorac Surg* 1978;25:91–98.

86. Marino M, Muller-Hermelink HK. Thymoma and thymic carcinoma. Relation of thymoma epithelial cells to the cortical and medullary differentiation of the thymus. *Virchows Arch* 1985;407:119–149.

87. Pescarmona E, Rendina EA, Venuta F, et al. The prognostic implication of thymoma histologic subtyping: a study of 80 consecutive cases. *Am J Clin Pathol* 1990;93:190–195.

88. Ricci C, Rendina EA, Pescarmona EO, et al. Correlations between histological type, clinical behaviour, and prognosis in thymoma. *Thorax* 1989;44:455–460.

89. Zerhouni EA, Scott WW, Baker RR, Wharam MO, Siegelman SS. Invasive thymomas: diagnosis and evaluation by computed tomography. *J Comput Assist Tomogr* 1982;6:92–100.

90. Scatarige JC, Fishman EK, Zerhouni EA, Siegelman SS. Transdiaphragmatic extension of invasive thymoma. *AJR Am J Roentgenol* 1985;144:31–35.

91. Kaplan I, Swayne LC, Widmann WD, Wolff M. Case report. CT demonstration of ''ectopic'' thymoma. *J Comput Assist Tomogr* 1988;12:1037–1038.

92. Korobkin M, Casano VA. Case report. Intracaval and intracardiac extension of malignant thymoma: CT diagnosis. *J Comput Assist Tomogr* 1989;13:348–350.

93. Asamura H, Morinaga S, Shimosato Y, Ono R, Naruke T. Thymoma displaying endobronchial polypoid growth. *Chest* 1988;94:647–649.

94. Maggi G, Giaccone G, Donadio M, et al. Thymomas. A review of 169 cases, with particular reference to results of surgical treatment. *Cancer* 1986;58:756–776.

95. Fujimura S, Kondo T, Handa M, et al. Results of surgical treatment for thymoma based on 66 patients. *J Thorac Cardiovasc Surg* 1987;93:708–714.

96. Krueger JB, Sagerman RH, King GA. Stage III thymoma: results of postoperative radiation therapy. *Radiology* 1988;168:855–858.

97. Mink JH, Bein ME, Sukov R, et al. Computed tomography of the anterior mediastinum in patients with myasthenia gravis and suspected thymoma. *AJR Am J Roentgenol* 1978;130:239–246.

98. McLoud TC, Wittenberg J, Ferrucci JT. Computed tomography of the thorax and standard radiographic evaluation of the chest: A comparative study. *J Comput Assist Tomogr* 1979;3:170–180.

99. Aita JF, Wannamaker WM. Body computerized tomography and the thymus. *Arch Neurol* 1979;36:20–21.

100. Baron RL, Lee JKT, Sagel SS, Levitt RG. Computed tomography of the abnormal thymus. *Radiology* 1982;142:127–134.

101. Keesey J, Bein M, Mink J. Detection of thymoma in myasthenia gravis. *Neurology* 1980;30:233–239.

102. Fon GT, Bein ME, Mancuso AA, et al. Computed tomography of the anterior mediastinum in myasthenia gravis. A radiologic-pathologic correlative study. *Radiology* 1982;142:135–141.

103. Ellis K, Austin JHM, Jaretzki A. Radiologic detection of thymoma in patients with myasthenia gravis. *AJR Am J Roentgenol* 1988;151:873–881.

104. Miller WT Jr. Thymoma mimicking a thyroid mass. *Radiology* 1992;184:75–76.

105. Kaye AD, Janssen R, Arger PH, et al. Mediastinal computed tomography in myasthenia gravis. *J Comp Assist Tomogr* 1983;7:273–279.

106. Endo M, Adachi S, Kusumoto M, et al. A study of the utility of the MR image for the diagnosis of thymic tumors: imaging and pathologic correlation [Japanese]. *Nippon Igaku Hoshasen Gakkai Zasshi* 1993;53:1–10.

107. Sakai F, Sone S, Kiyono K, et al. MR imaging of thymoma: radiologic-pathologic correlation. *AJR Am J Roentgenol* 1992;158:751–756.

108. Jaretzki A, Penn AS, Younger DS, et al. ''Maximal'' thymectomy for myasthenia gravis. *J Thorac Cardiovasc Surg* 1988;95:747–757.

109. Batra P, Herrmann C, Mulder D. Mediastinal imaging in myasthenia gravis: correlation of chest radiography, CT, MR, and surgical findings. *AJR Am J Roentgenol* 1987;148:515–519.

110. Quagliano PV. Thymic carcinoma: case reports and review. *J Thorac Imaging* 1996;11:66–74.

111. Hartman CA, Roth C, Minck C, Niedobitek G. Thymic carcinoma: report of five cases and review of the literature. *J Cancer Res Clin Oncol* 1990;116:69–82.

112. Do YS, Im JG, Lee BH, et al. CT findings in malignant tumors of thymic epithelium. *J Comput Assist Tomogr* 1995;19:192–197.

113. Doppman JL, Pass HI, Nieman LK, et al. Corticotropin-secreting carcinoid tumors of the thymus: diagnostic unreliability of thymic venous sampling. *Radiology* 1992;184:71–74.

114. Doppman JL, Nieman L, Miller DL, et al. Ectopic adrenocorticotropic hormone syndrome: localization studies in 28 patients. *Radiology* 1989;172:115–124.

115. Rosado-de-Christenson ML, Pugatch RD, Moran CA, Galobardes J. Thymolipoma: analysis of 27 cases. *Radiology* 1994;193:121–126.

116. Herrera L, Oz M, Lally J, Davies A. Thymolipoma simulating pulmonary sequestration. *J Pediatr Surg* 1982;17:313–315.

117. Shirkhoda A, Chasen MH, Eftekhari F, Goldman AM, Decaro L. MR imaging of mediastinal thymolipoma. *J Comput Assist Tomogr* 1987;11:364–365.

118. Yeh HC, Gordon A, Kirshner PA, Cohen BA. Computed tomography and sonography of thymolipoma. *AJR Am J Roentgenol* 1983;140:1131–1133.

119. Baron RL, Sagel SS, Baglan RJ. Thymic cysts following radiation therapy for Hodgkin disease. *Radiology* 1981;141:593–597.

120. Lewis CR, Manoharan A. Benign thymic cysts in Hodgkin's disease: report of a case and review of published cases. *Thorax* 1987;42:633–634.

121. Lindfors KK, Meyer JE, Dedrick CG, Hassell LA, Harris NL. Thymic cysts in mediastinal Hodgkin disease. *Radiology* 1985;156:37–41.

122. Gouliamos A, Striggaris K, Lolas C, et al. Case report. Thymic cyst. *J Comput Assist Tomogr* 1982;6:172–174.

123. Levine C. Case report. Cervical presentation of a large thymic cyst: CT appearance. *J Comput Assist Tomogr* 1988;12:656–657.

124. Jaramillo D, Perez-Atayde A, Griscom NT. Apparent association between thymic cysts and prior thoracotomy. *Radiology* 1989;172:207–209.

125. Heron CW, Husband JE, Williams MP. Hodgkin disease: CT of the thymus. *Radiology* 1988;167:647–651.

126. Luker G, Siegel MJ. Mediastinal Hodgkin disease in children: response to therapy. *Radiology* 1993;189:737–740.
127. Wernecke K, Vassallo P, Rutsch F, Peters PE, Potter R. Thymic involvement in Hodgkin disease: CT and sonographic findings. *Radiology* 1991;181:375–383.
128. Lagrange W, Dahm HM, Karstens J, Feichtinger J, Mittermayer C. Melanocystic neuroendocrine carcinoma of the thymus. *Cancer* 1987; 59:484–488.
129. Strollo DC, Rosado de Christenson ML, Jett JR. Primary mediastinal tumors. Part 1. Tumors of the anterior mediastinum. *Chest* 1997;112: 511–522.
130. Davis RD, Oldham HN, Sabiston DC. Primary cysts and neoplasms of the mediastinum: recent changes in clinical presentatin, methods of diagnosis, management, and results. *Ann Thorac Surg* 1987;44: 229–237.
131. Lee KS, Im JG, Han CH, et al. Malignant primary germ cell tumors of the mediastinum: CT features. *AJR Am J Roentgenol* 1989;153: 947–951.
132. Rosado-de-Christenson ML, Templeton PA, Moran CA. Mediastinal germ-cell tumors: radiologic and pathologic correlation. *Radiographics* 1992;12:1013–1030.
133. Moran CA, Suster S. Primary germ cell tumors of the mediastinum: 1. Analysis of 322 cases with special emphasis on teratomatous lesions and a proposal for histopathologic classification and clinical staging. *Cancer* 1997;80:681–690.
134. Moran CA, Suster S, Przygodzki RM, Koss MN. Primary germ cell tumors of the mediastinum: 2. Mediastinal seminomas—A clinicopathologic and immunohistochemical study of 120 cases. *Cancer* 1997;80:691–698.
135. Moran CA, Suster S, Koss MN. Primary germ cell tumors of the mediastinum: 3. Yolk sac tumor, embryonal carcinoma, choriocarcinoma, and combined nonteratomatous germ cell tumors of the mediastinum—A clinicopathologic and immunohistochemical study of 64 cases. *Cancer* 1997;80:699–707.
136. Knapp RH, Hurt RD, Payne WS, et al. Malignant germ cell tumors of the mediastinum. *J Thorac Cardiovasc Surg* 1985;89:82–89.
137. Dobranowski J, Martin LFW, Bennett WF. Case report. CT evaluation of posterior mediastinal teratoma. *J Comput Assist Tomogr* 1987;11: 156–157.
138. Weinberg B, Rose JS, Efremidis SC, Kirshner PA, Gribetz D. Posterior mediastinal teratoma (cystic dermoid): diagnosis by computerized tomography. *Chest* 1980;77:694–695.
139. Moeller KH, Rosado-de-Christensen ML, Templeton PA. Mediastinal mature teratoma: imaging features. *AJR Am J Roentgenol* 1997;169: 985–990.
140. Suzuki M, Takashima T, Itoh H, Choutoh S, Kanwamura I, Watamabe Y. Computed tomography of mediastinal teratomas. *J Comput Assist Tomogr* 1983;7:74–76.
141. Fulcher AS, Proto AV, Jolles H. Cystic teratoma of the mediastinum: demonstration of fat/fluid level. *AJR Am J Roentgenol* 1990;154: 259,260.
142. Seltzer SE, Herman PG, Sagel SS. Differential diagnosis of mediastinal fluid levels visualized on computed tomography. *J Comput Assist Tomogr* 1984;8:244–246.
143. Fulcher AS, Proto AV, Jolles H. Case report. Cystic teratoma of the mediastinum: demonstration of fat-fluid level. *AJR Am J Roentgenol* 1990;154:259–260.
144. Sasaka K, Kurihara Y, Nakajima Y, et al. Pictorial essay. Spontaneous rupture: complication of benign mature teratomas of the mediastinum. *AJR Am J Roentgenol* 1998;170:323–328.
145. Yeoman LJ, Dalton HR, Adam EJ. Case report. Fat-fluid level in pleural effusion as a complication of a mediastinal dermoid: CT characteristics. *J Comput Assist Tomogr* 1990;14:307–309.
146. Polansky SM, Barwick KW, Ravin CE. Primary mediastinal seminoma. *AJR Am J Roentgenol* 1979;132:17–21.
147. Shin MS, Ho KJ. Computed tomography of primary mediastinal seminomas. *J Comput Assist Tomogr* 1983;7:990–994.
148. Levitt RG, Husband JE, Glazer HS. CT of primary germ-cell tumors of the mediastinum. *AJR Am J Roentgenol* 1984;142:73–78.
149. Blomlie V, Lien HH, Fossa SD, Jawbsen AB, Stenwig AE. Computed tomography in primary non-seminomatous germ cell tumors of the mediastinum. *Acta Radiol* 1988;29:289–292.
150. Fox MA, Vix VA. Endodermal sinus (yolk sac) tumors of the anterior mediastinum. *AJR Am J Roentgenol* 1980;135:291–294.
151. Afifi HY, Bosl GJ, Burt ME. Mediastinal growing teratoma syndrome. *Ann Thorac Surg* 1997;64:359–362.

152. Park HM, Tarver RD, Siddiqui AR, Schauwecker DS, Wellman HN. Efficacy of thyroid scintigraphy in the diagnosis of intrathoracic goiter. *AJR Am J Roentgenol* 1987;148:527–529.
153. Glazer GM, Axel L, Moss AA. CT diagnosis of mediastinal thyroid. *AJR Am J Roentgenol* 1982;138:495–498.
154. Shahian DM, Rossi R. Posterior mediastinal goiter. *Chest* 1988;94: 599–602.
155. Sekiya T, Tada S, Kawakami K, et al. Clinical application of computed tomography to thyroid disease. *Comput Tomogr* 1979;3:185–193.
156. Machida K, Yoshikawa K. Case report. Aberrant thyroid gland demonstrated by computed tomography. *J Comput Assist Tomogr* 1979; 3:689–690.
157. Silverman PM, Newman GE, Korobkin M, Moore AV, Coleman RE. Computed tomography in the evaluation of thyroid disease. *AJR Am J Roentgenol* 1984;141:897–902.
158. Bashist B, Ellis K, Gold RP. Computed tomography of intrathoracic goiters. *AJR Am J Roentgenol* 1983;140:455–460.
159. Binder RE, Pugatch RD, J. FL, Kanter RA, Sawin CT. Case report. Diagnosis of posterior mediastinal goiter by computed tomography. *J Comput Assist Tomogr* 1980;4:550–552.
160. Morris UL, Colletti PM, Ralls PW, et al. Case report. CT demonstration of intrathoracic thyroid tissue. *J Comput Assist Tomogr* 1982;6: 821–824.
161. Radecki PD, Arger PH, Arenson RL, et al. Thyroid imaging: comparison of high-resolution real-time ultrasound and computed tomography. *Radiology* 1984;153:145–147.
162. Stark DD, Clark OH, Gooding GAW, Moss AA. High-resolution ultrasonography and computed tomography of thyroid lesions in patients with hyperparathyroidism. *Surgery* 1983;94:863–868.
163. Takashima S, Ikezoe J, Morimoto S, et al. Primary thyroid lymphoma: evaluation with CT. *Radiology* 1988;168:765–768.
164. Takashima S, Morimoto S, Ikezoe J, et al. Primary thyroid lymphoma: comparison of CT and US assessment. *Radiology* 1989;171:439–443.
165. Katz JF, Kane RA, Reyes J, Clarke MP, Hill TC. Thyroid nodules: sonographic-pathologic correlation. *Radiology* 1984;151:741–745.
166. Kier R, Silverman PM, Korobkin M, et al. Case report. Malignant teratoma of the thyroid in an adult: CT appearance. *J Comput Assist Tomogr* 1985;9:174–176.
167. deCertaines J, Herry JY, Lancien G, et al. Evaluation of human thyroid tumors by proton nuclear magnetic resonance. *J Nucl Med* 1982;23: 48–51.
168. Tennvall J, Biorklund A, Moller T, Olsen M, Persson B, Akerman M. Studies of NMR-relaxation-times in malignant tumours and normal tissues of the human thyroid gland. *Prog Nucl Med* 1984;8:142–148.
169. von Schulthess GK, McMurdo K, Tscholakoff D, et al. Mediastinal masses: MR imaging. *Radiology* 1986;158:289–296.
170. Gamsu G, Stark DD, Webb WR, Moore EH, Sheldon PE. Magnetic resonance imaging of benign mediastinal masses. *Radiology* 1984; 151:709–713.
171. Stark DD, Moss AA, Gamsu G, et al. Magnetic resonance imaging of the neck, part 1: normal anatomy. *Radiology* 1984;150:447–454.
172. Stark DD, Moss AA, Gamsu G, et al. Magnetic resonance imaging of the neck, part 2: pathologic findings. *Radiology* 1984;150:455–461.
173. Stark DD, Clark OH, Moss AA. Magnetic resonance imaging of the thyroid, thymus, and parathyroid glands. *Surgery* 1984;96: 1083–1091.
174. Higgins CB, McNamara MT, Fisher MR, Clark OH. MR imaging of the thyroid. *AJR Am J Roentgenol* 1986;147:1255–1261.
175. Higgins CB, Auffermann W. MR imaging of thyroid and parathyroid glands: a review of current status. *AJR* 1988;151:1095–1106.
176. Mountz JM, Glazer GM, Dmuchowski C, Sisson JC. MR imaging of the thyroid: comparison with scintigraphy in the normal and diseased gland. *J Comput Assist Tomogr* 1987;11:612–619.
177. Gefter WB, Spritzer CE, Eisenberg B, et al. Thyroid imaging with high-field strength surface-coil MR. *Radiology* 1987;164:483–490.
178. Noma S, Nishimura K, Togashi K, et al. Thyroid gland: MR imaging. *Radiology* 1987;164:495–499.
179. Noma S, Kanaoka M, Minami S, et al. Thyroid masses: MR imaging and pathologic correlation. *Radiology* 1988;168:759–764.
180. Charkes ND, Maurer AH, Siegel JA, Radecki PD, Malmud LS. MR imaging in thyroid disorders: correlation of signal intensity with Graves disease activity. *Radiology* 1987;164:491–494.
181. Auffermann W, Clark OH, Thurnher S, Galante M, Higgins CB. Recurrent thyroid carcinoma: characteristics on MR images. *Radiology* 1988;168:753–757.
182. Norris EH. The parathyroid adenoma: a study of 322 cases. *Int Abst Surg* 1947;84:1–41.

183. Clark OH. Mediastinal parathyroid tumors. *Arch Surg* 1988;123:1096–1100.
184. Kang YS, Rosen K, Clark OH, Higgins CB. Localization of abnormal parathyroid glands of the mediastinum with MR imaging. *Radiology* 1993;189:137–141.
185. Doppman JL, Brennan MF, Koehler JO, Marx SJ. Computed tomography for parathyroid localization. *J Comput Assist Tomogr* 1977;1:30–36.
186. Shimshak RR, Sundaram M, Eddelston B, Prendergast J. Diagnosis of parathyroid adenoma by computed tomography. *J Comput Assist Tomogr* 1979;3:117–119.
187. Whitley NO, Bohlman M, Connor TB, et al. Computed tomography for localization of parathyroid adenomas. *J Comput Assist Tomogr* 1981;5:812–817.
188. Wolverson MK, Sundaram M, Eddelston B, Prendergast J. Diagnosis of parathyroid adenoma by computed tomography. *J Comput Assist Tomogr* 1981;5:818–821.
189. Krudy AG, Doppman JL, Brennan MF, et al. The detection of mediastinal parathyroid glands by computed tomography, selective arteriography, and venous sampling. *Radiology* 1981;140:739–744.
190. Adams JE, Adams PH, Mantora H. Computed tomography in localization of parathyroid tumors. *Clin Radiol* 1981;32:251–254.
191. Ovenfors CO, Stark D, Moss A, et al. Localization of parathyroid adenoma by computed tomography. *J Comput Assist Tomogr* 1982;6:1094–1098.
192. Sommer B, Welter HF, Spelsberg F, Scherer U, Lissner J. Computed tomography for localizing enlarged parathyroid glands in primary hyperparathyroidism. *J Comput Assist Tomogr* 1982;6:521–526.
193. Doppman JL, Krudy AG, Brennan MF, et al. CT appearance of enlarged parathyroid glands in the posterior superior mediastinum. *J Comput Assist Tomogr* 1982;6:1099–1102.
194. Takagi H, Tominaga Y, Uchida K, et al. Preoperative diagnosis of secondary hyperparathyroidism using computed tomography. *J Comput Assist Tomogr* 1982;6:527–528.
195. Krudy AG, Doppman JL, Shawker TH, et al. Hyperfunctioning cystic parathyroid glands: CT and sonographic findings. *AJR Am J Roentgenol* 1984;142:175–178.
196. College D, Rohatgi RK. Mediastinal parathyroid cyst. *J Comput Assist Tomogr* 1983;7:140–142.
197. Lineaweaver W, Clore F, Mancuso A, Hill S, Rumley T. Calcified parathyroid glands detected by computed tomography. *J Comput Assist Tomogr* 1984;8:975–977.
198. Krubsack AJ, Wilson SD, Lawson TL, et al. Prospective comparison of radionuclide, computed tomographic, and sonographic localization of parathyroid tumors. *World J Surg* 1986;10:579–585.
199. Stark DD, Gooding GAW, Moss AA, Clark OH, Ovenfors CO. Parathyroid imaging: comparison of high-resolution CT and high-resolution sonography. *AJR Am J Roentgenol* 1983;141:633–638.
200. Cates JD, Thorsen K, Lawson TL, et al. CT evaluation of parathyroid adenomas: diagnostic criteria and pitfalls. *J Comput Assist Tomogr* 1988;12:626–629.
201. Lee VS, Spritzer CE, Coleman RE, et al. The complementary roles of fast spin-echo MR imaging and double-phase 99mTC-sestamibi scintigraphy for localization of hyperfunctioning parathyroid glands. *AJR Am J Roentgenol* 1996;167:1555–1562.
202. Miller DL, Doppman JL, Shawker TH, et al. Localization of parathyroid adenomas in patients who have undergone surgery. Part 1. Noninvasive imaging methods. *Radiology* 1987;162:133–137.
203. Satava RM, Beahrs OH, Scholz DA. Success rate of cervical exploration for hyperparathyroidism. *Arch Surg* 1975;110:625–627.
204. Shaha AR, Jaffe BM. Cervical exploration for primary hyperparathyroidism. *J Surg Oncol* 1993;52:14–17.
205. Perez-Monte JE, Brown ML, Shah AN, et al. Parathyroid adenomas: accurate detection and localization with Tc-99m sestamibi SPECT. *Radiology* 1996;201:85–91.
206. Weber CJ, Vansant J, Alazraki N, et al. Value of technetium 99m sestamibi iodine 123 imaging in reoperative parathyroid surgery. *Surgery* 1993;114:1011–1018.
207. Levin KE, Gooding GAW, Okerlund MD. Localizing studies in patients with persistent or recurrent hyperparathyroidism. *Surgery* 1987;102:917–925.
208. Kneeland JB, Krubsack AJ, Lawson TL, et al. Enlarged parathyroid glands: high-resolution local coil MR imaging. *Radiology* 1987;162:143–146.
209. Peck WW, Higgins CB, Fisher MR, et al. Hyperparathyroidism: comparison of MR imaging with radionuclide scanning. *Radiology* 1987;163:415–420.
210. Spritzer CE, Gefter WB, Hamilton R, et al. Abnormal parathyroid glands: high-resolution MR imaging. *Radiology* 1987;162:487–491.
211. Kier R, Blinder RA, Herfkins RJ, et al. MR imaging with surface coils in primary hyperparathyroidism. *J Comput Assist Tomogr* 1987;11:863–868.
212. Auffermann W, Gooding GAW, Okerlund MD, et al. Diagnosis of recurrent hyperparathyroidism: comparison of MR imaging and other imaging techniques. *AJR Am J Roentgenol* 1988;150:1027–1033.
213. Kang EH, Schiebler ML, Gefter WB, Kressel HY. Case report. MR demonstration of bilateral intrathyroidal parathyroid glands. *J Comput Assist Tomogr* 1988;12:349–350.
214. Krudy AG, Doppman JL, Marx SJ, et al. Radiographic findings in recurrent parathyroid carcinoma. *Radiology* 1982;142:625–629.
215. Miller DL, Doppman JL, Chang R, et al. Angiographic ablation of parathyroid adenomas: lessons from a 10-year experience. *Radiology* 1987;165:601–607.
216. Rouviere H. *Anatomie des lymphatiques de l'homme*. Paris: Masson et Cie, 1932.
217. Buy JN, Ghossain MA, Poirson F, et al. Computed tomography of mediastinal lymph nodes in nonsmall cell lung cancer: a new approach based on the lymphatic pathway of tumor spread. *J Comput Assist Tomogr* 1988;12:545–552.
218. Goss CM, ed. *Gray's Anatomy*. Philadelphia: Lea and Febiger, 1966.
219. Jochelson MS, Balikian JP, Mauch P, Liebman H. Peri- and paracardial involvement in lymphoma: a radiographic study in 11 cases. *AJR Am J Roentgenol* 1983;140:483–488.
220. Meyer JE, McLoud TC, Lindfors KK. CT demonstration of cardiophrenic angle lymphadenopathy in Hodgkin disease. *J Comput Assist Tomogr* 1985;9:485–488.
221. Scatarige JC, Fishman EK, Zinreich ES, Brem RF, Almaraz R. Internal mammary lymphadenopathy in breast cancinoma: CT appraisal of anatomic distribution. *Radiology* 1988;167:89–91.
222. Scatarige JC, Boxen I, Smathers RL. Interal mammary lymphadenopathy: imaging of a vital lymphatic pathway in breast cancer. *Radiographics* 1990;10:857–870.
223. Filly R, Blank N, Castellino R. Radiographic distribution of intrathoracic disease in previously untreated patients with Hodgkin's disease and non-Hodgkin's lymphoma. *Radiology* 1976;120:277.
224. Cho CS, Blank N, Castellino RA. CT evaluation of cardiophrenic angle lymph nodes in patients with malignant lymphoma. *AJR* 1984;143:719–721.
225. Aronberg DJ, Peterson RR, Glazer HS, Sagel SS. Superior diaphragmatic lymph nodes: CT assessment. *J Comput Assist Tomogr* 1986;10:937–941.
226. Sussman SK, Halvorsen RA, Silverman PM, Saeed M. Paracardiac adenopathy: CT evaluation. *AJR* 1987;149:29–34.
227. Vock P, Hodler J. Cardiophrenic angle adenopathy: update of causes and significance. *Radiology* 1986;159:395–399.
228. Schnyder PA, Gamsu G. CT of the pretracheal retrocaval space. *AJR* 1981;136:303–308.
229. Müller NL, Webb WR, Gamsu G. Paratracheal lymphadenopathy: radiographic findings and correlation with CT. *Radiology* 1985;156:761–765.
230. Platt JF, Glazer GM, Orringer MB, et al. Radiologic evaluation of the subcarinal lymph nodes: a comparative study. *AJR Am J Roentgenol* 1988;151:279–282.
231. Mountain CF. Revisions in the International System for Staging Lung Cancer. *Chest* 1997;111:1710–1717.
232. Mountain CF, Dresler CM. Regional lymph node classification for lung cancer staging. *Chest* 1997;111:1718–1723.
233. Beck E, Beattie EJ. The lymph nodes in the mediastinum. *J Int Coll Surgeons* 1958;29:247–251.
234. Glazer HS, Aronberg DJ, Sagel SS. Pictorial essay. Pitfalls in CT recognition of mediastinal lymphadenopathy. *AJR* 1985;144:267–274.
235. Mencini RA, Proto AV. The high left and main pulmonary arteries: A CT pitfall. *J Comput Assist Tomogr* 1982;6:452–459.
236. Quint LE, Glazer GM, Orringer MB, Francis IR, Bookstein FL. Mediastinal lymph node detection and sizing at CT and autopsy. *AJR Am J Roentgenol* 1986;147:469–472.

237. Moak GD, Cockerill EM, Farver MO, Yaw PB, Manfredi F. Computed tomography vs standard radiology in the evaluation of mediastinal adenopathy. *Chest* 1982;82:69–75.

238. Genereux GP, Howie JL. Normal mediastinal lymph node size and number: CT and anatomic study. *AJR Am J Roentgenol* 1984;142:1095–1100.

239. Klein JS, Webb WR. The radiologic staging of lung cancer. *J Thorac Imaging* 1991;7:29–47.

240. Daly BD, Faling LJ, Bite G, et al. Mediastinal lymph node evaluation by computed tomography in lung cancer. An analysis of 345 patients grouped by TNM staging, tumor size, and tumor location. *J Thorac Cardiovasc Surg* 1987;94:664–672.

241. Staples CA, Müller NL, Miller RR, Evans KG, Nelems B. Mediastinal nodes in bronchogenic carcinoma: comparison between CT and mediastinoscopy. *Radiology* 1988;167:367–372.

242. Lewis JW, Pearlberg JL, Beute GH, et al. Can computed tomography of the chest stage lung cancer? Yes and no. *Ann Thorac Surg* 1990;49:591–596.

243. Webb WR, Gatsonis C, Zerhouni EA, et al. CT and MR imaging in staging non-small cell bronchogenic carcinoma: report of the Radiologic Diagnostic Oncology Group. *Radiology* 1991;178:705–713.

244. Mori K, Yokoi K, Saito Y, Tominaga K, Miyazawa N. Diagnosis of mediastinal lymph node metastases in lung cancer. *Jpn J Clin Oncol* 1992;22:35–40.

245. McLoud TC, Bourgouin PM, Greenberg RW, et al. Bronchogenic carcinoma: analysis of staging in the mediastinum with CT by correlative lymph node mapping and sampling. *Radiology* 1992;182:319–323.

246. Andonopoulos AP, Karadanas AH, Drosis AA, et al. CT evaluation of mediastinal lymph nodes in primary Sjogren syndrome. *J Comput Assist Tomogr* 1988;12:199–201.

247. Aberle DR, Gamsu G, Lynch D. Thoracic manifestations of Wegener granulomatosis: diagnosis and course. *Radiology* 1990;174:703–709.

248. Bergin C, Castellino RA. Mediastinal lymph node enlargement on CT scans in patients with usual interstitial pneumonitis. *AJR Am J Roentgenol* 1990;154:251–254.

249. Glazer HS, Aronberg DJ, Sagel SS, Friedman PJ. CT demonstration of calcified mediastinal lymph nodes: a guide to the new ATS classification. *AJR Am J Roentgenol* 1986;147:17–20.

250. Lautin EM, Rosenblatt M, Friedman AC, et al. Calcification in non-Hodgkin lymphoma occurring before therapy: identification of plain films and CT. *AJR Am J Roentgenol* 1990;155:739–740.

251. Mallens WMC, Nijhuis-Heddes JMA, Bakker W. Calcified lymph node metastases in bronchioloalveolar carcinoma. *Radiology* 1986;161:103–104.

252. Panicek DM, Harty MP, Scicutella CJ, Carsky EW. Calcification in untreated mediastinal lymphoma. *Radiology* 1988;166:735–736.

253. Breatnach E, Myers JD, McElvein RB, Zorn GL. Roentgenogram of the month. Unusual case of a calcified anterior mediastinal mass. *Chest* 1986;89:113–115.

254. Gross BH, Schneider HJ, Proto AV. Eggshell calcification of lymph nodes: an update. *AJR Am J Roentgenol* 1980;135:1265–1268.

255. Mesisel S, Rozenman J, Yellin A, Apter S, Herczeg E, Knecht A. Castleman's disease. An uncommon computed tomographic feature. *Chest* 1988;93:1306–1307.

256. Stark P, Smith DC, Watkins GE, Chun KE. Primary intrathoracic extraosseous osteogenic sarcoma: report of three cases. *Radiology* 1990;174:725–726.

257. Groskin SA, Massi AF, Randall PA. Calcified hilar and mediastinal lymph nodes in an AIDS patient with *Pneumocystis carinii* infection. *Radiology* 1990;175:345–346.

258. Reede DL, Bergeron RT. Cervical tuberculous adenitis: CT manifestations. *Radiology* 1985;154:701–704.

259. Lee KS, Song KS, Lim TH, et al. Adult-onset pulmonary tuberculosis: findings on chest radiographs and CT scans. *AJR Am J Roentgenol* 1993;160:753–758.

260. Scatarige JC, Fishman EK, Kuhajda FP, Taylor GA, Siegelman SS. Low attenuation nodal metastases in testicular carcinoma. *J Comput Assist Tomogr* 1983;7:682–687.

261. Yousem DM, Scatariage JC, Fishman EK, Siegelman SS. Low-attenuation thoracic metastases in testicular malignancy. *AJR Am J Roentgenol* 1986;146:291–293.

262. Pombo F, Rodriquez E, Caruncho MV, et al. CT attenuation values and enhancing charateristics of thoraoabdominal lymphomatous adenopathy. *J Comput Assist Tomogr* 1994;18:59–64.

263. Hopper KD, Diehl LF, Cole BA, et al. The significance of necrotic mediastinal lymph nodes on CT in patients with newly diagnosed Hodgkin disease. *AJR Am J Roentgenol* 1990;155:267–270.

264. Samuels T, Hamilton P, Shaw P. Case report. Whipple disease of the mediastinum. *AJR Am J Roentgenol* 1990;154:1187–1188.

265. Shahidi H, Myers JL, Kvale PA. Castleman's disease. *Mayo Clin Proc* 1995;70:969–977.

266. Davis JM, Mark GJ, Greene R. Benign blood vascular tumors of the mediastinum. Report of four cases and review of the literature. *Radiology* 1978;126:581–587.

267. Hamper UM, Fishman EK, Khouri NF, et al. Typical and atypical CT manifestations of pulmonary sarcoidosis. *J Comput Assist Tomogr* 1986;10:928–936.

268. Kirks DR, McCormick VD, Greenspan RH. Pulmonary sarcoidosis: roentgenographic analysis of 150 patients. *AJR Am J Roentgenol* 1973;117:777–786.

269. Kuhlman JE, Fishman EK, Hamper WM, Knowles M, Siegelman SS. The computed tomographic spectrum of thoracic sarcoidosis. *Radiographics* 1989;9:449–466.

270. Castellino RA, Blank N, Hoppe RT, Cho C. Hodgkin disease: contributions of chest CT in the initial staging evaluation. *Radiology* 1986;160:603–605.

271. Castellino RA. Hodgkin disease: practical concepts for the diagnostic radiologist. *Radiology* 1986;157:305–310.

272. Castellino RA. Hodgkin disease: imaging studies and patient management. *Radiology* 1988;169:269–270.

273. Frija J, Bellin MF, Laval-Jeantet M. CT mediastinum examination in recurrent nerve paralysis. *J Comput Assist Tomogr* 1984;8:901–905.

274. Dooms GC, Hricak H, Crooks LE, Higgins CB. Magnetic resonance imaging of the lymph nodes: comparison with CT. *Radiology* 1984;153:719–728.

275. Dubray B, Grenier P, Carette MF, Frija G, Chastang C. Mediastinal lymph node involvement in bronchogenic carcinoma. CT and MRI evaluation using ROC methodology. *Rev Im Med* 1991;3:249–256.

276. Poon PY, Bronskill MJ, Henkelman RM, et al. Mediastinal lymph node metastases from bronchogenic carcinoma: detection with MR imaging and CT. *Radiology* 1987;162:651–656.

277. Laurent F, Drouillard J, Dorcier F, et al. Contribution and limits of x-ray computed tomography and magnetic resonance imaging in evaluating the extent of primary cancers of the bronchi. *Bull Cancer (Paris)* 1988;75:903–916.

278. Musset D, Grenier P, Carette MF, et al. Primary lung cancer staging: prospective comparative study of MR imaging with CT. *Radiology* 1986;160:607–611.

279. Dooms GC, Hricak H, Moseley ME, et al. Characterization of lymphadenopathy by magnetic resonance relaxation times: preliminary results. *Radiology* 1985;155:691–697.

280. de Geer G, Webb WR, Sollitto R, Golden J. MR characteristics of benign lymph node enlargement in sarcoidosis and Castleman's disease. *Eur J Radiol* 1986;6:145–148.

281. Glazer GM, Orringer MB, Chenevert TL, et al. Mediastinal lymph nodes: relaxation time/pathologic correlation and implications in staging of lung cancer with MR imaging. *Radiology* 1988;168:429–431.

282. Farmer DW, Moore E, Amparo E, et al. Calcific fibrosing mediastinitis: demonstration of pulmonary vascular obstruction by magnetic resonance imaging. *AJR Am J Roentgenol* 1984;143:1189–1191.

283. Rholl KS, Levitt RG, Glazer HS. Magnetic resonance imaging of fibrosing mediastinitis. *AJR Am J Roentgenol* 1985;145:255–259.

284. Batra P, Brown K, Steckel RJ, et al. MR imaging of the thorax: a comparison of axial, coronal, and sagittal imaging planes. *J Comput Assist Tomogr* 1988;12:75–81.

285. Webb WR, Jensen BG, Gamsu G, Sollitto R, Moore EH. Coronal magnetic resonance imaging of the chest: normal and abnormal. *Radiology* 1984;153:729–735.

286. Castellino RA. The non-Hodgkin lymphomas: practical concepts for the diagnostic radiologist. *Radiology* 1991;178:315–321.

287. Hoppe RT. The contemporary management of Hodgkin disease. *Radiology* 1988;169:297–304.

288. Hopper KD, Diehl LF, Lesar M, et al. Hodgkin disease: clinical utility of CT in initial staging and treatment. *Radiology* 1988;169:17–22.

289. Schomberg TJ, Evans RG, O'Connell MJ. Prognostic significance of mediastinal mass in adult Hodgkin's disease. *Cancer* 1984;53:324–328.

290. Kaplan HS. Hodgkin's disease: unfolding concepts concerning its nature, management and prognosis. *Cancer* 1980;45:2439.

291. Kadin ME, Glatstein EJ, Dorfman RE. Clinical pathologic studies in 177 untreated patients subjected to a laparotomy for the staging of Hodgkin's disease. *Cancer* 1977;27:1277.

292. Castellino RA, Hoppe RT, Blank N, et al. Computed tomography, lymphography and staging laporotomy: correlations with initial staging of Hodgkin's disease. *AJR Am J Roentgenol* 1984;143:37–41.

293. Castellino RA, Hilton S, O'Brien JP, Portlock CS. Non-Hodgkin lymphoma: contribution of chest CT in the intitial staging evaluation. *Radiology* 1996;199:129–132.

294. Khoury MB, Godwin JD, Halvorsen R, Hanum Y, Putman CE. Role of chest CT in non-Hodgkin's lymphoma. *Radiology* 1986;158:659–662.

295. Bragg DG, Colby TV, Ward JH. New concepts in the non-Hodgkin lymphomas: radiologic implications. *Radiology* 1986;159:289–304.

296. Wang Y. Classification of non-Hodgkin's lymphoma. *AJR Am J Roentgenol* 1986;147:205–208.

297. Kazerooni EA, Williams DM, Deeb GM. Thoracic periaortic lymphoma mimicking aortic dissection. *AJR Am J Roentgenol* 1992;159:705–707.

298. Fishman EK, Kuhlman JE, Jones RJ. CT of lymphoma: spectrum of disease. *Radiographics* 1991;11:647–669.

299. Neuman CH, Robert NJ, Canellos G, Rosenthal D. Computed tomography of the abdomen and pelvis in non-Hodgkin lymphoma. *J Comput Assist Tomogr* 1983;7:846–850.

300. Shaffer K, Smith D, Kirn D, et al. Primary mediastinal large-B-cell lymphoma: radiologic findings at presentation. *AJR Am J Roentgenol* 1996;167:425–430.

301. North LB, Fuller LM, Sullivan-Halley J, Hagemeister FB. Regression of mediastinal Hodgkin disease after therapy: evaluation of time interval. *Radiology* 1987;164:599–602.

302. Nyman RS, Rehn SM, Glimelius BLG, et al. Residual mediastinal masses in Hodgkin disease: prediction of size with MR imaging. *Radiology* 1989;170:435–440.

303. Libshitz HJ, Jing BS, Walace S, Logothetis CJ. Sterilized metastases: a diagnostic and therapeutic dilemma. *AJR Am J Roentgenol* 1983;140:14–19.

304. Chen JL, Osborne BM, Butler JJ. Residual fibrous masses in treated Hodgkin's disease. *Cancer* 1987;60:407–413.

305. Durkin W, Durant J. Benign mass lesions after therapy for Hodgkin's disease. *Arch Int Med* 1979;139:333–336.

306. Jochelson M, Mauch P, Balikian J, Rosenthal D, Canellos G. The significance of the residual mediastinal mass in treated Hodgkin's disease. *J Clin Oncol* 1985;3:637–640.

307. Radford JA, Cowan RA, Flanagan M, et al. The significance of residual mediastinal abnormality on the chest radiograph following treatment for Hodgkin's disease. *J Clin Oncol* 1988;6:940–946.

308. Stewart FM, Williamson BR, Innes DJ, Hess CE. Residual tumor masses following treatment for advanced histiocytic lymphoma. *Cancer* 1985;55:620–623.

309. Lee CKK, Bloomfield CD, Goldman AI, Levitt SH. Prognostic significance of mediastinal involvement in Hodgkin's disease treated with curative radiotherapy. *Cancer* 1980;46:2403–2409.

310. Mauch P, Goodman R, Hellman S. The significance of mediastinal involvement in early stage Hodgkin's disease. *Cancer* 1978;42:1039–1045.

311. North LB, Fuller LM, Hagemeister FB, Importance of initial mediastinal adenopathy in Hodgkin's disease. *AJR Am J Roentgenol* 1982;138:229–235.

312. Anderson H, Jenkins JPR, Brigg DJ, et al. The prognostic significance of mediastinal bulk in patients with stage IA-IVB Hodgkin's disease: a report from the Manchester Lymphoma Group. *Clin Radiol* 1985;36:449–454.

313. Tumeh SS, Rosenthal DS, Kaplan WD, English RJ, Holman BL. Lymphoma: evaluation with Ga-67 SPECT. *Radiology* 1987;164:111–114.

314. Israel O, Front D, Lam M, et al. Gallium 67 imaging in monitoring lymphoma response to treatment. *Cancer* 1988;61:2439–2443.

315. Webb WR. MR imaging of treated mediastinal Hodgkin disease (editorial). *Radiology* 1989;170:315,316.

316. Rahmouni A, Tempany C, Jones R, et al. Lymphoma: monitoring tumor size and signal intensity with MR imaging. *Radiology* 1993;188:445–451.

317. Nyman R, Rehn S, Glimelius B, et al. Magnetic resonance imaging for assessment of treatment effects in mediastinal Hodgkin's disease. *Acta Radiol* 1987;28:145–151.

318. Glazer HS, Lee JK, Levitt RG, et al. Radiation fibrosis: differentiation from recurrent tumor by MR imaging. *Radiology* 1985;156:721–726.

319. Rehn SM, Nyman RS, Glimelius BL, Hagberg HE, Sundström JC. Non-Hodgkin lymphoma: predicting prognostic grade with MR imaging. *Radiology* 1990;176:249–253.

320. Zerhouni EA, Fishman EK, Jones R, Siegelman SS, Soulen RL. MR imaging of sterilized lymphoma (abstr). *Radiology* 1986;161(P):207.

321. Rahmouni AD, Zerhouni EA. Role of MRI in the management of thoracic lymphoma. In: Zerhouni EA, ed. *CT and MRI of the thorax.* New York: Churchill-Livingstone, 1990.

322. Weller SA, Glatstein E, Kaplan HS, Rosenberg SA. Initial relapses in previously treated Hodgkin's disease: results of second treatment. *Cancer* 1976;37:2840–2846.

323. Schein PS, Chabner BA, Canellos GP, Young RC, de Vita VT. Non-Hodgkin's lymphoma: patterns of relapse from complete remission after combination chemotherapy. *Cancer* 1975;35:334–357.

324. Rostock RA, Giangreco A, Wharam MD, et al. CT scan modification in the treatment of mediastinal Hodgkin's disease. *Cancer* 1982;49:2267–2275.

325. Maile CW, Moore AV, Ulreich S, Putman CE. Chest radiographic-pathologic correlation in adult leukemic patients. *Invest Radiol* 1983;18:495–499.

326. Takasugi JE, Godwin JD, Marglin SI, Petersdorf SH. Intrathoracic granulocytic sarcomas. *J Thorac Imaging* 1996;11:223–230.

327. Keller AR, Hochholzer L, Castleman B. Hyaline-vascular and plasma-cell types of giant lymph node hyperplasia of the mediastinum and other locations. *Cancer* 1972;29:670–683.

328. Bragg DG, Chor PJ, Murray KA, Kjeldsberg CR. Lymphoproliferative disorders of the lung: histopathology, clinical manifestations, and imaging features. *AJR Am J Roentgenol* 1994;163:273–281.

329. Menke DM, Camoriano JK, Banks PM. Angiofollicular lymph node hyperplasia: a comparison of unicentric, multicentric, hyaline vascular, and plasma cell types of disease by morphometric and clinical analysis. *Mod Path* 1992;5:525–530.

330. Fiore D, Biondetti PR, Calabro F, Rea F. Case report. CT demonstration of bilateral Castleman's tumors in the mediastinum. *J Comput Assist Tomogr* 1983;7:719–720.

331. Ferreiros J, Leon NG, Mata MI, et al. Computed tomography in abdominal Castleman's disease. *J Comput Assist Tomogr* 1989;13:433–436.

332. Meisel S, Rozenman J, Yellin A, et al. Castleman's disease: an uncommon computed tomographic feature. *Chest* 1988;93:1306–1307.

333. Libson E, Fields S, Strauss S, et al. Widespread Castleman disease: CT and US findings. *Radiology* 1988;166:753–755.

334. Thompson GP, Utz JP, Rosenow EC, Myers JL, Swensen SJ. Pulmonary lymphoproliferative disorders. *Mayo Clin Proc* 1993;68:804–817.

335. Harris KM, Schwartz ML, Slasky BS, Nalesnik M, Makowka L. Post-transplantation cyclosporine-induced lymphoproliferative disorders: clinical and radiological manifestations. *Radiology* 1987;162:697–700.

336. McLoud TC, Kalisher L, Stark P, Greene R. Intrathoracic lymph node metastases from extrathoracic neoplasms. *AJR Am J Roentgenol* 1978;131:403–407.

337. Müller NL, Kullnig P, Miller RR. The CT findings of pulmonary sarcoidosis: analysis of 25 patients. *AJR Am J Roentgenol* 1989;152:1179–1182.

338. Bein ME, Putman CE, McLoud TC, Mink JH. A reevaluation of intrathoracic lymphadenopathy in sarcoidosis. *AJR Am J Roentgenol* 1978;131:409–415.

339. Rockoff SD, Rohatgi PK. Unusual manifestations of thoracic sarcoidosis. *AJR Am J Roentgenol* 1985;144:513–528.

340. Kushihashi T, Munechika H, Motoya H, et al. CT and MR findings in tuberculous mediastinitis. *J Comput Assist Tomogr* 1995;19:379–382.

341. Naidich DP, Garay SM, Goodman PC, Ryback BJ, Kramer EL. Pulmonary manifestations of AIDS. In: Federle M, Megibow A, Naidich DP, eds. *Radiology of acquired immune deficiency syndrome.* New York: Raven, 1988:47–77.

342. Hartman TE, Primack SL, Müller NL, Staples CA. Diagnosis of thoracic complications in AIDS: accuracy of CT. *AJR Am J Roentgenol* 1994;162:547–553.

343. Naidich DP, Tarras M, Garay SM, et al. Kaposi sarcoma: CT-radiographic correlation. *Chest* 1989;96:723–728.

344. Moon WK, Im JG, In KY, et al. Mediastinal tuberculous lymphadenitis: MR imaging appearance with clinicopathologic correlation. *AJR Am J Roentgenol* 1996;166:21–25.

345. Landay MJ, Rollins NK. Mediastinal histoplasmosis granuloma: evaluation with CT. *Radiology* 1989;172:657–659.

346. Loyd JE, Tillman BF, Atkinson JB, Des Prez RM. Mediastinal fibrosis complicating histoplasmosis. *Medicine* 1988;67:295–310.

347. Wieder S, Rabinowitz JG. Fibrous mediastinitis: a late manifestation of mediastinal histoplasmosis. *Radiology* 1977;125:305–312.

348. Weinstein JB, Aronberg DJ, Sagel SS. CT of fibrosing mediastinitis: findings and their utility. *AJR Am J Roentgenol* 1983;141:247–251.

349. Goodwin RA, Nickell JA, Des Pres RM. Mediastinal fibrosis complicating healed primary histoplasmosis and tuberculosis. *Medicine* 1972;51:227–246.

350. Kountz PD, Molina PL, Sagel SS. Fibrosing mediastinitis in the posterior thorax. *AJR Am J Roentgenol* 1989;153:489–490.

351. Sherrick AD, Brown LR, Harms GF, et al. Radiographic findings of fibrosing mediastinitis. *Chest* 1994;106:484–489.

352. Paling MR, Williamson BRJ. Epipericardial fat pad: CT findings. *Radiology* 1987;165:335–339.

353. Homer JM, Wechsler RJ, Carter BL. Mediastinal lipomatosis. *Radiology* 1978;128:657–661.

354. Koerner HF, Sun DIC. Mediastinal lipomatosis secondary to steroid therapy. *Am J Rad Ther* 1966;98:461–464.

355. Price JE, Rigler LG. Widening of the mediastinum resulting from fat accumulation. *Radiology* 1970;96:497–500.

356. Bein NE, Mancuso AA, Mink JH, Hansen GC. Computed tomography in the evaluation of mediastinal lipomatosis. *J Comput Assist Tomogr* 1978;2:379–383.

357. Glickstein MF, Miller WT, Dalinka MK, Lally JF. Paraspinal lipomatosis: a benign mass. *Radiology* 1987;163:79–80.

358. Streiter ML, Schneider HJ, Proto AV. Steroid-induced thoracic lipomatosis: paraspinal involvement. *Am J Roentgenol* 1982;139:679–681.

359. Keely JG, Vana AJ. Lipomas of the mediastinum, 1940–1955. *Int Abst Surg* 1956;103:312–322.

360. Truwit JD, Jacobs JK, Newman JH, Dyer EL. Roentgenogram of the month. Anterior mediastinal mass following pneumonectomy. *Chest* 1988;94:173–174.

361. Cohen WN, Seidelmann FE, Bryan PJ. Computed tomography of localized adipose deposits presenting as tumor masses. *Am J Roentgenol* 1977;128:1007–1011.

362. Rubin E. Case of the winter season. *Semin Roentgenol* 1978;13:5–6.

363. Schweitzer DL, Aguam AS. Primary liposarcoma of the mediastinum. *J Thorac Cardiovasc Surg* 1977;741:83–97.

364. Yang R, Elliston L, Peterson R, Sahmel R. Roentgenogram of the month. Dysphagia and cough in a patient with a posterior mediastinal mass. *Chest* 1987;92:529–530.

365. DeSantos LA, Ginaldi S, Wallace S. Computed tomography in liposarcoma. *Cancer* 1981;47:46–54.

366. Quinn SF, Monson M, Paling M. Case report. Spinal lipoma presenting as a mediastinal mass: diagnosis by CT. *J Comput Assist Tomogr* 1983;7:1087–1089.

367. Kim K, Koo BC, Davis JT, Franco-Saenz R. Primary myelolipoma of mediastinum. *CT* 1984;8:119–123.

368. Kline ME, Patel BU, Agosti SJ. Noninfiltrating angiolipoma of the mediastinum. *Radiology* 1990;175:737–738.

369. Fagelman D, Caridi JG. CT diagnosis of hernia of Morgagni. *Gastrointest Radiol* 1984;9:153–155.

370. Gale ME. Bochdalek hernia: prevalence and CT characteristics. *Radiology* 1985;156:449–452.

371. DeMartini WJ, House AJS. Partial Bochdalek's herniation: computed tomographic evaluation. *Chest* 1980;77:702–704.

372. Ginalski JM, Schnuder P, Moss AA, Brasch RC. Incidence and significance of a widened esophageal hiatus at CT scan. *J Clin Gastroenterol* 1984;6:467–470.

373. Yeager BA, Guglielmi GE, Schiebler ML, Gefter WB, Kressel HY. Magnetic resonance imaging of Morgagni hernia. *Gastrointest Radiology* 1987;12:296–298.

374. London J, Kim EE, Wallace S, et al. MR imaging of liposarcomas: correlation of MR features and histology. *J Comput Assist Tomogr* 1989;13:832–835.

375. Dooms GC, Hricak H, Sollitto RA, Higgins CB. Lipomatous tumors and tumors with fatty component: MR imaging potential and comparison of MR and CT results. *Radiology* 1985;157:479–483.

376. Fitch SJ, Tonkin ILD, Tonkin AK. Imaging of foregut duplication cysts. *Radiographics* 1986;6:189–201.

377. Panicek DM, Heitzman ER, Randall PA, et al. The continuum of pulmonary developmental anomalies. *Radiographics* 1987;7:747–772.

378. Pugatch RD, Faling LJ, Spira R. CT diagnosis of benign mediastinal abnormalities. *AJR Am J Roentgenol* 1980;134:685–694.

379. Marvasti MA, Mitchell GE, Burke WA, Meyer JA. Misleading density of mediastinal cysts on computerized tomography. *Ann Thorac Surg* 1981;31:167–170.

380. Nakata H, Nakayama C, Kimoto T, et al. Computed tomography of mediastinal bronchogenic cysts. *J Comput Assist Tomogr* 1982;6:733–738.

381. Mendelson DS, Rose JS, Efremidis SC, Kirschner PA, Cohen BA. Bronchogenic cysts with high CT numbers. *AJR Am J Roentgenol* 1983;140:463–465.

382. Nakata H, Sato Y, Nakayama T, Yoshimatsu H, Kobayashi T. Bronchogenic cyst with high CT number: analysis of contents. *J Comput Assist Tomogr* 1986;10:360–362.

383. Yemault JC, Kuhn G, Dumortier P, et al. "Solid" mediastinal bronchogenic cyst: mineralogic analysis. *J Comput Assist Tomogr* 1986;146:73–74.

384. Dahmash NS, Chen JTT, Ravin CE, Reed JC, Pratt PC. Unusual radiologic manifestations of bronchogenic cyst. *South Med J* 1984;77:762–764.

385. Reed JC, Sobonya RE. Morphologic analysis of foregut cysts in the thorax. *AJR Am J Roentgenol* 1974;120:851–860.

386. Volpi A, Cavalli A, Maggioni AP, Pieri-Nerli F. Left atrial compression by a mediastinal bronchogenic cyst presenting with paroxysmal atrial fibrillation. *Thorax* 1988;43:216–217.

387. Bankoff MS, Daly BDT, Johnson HA, Carter BL. Case report. Bronchogenic cyst causing superior vena cava obstruction: CT appearance. *J Comput Assist Tomogr* 1985;9:951–952.

388. Kuhlman JE, Fishman EK, Wang KP, Zerhouni EA, Siegelman SS. Mediastinal cysts: diagnosis by CT and needle aspiration. *AJR Am J Roentgenol* 1988;150:75–78.

389. Haller JA, Golladay ES, Pickard LR, Tepas JJ, Shorter NA, Shermeta DW. Surgical management of lung bud anomalies: lobar emphysema, bronchogenic cyst, cystic adenomatoid malformation, and intralobar pulmonary sequestration. *Ann Thorac Surg* 1979;28:33–43.

390. Schwartz DB, Beals TF, Wimbish KJ, Hammersley JR. Transbronchial fine needle aspiration of bronchogenic cysts. *Chest* 1985;88:573–575.

391. Zimmer WD, Kamida CB, McGough PF, Rosenow EC. Mediastinal duplication cyst. Percutaneous aspiration and cystography for diagnosis and treatment. *Chest* 1986;90:772–773.

392. Kuhlman JE, Fishman EK, Wang KP, Siegelman SS. Esophageal duplication cysts: CT and transesophageal aspiration. *AJR Am J Roentgenol* 1985;145:531,532.

393. Wittich GR, Karnel F, Schurawitzki H, Jantsch H. Percutaneous drainage of mediastinal pseudocysts. *Radiology* 1988;167:51–53.

394. Kawashima A, Fishman EK, Kuhlman JE, Nixon MS. CT of posterior mediastinal masses. *Radiographics* 1991;11:1045–1067.

395. Weiss LM, Fagelman D, Warhit JM. CT demonstration of an esophageal duplication cyst. *J Comput Assist Tomogr* 1983;7:716–718.

396. Maroko I, Hirsch M, Sharon N, Benharroch D. Calcified mediastinal enterogenous cyst. *Gastrointest Radiol* 1984;9:105–106.

397. Rogers CI, Seymour Q, Brock JG. Case report. Atypical pericardial cyst location: the value of computed tomography. *J Comput Assist Tomogr* 1980;4:683–684.

398. Patel BK, Markivee CR, George EA. Pericardial cyst simulating intracardiac mass. *AJR Am J Roentgenol* 1983;141:292–294.

399. Pugatch RD, Braver JH, Robbins AH, Faling J. CT diagnosis of pericardial cysts. *AJR Am J Roentgenol* 1978;131:515–516.

400. Brunner DR, Whitley NO. A pericardial cyst with high CT numbers. *AJR Am J Roentgenol* 1984;142:279–280.

401. Parienty RA, Fontaine Y, Guillemette D. Transformation of a pericardial cyst observed on long-term follow-up. *CT* 1984;8:125–128.

402. Winer-Muram HT, Gold RE. Effusion in the superior pericardial recess simulating a medistinal mass. *AJR Am J Roentgenol* 1990;154:69–71.

403. Terrier F, Revel D, Pajannen H, et al. MR imaging of body fluid collections. *J Comput Assist Tomogr* 1986;10:953–962.

404. Naidich DP, Rumancik WM, Ettenger NA, et al. Congenital anomalies of the lungs in adults: MR diagnosis. *AJR Am J Roentgenol* 1988;151:13–19.

405. Stark DD, Higgins CB, Lanzer P, et al. Magnetic resonance imaging of the pericardium: normal and pathologic findings. *Radiology* 1984;150:469–474.

406. Barakos JA, Brown JJ, Brescia RJ, Higgins CB. High signal intensity lesions of the chest in MR imaging. *J Comput Assist Tomogr* 1989;13:797–802.

407. Siegel MJ, Nadel SN, Glazer HS, Sagel SS. Mediastinal lesions in children: comparison of CT and MR. *Radiology* 1986;160:241–244.

408. Winsett MZ, Amparo EG, Fagan CJ, et al. MR imaging of mediastinal pseudocyst. *J Comput Assist Tomogr* 1988;12:320–322.

409. Murayama S, Murakami J, Watanabe H, et al. Signal intensity characteristics of mediastinal cystic masses on T1-weighted MRI. *J Comput Assist Tomogr* 1995;19:188–191.

410. Lyon RD, McAdams HP. Mediastinal bronchogenic cyst: demonstration of a fluid-fluid level at MR imaging. *Radiology* 1993;186:427–428.

411. Shaffer K, Rosado-de-Christenson ML, Patz EFJr, Young S, Farver CF. Thoracic lymphangioma in adults: CT and MR imaging features. *AJR* 1994;162:283–289.

412. Brown LR, Reiman HM, Rosenow EC, Gloviczki PM, Divertie MB. Intrathoracic lymphangioma. *Mayo Clin Proc* 1986;61:882–892.

413. Miyake H, Shiga M, Takaki H, et al. Mediastinal lymphangiomas in adults: CT findings. *J Thorac Imaging* 1996;1:83–85.

414. Pilla TJ, Wolverson MK, Sundaram M, Heiberg E, Shields JB. CT evaluation of cystic lymphangiomas of the mediastinum. *Radiology* 1982;144:841–842.

415. Pannell TL, Jolles H. Adult cystic mediastinal lymphangioma simulating a thymic cyst. *J Thorac Imaging* 1991;7:86–89.

416. Angtuaco EJC, Jiminez JF, Burrows P, Ferris E. Case report. Lymphatic-venous malformation (lymphangiohemangioma) of the mediastinum. *J Comput Assist Tomogr* 1983;7:895–897.

417. Shaked A, Raz I, Gottehrer A, Romanoff H. Aymptomatic, highly vascularized superior mediastinal mass. *Chest* 1984;86:621,622.

418. Cohen AJ, Sbaschnig RJ, Hochholzer L, Lough FC, Albus RA. Mediastinal hemangiomas. *Ann Thorac Surg* 1987;43:656–659.

419. Halber MD, Daffner RH, Thompson WM. CT of the esophagus: normal appearance. *AJR* 1979;133:1047–1050.

420. Noh HM, Fishman EK, Forastiere AA, Bliss DF, Calhoun PS. CT of the esophagus: spectrum of diseaase with emphasis on esophageal carcinoma. *Radiographics* 1995;15:1113–1134.

421. Boring CC, Squires TS, Tong T, Montgomery S. Cancer statistics 1994. *CA Cancer J Clin* 1994;44:7–26.

422. Kressel HY, Callen PW, Montagne JP, et al. Computed tomographic evaluation of disorders affecting the alimentary tract. *Radiology* 1978;129:451–455.

423. Agostini S, Salducci J, Clement JP. Case report. Idiopathic muscular hypertrophy of the esophagus: CT features. *J Comput Assist Tomogr* 1988;12:1041–1043.

424. Mori S, Kasai M, Watanabe T. Preoperative assessment of resectability for carcinoma of the thoracic esophagus. *Ann Surg* 1979;190:100–105.

425. Beahrs OH, Meyers MH, eds. *Manual for staging of cancer*, 2nd ed. Philadelphia: JB Lippincott, 1983.

426. Moss AA, Schnyder P, Thoeni RF, Margulis AR. Esophageal carcinoma: pretherapy staging by computed tomography. *AJR Am J Roentgenol* 1981;136:1051–1056.

427. Reinig JW, Stanley JH, Schabel SI. CT evaluation of thickened esophageal walls. *AJR Am J Roentgenol* 1983;140:951–958.

428. Schneekloth G, Terrier F, Fuchs WA. Computed tomography in carcinoma of esophagus and cardia. *Gastrointest Radiol* 1983;8:193–206.

429. Samuelson L, Hambraeus GM, Mercke EC. CT staging of esophageal carcinoma. *Acta Radiol Diag* 1984;25:7–11.

430. Terrier F, Schapira CL, Fuchs WA. CT assessment of operability in carcinoma of the esophagogastric junction. *Eur J Radiol* 1984;4:114–117.

431. Daffner RH, Halber MD, Postlethwait RW, Korobkin M, Thompson WM. CT of the esophagus. Part 2. Carcinoma. *AJR Am J Roentgenol* 1979;133:1051–1055.

432. Thompson WM, Halvorsen RA, Foster WL, et al. Computed tomography for staging esophageal and gastroesophageal cancer: reevaluation. *AJR Am J Roentgenol* 1983;141:951–958.

433. Kron IL, Cantrell RW, Johns ME, Joob A, Minor G. Computerized axial tomography of the esophagus to determine the suitability for blunt esophagectomy. *Ann Surg* 1984;49:173,174.

434. Quint LE, Glazer GM, Orringer MB, Gross BH. Esophageal carcinoma: CT findings. *Radiology* 1985;155:171–175.

435. Freeny PC, Marks WM. Adenocarcinoma of the gastroesophageal junction: barium and CT examination. *AJR Am J Roentgenol* 1982;138:1077–1084.

436. Picus D, Balfe DM, Koehler RE, Roper CL, Owen JW. Computed tomography in the staging of esophageal carcinoma. *Radiology* 1983;146:433–438.

437. Moss AA. Critical reviews. Esophageal carcinoma: CT findings. *Invest Radiol* 1987;22:84–87.

438. Quint LE, Glazer GM, Orringer MB, Gross BH. Esophageal imaging by MR and CT: study of normal anatomy and neoplasms. *Radiology* 1985;156:727–731.

439. Halvorsen RA, Magruder-Habib K, Foster WL, et al. Esophageal cancer staging by CT: long-term follow-up study. *Radiology* 1986;161:147–151.

440. Halvorsen RA, Thompson WM. Computed tomographic staging of gastrointestinal tract malignancies. Part 1. Esophagus and stomach. *Invest Radiol* 1987;22:2–16.

441. Vilgrain V, Mompoint D, Palazzo L, et al. Staging of esophageal carcinoma: comparison of results with endoscopic sonography and CT. *AJR Am J Roentgenol* 1990;155:277–281.

442. Iizuka T, Isono K, Kakegawa T, Watanabe H. Parameters linked to ten-year survival in Japan of resected esophageal carcinoma. Report of the Japanese Committee for Registration of Esophageal Carcinoma Cases. *Chest* 1989;96:1005–1011.

443. Maerz LL, Deveny CW, Lopez RR, McConnell BD. Role of computed tomographic scans in the staging of esoph ageal and proximal gastric malignancies. *Am J Surg* 1993;165:558–560.

444. Wippold FJ, Schnapf D, Bennet LL, Friedman AC. Case report. Esophago-subarachnoidal fistula: an unusual complication of esophageal carcinoma. *J Comput Assist Tomogr* 1982;6:147–149.

445. Reddy SC. Esophagopleural fistula. *J Comput Assist Tomogr* 1983;7:376–378.

446. Cornwell J, Walden C, Ghahremani GG. Case report. CT demonstration of fistula between esophageal carcinoma and spinal canal. *J Comput Assist Tomogr* 1986;10:871–873.

447. Heiken JP, Balfe DM, Roper CL. CT evaluation after esophagogastrectomy. *AJR Am J Roentgenol* 1984;143:555–560.

448. Gross BH, Agha FP, Glazer GM, Orringer MB. Gastric interposition following transhiatal esophagectomy: CT evaluation. *Radiology* 1985;155:177–179.

449. Recht MP, Coleman BG, Barbot DJ, et al. Recurrent esophageal carcinoma at thoracotomy incisions: diagnostic contributions of CT. *J Comput Assist Tomogr* 1989;13:58–60.

450. Glickstein MF, Gefter WB, Low D, Stephenson LW. Case report. Esophageal mucocele after surgical isolation of the esophagus. *AJR Am J Roentgenol* 1987;149:729–730.

451. Shaer AH, Bashist B. Case report. Computed tomography of bronchial artery aneurysm with erosion into the esophagus. *J Comput Assist Tomogr* 1989;13:1069–1071.

452. Webb WR, Gamsu G, Speckman JM, et al. CT demonstration of mediastinal aortic arch anomalies. *J Comput Assist Tomogr* 1982;6:445–451.

453. Day DL. Aortic arch in neonates with esophageal atresia: preoperative assessment using CT. *Radiology* 1985;155:99–100.

454. Williford ME, Thompson WM, Hamilton JD, Postlethwait RW. Esophageal tuberculosis: findings on barium swallow and computed tomography. *Gastrointest Radiol* 1983;8:119–122.

455. Im KG, Kim JH, Han MC, Kim CW. Computed tomography of esophagomediastinal fistula in tuberculous mediastinal lymphadenitis. *J Comput Assist Tomogr* 1990;14:89–92.

456. Pakter RL, Fishman EK. Metastatic osteosarcoma to the heart and mediastinum presenting as esophageal obstruction. *J Comput Assist Tomogr* 1983;7:1114–1115.

457. Gale ME, Birnbaum SB, Gale DR, Vincent ME. Esophageal invasion by lung cancer: CT diagnosis. *J Comput Assist Tomogr* 1984;8:694–698.

458. Clark KE, Foley WD, Lawson TL, Berland LL, Maddison FE. CT evaluation of esophageal and upper abdominal varices. *J Comput Assist Tomogr* 1980;4:510–515.

459. Balthazar EJ, Naidich DP, Megibow AJ, Lefleur RS. CT evaluation of esophageal varices. *AJR Am J Roentgenol* 1987;148:131–135.

460. Hirose WJ, Takashima T, Suzuki M, Matsui O. Case report. "Downhill" varices demonstrated by dynamic computed tomography. *J Comput Assist Tomogr* 1984;8:1007–1009.

461. Halden WJ, Harnsberger HR, Mancuso AA. Computed tomography of esophageal varices after sclerotherapy. *AJR Am J Roentgenol* 1983;140:1195–1196.

462. Mauro MA, Jaques PF, Swantkowski TM, Staab EV, Bozymski EM. CT after uncomplicated esophageal sclerotherapy. *AJR Am J Roentgenol* 1986;147:57–60.

463. Saks BJ, Kilby AE, Dietrich PA. Pleural and mediastinal changes following endoscopic injection sclerotherapy of esophageal varices. *Radiology* 1983;149:639–642.

464. Callen PWQ, Filly RA, Korobkin M. Computed tomographic evaluation of the diaphragmatic crura. *Radiology* 1978;126:413–416.

465. Naidich DP, Megibow AJ, Ross CR, Beranbaum ER, Siegelman SS. Computed tomography of the diaphragm: normal anatomy and variants. *J Comput Assist Tomogr* 1983;7:633–640.

466. Thompson WM, Halvorsen RA, Williford ME, Foster WL, Korobkin M. Computed tomography of the gastroesophageal junction. *Radiographics* 1982;2:179–193.

467. Govoni AF, Whalen JP, Kazam E. Hiatal hernia: a relook. *Radiographics* 1983;3:612–644.

468. Marks WM, Callen PW, Moss AA. Gastroesophageal region: Source of confusion on CT. *AJR Am J Roentgenol* 1981;136:359–362.

469. Thompson WM, Halvorsen RA, Foster W, Roberts L, Korobkin M. Computed tomography of the gastroesophageal junction: value of the left lateral decubitus view. *J Comput Assist Tomogr* 1984;8:346–349.

470. Godwin JD, MacGregor JM. Case report. Extension of ascites into the chest with hiatal hernia: visualization on CT. *AJR Am J Roentgenol* 1987;148:31–32.

471. Lindell MM, Bernadino ME. Diagnosis of hiatus hernia by computed tomography. *Comput Radiol* 1981;5:16–19.

472. Pupols A, Ruzicka FF. Hiatal hernia causing a cardia pseudomass on computed tomography. *J Comput Assist Tomogr* 1984;8:699–700.

473. Carrol CL, Jeffrey RB, Federle MP, Vernacchia FS. CT evaluation of mediastinal infections. *J Comput Assist Tomogr* 1987;11:449–454.

474. Breatnach E, Nath PH, Delany DJ. The role of computed tomography in acute and subacute mediastinitis. *Clin Radiol* 1986;37:139–145.

475. Morgan DE, Nath H, Sanders C, Hasson JH. Mediastinal actinomycosis. *AJR Am J Roentgenol* 1990;155:735–737.

476. Kay HR, Goodman LR, Teplick SK, Mundth ED. Use of computed tomography to assess mediastinal complications after median sternotomy. *Ann Thorac Surg* 1983;36:706–714.

477. Jolles H, Henry DA, Roberson JP, Cole TJ, Spratt JA. Mediastinitis following median sternotomy: CT findings. *Radiology* 1996;201:463–466.

478. Wechsler RJ, Steiner RM, Goodman LR, et al. Iatrogenic esophageal-pleural fistula: subtlety of diagnosis in the absence of mediastinitis. *Radiology* 1982;144:239–243.

479. Glenny RW, Fulkerson WJ, Ravin CE. Occult spontaneous esophageal perforation. Unusual clinical and radiographic presentation. *Chest* 1987;92:562–565.

480. Pezzulli FA, Aronson D, Goldberg N. Case report. Computed tomography of mediastinal hematoma secondary to unusual esophageal laceration: a Boerhaave variant. *J Comput Assist Tomogr* 1989;13:129–131.

481. Brown BM. Case report. Computed tomography of mediastinal abscess secondary to posttraumatic esophageal laceration. *J Comput Assist Tomogr* 1984;8:765–767.

482. Berkmen YM, Auh YH. CT diagnosis of acquired tracheoesophageal fistula in adults. *J Comput Assist Tomogr* 1985;9:302–304.

483. Kronthal AJ, Heitmiller RF, Fishman EK, Kuhlman JE. Mediastinal seroma after esophagogastrectomy. *AJR Am J Roentgenol* 1991;156:715–716.

484. Gobien RP, Stanley JH, Gobien BS, Vujic I, Pass HI. Percutaneous catheter aspiration and drainage of suspected mediastinal abscesses. *Radiology* 1984;151:69–71.

485. Efremidis SC, Dan SJ, Cohen BA, Mitty HA, Rabinowitz JG. Displaced paraspinal line: role of CT and lymphography. *AJR Am J Roentgenol* 1981;136:505–509.

486. Black WC, Armstrong P, Daniel TM, Cooper PH. Case report. Computed tomography of aggressive fibromatosis in the posterior mediastinum. *J Comput Assist Tomogr* 1987;11:153–155.

487. Tarr RW, Glick AG, Shaff MI. Case report. Benign hemangioendothelioma involving posterior mediastinum: CT findings. *J Comput Assist Tomogr* 1986;10:865–867.

488. Ribet ME, Cardot GR. Neurogenic tumors of the thorax. *Ann Thor Surg* 1994;58:1091–1095.

489. Reed JC, Hallet KK, Feigin DS. Neural tumors of the thorax: subject review from the AFIP. *Radiology* 1978;126:9–17.

490. Ross CR, McCauley DI, Naidich DP. Intrathoracic neurofibroma of the vagus nerve associated with bronchial obstruction. *J Comput Assist Tomogr* 1982;6:406–412.

491. Kumar AJ, Kuhajda FP, Martinez CR, et al. CT of extracranial nerve sheath tumors. *J Comput Assist Tomogr* 1983;7:857–865.

492. Biondetti PR, Vigo M, Fiore D, et al. CT appearance of generalized von Recklinghausen neurofibromatosis. *J Comput Assist Tomogr* 1983;7:866–869.

493. Bourgouin PM, Shepard JO, Moore EH, McLoud TC. Plexiform neurofibromatosis of the mediastinum: CT appearance. *AJR Am J Roentgenol* 1988;151:461–463.

494. Joseph SG, Tellis CJ. Posterior mediastinal mass with intraspinous extension. *Chest* 1988;93:1101–1103.

495. Aughenbaugh GL. Thoracic manifestations of neurocutaneous diseases. *Radiol Clin North Am* 1984;22:741–756.

496. Coleman BG, Arger PH, Dalinka MK, et al. CT of sarcomatous degeneration in neurofibromatosis. *AJR Am J Roentgenol* 1983;140:383–387.

497. Levine E, Huntrakoon M, Wetzel LH. Malignant nerve-sheath neoplasms in neurofibromatosis: distinction from benign tumors by using imaging techniques. *AJR Am J Roentgenol* 1987;149:1059–1064.

498. Feinstein RS, Gatewood OMB, Fishman EK, Goldman SM, Siegelman SS. Computed tomography of adult neuroblastoma. *J Comput Assist Tomogr* 1984;8:720–726.

499. Cohen LA, Schwartz AM, Rockoff SD. Benign schwannomas: pathologic basis for CT inhomogeneities. *AJR Am J Roentgenol* 1986;147:141–143.

500. Healy JF, Wells MV, Carlstom T, Rosenkrantz H. Lateral thoracic meningocele demonstrated by computerized tomography. *Comput Tomogr* 1980;4:159–163.

501. Moon WK, Im IJ, Han MC. Malignant schwannomas of the thorax: CT findings. *J Comput Assist Tomogr* 1993;17:274–276.

502. Burk DLJr, Brunberg JA, Kanal E, Latchaw RE, Wolf GL. Spinal and paraspinal neurofibromatosis: surface coil MR imaging at 1.5 T. *Radiology* 1987;162:797–801.

503. Dietrich RB, Kangarloo H, Lenarsky C, Feig SA. Neuroblastoma: the role of MR imaging. *AJR Am J Roentgenol* 1987;148:927–942.

504. Cohen MD, Weetman R, Provisor A. Magnetic resonance imaging of neuroblastoma with 0.15-T magnet. *AJR Am J Roentgenol* 1984;143:1241–1248.

505. Sakai F, Sone S, Kiyono K, et al. Intrathoracic neurogenic tumors: MR-pathologic correlation. *AJR Am J Roentgenol* 1992;159:279–283.

506. Armstrong EA, Harwood-Nash DCF, Ritz CR, et al. CT of neuroblastomas and ganglioneuromas in children. *AJR Am J Roentgenol* 1982;139:571–576.

507. Frances IR, Glazer GM, Shapiro B, Sisson JC, Gross BH. Complementary roles of CT and 131-I-MIBG scintigraphy in diagnosing pheochromocytoma. *AJR Am J Roentgenol* 1983;141:719–725.

508. Swensen SJ, Brown ML, Sheps SG, et al. Use of 13I-MIBG scintigraphy in the evaluation of suspected pheochromocytoma. *Mayo Clin Proc* 1985;60:299–304.

509. Miles J, Pennybacker J, Sheldon P. Intrathoracic meningocele. Its development and association with neurofibromatosis. *J Neurol Neurosurg Psychiatry* 1969;32:99.

510. Gumbs RV, Higginbotham-Ford EA, Teal JS, Kletter GG, Castro O. Thoracic extramedullary hematopoiesis in sickle-cell disease. *AJR Am J Roentgenol* 1987;149:889–893.

511. Long JA, Doppman JL, Nienhuis AW. Computed tomographic studies of thoracic extramedullary hematopoiesis. *J Comput Assist Tomogr* 1980;4:67–70.

512. Danza FM, Falappa P, Leone G, Pincelli G. Extramedullary hematopoiesis (letter). *AJR Am J Roentgenol* 1982;139:837–838.

513. Kirchner SG, Heller RM, Smith CW. Pancreatic pseudocyst of the mediastinum. *Radiology* 1977;123:37–42.

CHAPTER 3

Airways

TECHNIQUE

The introduction of volumetric (helical/spiral) computed tomography (CT) has profoundly altered our approach to scanning the airways. This is because no single set of optimal scan parameters currently suffices for all applications. Rather, certain protocols may be used to reflect a variety of clinical indications (Tables 3-1–3-3). Most often, these indications include one of the following three broad categories: (a) occult disease; this category includes patients presenting with hemoptysis and a normal or nonlocalizing radiograph and patients with suspected bronchogenic carcinoma presenting with normal radiographs and evidence of extrathoracic metastases to the brain or the adrenal glands; (b) airway patency; in addition to patients with radiographic evidence of atelectasis, this category also includes patients with slowly resolving infiltrates; and (c) inflammatory airway disease; included in this category are patients with suspected bronchiectasis, as well as bronchiolar inflammation occurring, for example, in patients who are immunocompromised, who have undergone organ transplantation, or who are human immunodeficiency virus (HIV) positive, among others. As discussed later, in each of these settings, optimal CT evaluation requires separate protocols.

Scan Acquisition

Many of the basic principles that pertain to the performance of conventional CT of the airways also pertain to volumetric CT. In our experience, it is helpful to visualize the chest as divided into three zones whenever the airways are the principle focus of the CT examination (Fig. 3-1). These include the following: (a) an apical zone, extending from the thoracic inlet to just above the carina; (b) a hilar zone, extending from just above the carina to the level of the inferior pulmonary veins; and (c) a basilar zone, extending from the inferior pulmonary veins to the base of the lungs. This method was initially proposed for evaluating patients presenting with hemoptysis by means of sequential axial images (1), and it is easily adapted to helical or spiral scanning. Emphasizing adaptability, individual axial or helical scans or variable combinations of both can be obtained. When intravenous contrast is indicated, administration may be optimized by timing the bolus of contrast agent to coincide with scanning of a particular region, for example, through the hilum in patients presenting with lobar or segmental atelectasis (2).

Although some evidence suggests that for routine applications there is little difference among 3-, 5-, and even 10-mm collimation techniques, provided overlapping reconstructions are used (3), nonetheless, it is our practice to

TABLE 3-1. *Occult airway disease (hemoptysis): helical CT protocol*

Collimation	Axial, 1 mm; helical, 3 and 5 mm
Pitch	1.6–2
Helical exposure time	Multiple sequential acquisitions
Reconstruction interval	3's q2; 5's q4
Section sequences	3-phase aquisition 1. Initial 5-mm collimation (helical acquisition from the level of the true cords (C5) to 1 cm above the carina), followed by: 2. 3-mm collimation for the duration of a single breath-hold period (pitch, 2), and then: 3. 1-mm routine axial high-resolution CT images q10 mm to the lung bases
Intravenous contrast	Optional: 125 mL/60%, 2.5 mL/sec, timed to coincide with the 3-mm sections Scan delay: 20 sec

obtain scans using collimation matched to the size of the airways to be evaluated (Fig. 3-2). In most cases, the central airways, from the carina through the origins of the basilar segmental airways, can be adequately studied using 5-mm collimation. This includes patients with evidence of airway obstruction (see Table 3-2). However, when the main indication for scanning is identification of occult airway disease, 3-mm collimation should be used, with a reconstruction interval of 2 mm (see Table 3-1). Scanning should begin approximately 2 cm above the carina and should extend below the origins of the basilar segmental airways (at a minimum

TABLE 3-2. *Airway patency (atelectasis, stenoses, hilar masses): helical CT protocol*

Collimation	3 and 5 mm
Pitch	1.6–2
Helical exposure time	Single or multiple sequential acquisitions as needed
Reconstruction interval	3's q2; 5's q4
Scan sequences	Two options Single-phase acquisition 5-mm collimation; 4-mm reconstruction interval from the thoracic inlet to the hemidiaphragms, or: 3-phase acquisition 1. Initial 5-mm collimation from the apices to 2 cm above the carina, followed by: 2. 3-mm collimation for duration of single breath-hold period, then: 3. 5-mm collimation to the level of the diaphragms
Intravenous contrast	Optional: 125 mL/60%/2.5 mL/sec Scan delay: 20 sec

TABLE 3-3. *Inflammatory airway disease: helical CT protocol*

Collimation	Axial, 1 mm; helical, 3 mm
Pitch	2
Helical exposure time	Multiple sequential acquisitions
Reconstruction interval	q2mm (3-mm collimation only)
Section sequences	3-Phase aquisition: 1. Initial 1-mm routine axial high-resolution CT images q10mm from the thoracic inlet to 2 cm above the carina, followed by: 2. 3-mm sections for duration of a single breath-hold period (pitch, 2), followed by: 3. 1-mm routine axial high-resolution CT images q10mm to the lung bases
Intravenous contrast	None
Comments	Additional expiratory images using either 1- or 3-mm collimation at selected levels may be of value for detecting bronchiolar disease, with or without low-dose technique Images acquired with an angled gantry may be of value in select cases in which assessment of obliquely oriented airways proved problematic

Adapted from ref. 9, with permission.

to the level of the inferior pulmonary veins). Use of 3-mm collimation is especially recommended when multiplanar reconstructions (MPRs) are desired, even though these will exclude most of the trachea if the technique outlined earlier is followed (3). In distinction, adequate evaluation of the peripheral airways usually requires high-resolution 1-mm collimation, although 3-mm sections may be of value, especially in patients with mild cylindric bronchiectasis (see Table 3-3) (4). As discussed in greater detail later, adequate evaluation of small airways disease also often requires use of both inspiratory and expiratory scans to assess for possible air trapping.

The largest possible pitch should be used to cover as large a volume as possible. In our experience, pitch as great as 1.6 to 2 can be used without significant degradation in image quality. The introduction of scanners with the ability to acquire data with a pitch even greater than 2 no doubt will lead to further modifications of our current concepts of optimal technique. When MPRs or other retrospective reconstructions are indicated, provided that multiple breath-held acquisitions may still be acquired, slice thickness and field-of-view must remain constant (1). In select cases, this may require that additional scans be obtained through select regions of interest to accommodate this requirement.

Volumetric CT can also be performed using an angled gantry (20 degrees cephalad in most cases). This may be advantageous in select cases to assess airways that course

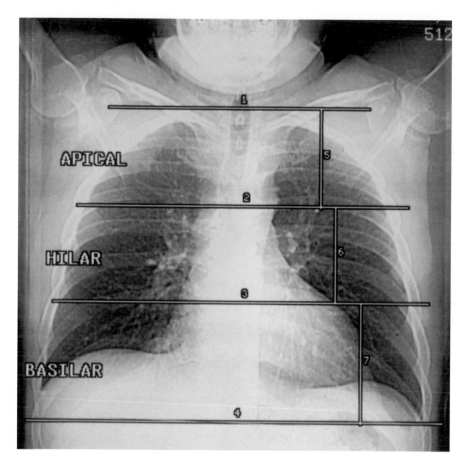

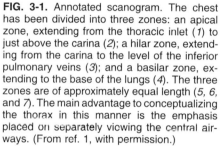

FIG. 3-1. Annotated scanogram. The chest has been divided into three zones: an apical zone, extending from the thoracic inlet (*1*) to just above the carina (*2*); a hilar zone, extending from the carina to the level of the inferior pulmonary veins (*3*); and a basilar zone, extending to the base of the lungs (*4*). The three zones are of approximately equal length (*5, 6,* and *7*). The main advantage to conceptualizing the thorax in this manner is the emphasis placed on separately viewing the central airways. (From ref. 1, with permission.)

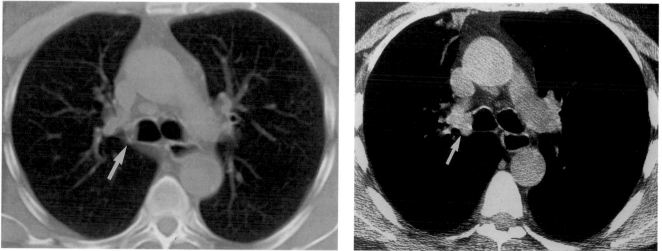

A   B

FIG. 3-2. Occult bronchial tumor: value of 3-mm versus 10-mm collimation. **A:** A 10-mm section imaged with lung windows at the level of the carina initially interpreted as normal. Slight increased density along the lateral bronchial wall on the right (*arrow*) was attributed to secretions. **B:** Follow-up 3-mm section obtained a few weeks after **A** in this patient with persistent hemoptysis clearly shows the presence of a soft tissue mass involving the lateral wall of the right main stem bronchus (*arrow*). This case illustrates the advantage of using appropriate collimation to evaluate the central airways.

obliquely, in particular, the middle lobe or lingular bronchi (4). As emphasized by Perhomaa and colleagues (3), however, use of either cephalad or caudad angulation does pose problems in ensuring that all segmental airways will be imaged in a single breath-hold period. In most cases, this problem can be obviated by use of a greater pitch.

Another potential volumetric CT technique is that of "physiologic scanning." To date, this type of study has generally been performed using only dynamic or fast electron-beam CT scanners with images typically obtained at a single level during various phases of respiration (5,6). Because volumetric CT data can be acquired through a broad region of

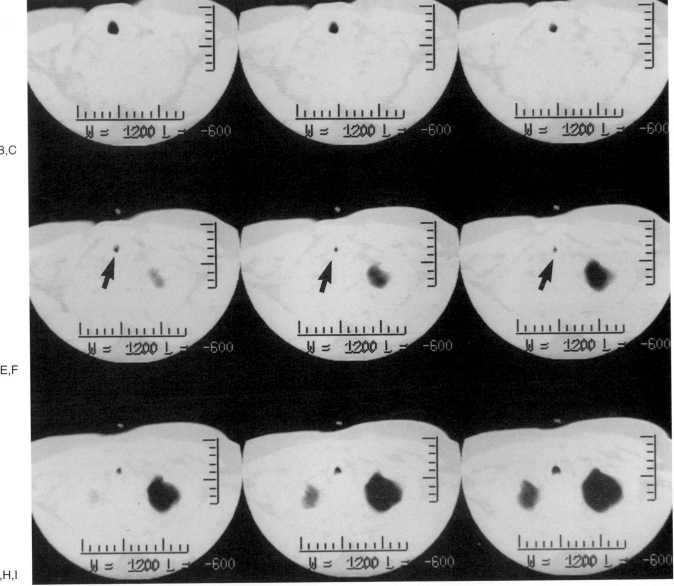

A,B,C

D,E,F

G,H,I

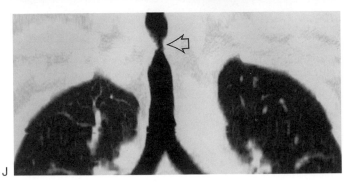

J

FIG. 3-3. Tracheal stenosis: evaluation with multiplanar reconstructions (MPRs). **A–I:** Sequential 5-mm sections through the lower neck and thoracic inlet show marked focal narrowing of the trachea in a patient with postintubation tracheal stenosis (*arrows in* **D–F**). **J:** Coronal MPR shows to better advantage the true location and extent of the focal tracheal stenosis (*arrow*). This technique is of value in presurgical assessment. (From ref. 323, with permission.)

interest during two separate breath-holds, misregistration can be eliminated allowing an accurate assessment of tracheobronchial dynamics through direct comparison of identical sections at various lung volumes. Radiation dose can be minimized without sacrificing anatomic detail by use of low-dose (50–80 mA) technique.

Retrospective Reconstructions

Although routine axial images remain the standard for identifying airway disease, this method has important limitations, including the following: (a) an inability to identify mucosal disease; (b) limited accuracy in identifying submucosal disease, especially central extension of neoplasm; (c) limited accuracy in the estimation of the length of tracheal and bronchial stenoses; and (d) limited assessment of obliquely coursing airways (7–9). Endobronchial lung cancers, even those located in the central airways, can be missed on conventional CT, particularly when 10-mm sections only are acquired (see Fig. 3-2) (10,11).

With the introduction of volumetric CT, various high-quality reconstruction techniques have become routinely available. These include the following: (a) MPRs, including curved multiplanar reformations; (b) multiplanar volume reconstructions (MPVRs); (c) external rendering with three

dimensional shaded-surface displays; and (d) internal rendering, or so-called virtual bronchoscopy (12). As these techniques have been described in Chapter 1, the current discussion will focus on their use for imaging airway disease.

Multiplanar Reconstructions

MPRs are typically 1 voxel thick two dimensional "tomographic" sections interpolated along an arbitrary plane or curved surface (Figs. 3-3–3-5). Thicker sections using more than 1 pixel may also be obtained and often have the advantage of a smoother appearance. With conventional CT scanners, MPRs were of limited value because of the prolonged imaging times needed to acquire a sufficient number of sections to generate high-quality reconstructions, difficulties largely overcome with helical CT.

Compared with other reconstruction techniques, the main advantage of MPRs is that they require only a few seconds to perform. Therefore, the examiner can obtain a series of single oblique reconstructions derived from corresponding axial sections interactively, thus allowing individual airways to be displayed to best advantage along their nearest long axes. It is also possible to generate double-obliquity MPRs perpendicular to previously reconstructed three dimensional images (13). Although this technique allows

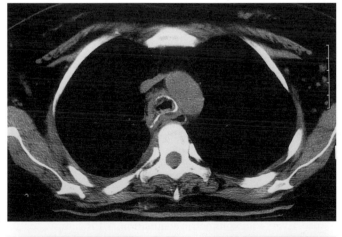
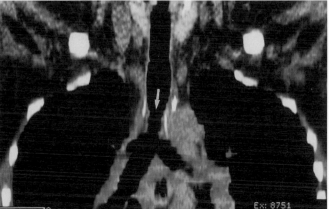
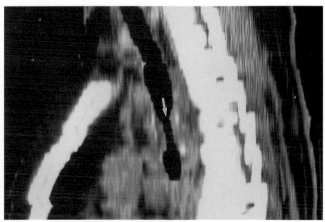

FIG. 3-4. Tracheal stenosis: postoperative assessment. **A:** Axial 5-mm section through the midtrachea in a patient after repair of tracheal stenosis. Note the presence of sutures with marked narrowing of the trachea. **B,C:** Coronal and sagittal multiplanar reconstructions, respectively, show to much better advantage the extent of postsurgical narrowing (*arrows*). (**A** and **B** from ref. 9, with permission.)

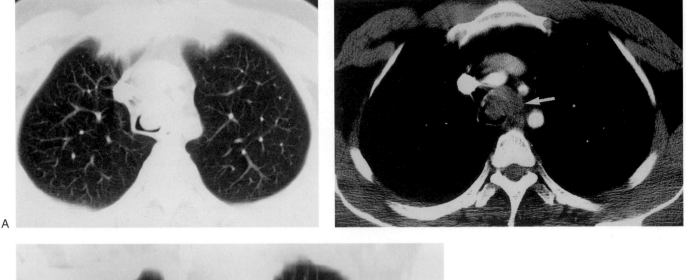

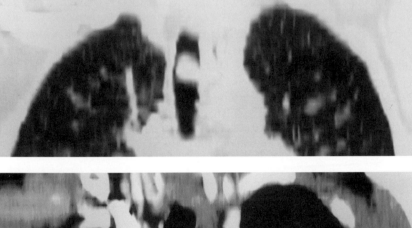

FIG. 3-5. Adenoid-cystic carcinoma of the trachea. **A,B:** 5-mm sections through the mid-trachea after a bolus of intravenous contrast, imaged with wide and narrow windows, respectively. A soft tissue mass nearly occludes the trachea with extension into the adjacent mediastinum (*arrow* in **B**). **C,D:** Coronal and parasagittal multiplanar reconstructions imaged with wide and narrow windows, respectively, show to better advantage than axial images both the true intraluminal and extraluminal extent of tumor. Despite mediastinal invasion, tumor is clearly separable from adjacent mediastinal structures, including the aorta and left subclavian artery (*arrows* in **D**). This tumor proved resectable. (From ref. 323, with permission.)

true orthogonal planar reformations to be obtained through any segmental bronchus, providing so-called lesion oriented multiplanar reformations, this particular application takes considerable time and is not available on all scanners (13,14).

Curved reformations are another variant of MPRs that have the effect of rendering complex three dimensional structures in a single, flat tomographic plane (Fig. 3-6). Although these require that a user-defined trace be applied, curved reformations only take minimal additional time to reformat compared with routine MPRs. Unfortunately, although they are of occasional value for demonstrating extremely tortuous airways, they are particularly susceptible to partial volume averaging, which leads to considerable anatomic distortion and renders them of only limited clinical

use. Even with volumetric acquisition, MPRs are susceptible to stair-step artifacts, which limit interpretation. Typically, these artifacts manifest as irregularities along the surfaces of airways that course obliquely. They are directly related to pitch and are independent of collimation or reconstruction algorithm (15).

A variant of MPRs, MPVRs allow the definition of a three dimensional slab to be obtained from the original data set at any angle from which average, maximum, or minimum intensity projection images may be derived. When obtained in the axial plane, these images simulate routine cross-sectional images. This method of reconstruction was first introduced by Napel (16) as a technique for improving visualization of blood vessels and airways in the parenchyma of the lung, so-called sliding thin-slab maximum intensity projection images. Use of the lowest attenuation values within the slab (minimum intensity projection imaging) yields images in which the bronchial lumen is accentuated at the expense of the bronchial wall (Fig. 3-7). In distinction, use of the highest available attenuation values within the slab (maximum intensity projection imaging) accentuates the bronchial wall at the expense of the bronchial lumen. In both cases, the result is to distort the normal cross-sectional appearance of the airways by accentuating only a portion of airway anatomy (9,12).

External Rendering

External rendering allows visualization of structures from an external vantage point, most often using a simulated light source (Figs. 3-8 and 3-9). This can be accomplished using either surface thresholding or volume rendering techniques. In the former, a single threshold is applied, rendering only a few voxels visible; with volume rendering, each voxel is assigned a percentage value, and all are potentially visible (17).

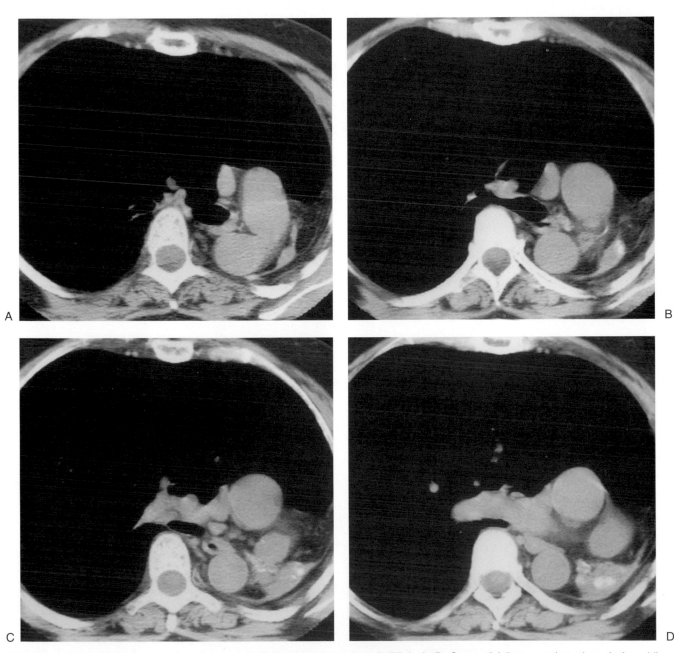

FIG. 3-6. Autopneumonectomy: value of curved multiplanar reconstructions (MPRs). **A–D:** Sequential 5-mm sections through the midlung imaged with narrow windows shows marked displacement of the mediastinum into the posterior left hemithorax: the left lung is shrunken and calcified—the CT equivalent of an autopneumonectomy—as a result of long-standing tuberculosis. *(continues)*

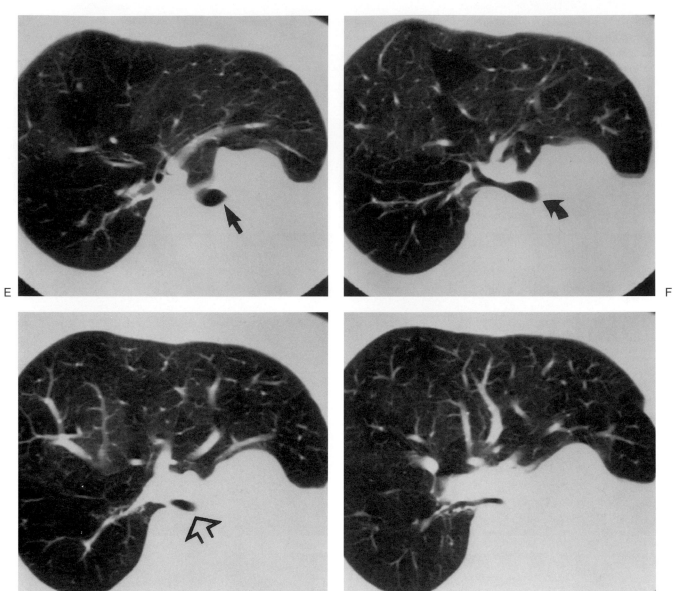

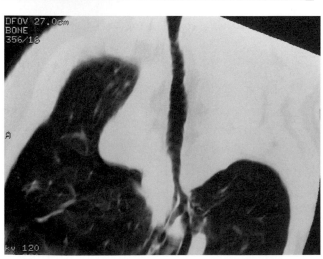

FIG. 3-6. *Continued.* **E–H:** Identical sections as in **A–D,** imaged with lung windows, show marked posterior and lateral displacement of the distal trachea (*arrow*), right upper lobe bronchus (*curved arrow*), bronchus intermedius (*open arrow*), and right lower lobe bronchus, respectively. The marked mosaic attenuation throughout visualized portions of the right lung is consistent with associated bronchiolitis. **I:** Curved MPR allows visualization of the entire length of the trachea and proximal right-sided airways in a single plane. Although curved MPRs are of value in cases with marked anatomic distortion, they are particularly susceptible to partial volume averaging leading to potentially misleading diagnoses of airway obstruction or narrowing. (**A–D,** from ref. 9, with permission.)

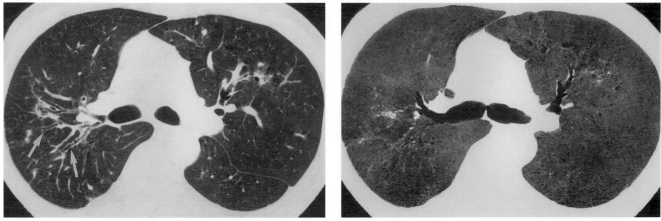

FIG. 3-7. Bronchial assessment with minimum intensity projection images (MiNIP). **A:** A 1-mm section through the right upper lobe shows moderately severe dilatation and bronchial wall thickening of right upper lobe airways (*arrows*). **B:** MiNIP derived from a series of five contiguous 1-mm sections centered at the same level as **A**. With minimum projection imaging, only those voxels with the lowest density are preserved; the result is that walls of airways and vessels are subtracted from the image (compare with **A**). This case vividly shows the necessity of visualizing bronchial walls to diagnose bronchiectasis. (From ref. 9, with permission.)

Three dimensional reconstructions are most often generated using a shaded-surface display (18). Despite the striking visual appearance of these images, external rendering techniques usually require time-consuming editing to create appropriate subvolumes for analysis using either manual trace or connectivity-based editing techniques. In addition, the use of a single threshold makes shaded-surface techniques susceptible to both noise and to artifacts related to partial volume averaging; this causes surface discontinuities or "holes," jagged edges, and "floating pixels." Furthermore, focal areas of high density (bronchial stents, bronchial cartilage calcifications, or broncholiths) may be completely obscured (15).

In distinction, volume rendering uses linear or continuous scaling techniques in which every voxel within the original data set is assigned a proportional value based on the full range of tissue densities represented. This approach results in fewer artifacts and allows a greater range of possible three dimensional images (including the ability to create transparent tissue planes allowing anatomic structures to be viewed at various depths). Although limited until recently by the need for extensive, time-consuming image processing (12,17), investigators have shown that three dimensional CT can be performed using real-time interactive volume rendering, thereby opening the potential for more general use (19).

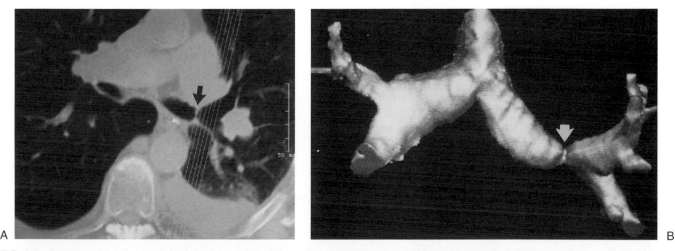

FIG. 3-8. Posttransplantation bronchial stricture: value of three dimensional shaded-surface rendering. **A:** Axial section through the left upper lobe bronchus in a patient after recent left lung transplantation shows focal narrowing at the anastomotic site, identifiable as a thin line (*arrow*). **B:** Three dimensional shaded-surface rendering shows to better advantage than **A** the location and extent of anastomotic stricturing (*arrow*). (Courtesy of Warren Gefter M.D., University of Pennsylvania, Philadelphia, PA.)

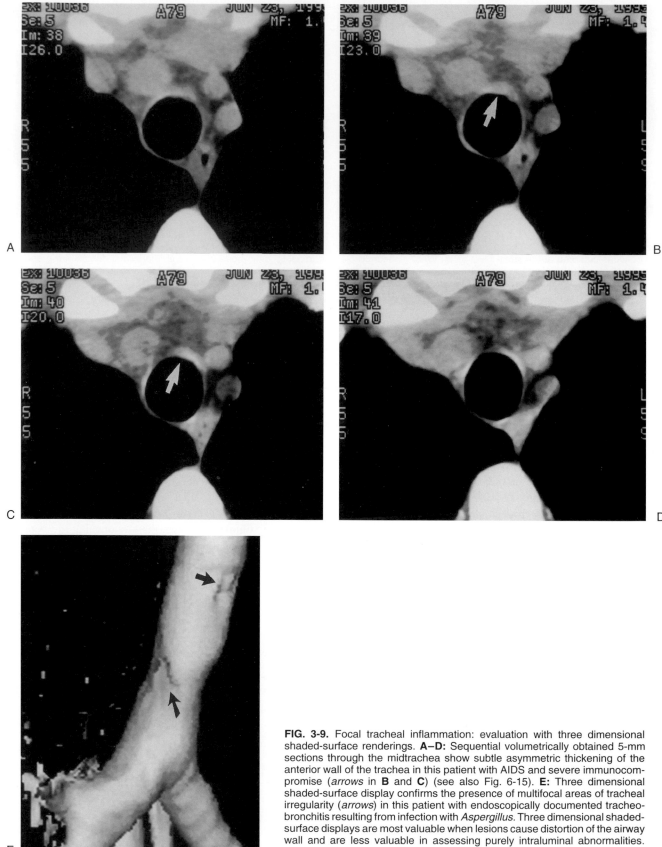

FIG. 3-9. Focal tracheal inflammation: evaluation with three dimensional shaded-surface renderings. **A–D:** Sequential volumetrically obtained 5-mm sections through the midtrachea show subtle asymmetric thickening of the anterior wall of the trachea in this patient with AIDS and severe immunocompromise (*arrows* in **B** and **C**) (see also Fig. 6-15). **E:** Three dimensional shaded-surface display confirms the presence of multifocal areas of tracheal irregularity (*arrows*) in this patient with endoscopically documented tracheobronchitis resulting from infection with *Aspergillus.* Three dimensional shaded-surface displays are most valuable when lesions cause distortion of the airway wall and are less valuable in assessing purely intraluminal abnormalities. (From ref. 156, with permission.)

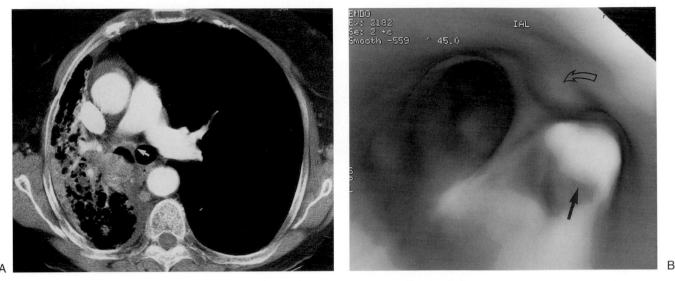

FIG. 3-10. Endobronchial tumor: evaluation with internal rendering (virtual bronchoscopy). **A:** Contrast-enhanced CT section shows obstruction of the right main stem bronchus by tumor with resultant volume loss and consolidation of the right lung. Note the slight thickening of the anterior carina (*arrow*). **B:** Internal rendering of the carina oriented to correlate with appearance at flexible bronchoscopy shows occlusion of the right main stem bronchus (*straight arrow*) and nodular thickening of the anterior carina (*curved arrow*), precisely corresponding to **A.**

Internal Rendering

Internal rendering or "virtual" bronchoscopy allows visualization of the airways internally from a point source at a finite distance, simulating human perspective as seen through a bronchoscope (Figs. 3-10–3-13). Images are then viewed through the tip of a cone with either a narrow (15-degree) or a wide (60-degree) field-of-view. A flight path of sequential images can also be constructed and navigated either sequentially or in a cine loop, further simulating endoscopy (12,20).

Although a detailed description of the various methods for obtaining these images is beyond the scope of this chapter, a brief description is in order. Virtual bronchoscopic images can be obtained using either three dimensional surface-shaded reconstructions (see Figs. 3-10–3-12) or volumetric rendering (see Fig. 3-13) (20,21). In the former, image segmentation (the process of computer identification of specific anatomic regions within a volume of data) is usually obtained using region-growing algorithms in which a single voxel within the airway lumen is first selected, with each

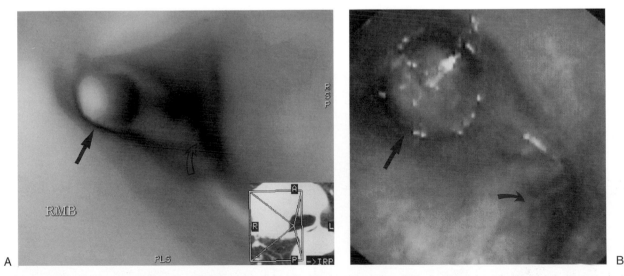

FIG. 3-11. Endobronchial tumor: correlation between virtual and flexible bronchoscopy (FB). **A:** Internal rendering of a patient viewed from within the right main bronchus shows tumor occluding the bronchus intermedius (*arrow*) and narrowing of the right upper lobe bronchus (*curved arrow*) resulting from extrinsic compression from extensive hilar adenopathy. This image is oriented to correspond with FB, with right-sided airways shown on the right side. **B:** Image obtained at bronchoscopy confirms the presence of an endobronchial mass occluding the bronchus intermedius (*arrow*) and extrinsic narrowing of the right upper lobe bronchus (*curved arrow*). Despite close correlation between gross abnormalities identified in **A** and appearance at FB, note the lack of any mucosal detail on the virtual bronchoscopic rendering.

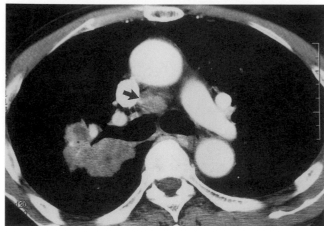

A

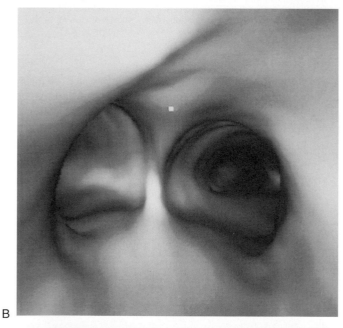

B

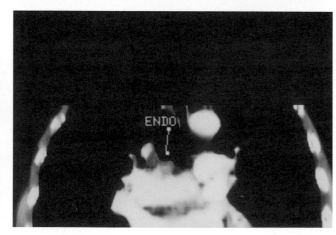

C

D

E

FIG. 3-12. Virtual bronchoscopy: correlation with transbronchial needle aspiration (TBNA). **A:** Contrast-enhanced CT section through the right upper lobe shows a large tumor mass in the right hilum extending behind the right upper lobe bronchus (*arrow*). Note the presence of enlarged precarinal nodes. **B–E:** Internal rendering (**B**) from within the distal trachea looking inferiorly toward the carina with simultaneous axial (**C**), sagittal (**D**), and coronal (**E**) reformations corresponding to the same plane as **A**. This format allows instantaneous evaluation of both the intraluminal appearance of the airways as well as corresponding findings in the adjacent soft tissues surrounding airways. The *square white cursor* placed on the anterior carina in **B** appears instantaneously on the corresponding axial, sagittal, and coronal windows. This guide is of obvious benefit in cases such as this in which TBNA of mediastinal nodes is planned.

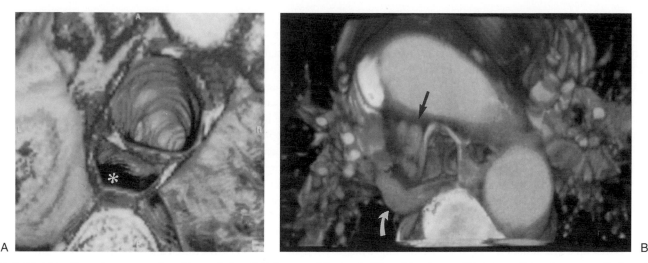

FIG. 3-13. Virtual bronchoscopy: volumetric rendering. **A,B:** Images at the level of the midtrachea and just above the carina, respectively, using volumetric rendering allow simultaneous depiction of both the internal appearance of airways as well as surrounding anatomic structures. In this case, note the simultaneous internal rendering of the esophagus in **A** (*asterisk*), and the appearance of enlarged right paratracheal nodes (*straight arrow* in **B**) medial to the azygos vein (*curved arrow* in **B**). With the introduction of on-line volumetric rendering, this will probably become the preferred method for internal airway rendering.

neighboring voxel subsequently examined to determine whether it satisfies an acceptance criterion typically defined as a range of Hounsfield units (HU) (21,22). An isosurface algorithm is then used to generate a wire-frame model of the airway surface (14,23). In this model, the choice of thresholds is clearly defining. In distinction, volume rendering displays all voxel data simultaneously by assigning both a color and an opacity to each voxel (14,17). This allows targeted anatomy to be highlighted while undesired structures are rendered transparent.

The advantages of three dimensional shaded-surface reconstructions over volume rendering techniques include greater speed and the ability to generate images using currently available work stations. Three dimensional shaded-surface techniques are limited, however, by their greater susceptibility to noise and partial volume averaging; this can result in surface discontinuities, jagged edges, and floating pixels (Fig. 3-14). In our experience, these artifacts typically occur only when attempting to visualize distal airways and may be limited by use of a standard rather than an edge-

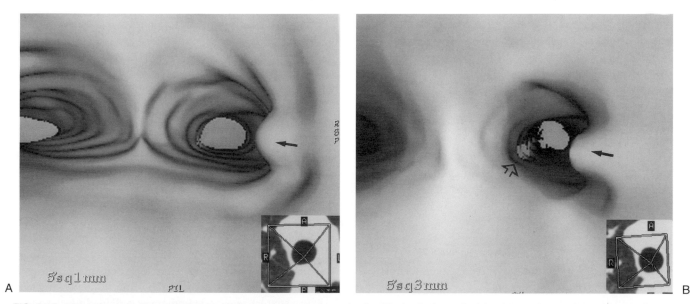

FIG. 3-14. Virtual bronchoscopy: limitations. **A,B:** Internal renderings of a focal lesion in the wall of the right main stem bronchus (*solid arrows* in **A** and **B**) using 5-mm collimation, with reconstruction intervals (RIs) of 1 and 3 mm, respectively. Note the presence of jagged holes in the medial wall of the bronchus intermedius with an RI of 3 mm (*open arrow* in **B**). This results from a combination of noise and partial volume averaging and is a limitation of shaded-surface techniques for internal rendering. Although an RI of 1 mm effectively eliminates this artifact, curvilinear densities apparent in both the right and left main stem bronchi unfortunately represent spiral artifacts, not bronchial cartilage. (From ref 9, with permission.)

enhancing algorithm coupled with thin collimation and small reconstruction intervals.

Volumetric rendering has the advantage over shaded-surface techniques of allowing peribronchial tissues to be seen through or alongside bronchial walls, but shaded-surface reconstructions also allow precise localization of peribronchial tissues by means of certain navigational aids now available for real-time virtual bronchoscopy. As ingeniously elaborated by Summers and associates (23), these include the following, among others: simultaneous annotated displays of corresponding axial, coronal, and sagittal images oriented to conform to any given plane identified from the endoluminal display; orthogonal axes to indicate anterior, posterior, or superior direction, as desired; three dimensional global images of the airways rendered semitransparent on which "trail" markers indicating position and direction can be measured; simultaneous "rearview" imaging, allowing simultaneous depiction of a virtual endoscopic image pointing backward from any given location; and even automated methods to avoid collisions with the bronchial wall to ensure that the "virtual endoscope" does not inadvertently pass through the bronchial wall (23). One can even generate true stereoscopic displays of airway anatomy using specialized liquid crystal display (three dimensional) glasses. Perhaps most important, one can also precisely measure the distance from any fixed point within the airways to any other point using trail markers, analogous to the distance markers present on real fiberoptic bronchoscopes (23).

Regardless of the reconstruction technique used, internal rendering results in the creation of artifactual stripes or ribbing, findings that should not be confused with actual cartilaginous rings. These stripes result from slight changes in the caliber of the airways; every other slice appears slightly different, especially when 180-degree linear-interpolation algorithms are employed. This accounts for the unexpected finding that the stripes become more apparent the smaller the reconstruction interval (see Fig. 3-14).

Clinical Indications

Given the diversity of potential reconstructions available from volumetric scan acquisitions, it remains to be determined which of these, if any, are worth the time and effort necessary to obtain them.

Multiplanar Reconstructions

To date, the most useful retrospective imaging technique has been MPRs. These have proved of greatest value for assessing focal airway stenoses, particularly those after prolonged tracheal intubation or lung transplantation (see Fig. 3-3) (24,25). Quint and associates (24) evaluated 27 patients after lung transplantation (3-mm collimation; pitch, 1; 1.5-mm reconstruction interval) and found that MPRs in con-

junction with axial images allowed accurate identification in 94% of cases. Although this result represented only a marginal improvement over axial imaging alone, which identified 91% of stenoses, in the opinion of these investigators, the addition of MPRs allowed more precise and unequivocal assessment of the true length of stenoses (24). As shown by McAdams and colleagues (26), MPRs are also of considerable value by more accurately depicting normal postoperative changes such as the presence of diverticula resulting from redundant mucosal folds and endoluminal flaps and linear air collections resulting from bronchial invagination from the more ominous findings of dehiscence and bronchial fistulization (26).

MPRs have also been shown to be of value in selected patients with central lung cancer (27). In this setting, MPRs may allow more precise visualization of airway involvement, especially along obliquely coursing airways such as the left main stem bronchus. Additional information regarding nodal involvement in otherwise difficult to interpret regions such as the aorticopulmonary window and subcarinal space can also be occasionally obtained using MPRs (see Fig. 3-5).

In distinction, MPVRs have proved of less value than routine MPRs. MPVRs using minimum intensity projection images have been employed to evaluate the central airways, specifically bronchial changes after lung transplantation (25). The technique is limited, however, because endobronchial lesions of soft tissue attenuation are difficult to identify (16). MPVRs using minimum intensity projection imaging also may allow visualization of dilated or tortuous peripheral airways otherwise obscured by increased reticular markings, especially in patients with underlying fibrosis. In most cases, however, evaluation of peripheral airways using minimum intensity projection images is extremely limited because identification of dilated airways requires visualization of bronchial walls (see Fig. 3-7) (28). These airways all but disappear with minimum intensity projection imaging when MPVRs reach 8 to 10 mm in thickness. In distinction, MPVRs using maximum intensity projection images may be of limited value in patients with infectious forms of bronchiolitis in which the predominant abnormality consists of nodular densities resulting from mucoid impaction of distal small airways.

Three-Dimensional Surface Rendering

Like MPRs, three dimensional surface rendering techniques have most often been used to identify bronchial stenoses, particularly in patients after lung transplantation (see Fig. 3-9) (18,29). As documented by Kauczor and associates (18) in a study using a test phantom as well as clinical evaluations in 36 patients, three dimensional helical CT proved a reliable method for assessing the trachea, main stem, and proximal segmental airways in all cases. Advantages of three dimensional shaded-surface renderings compared with bronchoscopy included accurate assessment of both the presence and the length of central stenoses ($n = 36$) as well as the ability to characterize distal airways that could not otherwise be visualized bronchoscopically. Unfortunately, three dimensional shaded-surface renderings proved less reliable for detecting peripheral (segmental) airway stenoses, a problem not encountered with routine MPRs (18).

Three dimensional images also have been anecdotally reported of value in certain disparate conditions including congenital airway abnormalities such as anomalous cardiac bronchi, abnormalities associated with vascular malformations or rings, acquired tracheomalacia, and even bronchopleural fistulas (30–32). In these instances, the ability to visualize the external contour of airways has proved of value, especially when visualization of the three dimensional configuration of airways is difficult based solely on cross-sectional appearance. In our experience, given limitations in spatial resolution, inability to detect disease that is not causing marked topographic alterations, and the need for extensive image editing, three dimensional surface rendering at present should be considered less valuable than MPRs for assessing the central airways.

Virtual Bronchoscopy

Despite initial enthusiasm, certain important limitations currently affect practical application of internal rendering techniques. Insufficient clinical data are available to judge the efficacy of endoluminal imaging. Vining and colleagues (22), in a preliminary study using volumetric rendering, used an initial volumetric CT (VCT) data set with 3-mm collimation, a pitch of 2, and a 1-mm reconstruction interval to generate "virtual bronchoscopy" images and compared these to bronchoscopic findings in 20 patients. Although virtual bronchoscopy accurately identified endobronchial tumor with obstruction in 5 patients, airway distortion or ectasia in 4, and an accessory bronchus in the remaining case, suboptimal examinations limited evaluation in 50% of cases.

Summers and colleagues (14), employing a specialized segmentation method to enhance identification of bronchial walls, used virtual bronchoscopy to assess 14 patients with a variety of airway abnormalities. Using 3-mm sections, a field-of-view of 26, sequential 15 second breath-holds, a high-frequency reconstruction algorithm, a pitch of 2, and 1-mm reconstruction intervals, these authors found that "virtual bronchoscopy" depicted up to third-order bronchi in 90% of cases. However, only 82% of lobar and 76% of segmental airways were identified; as expected, the middle lobe and lingular bronchi were most difficult to visualize. Axial CT and the "virtual" images were of equal accuracy in estimating the maximal luminal diameter and cross-sectional area of the central airways (when the airways could be identified).

Similar findings have been reported by Ferretti and associates (33). In their study of 29 patients with central airway stenoses evaluated with virtual bronchoscopic simulations using surface-shaded reconstructions, these authors noted that, whereas virtual bronchoscopy identified stenoses in 39 of 41 cases, with good-quality images obtained in 27 of 29 patients, in no case did virtual bronchoscopy add information not available on the axial source images (33).

Indeed, virtual bronchoscopy appears to be a technique in search of an application. To date, speculation on possible clinical applications has focused primarily on use of virtual bronchoscopy either as a potential screening modality or as a guide to bronchoscopy (see Fig. 3-12). Use of this technique as a potential screening modality is currently precluded by the length of time necessary to generate or navigate these images; in addition, although the sensitivity of this technique has not been established, it is unlikely to be sufficient to obviate fiberoptic bronchoscopy (FB). The standard reconstruction algorithm, essential to minimize noise, means that small lesions may be missed because of excessive smoothing. Of greater significance is the problem of false-positive findings resulting either from artifacts or from the presence of retained secretions. Pending prospective documentation of the accuracy of endoluminal imaging, therefore, its use as a screening test remains at best speculative.

Although seemingly more promising, the use of virtual bronchoscopy as a guide for bronchoscopy also appears limited. In most cases, routine axial images perform this function (see Fig. 3-12) (1). A more extensive or elaborate depiction of bronchial and peribronchial disease than that afforded by axial images is not necessary because endoscopically the number of sites practically accessible for aspiration or biopsy is sharply circumscribed (see Chapter 5) (34).

TRACHEA

Anatomy

The trachea is a cartilaginous and fibromuscular tube extending from the inferior aspect of the cricoid cartilage (at the level of the sixth cervical vertebra) to the carina (at the level of the fifth thoracic vertebra). It measures from 10 to 12 cm in length (35,36). The trachea is divided into extrathoracic and intrathoracic portions; the trachea can be considered intrathoracic at the point at which it passes posterior to the manubrium (Fig. 3-15). In a CT study of 50 anatomically normal persons (35), the extrathoracic trachea measured 2 to 4 cm in length, whereas the intrathoracic trachea measured 6 to 9 cm in length (mean, $7.5 + 0.8$ cm).

The trachea contains 16 to 22 cartilaginous "rings," which are in fact horseshoe shaped and incomplete posteriorly (see Fig. 3-15; Fig. 3-16). These help to support the tracheal wall and to maintain an adequate tracheal lumen during forced expiration. The posterior portion of the tra-

tracheal cartilage

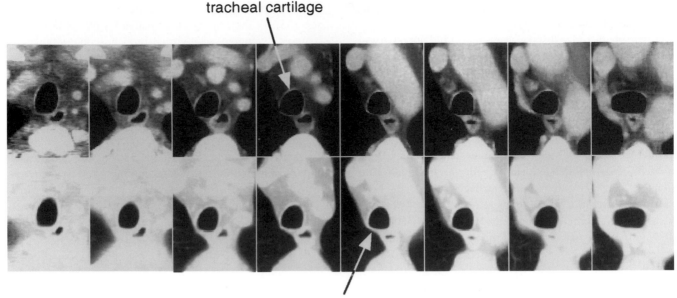

posterior tracheal membrane

FIG. 3-15. Normal trachea: scans with 7-mm collimation at 7-mm intervals from the level of the extrathoracic trachea (*left*) to a level just above the carina (*right*), shown with mediastinal (*above*) and lung windows (*below*). The shape of the trachea is different at different levels, being more ovoid superiorly. The horseshoe-shaped tracheal cartilages give the anterior trachea a rounded appearance (*arrow, top row*). The posterior trachea represents the posterior tracheal membrane and often appears flattened (*arrow, bottom row*).

cheal wall, lying between the open ends of the tracheal cartilages, is a thin fibromuscular membrane termed the posterior tracheal membrane (see Figs. 3-15 and 3-16). The blood supply to the trachea is lateral and tenuous (37). Superiorly, blood is supplied from branches of the inferior thyroid arteries and the extreme right intercostal artery, whereas inferiorly, the trachea is supplied by branches of the bronchial arteries and the third intercostal artery.

There is marked variability in the cross-sectional appearance of the trachea, which may appear rounded, oval, or horseshoe shaped (see Fig. 3-15; Fig. 3-17). The posterior tracheal membrane may appear convex posteriorly, flat, or convex anteriorly (35,38). In a study of anatomically normal persons (35), the trachea most often appeared round or oval; a horseshoe-shaped trachea with a flat posterior membrane was present in nearly 25%, whereas an inverted pear-shape or square appearance can also be seen.

Tracheal diameter can vary widely in anatomically normal persons. In men, tracheal diameter averages 19.5 mm and ranges from 13 to 25 mm (mean, ±3 standard deviations) in the coronal plane and 13 to 27 mm in the sagittal plane (39). In women, tracheal diameter is slightly less, averaging 17.5 mm and ranging from 10 to 21 mm in the coronal plane and 10 to 23 mm in the sagittal plane (39). In children, tracheal diameter increases as the child grows, and tracheal cross-sectional area correlates most closely with height (40,41). In adults, slight tracheal narrowing is often seen at the level of the aortic arch. In children, variation in tracheal dimensions at different levels is as much as 20% (40,41).

The shape of the intrathoracic trachea can change dramatically with expiration or dynamic respiratory maneuvers (Fig. 3-18). Most commonly, invagination of the posterior membrane occurs with forced expiration, resulting in a crescent-moon or horseshoe-shaped lumen (6). Marked anterior bowing of the posterior tracheal membrane can be used on expiratory CT as a marker of forced expiration. Slight side-to-side narrowing of the trachea also occurs during expiration, a finding accentuated in the presence of tracheomalacia. In a study of dynamic CT during forced expiration, the sagittal tracheal diameter decreased an average of 32%, from 19.6 ± 2.3 to 13.3 ± 3.5 mm. In the coronal plane, mean tracheal diameter decreased 13%, from 19.4 ± 2.7 to 16.9 ± 2.6 mm during forced expiration (6). The extrathoracic trachea can increase in diameter slightly during forced expiration or during a Valsalva maneuver.

Despite some variability, the tracheal wall almost always appears as a thin (1–2 mm) soft tissue stripe, well defined internally by air in the tracheal lumen and usually as well delineated externally by the presence of mediastinal fat (see Figs. 3-15–3-18; Figs. 3-19 and 3-20). Cartilage calcification can be seen in older subjects, particularly in women. The tracheal wall normally appears thinner posteriorly, where cartilage is lacking.

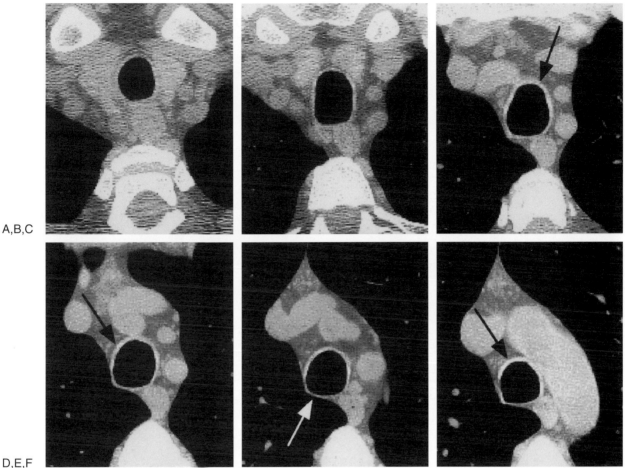

A,B,C

D,E,F

FIG. 3-16. A–F: Normal trachea: high-resolution CT sections through the trachea, obtained at 1-cm intervals. The tracheal wall is well defined internally by air in the tracheal lumen and is well defined externally by mediastinal fat. Tracheal cartilage within the anterior and lateral tracheal walls appears a few millimeters thick; calcification (*black arrows*) is often present in older patients, more commonly in women. The posterior tracheal wall represents the posterior tracheal membrane (*white arrow*) and is relatively thin. In this patient, it is sharply outlined by lung. The posterior tracheal membrane appears flattened, whereas the cartilage anteriorly gives the trachea a rounded or horseshoe shape.

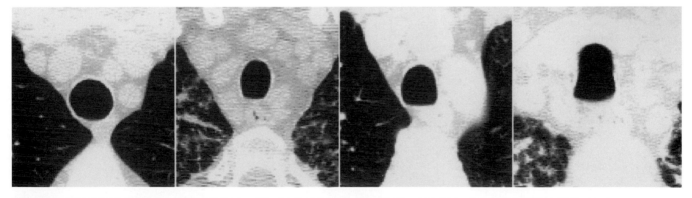

FIG. 3-17. Variability in the cross-sectional shape of the trachea in four anatomically normal persons. From *left* to *right,* the trachea may appear round, oval, horseshoe shaped, or square. The posterior tracheal membrane may appear convex posteriorly, flat, or convex anteriorly in anatomically normal persons.

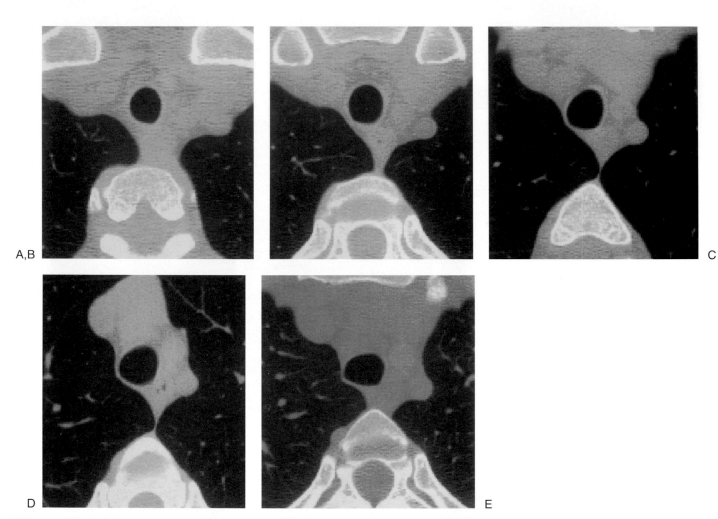

A,B

C

D

E

FIG. 3-18. Cross-sectional shape of the trachea in a healthy person on inspiratory (**A–D**) and expiratory (**E**) scans. The expiratory scan (**E**) is matched to its closest inspiratory level (**C**). Expiration results in some flattening of the tracheal contour, with a decrease in sagittal diameter and an increase in coronal diameter.

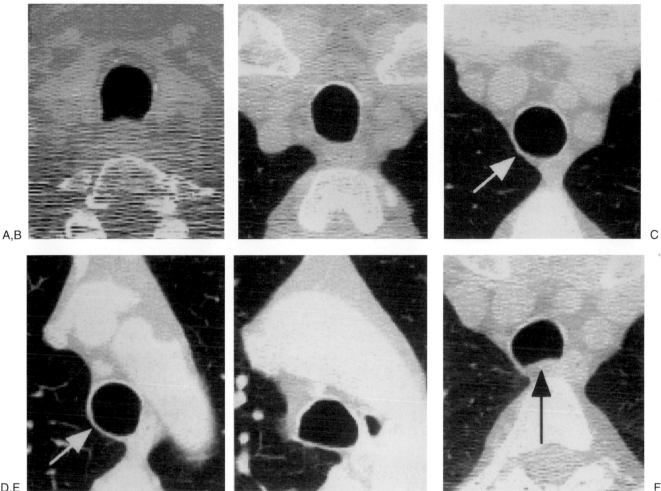

FIG. 3-19. Cross-sectional shape of the trachea in a healthy person on inspiratory (**A–E**) and expiratory (**F**) scans. The right posterolateral tracheal wall (*white arrows,* **C** and **D**) is clearly outlined by lung. The expiratory scan is matched to its most similar inspiratory level (**C**). In this person, expiration results in anterior bowing of the posterior tracheal membrane (*black arrow,* **F**). This appearance on expiration is common. In addition, the extrathoracic trachea (**A**) shows anterior bowing of the posterior tracheal membrane on the inspiratory scan caused by the esophagus.

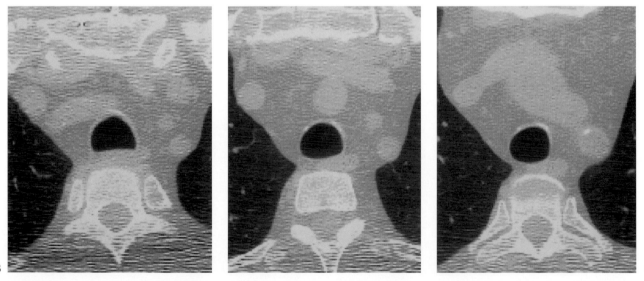

FIG. 3-20. Cross-sectional shape of the trachea in a healthy person on inspiratory (**A–E**) and expiratory (**F**) scans. The expiratory scan is matched to its most similar inspiratory level (**D**). In this person, expiration has resulted in more marked anterior bowing of the posterior tracheal membrane (*arrow*) than seen in Figure 3-19. (*continues*)

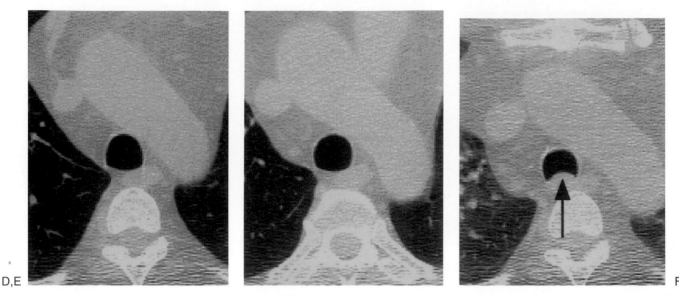

D,E

F

FIG. 3-20. *Continued.*

The position of the trachea within the mediastinum varies, depending on the level of the section. It angles posteriorly from its position at the thoracic inlet and appears at progressively more posterior at more caudal levels (see Fig. 3-15). Along most of its length, the right wall of the trachea is in contact with the pleural reflection of the right upper lobe (see Figs. 3-15–3-20), resulting in the right paratracheal stripe seen on routine posteroanterior chest radiographs. The lung also frequently contacts the posterolateral tracheal wall, in close association with the esophagus, in what is termed the retrotracheal recess. When the posterior tracheal wall is visible on the lateral chest radiograph, it is termed the posterior tracheal band (38).

''Saber-sheath'' trachea is a common variation in tracheal morphology (Fig. 3-21), in which the internal side-to-side diameter of the trachea is decreased to half or less the corresponding sagittal diameter. It is almost always associated with chronic obstructive pulmonary disease (42). Although this condition is classically described as a static deformity, further narrowing of the tracheal lumen can be documented when patients are examined using CT obtained during forced expiration or a Valsalva maneuver (35,36,43,44).

True anatomic variants are unusual. Most frequent is tracheal bronchus, which has an incidence as high as 1% (Fig. 3-22). A tracheal bronchus usually arises from the right tracheal wall, at or within 2 cm of the tracheal bifurcation, and typically supplies a variable portion of the medial or apical right upper lobe (45–47). A tracheal bronchus may be supernumerary or may represent a replaced segment or subsegment of the right upper lobe. Recurrent infection or bronchiectasis may result from narrowing at the origin of the bronchus; in intubated patients, particularly children, it may result in persistent

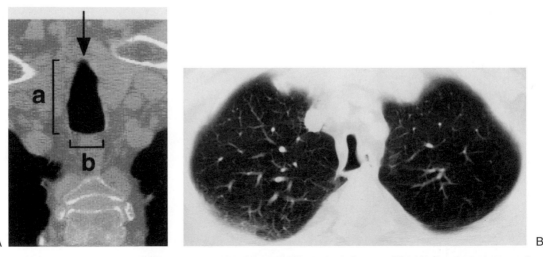

A

B

FIG. 3-21. Saber-sheath trachea. **A:** A sagittal tracheal diameter (*a*) twice the coronal diameter (*b*) indicates the presence of a saber-sheath trachea. This deformity only involves the intrathoracic trachea and, as in this patient, is first recognized at the thoracic inlet. The trachea may assume a triangular shape (*arrow*) because of weakness of the anterior tracheal cartilage. **B:** Section through the midtrachea in another patient again shows characteristic appearance of a saber-sheath trachea.

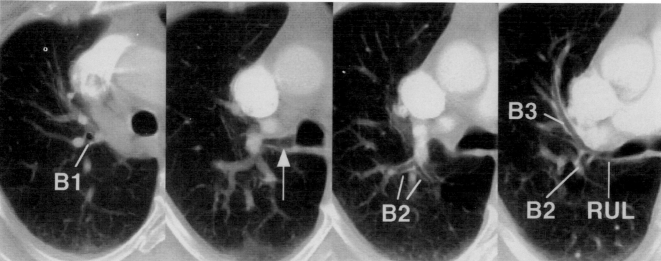

A,B

C,D

FIG. 3-22. Tracheal bronchus: Four images (**A–D**) at contiguous levels in a patient with a tracheal bronchus, obtained with spiral technique, 7-mm collimation, and reconstruction at 7-mm intervals. The tracheal bronchus (*arrow,* **B**) arises from the lateral tracheal wall. It supplies the apical segment of the right upper lobe (*B1*), seen in cross section in **A.** The right upper lobe bronchus (*RUL*) gives rise to the anterior (*B3*) and posterior (*B2*) segmental bronchi.

right upper lobe atelectasis (48). Associated vascular and tracheobronchial anomalies have also been reported.

Rarely, an outpouching or diverticulum may be identified involving the posterolateral tracheal wall, a so-called tracheocele (49,50). Resulting from foci of muscular weakness within the trachealis muscle, tracheoceles have been divided into two groups: those with wide mouths, likely acquired; and those with narrow mouths, likely congenital in origin (Fig. 3-23). These lesions may grow to be capacious and thus may serve as reservoirs for debris, leading to dumping of their contents into the tracheobronchial tree.

Until recently, magnetic resonance (MR) offered the unique advantage of allowing the trachea to be imaged in both coronal and sagittal planes. However, coronal, sagittal, and three dimensional reconstructions of volumetric spiral CT appear to be of greater clinical utility. CT and MR allow evaluation of the tracheal wall and the tracheal lumen, as well as the assessment of extraluminal disease. In patients with tracheal tumors, both primary and secondary, MR appears comparable to CT in identification of the extent of disease (Fig. 3-24).

Clinical Applications

Identification of tracheal disease is notoriously difficult: clinically, it has been estimated that lesions need to occlude more than 75% of the lumen before the development of symptoms related to airway obstruction, and even then these are frequently mistaken as being due to asthma. Early diagnosis is rare and usually occurs as a result of hemoptysis. Radiographically, the trachea has been described as the blind spot in the chest, with lesions characteristically identified only when large (51). For descriptive purposes, this section addresses first focal and then diffuse tracheal abnormalities, with an acknowledgment that this distinction may be arbitrary (Table 3-4).

Focal Tracheal Disease

Tracheal Stenosis

Benign airway strictures may be either congenital or acquired. In either case, accurate evaluation requires that the precise length and degree of stenosis be assessed along with associated peritracheal or bronchial abnormalities. Among acquired strictures, the most common cause is iatrogenic injury resulting from intubation. Although investigators have estimated that complications occur in up to 10% to 15% of patients after intubation, and in up to 40% of patients after tracheotomies, the incidence of serious complications after intubation has decreased dramatically since the introduction of high-volume/low-pressure tubes (52). The two principal sites of postintubation stenosis are at the stoma or at the level of the endotracheal tube or tracheostomy tube balloon (37). In both cases, strictures result from pressure necrosis, which causes ischemia and subsequent scarring. Stenosis also may be due to inflammation with subsequent thinning and weakening of the tracheal wall (tracheomalacia) in the segments between the stoma and the cuff; narrowing may also be caused by granulation tissue resulting from direct tracheal injury by the endotracheal or tracheostomy tube tip (37). Other complications of intubation include tracheal rupture and tracheobrachiocephalic artery or tracheoesophageal fistulas, the latter usually occurring in the presence of combined tracheal and esophageal intubation.

In addition to postintubation stenoses, tracheobronchial strictures also occur as a result of infection, in particular tuberculosis and histoplasmosis, and after lung transplantation. After lung transplantation, complications commonly occur at the level of the bronchial anastomosis and include dehiscence, necrosis, and stenosis from malacia, fibrous stricture, prominent granulation tissue formation, or a combination of these conditions (53–57).

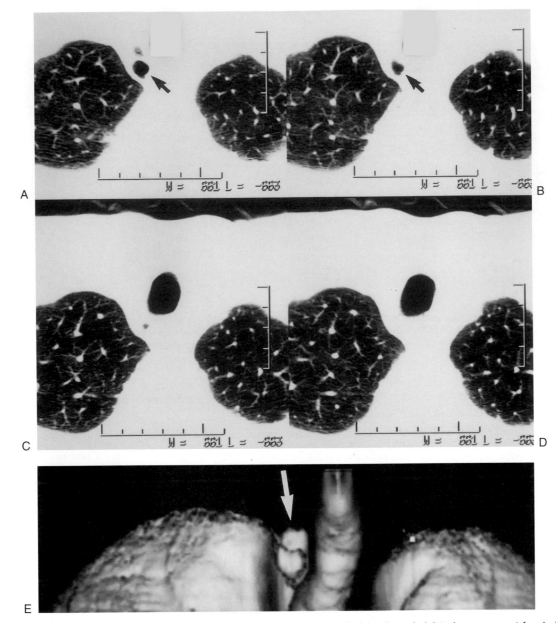

FIG. 3-23. Tracheocele. A–D: Sequential sections through the trachea at the level of the thoracic inlet show apparent focal air collection to the right (*arrows* in **A** and **B**). **E:** Three dimensional surface rendering derived shows focal outpouching arising from the lateral tracheal wall (*arrow*) characteristic of a tracheocele.

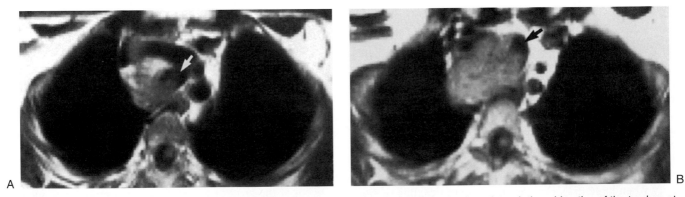

FIG. 3-24. Central tumor: MR evaluation. A,B: Sequential, every-beat-gated, axial spin-echo sections through the midportion of the trachea at the level of the great vessels. On these relatively T1-weighted images, tumor is easily identified as a lobular mass of intermediate signal intensity, distinct from adjacent mediastinal fat, clearly narrowing and invading the trachea (*arrows*).

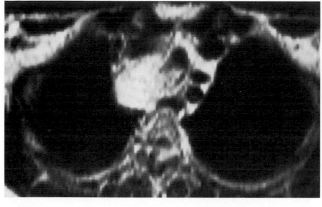

C

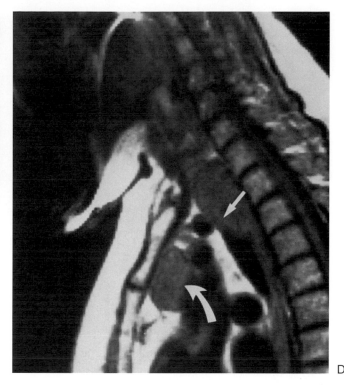

D

FIG. 3-24. *Continued.* **C:** Every-third-beat-gated axial SE image at approximately the same level as shown in **B.** With T2 weighting, the tumor is no longer as distinct as in **A** and **B. D:** Sagittal image through the trachea obtained with the same technique as in **A.** Tumor is again easily identified as lobular masses of intermediate signal causing apparent total obstruction of the trachea (*straight arrow*), as well as anterior mediastinal adenopathy (*curved arrow*). The patient has biopsy-proved metastatic medullary carcinoma of the thyroid.

Regardless of the cause of a stricture, CT, especially when performed using the helical technique, has proved a reliable method for assessing tracheobronchial strictures (see Fig. 3-3). As documented by Whyte and colleagues (58), in their study of 25 patients with known or suspected stenosis, CT with MPRs demonstrated the site and degree of tracheal or main bronchial stenoses with a sensitivity of 93% and a specificity of 100%. CT has also proved of value in assessing patients with tracheobronchial tears, after either intubation or blunt trauma. In the case of blunt trauma, likely mechanisms for tracheobronchial rupture include compression between the sternum and the vertebral column and shearing forces from sudden decompression (37). Most cases involve the carina or proximal main stem bronchi because these represent points of airway fixation and result in linear splitting. Radiologic findings in patients with blunt tracheal rupture have been described: for the most part, these are nonspecific and include pneumothoraces (both unilateral and bilateral, with or without tension pneumothorax), pneumomediastinum, and subcutaneous emphysema (59). More specific signs include orientation of the endotracheal tube to the right associated with an overdistended balloon cuff with subsequent migration of the balloon toward the endotracheal tube tip (59) and the so-called "fallen lung" sign, indicative of central bronchial disruption. In comparison with radiographic findings, CT allows more precise evaluation of the presence of peritracheal or bronchial air and is more accurate in assessing sternal or other osseous injuries that may also be present (52,59–62).

TABLE 3-4. *Classification of diseases of the trachea and main stem bronchi*

Focal disease
  Tracheal Strictures
    Congenital
    Acquired
      Postintubation
      Infection (tuberculosis, fungal disease)
  Benign Neoplasms
    Commonest:
      Squamous cell papilloma (solitary)
      Laryngotracheobronchial papillomatosis
  Primary Malignant Neoplasms
    Commonest:
      Squamous cell carcinoma
      Adenoid-cystic carcinoma
      Carcinoid tumors
  Secondary malignant neoplasms
Diffuse disease
  Increased diameter
    Tracheobronchomegaly
  Decreased diameter
    Relapsing polychondritis; amyloidosis; sarcoidosis; Wegener's granulomatosis; tracheopathia osteochondrolytica; ulcerative colitis; saber-sheath trachea; infection

Adapted from ref. 43, with permission.

Tracheal Neoplasia

Etiology. Although many different tracheal tumors, both benign and malignant, have been reported, primary tracheal neoplasia is rare. These tumors include both primary epithelial and mesenchymal neoplasms and secondary neoplasia

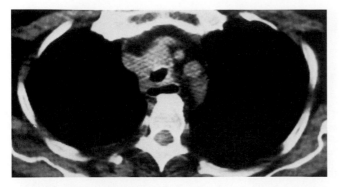

FIG. 3-25. Squamous cell carcinoma of the trachea: Section through the trachea at the level of the great vessels. The trachea wall is thickened, and the lumen appears circumferentially and irregularly narrowed. A soft tissue mass can be identified in infiltrating deeply into the mediastinum, obliterating the normal fascial planes surrounding the brachiocephalic artery and medial wall of the right brachiocephalic vein. As compared with the appearance of the trachea shown in Figure 3-26, this tumor proved unresectable.

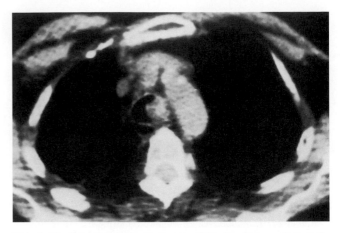

FIG. 3-26. Adenoid-cystic carcinoma of the trachea: section at the level of the aortic arch shows a focal, well-defined soft tissue mass arising from the left lateral wall of the trachea. Although the mass extends outside the wall into mediastinum, one sees a clear plane of separation between the mass and adjacent mediastinal structures, indicating potential resectability, later confirmed surgically.

due to either metastases or, more commonly, direct tracheal invasion by adjacent mediastinal neoplasms, especially carcinomas arising from the lung, thyroid, and esophagus (63). In fact, only a few lesions occur with any frequency, with squamous cell carcinomas and adenoid-cystic carcinomas together accounting for up to 86% of cases (64).

Squamous cell carcinoma most often occurs in middle-aged male smokers, and not surprisingly it has been found to be associated with other malignant diseases of the respiratory tract in as many as one-third of patients (Fig. 3-25) (64). In approximately 10% of cases, these tumors prove to be multifocal and are frequently found to extend into the main stem bronchi or adjacent esophagus, resulting in malignant esophageal-bronchial fistulas (63).

Adenoid-cystic carcinomas arise from the tracheobronchial mucous glands, most frequently on the posterolateral wall of the trachea (see Fig. 3-5; Fig. 3-26). Previously classified along with carcinoid tumors and mucoepidermoid tumors as "bronchial adenomas," these lesions all represent low-grade malignant tumors and, along with squamous cell carcinomas, show a marked propensity for local, especially submucosal invasion. For this reason, the term "bronchial adenoma" should be considered a misnomer and should no longer be used. Most often, adenoid-cystic carcinomas present as either broad or pedunculated polypoid lesions, although circumferential involvement of the trachea and bronchus in the absence of a distinct mass has been described (62). Unlike squamous cell carcinomas, but in common with mucoepidermoid tumors and carcinoids, no known association between exists adenoid-cystic carcinomas and cigarette smoking, nor is there any predilection for either sex.

The most common benign tracheal neoplasm is squamous

cell papilloma. Although, like squamous cell carcinomas, these most often occur in middle-aged male smokers, squamous cell papillomas typically involve the larynx or bronchi, with tracheal involvement uncommon: more important, involvement is limited to the tracheal wall (63). Laryngotracheobronchial papillomatosis refers to a condition associated with multiple papillomas (Fig. 3-27). Histologically similar to solitary papillomas, this condition most often occurs in children younger than 5 years of age and usually is restricted to the larynx, with spontaneous resolution noted in most cases. Furthermore, papillomatosis has been shown to be etiologically linked to infection with human papillomavirus, either contracted at birth or acquired through sexual transmission. Papillomatosis has been noted to occur in patients with acquired immunodeficiency syndrome (AIDS) (see Fig. 3-27). Widespread disease occurs in a few patients. As shown by Kramer and associates (65) in a literature review of 532 patients, tracheal and bronchial involvement occurs in only approximately 5% of cases, whereas pulmonary parenchymal disease occurs in less than 1%. Unfortunately, in this population, spontaneous remission is unusual, with malignant transformation to squamous cell carcinoma reported in adults. The origin of parenchymal disease is controversial. Because tracheobronchial and parenchymal disease is rarely encountered without coexistent laryngeal disease, investigators have postulated that spread is by endobronchial dissemination. An association between distal spread and prior tracheostomy further supports this cause. Typically, lesions appear first as well-defined nodules, occasionally identifiable as centrilobular, that subsequently undergo central necrosis resulting in multiple thin-walled cavities. Bronchiectasis, with or without parenchymal consolidation and atelectasis, is often identified in association with nodular

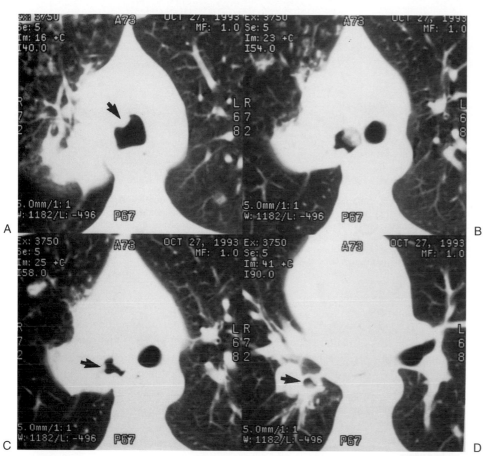

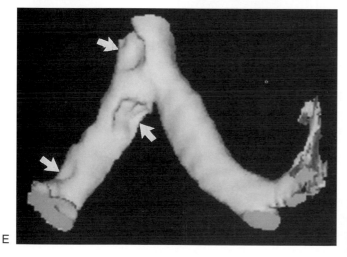

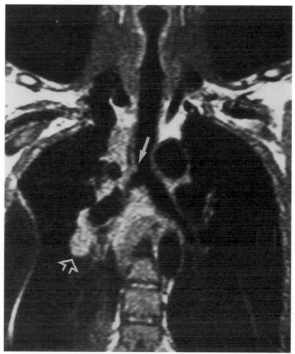

FIG. 3-27. Laryngotracheobronchial papillomatosis. **A–D:** Enlargements of select 5-mm sections through the distal trachea, carina, bronchus intermedius, and right lower lobe bronchus, respectively, show multiple irregular filling defects in an AIDS patient with documented tracheobronchial papillomatosis (*arrows* in **A, C,** and **D**). **E:** Three dimensional surface rendering shows multiple areas of tracheal and bronchial narrowing corresponding to multiple papillomas. **F:** Coronal T1-weighted MR image through the carina also show nodular soft tissue lesions of intermediate signal intensity along the right tracheal wall (*arrow*) and partially occluding the bronchus intermedius (*open arrow*). (*continues*)

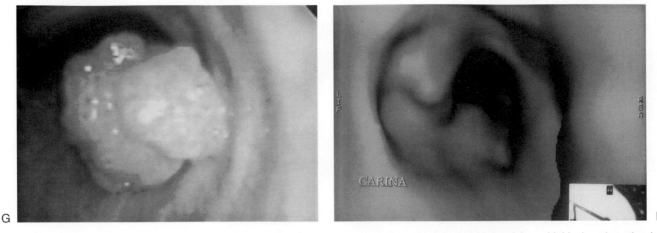

G   H

FIG. 3-27. *Continued.* **G:** Image obtained at flexible bronchoscopy confirms the presence of an irregular endobronchial lesion along the right lateral tracheal wall. In this case, the bronchoscope could not be safely passed beyond the proximal tracheal lesion limiting endoscopic evaluation of the distal airways. **H:** Internal rendering from within the right main stem bronchus looking caudally shows numerous large endoluminal masses partially obstructing the airway. The ability to visualize airways distal to points of obstruction otherwise limiting bronchoscopy has been touted as a potential advantage of virtual bronchoscopy. In this case, lesions throughout the airways are also well visualized on routine axial images as well as three dimensional surface renderings and coronal MR (compare with **A–F**).

densities, presumably the result of bronchial occlusion and subsequent inflammation or infection (Fig. 3-28).

CT Findings. Not surprisingly, the CT appearances of tracheal neoplasms overlap. Indeed, regardless of cell type, these tumors have in common the finding of an endobronchial soft tissue mass or asymmetric tracheal or bronchial wall thickening causing eccentric narrowing of the tracheal or carinal lumen (see Figs. 3-24–3-27). Asymmetric tracheal or bronchial wall thickening may be exceedingly subtle, especially in patients with benign lesions such as papillomas. Because retained secretions may also have this appearance, the examiner often needs to acquire additional images after requesting patients to cough (Fig. 3-29). Although the presence of calcification should raise the suspicion of a mesenchymal tumor, especially chondromatous lesions, definitive diagnosis still requires histologic evaluation in cases of focal tracheal disease. However, whereas endoscopic biopsy can

reliably establish the diagnosis, adequate preoperative evaluation requires accurate definition of the extent of extraluminal involvement if present. This is especially important because as much as one-half the length of the trachea may be successfully resected in the absence of mediastinal invasion (37).

Tuberculosis of the Trachea and Main Stem Bronchi

Tuberculosis typically involves the distal trachea and proximal main stem bronchi: isolated tracheal disease is rare (66,67). Active inflammation causes irregular circumferential bronchial wall thickening, resulting in narrowed or even obstructed airways (Fig. 3-30). Enhancement of the tracheal wall has been reported in patients with acute inflammation after the administration of intravenous contrast material (67). In most cases, active infection results

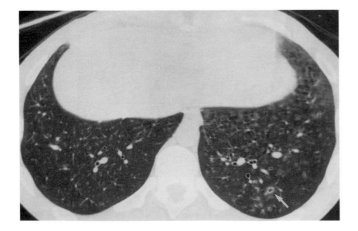

FIG. 3-28. Pulmonary involvement with tracheobronchial papillomatosis: section through the lung bases shows multiple ill-defined centrilobular nodules, some of which show evidence of early cavitation (*arrow*). The patient has histologically documented tracheobronchial papillomatosis. (Courtesy of James Gruden, M.D., NYU Medical Center, New York.)

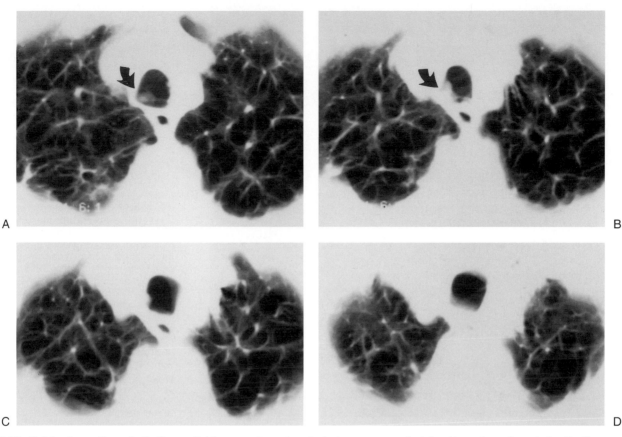

FIG. 3-29. Retained secretions. **A–D:** Sequential 5-mm sections show typical appearance of retained secretions characterized by the presence of a mottled, irregular intraluminal density (*arrows* in **A** and **B**). In equivocal cases, repeat scans through the same region showing disappearance of these filling defects may be of value after the patient coughs. (From ref. 9, with permission.)

from extension from peribronchial lymphatic disease, although endobronchial implantation from contaminated sputum has also been postulated as a potential mechanism (66,67). Evidence of associated mediastinal inflammation, in the form of diffuse increased density of mediastinal fat or enlarged mediastinal or pericarinal nodes, may also be identified (67,68). If this condition is untreated, ulceration with resulting fistulas between nodes and adjacent airways may develop (Fig. 3-31). With appropriate therapy, these changes are usually, although not invariably, reversible. Unlike active infection, fibrotic tuberculosis results in smoothly narrowed airways without evidence of either wall thickening or active peribronchial inflammation (66,67). Unlike active infection, which involves both main stem bronchi equally, fibrotic tuberculosis usually involves the left main bronchus, perhaps because of its greater length. CT findings in patients with central airway tuberculosis are rarely specific. As noted by Moon and colleagues (67), findings that help to differentiate tuberculous disease from bronchogenic carcinoma include longer circumferential involvement and the absence of an intraluminal mass. Notwithstanding these distinctions, accurate diagnosis usually requires histologic evaluation.

Diffuse Tracheal Disease

In addition to tracheal tumors, many different inflammatory abnormalities, both infectious and noninfectious, diffusely affect the trachea and main stem bronchi. These include both primary tracheal abnormalities and those resulting from spread of adjacent mediastinal inflammation, and they may manifest as either diffuse narrowing or dilatation.

Diffuse Tracheal Widening or Tracheobronchomegaly

Also referred to as Mounier-Kuhn syndrome, the term tracheobronchomegaly refers to a heterogeneous group of patients who have marked dilatation of the trachea and main stem bronchi, frequently in association with tracheal diverticulosis, recurrent lower respiratory tract infections and bronchiectasis (69–71). The etiology of this disorder is controversial. Findings in favor of a congenital etiology include histopathologic evidence of deficiency of tracheobronchial muscle fibers and absence of the myenteric plexus as well as an association with other congenital or connective tissue disorders including ankylosing spondylitis, Marfan's syndrome, cystic fibrosis, Ehlers-Danlos syndrome and cutis laxa in children (72,73). In distinction, findings in favor of

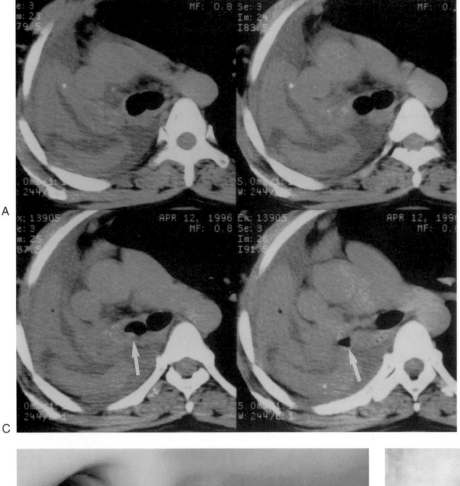

FIG. 3-30. Tuberculous bronchial stenosis. A–D: Sequential 5-mm helically obtained images (pitch, 1; reconstruction interval, 4 mm) show marked narrowing of the right main stem bronchus and bronchus intermedius (*arrows* in C and D) associated with extensive atelectasis and loculated pleural fluid. Evaluation of the presence and extent of a stricture in this case is limited when assessing axial images only. E: Endoscopic projection image looking down the right main stem bronchus shows complete bronchial occlusion (*arrow*). F: Corresponding view obtained at the time of bronchoscopy confirms the presence of stenosis (*arrow*) (compare with E). G: Coronal multiplanar reconstruction shows only a short segment stenosis (*arrow*), beyond which the distal bronchus intermedius is patent. In this case, the advantages of multiplanar reconstructions in determining the length of bronchial narrowing as compared with direct bronchoscopic evaluation are apparent. Despite the appearance of irreversible stenosis and the expectation that this appearance would result in cicatrization atelectasis of the entire right lung, airway patency with resultant reexpansion of the right lung was reestablished after surgical resection of the stricture (compare with Fig. 3-6). H: Follow-up chest radiograph confirming near complete reexpansion of the right lung. Note the presence of surgical clips in right hilum. (A–G from ref. 9, with permission.)

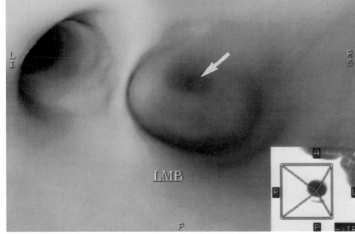

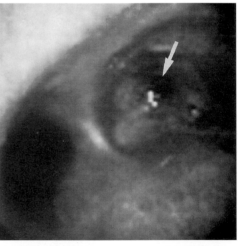

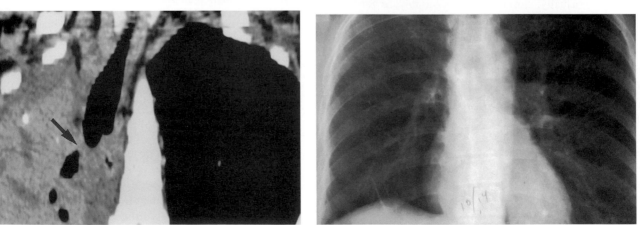

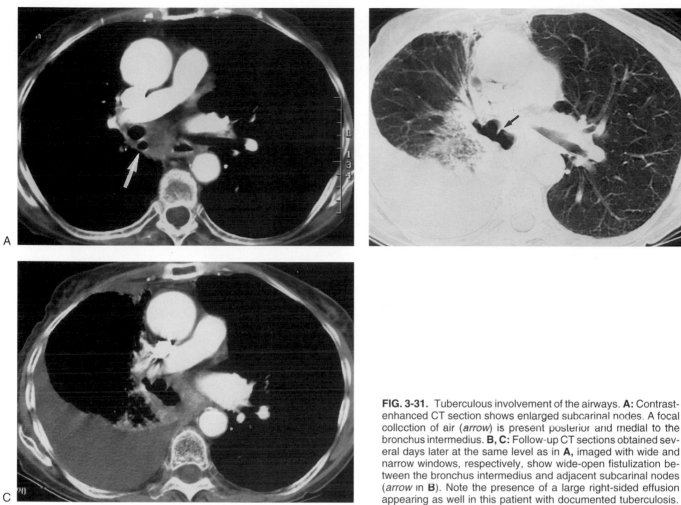

FIG. 3-31. Tuberculous involvement of the airways. **A:** Contrast-enhanced CT section shows enlarged subcarinal nodes. A focal collection of air (*arrow*) is present posterior and medial to the bronchus intermedius. **B, C:** Follow-up CT sections obtained several days later at the same level as in **A,** imaged with wide and narrow windows, respectively, show wide-open fistulization between the bronchus intermedius and adjacent subcarinal nodes (*arrow* in **B**). Note the presence of a large right-sided effusion appearing as well in this patient with documented tuberculosis.

an acquired etiology include the fact that tracheobroncho-megaly most often is diagnosed in men in their third and fourth decades without an antecedent history of respiratory tract infection, often in association with chronic cigarette smoking (72,73). An association between tracheomegaly and diffuse pulmonary fibrosis has also been reported, presumably the result of increased traction on the tracheal wall due to increased elastic recoil pressure in both lungs exerting opposing force (72,73).

CT findings in patients with tracheobronchomegaly have been described (43,74). Using a tracheal diameter of greater than 3 cm measured 2 cm above the aortic arch, and diameters of 2.4 and 2.3 cm for the right and left main bronchi, respectively, the diagnosis of tracheobronchomegaly is relatively straightforward (74). Additional findings include tracheal scalloping or diverticula, the latter especially common along the posterior tracheal wall. Also common is the finding of a marked tracheal flaccidity identifiable as a marked decrease in the diameter of the trachea on expiration, even to the point of airway occlusion, indicative of tracheomalacia (Fig. 3-32) (6).

The importance of tracheomegaly lies in its association with distal airway inflammation. In a study of 75 consecutive patients referred for CT evaluation of possible bronchiectasis, Roditi and Weir (72) found that, overall, 12% of their patients proved to have dilated tracheas, including 7 (17%) of 42 patients with CT evidence of bronchiectasis as well as 3 (6%) of 32 without. These data suggest that tracheomegaly may play a causative role in the development of bronchiectasis as a result of a predisposition to infection resulting from abnormal mucus clearance in patients with inefficient cough and stagnant mucus (Fig. 3-33).

Diffuse Tracheal Narrowing

Included in the group of patients with diffuse narrowing are those with infectious disorders, including bacterial, viral, and fungal infections either primary or secondary resulting from adjacent mediastinitis, as well as patients with a variety of noninfectious disorders including tracheopathia osteochondrolytica, relapsing polychondritis, Wegener's granulomatosis, amyloidosis, sarcoidosis, and ulcerative colitis

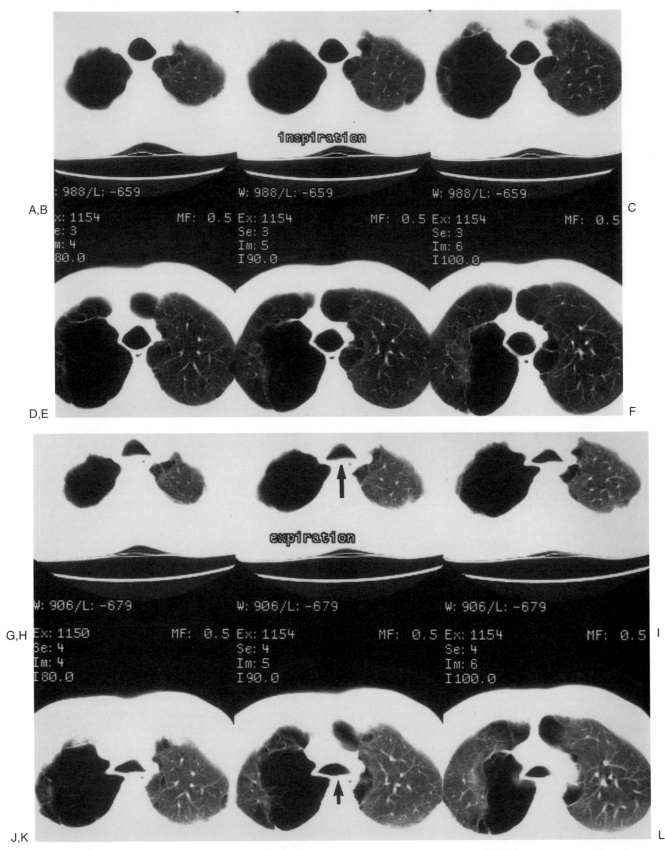

FIG. 3-32. Tracheobronchomegaly. **A–F:** Select 5-mm sections obtained in deep inspiration show marked diffuse enlargement of the tracheal lumen. Note the presence of extensive bilateral bullous emphysema as well. **G–L:** Images obtained at the same levels as shown in **A–F,** imaged at end-expiration show marked diffuse tracheal narrowing (*arrows*) (compare with **A–F**). Tracheomalacia is usually present in patients with diffuse tracheomegaly, easily confirmed with expiratory scans.

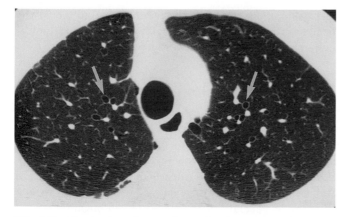

FIG. 3-33. Tracheobronchomegaly: section through the upper lobes shows marked enlargement of the tracheal lumen consistent with tracheomegaly. Note the presence of mild cylindric bronchiectasis in both upper lobes (*arrows*). A causative association between tracheomegaly and the development of bronchiectasis has been postulated.

(43,69). Although many of these have similar appearances in cross section, some are sufficiently distinctive to allow a definitive diagnosis with appropriate clinical correlation.

Tracheobronchopathia Osteochondroplastica

Tracheobronchopathia osteochondroplastica is a rare disorder involving the trachea and main bronchi in which multiple submucosal nodules representing bone, cartilage, or calcified acellular protein matrix may be identified resulting in diffuse narrowing of the airway lumen (Fig. 3-34). Characteristically, these nodules spare the membranous posterior wall of the trachea. Often asymptomatic, tracheopathia osteochondrolytica has been reported to cause hemoptysis in as many as 25% of cases (75). Other symptoms including cough, dyspnea, hoarseness, stridor, and recurrent lower respiratory tract infections have also been noted. Typically occurring in middle-aged men, the course of this disease is generally benign, and in most cases the diagnosis is made only at autopsy.

The origin of this disease is unknown. Thought by Virchow to represent enchondroses and exostoses arising from the perichondrium of cartilage rings, calcified nodules alternatively have been attributed to cartilaginous and bony metaplasia involving elastic tissue (76). Although investigators have postulated that tracheopathia osteochondrolytica represents an end stage of tracheal amyloid, to date, the presence of amyloid has been reported in only a handful of cases.

Radiologically, the diagnosis is difficult unless the patient has marked nodularity and narrowing of the trachea. Bronchoscopically, these lesions appear as multiple yellowwhite, hard papillary nodules that may be difficult to sample for biopsy because of their bony nature. In distinction, numerous reports have documented a characteristic CT appearance of calcified nodules measuring between 3 and 8 mm in diameter resulting in irregular narrowing of the lower trachea and main stem bronchi with sparing of the posterior tracheal wall (43,76–78).

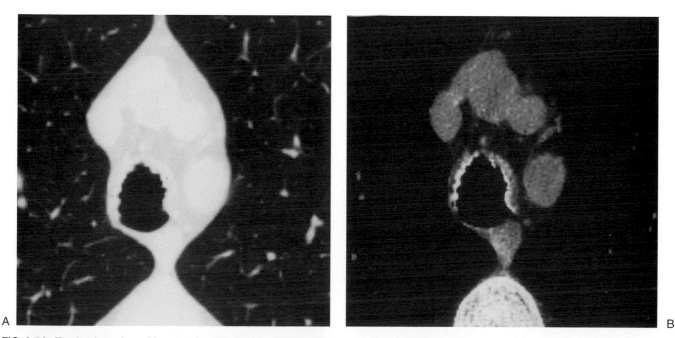

FIG. 3-34. Tracheobronchopathia osteochondroplastica. **A, B:** Sections through the midtrachea imaged with wide and narrow windows, respectively, show marked nodularity of the anterior and lateral walls of the trachea with extensive calcifications causing slight narrowing of the tracheal lumen. Note the sparing of the posterior wall of the trachea, characteristic of this entity.

Relapsing Polychondritis

Relapsing polychondritis is a rare disorder that results in destruction of cartilage within the pinna of the ear, nose, joints, and upper airways, including the larynx and subglottic trachea (43,69). Thought to be related to abnormal acid mucopolysaccharide metabolism, an association has also been noted in approximately 25% of cases with autoimmune vasculitis (79). Although nonerosive polyarteritis, nasal deformity, and auricular chondritis are characteristic, they need not be present in all cases. Arteritis resulting in aortitis and aortic insufficiency, mitral insufficiency, and aneurysms involving medium-sized arteries have also been reported (80). Histologically, one sees evidence of chondritis with perichondral inflammation, loss of basophilic staining of cartilage matrix, and ultimately fibrous replacement of involved cartilage.

Characterized by episodic inflammation, relapsing polychondritis results in diffuse tracheal and bronchial narrowing in approximately 50% of cases, secondary to a combination of edema, granulation tissue, cartilage destruction, and ultimately fibrosis of the tracheal wall (79). When severe, this disease may result in airway obstruction and recurrent episodes of atelectasis and pneumonia. CT findings in this disease have been reported and include tracheal narrowing resulting from thickening of the anterior and lateral tracheal walls with characteristic sparing of the posterior tracheal wall (43,62,79,80). Because this disorder is often indistinguishable from other causes of diffuse tracheal narrowing, the diagnosis rests on a combination of pathologic, clinical, and radiologic findings, especially the presence of abnormal calcifications in the pinna of the ear (Fig. 3-35) (80). As documented by Im and colleagues (79), CT may be of partic-

ular value in documenting a response to steroid therapy by demonstrating decreased tracheal wall thickening, potentially obviating more invasive follow-up procedures.

Wegener's Granulomatosis

Wegener's granulomatosis is a systemic necrotizing vasculitis typically involving middle-aged adults (69). Although characteristically described by the classic triad of upper respiratory tract, lung, and renal involvement with glomerulonephritis, the disease also often involves skin and joints as well as the middle ear, eye, and nervous system (81). In 90% of cases of generalized Wegener's granulomatosis, serum antineutrophil cytoplasmic antibodies characterized by a diffuse granular cytoplasmic immunofluorescent staining pattern (C-ANCA) may be detected: these are thought to be highly specific for the disease, although false-positive test results have been noted in patients with a variety of both inflammatory and neoplastic diseases (81).

Within the lungs, Wegener's granulomatosis usually manifests either as multiple parenchymal nodules or as areas of focal consolidation, frequently with evidence of cavitation. Although airway involvement in Wegener's granulomatosis has been estimated to occur in between 15% and 25% of cases (82), if obtained, transbronchial biopsy reveals evidence of airway inflammation in nearly all cases. Lesions may be either focal or diffuse and may involve any portion of the airways from the hypopharynx to the lobar bronchi (Fig. 3-36). Involvement of segmental bronchi may result in atelectasis or infection. Typically, the disease causes diffuse wall thickening resulting in circumferential narrowing of the airway lumen. Although it is uncommon, mediastinal or hilar adenopathy may also be identified. As noted by Aberle and

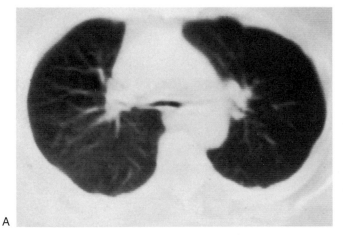

A

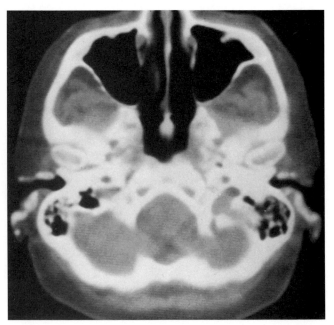

B

FIG. 3-35. Relapsing polychondritis. **A:** Section through the carina shows marked narrowing of the right and left main stem bronchi, as well as the right upper lobe bronchus. The lung fields appear normal. **B:** Scan through the base of the skull shows diffuse calcifications of the pinnae of both ears. This combination of findings is pathognomonic of relapsing polychondritis. (Case courtesy of Burton Cohen, M.D., Mt. Sinai Hospital, New York.)

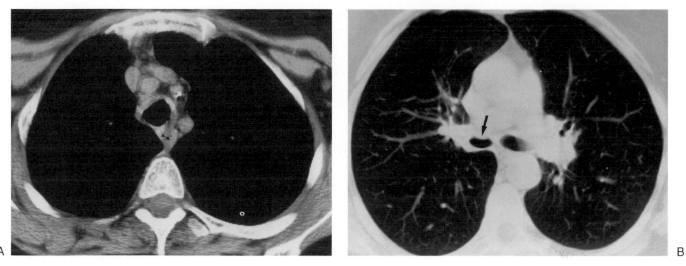

FIG. 3-36. Wegener's granulomatosis. **A:** Section shows asymmetric, circumferential thickening of the tracheal wall associated with a few shotty mediastinal nodes. **B:** Section through the carina in the same patient as in **A** imaged with wide windows shows involvement of the right main stem bronchus, which is clearly narrowed in comparison with the left main stem bronchus (*arrow*). Note the absence of parenchymal disease. Airway involvement with Wegener's granulomatosis may be either focal or, as in this case, diffuse and is often present in the absence of associated parenchymal abnormalities.

colleagues (83), whereas airway narrowing is an infrequent presenting manifestation of disease, airway lesions often occur in the course of therapy, possibly because of prolonged survival with use of cytotoxic agents. In their series of 19 patients, airway lesions occurred in 5 patients in the course of 8 relapses and always proved symptomatic, manifest as hoarseness, cough, or stridor (83). In selected cases, CT may prove invaluable by demonstrating optimal sites for tracheostomy as well as by defining the true extent of disease when bronchial narrowing precludes complete bronchoscopic evaluation. The use of cine CT has also been recommended to evaluate tracheal mechanics more precisely (83,84).

Amyloidosis

Amyloid infiltration of the airways and lungs may occur as an isolated phenomenon or as part of diffuse systemic disease. Three forms of respiratory amyloid have been described: diffuse alveolar septal, nodular pulmonary, and tracheobronchial (81). Tracheobronchial amyloidosis is rare and is generally confined to the trachea without evidence of concurrent parenchymal disease. Deposits may be either solitary or multiple, with or without calcification, and if sufficiently large, they can lead to hemoptysis or airway obstruction with resultant atelectasis or recurrent pulmonary infection (85). Histologically, amyloid appears as amorphous, submucosal eosinophilic material when stained with hematoxylin and eosin, and it is apple green when stained with Congo red (81).

The CT appearance of tracheobronchial amyloid has been described (43,62,86). In its nodular form, amyloid appears as a focal mass partially or completely occluding airways with infiltration of the adjacent peritracheal or bronchial tissues, often with foci of calcification. In this form, it may mimic the appearance of both benign and malignant tracheal neoplasms (86). In its more diffuse form, tracheal amyloid leads to concentric nodular thickening of the tracheal wall.

Ulcerative Colitis

Although this manifestation is rare, changes involving both large and small airways have been reported to occur in patients with ulcerative colitis. Within small airways, findings consistent with constrictive bronchiolitis have been described reminiscent of sclerosing cholangitis, although the two diseases rarely coexist (87). Similar findings of submucosal fibrosis and airway narrowing have also been described within the larger airways, including the trachea, often in association with bronchiecatsis (87). To date, no apparent relationship has been established between disease activity within the colon and airway abnormalities: in fact, airway disease may occur even years after colectomy (87). On CT, the tracheobronchial walls appear thickened, resulting in irregular narrowing indistinguishable from the other causes of diffuse airway narrowing described earlier (Fig. 3-37) (43).

LOBAR AND SEGMENTAL BRONCHI

Anatomy

As with the trachea, the bronchi are composed of both cartilaginous and fibromuscular elements. However, the distinction between parts of the bronchial lumen supported by cartilage and those that are not is less clear-cut than in the trachea. For a short distance, the main bronchi contain horseshoe-shaped cartilage plates, as does the trachea, but the

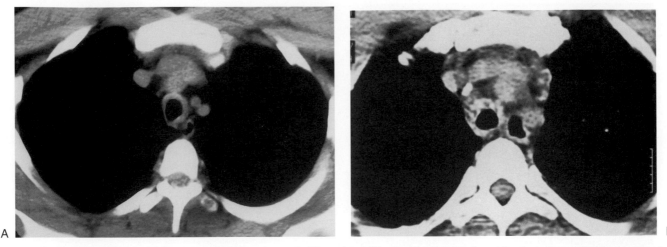

FIG. 3-37. Diffuse tracheal narrowing: miscellaneous causes. **A:** Ulcerative colitis. Section through the midtrachea shows slightly asymmetric, circumferential thickening of the tracheal wall in a patient with documented ulcerative colitis. In the absence of clinical or histologic correlation, this appearance is nonspecific (compare with Fig. 3-36). **B:** Tracheal sarcoid. Section through the aortic arch. The trachea is circumferentially thickened; the tracheal lumen is narrowed. Enlarged mediastinal nodes are present as well. Biopsy confirmed tracheal sarcoid. This appearance may be indistinguishable from other infiltrative–inflammatory diseases of the tracheal wall.

cartilage plates become less regularly shaped at more peripheral levels. On dynamic expiratory scans, some posterior invagination of the walls of the central bronchi is often visible on CT, as in the trachea, reflecting this anatomy.

Airways divide by dichotomous branching, with approximately 23 generations of branches from the trachea to the alveoli. The wall thickness of conducting bronchi and bronchioles is approximately proportional to their diameter, at least for bronchi distal to the segmental level. In general, the thickness of the wall of a bronchus or bronchiole less than 5 mm in diameter should measure $\frac{1}{6}$ to $\frac{1}{10}$ of its diameter (Table 3-5) (88); however, precise measurement of the wall thickness of small bronchi or bronchioles is difficult because wall thickness approximates pixel size.

Because bronchi taper and become thinner walled as they branch, they are progressively more difficult to see in the peripheral lung. Bronchi less than 2 mm in diameter and closer than 2 cm to the pleural surface are not normally visible on high-resolution CT (HRCT) (89,90). Because a bronchus is usually recognized only when its walls are visible, one cannot see bronchi with a wall thickness of less than 300 μm on CT or HRCT. This corresponds to bronchi

TABLE 3-5. *Relation of airway diameter to wall thickness*

	Diameter (mm)	Wall thickness (mm)
Lobar and segmental bronchi	5–8	1.5
Subsegmental bronchi/ bronchiole	1.5–3	0.2–0.3
Lobar bronchiole	1	0.15
Terminal bronchiole	0.7	0.1
Acinar bronchiole	0.5	0.05

Adapted from ref. 88, with permission.

of about 1.5 to 2 mm in diameter and closer than 2 cm to the pleural surface, equivalent to between the seventh and ninth generation of airways (89,90). Rarely, smaller bronchi approximately 1 mm in diameter can be recognized coursing perpendicularly within the plane of a thin section by virtue of their lower density and their proximity to an adjacent pulmonary artery, even though their walls cannot be individually resolved.

CT Identification of Bronchial Anatomy

Accurate evaluation of the airways necessitates both a detailed knowledge of normal anatomy and variants and careful attention to technique (Table 3-6). Using spiral CT technique and collimation of 3 to 5 mm, all segmental bronchi should be visible, but this is not always possible with thicker collimation or conventional CT technique. In a study of 50 patients with normal chest radiographs evaluated using contiguous 10-mm thick sections, Osborne and colleagues (91) found that only 70% of segmental bronchi could be reliably identified. Similar results have been reported by others (92).

The ability of CT to image a particular bronchus depends on its size and orientation relative to the scan plane (93–95). The main bronchi and bronchus intermedius are easily seen and are always visible because of their large size. The origin and proximal portion of lobar and segmental bronchi lying in the scan plane should be identifiable in virtually all cases on CT. Bronchi oriented in or near the scan plane include the right upper lobe bronchus (including both the anterior and posterior segmental bronchi), the left upper lobe bronchus (including the anterior segmental bronchus), the middle lobe bronchus (generally including some portion of both medial and lateral segmental bronchi), and the superior segmen-

TABLE 3-6. *Segmental and subsegmental bronchi: nomenclature and variants*

Bronchi and segments	Subsegments	Most common variants/comments[a]
Right lung		
Right upper lobe		
B1, apical	a, apical	B1 origin from B3 or less likely B2
	b, anterior	
B2, posterior	a, apical	B2 arising cephalad to B3 (56%), at same level
	b, posterior	as B2 or B2b (44%)
B3, anterior	a, lateral	axillary subsegment formed by B2a and B3b (or
	b, anterior	both)
Middle lobe		
B4, lateral	a, lateral	B4 and B5 equivalent in size (44%)
	b, medial	trifurcation B4a, B4b, B5 (13%)
B5, medial	a, superior	B5 larger than B4 (27%)
	b, inferior	
Right lower lobe		
B6, superior segmental bronchus	a, medial	B6c, B6a + b bifurcation (60%)
	b, superior	
	c, lateral	
B*, subsuperior bronchus		variable, arises between B6 and B7 (30%)
truncus basalis		bronchial trunk caudal to B6 giving rise to basal
		segments
B7, medial basilar bronchus	a, anterior	B7a + b anterior to the right inferior pulmonary
	b, medial	vein (60%)
B8, anterior	a, lateral	rudimentary B8 (10%)
	b, basilar	
B9, lateral	a, lateral	B8, B9 + 10 bifurcation (60%)
	b, basilar	B8, B9, B10 trifurcation (15%)
B10, posterior basilar bronchi	a, posterior	
	b, lateral	
	c, basilar	
Left lung		
Left upper lobe		bifurcation into superior (B1 + 2, B3) and inferior
		trunks (B4, B5) (75%)
		trifurcation of left upper lobe into B1 + 2, B3,
		B4 + 5 (16–25%)
B1 + 2, apicoposterior	a, apical	
	b, posterior	
	c, lateral	variation in origin of B1 + 2c common
B3, anterior	a, lateral	B3 may arise anywhere between B1 + 2 and
	b, medial	B4 + 5
	c, superior	B3 poorly defined (25%)
B4, superior lingular bronchus	a, lateral	well-developed B4a (40%); size varies
	b, anterior	depending on distribution of B3
B5, inferior lingular bronchus	a, superior	
	b, inferior	
Left lower lobe		
B6 +, superior bronchus	a, medial	B6a, B6b + c bifurcation (45%)
	b, superior	
	c, lateral	
B*, subsuperior bronchus		variable, arises between B6 and B7, a single
truncus basalis		stem (30%)
		bronchial trunk giving rise to basal segments,
		longer than on right
B7 + 8, anteromedial bronchus	B7a, medial	separate origin of B7 (<5%)
	B7b, lateral	B7 + 8, B9–10 bifurcation (45%)
	B8a, lateral	B7 + 8, 9, 10 trifurcation (15%)
	B8b, basilar	
B9, lateral basilar bronchus	a, lateral	
	b, basilar	
B10, posterior basilar bronchus	a, lateral	
	b, basilar	

[a] Percentages shown are approximate.

tal bronchi of both lower lobes. Bronchi having a vertical course and seen only in cross section appear as circular lucencies, and are also clearly seen on CT. Such bronchi include the apical segmental bronchus of the right upper lobe, the apical-posterior segmental bronchus of the left upper lobe, proximal portions of both lower lobe bronchi (below the takeoff of the superior segmental bronchi), and the medial and posterior basal lower lobe segments. The most difficult bronchi to visualize are those oriented obliquely relative to the scan plane, including the superior and inferior lingular bronchi, the lateral and medial segmental bronchi of the middle lobe, and the anterior and lateral basal lower lobe segments. Such bronchi appear elliptic when viewed in cross section.

Depending on their orientation, subsegmental bronchi can sometimes be identified. For example, using thin collimation, subsegmental bronchi can be seen in the basal segments of the right and left lower lobes in 56% and 35% of cases, respectively (96). Nearly all subsegmental bronchi in the upper lobes are also identifiable using thin-section CT (97,98).

Nomenclature for describing segmental lung anatomy has undergone several changes, but that described by Jackson and Huber in 1943 (99) has been generally adopted. Bronchi are also designated using a numeric system popularized by Boyden (100), in which segments are designated by B followed by a number (e.g., B1) and subsegments are indicated by the segmental number followed by a small letter (e.g., B1a). The numbering of segments is roughly in their order of origin from the airway as one progresses most distally from the trachea.

Some confusion has arisen because the numbering system described by Boyden underwent a change during the course of his publications, as a result of international agreement (100–102). Upper lobe bronchial segments were initially designated by Boyden as B1 (apical segment), B2 (anterior segment), and B3 (posterior segment), with the left apical-posterior segment being B1-3. In 1961 (100), numbers for the anterior and posterior upper lobe segments were switched, with the posterior segment becoming B2, the anterior segment becoming B3, and the left apical-posterior segment becoming B1-2. Standard nomenclature and 1961 revisions in letter-number codes are used in this book (see Table 3-6) (96,98–100,103–105).

The right and left bronchial trees are considered independently. Although each lobar and segmental bronchus and its segments are described, emphasis is placed on recognition of characteristic sections (Fig. 3-38). Some variability in the cross-sectional appearance of the airways is to be anticipated; this often is the result of variation in the relationship of bronchi to the plane of the scan rather than true anatomic variation. As already discussed, accurate visualization of bronchi requires meticulous technique: it is easy to distort

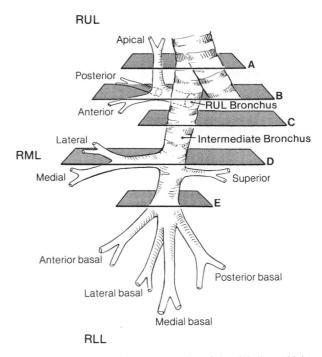

FIG. 3-38. Diagrammatic representation of the right bronchial tree in a steep oblique projection. Levels *A–E* represent key levels. *RUL*, right upper lobe; *RML*, right middle lobe; *RLL*, right lower lobe. Anatomic detail corresponding to the basilar segmental bronchi in particular is more accurately shown in Figure 3-51.

the normal appearance of a horizontally oriented bronchus if sections are not obtained through its center. Variations in subsegmental bronchi are common (see Table 3-6).

Right Lung Bronchial Anatomy

The right main bronchus is relatively short, dividing into the right upper lobe bronchus and bronchus intermedius. Often, the carina, right main bronchus, and right upper lobe bronchus are visible on a single scan.

Right Upper Lobe Bronchus. The right upper lobe bronchus arises at or just below the carina and courses laterally for a distance of 1 to 2 cm before dividing into its three segmental branches (i.e., apical, anterior, and posterior). Although the precise branching pattern of the right upper lobe bronchus is variable, the three upper lobe segments are easily identified because of their characteristic appearances and relative locations (Figs. 3-39–3-43) (98).

Frequently, the precise point of origin of the right upper lobe bronchus can be identified as a faint curvilinear density marginating the lateral wall of the right main bronchus. At the level of the origins of the segmental airways, in particular the anterior and posterior segmental bronchi, either a thin septum or a triangular wedge of tissue along the edge of a bronchus can be identified: anatomically, these images cor-

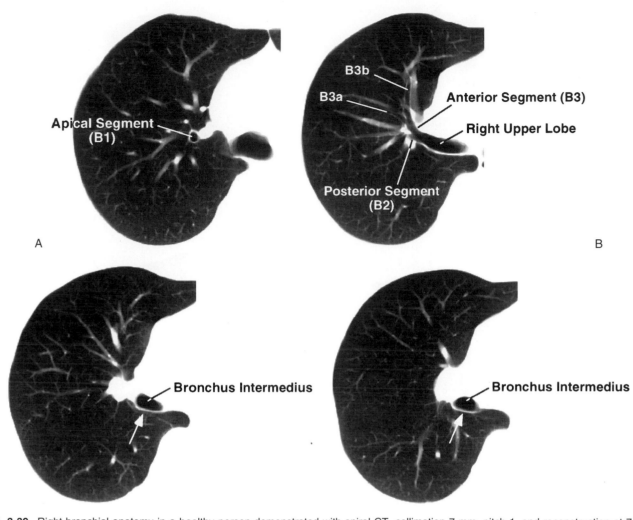

FIG. 3-39. Right bronchial anatomy in a healthy person demonstrated with spiral CT, collimation 7 mm, pitch 1, and reconstruction at 7-mm intervals. **A:** Apical segmental bronchus of the right upper lobe (see Fig. 3-38, level A). CT at the level of the carina shows the apical segmental bronchus of the right upper lobe (*B1*) in cross section at its point of bifurcation into its apical (*B1a*) and anterior (*B1b*) subsegments. **B:** Right upper lobe bronchus (see Fig. 3-38, level B). The right upper lobe bronchus is visible along its length. The anterior segmental bronchus (*B3*) lies in the plane of scan and can be seen to divide into its lateral (*B3a*) and anterior (*B3b*) branches. Only the origin of the posterior segmental bronchus (*B2*) is visible. The posterior wall of the upper lobe bronchus appears smooth and is about 2 mm in thickness. **C, D:** Bronchus intermedius (see Fig. 3-38, level C). The bronchus intermedius is visible as an oval lucency, with its posterior wall sharply outlined by lung (*arrows*). The posterior bronchial wall appears thin and sharply defined. The bronchus intermedius is typically seen at two or three levels, because of its length. (*continues*)

respond to spurs (93). Identification of these sites of bronchial bifurcation is critical because the spurs serve as precise anatomic landmarks and because bronchial bifurcations are frequent sites of bronchial disease, including bronchogenic carcinoma.

Apical segment bronchus. At the level of the distal trachea, the apical segmental bronchus of the right upper lobe is the first branch of the right upper lobe that is identified when scans are viewed in a cephalocaudal fashion. It is seen in cross section, appearing as a circular lucency in close proximity to the accompanying branches of the right upper lobe pulmonary artery and right superior pulmonary vein. Subsegments are commonly seen (see Figs. 3-42 and 3-43).

The right upper lobe bronchus is always found at or just below the level of the tracheal carina (see Figs. 3-22, 3-39B, and 3-40–3-43). The carina is easily identified as a thin septum separating the right from the left main stem bronchi. The right upper lobe bronchus originates more cephalad than the left upper lobe bronchus, above the level of the right main pulmonary artery. Characteristically, the posterior wall of the right upper lobe bronchus is in direct contact with air in either the posterior segment of the right upper lobe or the superior segment of the right lower lobe, depending on the position of the major fissure (see Figs. 3-39B and 3-40–3-43).

The right upper lobe bronchus courses horizontally: the origins and proximal portions of the anterior and posterior segmental bronchi are almost always seen when appropriate

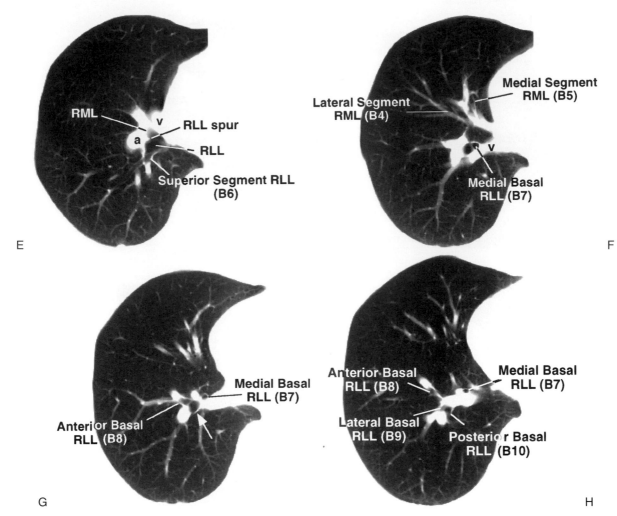

FIG. 3-39. *Continued.* **E:** Right middle lobe (*RML*) bronchus (see Fig. 3-38, level D). The RML bronchus arises anteriorly and extends anteriorly and laterally at an angle of about 45 degrees. Because it is also angled caudally, only a short segment of its lumen is visible. The superior segmental bronchus of the lower lobe (*B6*) arises posterolaterally at the same level, as is common. The superior pulmonary veins (*v*) lie anterior and medial to the middle lobe bronchus at this level, whereas the descending (interlobar) branch of the right pulmonary artery (*a*) lies beside and behind it. The carina or spur posterior to the origin of the middle lobe bronchus marks the origin of the lower lobe bronchus. **F:** Middle lobe segments and basal right lower lobe (*RLL*) bronchi (see Fig. 3-38, level E). The lateral (*B4*) and medial (*B5*) segments of the RML are visible below the level of its origin. The truncus basalis of the lower lobe (the lower lobe bronchus below the origin of the superior segment) has divided into two branches, the most anterior of which represents its medial basal segment (*B7*) branch. The inferior pulmonary vein (*v*) is posterior and medial, and pulmonary artery branches accompany the bronchi. **G:** The medial basal segmental bronchus (*B7*) of the RLL is most medial and lies anterior to the inferior pulmonary vein. The anterior segmental bronchus (*B8*) is anterior and lateral to the medial segment. The lateral and posterior segments are yet to arise as separate branches from their common bronchial trunk (*arrow*). **H:** The four basal segmental branches of the RLL are all visible at this level. The medial and posterior segmental bronchi are imaged more nearly in cross section than the anterior and lateral bronchi, which are more obliquely oriented.

FIG. 3-40. Variations in branching of right upper lobe bronchus (*RUL*) in four patients (**I–IV**). In each patient, scans obtained with 7-mm collimation and reconstructed at 7-mm intervals are displayed in a cephalocaudal direction from left (**A**) to right (**C**). *B1,* apical segment; *B2,* posterior segment; *B3,* anterior segment. For identification of subsegmental anatomy, refer to Table 3-6. The RUL bronchus originates from the lateral aspect of the right main stem bronchus at or just below the carina (corresponding to level B in Fig. 3-38). The RUL bronchus courses horizontally. Posteriorly, air within either the posterior segment of the RUL or the superior segment of the right lower lobe comes in contact with the posterior wall of the RUL bronchus, which is uniformly smooth; occasionally, a prominent azygos vein is identifiable posteromedially (*Ic*). The anterior (*B2*) and posterior (*B3*) segmental bronchi also have a horizontal configuration in many cases, making their identification easy. However, the posterior segmental bronchus may be best seen slightly cephalad to the anterior segment. The origin of B1 is variable; it may arise at a trifurcation of the right upper lobe bronchus (*Ib*) or in association with B3 (**IIB** and **IVB2**). As a rule, sections through the anterior segmental bronchus allow identification of both third- and sometimes fourth-order subsegmental divisions (**IIC** and **IVC**). As elsewhere within the bronchial tree, the origins of particular airways are marked by the presence of spurs. These are soft tissue divisions among contiguous airways, easily identified as thin lines or, when sectioned obliquely, triangular densities. Prominent spurs can be identified in IIc, separating the origins of B2 from B3, as well as the origins of two third-order subdivisions of B3. Sections also show the proximal portion of the apical segmental bronchus (*B1*) arising from the superior aspect of the RUL bronchus (corresponding to level A in Fig. 3-38) and quickly subdividing into anterior and posterior subsegments (**IIA** and **IIIA**). As a general rule, branches of the pulmonary artery to the RUL, the truncus anterior, lie medial to B1. The arteries and veins of the apical segment have a vertical orientation, whereas vessels to the anterior and posterior segments course more horizontally.

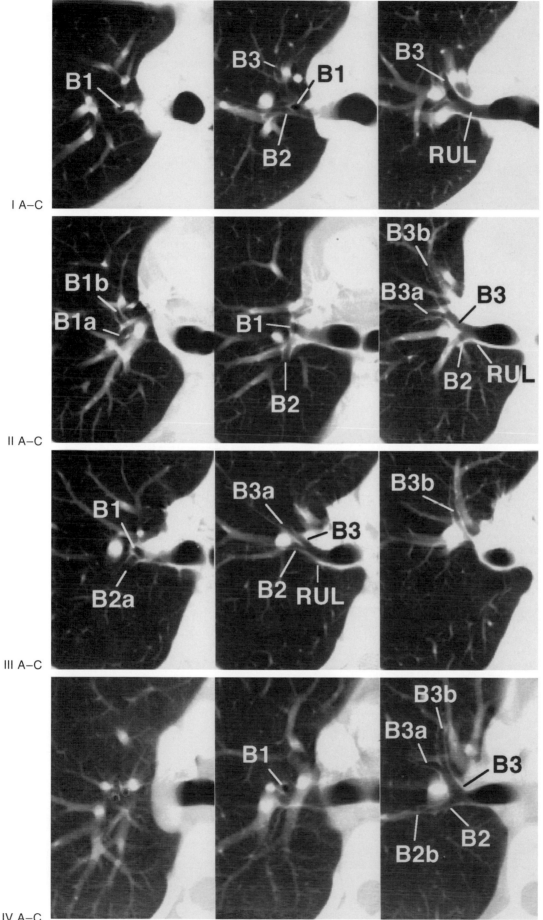

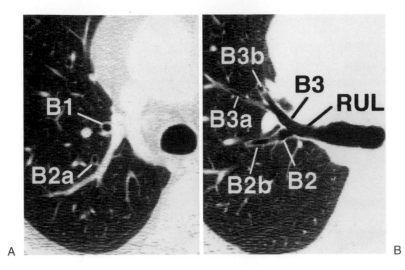

A

B

FIG. 3-41. A,B: High-resolution CT (1-mm collimation) scans through the right upper lobe bronchus. Segmental and subsegmental anatomy of the right upper lobe, as described in Table 3-6, is well defined. *RUL,* right upper lobe.

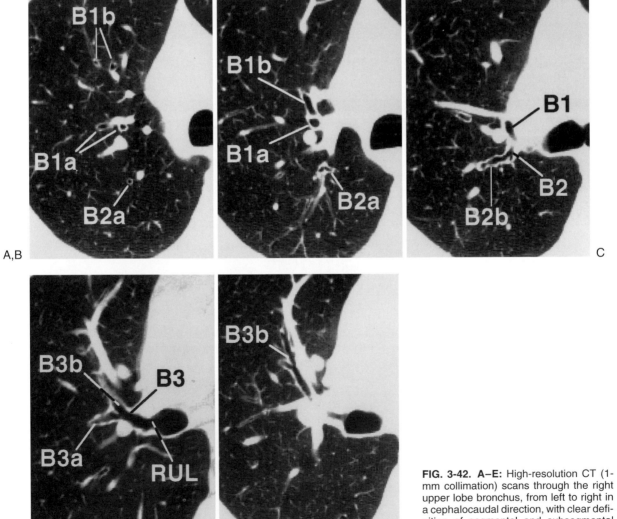

A,B

C

D,E

FIG. 3-42. A–E: High-resolution CT (1-mm collimation) scans through the right upper lobe bronchus, from left to right in a cephalocaudal direction, with clear definition of segmental and subsegmental anatomy. *RUL,* right upper lobe.

CT technique is used (see Figs. 3-39–3-43). Displacement (with or without displacement of the right main stem bronchus or bronchus intermedius) is a sensitive indicator of volume loss within the right upper lobe as a result of scarring, as occurs most often in patients with tuberculosis (see the section later on cicatrization atelectasis).

The anterior segment bronchus (B3) almost always lies in the plane of scan and is most easily seen. The posterior segmental bronchus (B2) may have a similar appearance (see Figs. 3-40IVC and 3-41B), but it often angles slightly cephalad from its origin and is usually visible at progressively higher levels as it courses posteriorly (see Figs. 3-39B, 3-40A–C, and 3-42): this pattern was visible in 56%

of cases studied by Lee and associates (97). Only its point of origin may be visible at the level of the anterior segmental bronchus (see Fig. 3-39B). Subsegments of the anterior and posterior segmental bronchi are commonly visible (see Figs. 3-39B and 3-40–3-43).

The origin of the apical segment (B1) of the right upper lobe bronchus can often be visualized as a rounded area of lucency superimposed on the distal portion of the right upper lobe bronchus (see Fig. 3-40A), at or just above the origins of the anterior and posterior segments. In many patients, a trifurcation of the upper lobe bronchus is present. In others, the apical segmental bronchus arises from the proximal anterior or posterior segmental bronchus (see Fig. 3-40B, D).

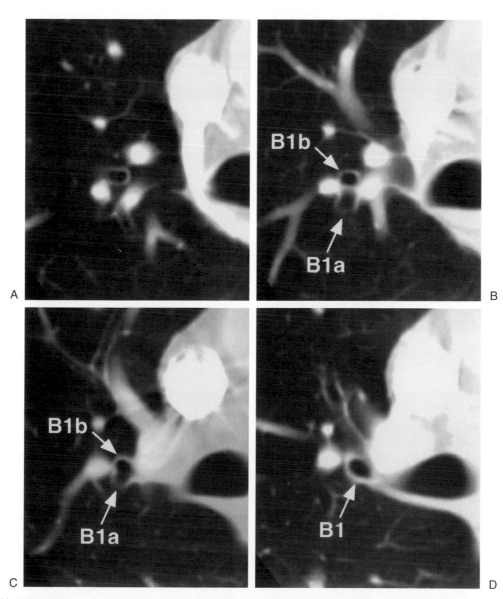

FIG. 3-43. A–H: Variation in the origin of the anterior and posterior segments of the right upper lobe on scans obtained with 5-mm collimation and reconstructed at 2.5-mm intervals. The anterior segmental bronchus (*B3*) arises above the level of the posterior segmental bronchus (*B2*). B2 appears to arise as a trunk from the undersurface of the right upper lobe bronchus (**G**). (*continues*)

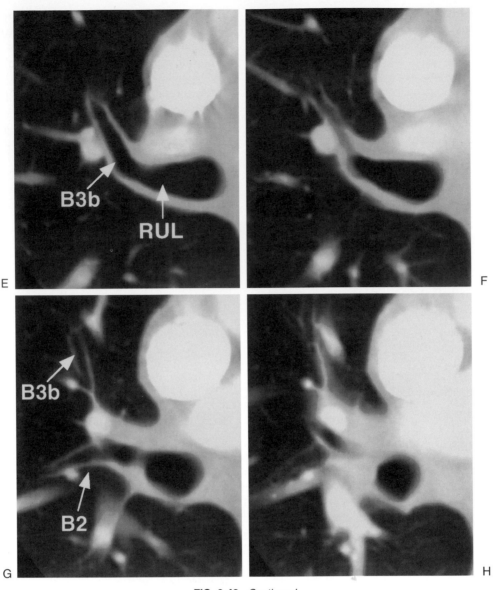

FIG. 3-43. *Continued.*

On scans obtained through both the anterior and posterior segmental bronchi and their subsegmental divisions, Mac-Gregor and colleagues (106) noted that an independent ramus of the posterior segmental bronchus of the right upper lobe can be recognized in about 15% of anatomically normal patients, supplying a discrete axillary subsegment. More often, this actually represents a prominent subsegmental division of the posterior (B2b) segment.

Although some variation exists in the origins of the right upper lobe segments and subsegments (see Fig. 3-43) (98), true anatomic variants are unusual.

The posterior wall of the right upper lobe bronchus is an important anatomic landmark (see Figs. 3-39 and 3-40–3-43). Although some variability exists in its overall thickness,

the upper limits of normal for the posterior wall of the right upper lobe bronchus should be about 5 mm. The posterior bronchial wall should be uniform in thickness, but a prominent azygos arch can result in apparent bronchial wall thickening (95,107). Analysis of scan sections just above and below this level should establish the presence of a prominent azygos vein as the cause of the prominent bronchial wall. If doubt persists, scans taken after a Valsalva maneuver should show marked decrease in the size of the azygos vein.

Bronchus Intermedius. The bronchus intermedius is 3 to 4 cm long, begins at the level of the right upper lobe bronchus, and gives rise to the middle lobe and lower lobe bronchi (see Figs. 3-38 and 3-39). Because of its length, it is characteristically seen on several adjacent sections.

The bronchus intermedius lies directly posterior to the

right main pulmonary artery and, at a slightly lower level, just medial to the right interlobar pulmonary artery. Because it courses obliquely, on CT it appears oval in cross section. The entire posterior wall of this bronchus is in contact with the superior segment of the right lower lobe, and thus, it is sharply outlined by air-containing lung (Fig. 3-44); the posterior bronchial wall should be thin and of uniform thickness (93,94,95). Pulmonary parenchyma may also extend posteromedial to the bronchus intermedius, in the aptly named azygoesophageal recess, the medial border of which is closely associated with the azygos vein and esophagus.

Cardiac bronchus. A rare congenital anomaly of the tracheobronchial tree, the accessory cardiac bronchus is the only true supernumerary anomalous bronchus, with an incidence of less than 0.5% (30). It arises from the medial wall of the bronchus intermedius before the origin of the superior segmental bronchus to the right lower lobe and usually before the origin of the middle lobe bronchus (Fig. 3-45). The bronchus is then directed caudally toward the mediastinum, hence the "cardiac" appellation. The length of the cardiac bronchus is variable, ranging from a short, blind-ending diverticulum to a longer, branching structure. The short type is usually a simple bronchial stump without associated alveolar tissue, whereas the longer subtype has been noted both with and without associated rudimentary alveolar tissue (30). Investigators have speculated that this anomaly, in fact, represents a rudimentary accessory lobe. Rarely, this blind-ending airway may serve as a potential reservoir for infectious material, with symptoms resulting from retained secretions with resultant inflammation.

Middle Lobe Bronchus. The middle lobe bronchus arises from the anterolateral wall of the bronchus intermedius and extends anteriorly and laterally (see Figs. 3-38 and 3-39E;

Figs. 3-46–3-49). The level of the middle lobe bronchus also marks the point of origin of the right lower lobe bronchus. Although a thin septum of tissue may be identified separating the orifices of these two airways, more frequently only the lateral aspect of the spur can be seen (see Figs. 3-44 and 3-49) (93). This is identified as a triangular wedge of tissue just lateral to the bronchial bifurcation. Identification of such bronchial spurs can be important, serving as convenient landmarks. Furthermore, spurs are frequent sites of bronchial disease, including bronchogenic carcinoma.

Lateral (B4) and medial (B5) segments. The middle lobe bronchus extends for a distance of about 1 to 2 cm before dividing into its lateral (B4) and medial (B5) segmental branches (see Figs. 3-38, 3-39E, and 3-46–3-49). Because the middle lobe bronchus courses caudally, it is obliquely oriented relative to the scan plane, and in many cases, only a short segment of the bronchus is seen on each CT. The main portion of the middle lobe bronchus and its lateral and medial segments are often seen at a level 1 to 2 cm below the origin of the middle lobe. In select cases, bronchi that course in an oblique plane, such as the middle lobe bronchus, may be visualized to better advantage when the gantry is tilted 20 degrees cranially, thus making it more nearly parallel to its course (Fig. 3-50) (108).

In about half of patients, the middle lobe bronchus divides into medial and lateral segmental branches of equal size (see Fig. 3-48). In most of the remaining patients, the medial segmental bronchus predominates and can be recognized as larger on CT. Less commonly, the middle lobe bronchus trifurcates into the medial segment and two lateral subsegments. None of these variations should cause confusion when scans are viewed sequentially.

Although both middle lobe segmental bronchi are directed

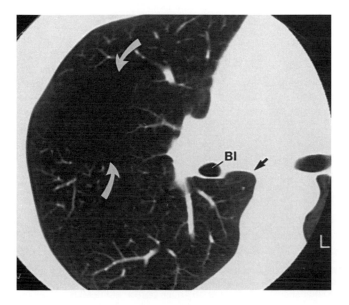

FIG. 3-44. Bronchus intermedius (*BI*). The BI lies immediately posterior and medial to the right main and interlobar pulmonary arteries. Typically, a portion of the superior segment of the right lower lobe extends medially to form a convexity—the azygoesophageal recess (*arrow*). The circular hypovascular region on the right is caused by the minor fissure, the so-called right midlung window (*curved arrows*).

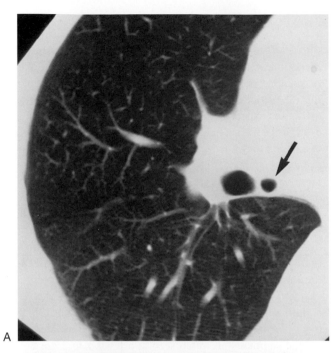

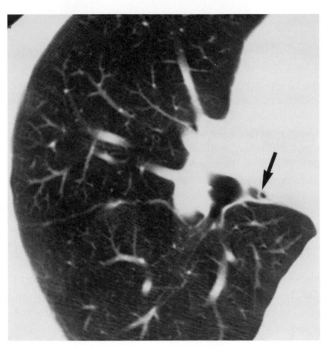

A

B

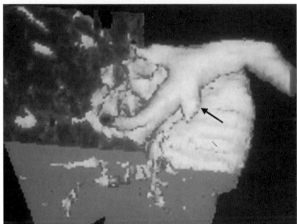

C

FIG. 3-45. A,B: Enlargements of select 5-mm sections show a discrete air collection medial to the bronchus intermedius (*arrow* in **A**) within which is a suggestion of an ill-defined filling defect (*arrow* in **B**). Note the close proximity of this airway to the origins of both the middle lobe (*open arrow*) and superior segmental bronchi. **C:** Three dimensional surface rendering shows presence of a diverticulum arising from the medial wall of the bronchus intermedius (*arrow*); this represents a true supernumerary bronchus. Given its close proximity to the origin of the middle lobe bronchus, retained secretions within cardiac bronchi may result in recurrent episodes of aspiration within the middle lobe.

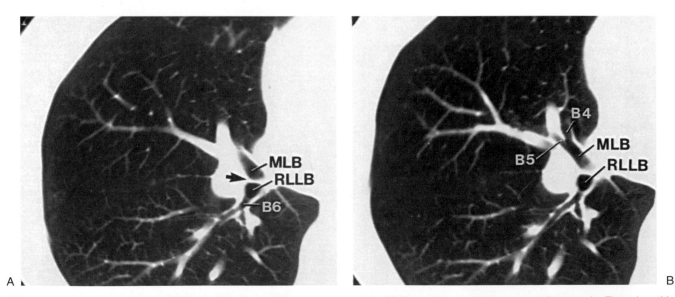

A

B

FIG. 3-46. Middle lobe bronchus (*MLB*). **A:** CT section shows the origin of the MLB coursing anteriorly on an oblique angle. There is a thin line, or septum, separating the MLB anteriorly from the right lower lobe bronchus (*RLLB*); this represents the middle lobe spur (*arrow*). *B6*, superior segmental bronchus of the right lower lobe. **B:** Section just caudal to that shown in **A,** through the main portion of the MLB as well as the origins of the medial (*B4*) and lateral (*B5*) segmental bronchi.

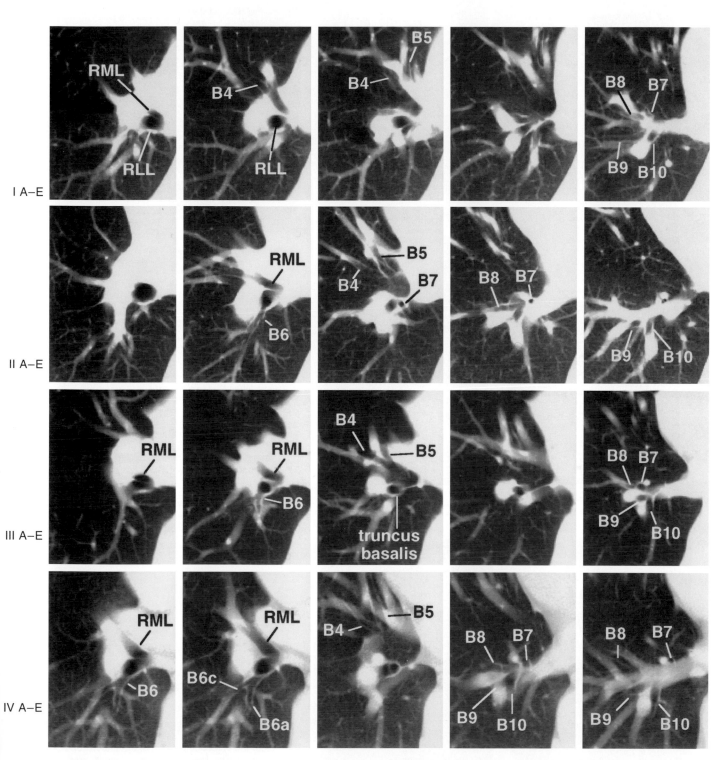

FIG. 3-47. Right middle lobe (*RML*) and right lower lobe (*RLL*) bronchial anatomy in four patients (**I–IV**). In each patient scans obtained with 7-mm collimation and reconstructed at 7-mm intervals are displayed in a cephalocaudal direction from left (**A**) to right (**E**). *B4,* lateral segment of RML; *B5,* medial segment of RML; *B6,* superior segment of RLL; *B7,* medial basal segment of RLL; *B8,* anterior basal segment of RLL; *B9,* lateral basal segment of RLL; *B10,* posterior basal segment of RLL. For subsegments, see Table 3-6.

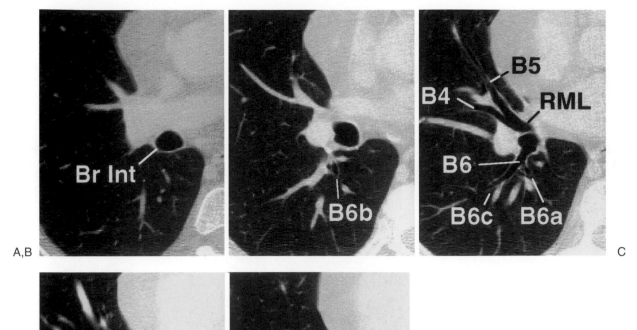

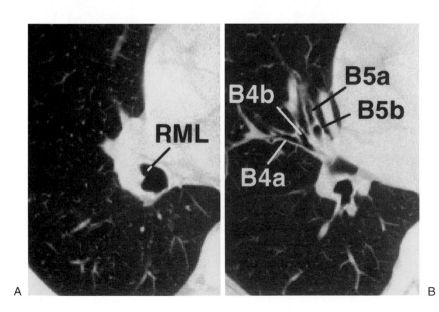

FIG. 3-48. Right middle lobe (*RML*) and right lower lobe (*RLL*) bronchial anatomy shown using spiral CT with 5-mm collimation and reconstruction at 5-mm intervals (**A–E**). A clearly defined spur separates the RML bronchus from the lower lobe bronchus. *Br Int*, bronchus intermedius; *B4,* lateral segment of RML; *B5,* medial segment of RML; *B6,* superior segment of RLL; *B7,* medial basal segment of RLL; *B8,* anterior basal segment of RLL; *B9,* lateral basal segment of RLL; *B10,* posterior basal segment of RLL. For subsegments, see Table 3-6.

FIG. 3-49. Subsegmental anatomy of the right middle lobe show using thin collimation. **A:** Scan at the level of the origin of the middle lobe bronchus. The bronchial spur is visible. *RML*, right middle lobe. **B:** At a more caudad level, segmental and subsegmental branches of the middle lobe are clearly seen. For subsegmental bronchi, refer to Table 3-6.

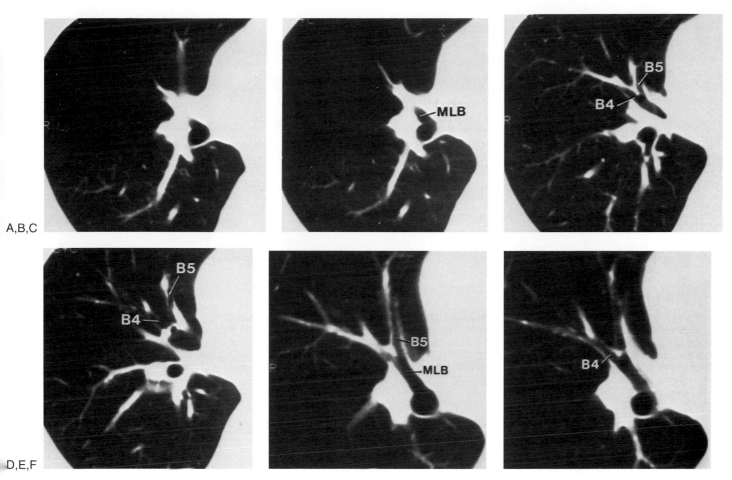

FIG. 3-50. Middle lobe bronchus (*MLB*): 20-degree angulation. **A–D:** Sequential 5-mm thick sections through the MLB and its subdivisions, B4 and B5. **E, F:** Sequential 5-mm thick sections through the MLB in the same patient as **A–D,** obtained with 20-degree cephalic angulation of the gantry. Because of its oblique orientation, the MLB is seen along its entire length, as are the lateral (*B4*) and medial (*B5*) segmental bronchi, when the gantry is tilted 20 degrees. In selected cases, this technique may allow easier interpretation.

inferiorly, the lateral segmental bronchus lies closer to the scan plane and is imaged over a greater distance on each scan. The medial segmental bronchus has a more oblique course. The middle lobe segmental bronchi are not always seen with 1-cm collimation, but they are reliably seen using thinner collimation. Subsegmental branches can sometimes be seen, particularly when thin collimation is used (see Fig. 3-49).

Lower Lobe Bronchus. The undivided lower lobe bronchus is short; near its origin, it gives rise to the superior segmental bronchus (B6) of the lower lobe from its posterior wall (see Figs. 3-38, 3-39E, and 3-46–3-48; Figs. 3-51 and 3-52). Distal to the origin of the superior segment, the basal lower lobe trunk (truncus basalis) is often visible, extending for a short distance before dividing into four basal segmental branches of the right lower lobe (see Figs. 3-38 and 3-47) (i.e., the medial, anterior, lateral, and posterior segments).

Superior segment (B6). The superior segmental bron-

chus of the right lower lobe may arise at the same level as, or slightly caudad to, the origin of the middle lobe bronchus (see Figs. 3-38, 3-39E, 3-46–3-48, 3-51, and 3-52). In an occasional case, the superior segmental bronchus appears to arise at a level cephalad to the origin of the middle lobe.

The superior segmental bronchus, which is about 1 cm in length, courses posteriorly within the scan plane. Typically, it divides into two subsegments, although trifurcation into medial, superior, and lateral subsegments is not unusual (see Fig. 3-47, 3–48, and 3–52). In some patients, two superior segmental bronchi may be present (Fig. 3-53).

Truncus basalis and basal segments. Below the origin of the superior segmental bronchus, the lower lobe bronchus continues for about 5 to 10 mm as the truncus basalis (see Figs. 3-39, 3-40, 3-48, and 3-51), oriented perpendicular to the scan plane and visualized as a circular lucency. The anterior wall of the basal bronchial trunk (truncus basalis) is commonly outlined by lung.

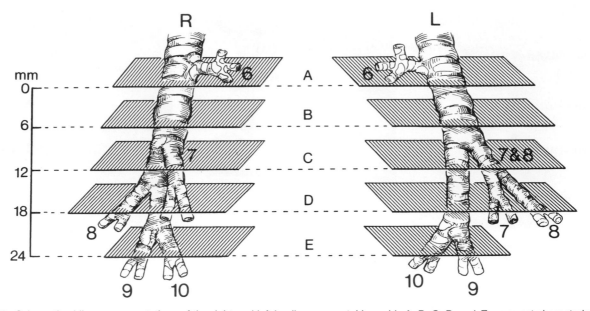

FIG. 3-51. Schematic oblique representations of the right and left basilar segmental bronchi. *A, B, C, D,* and *E* represent characteristic levels through the origins of the superior segmental bronchi (*B6*) (level *A*); the truncus basalis (level *B*); the medial basilar segmental bronchus (*B7*) on the right, and the anteromedial basilar segmental bronchus (*B7* and *B8*) on the left (level *C*); the anterior basilar segmental bronchus (*B8*) on the right, and the medial (*B7*) and anterior (*B8*) basilar segmental bronchi on the left (level *D*); and the origins of the lateral (*B9*) and posterior (*B10*) basilar segmental bronchi from their common trunks (level *E*), respectively. The scale on the *right* indicates approximate distances among these levels, given a wide range of variations encountered.

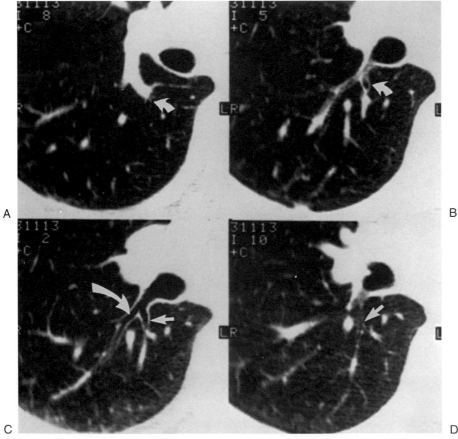

FIG. 3-52. Superior segmental bronchus (*B6*). **A–D:** Enlargements of sequential 1.5-mm thick sections through the superior segmental bronchus, obtained every 3 mm. The origin of the superior segmental bronchus is clearly seen originating from the posterolateral wall of the distal bronchus intermedius. The superior segmental bronchus on the right typically bifurcates into a prominent lateral subsegment (*B6c*) (*curved arrow* in **C**) and a common trunk for the medial (*B6a*) (*small arrows* in **C** and **D**) and superior (*B6b*) (*small curved arrows* in **A** and **B**) subsegmental bronchi. Note how far superiorly the superior subsegmental bronchus can be traced.

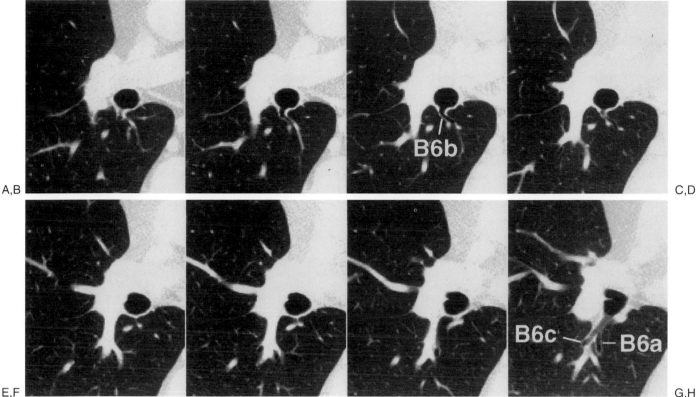

FIG. 3-53. Superior segment bronchus of the right lower lobe: variation. High-resolution scans with 1-mm collimation at 1-mm intervals (**A–H**). The superior segment is supplied by two branches. The most superior (**C**) arises from the posterior wall of the bronchus intermedius and supplies the superior subsegment (*B6b*). The main portion of the superior segment bronchus arises at the level of the origin of the right middle lobe bronchus (**H**), and gives rise to medial (*B6a*) and lateral (*B6c*) subsegments.

Despite considerable variability in the cross-sectional appearance of the basilar segmental bronchi, each can usually be identified, provided 1- to 5-mm thick sections are obtained (92,96). As with other airways, identification of individual basilar segmental and subsegmental bronchi is facilitated by reference to characteristic sections (see Fig. 3-51). Typically, the medial basilar segmental bronchus (B7) arises first, lying just anterior to the inferior pulmonary vein. Although variable in appearance, the anterior (B8), lateral (B9), and posterior basilar (B10) bronchi may all be identified because of their positions relative to one another and because they each course toward the segments they supply (see Fig. 3-39F–H, 3-47, and 3-48). This feature makes identification of normal variants and anomalies relatively easy (Figs. 3-54 and 3-55). In general, the medial and posterior segmental bronchi are imaged more nearly in cross section than the anterior and lateral, which are more obliquely oriented (see Figs. 3-39F–H, 3-47, and 3-48). Anatomic variation in the origins of these segments is common. In about 20% of cases, the branching pattern is variable; Naidich and associates (96) found six patterns of branching. The lower lobe bronchi always lie medial and anterior to the corresponding lower lobe pulmonary arteries.

Left Lung Bronchial Anatomy

The left main bronchus is much longer than the right and is typically seen on three to four contiguous 1-cm thick sections below the carina. It divides into upper and lower lobe branches (Fig. 3-56).

Left Upper Lobe Bronchus. The upper lobe bronchus is 2 to 3 cm long (see Fig. 3-56; Figs. 3-57 and 3-58). In about 75% of persons, the left upper lobe bronchus branches into superior and lingular divisions (Fig. 3-59) (93,109). The superior division is about 1 cm in length, giving rise to the apical-posterior (B1-2) and anterior (B3) segmental bronchi (see Figs. 3-57–3-59). In 25% of cases, the left upper lobe bronchus trifurcates into the apical-posterior (B1q-2) segmental bronchus, anterior (B3) segmental bronchus, and lingular bronchus (see Fig. 3-59). When the left upper lobe bronchus trifurcates in this manner, the anterior segmental bronchus arises in close proximity to the origin of the apical-posterior segmental bronchus or the lingular bronchus. A trifurcation branching pattern was identified in 16% of cases reported by Lee and associates (97). Thin collimation can be valuable in distinguishing the anterior segmental and lingular bronchi when a trifurcation pattern is present (Figs. 3-60 and 3-61).

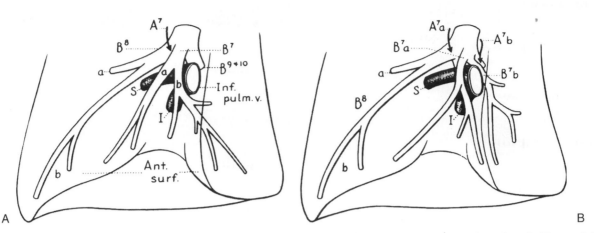

FIG. 3-54. Schematic representations of the two commonest variations in the subdivision of the medial basilar bronchus. **A:** The medial basilar segmental bronchus (*B7*) generally subdivides into an anterior (*B7a*) and a medial (*B7b*) ramus. Characteristically, these two subsegmental bronchi lie anterior to the right inferior pulmonary vein (*Inf.pulm. v.*). In approximately one-third of cases, B7b extends solely to the anterior surface of the right lower lobe (*Ant. Surf.*), whereas in approximately one-fifth of cases, a subdivision extends to the paravertebral surface of the medial basilar segment inferiority. *A7,* medial basilar segmental artery; *S,* superior; *I,* interior rami of the right inferior pulmonary vein; *B8* (*a* and *b*), subdivisions of the anterior basilar segmental bronchus. **B:** Diagrammatic representation of the most common variation in the subdivision of the medial basilar segmental bronchus. In approximately one-fourth of cases, the medial ramus (*B7b*) courses posterior to the right interior pulmonary vein, unlike the anterior ramus (*B7a*), which remains anteriorly oriented. Knowledge of this variation is significant, especially to surgeons attempting medial basilar segmental resections. *A7a* and *A7b,* corresponding arterial rami supplying the medial basilar segment.

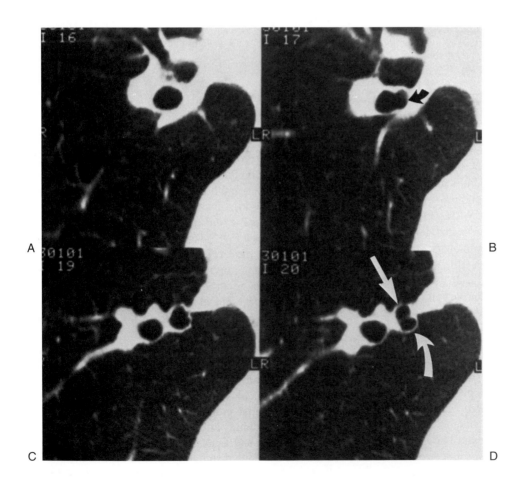

FIG. 3-55. B7 variant/B*-subsuperior bronchus. **A–H:** Sequential 1.5-mm thick sections obtained through the origin of the medial segmental bronchus (*B7*) and its anterior (*B7a*) and medial (*B7b*) subdivisions. The origin of B7 is easily identified, arising characteristically from the anteromedial surface of the truncus basalis (*curved black arrow* in **B**). B7a (*white arrow* in **D**) and B7b (*curved white arrow* in **D**) originate as equivalent sized trunks, which then split around the inferior pulmonary vein (*v* in **E**). B7a and its subdivisions are easily defined, coursing anterior to the vein (*single white arrows* in **E** and **F**), whereas B7b courses posteriorly (*curved white arrows* in **E** and **F**). Note the position and origin of the anterior segmental bronchus (*white arrowhead* in **E**), the point of origin of the lateral (*B9*) and posterior (*B10*) segmental bronchi from a common trunk (*B9–10*) (*black arrow* in **F**) as well as the subsuperior segmental bronchus (*B*; double white arrows* in **E** and **F**).

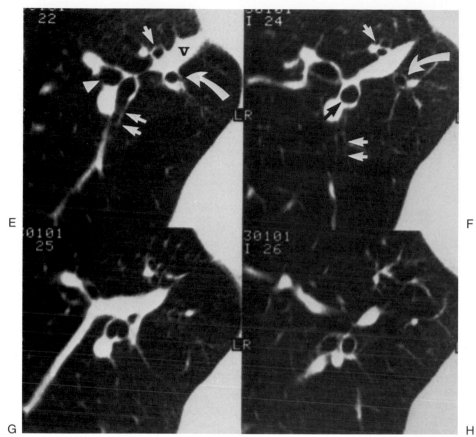

E   F

G   H   **FIG. 3-55.** *Continued.*

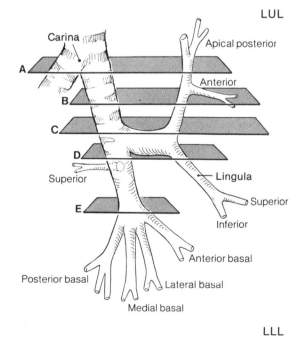

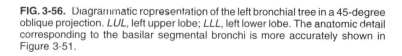

FIG. 3-56. Diagrammatic representation of the left bronchial tree in a 45-degree oblique projection. *LUL*, left upper lobe; *LLL*, left lower lobe. The anatomic detail corresponding to the basilar segmental bronchi is more accurately shown in Figure 3-51.

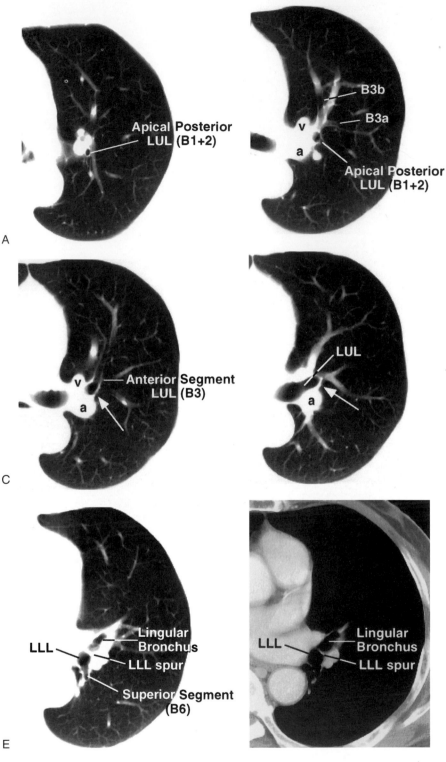

FIG. 3-57. Left bronchial anatomy in a healthy person demonstrated with spiral CT, collimation 7 mm, pitch 1, and reconstruction at 7-mm intervals. This is the same patient as shown in Figure 3-39. **A:** Apical-posterior segmental bronchus of the left upper lobe (see Fig. 3-56, level A). CT near the level of the carina shows the apical posterior segmental bronchus of the left upper lobe (*B1+2*) in cross section, along with its associated arteries and veins. **B:** Apical-posterior segmental bronchus of the left upper lobe (see Fig. 3-56, level A). The apical-posterior segment is seen in cross section as a rounded lucency. The lateral (*B3a*) and medial (*B3b*) subsegmental branches of the anterior segmental bronchus are visible at this level. The bronchi lie lateral to the main branch of the left pulmonary artery (*a*), which produces a convexity in the posterior hilum, and the superior pulmonary vein (*v*), which results in an anterior convexity. **C:** Anterior segmental bronchus (see Fig. 3-56, level B). The origin of the anterior segmental bronchus (*B3*) of the left upper lobe is well seen. The bronchus seen in cross section (*arrow*), giving rise to the anterior segment represents the superior bronchial trunk arising from the left upper lobe bronchus (between levels B and C, Fig. 3-56). The left main bronchus is medial. As at the level above, the pulmonary vein (*v*) is anterior, and the pulmonary artery (*a*) is posterior. **D:** Upper portion of left upper lobe bronchus (*LUL*) (see Fig. 3-56, level C). The main left upper lobe bronchus is visible at this level; it is usually seen along its axis, extending anteriorly and laterally from its origin. Its posterior wall is slightly concave because of the interlobar pulmonary artery (*a*) posterior to it. The oval lucency laterally (*arrow*) represents the origin of the superior trunk of the left upper lobe bronchus. The left superior pulmonary vein is anterior to the bronchus, and the descending branch of the left pulmonary artery is posterior and lateral to it. The left posterior bronchial wall, the "left retrobronchial stripe," is typically outlined by lung at this level. **E,F:** Lower left upper lobe bronchus, bronchial spur, and lingular bronchus (see Fig. 3-56, level D) shown at lung (**E**) and tissue windows (**F**). The lingular bronchus arises anteriorly and extends anteriorly and laterally at an angle of about 45 degrees. Because it is also angled caudally, only a short segment of its lumen is visible. The superior segmental bronchus of the lower lobe (*B6*) arises posterolaterally at this same level, as is common. The carina or spur posterior to the origin of the lingular lobe bronchus marks the origin of the left lower lobe bronchus (*LLL*); in this patient, it is better shown with a soft tissue window (**F**).

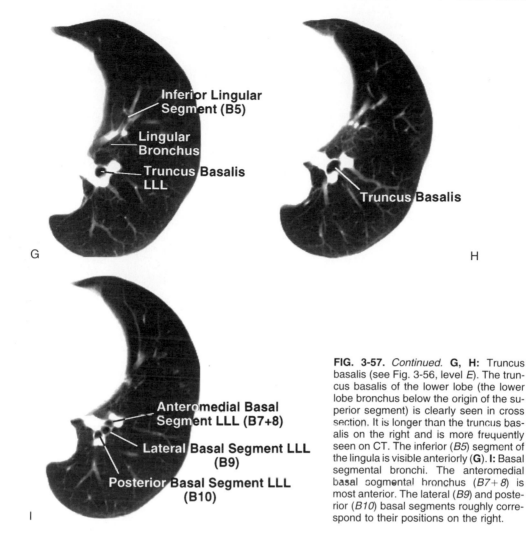

FIG. 3-57. *Continued.* **G, H:** Truncus basalis (see Fig. 3-56, level *E*). The truncus basalis of the lower lobe (the lower lobe bronchus below the origin of the superior segment) is clearly seen in cross section. It is longer than the truncus basalis on the right and is more frequently seen on CT. The inferior (*B5*) segment of the lingula is visible anteriorly (**G**). **I:** Basal segmental bronchi. The anteromedial basal segmental bronchus (*B7+8*) is most anterior. The lateral (*B9*) and posterior (*B10*) basal segments roughly correspond to their positions on the right.

The lingular bronchus extends anteriorly and inferiorly for 2 to 3 cm before dividing into its superior and inferior segmental branches (see Fig. 3-58). The superior segmental bronchus of the lingula is directed more laterally than the inferior segment, analogous to the pattern of branching of the medial and lateral segments of the middle lobe.

Because of its complexity, the appearance of the left upper lobe bronchus and of its branches is described at three specific levels, the levels of the apical-posterior and anterior segments, the upper portion of the left upper lobe bronchus, and the lower portion of the left upper lobe bronchus and lingula.

Apical-posterior (B1-2) and anterior (B3) segmental bronchi. Because of the variable origin of the anterior segmental bronchus, its identification is important in defining left upper lobe bronchial anatomy. The anterior segmental bronchus roughly lies in the plane of scan and is oriented almost directly anteriorly (see Figs. 3-56, 3-57B, C, and 3-58): it is usually visible over several centimeters and is accompanied by the anterior segmental artery (see Figs. 3-58 and 3-60). Sequential sections through the lower trachea and carina are shown in Figure 3-28, corresponding to levels A and B in Figure 3-14. These two levels are grouped together because they both represent sections through the apical-posterior segmental bronchus of the left upper lobe.

The apical-posterior segmental bronchus is visible as a circular lucency at and above the origin of the anterior segment bronchus (see Figs. 3-56–3-58). If a bronchus is seen in cross section below the anterior segment and above the left upper lobe bronchus, it represents the short superior division of the left upper lobe bronchus described earlier (see Fig. 3-58); although similar in appearance to the apical-posterior segment, and following the same course, it is larger. In Figures 3-57 and 3-58, the apical-posterior segmental bronchus is seen as a circular lucency surrounded medially and laterally by main branches of the left upper lobe pulmonary artery and vein. The branching pattern of the left upper lobe segments and subsegments is more variable than that of the right upper lobe. Four patterns of segmental and subsegmental branching of the left upper lobe have been reported by Lee and associates (97).

Upper portion of the left upper lobe bronchus. The left upper lobe bronchus originates at a level lower than the right upper lobe bronchus and forms a "sling" over which the

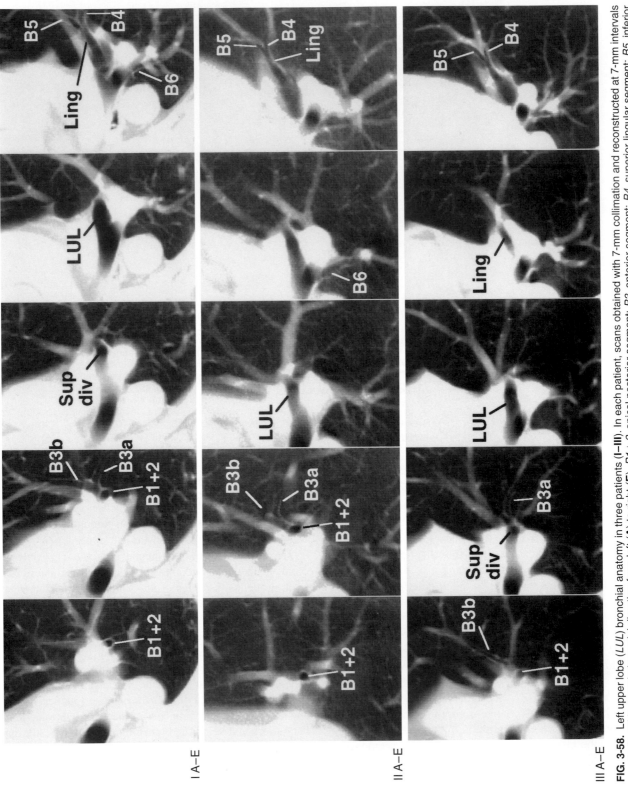

FIG. 3-58. Left upper lobe (*LUL*) bronchial anatomy in three patients (**I–III**). In each patient, scans obtained with 7-mm collimation and reconstructed at 7-mm intervals are displayed in a cephalocaudal direction from left (**A**) to right (**E**). *B1+2*, apical posterior segment; *B3*, anterior segment; *B4*, superior lingular segment; *B5*, inferior lingular segment; *B6*, superior segment left lower lobe; *Ling*, lingula; *Sup div*, superior division of the left upper lobe bronchus. In patients I and III, a bifurcation pattern of the left upper lobe bronchus is visible, with the main upper lobe bronchus dividing into superior and inferior (lingular) branches.

I A–E

II A–E

III A–E

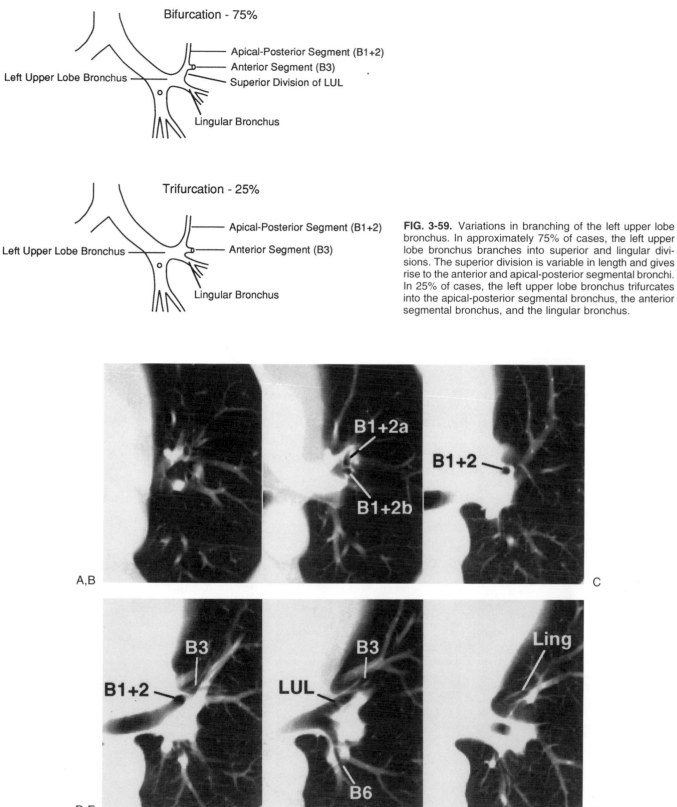

FIG. 3-59. Variations in branching of the left upper lobe bronchus. In approximately 75% of cases, the left upper lobe bronchus branches into superior and lingular divisions. The superior division is variable in length and gives rise to the anterior and apical-posterior segmental bronchi. In 25% of cases, the left upper lobe bronchus trifurcates into the apical-posterior segmental bronchus, the anterior segmental bronchus, and the lingular bronchus.

FIG. 3-60. Left upper lobe anatomy: trifurcation pattern. Helical CT (7-mm collimation and 7-mm interval reconstruction). **A–C:** Scans superiorly show the apical posterior bronchus (*B1—2*) and its subsegmental branches. **D:** The anterior segmental bronchus (*B3*) arises near the origin of the apical posterior segment. Its course is approximately in the plane of scan. **E:** Scan through the upper lobe bronchus shows the origin of the anterior segmental bronchus (*B3*). The superior segmental bronchus also arises at this level. **F:** The lingular bronchus (*Ling*) courses inferiorly, below the level of the anterior segment. In this subject, the anterior segment of the left upper lobe and the lingular segment arise at similar levels and may be confused (see Fig. 3-61 for high-resolution scans through these bronchi).

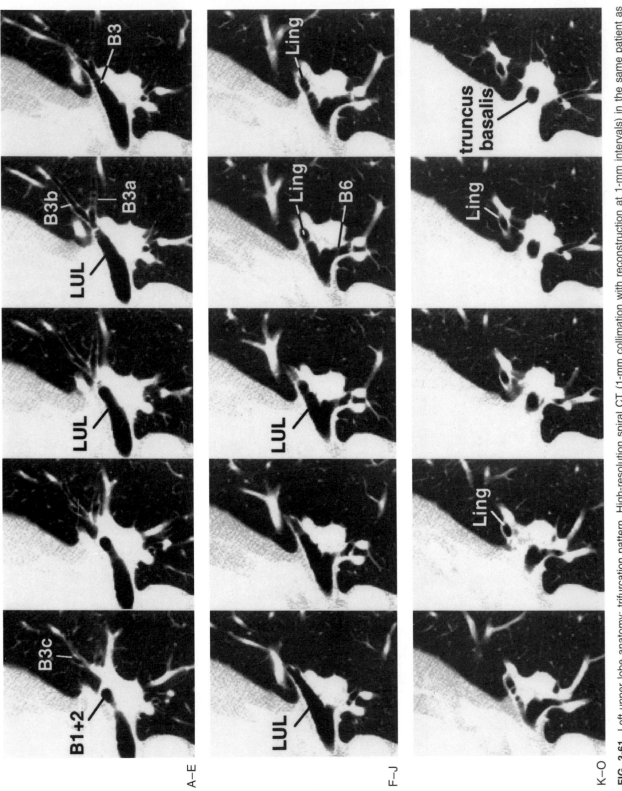

FIG. 3-61. Left upper lobe anatomy: trifurcation pattern. High-resolution spiral CT (1-mm collimation with reconstruction at 1-mm intervals) in the same patient as shown in Figure 3-60. Sequential images in a caudal direction from the top left (**A**) to bottom right (**O**). High-resolution scans allow the clear distinction of the anterior segment bronchus (*B3*), arising from the superior aspect of the upper lobe bronchus, from the lingular bronchus (*Ling*), arising from its inferior aspect. In addition, the course of the anterior segment bronchus is roughly in the plane of scan, whereas the lingular bronchus angles caudally. *B1 + 2*, apical posterior segment; *B3*, anterior segment bronchus; *B6*, superior segment of left lower lobe; *Ling*, lingular bronchus; *LUL*, left upper lobe bronchus. For identified subsegments, see Table 3-6.

left pulmonary artery passes. The key to understanding the anatomy of the left upper lobe bronchus and its branches is to realize that the left upper lobe bronchus is large, and it is therefore possible to obtain sections through both the upper and lower portions of this bronchus. Each has a characteristic appearance (see Figs. 3-57D,E and 3-60D,E).

In a section through the "upper" portion of the left upper lobe bronchus (see Figs. 3-57E and 3-60D), the posterior wall of the left upper lobe bronchus is smooth and slightly concave; this concavity is caused by the left pulmonary artery as it passes above and then posterior to the left upper lobe bronchus. At this level, the origin of the apical-posterior segmental bronchus, or the superior bronchial division that gives rise to the apical posterior and anterior segmental bronchi, can be recognized as a rounded area of increased lucency superimposed on the distal portion of the left upper lobe bronchus (see Figs. 3-57E and 3-60D). When the left upper lobe bronchus trifurcates (see Figs. 3-60D and 3-61), the anterior segmental bronchus arises in close proximity to the apical-posterior segmental bronchus or the lingular bronchus. In this case, the anterior segment arises near the upper margin of the upper lobe bronchus, whereas the lingular bronchus arises at or below the level of the lower lobe spur.

Just posterior to the medial portion of the left upper lobe bronchus, air in the superior segment of the left lower lobe abuts the posteromedial bronchial wall. This tongue of lung extends between the descending aorta and the left interlobar pulmonary artery, outlining the so-called left "retrobronchial stripe" (see Fig. 3-57D; Fig. 3-62) (110). Adenopathy

or a hilar mass effaces this segment of lung, similar to the effacement of the azygoesophageal recess on the right side caused by subcarinal adenopathy (Fig. 3-63). Thickening or nodularity of the left "retrobronchial stripe" is a sensitive sign for tumor infiltration or adenopathy in the left hilum, and the examiner should search for it. However, in about 10% of anatomically normal persons, close approximation of the descending left pulmonary artery and aorta prevents the retrobronchial stripe from being seen (Fig. 3-64).

Lower portion of the left upper lobe bronchus and lingular bronchi. The most important anatomic landmark for identifying a scan as being through the lower portion of the left upper lobe bronchus is the left upper lobe spur (see Fig. 3-57E, F) (93). This spur marks the point of origin of the left lower lobe bronchus and is also referred to as the "secondary carina." This spur can be recognized as a triangular density separating the lower portion of the left upper from the left lower lobe bronchus and appears similar to the middle lobe spur of the right side (compare with Figs. 3-39E and 3-46–3-49).

The lingular bronchus arises from the undersurface of the distal portion of the left upper lobe bronchus and has an oblique course inferiorly (see Figs. 3-57E–G, 3-58, 3-60, and 3-61). The origin of the lingular bronchus can be identified as a circular area of increased lucency superimposed on the distal portion of the left upper lobe bronchus, in much the same manner as the origin of the apical-posterior segmental bronchus. The key to differentiating the origin of the lingular bronchus from the apical-posterior and anterior segmental

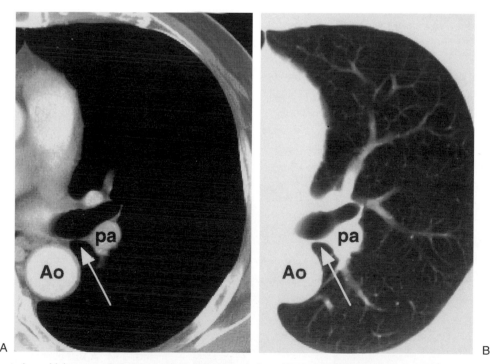

FIG. 3-62. Normal retrobronchial recess. Soft tissue (**A**) and lung (**B**) windows in a healthy person. Lung contacts the posterior left main or left upper lobe bronchial wall (*arrows*) between the aorta (*Ao*) and the interlobar pulmonary artery (*pa*). The bronchial wall appears thin and sharply defined.

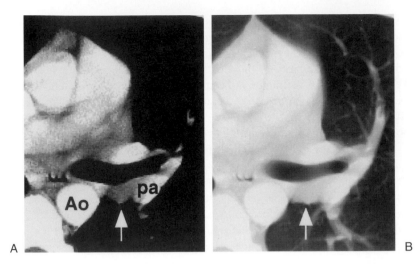

FIG. 3-63. Abnormal retrobronchial recess in a patient with hilar lymph node enlargement. Soft tissue (**A**) and lung (**B**) windows. An enlarged lymph node (*arrows*) separates lung from bronchial wall between the aorta (*Ao*) and the interlobar pulmonary artery (*pa*).

bronchi is identification of the left upper lobe bronchial spur (see Fig. 3-57E,F), which confirms that the section shows the lower portion of the left upper lobe bronchus.

The lingular bronchus courses inferiorly, anteriorly, and laterally on an oblique path, roughly analogous to that of the middle lobe bronchus. In cross section, the lingular bronchus is oval or elliptic. If sections are obtained just below the left upper lobe bronchus, the lingular bronchus will appear as a discrete oval lucency separated from the left lower lobe bronchus. Sequential sections obtained below the origin of the lingular bronchus show progressively wider separation between the lingular bronchus anteriorly and the left lower lobe bronchus posteriorly.

The superior (B4) and, especially, the inferior (B5) divisions of the lingular bronchus are infrequently seen on CT when standard 8- to 10-mm thick sections are used. These segmental bronchi tend to originate at a considerable distance from the origin of the lingular bronchus and may be too small and peripheral to be visualized with standard technique. However, their identification is significantly en-

hanced with use of 1.5- to 5-mm thick sections and spiral technique (see Figs. 3-57E–G, 3-58, 3-60, and 3-61). As noted previously, in select cases, 20-degree angulation of the gantry, roughly parallel to the course of the bronchus, may be beneficial (108).

Left Lower Lobe Bronchus. The left lower lobe bronchus usually conforms to the same general branching pattern as the right lower lobe bronchus, although only three basal segments are generally present: anteromedial, lateral, and posterior (see Figs. 3-51 and 3-56) (92,96).

Superior segment (B6). The superior segmental bronchus of the left lower lobe arises within 1 cm of the origin of the left lower lobe bronchus and is identical in shape and configuration to the same bronchus on the right side (see Figs. 3-57E, 3-58, and 3-60).

Truncus basalis and basal segments. The truncus basalis, the lower lobe bronchus giving rise to the basal lower lobe segments, is visible below the origin of the superior segment for a distance of 1 to 2 cm (see Figs. 3-56, 3-57G, H, 3-63; Fig. 3-65). It is generally longer than the truncus basalis on

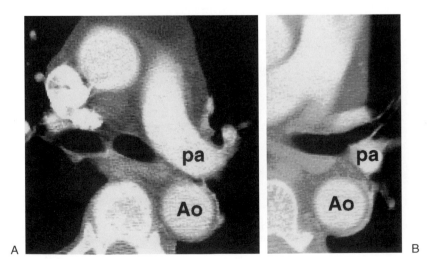

FIG. 3-64. **A,B:** Retrobronchial recess: variant. In about 10% of healthy persons, the aorta (*Ao*) and the interlobar pulmonary artery (*pa*) contact each other, and a retrobronchial recess is not visible.

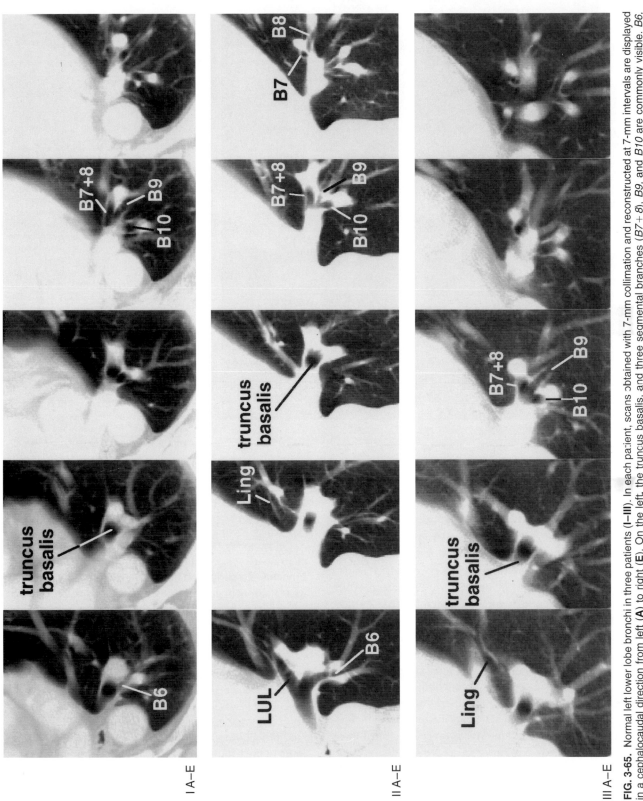

FIG. 3-65. Normal left lower lobe bronchi in three patients (**I–III**). In each patient, scans obtained with 7-mm collimation and reconstructed at 7-mm intervals are displayed in a cephalocaudal direction from left (**A**) to right (**E**). On the left, the truncus basalis, and three segmental branches (*B7+8*), *B9*, and *B10* are commonly visible. *B6*, superior segment; *ling*, lingula; *LUL*, left upper lobe.

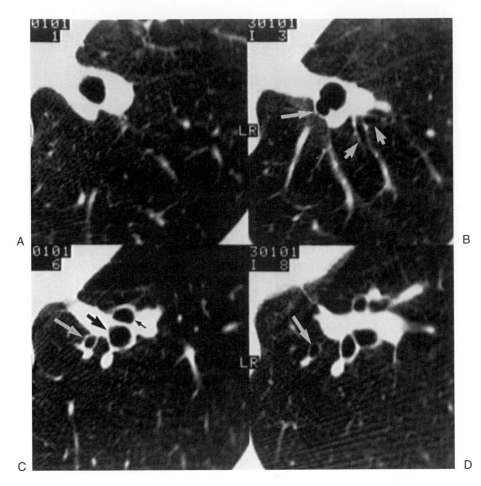

FIG. 3-66. B*-subsuperior segmental bronchus: left lower lobe (LLL). **A–D:** Sequential 1.5-mm thick sections obtained through the proximal divisions of the LLL basilar segmental bronchi. An anomalous bronchus can be defined originating off the posteromedial aspect of the truncus basalis (*white arrow* in **B**), which then extends inferomedially (*white arrows* in **C** and **D**). This subsuperior bronchus is easily differentiated from the anteromedial segmental bronchus (B7 + 8) (*small black arrow* in **C**), as well as a common trunk of the lateral and posterior segmental bronchi (B9 and 10) (*large black arrow* in **C**). Note that superiorly, inferior branches of the superior segmental bronchus (B6) can be identified (*short white arrows* in **B**), distinct from the subsuperior bronchus.

the right. As on the right, the anterior wall of the basal trunk may be outlined by lung.

The basilar segmental bronchi are essentially mirror images of the right lower lobe basilar bronchi, except on the left side, the medial and anterior basilar bronchi characteristically originate together as a common trunk (B7-8) (see Figs. 3-56, 3-57, and 3-65). The lateral (B9) and posterior (B10) basal segments resemble those on the right side.

As on the right, the key to identification of the basal segmental bronchi is to note their relative positions as they course to their corresponding basilar lung segments. Basal segmental and even subsegmental bronchi have characteristic cross-sectional appearances. Familiarity with these characteristic sections allows easy identification, even in the presence of anatomic variation. This is especially true if thin sections are obtained. As shown in a study of the basilar segmental bronchi of 31 patients in which the investigators used thin sections, in each case all segmental bronchi could be identified, regardless of variations in origin and course; in a majority of cases, most subsegmental airways could be identified as well (Fig. 3-66) (96). Five branching patterns of the lower lobe segments have been identified.

CENTRAL AIRWAYS: PRINCIPLES OF INTERPRETATION INCLUDING CT/ BRONCHOSCOPIC CORRELATIONS

For purposes of analysis, the airways can be divided into central airways, extending from the trachea to the segmental bronchi, and peripheral airways, extending from the subsegmental bronchi to the bronchioles. This approach has the advantage of correlating with the approximate range of visualization of the airways by FB, as well as reemphasizing the need for selective imaging strategies.

The accuracy of CT to evaluate the central airways is well established (111–116). Nonetheless, the precise role of CT in relation to bronchoscopy, both rigid bronchoscopy and especially FB, is still to be defined (1). Bronchoscopic evaluation of the airways has numerous advantages. Most important, bronchoscopy allows direct visualization of airway lumina to the fifth generation enabling identification of subtle mucosal, submucosal, and endobronchial abnormalities (see Fig. 3-11). Bronchoscopy also allows acquisition of bacteriologic, cytologic, and histologic material from endobronchial, peribronchial, and parenchymal sites with minimal risk (117). In select cases, bronchoscopy may provide localization of bleeding sites before surgery. In addition, an increas-

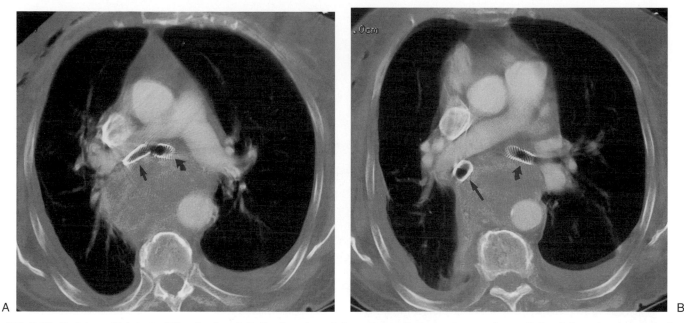

FIG. 3-67. Endobronchial stents: CT evaluation. **A, B:** Sections through the carina and bronchus intermedius and left main bronchus, respectively, in a patient with known nonsmall cell lung cancer after radiation therapy show the following placement of three separate stents: one within the right main stem bronchus (*straight arrow* in **A**), one in the left main stem and left upper lobe bronchus (*curved arrows* in **A** and **B**), and another in the bronchus intermedius open (*straight arrow* in **B**) in this patient with extensive mediastinal nodal metastases.

ing number of therapeutic interventions may now be performed endoscopically, including traditional procedures, such as removal of mucus plugs or foreign bodies, as well as a growing number of more sophisticated applications, including the use of various stents to provide airway patency (Fig. 3-67). Despite these advantages, the value of bronchoscopy has important limitations, especially for those patients without evidence of endobronchial disease in whom a specific histologic diagnosis is sought (117,118).

In comparing CT with FB, terminology appropriate for bronchoscopic evaluation may not be appropriate for CT. Descriptive terms such as mucosal or submucosal, in particular, may be misleading (115,119). CT evidence of smooth airway narrowing, for example, may be associated endoscopically with endobronchial, submucosal, or peribronchial disease (Figs. 3-68–3-71). In fact, as a general rule, CT is imprecise in characterizing abnormalities identified bronchoscopically (115). An exception is the finding of a discrete, calcific endobronchial filling defect, as may occur, for example, in patients with aspirated foreign bodies or broncholiths, or the rare patient with an endobronchial hamartoma within which fat can be identified (Figs. 3-72–3-74). In the case of broncholithiasis, CT may prove more sensitive than FB by identifying both intraluminal and peribronchial calcifications distal to inflamed and narrowed airways rendered inaccessible to bronchoscopy. As documented by Conces and colleagues (120) in a study of 15 patients with proved broncholithiasis, whereas CT correctly localized 6 of 10 endobronchial lesions and 4 of 5 calcified peribronchial nodes, the diagnosis of broncholithiasis was established endoscopically in only 5 cases.

To date, CT has proved of greatest value in bronchoscopy by defining the precise location and extent of disease within and surrounding the central airways in patients with known or suspected lung cancer. In patients with central airway obstruction, CT allows distinction between central tumor and peripheral atelectasis (2,121). In patients with evidence of direct invasion of adjacent mediastinal organs, CT can identify those with unresectable tumor (see Fig. 3-68). CT also allows visualization of distal airways that otherwise cannot be evaluated bronchoscopically because of proximal airway obstruction (see Figs. 3-27 and 3-30). Additionally, in patients with central obstructing tumors, CT can be used to predict which patients will benefit from laser therapy by identifying those lesions with less extensive peribronchial tumor (122,123). Of even greater potential value is the use of CT to guide transbronchial needle aspiration and biopsy (TBNA) (124–129). In select cases, TBNA may obviate more invasive surgical staging procedures including mediastinoscopy by providing cytologic or histologic samples of peribronchial tissues.

Adequate use of TBNA necessitates prior evaluation with CT (34). This requires not only thorough familiarity with bronchial anatomy, but also awareness from a bronchoscopic viewpoint of which nodes are most likely to undergo successful biopsy using a transbronchial approach (see Chapter 5, Fig. 5-16) (34). A more extensive or elaborate depiction of bronchial and peribronchial disease than that afforded by axial images is not necessary in most cases because the numbers of sites practically accessible for aspiration or biopsy at bronchoscopy are limited (34). Contrary to popular opinion, precise localization of peribronchial vessels is also

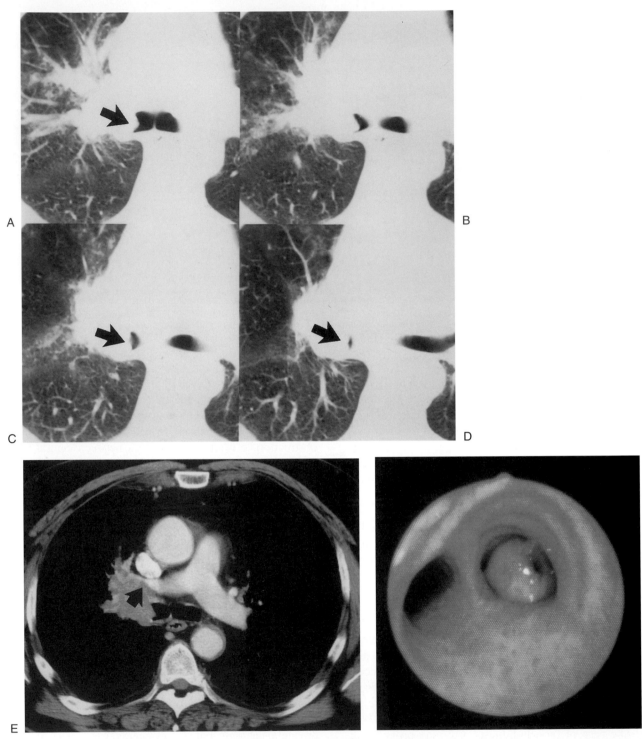

FIG. 3-68. CT–bronchoscopic correlation: central endobronchial tumor. **A–D:** Sequential 5-mm sections through the carina and proximal portions of the bronchus intermedius show a well-defined intraluminal filling defect in the right main stem bronchus causing obstruction of the right upper lobe bronchus that cannot be identified and marked narrowing of the proximal bronchus intermedius (*arrows* in **A, C,** and **D**). **E:** Contrast-enhanced section shows extensive tumor infiltrating the mediastinum encasing the right main pulmonary artery (*arrow*). **F:** Image obtained at flexible bronchoscopy (*FB*) confirms the presence of a well-defined endobronchial mass in the right main stem bronchus diagnosed as nonsmall cell lung cancer by transbronchial biopsy. This case clearly demonstrates the complementary nature of CT and FB: whereas the endoluminal component of the tumor is easily assessed endoscopically, CT is more accurate in assessing the true extent of disease. In this case, both proved necessary for accurate presurgical assessment. (From ref. 1, with permission.)

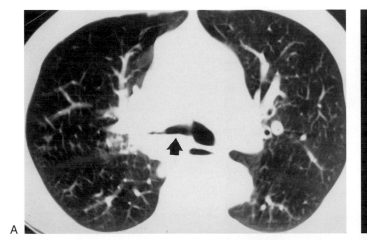

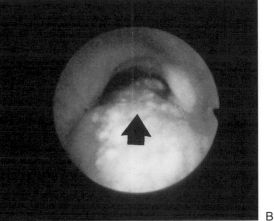

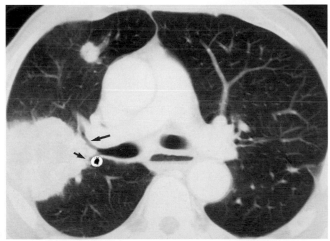

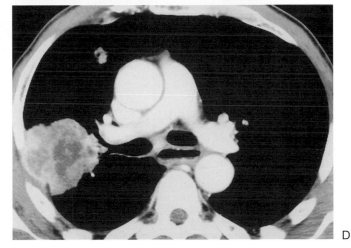

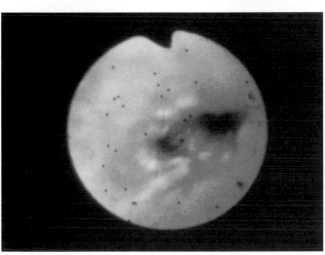

FIG. 3-69. CT–bronchoscopic correlation: submucosal disease. **A:** A 5-mm section through the carina shows nodular thickening and narrowing of the right main stem bronchus (*arrow*). **B:** Corresponding bronchoscopic view of the carina shows marked submucosal involvement of the posterior wall of the distal trachea and main stem bronchi resulting from extensive submucosal tumor (*arrow*). In this case, CT findings closely correlate with bronchoscopic appearance (compare with **A**). **C,D:** Identical 5-mm sections through the right upper lobe in a different patient from **A** and **B** imaged with wide and narrow windows, respectively, shows extensive tumor in the right upper lobe extending to the right hila. Despite enlargement of the right upper lobe spur, the proximal portions of the anterior and posterior segmental bronchi are grossly normal in caliber (*arrows* in **C**). **E:** Corresponding bronchoscopic view of the right upper lobe spur shows nodular thickening of both the anterior and posterior segmental bronchi resulting from submucosal infiltration with tumor. In this case, the CT appearance of these airways was not predictive of bronchoscopic findings. (From ref. 1, with permission.)

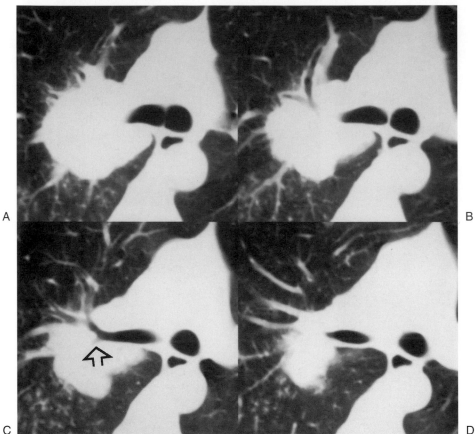

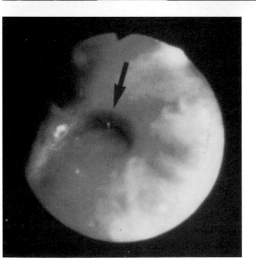

FIG. 3-70. CT–bronchoscopic correlation: extrinsic compression. **A–D:** Sequential coned-down 5-mm sections through the right upper lobe bronchus shows a large right hilar mass with amputation of the posterior segmental bronchus just past its origin (*arrow* in **C**). This appearance should not be interpreted as evidence of endobronchial disease. **E:** Corresponding bronchoscopic view of the right upper lobe segmental bronchi shows marked extrinsic narrowing of the posterior segmental bronchus without evidence of an endobronchial lesion (*arrow*). (From ref. 1, with permission.)

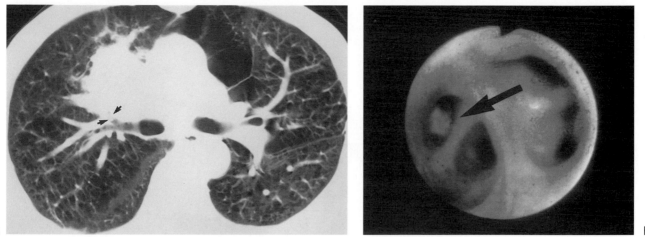

FIG. 3-71. CT–bronchoscopic correlation: endobronchial tumor. **A:** A 5-mm section through the right upper lobe bronchus shows an approximately 3-mm filling defect in the anterior segmental bronchus (*arrows*) in association with an extensive mass in the right upper lobe. **B:** Corresponding bronchoscopic view shows a well-defined endobronchial lesion in the anterior segmental bronchus (*arrow*). This represents the smallest endobronchial lesion likely to be identified with any certainty using CT.

unimportant; inadvertent needle placement into the pulmonary arteries and even the aorta results in no increased morbidity or mortality (34). In this regard, investigators have argued that the utility of TBNA will be enhanced by use of virtual bronchoscopic techniques as a means for more precise mapping of mediastinal lymph nodes for the bronchoscopist before FB (21). Although the use of virtual bronchoscopy does allow visualization of peribronchial tissues through the bronchial wall, in our experience, this information is always available from close scrutiny of the transaxial images source images. Similar claims have also been made for use of ultrasound-guided TBNA (130,131), as well as for the use of CT (132). Indeed, in selected cases, one can perform TBNA under direct CT guidance, with or without

CT fluoroscopy (Fig. 3-75). Unfortunately, in our experience, even confirmation of the precise location of the needle tip under CT guidance does not necessarily translate to a successful biopsy; presumably, this is due to factors relating both to the nature of the underlying tumor and to the technique itself.

Using CT as a guide, TBNA has proved diagnostic in up to 80% of patients with enlarged mediastinal nodes (127). In patients with extensive adenopathy, in the absence of a clearly defined peripheral lesion, CT may also be of value by suggesting a diagnosis of small cell lung cancer. In this setting, because endobronchial forceps biopsy specimens may be difficult to evaluate because of the presence of extensive crush artifacts, CT findings may be a clue to perform

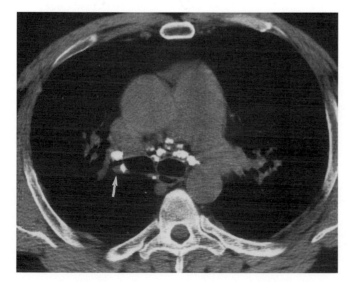

FIG. 3-72. Broncholithiasis. CT section through the carina in a patient presenting with recurrent episodes of hemoptysis shows extensive mediastinal and hilar nodal calcifications resulting from prior granulomatous infection. Within the posterior wall of the right upper lobe bronchus is a focal calcification associated with a soft tissue density (*arrow*) causing marked narrowing of the airway. CT may prove more sensitive than bronchoscopy by identifying both intraluminal or peribronchial calcification otherwise obscured by bronchial wall inflammation.

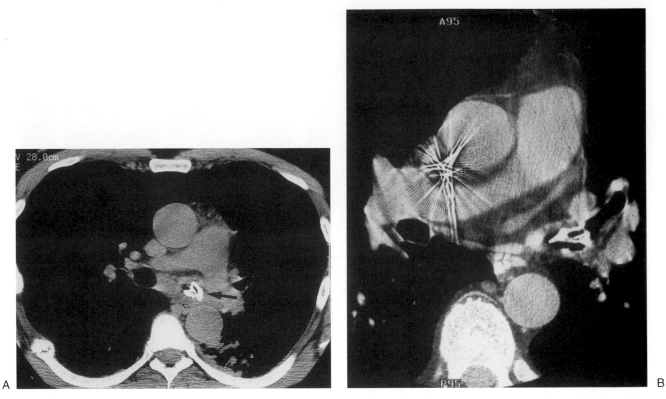

FIG. 3-73. Calcified foreign body. **A:** Section through the left main stem bronchus shows calcific density within the left upper lobe bronchus (*arrow*). This has a branching, tubular configuration—findings consistent with an aspirated soup bone. **B:** Section through the left upper lobe bronchus in a different patient from **A** shows a similar appearance of an aspirated bone partially occluding the left upper lobe bronchus.

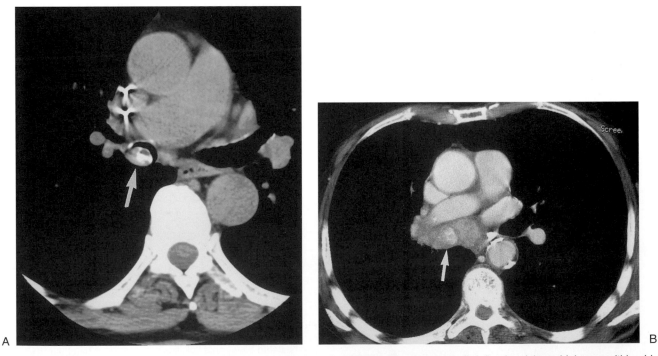

FIG. 3-74. Calcified endobronchial tumors. **A:** Section through the bronchus intermedius shows a well-defined endobronchial mass within which foci of both calcification and fat (*arrow*) can be identified. This lesion is a histologically proved endobronchial hamartoma. **B:** Section through the bronchus intermedius in a different patient (same as shown in Fig. 3-11) also shows a calcified endobronchial mass (*arrow*). In this case, the finding of tumor in the subcarinal space and right hilum is key to identifying this as a malignant tumor. Biopsy proved this tumor to be a papillary adenocarcinoma.

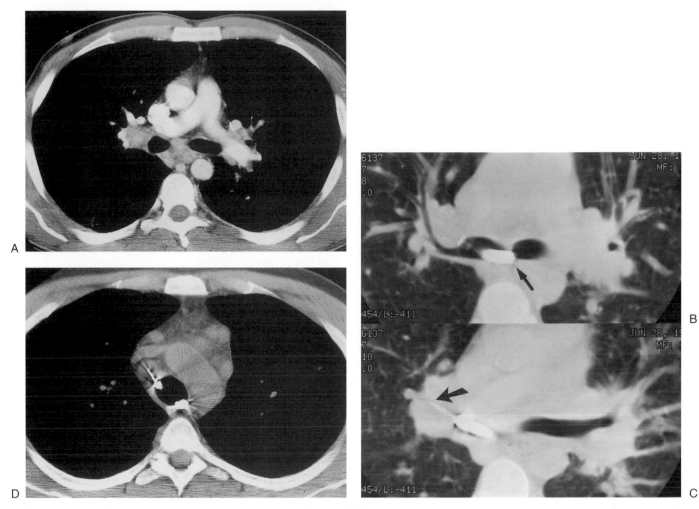

FIG. 3-75. CT-guided transbronchial needle aspiration and biopsy (TBNA). **A:** Contrast-enhanced CT section shows extensive bilateral hilar and subcarinal adenopathy. **B, C:** Images obtained during TBNA show the tip of the bronchoscope up against the posterior wall of the right main stem bronchus (*arrow* in **B**). The needle tip is clearly identifiable within the right hilum (*arrow* in **C**). Histologic evaluation of specimen showed noncaseating granulomas, consistent with a clinical diagnosis of sarcoidosis. **D:** CT section in a different patient from **A–C**, obtained during TBNA shows the tip of the needle within enlarged right paratracheal nodes. Despite histologic evidence of lymphocytes confirming the location of the needle tip within nodal tissue, no diagnosis could be made. Subsequent mediastinoscopy confirmed the presence of nonsmall cell lung cancer. In our experience, precise localization of the needle tip does not ensure adequate histologic or cytologic sampling.

endobronchial needle biopsies instead (133). CT is also invaluable by identifying cases for which TBNA is not indicated. This includes patients with negative CT scans, for whom the yield has been shown to be sufficiently low to obviate TBNA (126), as well as those in whom CT can identify parenchymal tumors that abut the central airways, making TBNA staging unreliable, as may occur in patients with lesions in the medial portion of the right upper lobe simulating right paratracheal adenopathy (134).

Less well appreciated is the fact that CT also may be of value as a guide to TBNA in patients with benign mediastinal or hilar disease. Morales and associates (135), in a study of 51 consecutive patients with suspected sarcoidosis who underwent both transbronchial lung biopsy and flexible TBNA of mediastinal or hilar nodes, showed that 23% of patients with stage 1 disease and 10% of patients with stage 2 disease had their diagnoses established only with TBNA.

Overall, the combined use of transbronchial lung biopsy and TBNA allowed a histologic diagnosis in 83% of these cases. In patients for whom TBNA is contemplated, CT may also prove cost-effective. In the same study, 9 of 51 patients who would otherwise have required surgical assessment to obtain a definitive diagnosis had a successful diagnosis by TBNA; thus, in the judgment of these investigators, the results more than financially justify the routine prebronchoscopic use of HRCT (135).

CT has also been documented to be of particular value in patients with AIDS. In immunocompromised patients, the finding of low-density mediastinal or hilar lymph nodes, in particular, strongly correlates with active mycobacterial infection (136). In these patients, TBNA may represent the least invasive means of obtaining diagnostic material, especially when sputum smears prove nondiagnostic. As documented by Harkin and associates (137), TBNA proved diagnostic in 23 (51%) of 45 procedures performed in 42 HIV-positive patients. This included identification of 21 of 23 documented cases of mycobacterial infection, of which TBNA provided the only diagnostic specimen in 13 (57%) (137).

Although CT is of value in assessing central airway disease, important limitations with regard to bronchoscopy have also been noted. CT is of limited value, for example, in the detection of endobronchial lesions smaller than 2 to 3 mm (see Fig. 3-71). Subtle irregularities of the airway walls, often the result of prominent bronchial cartilage, or partial volume averaging in airways coursing obliquely, also limit diagnostic accuracy. Finally, as mentioned previously, accurate interpretation requires thorough familiarity with normal bronchial anatomy and variants. In this regard, even among experienced observers, substantial interobserver variability may exist. As documented by Webb and associates (138) in a study of 40 randomly chosen cases of documented non-small cell lung cancer, the average agreement among 4 separate readers for detecting bronchial involvement was only 80% (139).

The relationship between FB and tumor size of radiographically occult squamous cell carcinomas has been evaluated (140). In a prospective study of 105 lesions in 98 patients with radiographically occult squamous cell carcinoma identified on the basis of positive sputum cytology, Usuda and colleagues (140) showed that although 55 (53%) of these lesions were larger than 2 mm (including 22 characterized as either polypoid or nodular, with the remainder appearing flat or as focal areas of bronchial irregularity), 27 lesions (26%) proved to be smaller than 2 mm, and 23 lesions (22%) were endoscopically invisible, being identified by bronchial brushings alone. From these data, it is unlikely that CT, even optimally performed, would have identified more than 20% of these lesions, rendering CT of limited value in routine screening of the central airways in patients with positive sputum cytology.

Although FB can detect subtle endobronchial disease not identifiable with CT, one should not assumed that all such lesions are significant. Even in patients presenting with hemoptysis, investigators have shown that many such lesions are nonspecific. McGuinness and associates (114), in a prospective study evaluating both CT and FOB in 57 consecutive patients presenting with hemoptysis, found that focal endobronchial lesions could be identified bronchoscopically in a total of 18 (32%) cases. Although 6 of these lesions proved to be due to bronchogenic carcinoma, all prospectively identified by CT, in the remaining 12 cases, transbronchial biopsies proved diagnostic in only 1, a patient with mucosal Kaposi's sarcoma.

LOBAR ATELECTASIS

Evaluation of patients with radiographic evidence of lobar or segmental atelectasis represents one of the most important indications for the use of CT. The radiographic patterns of lobar atelectsis have been extensively reviewed (121, 141–143). A wide range of abnormalities has been described characterizing the appearance of the atelectatic lobe as well as secondary, compensatory changes, including shifts of mediastinal structures, the hila, the hemidiaphragms, and the fissures.

Lobar atelectasis results from certain variably categorized mechanisms (141,144). These include the following: (a) resorption or obstructive atelectasis, resulting from endobronchial obstruction; (b) compression or passive atelectasis, which is collapse caused by extrinsic compression, such as from pleural fluid or air, or the presence of any space-occupying intrathoracic lesion resulting in extrinsic compression of adjacent parenchyma; (c) cicatrization atelectasis, resulting from parenchymal fibrosis; and (d) adhesive atelectasis, which is collapse resulting from loss of surfactant.

CT has proved to be an essential adjunct to routine radiography in the evaluation of atelectasis (2,145–150). This is primarily because CT can accurately identify and localize the presence of an obstructing lesion (113,115,150,151). CT is especially valuable in patients with unusual combinations of lobar atelectasis, as occurs, for example, in patients with combined middle and lower lobe atelectasis, or even right upper and lower lobe atelectasis (121,152). In the absence of bronchial obstruction, characteristic alterations in the normal appearance of the airways consequent to volume loss with resultant changes in the caliber and position of airways may also be identified far more accurately with CT than on corresponding chest radiographs.

Proper CT technique for evaluating the central airways in patients with atelectasis requires some modifications compared with techniques geared to identifying radiographically occult central airway disease (153). In particular, adequate assessment requires not only precise visualization of the airways, but also detailed examination of the atelectatic lung itself, as well as evaluation of the hilum and mediastinum. In most cases, this requires use of a bolus of intravenous contrast (see Table 3-2). As discussed in greater detail later, in addition to allowing differentiation between central tumor and peripherally collapsed lung, contrast administration also allows for more precise staging of central tumors by allowing more accurate assessment both of nodal disease as well as direct mediastinal invasion. Additionally, administration of contrast often provides detailed evaluation of parenchymal changes within the atelectatic lung itself, including the presence of generalized or focal infection, as well as more precise delineation of accompanying pleural fluid, especially when loculated.

Resorption Atelectasis

Mechanisms and Causes

Most commonly the result of primary bronchogenic carcinoma, otherwise indistinguishable endobronchial masses have been reported to represent a wide range of benign and malignant lesions (Table 3-7).

TABLE 3-7. *Resorption atelectasis: causes*

Endobronchial neoplasms
  Common
    Bronchogenic carcinoma
    Bronchial carcinoid/adenoid cystic carcinoma
    Metastases (kidney, breast, colon, melanoma)
    Lymphoma
    Kaposi's sarcoma
  Rare
    Benign neoplasms
    Hamartoma, papilloma, granular cell myoblastoma
Nonneoplastic endobronchial lesions
  Common
    Mucus plugs
    Aspirated foreign bodies
    Inflammatory strictures
    Tuberculous/fungal infection
    Broncholithiasis
  Rare
    Bronchial laceration
    Bronchial torsion
    Wegener's granulomatosis
    Amyloidosis
    Sarcoidosis
Extrinsic bronchial obstruction
  Common
    Enlarged hilar nodes tuberculosis, sarcoidosis
    Aortic aneurysm

Adapted from ref. 144, with permission.

Endobronchial Tumors. In addition to metastases, most commonly of breast, colon, kidney and thyroid carcinoma, and melanoma, but also including those of uterine, prostatic, testicular, and adrenal malignancies (154), other neoplastic lesions to be considered include carcinoid tumors (155), lymphoma (156), and, in patients with AIDS, Kaposi's sarcoma (157). As discussed in greater detail later, malignant lesions are generally more likely to be associated with extraluminal soft tissue masses, usually identifiable after administration of intravenous contrast medium. Benign tumors involving the tracheobronchial tree are less common than malignant lesions and, with the exception of amyloidomas (which are of unknown origin), originate from a large number of diverse cell lines including papillomas (epithelial gland origin), myoblastomas (neural cell origin), and, most commonly, hamartomas and chondromas (connective tissue origin) (158). Rarely, specific features such as the presence of calcium, as occurs in patients with central carcinoid tumors, or fat with or without calcification (see Fig. 3-74), as may be seen in patients with endobronchial hamartomas, allow a specific diagnosis.

Nontumoral Obstruction. Endobronchial obstruction may also result from certain nonneoplastic causes, including the following: retained secretions; blood clots; inflammatory strictures, in particular those secondary to granulomatous infections, with or without associated broncholithiasis; aspirated foreign bodies; and bronchial trauma.

Obstruction commonly results from retained secretions. Although this disorder may cause confusion with central endobronchial masses, in general, inspissated secretions may be identified either because of demonstrable fluid density (including the presence of an air-fluid level) or because of the finding of a clear separation between irregular intraluminal densities and the adjacent bronchial wall (especially when viewed with narrow, mediastinal windows). This appearance should be differentiated, of course, from the finding of fluid-filled, distended bronchi within the peripheral portions of lobes obstructed by central tumors (159). The finding of intraluminal blood, on the other hand, may indeed mimic the appearance of an endoluminal soft tissue mass (160). This finding, however, in our experience, is sufficiently rare in the absence of central tumor to obviate concern in most cases (114). Atelectasis secondary to bronchial strictures also may mimic the appearance of discrete central endobronchial lesions, especially as a result of tuberculosis (see Fig. 3-30) (66,67). In these cases, the use of MPRs (24) and of three dimensional reconstructions (66) may be of value by demonstrating the true extent and configuration of the lesions. Often, these lesions are associated with extraluminal nodal calcifications, thereby simplifying the differential diagnosis.

The accuracy of CT for detecting endobronchial obstructing lesions nears 100% when proper attention is paid to CT technique. In a retrospective analysis of 50 patients with segmental or lobar atelectasis, Woodring (161) compared the accuracy of chest radiographs with CT in identifying patients with central obstructing tumors. Using the findings of bronchial obstruction and a central mass causing a contour abnormality, unlike chest radiographs, which were diagnostic in 24 (89%) of 27 patients, CT proved 100% sensitive, correctly identifying all 27 obstructing carcinomas. In 3 cases (10%), CT findings led to false-positive diagnoses: in each, benign causes of bronchial obstruction led to the false assumption of central tumor. Importantly, in no case in which the proximal airways were shown to be patent was tumor ultimately found. A similar degree of accuracy using CT to detect central tumors has been documented by other investigators (113,115,145). The finding of peripheral air bronchograms in themselves does not exclude central obstruction, especially in patients with more peripheral, segmental occlusion. CT air bronchograms may be seen within otherwise obstructed segments or lobes because central obstruction is of recent onset, because it is incomplete, or because the effects are mitigated by collateral air drift. As documented by Woodring (161), in 32 cases in which peripheral air bronchograms could be identified with CT, a central obstructing tumor was present in 11 (34%).

As noted previously, most malignant endobronchial lesions are associated with extraluminal soft tissue masses (see Figs. 3-2, 3-5, 3-11, 3-12, 3-25, 3-68, and 3-74). Although in many cases these lesions may be outlined as distinct from the postobstructive pneumonitis and atelectasis by administration of a bolus of intravenous contrast medium (to be discussed later), the accuracy of this approach depends on technique (145,149,153,162). In a retrospective study of 25 cases of postobstructive lobar atelectasis, Khoury and colleagues (149), administering first an intravenous bolus and then a rapid drip of contrast material using routine axial imaging with contiguous 1-cm sections, found that differential enhancement separated tumor from collapsed lung in only 2 of 8 patients. In distinction, Tobler and associates (162), in their evaluation of 18 patients with proximal bronchogenic carcinoma and postobstructive lobar atelectasis, found that in 8 (80%) of 10 patients evaluated with a bolus of intravenous contrast, differentiation of tumor from adjacent lung was possible. In this study, unlike that described by Khouri, the authors used a dynamic-static sequence of images in which 6 scans of 3 seconds each were obtained with a 2-second interscan delay, providing 6 sequential images all at the same level with variable degrees of contrast enhancement. Interestingly, in the 2 cases in this study evaluated with a dynamic-incremental technique after first a bolus and then a rapid drip infusion of contrast, central tumor could not be differentiated from peripheral collapse with either technique. These findings suggest that the timing of scan acquisition is a critical determinant of the ability of CT to differentiate tumor from atelectatic lung. Ideally, images should be obtained early to assess the bronchial arterial component of tumor enhancement, optimally at a minimum of 30 to 40 seconds after initiation of contrast administration, followed by delayed images up to 2 minutes after equilibration to help to differentiate the relatively lower attenuation of most tumors compared with the higher attenuation noted within peripheral atelectatic lung, the consequence of delayed tissue perfusion (153). Although one may anticipate that assessment of central tumors would be preferentially evaluated using helical scan techniques, to date, an optimal method using spiral CT has yet to be described. That variable findings should be reported using intravenous contrast to differentiate tumor from atelectasis is not surprising. Differentiation is based on numerous factors, most importantly including tumor vascularity, the presence, and extent of tumor necrosis, evidence of pulmonary artery obstruction, and the state of the atelectatic lung, including the presence or absence of infection (163).

CT Appearance

Endobronchial obstruction causes a spectrum of radiologic abnormalities, reflecting both the nature and the extent of the disease process within the affected lung, as well as compensatory changes involving adjacent lung, mediastinum, hilum, diaphragm, and chest wall, and therefore should be viewed as a dynamic process accounting for a wide variability of appearances.

Bronchial obstruction usually causes increased density within the affected segment or lobe, secondary to the presence of intraalveolar fluid. The amount of fluid present within the obstructed lung is generally a function of both the degree of obstruction and time. Occasionally, in the presence of endobronchial obstruction, the affected lung may contain air and may appear relatively normal in density, especially in the presence of an incomplete fissure. In these cases, CT may be especially valuable by detecting otherwise occult tumors (Fig. 3-76).

As documented by Burke and Fraser (163) in their study of 50 consecutive patients undergoing pulmonary resection for bronchogenic carcinomas, a wide spectrum of histologic changes can be identified within atelectatic lung when atelectasis occurs over a prolonged time interval. Initially, histologic changes reflect noninfectious processes including mucoid impaction and dilatation of the airways, frequently associated with lymphocytic infiltration of bronchial walls, and the presence of edema fluid and eosinophilic proteinaceous material within airspaces, representing, at least in part, retained surfactant. Subsequently, aggregates of lipid-laden macrophages accumulate, and progressive lymphocytic infiltration and collagen deposition occur within the pulmonary interstitium (so-called lipid pneumonia). Finally, with sufficient time, interstitial fibrosis supervenes. Surprisingly, in the foregoing series, infection proved relatively rare and, when present, appeared either as focal bronchitis or as bronchiolitis, with only minimal or absent parenchymal involvement. Despite great variability, the various causes of lobar atelectasis form discrete and usually easily identifiable subsets in cross section, typical identifying features of which are described in Table 3-8.

Right Upper Lobe Atelectasis. The right upper lobe is bordered medially by the mediastinum, superiorly by the chest wall, inferiorly by the minor fissure, and posterolaterally by the superior portion of the oblique fissure. When collapsed as a result of endobronchial obstruction, the right upper lobe progressively "pancakes" against the mediastinum and maintains its connection to the hilum by a tongue of tissue referred to as the mediastinal wedge (Figs. 3-77 and 3-78).

The lower and middle lobes undergo compensatory overinflation (see Fig. 3-78); the result is upward displacement of the minor fissure and anterior displacement of the upper portion of the oblique fissure. As the right upper lobe collapses toward the midline, the middle lobe, especially the lateral segment, insinuates itself laterally between the chest wall and the lateral portion of the collapsing right upper lobe. With hyperaeration and expansion, the pulmonary vessels within the middle and lower lobes appear abnormally spaced. Compensatory hyperexpansion of the right lower lobe, especially the superior segment, may lead to visualization of a sliver of lung invaginating between the mediastinum medially and the posterior aspect of the collapsed right upper lobe laterally. This situation results in a sharp lucent interface between the atelectatic lobe and the mediastinum on the chest radiograph, a phenomenon known as the Luftsichel sign, and in a triangular configuration of the posteroinferior portion of the collapsed right upper lobe (see Fig. 3-78) (149). Luftsichel is far more commonly seen with left upper

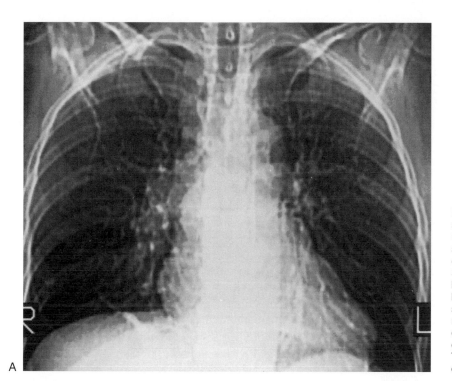

FIG. 3-76. Endobronchial obstruction: metastatic renal cell carcinoma. **A:** Scanogram. A nodular density is present in the right lower lobe. A subcarinal mass is present as well. There is no evidence of volume loss on the right side. **B–E:** Sequential images through the right upper lobe bronchus, bronchus intermedius, right lower lobe bronchus, and right lower lobe, respectively. A small density can be seen within the lumen of the right upper lobe bronchus. The bronchus intermedius is obliterated. Despite this situation, aeration of the middle and right lower lobes is normal. Total obstruction was confirmed bronchoscopically.

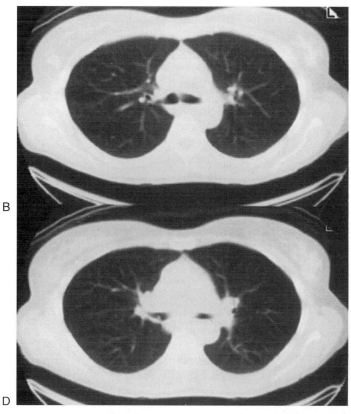

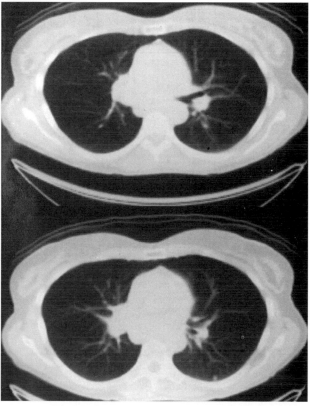

TABLE 3-8. *CT of lobar atelectasis: primary findings*

• Endobronchial tumor causes irregular narrowing or occlusion of airways; patent central bronchi are usually identified with other causes of collapse.

• With endobronchial obstruction, the involved lobe becomes wedge shaped rather than hemispheric, with the proximal portion of the lobe usually assuming a V shape, with the apex situated at the origin of the affected bronchus. Loss of volume typically results in a reduced zone of contact between the pleural surface and the chest wall unless the patient has preexisting pleural adhesions.

• Large tumor masses produce a bulge in the contour of the collapsed lobe (S sign of Golden) and may by identified separately from the remaining collapsed lobe in most cases after a bolus of intravenous contrast. Characteristically, central tumor masses have lower attenuation than collapsed peripheral lung.

• Lucencies within atelectatic lobes typically result from bronchiectasis and are only rarely seen in patients with endobronchial tumors. Abscesses are relatively less common and again usually occur in the setting of long-standing nonobstructive collapse. In distinction, fluid distending peripheral airways within atelectatic segments is often identified in patients with endobronchial obstruction (so-called fluid bronchogram sign).

• Rarely, most of an entire lobe may be replaced by tumor; this results in a lobular rather than a wedge-shaped appearance to the collapsed lobe with or without central bronchial obstruction.

lobe collapse. Ancillary changes, such as shift to the right of the trachea and mediastinum and elevation of the right hemidiaphragm, may occur, but they are less common.

CT findings in right upper lobe collapse are summarized in Table 3-7 and are shown in Figure 3-77; the importance

of intravenous contrast media in imaging right upper lobe atelectasis is presented in Figures 3-79–3-81.

Left Upper Lobe Atelectasis

The left upper lobe is bounded medially by the mediastinum and more inferiorly by the left heart border, superiorly and laterally by the chest wall, and posteriorly by the major fissure. With atelectasis, the left upper lobe moves anterosuperiorly. Unlike the right upper lobe, which collapses against the mediastinum along its entire length, the left upper lobe generally retains more contact with the anterior and lateral chest wall as it collapses. Superiorly, the left upper lobe may be displaced from the mediastinum by overinflation of the superior segment of the left lower lobe. This accounts for the frequent finding of periaortic lucency or Luftsichel on posteroanterior radiographs after left upper lobe collapse (Fig. 3-82). Inferiorly, the left upper lobe, like the right upper lobe, marginates the mediastinum and is connected to the left hilum by a wedge of collapsed tissue.

Superiorly, the collapsed upper lobe has a wedge-shaped, triangular configuration, with the apex pointing posteriorly. This configuration is caused by the general anterosuperior direction of collapse; the broad base of the triangular collapsed lobe retains its connection to the anterior chest wall. Posteriorly, this V-shaped contour is caused by anterior displacement of the superior segment of the left lower lobe along both the medial and lateral limbs of the V (149). Hyperinflation of the left lower lobe and right lung, which crosses the midline, is greater than that seen in right upper lobe collapse, probably because the left upper lobe has a much greater volume. Superiorly, the overinflated left lower

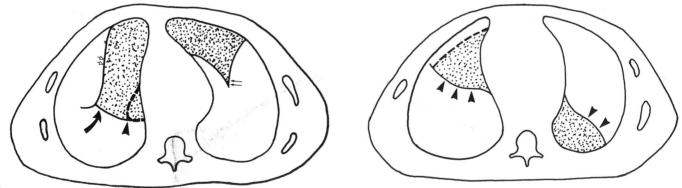

A   B

FIG. 3-77. Schematic representation of collapse. **A:** Cross-sectional appearance of idealized collapse of the right and left upper lobes secondary to central obstructing tumors. The right upper lobe (*stippled area* on the left side of the image) typically collapses anteromedially against the mediastinum. The middle lobe fissure rotates anteromedially as the hyperinflated middle lobe insinuates between the collapsed lobe medially and the lateral chest wall (*open arrows*). The major fissure is shifted slightly anteriorly (*curved arrow*). Rarely, a small portion of the superior segment invaginates between the collapsed lung laterally and the mediastinum, so-called Luftsichel (*dashed lines*), giving a triangular appearance to the posterior aspect of the collapsed right upper lobe (*arrowhead*). Unlike right upper lobe collapse, left upper lobe collapse (*stippled area* on the right side of the image) typically is anterosuperior, and the posterior portion of the collapsed lobe is more characteristically V-shaped (*double arrows*). This appearance is caused by pronounced medial insinuation of the hyperaerated superior segment of the left lower lobe. **B:** Cross-sectional appearance of idealized collapse of the middle lobe and left lower lobe, secondary to central obstructing tumors. The middle lobe characteristically collapses anteromedially against the right heart border (*stippled area* on the left side of the image). The major fissure rotates anteriorly (*triple arrowheads*) and is typically sharply defined. The minor fissure is deviated inferiorly (*dotted lines*) and is usually indistinct because of its oblique orientation. The lower lobes collapse posteromedially against the spine. As a consequence, the major fissure is displaced posteriorly (*double arrowhead*).

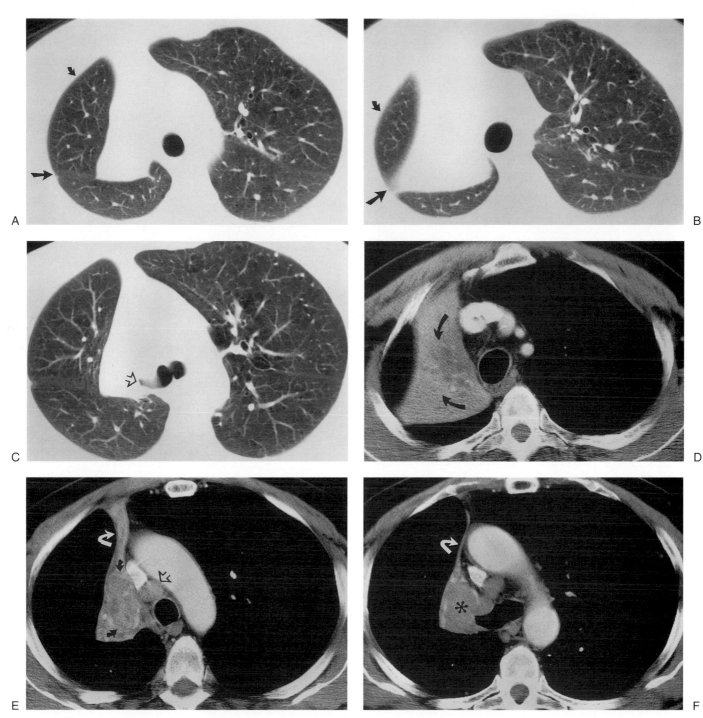

FIG. 3-78. Right upper lobe atelectasis. Central airway obstruction. **A–C:** Sequential images through the middle and lower trachea and right upper lobe bronchus, respectively. The collapsed right upper lobe can be identified as a wedge extending along the mediastinum to the anterior chest wall. Hyperinflation of the middle and lower lobes can be clearly separated by identification of the lateral margin of the oblique fissure (*straight arrows* in **A** and **B**). The middle lobe is insinuated between the collapsed upper lobe medially and the lateral chest wall (*curved arrows* in **A** and **B**). Note the abrupt obstruction of the distal portion of the right upper lobe bronchus (*arrow* in **C**). **D–F:** Identical images as in **A–C**, imaged with narrow windows. After intravenous contrast administration, one can differentiate the central tumor mass (*curved arrows* in **D**; asterisk in **F**) from the peripherally collapsed right upper lobe (*curved arrows* in **E** and **F**) because of subtle differences in attenuation between tumor tissue and atelectatic lung. Note the presence of markedly enlarged mediastinal nodes (*open arrow* in **E**). (*continues*)

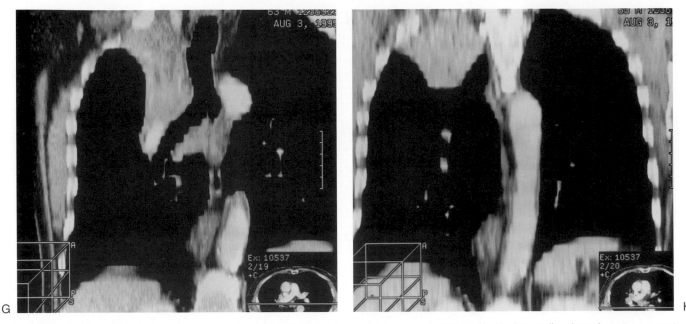

FIG. 3-78. *Continued.* **G,H:** Coronal reconstructions through the carina and more posteriorly through the descending thoracic aorta convey to better advantage the three dimensional appearance of right upper lobe collapse, in particular the location of the major and minor fissures.

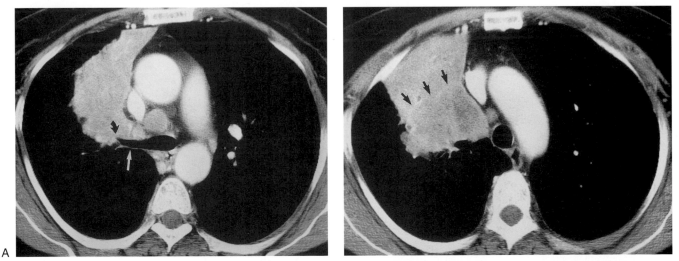

FIG. 3-79. Right upper lobe atelectasis. **A:** Section shows narrowing of the right upper lobe bronchus (*black arrow*) and apparent obstruction of the anterior segmental bronchus (*white arrow*). Unlike the case illustrated in Figure 3-78, the lateral border of the collapsed right upper lobe is irregular, and the fissure is not clearly identifiable. **B:** Section through the lower trachea imaged with narrow windows after intravenous contrast administration shows subtle differentiation between central tumor (*arrows*) and peripheral lung (compare with Fig. 3–78D–F). In this case, tumor is extending along the anterior border of the right upper lobe bronchus consistent with submucosal extension of disease, subsequently confirmed at bronchoscopy: enlarged mediastinal nodes are also present. This patient has histologically proved nonsmall cell lung cancer.

FIG. 3-81. Combined right upper and middle lobe atelectasis. **A,B:** Posteroanterior and lateral radiographs, respectively, show an ill-defined hazy density obscuring the right hilum on the posteroanterior radiograph with apparent displacement of the entire length of the major fissure (*arrows* in **B**), a pattern more consistent with left rather than right upper lobe collapse. **C, D:** Contrast-enhanced CT sections through the right upper and middle lobes, respectively, show that both these airways are obstructed by tumor (*arrows*), with resultant combined upper and middle lobe atelectasis. In this case, despite the use of contrast, differentiation between tumor and atelectatic lung is difficult. At endoscopy, obstructing endobronchial lesions with identical histologic features were identified in both the right upper and middle lobe bronchi. Combined right upper and middle lobe collapse account for the apparent left upper lobe pattern of collapse seen on the corresponding posteroanterior and lateral chest radiographs shown in **A** and **B**.

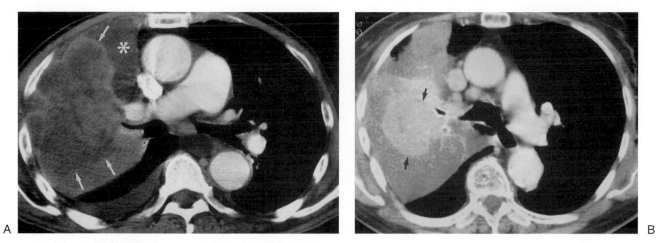

FIG. 3-80. Right upper lobe atelectasis: value of intravenous contrast administration. **A:** Section at the level of the right upper lobe bronchus after intravenous contrast administration shows evidence of tumor replacing most of the right upper lobe (*arrows*) in addition to obstructing the right upper lobe bronchus; only a small volume of atelectatic lung is still identifiable (*asterisk*). A small right pleural effusion is also present. **B:** Section through the right upper lobe in a different patient from **A**. In this case, tumor is located centrally (*arrows*) and is surrounded by lung within which normal branching vessels can still be identified. Posterior bulging of the major fissure is noted. These findings are consistent with so-called "drowned lung" secondary to central bronchial obstruction (compare with **A** and Figs. 3-78 and 3-79). These cases illustrate the importance of administering intravenous contrast media to identify the presence and extent of tumor accurately.

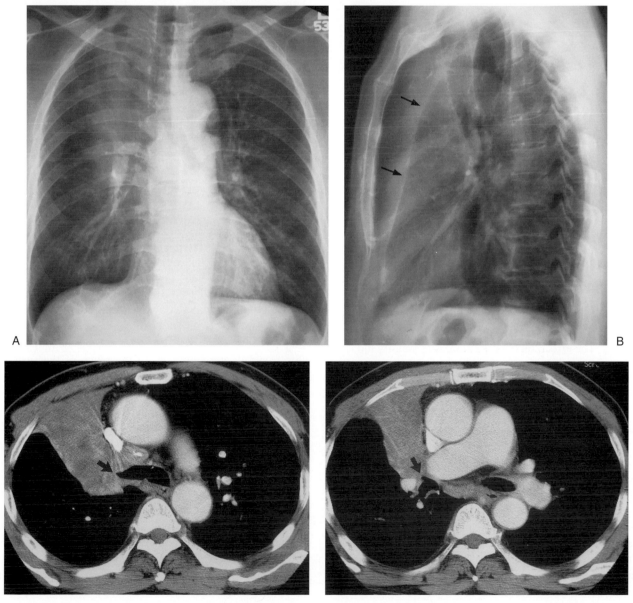

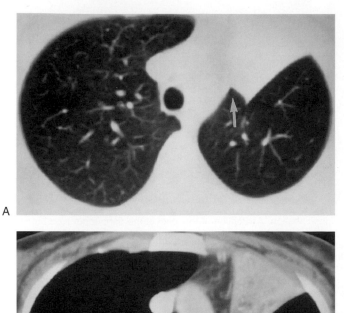

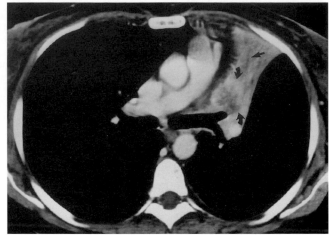

FIG. 3-82. Left upper lobe atelectasis. **A, B:** Section through the midtrachea imaged with wide and narrow windows, respectively, shows characteristic appearance of left upper lobe collapse resulting from central airway obstruction. The collapsed left upper lobe forms a sharply defined triangular density, with the apex pointing posteriorly. The hyperinflated left lower lobe lies between the collapsed upper lobe and the mediastinum (*arrow* in **A**), accounting for the characteristic radiographic finding of periaortic lucency after left upper lobe collapse. **C:** Section shows obstruction of the left upper lobe bronchus by a clearly identifiable low-density tumor mass (*curved arrows*). Note the presence of fluid-filled bronchi in the peripheral, atelectatic lung (*straight arrow*).

lobe insinuates itself between the aorta and mediastinum medially and the atelectatic upper lobe laterally.

Depending on the degree of atelectasis, the left hilum becomes elevated. The degree of elevation of the left hilum and the subsequent rotation of the left bronchial tree are of lesser magnitude on the left side, compared with changes accompanying right upper lobe collapse, because the left upper lobe bronchus is anchored by the left pulmonary artery superiorly. The effect, on cross section, is to identify the left main bronchus at the same level as the right upper lobe bronchus, rarely any higher with endobronchial obstruction (see Fig. 3-82). As discussed later, greater elevation of the left upper lobe bronchus typically requires long-standing scarring within the left upper lobe itself, rarely identified in patients with endobronchial tumors. Again, identification of tumor versus periphereal, atelectatic lung is facilitated by use of intravenous contrast (Fig. 3-83).

Although lesions involving the left upper lobe bronchus generally cause collapse of the entire lobe, occasionally atelectasis is more pronounced in one of the segments. Lingular atelectasis results in increased density adjacent to the left heart border, causing marked anteromedial displacement of the major fissure. CT findings in left upper lobe atelectasis are reviewed in Table 3-8 and are illustrated in Figure 3-77.

Middle Lobe Atelectasis

The middle lobe is bounded medially by the right heart border, anteriorly and laterally by the chest wall, posteriorly by the major fissure, and superiorly by the minor fissure. As the middle lobe collapses, the two fissures begin to approximate one another; that is, downward shift of the minor fissure and forward displacement of the oblique fissure occur. The major fissure is clearly seen with CT because the axis of this fissure is perpendicular to the plane of the scan. The minor fissure, parallel to the plane of the scan, is not as sharply defined. As the middle lobe loses volume, it collapses medially against the right heart border. This phenomenon accounts for the silhouette sign on posteroanterior radiographs. The middle lobe normally has a triangular or wedge-shaped configuration; this becomes accentuated as the lobe collapses, with the apex of the triangle directed toward the hilum. Because of the relatively smaller volume of the middle lobe, compared with the other lobes, compensatory changes such as shift of the mediastinum and hyperaeration of the remainder of the lung tend to be less pronounced (Fig. 3-84). This remains true even in extreme degrees of volume loss within the middle lobe, as occurs in patients with the so-called middle lobe syndrome, which is discussed later.

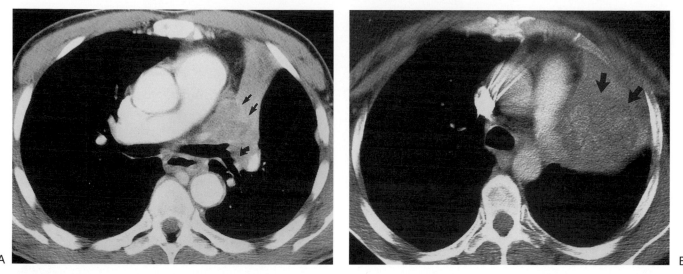

FIG. 3-83. Left upper lobe atelectasis: value of intravenous contrast administration. **A:** Contrast-enhanced section shows obstruction of the left upper lobe bronchus. A large mass can be identified by the subtle difference in attenuation between the mass and peripheral atelectatic lung (*arrows*). This tumor extends into the left hilum and displaces the left interlobar pulmonary artery (*curved arrow*), as well as medially causing partial obstruction of the left superior pulmonary vein. **B:** Contrast-enhanced section through the lower trachea in a different patient from **A** shows a large tumor mass occupying most of the left upper lobe at this level (*arrows*) within which subtle dystrophic calcification can be identified. This patient has bronchoscopically confirmed metastatic mucinous carcinoma of the colon.

The typical configuration of middle lobe collapse, as in any other form of lobar collapse, is altered in the presence of pleural adhesions. This complication may result in unusual appearances that may be difficult to interpret on the chest radiograph; in this setting, CT may prove invaluable. Similarly, in complex patterns of collapse, such as occurs in patients with combined middle and lower lobe collapse, in which radiographs are frequently confusing, CT also may be indispensable (see Fig. 3-81) (164). CT findings of middle lobe collapse resulting from endobronchial obstruction are summarized in Table 3-8 and are shown in Figure 3-77.

Lower Lobe Atelectasis

The lower lobes should be considered together because anatomically they appear identical in the collapsed state. The lower lobes are bordered inferiorly by the hemidiaphragms, posteriorly and laterally by the chest wall, medially by the heart and mediastinum, and anteriorly by the major fissure. The lower lobes collapse medially toward the mediastinum, generally maintaining contact with the hemidiaphragms. These changes reflect the attachments of the inferior pulmonary ligaments. The major fissure, especially the lateral portion, moves posteriorly. This phenomenon accounts for the usually sharp interface between the lateral portion of the collapsed lobe in patients with left lower lobe collapse (Figs. 3-85 and 3-86). Occasionally, the attachments between the lower lobes and the pulmonary ligaments are incomplete. In this case, collapse of the lower lobes may assume an unusual or rounded configuration.

Right lower lobe atelectasis mimics the appearance of left lower lobe collapse in cross section. Collapse is generally posteromedial against the posterior mediastinum and spine.

The lateral contour of the atelectatic lobe is convex laterally when atelectasis is secondary to central tumor. Occasionally, a central tumor causes atelectasis of the superior segment alone. Isolated from the remainder of the basilar segmental bronchi, a strategically placed tumor can obstruct the superior segmental orifice without compromising the main portion of the right lower lobe bronchus. Although this appearance may cause confusion on plain radiographs, identification of isolated superior segmental collapse is straightforward on the cross-sectional CT image (Fig. 3-87). CT findings of lower lobe atelectasis resulting from endobronchial obstruction are summarized in Table 3-8 and are shown in Figure 3-77.

Nonobstructive Atelectasis

Mechanisms of nonobstructive atelectasis have been described and include cicatrization atelectasis, passive atelectasis, and adhesive atelectasis (146). Table 3-9 presents their various causes.

Cicatrization (Cicatricial) Atelectasis

Cicatrization atelectasis results from scarring and fibrosis consequent to long-standing inflammatory disease. Often the result of chronic granulomatous infection, similar changes may be identified in a nonanatomic distribution in patients with radiation fibrosis and more diffusely in patients with interstitial pulmonary fibrosis (144).

Cicatrization atelectasis may be differentiated from other forms of lobar atelectasis, especially obstructive causes, by recognition of the following criteria: (a) endobronchial obstruction is typically absent; with careful scan technique, patency of the bronchial tree subtending the involved seg-

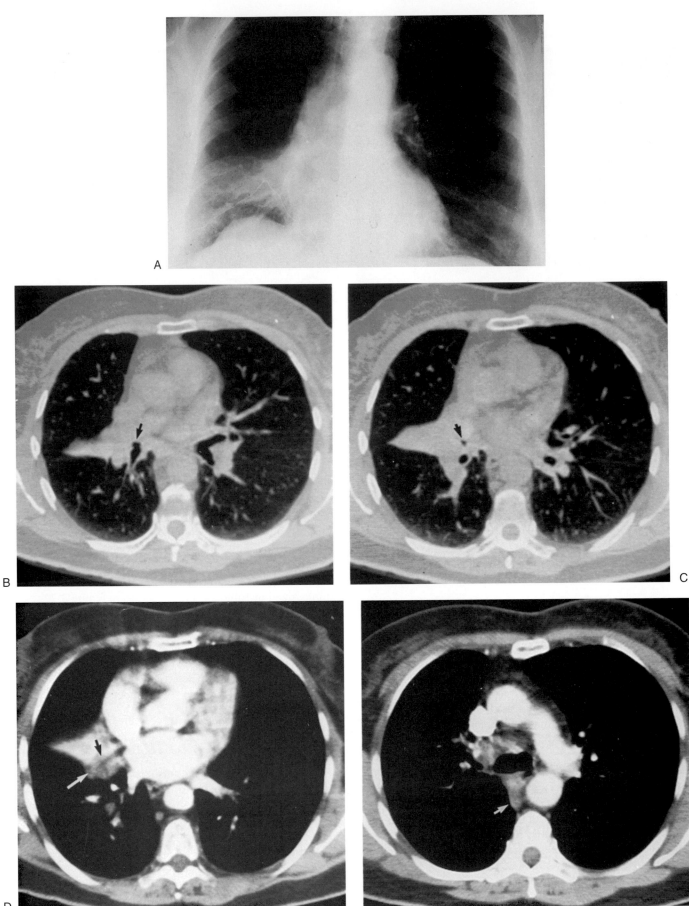

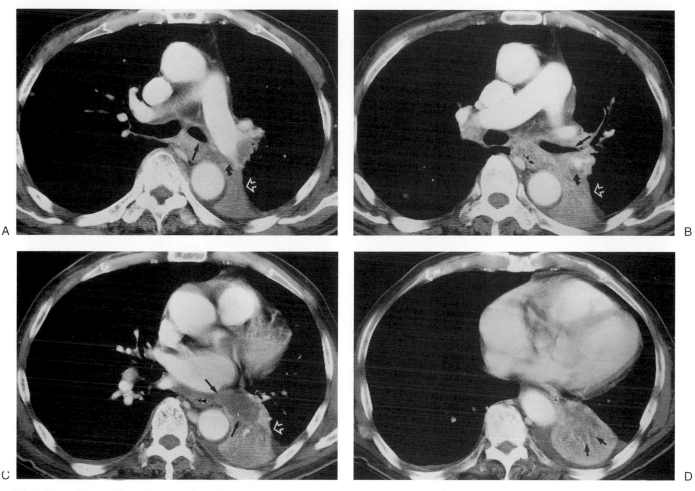

FIG. 3-85. Left lower lobe atelectasis. **A–D:** Select contrast-enhanced images in a patient with left lower lobe atelectasis. The marked narrowing of the left main stem (*arrow* in **A**) and left upper lobe bronchi (*arrow* in **B**) is consistent with submucosal and peribronchial tumor infiltration; the left lower lobe bronchus is obstructed at its origin. Tumor also infiltrates the left hilum and narrows the left interlobar pulmonary artery (*curved arrows* in **A** and **B**). A large, necrotic tumor mass is identifiable distinct from atelectatic lung (*arrows* in **C**): fluid-filled bronchi are present in the lower lobe (*arrows* in **D**). There is marked posterior and medial displacement of the major fissure (*open arrows* in **A–C**). A small quantity of pleural fluid is also present. This patient has bronchoscopically confirmed nonsmall cell lung cancer.

FIG. 3-84. Middle lobe collapse: squamous cell carcinoma. **A:** Posteroanterior radiograph showing increased density inferiorly on the *right,* suggestive of collapse of the middle lobe. **B, C:** Sections through and just below the origin of the middle lobe bronchus, imaged with wide windows. The middle lobe bronchus is patent at its origin (*arrow* in **B**); just below, however, the distal portion of the middle lobe bronchus is significantly narrowed (*arrow* in **C**). The apex of the middle lobe can be defined as a small airless wedge extending laterally from the hilum toward the lateral chest wall, defined posteriorly by the right lower lobe and anteriorly by the hyperinflated upper lobe. **D:** Section at almost the same level as **B,** imaged with narrow windows, after administration of a bolus of intravenous contrast medium through a power injector, imaged with narrow windows. Central tumor can be identified as an area of low attenuation, easily differentiated from the uniformly enhancing collapsed middle lobe (*arrows*). **E:** Section through the carina shows extensive precarinal lymphadenopathy, as well as extensive posterior lymph nodes (*arrow*), which on more inferior scans proved to be continuous with markedly enlarged subcarinal lymph nodes (not shown).

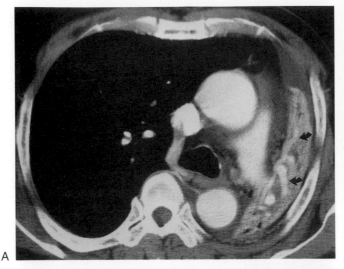

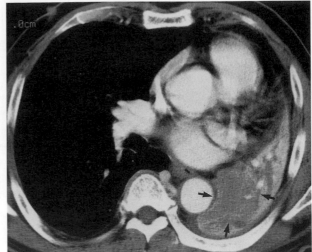

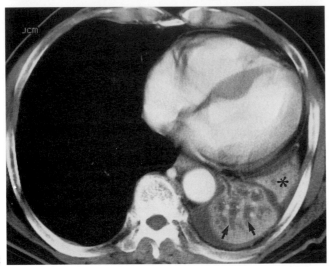

FIG. 3-86. Combined left upper and lower lobe atelectasis. **A–C:** Select contrast-enhanced images show complete atelectasis of the left lung. Central tumor is again identifiable as an irregular area of low density (*arrows* in **B**) easily distinguished from atelectatic lung within which enhancing vessels (*curved arrows* in **A**) and fluid-filled bronchi (*arrows* in **C**) can be identified. The lingula is clearly distinct from the left lower lobe (*asterisk in* **C**).

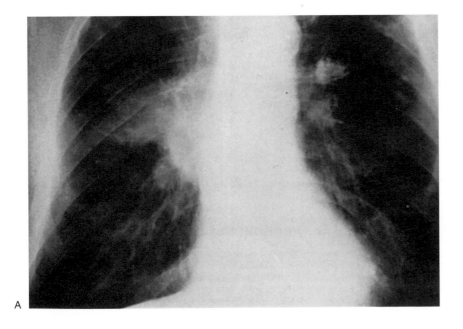

FIG. 3-87. Superior segmental collapse: bronchogenic carcinoma. **A:** Posteroanterior radiograph shows increased density in the region of the right hilum. **B, C:** Sections through the right upper lobe bronchus and 1 cm below, respectively, imaged with narrow, mediastinal windows after a bolus of intravenous contrast. The superior segment is collapsed medially against the spine (*arrows* in **B** and **C**). A necrotic tumor can be seen within the apical portions of the superior segment, identifiable as an ill-defined area of low attenuation (*curved arrows* in **C**), distinct from the otherwise uniform enhancement present in the remainder of the atelectatic lobe uninvolved by tumor.

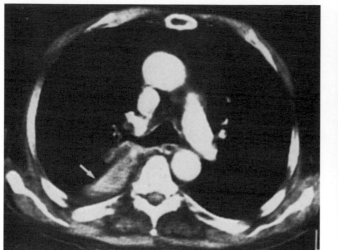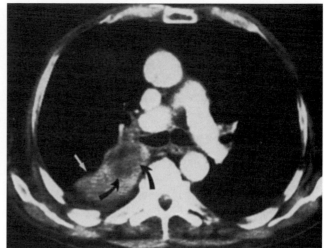

B

C

FIG. 3-87. *Continued.*

ment or lobe can be confirmed (Figs. 3-88–3-91); (b) inflammatory changes in the lobar bronchi often result in airway irregularity, narrowing, or distortion; bronchiectatic changes are frequently present within the involved lobe peripherally and further help to identify collapse as the result of chronic inflammation and fibrosis (see Figs. 3-88–3-91); (c) lobar bronchi are displaced to a far greater degree than typically seen in patients with obstructive forms of atelectasis; in the case of the right upper lobe, the right upper lobe bronchus is characteristically displaced posteriorly, with resultant posterior orientation of the right main bronchus and bronchus intermedius (see Fig. 3-88); in the extreme form, lobar airways may appear to lie in a paramediastinal location (see

Fig. 3-89); (d) the degree of volume loss, in general, is more marked in cicatrization atelectasis than in collapse secondary to endobronchial obstruction, presumably as a reflection of the longer time course over which cicatrization atelectasis occurs; (e) finally, especially in patients with chronic tuberculosis, calcified hilar or mediastinal nodes with or without punctate parenchymal calcifications are frequently identifiable; rarely, an entire lobe or even lung may calcify (see Fig. 3-89). The term "autolobectomy" or "autopneumonectomy" seems appropriate for these cases of extreme volume loss, with or without diffuse calcification, analogous to the changes seen in patients with long-standing renal tuberculosis (see Figs. 3-6 and 3-89–3-91).

The chronic middle lobe syndrome best typifies cicatrization atelectasis (see Fig. 3-90). This syndrome occurs most commonly in middle-aged women with histories of chronic cough and chest pain, and it usually involves the middle lobe or the inferior lingular segments (165). As detailed by Kwon and colleagues (166) in a clinicopathologic study of 21 patients, middle lobe syndrome can result from a wide range of both neoplastic and nonneoplastic causes. These include extrinsic causes of bronchial obstruction, usually from enlarged peribronchial nodes and often the result of prior granulomatous infection, from intrinsic bronchial obstruction, as may occur in chronic foreign body aspiration or broncholithiasis, and from nonobstructing conditions, in particular bronchiectasis (166). Pathologically, a combination of bronchiectasis and bronchiolitis is most commonly seen, frequently in association with secondary findings of organizing pneumonia. The finding of granulomas histologically is also common and should suggest the possibility of atypical mycobacterial infection, especially when it is associated with small, ill-defined nodules on HRCT. Pathologic changes in patients with middle lobe syndrome have been attributed both to lack of normal collateral ventilation in these rela-

TABLE 3-9. *Nonobstructive atelectasis: causes*

Cicatrization atelectasis (localized)
 Common
  Tuberculosis or fungal infection
  Bronchiectasis
  Radiation fibrosis
Compressive (passive) atelectasis
 Common
  Pleural effusion
   Malignant
   Benign (especially empyema)
  Pneumothorax
  Diaphragm dysfunction or elevation
  Aortic aneurysm (especially left lower lobe)
 Rare
  Pleural tumors
  Emphysematous bullae
Adhesive atelectasis (localized)
 Common
  Acute radiation pneumonitis
 Rare
  Pulmonary embolism

Adapted from ref. 144, with permission.

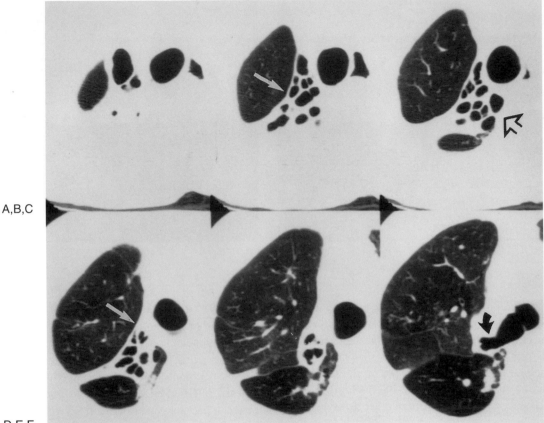

A,B,C

D,E,F

FIG. 3-88. Cicatrization atelectasis: right upper lobe. **A–F:** Selected 5-mm sections show typical appearance of cicatrization of the RUL. Cicatrization atelectasis is characterized by marked posterior displacement of the right main stem and right upper lobe bronchi (*RULB*) *(curved arrow* in **F**) in the absence of endobronchial mass or central airway. This appearance is distinct from the pattern seen in postobstructive atelectasis in which one sees little if any displacement of the RULB (compare with Figs. 3-78–3-81). The collapsed RUL is sharply marginated laterally by hyperinflated middle lobe (*arrows* in **B** and **D**) and posteriorly by the superior segment of the right lower lobe. Extensive bronchiectasis is apparent (*open arrow* in **C**), indicative of long-standing fibrosis.

tively isolated lung segments and to poor drainage because of the oblique orientation of these smaller and shorter lobar airways.

Despite the reported association between middle lobe syndrome and bronchial obstruction, in most cases, classic middle lobe atelectasis develops in the presence of a widely patent lobar bronchi (165). In the study reported by Kwon and associates (166), for example, 20 of 21 patients with documented middle lobe syndrome were found to have patent central airways, with the sole exception of a case with bronchoscopically identified broncholithiasis.

Although typically lobar or segmental in distribution, cicatrization atelectasis may result in the destruction and shrinkage of an entire lung (see Figs. 3-6 and 3-88–3-91). In these cases, again usually the result of long-standing mycobacterial infection, cicatrization atelectasis may result in significant compromise of respiratory function as a result of compensatory spatial rearrangements affecting otherwise uninvolved portions of the lung, findings commonly apparent on routine chest radiographs.

Compressive (Passive) Atelectasis

Compressive atelectasis denotes volume loss secondary to extrinsic compression of adjacent lung. Although a distinction may be made between compressive and passive atelectasis, defined as loss of volume resulting from interruption of the normal balance between elastic recoil of the lung and the opposing outward pull of the chest wall and diaphragm, from the standpoint of CT interpretation, this distinction is arbitrary and of no clinical significance. Most often, both compressive atelectasis and passive atelectasis result from the presence of fluid (benign or malignant) or air (with or without tension pneumothorax) within the pleural space (Figs. 3-92–3-94). Less frequently, compressive atelectasis is caused by space-occupying lesions arising from the pleura, chest wall, or mediastinum, including, as reported by Gierada and colleagues (167), atelectasis resulting from severe bullous emphysema.

Fluid within the pleural space is easily identified, distinct from underlying lung, especially after the administration of intravenous contrast media (see Fig. 3-92). Pleural fluid,

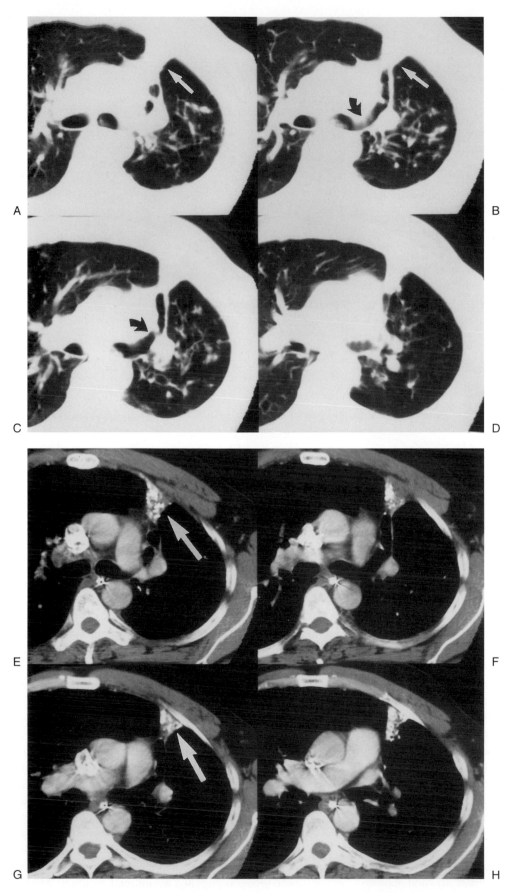

FIG. 3-89. Cicatrization atelectasis: left upper lobe (*LUL*). **A–D:** Select 5-mm sections show marked volume loss in the left upper lobe which is sharply outlined laterally by the displaced major fissure (*arrows* in **A** and **B**). The left upper lobe bronchus is markedly dilated and displaced medially (*curved arrows* **B** and **C**). There is marked hyperinflation of the right upper lobe that crosses the midline anteriorly. **E–H:** Identical sections as in **A–D,** imaged with narrow windows shows extensive calcifications (*arrows* in **E** and **G**) present throughout the shrunken left upper lobe, consistent with clinical history of prior treated tuberculosis.

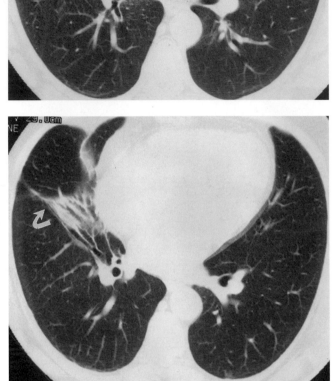

A

FIG. 3-90. Cicatrization atelectasis: middle lobe *(ML)*. **A–C:** Sequential 5-mm sections show typical appearance of cicatrization atelectasis of the ML with a patent middle lobe bronchus *(arrow* in **A)** leading to a markedly shrunken middle lobe within which dilated, bronchiectatic airways are apparent *(arrow* in **B).** The major fissure is displaced anteromedially *(curved arrow* in **C);** in distinction, the minor fissure is more difficult to identify due to partial volume averaging.

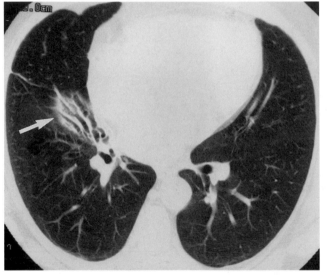

B

C

when sufficiently massive, distorts the usual configuration of collapsed lobes seen in patients with endobronchial lesions. Although investigators have reported that exclusion of tumor in patients with atelectatic lobes may be difficult (161), if the lobar bronchi are patent and air bronchograms can be defined in every portion of the atelectatic lobe, tumor can be confidently excluded. Also strongly suggestive of a lack of tumor within collapsed lung is the finding of a markedly shrunken lobe surrounded by or floating within pleural fluid (see Figs. 3-92 and 3-93). In our experience, this degree of collapse excludes the possibility of an infiltrative tumor because only a relatively spongy lobe not fixed or infiltrated by tumor can collapse to this degree. In patients with pleural effusions, CT is also of value by identifying malignant changes along pleural surfaces. As discussed in greater detail in Chapter 9, the diagnosis of a malignant effusion depends on recognition of an abnormal parietal pleura, identifiable

either as nodular foci of soft tissue density or as an enveloping rind of thickened nodular pleura, usually in association with loculated areas of pleural fluid (146).

Unusual configurations of collapse may result when air, fluid, or both are present in the pleural space. The magnitude of pressure exerted on lung by adjacent pleural fluid or air may be great; the result may be initially confusing radiographically. Of particular interest is the phenomenon of lung torsion (168–170). Torsion has been noted to occur spontaneously, usually in association with some other pulmonary abnormality, such as pneumonia or tumor, after traumatic pneumothorax, and especially as a complication of surgery. Radiographically, the hallmark of this entity is the finding of a collapsed lobe, almost always either the right or the left upper lobe, less commonly the middle lobe, and only rarely the lower lobes, occupying an unusual position. Marked change in position of the collapsed lobe on sequential radio-

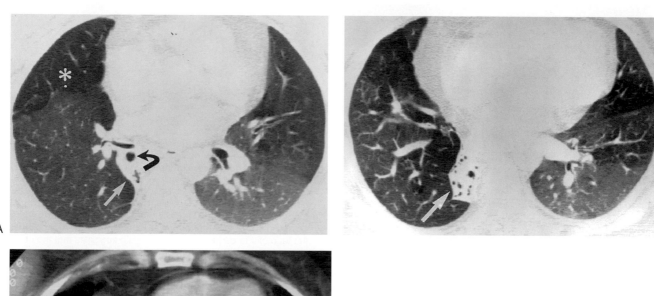

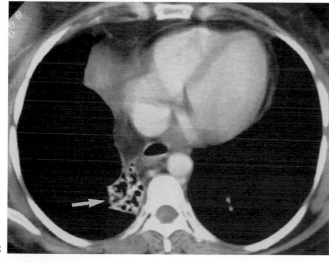

FIG. 3-91. Cicatrization atelectasis: right lower lobe (*RLL*). **A,B:** Selected 5-mm sections imaged with wide windows show a shrunken right lower lobe outlined laterally by the markedly displaced major fissure (*arrows* in **A** and **B**). Note the patency of the right lower lobe bronchus (*curved arrow* in **A**) and posterior displacement of the middle lobe bronchus, associated with extensive bronchiectasis. In this case, one sees evidence of a marked difference in lung density between the right upper lobe (*asterisk*) and lingula versus the right middle lobe and left lower lobe, likely the result of associated small airways disease in the upper lobes. **C:** Identical section as **B,** imaged with narrow windows shows that bronchiectatic airways fill the shrunken right lower lobe (*arrow*).

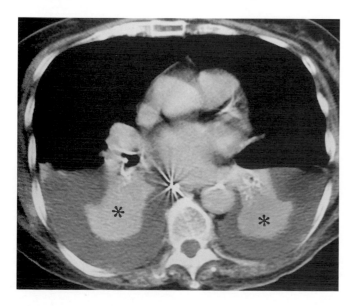

FIG. 3-92. Compression atelectasis. Contrast-enhanced CT section shows bilateral pleural effusions associated with bilateral lower lobe compression atelectasis (*asterisks*). In this case, the degree of collapse coupled with homogeneous enhancement suggests that the underlying lung is grossly normal: lung infiltrated with tumor or stiffened by inflammation is unlikely to have this appearance.

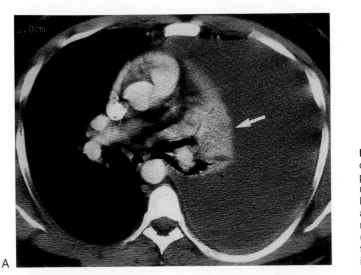

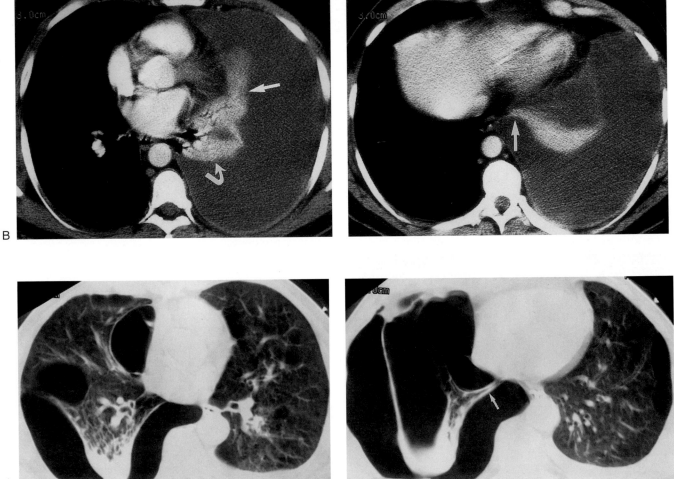

FIG. 3-93. Compression atelectasis. **A–C:** Selected 5-mm sections obtained after intravenous contrast administration show large left pleural effusion causing compression atelectasis of the entire left upper lobe (*arrow* in **A**) as well as the lingula (*arrow* in **B**) and left lower lobe (*curved arrow* in **B**). With the exception of the central airways and pulmonary vessels, the atelectatic lung appears homogenous in density. Medially, the inferior pulmonary ligament (*arrow* in **C**) tethers the left lower lobe. This degree of collapse in the face of a large pleural effusion again suggests that the underlying lung is grossly normal (compare with Fig. 3-92).

FIG. 3-94. Compression atelectasis. **A, B:** Select images show the presence of a hydropneumothorax causing compression atelectasis of the right lower and, to a lesser degree, middle lobe. The inferior pulmonary ligament (*arrow* in **B**) tethers the right lower lobe medially and inferiorly. Increased density in the posterior portion of the right lower lobe is consistent with more severe focal atelectasis. In this case, pneumothorax is secondary to underlying bullous emphysema, present as well in the left lung.

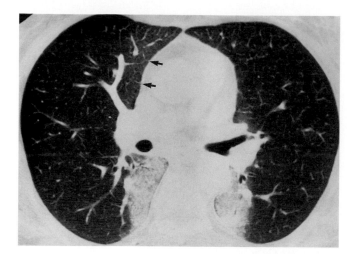

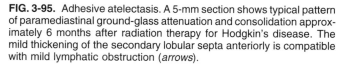

FIG. 3-95. Adhesive atelectasis. A 5-mm section shows typical pattern of paramediastinal ground-glass attenuation and consolidation approximately 6 months after radiation therapy for Hodgkin's disease. The mild thickening of the secondary lobular septa anteriorly is compatible with mild lymphatic obstruction (*arrows*).

graphs is considered characteristic. Although the condition is rare, the diagnosis is significant, especially in postoperative patients, because unrecognized torsion is associated with a high mortality from resultant pulmonary infarction.

Adhesive Atelectasis

Adhesive atelectasis refers to atelectasis resulting from an absence of surfactant and may be thought of as a form of resorption atelectasis occurring without bronchial obstruction. The prototype for this form of atelectasis is acute radiation pneumonitis (Figs. 3-95 and 3-96). The changes seen in the thorax consequent to radiation therapy have been described (171–173). In patients with acute radiation pneumonitis, the predominant finding is ground glass attenuation, typically conforming to known radiation ports. With time, fibrosis ensues with resultant cicatricial atelectasis.

MR Evaluation

The role of MR for evaluating pulmonary collapse is limited (162,174,175). Studies performed have shown that T2 weighting may allow differentiation between central obstructing tumor and peripheral collapsed lung (Figs. 3-97 and 3-98) (175). Herold and associates (176), in a comparison of routine spin-echo MR imaging of 17 patients with obstructive atelectasis and 25 patients with nonobstructive atelectasis, found that all 17 patients with obstructive atelectasis had increased signal using T2 weighting, whereas in distinction, 22 of 25 cases with nonobstructive atelectasis showed no evidence of increased signal ($p < .0001$). The authors attributed this difference to the presence of retained secretions or fluid in lung distal to proximal airway obstruction.

The relationship between MR and CT to assess patients with lobar atelectasis has been explored (see Fig. 3-97). In a retrospective study of 18 patients with proximal broncho-

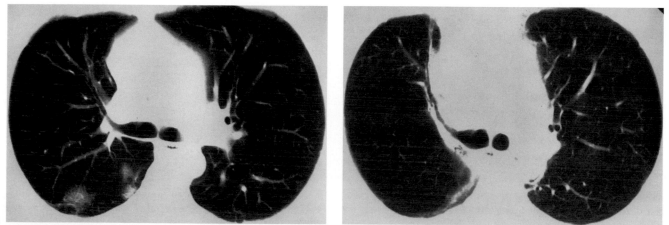

FIG. 3-96. Adhesive atelectasis. **A:** A 5-mm section through the midlung shows patchy areas of nodular ground glass attenuation in the posterior portion of the right upper lobe and the apex of the superior segment of the right lower lobe approximately 6 months after radiation therapy for mediastinal lymphoma. This appearance was initially mistaken as possibly resulting from infection or even tumor infiltration of the lung. **B:** Section at the same approximate level as shown in **A,** 5 months later, shows extensive adhesive atelectasis resulting from radiation.

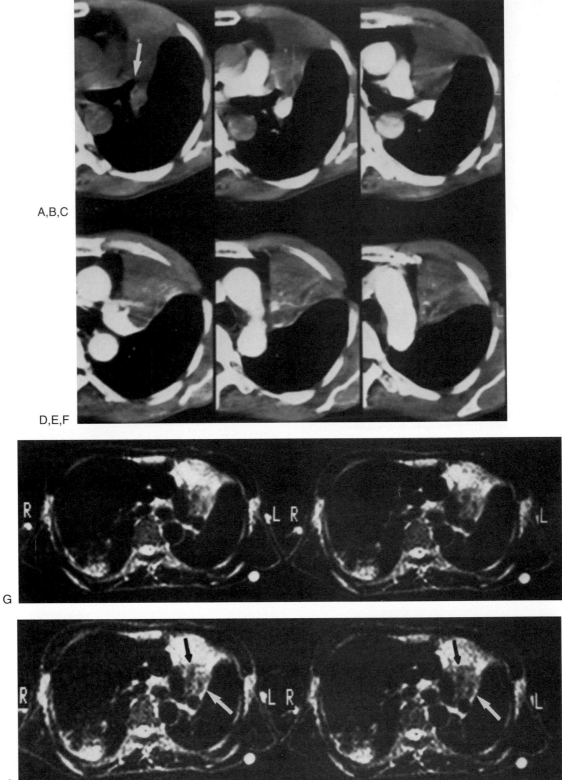

FIG. 3-97. Left upper lobe collapse: CT–MR correlation. **A–F:** Dynamic incremental CT sections through the left upper lobe obtained after a bolus of 60 mL of 60% iodinated contrast medium injected at a rate of 2 mL/sec using a power injector. The left upper lobe bronchus is obstructed (*arrow* in **A**). Despite good opacification of vessels, differentiation of tumor from collapsed lung is impossible. **G–J:** MR images obtained at eye level of the left main pulmonary artery (compare with **C**), utilizing a single-level, multiple-echo technique. With progressively longer TEs (150, 180, 210, and 240 msec, respectively), central tumor is easily differentiable from peripheral collapse as an area of relatively lower signal intensity (*arrows* in **I** and **J**). Abnormal signal is also present in the right lower lobe corresponding to a documented aspiration pneumonia.

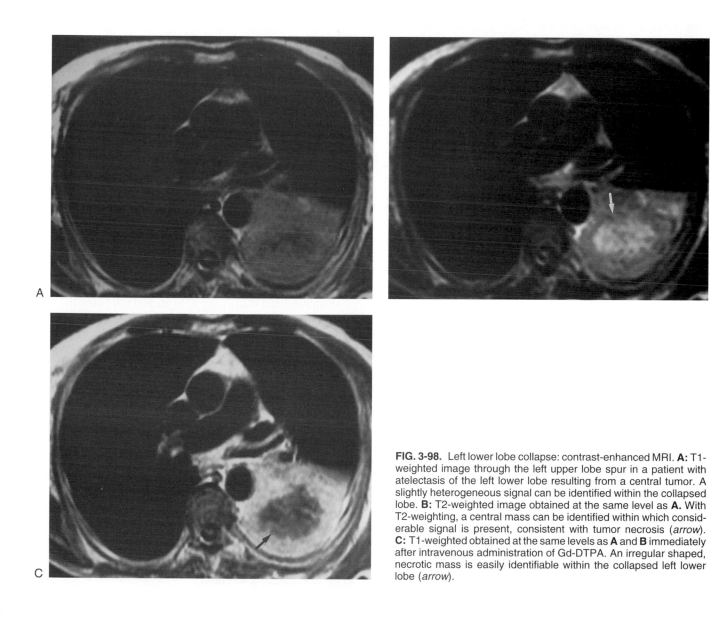

FIG. 3-98. Left lower lobe collapse: contrast-enhanced MRI. **A:** T1-weighted image through the left upper lobe spur in a patient with atelectasis of the left lower lobe resulting from a central tumor. A slightly heterogeneous signal can be identified within the collapsed lobe. **B:** T2-weighted image obtained at the same level as **A.** With T2-weighting, a central mass can be identified within which considerable signal is present, consistent with tumor necrosis (*arrow*). **C:** T1-weighted obtained at the same levels as **A** and **B** immediately after intravenous administration of Gd-DTPA. An irregular shaped, necrotic mass is easily identifiable within the collapsed left lower lobe (*arrow*).

genic carcinomas and postobstructive lobar atelectasis evaluating both with dynamic contrast-enhanced CT and MR, Tobler and associates (162) reported that the use of T2-weighted sequences showed different signal intensities of tumor and collapsed lung in only 5 (50%) of 10 patients with MR, whereas dynamic CT differentiated tumor from collapsed lung in 8 (80%) of 10 patients. Of 18 patients evaluated with T1-weighted sequences, MR accurately differentiated tumor from collapse in only 1 patient (5%). Despite these differences, the authors of this study concluded that no significant statistical difference existed between the modalities. Of particular interest was the finding that CT and MR were apparently complementary in that, in 2 cases in which differentiation was not possible with dynamic CT scanning, MR was successful.

Experimental verification of improved delineation of tumor versus collapsed lung using T2-weighted sequences in both animals and human tissue samples has been reported, and it has been presumed, at least in part, to be due to differences in total water content of tumor and lung (174,175).

As previously discussed, atelectasis resulting from endobronchial obstruction results in a wide and sequential spectrum of gross and histologic changes from an initial appearance of dilated and mucoid-impacted proximal airways with accumulation of proteinaceous material within distal airspaces, to the later accumulation of lipid-laden macrophages with progressive lymphocytic infiltration and collagen deposition within the pulmonary interstitium (so-called lipid pneumonia), and finally to interstitial fibrosis (163). These factors clearly have implications for MR evaluation. When MR signal intensity ratios of tumor to fat and collapsed lung to fat are calculated using T2-weighted sequences, at least in one study, tumor could be differentiated from collapsed lung only in patients with ratios of collapsed lung to fat that were higher than 1. These preliminary findings suggest that MR may be most useful in the subacute stage of atelectasis, in which lipid-laden macrophages are most conspicuous (162).

Another form of atelectasis that has been evaluated with MR is adhesive atelectasis secondary to pulmonary irradiation (177). On the assumption that, with time, radiated lung becomes fibrotic, investigators have suggested that T2-weighted sequences may be of value in differentiating fibrosis from residual or recurrent tumor, or areas of radiation-induced pneumonitis. Unfortunately, at least in our experience, considerable signal is almost always present within areas of irradiated lung, even when these areas have been stable radiographically over a prolonged time interval. This signal presumably reflects either residual pneumonitis or, more likely, the presence of retained secretions within dilated, damaged airways, resulting from decreased mucociliary clearance.

PERIPHERAL AIRWAYS

Bronchiectasis

Bronchiectasis is defined as localized, irreversible dilatation of the bronchial tree. Although many different disorders have been associated with bronchiectasis, it most commonly results from acute, chronic, or recurrent infection (Table 3-10) (112,178,179). Clinically, the diagnosis of bronchiectasis is usually made only in patients with severe disease (180). Patients can present with a history of recurrent pulmonary infections, persistent cough productive of large or small amounts of sputum, or hemoptysis. Hemoptysis also is frequent, occurring in up to 50% of cases, and it may be the only clinical finding (179,181,182).

Bronchiectasis most often results from necrotizing infections such as those caused by *Staphylococcus, Klebsiella,* or *Bordetella pertussis* (112). Granulomatous infections, including those caused by *Mycobacterium tuberculosis* (183), atypical mycobacteria, especially *M. avium-intracellulare* complex (MAC) (184–186), and fungal organisms such as *Histoplasma,* are also associated with bronchiectasis. Bronchiectasis is increasingly frequently identified in HIV-positive patients (187). Mechanisms have been proposed to account for accelerated bronchial wall destruction in these patients, including the finding of both bronchiolitis obliterans and, more commonly, lymphocytic interstitial pneumonitis in patients with AIDS (188,189). King and colleagues (190) showed that the finding of bronchial dilatation in HIV-positive patients is associated with elevated levels of neutro-

TABLE 3-10. *Bronchiectasis: causes*

Postinfectious causes
Bacterial
  Granulomatous
Viral (Swyer-James syndrome)
Congenital abnormalities
Immunodeficiency syndrome
Cystic fibrosis
Dyskinetic cilia syndrome
Mounier-Kuhn syndrome
Williams-Campbell syndrome
Bronchopulmonary sequestration
Congenital cystic bronchiectasis
Acquired immunodeficiency
AIDS
Acquired hypogammaglobulinemia
Postobstructive causes
Intrinsic
  Neoplasm; foreign body; mucus plug; stricture
Extrinsic (lymphadenopathy; mass)
Posttransplant complications
Inflammatory causes
Allergic bronchopulmonary aspergillosis
Asthma

Adapted from ref. 336, with permission.

phils in bronchoalveolar lavage fluid, in distinction to HIV-positive patients with normal airways on HRCT. Neutrophil elastase is associated with airway destruction in patients with alpha-1-antitrypsin deficiency, and similarly may be an early mediator of bronchial wall destruction, even in asymptomatic patients.

Bronchiectasis may occur in association with a variety of genetic abnormalities, generally associated with abnormal mucociliary clearance, immunodeficiency, or structural abnormalities of the bronchi or bronchial wall. This group includes patients with cystic fibrosis, as well as those with the dyskinetic cilia syndrome and Young's syndrome. Bronchiectasis is also frequently identified in patients with α_1-antitrypsin deficiency. King and colleagues (191), in a study of 14 patients with α_1-antitrypsin deficiency, found evidence of bronchiectasis in 6 (43%). This correlates well with the finding that approximately 50% of patients with this deficiency manifest symptoms of airway disease, in particular chronic sputum production. Surprisingly, documentation of a frequent association between bronchiectasis and other forms of emphysema has not been well documented (191). Patients with Williams-Campbell syndrome (congenital deficiency of bronchial cartilage) have defective cartilage in the fourth- to sixth-order bronchi often in association with distal air trapping (192,193). Bronchiectasis is also associated with Mounier-Kuhn syndrome (congenital tracheobronchomegaly), with immunodeficiency syndromes, including Bruton's hypogammaglobulinemia and immunoglobulin A (IgA) and combined IgA-IgG subclass deficiencies, and with the yellow nail syndrome (yellow nails, lymphedema, and pleural effusions). Although the cause of bronchiectasis in these conditions varies, bronchial obstruction, abnormal mucociliary clearance, and chronic infection are often present.

Other noninfectious diseases that result in airway inflammation, mucus plugging, and bronchiectasis include allergic bronchopulmonary aspergillosis (ABPA) (194,195) and asthma (192). Bronchiectasis also has been noted to occur in patients with obliterative bronchiolitis, especially in patients with chronic rejection after heart-lung or lung transplantation (55,57,196–200) or bone marrow transplantation, as a result of rejection or chronic graft-versus-host disease (201).

Although the incidence of bronchiectasis is generally cited as decreasing in the United States, the true incidence of bronchiectasis has probably been underestimated (202). Documentation of this disease has traditionally relied on bronchography, which is rarely performed, and it has not taken into account the significant impact of CT on the diagnosis of mild or unsuspected disease.

The radiographic manifestations of bronchiectasis have been well described (203). They include a loss of definition of vascular markings in specific lung segments, presumably secondary to peribronchial fibrosis and volume loss, evidence of bronchial wall thickening, and, in more severely affected patients, the presence of discrete cystic masses occasionally containing air-fluid levels. Most of these findings are nonspecific; a definitive diagnosis of bronchiectasis can seldom be made radiographically (180).

Bronchographic findings indicative of bronchiectasis include proximal or distal bronchial dilatation, pruning or lack of normal tapering of peripheral airways, and luminal filling defects. Although bronchography has traditionally been considered the standard, the reliability of bronchography in the diagnosis of bronchiectasis has been called into question. Currie and associates (180), in a study of 27 patients with chronic sputum production evaluated bronchographically, showed significant interobserver variability when studies were interpreted by two well-trained bronchographers. Agreement was only reached on 19 of 27 (70%) of patients and 94 of 448 (21%) of bronchopulmonary segments. Bronchiectasis was identified in a further 2 patients (7%) by 1 radiologist only. These findings suggest that bronchography may be more limited in its utility than previously thought, and it should not be considered an absolute standard for diagnosis.

CT Evaluation: Diagnostic Criteria

Bronchiectasis traditionally has been classified as cylindric, varicose, or cystic (204). Although differentiation among these categories is useful in assessing disease severity and occasionally may be of value in the differential diagnosis, these distinctions are less important clinically than defining the presence and extent of disease. Evaluating the extent of bronchiectasis is particularly important, because surgery is only rarely performed in patients with involvement of multiple lung segments (178,179,205).

Various descriptive terms have been used to identify bronchiectasis. These include "tram tracks" to describe dilated airways coursing within the scan plane, "signet rings" to describe vertically coursing dilated airways adjacent to eccentrically located pulmonary artery branches, and both "string of pearls" and "cluster of grapes" to describe the appearance of saccular airways seen either along their length or in atelectatic lung segments, respectively (206). Of interest as purely descriptive terms, they are of only limited value for CT interpretation.

HRCT is the imaging modality of choice for evaluating bronchiectasis and all but eliminates the need for bronchography (Fig. 3-99) (207). Currently, the CT diagnosis of bronchiectasis is based on recognition of a variety of findings, both direct and indirect. Direct findings include bronchial dilatation, lack of normal bronchial tapering, and visibility of airways in the peripheral lung zones (Fig. 3-100). Indirect signs include bronchial wall thickening and irregularity, as well as the presence of mucoid impaction. Ancillary signs have also been described and include tracheomegaly, focal

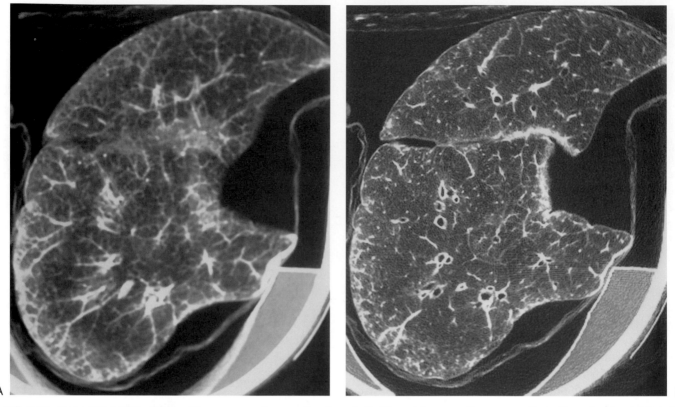

FIG. 3-99. Normal bronchial anatomy: 10-mm versus 1-mm collimation. **A, B:** 10- and 1-mm sections, respectively, through a fixed, inflated lung specimen. Airways easily identifiable on the high-resolution CT image are nearly invisible on the 10-mm section. Normally, airways are only visualized in the central portions of lobes: visualization of airways in the peripheral portions of the lungs in the absence of parenchymal consolidation is reliable evidence of abnormality.

air trapping (as a manifestation of small airways disease identifiable on expiration scans), and emphysema (see Fig. 3-100; Fig. 3-101). Although a combination of these findings enables accurate diagnosis in most cases, wide variations exist in their definitions as currently used.

Bronchial Dilatation

Recognition of bronchial dilatation is key to the CT diagnosis of bronchiectasis. Unfortunately, to date, no absolute CT criteria of normal bronchial diameter have been determined, and the HRCT diagnosis of bronchial dilatation remains controversial (Table 3-11) (208–212).

Bronchoarterial Ratios. In most cases, bronchiectasis is considered to be present when the internal diameter of a bronchus is greater than the diameter of the adjacent pulmonary artery branch (see Fig. 3-100A, C, D) (213). The accuracy of this bronchoarterial relationship has been validated in certain studies comparing CT with bronchography in patients with bronchiectasis (214–217). In patients with bronchiectasis, the bronchial diameter is often much larger that the pulmonary artery diameter, a finding that reflects not only the presence of bronchial dilatation, but also some reduction in pulmonary artery size, likely a consequence of

hypoxia in regions of bronchiectasis resulting in decreased lung perfusion and a corresponding decrease in pulmonary artery size (211). Another potential limitation of the use of bronchoarterial ratios is the necessity to identify airways and accompanying vessels. This may not always be possible, especially in patients with coexisting parenchymal consolidation (209). Kang and associates (209), in a study of 47 resected lobes with documented bronchiectasis, failed to identify 3 cases in which bronchoarterial ratios could not be assessed because of the presence of parenchymal consolidation. These findings reinforce the recommendation that the diagnosis of bronchiectasis should only be considered in patients who have no evidence of active parenchymal consolidation (218).

Unfortunately, the reliability of bronchoarterial ratios in the diagnosis of bronchiectasis is limited (209,211,219,220). Lynch and colleagues (208), in an assessment of 27 healthy subjects living in Denver, Colorado, found that 37 (26%) of 142 bronchi (or 59% of study subjects) evaluated had abnormal bronchoarterial ratios. Similarly, Kim and associates (211) also documented the unreliability of abnormal bronchoarterial ratios in the diagnosis of bronchiectasis, especially for persons living at high altitudes. In this study, 9 of 17 (53%) of healthy persons living at an altitude of 1,600

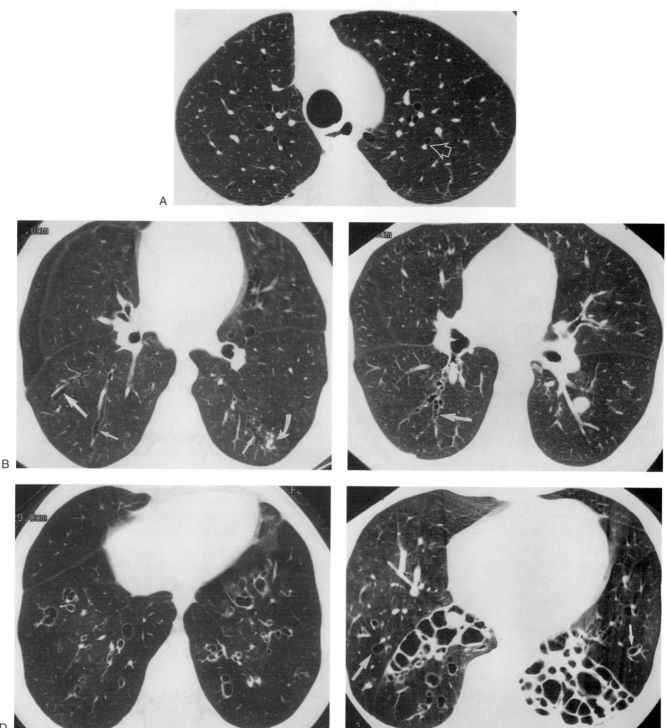

FIG. 3-100. Bronchiectasis: high-resolution CT findings. **A:** Cylindric bronchiectasis. Section shows moderate dilatation of thin-walled airways in both upper lobes. Airways oriented vertically appear as circular or oval lucencies: when dilated, these appear larger than their adjacent pulmonary artery branches (the so-called signet ring sign) (*arrow*). Note the association in this case with marked tracheomegaly. **B:** Cylindric bronchiectasis. Section through the superior segments of both lower lobes shows moderate dilatation of thin-walled airways bilaterally (*arrows*). Airways coursing in the plane of the section are seen along their length: when dilated, these extend into the lung periphery and characteristically show a lack of tapering. In this case, one also sees evidence of mild bronchial impaction resulting in a cluster of small centrilobular nodules adjacent to a peripherally dilated airway (*curved arrow*). **C:** Varicose bronchiectasis. Section through the superior segments shows moderately severe varicose bronchiectasis on the right (*arrow*). Varicose bronchiectasis results in a beaded appearance that is only reliably identified when airways course in the same plane as the CT section. **D:** Cystic bronchiectasis: section through the lower lobes in the same patient as shown in **B.** Cystic bronchiectasis results in a ballooning of the airways: when moderate (as in this case), relationships between airways and adjacent pulmonary artery branches are maintained. Cystic bronchiectasis may result in either thin-walled or thick-walled airways. **E:** Cystic bronchiectasis. When severe, cystic bronchiectasis results in a cluster of thick-walled cystic spaces (so-called cluster of grapes), usually in association with moderate to marked volume loss (in this case resulting in posterior displacement of both major fissures). Although this appearance may superficially mimic honeycombing, note the absence of reticular densities in aerated portions of lung always present in patients with underlying parenchymal fibrosis. In this case, less severe foci of bronchiectasis are also clearly discernible within both upper lobes and in the right lower lobe (*arrows*).

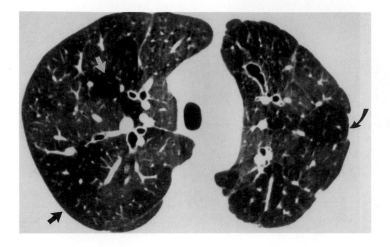

FIG. 3-101. Bronchiectasis: value of expiratory scanning. 1.5-mm axial image obtained at expiration in a patient with bilateral upper lobe bronchiectasis. Air trapping (*arrows*) is considerable, particularly in regions without bronchiectasis resulting in focal areas of hyperlucent lung. Note the relative paucity and attenuation of vessels in these regions, presumably resulting from vasoconstriction secondary to hypoxia. Investigators have postulated that air trapping in patients with bronchiectasis is a manifestation of associated small airways disease. (From ref. 336, with permission.)

m had evidence of at least one bronchus equal to or greater in size than the adjacent pulmonary artery; of greater import, these same authors found that 2 of 16 (12.5%) persons living at sea level similarly showed evidence of at least one abnormally dilated airway. Furthermore, and surprisingly, evaluation of the distribution of these abnormal airways failed to identify any significant difference in the likelihood of abnormal bronchoarterial ratios in airways either by lobe or by anteroposterior location within the lungs (211). A similar lack of variation by segments, lobes, or lungs has also been reported by Kim and colleagues (221).

The definition of an abnormal bronchoarterial ratio varies widely among reported series (see Table 3-11) (209,210, 212,213,220,221). In addition to variations in size criteria, with a range as great as one to two times the diameter of the adjacent pulmonary artery, as well as the use of internal versus external bronchial diameters, important differences may be also attributable to the use of visual inspection versus objective measurements of bronchial and arterial dimensions (Fig. 3-102). As emphasized by Kim and associates (211), visual inspection alone may lead to overestimation of bronchoarterial ratios because of a subtle optical illusion in which the diameter of hollow circles appears larger than that of solid circles despite their identical size.

Despite potential variability in normal bronchial size, CT measurements of bronchial diameter have proved remarkably consistent (222,223). Desai and associates (222) evalu-

ated both interobserver and intraobserver variation in CT measurements of bronchial wall circumference in 61 subsegmental bronchi and found the reproducibility of these measurements sufficiently significant to be clinically useful in demonstrating the progression of bronchiectasis. Unfortunately, these time-consuming measurements are unlikely to be of routine clinical use. As emphasized by Diederich and associates (212), visual inspection remains the mainstay for assessing bronchial dilatation because obtaining objective measurements (with or without the use of calipers) is time consuming and often clinically impracticable. In this regard, visual inspection has been shown to have acceptable interobserver variability. Using visual inspection only, Diederich and colleagues (212) found close agreement among 3 readers in both the detection ($\kappa = 0.78$) and the assessment of the severity ($\kappa = 0.68$) of bronchiectasis.

Lack of Bronchial Tapering. Lack of bronchial tapering has come to be increasingly recognized as a critical means for diagnosing bronchiectasis, in particular subtle cylindric bronchiectasis (see Fig. 3-100B,C; Fig. 3-103). First emphasized by Lynch and colleagues (224) as a necessary finding, the lack of bronchial tapering has been reported by some investigators to be the most sensitive means for diagnosing bronchiectasis. Kang and associates (209), for example, in an assessment of 47 lobes with pathologically proved bronchiectasis, found lack of tapering of bronchial lumina in 37 (79%) cases as compared with abnormal bronchioarterial

FIG. 3-102. Airway imaging: electronic windowing. **A–D:** Effect of varying window widths. Enlargements of identical sections through the right lower lobe, imaged with window widths of 1,600, 1,200, 1,000, and 850 HU, respectively, using a constant window level of −650 HUs. With decreasing window width, contrast resolution is improved, resulting in easier identification of focal emphysema (*arrows* in **A** and **D**) at the cost of a significant increase in the apparent size of vessels (*curved arrows* in **A** and **D**) and, to a lesser degree, bronchial wall thickness. **E–H:** Effect of varying window levels: identical section as shown in **A–D,** imaged with window levels of −700, 600, 500, and 400 HU, respectively, using a constant window width of 1,200 HU. With decreasing window levels, the marked loss of contrast resolution renders focal areas of emphysema all but unidentifiable (*arrows* in **E** and **H**). Other then rendering them more difficult to identify, little change is noted in apparent vessel size or bronchial wall thickness. This series of images (**A–H**) emphasizes the need to use a range of window levels and widths selectively, depending on the nature of the pathologic or anatomic features to be evaluated. Although narrower windows have the effect of rendering soft tissue structures slightly larger, in most cases, this is more than offset by enhanced visualization of parenchymal detail.

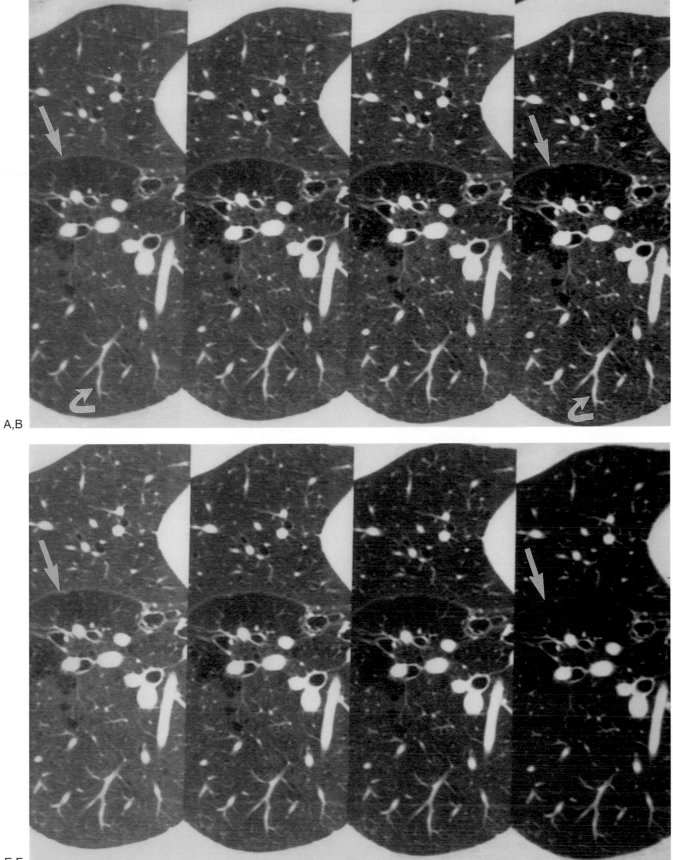

A,B

C,D

E,F

G,H

TABLE 3-11. *Bronchietasis: CT criteria*

Bronchial dilatation
  ID bronchus > adjacent PA (214)
  OD bronchus > adjacent PA (222)
    Minimum ID > 110% (211, 213)
    Minimum ID > 150% (210)
    Grade 1, <2× diameter adjacent PA; grade 2, 3×; grade
      3, >3× (223)
  Lack of Tapering
    Visual inspection (194, 209)
    Maintains same diameter >2 cm after branching (221)
  Peripheral bronchial dilatation
    Peripheral ½ of lung (223)
    Peripheral ⅓ of lung (194, 211, 336)
    Within 1 cm of costal/mediastinal pleura (210)
    Abutting mediastinal pleura (210)
Bronchial wall thickening
  Subjective (191, 194, 210)
  Bronchial wall 2× thickness normal adjacent bronchi (230)
  Minimum > diameter adjacent PA (229)
  Grade 1, 0.5 diameter adjacent PA; grade 2, 0.5–1.0; grade
    3>1× (223)
  ID <80% total outside diameter (213)
Mucoid impaction
  Tubular or Y-shaped structures ± branching or rounded
  opacities in cross section differentiated from blood vessels
  by position relative to adjacent patent bronchi (229)

ID, internal diameter; OD, outer diameter; PA, pulmonary artery.

ratios seen in only 28. Accurate assessment of this finding is difficult in the absence of contiguous sections, especially for vertically or obliquely oriented airways. Despite frequent citation, the value of this sign in studies in which noncontiguous, high-resolution 1- to 3-mm sections only are obtained is doubtful. Use of contiguous images is especially critical when identification requires that the diameter of airways remain unchanged for at least 2 cm after branching (220). As discussed later, these findings have clear implications for optimizing scan technique in patients with suspected inflammatory airway disease.

Visualization of Peripheral Airways. Another frequently cited manifestation of bronchiectasis is identification of airways in the lung periphery (see Fig. 3-99). Variously defined as the ability to identify airways in the peripheral one-half to one-third of the lung, this finding has proved useful because normally, even with HRCT technique, airways are rarely identifiable in the outer portions of the lung parenchyma. Kim and colleagues (220) more precisely characterized the value of this sign by differentiating between airways near the costal pleura and those near the mediastinal pleura. Using 1 cm from the pleural surface as indicative of bronchial dilatation, these authors found that visualization of bronchi within 1 cm of the pleura could be identified in 81% and 53% of patients with clinical or pathologic evidence of cylindric bronchiectasis, respectively. Most important, although bronchi were identified within 1 cm of the mediastinal pleura in

40% of anatomically normal persons, in no case was a bronchus identified within the same distance from the costal pleura in any anatomically normal person (220). Although bronchi normally may be seen within 1 cm of the mediastinal pleura, bronchi abutting the mediastinal pleura were always abnormal.

Bronchial Wall Thickening

In distinction to bronchial dilatation, the finding of bronchial wall thickening is not specific for bronchiectasis. Not surprisingly, however, bronchial wall abnormalities are commonly found in patients with bronchiectasis, thus making identification of this finding important (Fig. 3-104). Unfortunately, as with definitions of bronchial dilatation, precise measurements of bronchial wall thickness on CT have not been established.

As reported by Weibel (225), 2nd- to 4th-generation segmental airways have mean diameters of between 5 and 8 mm with walls measuring approximately 1.5 mm; 6th- to 8th-generation airways have mean diameters measuring between 1.5 and 3 mm with walls of approximately 0.3 mm; and 11th- to 13th-generation airways have diameters measuring 0.7 to 1 mm with walls of 0.1 to 0.15 mm. Because a bronchus is usually recognized only when its walls are visualized, one cannot resolve bronchi with a wall thickness of less than 300 μm. This corresponds to bronchi of about 1.5 to 2 mm in diameter, equivalent to the 7th to 9th generations of airways. Rarely, smaller bronchi, approximately 1 mm in diameter, can be recognized coursing perpendicularly with the plane of a 1-mm thick section by virtue of their lower density and proximity to an adjacent pulmonary artery, even though their walls cannot be resolved (226,227).

To date, identification of thickened bronchial walls has been largely subjective (see Fig. 3-104) (194,209). Attempts to define bronchial wall thickening more precisely have largely involved visually assessing or measuring ratios between bronchial walls and adjacent pulmonary arteries or nearby normal airways (see Table 3-11) (212,220,228,229). Because bronchiectasis and bronchial wall thickening are often multifocal rather than diffuse and uniform, a comparison of one lung region with another can be helpful in making this diagnosis. Objective measurements are cumbersome and have little use in general clinical practice. However, using a visual estimation of the internal diameter of airways as being either between 50% and 80% or more than 50% of the diameter of the adjacent pulmonary artery (indicative of mild or severe bronchial wall thickening, respectively), Diederich and associates (213) found acceptable levels of agreement among three readers ($\kappa = 0.64$), a finding suggesting that visual assessment of bronchial wall thickening is a reproducible and hence valuable sign for evaluating airways, especially on sequential studies (212).

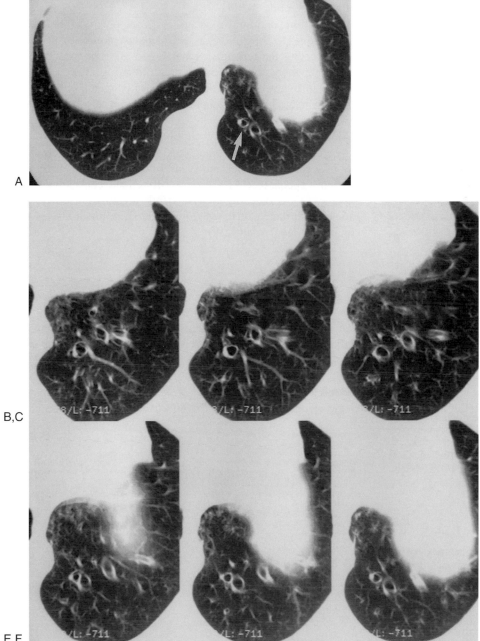

FIG. 3-103. Bronchiectasis: evaluation with helical CT. **A:** A 1-mm axial section shows dilated peripheral bronchi (*arrow*) in the left lower lobe. **B–G:** Enlargements of sequential 3-mm helical sections reconstructed every 2 mm obtained through the same anatomic region of the left lower lobe as shown in **A,** using a pitch of 2. In comparison with routine axial images, volumetric acquisition allows each individual airway to be evaluated sequentially as it extends toward the periphery. This technique may be of particular value in assessing subtle lack of tapering in oblique or vertically oriented. (From ref. 9, with permission.)

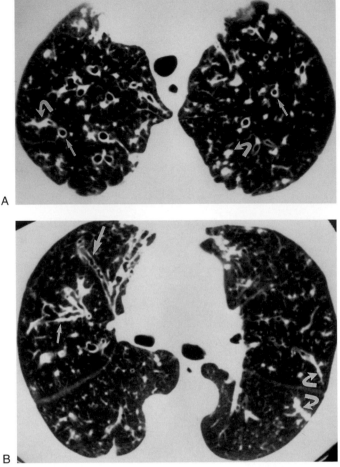

A

B

FIG. 3-104. Bronchiectasis: evaluation of bronchial wall thickening. **A, B:** Selected 1- and 5-mm sections show markedly dilated airways throughout both lungs. In this case, bronchial wall thickening is clearly apparent both in airways coursing vertically (*straight arrows* in **A**) as well as in the plane of the CT section (*straight arrows* in **B**) (compare with Fig. 3–100A, B). Although this finding is often subjective and subject to influence by variations in electronic windowing, in most cases, bronchial wall thickening is readily apparent. In this case, numerous peripheral nodular and branching densities are also apparent, consistent with mucoid impaction (*curved arrows* in **A** and **B**).

Mucoid Impaction

The appearance of fluid- or mucus-filled airways depends on both their size and orientation relative to the CT scan plane. Larger fluid-filled airways result in abnormal lobular or branching structures when they lie in the same plane as the CT scan (Figs. 3-105–3-107). Although confusion between fluid-filled branching airways and abnormally dilated vessels is possible, especially in studies performed without intravenous contrast administration, in nearly all cases, recognition of mucoid-impacted airways is straightforward. The diagnosis is usually simplified by the identification of other foci of bronchiectasis (see Fig. 3-105). In problematic cases, the distinction between larger fluid-filled bronchi and dilated blood vessels is easily made by repeat scanning of patients after a bolus of intravenous contrast medium.

The finding of dilated, mucous-filled airways, especially when central or predominantly segmental or lobar in distribution, should alert one to the possibility of central endobronchial obstruction, resulting either from tumor (especially carcinoid tumors) or from foreign body aspiration (see Figs. 3-106 and 3-107). As previously discussed, the use of intravenous contrast media in this setting may allow differentiation between central tumor and fluid-filled peripheral airways (see Fig. 3-107).

Mucoid impaction also occurs as a component of the sequestration spectrum, either as an isolated phenomenon, usually affecting the left upper lobe (Fig. 3-108), or typically as a component of intralobar sequestration (Fig. 3-109). As shown in Figure 3-108, combinations of congenital abnormalities related to the sequestration spectrum also may be encountered.

Fluid-filled small airways in the peripheral lung are usually identifiable either as branching structures within the center of secondary lobules, aptly described as having a "tree-in-bud" appearance (183), or as ill-defined centrilobular nodules (230–232): these are frequently identified in association with bronchiectasis (see Fig. 3-100B) and are discussed in greater detail later (233).

Ancillary Signs: Bronchiolar Disease

As CT has become established as the modality of choice for assessing bronchiectasis, investigators have become increasingly aware that, in addition to signs of large airway inflammation, most patients also have evidence of small airways disease (see Figs. 3-100B, 3-101, and 3-104). Kang and colleagues (209), for example, in their study of 47 resected lobes with documented bronchiectasis, found pathologic evidence of bronchiolitis in 85%. Results included 6

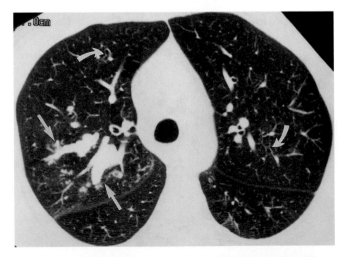

FIG. 3-105. Mucoid impaction central airways: 1-mm section of tubular, branching structures in the right upper lobe (*arrows*) characteristic of mucoid impaction. In this case, the presence of additional scattered foci of bronchiectasis (*curved arrows*) further simplifying the diagnosis.

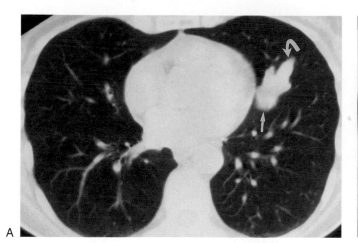
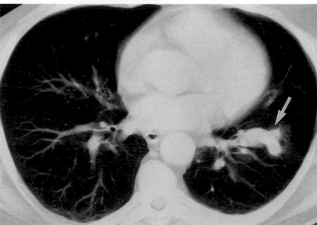
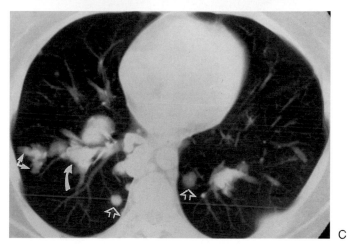

FIG. 3-106. Mucoid impaction secondary to bronchial obstruction. **A:** Section through the lingula shows a rounded density (*arrow*) associated with peripheral tubular, branching densities (*curved arrow*). This appearance should suggest the possibility of a central tumor mass, in this case resulting from a bronchoscopically verified carcinoid tumor. **B:** Section through the lower lobes in a different patient from **A** shows a tubular branching structure in the anterior portion of the left lower lobe (*arrow*). Although initially interpreted as representing mucoid impaction only, at bronchoscopy, a carcinoid tumor was identified obstructing the anterobasilar segmental bronchus. **C:** A 1.5-mm section through the lung bases shows the typical appearance of hematogenous metastases (*open arrows*) in this patient with documented metastatic renal cell carcinoma. Tubular branching densities can be identified in the anterobasilar segment of the right lower lobe (*forked arrow*) associated with central bronchial obstruction (*curved arrow*). At bronchoscopy, an endoluminal tumor was identified. (**C,** from ref. 336, with permission.)

lobes with obliterative bronchiolitis, 18 with inflammatory or suppurative bronchiolitis, and 16 with both obliterative and inflammatory bronchiolitis. Of these, CT findings consistent with bronchiolitis were identified in 30 (75%) of 47 lobes, including a pattern of mosaic attenuation (*n* = 21), bronchiolectasis (*n* = 17), centrilobular nodular, or branching opacities (*n* = 10) and consolidation (*n* = 8) (209).

The finding of mosaic attenuation or focal air trapping on expiratory scans, in particular, may prove of special interest as an early manifestation of bronchiectasis (see Fig. 3-101). In one study of 70 patients (234) with CT evidence of bronchiectasis visible in 52% of lobes evaluated, areas of decreased attenuation (mosaic perfusion) were visible on inspiratory scans in 20% of lobes and on expiration (air trapping) in 34%. Although areas of decreased attenuation on expiratory scans were more prevalent in lobes with severe (59%) or localized (28%) bronchiectasis, in 17% of lobes, air trapping could be identified in the absence of associated bronchiectasis. This finding has led to speculation that evidence of bronchiolar disease may, in fact, precede and even lead to the development of bronchiectasis (234). In this same study, the presence of decreased attenuation on expiratory scans was also associated with mucoid impaction, seen in 73% of lobes with large mucus plugs and in 58% of those with centrilobular mucus plugs. These same authors noted a correlation (*r* = 0.40, *p* < .001) between the total extent and severity of bronchiectasis and the extent of decreased attenuation shown on expiratory CT. Not surprisingly, in 55 patients who had pulmonary function tests, the extent of expiratory attenuation abnormalities proved inversely related to measures of airway obstruction such as forced expiratory volume in 1 second and the ratio of that parameter to forced vital capacity (FEV$_1$/FVC) (234).

Extent and Severity

Analogous to the lack of standardization for estimating both bronchial dilatation and wall thickening, little consensus exists on the best method for estimating extent and severity of disease in patients with bronchiectasis (191,210,220, 228,235). Although of only limited value in distinguishing among the various causes of bronchiectasis (220), assessing disease extent and severity is important, especially in patients for whom sequential CT studies are to be used to

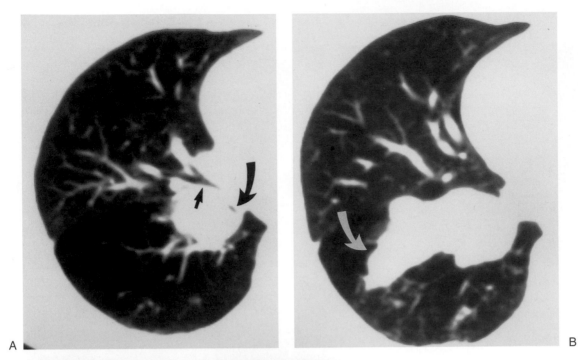

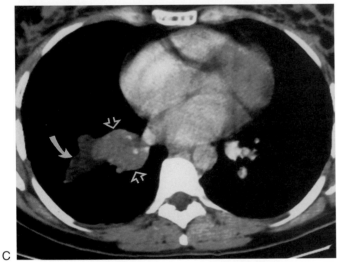

FIG. 3-107. Mucoid impaction: value of contrast enhancement. **A, B:** Magnified CT scans at (**A**) and just below (**B**) the origin of the middle lobe bronchus shows marked narrowing of both middle lobe (*straight arrow* in **A**) and proximal right lower lobe (*curved arrow* in **A**) bronchi. A branching density can be identified within the right lower lobe (*arrow* in **B**), associated with hyperlucency of peripheral aerated portions of lower lobe, best seen in **A**. These findings strongly suggest the presence of a central tumor mass with associated mucoid impaction and peripheral air trapping. **C:** Contrast-enhanced CT scan at same level as **B** shows a large central tumor mass (*open arrows*) that is easily distinguished from more peripheral lower density mucus-impacted airways (*curved arrow*). Identification of central obstructing lesions typically is made easier by intravenous administration of contrast material. A central carcinoid tumor with associated peripheral mucoid impaction was proved surgically.

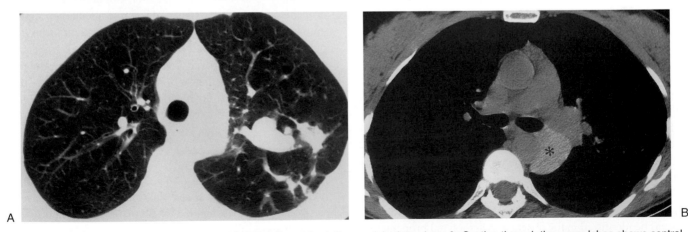

FIG. 3-108. Complex congenital disease: mucoid impaction of the left upper lobe bronchus. **A:** Section through the upper lobes shows central tubular branching structure on the left side, associated with extensive emphysema throughout the left upper lobe in a patient with congenital mucoid impaction of the left upper lobe bronchus. **B:** Noncontrast-enhanced section in the same patient as **A** shows a uniform high-density mass (*asterisk*). The finding that this lesion has insinuated itself between the descending aorta and left main pulmonary artery and the posterior wall of the left main stem bronchus is consistent with the diagnosis of a bronchogenic cyst. In this case, high density within the cyst presumably is due to either proteinaceous secretions or prior hemorrhage.

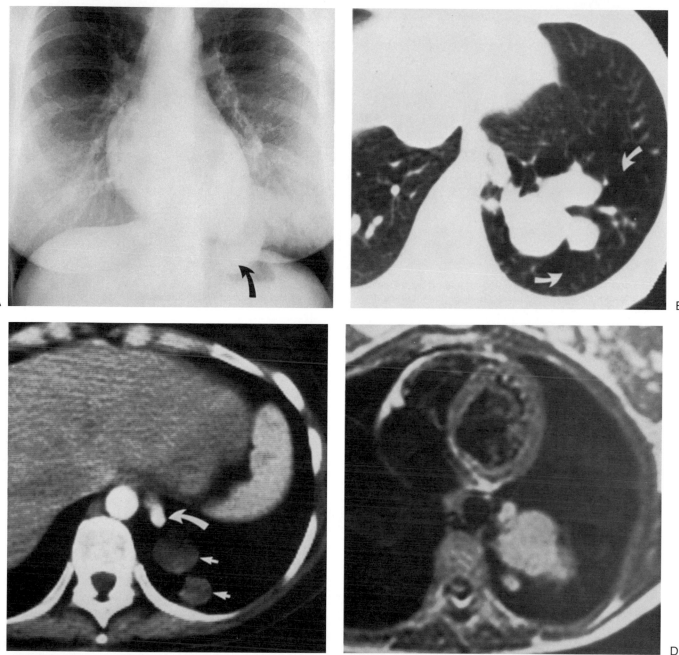

FIG. 3-109. Intralobar pulmonary sequestration. **A:** PA radiograph shows serpiginous densities at the left lung base, suggestive of pulmonary sequestration (*curved arrow*). **B:** CT scan through the left lung base, imaged with lung windows, shows characteristic appearance of dilated, branching densities surrounded by hyperaerated, emphysematous pulmonary parenchyma (*arrows*). **C:** Section through the lung bases following a bolus of intravenous contrast media. An anomalous vessel can be identified (*curved arrow*) coursing within the LLL, showing the same degree of opacification as the descending aorta, confirming this as arterial. Note the lack of enhancement within fluid-filled, dilated airways (*small arrows*). **D:** Every-beat gated, axial MR section through the LLL shows dilated, mucoid impacted bronchi, easily identified due to their characteristic, branching configuration (compare with **B** and **C**). Considerable signal is present within these airways, even on this relatively T1-weighted sequence, presumably due to the high protein content of the bronchial secretions. Note that unlike the corresponding CT scan, emphysematous changes within the LLL cannot be identified (compare with **B**). (*continues*)

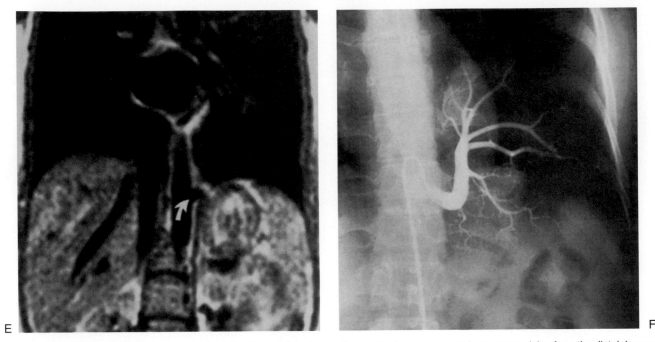

FIG. 3-109. *Continued.* **E:** ECG-gated coronal section through the descending aorta shows an anomalous artery arising from the distal descending aorta, clearly originating above the diaphragm (*curved arrow*). **F:** Coned-down view following selective catheterization of the anomalous vessel.

evaluate response to therapy and progression of disease (228,235).

In general, attempts have focused on the use of grading systems designed to assess the number of either segments or lobes, with corresponding correlation with disease severity. Bhalla and associates (228), in the most detailed method to date, used nine separate variables including extent of mucus plugging, peribronchial thickening, generations of bronchial divisions involved, the number of bullae, and the presence of emphysema, in addition to a 3-point severity scale to calculate a global CT score based on 25 points to correspond with prior radiographic scoring systems. Based on this approach, these authors found CT to be a valuable tool for objectively evaluating the extent and severity of bronchiectasis in patients with cystic fibrosis. Unfortunately, this system is extremely time consuming and is not of value for routine clinical assessment. Smith and colleagues (210), using a modification of the scoring system recommended by Bhalla and colleagues, replaced the assessment of segments (which are often difficult to identify) with that of lobes using a 5-point scale based on a visual assessment of the number of abnormal bronchi as less than 25%, 25% to 49%, 50% to 74%, or more than 75%, respectively. Although this approach has the benefit of relative simplicity, it has not proved extremely reliable. Using this same system, Diederich and associates (212) found only moderate interobserver agreement among 3 readers ($\kappa = 0.58$) for assessing disease severity in a study of 88 patients with suspected bronchiectasis. Based on these findings, in our opinion, when precise assessment of disease severity is clinically warranted, a more detailed scoring system is requisite (228,235).

CT Technique

Given the range and subtlety of CT findings present in patients with bronchiectasis, it is hardly surprising that accurate diagnosis requires meticulous attention to scan technique (See Table 3-3) (215,216,236–238). Grenier and associates (239), in a landmark article comparing CT and bronchography in 44 lungs in 36 patients, found that CT confirmed the diagnosis of bronchiectasis with a sensitivity of 97% and a specificity of 93%. Numerous other investigators have reported similar results. Young and colleagues (217) also assessed the reliability of HRCT in the assessment of bronchiectasis, as compared with bronchography, in 259 segmental bronchi from 70 lobes of 27 lungs. Results of HRCT were positive in 87 of 89 segmental bronchi shown to have bronchiectasis (sensitivity, 98%). Results of HRCT were negative in 169 of 170 segmental bronchi without bronchiectasis at bronchography (specificity, 99%). Similar results have been reported by Giron and associates (240).

Nonetheless, over the past decade, increasing awareness of the variety and limitations of CT criteria used for assessing bronchiectasis, as well as technologic improvements, including the appearance of both ultrafast and helical CT techniques, have clearly altered our concepts of optimal scan technique. To date, certain techniques have been suggested to improve diagnosis both of large and small airways disease. These techniques include the use of both inspiratory and expiratory scans to assess small airways disease, as well as angled gantries to assess obliquely oriented airways, and low-dose techniques to minimize radiation exposure, especially in younger patients, with or without use of helical or ultrafast CT scanners.

Helical CT

Reports have suggested a role for helical scanning for evaluating bronchiectasis (see Fig. 3-103). Van der Bruggen-Bogaarts and colleagues (241), in an evaluation of 31 patients with suspected bronchiectasis, found that spiral CT with 5-mm collimation was only slightly less sensitive than HRCT imaging in the detection of bronchiectasis. As documented by Engeler and colleagues (242), in a study of 50 consecutive patients using helical CT at 4 preselected levels through the thorax, volumetric data acquisition proved especially helpful in comparison with HRCT scans when assessing the lung bases. In the most definitive study performed to date, Lucidarme and associates (4) compared 1.5-mm sections obtained at 10-mm intervals with a single 24-second volumetric acquisition using 3-mm collimation, a pitch of 1.6, image reconstruction at 2-mm intervals, and an angled gantry in 50 consecutive patients. Helical CT was more accurate than routine HRCT in the identification of bronchiectasis; interobserver variability was also considerably better for helical CT in the assessment of segmental airways. Although helical CT failed to identify bronchiectasis in 7 segments in which the disease was diagnosed with HRCT, in 4 cases, including 3 with middle lobe disease, a diagnosis of subsegmental cylindric bronchiectasis was made only with helical CT. In comparison, in no patients was a diagnosis of bronchiectasis established by HRCT alone.

These data contradict previous reports in which axial 3-mm sections were assessed. As documented by Munro and associates (243) in their study of the accuracy of CT with 3-mm collimation versus bronchography, overall, the sensitivity of CT was 84% and its specificity was 82%, compared with bronchography. The differences in accuracy noted between this study and that of Lucidarme likely relate to the use of volumetric data acquisition in conjunction with select 1-mm sections.

In our opinion, the ability to acquire data volumetrically represents an important advance in the diagnosis of bronchiectasis, especially cases of mild cylindric bronchiectasis, and this technique should be routinely incorporated whenever possible. Despite reports to the contrary, evaluation of a lack of bronchial tapering in particular using noncontiguous 1-mm sections effectively reduces the value of this sign to those bronchi that course only within the plane of the CT scan (see Fig. 3-103). Despite the excellent sensitivity of HRCT, bronchiectasis may be focal and exceedingly subtle on HRCT scans. Cylindric bronchiectasis, in particular, can be missed on HRCT, especially if care is not taken to obtain images in deep inspiration (239,240,244). Giron and associates (240), in a study of 54 patients with bronchographic evidence of bronchiectasis, found that by using 1-mm sections every 10 mm, 3 cases were missed, all with mild cylindric bronchiectasis.

Based on these reports, our current recommendation, modified from that proposed by Lucidarme and colleagues (4), calls for an initial sequence of 1-mm sections through the upper lobes, followed by 3-mm sections through the central airways with a pitch of 2 reconstructed every 2 mm, followed by 1-mm axial images through the lung bases. A pitch of 2 ensures that the largest possible lung volume is scanned helically with minimal loss of spatial resolution in the Z axis (9).

Expiratory Scanning

Given increasing awareness of the high incidence of bronchiolar disease in patients with bronchiectasis, the use of expiration scans to identify focal air trapping also may be of benefit in selected cases. Although this is most easily accomplished by use of selected axial images acquired in expiration, one may also acquire data using either ultrafast or helical CT techniques (9,234,245). One of two methods may be used. In the first, most applicable to ultrafast CT scanners, images are repeatedly acquired at one preselected level throughout the respiratory cycle. Although this technique has the advantage of allowing detailed physiologic evaluation of airway mechanics, it is limited by acquiring data in a single plane only, resulting as well in considerable radiation exposure. In distinction, one can obtain two separate volumetric acquisitions, first in deep inspiration and then through the same region in expiration (5,6,176). This approach has the clear advantage of providing evaluation of a considerably larger portion of the airways and lung. In either case, the result is a series of dynamic images allowing identification of focal areas of air trapping as well as evaluation of airway mechanics.

Despite obvious improvement in detecting focal air trapping provided by expiratory scanning, whether or not these techniques need to be used in all cases remains unclear. In our experience, especially when extensive bronchiectasis is apparent, expiratory scans are of only limited diagnostic utility. In distinction, in patients with more subtle disease, especially those with equivocal findings of mild bronchiectasis, the addition of a few expiratory scans through selected regions of interest is likely to prove beneficial. The advantages of expiratory images in patients with suspected bronchiectasis have yet to be validated.

Angled Gantry and Low-Dose Scanning

As suggested by Remy-Jardin and Remy (8), visualization of bronchiectatic segments also may be enhanced by use of 20-degree cranial angulation of the CT gantry. This technique may be of value in equivocal cases, especially for those airways that normally course obliquely, such as the middle lobe and lingular bronchi. Also of interest is the potential use of low-dose HRCT scans for performing routine follow-up scans in patients with severe chronic disease (228,246). Bhalla and associates (228), evaluating scans obtained using both 70 and 20 mA, showed that high-quality HRCT images of bronchiectatic airways could be obtained in patients with cystic fibrosis.

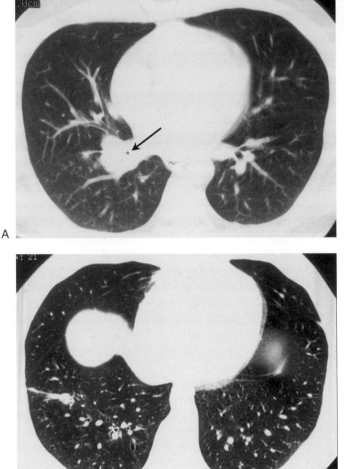

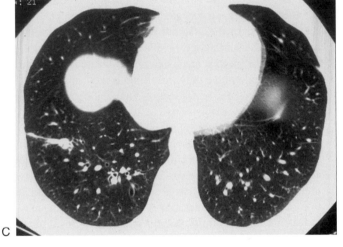

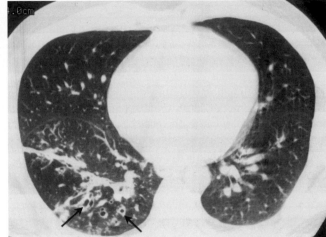

FIG. 3-110. Reversible bronchiectasis. **A, B:** Sections through the lower lobes show marked narrowing of the right lower lobe bronchus (*arrow* in **A**) associated with consolidation and bronchial dilation throughout the basilar segments of the right lower lobe (*arrows* in **B**). This finding was initially interpreted as likely due to central tumor with peripheral infection. **C:** Section at approximately the same level as **B** obtained several weeks after bronchoscopic extraction of a foreign body lodged within the right lower lobe bronchus at the same level as shown in **A**. After antibiotic therapy, one sees marked clearing of the pneumonia, and the airways have returned to a near-normal appearance. In this case, apparent bronchiectasis was due to reversible inflammation only.

Pitfalls in Diagnosis

Despite the overall accuracy of CT for diagnosing bronchiectasis, certain potential pitfalls have been described (218). Particularly frequent are those due to motion artifacts, both respiratory and cardiac (247). Respiratory artifacts, in particular, result in ghosting that can closely mimic the appearance of tram tracks.

Bronchiectasis is especially difficult to diagnose in patients with either parenchymal consolidation or atelectasis because CT often discloses dilated peripheral airways that will revert to normal after resolution of the lung disease, so-called "reversible bronchiectasis" (Fig. 3-110). Another potential pitfall related to consolidation is that, as discussed previously, consolidation may obscure vascular anatomy and thus may render interpretation of bronchoarterial ratios difficult or impossible (209).

Rarely, the appearance of cavitary nodules in patients with widespread bronchoalveolar cell carcinoma, cavitary metastases, or even cystic *Pneumocystis carinii* pneumonia or Langerhans' cell histiocytosis may result in "pseudobronchiectasis" (Fig. 3-111). In patients with Langerhans' cell histiocytosis, bizarrely shaped cysts are often seen, especially in the upper lobes. Because these cysts may be appear to branch, their appearance may be suggestive of bronchiectasis. In fact, pathologically, some of these cystic abnormalities do indeed represent abnormally dilated bronchi, ostensibly the result of peribronchiolar inflammation.

Most important, bronchial dilatation may occur as a component of diffuse fibrotic lung disease. The result is so-called "traction bronchiectasis" (Fig. 3-112). In most cases, this condition is easily identified because peripheral bronchi appear irregularly thick walled or corkscrewed and are invaria-

FIG. 3-112. Traction bronchiectasis. **A:** Enlargement of a section through the right lower lobe shows corkscrewed bronchi associated with marked architectural distortion and diffuse course reticulation. These findings are characteristic of parenchymal fibrosis in a patient with documented interstitial pulmonary fibrosis, with resulting traction bronchiectasis. **B:** Enlargement of a section through the right upper lobe in a patient with documented stage 3 sarcoidosis. In this case, parenchymal distortion is most marked in the central portion of the upper lobes (compare with **A**), resulting in characteristic corkscrewing and dilatation of upper lobe airways (*arrow*).

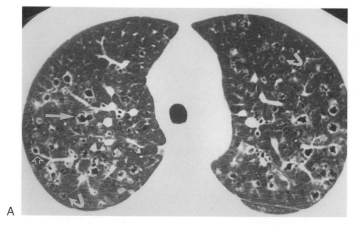

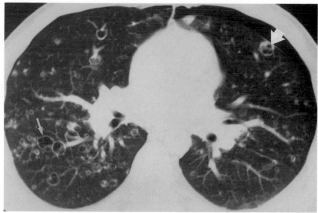

A

B

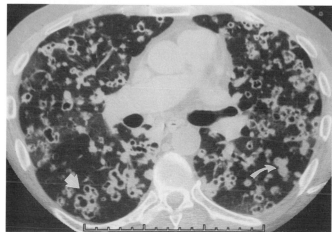

C

FIG. 3-111. Pitfalls in the diagnosis of bronchiectasis: diffuse cystic lung disease. **A:** Langerhans' cell histiocytosis. Section through the midlungs shows scattered, thick-walled cystic lesions. Although some appear to be branching (*arrow*), others are unrelated to any accompanying artery (*curved arrows*), whereas others appear to have feeding vessels (*open arrow*). Note also the presence of few ill-defined subpleural nodules. This constellation of findings is characteristic of Langerhans' cell histiocytosis. Although most of these cystic lesions represent cavitating nodules, some likely actually represent abnormally dilated airways. **B:** Cystic *Pneumocystis carinii* pneumonia. Section through the midlungs shows scattered thin-walled and thick-walled cysts, some with an apparent branching configuration (*small arrow*). Many of these cysts are unrelated to adjacent arteries, whereas others are clearly subpleural (*large arrow*), accounting in this case for the presence of a small anterior pneumothorax on the left side. **C:** Metastatic adenocarcinoma: 1-mm section in a patient with adenocarcinoma metastatic to the airways. The bronchi are dilated diffusely and are thick-walled (*arrow*), without central obstruction. Solid lobular densities (*curved arrow*) represent impacted bronchi. (From ref. 218, with permission.)

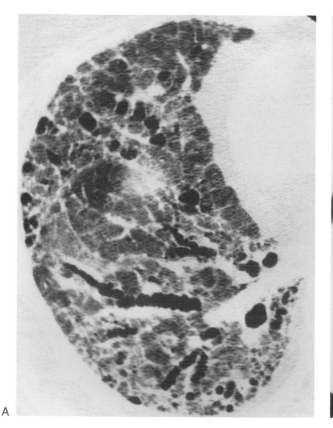

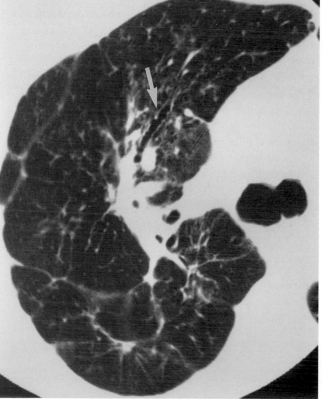

A

B

bly found in association with diffuse reticular changes or with honeycombing (see Fig. 3-112) (248).

Specific Causes

The CT appearances of several diseases associated with bronchiectasis have been described. In many of these diseases, such as hypogammaglobulinemia (249), the appearances of bronchiectasis are as described earlier. However, a few conditions associated with bronchiectasis have been reported to have distinctive HRCT appearances that can aid in their diagnosis. The most important of these diseases are nontuberculous mycobacterial infection, cystic fibrosis, and ABPA.

Atypical Mycobacterial Infection

Bronchiectasis in association with ill-defined clusters of centrilobular lung nodules on CT is characteristic of nontuberculous mycobacterial infection resulting from nontuberculous *Mycobacterium* (NTMB), in particular by MAC and *M. kansasii* (184–186,250). NTMBs are obligatory aerobic gram-positive rods with variable acid-fast staining that are ubiquitous organisms widely distributed throughout the environment resulting in widespread human exposure. NTMBs are typically low-grade pathogens that infrequently result in clinical infection (250).

Given the indolent nature of infection in most cases, the diagnosis is often difficult to establish. To distinguish definite infection from colonization, therefore, the following diagnostic criteria have been proposed: (a) isolation of NTMB from lung biopsy specimens; (b) identification of granulomas or acid-fast bacilli on transbronchial biopsy specimens in association with a positive culture from other respiratory secretions; (c) four or more sputum cultures demonstrating heavy growth of NTMB; (d) bronchoscopic washings demonstrating *M. kansasii,* because this organism is only rarely present as a contaminant; and (e) positive cultures obtained from bronchoscopic washings in association with positive blood or marrow cultures in AIDS patients only (251). Lesser degrees of diagnostic certainty result either in patients with bronchoscopic brushings demonstrating acid-fast bacilli with positive cultures obtained from bronchoalveolar lavage or in patients with two or three positive sputum cultures in association with radiographic evidence of pulmonary infiltrates or nodules (250,251). Definite diagnosis is requisite because patients usually require a prolonged course of multidrug therapy.

Three groups of patients have been identified to be at risk for pulmonary infection. Most commonly, NTMB affects elderly white men in their 60s who have preexisting lung disease, usually emphysema. Other predisposing factors include diabetes, alcoholism, and nonpulmonary malignant diseases. Infection in these patients results in a spectrum of radiographic findings indistinguishable from those seen in patients with tuberculosis, including linear and nodular den-

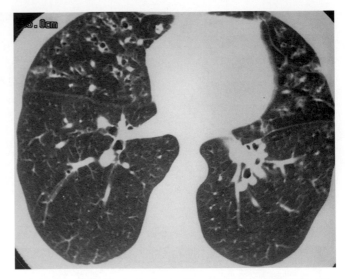

FIG. 3-113. Bronchiectasis due to *Mycobacterium avium-intercellulare* complex. Section through the midlungs show extensive bronchiectasis, primarily involving the middle lobe and lingula with only minimal changes of mild bronchiolar inflammation noted in the anterobasilar segment of the left lower lobe. This distribution of disease is characteristic of this infection, especially in elderly women.

sities most often involving the upper lobes and superior segments of the lower lobes, with or without evidence of cavitation and endobronchial spread. The second group of patients at risk are elderly women, typically without underlying predisposing factors. Radiographic findings in this group include scattered nodular densities associated with bronchiectasis, preferentially involving the lingular and middle lobes. This presentation is especially striking on CT (Fig. 3-113). Finally, also at risk are immunocompromised patients, especially those with AIDS (see Chapter 7). Unlike the preceding two groups, radiographs are typically normal in these patients. To date, MAC infection has been identified in up to 20% of AIDS patients, with estimates as high as 50% of patients infected at autopsy (250).

CT findings in patients with NTMB infection often are indistinguishable from those seen in patients with tuberculosis. However, as noted previously, a distinct pattern of involvement predominantly affecting the middle lobe and lingula has been identified in elderly women (185,186). As documented by Tanaka and colleagues (252) in a prospective study of 26 patients evaluated over a 4-year period with findings on CT suggestive of MAC pulmonary disease, including clusters of small nodules in the lung periphery and bronchiectasis, 13 (50%) of these patients proved to have positive MAC cultures from bronchial washings. Of these patients, epithelioid granulomas were demonstrated in 8 of 13. These findings are nearly identical to those reported by Swensen and associates (185), who also reported an approximately 50% rate of positive cultures in patients with bronchiectasis and nodules on CT. These nodules have a distinct appearance, identifiable as clustered around peripheral vessels and airways frequently having a tree-in-bud configuration (see Fig. 3-113). Histologically, this pattern is due either to impaction of peripheral bronchioles or to peribronchiolar granulomas (185). The finding of granulomas is especially significant in this population because it constitutes evidence that bronchiectasis, instead of being a precursor, is likely the result of chronic infection (186,252).

Cystic Fibrosis

Cystic fibrosis is a multisystem autosomal recessive disease in which a structural defect of the cystic fibrosis transmembrane regulator protein leads to abnormal chloride transport across epithelial membranes. This phenomenon leads to an abnormally low water content of airway mucus, resulting in decreased mucus clearance and mucus plugging and eventually to an increased incidence of bacterial infections, in particular due to *Pseudomonas*. Bronchial wall inflammation, progressing to widespread and severe bronchiectasis, is universal in patients with long-standing disease, and these features are commonly visible even on routine chest radiographs (253).

CT findings in patients with cystic fibrosis have been well described. The hallmark of disease is the finding of diffuse bronchiectasis, although an upper lobe distribution is often present (219,228,235,254). The central airways are also frequent sites of involvement, with bronchiectasis limited to the central airways in up to one-third of cases. These findings mimic those seen in patients with ABPA, a frequent complication in patients with cystic fibrosis.

Reports of the severity of bronchiectasis have varied. In one study, cylindric bronchiectasis was noted to predominate in 94% of lobes, compared with cystic bronchiectasis, identified in only 34% of lobes (235). This result compares with findings reported by Bhalla and associates (228), in which 8 of 14 (57%) of patients had evidence of cystic bronchiectasis or abscess cavities. No doubt, these differences reflect a combination of factors including disease severity and duration.

Bronchial wall or peribronchial interstitial thickening is also commonly present in patients with cystic fibrosis, especially early in the course of disease (228,254,255). Thickening of the wall of proximal right upper lobe bronchi was the earliest abnormal feature visible on HRCT in one study of patients with mild cystic fibrosis (254). Mucus plugging is also common, evident in 10 of 14 patients in one study, and it may be visible in all lobes (225,228). Other parenchymal findings include consolidation or atelectasis, with volume loss identified in up to 20% of lobes in patients with advanced disease (219,228,235,255). Also frequently noted, especially early in the course of disease, are findings indicative of small airways disease or bronchiolitis. These features include branching or nodular centrilobular opacities (so-called tree-in-bud secondary to the presence of bronchiolar dilatation with associated mucus impaction, infection, or peribronchiolar inflammation), as well as focal geographic areas of decreased lung attenuation resulting from regional

air trapping (219). These areas are best appreciated on expiratory scans, which should be obtained in all patients with suspected cystic fibrosis (235,245).

In addition to findings of bronchiectasis and bronchiolectasis, cystic or bullous lung lesions can also be identified, and they typically predominate in the subpleural regions of the upper lobes (228,235). Hilar or mediastinal lymph node enlargement and pleural abnormalities can also be seen, largely reflecting chronic infection. Pulmonary artery dilatation resulting from pulmonary hypertension can also be noted in patients with long-standing disease.

HRCT can demonstrate morphologic abnormalities in patients with early cystic fibrosis, even those whose pulmonary function tests and radiographs are normal. Santis and colleagues (254), in a study of 38 patients with mild cystic fibrosis, showed that chest radiographs were normal in nearly one-half; in distinction, HRCT disclosed evidence of bronchiectasis in 77% of these same patients and in 65% of those with normal chest radiographs (254). Similar findings have been reported by Lynch and colleagues (219), including HRCT evidence of bronchial wall thickening, bronchiectasis, centrilobular small airway abnormalities, and lobular or segmental inhomogeneities representing mosaic perfusion or air trapping all in patients with normal chest radiographs. Even in patients with more extensive disease, CT may be of value by disclosing otherwise unsuspected sites of disease. As reported by Bhalla and associates (218) in a study of 14 patients with cystic fibrosis, of a total of 162 segments assessed, bronchiectasis was detected in 124 segments using HRCT, compared with only 71 segments identified radiographically. Similar findings have been reported by Hansell and Strickland (235).

These data have led to the development of CT scoring systems (228,256). Based on an assessment of the degree and extent of bronchiectasis, bronchial wall thickening, mucus plugging, atelectasis, and emphysema, Bhalla and colleagues (225) showed a statistically significant correlation between CT scores and the percent ratios of FEV_1/FVC ($r = 0.69$, $p = .006$). In another study based on assessment of bronchiectasis and mucus plugging (256), CT scores correlated highly with clinical ($r = 0.88$, $p < .0001$) and chest radiographic ($r = 0.93$, $p < .0001$) scores, as well as pulmonary function tests.

Allergic Bronchopulmonary Aspergillosis

ABPA is a hypersensitivity reaction to *Aspergillus* species commonly found in the soil. It occurs almost exclusively in patients with either asthma or cystic fibrosis, in 1% to 2% of patients with asthma and in about 10% of patients with cystic fibrosis (257). The disease is the result of immunologic responses to the endoluminal growth of fungal species. The diagnosis of ABPA is based on a constellation of both primary and secondary diagnostic clinical, laboratory, and radiologic criteria. The acronym ARTEPICS has been suggested for the primary criteria, which include A (asthma), R (radiologic evidence of pulmonary infiltrates), T (positive skin test for *A. fumigatus*), E (eosinophilia), P (precipitating antibodies to *A. fumigatus*), I (elevated IgE), C (central bronchiectasis), and S (elevated *A. fumigatus* serum-specific IgE and IgG) (257). A diagnosis of ABPA is nearly certain when six of these eight criteria are fulfilled. Secondary criteria include the presence of *A. fumigatus* in sputum, a history of expectoration of mucus plugs, and delayed cutaneous reactivity to *Aspergillus* antigen (257).

Many of these findings are nonspecific: up to 10% of asthmatic patients, for example, have serum precipitating antibodies to *A. fumigatus,* and up to 25% demonstrate cutaneous hypersensitivity (194). Similarly, although peripheral blood eosinophilia and elevated levels of serum IgE are suggestive of the infection, they are hardly pathognomonic. Central bronchiectasis, thought essential to the diagnosis in most series, likely represents an advanced form of the disease resulting from chronic inhalation and growth of *A. fumigatus* spores within the bronchial tree (194).

Investigators have suggested that disease progression be divided into five separate phases. These are as follows: (a) an acute phase; (b) resolution, during which time pulmonary infiltrates clear and serum IgE declines; (c) remission, when all diagnostic criteria recur; (d) a phase of dependence on corticosteroids; and (e), finally, in some cases, diffuse pulmonary fibrosis (257).

CT findings in patients with ABPA have been reported in several studies (180,194,195,258–262). Neeld and associates (194), in a comparative study of 8 patients fulfilling clinical criteria of ABPA and 7 asthmatic patients evaluated with CT, identified bronchial dilatation in 19 (41%) of 46 lobes in the patients with ABPA, as compared with 15% in the patients with asthma. Moreover, in this same study, patients with APBA tended to have more severe forms of bronchiectasis in comparison with asthmatic patients, in whom cylindric bronchiectasis only could be identified. In this re-

gard, CT may be valuable in the early identification of lung damage in patients with ABPA and thus may help in planning treatment (180,258). Small airway abnormalities, with dilatation of mucus or fluid-filled centrilobular bronchioles, can also be seen on HRCT, resulting in a "tree-in-bud" appearance (263). Abnormalities of lung attenuation reflecting mosaic perfusion and air trapping on expiratory CT scans can also be seen.

In addition to central bronchiectasis, APBA also results in a variety of parenchymal and pleural abnormalities. As reported by Panchal and associates (262), in their assessment of 23 patients with ABPA, in addition to central bronchiectasis identified in all patients, parenchymal abnormalities could be identified in 43% of cases and included consolidation, collapse, cavitation, bullae, and parenchymal scarring, all of which were most pronounced in the upper lobes. An identical percentage of cases also had evidence of pleural abnormalities, especially focal pleural thickening.

The significance of central bronchiectasis as a specific marker for ABPA is disputed (194,220). As noted by Neeld and colleagues (194), central bronchiectasis is less likely a specific marker for ABPA as much as it is indicative of long-standing, severe bronchial inflammation (Fig. 3-114). Supportive data have been reported by Reiff and colleagues (264), who also found that although central bronchiectasis was more widespread and severe than idiopathic bronchiectasis, the finding of central bronchiectasis itself proved to have a sensitivity of only 37%. More specific is the finding of high-attenuation mucoid impaction (Fig. 3-115) (265,266). First described in association with chronic fungal sinusitis, high-density mucus presumably represents the presence of calcium or metallic ions within viscous mucus (267). The prevalence of this finding has been noted to be as high as 28% in one series, and when it is present, it should be considered characteristic (266).

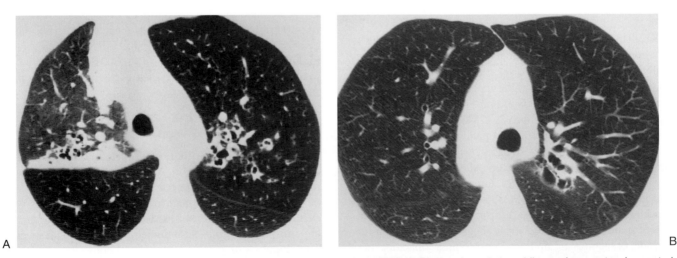

A   B

FIG. 3-114. Central bronchiectasis. **A:** Allergic bronchopulmonary aspergillosis (ABPA). Section through the midlungs shows extensive central bronchiectasis on the right side associated with focal consolidation or atelectasis of the posterior portion of the right upper lobe in a patient with documented ABPA. Although suggestive, the finding of a central distribution is not specific for ABPA (see Fig. 3–114B). **B:** Section through the midlungs shows central bronchiectasis on the left side associated with a right aortic arch in this patient with documented Kartagener's syndrome.

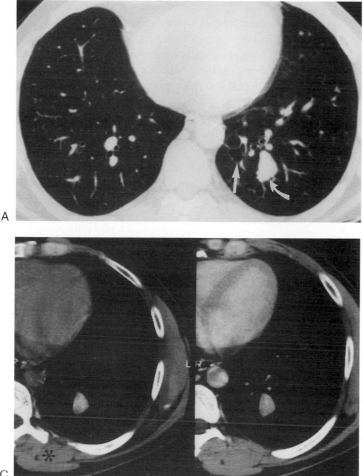

A

B,C

FIG. 3-115. High-density mucoid impaction: allergic bronchopulmonary aspergillosis (ABPA). **A:** Section through the lower lobes shows tubular density (*curved arrow*) in the left lower lobe associated with scattered foci of bronchiectasis (*straight arrow*) in this patient with documented ABPA. **B, C:** Precontrast- and contrast-enhanced CT sections at the same level as **A** shows the presence of high-density, nonenhancing fluid within the tubular density identified in **A,** consistent with high-density mucoid material in a focal area of mucoid impaction. Investigators have suggested that this finding is specific for ABPA. (From ref. 218, with permission.)

ABPA, a hypersensitivity reaction in which organisms remain within the airway lumen, should be differentiated from the distinct entity of invasive aspergillosis (268). This latter entity is defined as either angioinvasive or airway-invasive and almost always occurs in immunosuppressed persons (see Fig. 3-9; Fig. 3-116). In the airway-invasive form of the disease, organisms can be identified deep to the airway basement membrane. Clinically, in distinction to the angioinvasive form of disease, airway-invasive aspergillosis may occur even when the degree of immunosuppression is mild. Radiologically, airway-invasive aspergillosis most often manifests as patchy areas of parenchymal consolidation. On CT scans, most patients have been reported to have a distinct peribronchial or peribronchiolar distribution of disease, ranging from patchy areas of consolidation to poorly defined centrilobular nodules (268). In one study, sequential

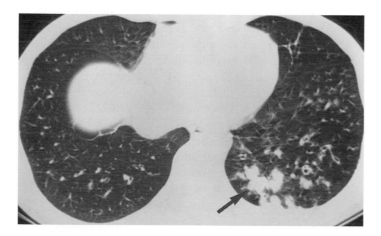

FIG. 3-116. AIDS-associated bronchiectasis: 1.5-mm axial image in a 32-year-old AIDS patient with productive cough and left lower lobe infiltrate. Evidence of focal rounded and tubular densities in the posterobasilar segment of the left lower lobe (*arrow*) is consistent with mucoid impaction in the absence of parenchymal consolidation. At bronchoscopy, the bronchial mucosa was inflamed, and the lumen was packed with inflammatory material and hyphae, identified as *Aspergillus.* (From ref. 218, with permission.)

CT studies showed that airway-invasive aspergillosis resulted in bronchiectasis in patients without prior airway dilatation (268).

In addition to immunosuppression related to leukemia, bone marrow or renal transplantation, or other immunosuppressive therapies, approximately 10% of patients with AIDS may show evidence of aspergillosis of the airways (157). Various descriptive terms have been used, including invasive aspergillosis, necrotizing tracheitis, obstructing bronchopulmonary aspergillosis, and chronic cavitary parenchymal aspergillosis (see Figs. 3-9 and 3-116; see Fig. 6-15). Involvement of the airways leads to certain abnormalities ranging from subtle nodular irregularity of airway walls to complete airway obstruction. In the latter case, obstructing bronchial aspergillosis has been reported to represent a stage before frank tissue invasion and is characterized by an acute onset of symptoms including fever, dyspnea, and cough associated with expectoration of bronchial casts laden with fungi (157).

Bronchiolitis

Clinicopathologic Classification

By definition, bronchiolitis is a generic term used to describe bronchiolar inflammation of various causes. To date, several clinicopathologic classifications have been proposed, but unfortunately, none has gained widespread acceptance (269). In part, this confusion is due to a bewildering array of redundant or even misleading descriptive terms that have been applied to this group of diseases, in particular, bronchiolitis obliterans. Further complicating this subject is the concept of small airways disease. First proposed by Hogg and associates (270) to describe inflammatory changes in peripheral airways of smokers resulting in moderate to severe airflow obstruction, this term was subsequently refined by Macklem and colleagues (271) to indicate an idiopathic syndrome of chronic airflow obstruction in patients without evidence of underlying emphysema or chronic bronchitis. As such, the concept of small airways disease is essentially physiologic, resulting from abnormalities involving airways between 2 and 3 mm in size. Although this category includes airways larger than bronchioles, the concept of small airways disease has now acquired the status of general usage as a general synonym for bronchiolar disease.

Histologically, two broad categories of bronchiolitis obliterans are generally described. The first is defined by the presence of bronchiolar and peribronchiolar inflammation resulting in organizing intraluminal exudate or granulation tissue polyps (so-called Masson bodies). This form is referred to as bronchiolitis obliterans with organizing pneumonia (BOOP), cryptogenic organizing pneumonia, or proliferative bronchiolitis (Fig. 3-117). In most cases, the predominant histologic abnormality in these patients is the presence of organizing pneumonia. Therefore, the terms BOOP and cryptogenic organizing pneumonia are preferable

to proliferative bronchiolitis. Reflecting not only the presence of intraluminal fibrotic buds but also more extensive inflammatory changes involving alveolar ducts and alveoli, BOOP characteristically results in predominantly restrictive lung disease manifest radiographically as ill-defined areas of parenchymal consolidation (81,272,273). Most often idiopathic, BOOP also may be associated with infection, toxic fume inhalation, or certain clinical syndromes resulting in a wide range of diffuse interstitial lung diseases, including idiopathic pulmonary fibrosis, connective tissue diseases, and vasculitides (269).

The second broad category of bronchiolitis obliterans is defined by the presence of concentric fibrosis resulting in marked narrowing of bronchioles in the absence of intraluminal granulation tissue polyps or surrounding parenchymal inflammation. This form of bronchiolitis obliterans is usually referred to as constrictive bronchiolitis or obliterative bronchiolitis (Fig. 3-118). Clinically, constrictive bronchiolitis is associated with marked airflow obstruction usually not responsive to steroid therapy (81,273). Radiographically, little if any abnormality apart from mild hyperinflation is apparent. Conditions associated with constrictive bronchiolitis include, most importantly, chronic allograft rejection associated with heart-lung or lung transplantation and graft-versus-host disease associated with bone marrow transplantation. Other associated conditions include collagen vascular diseases, drug toxicity, and childhood infections (Swyer-James or Macleod syndrome).

With the introduction of HRCT, a method is now available for classifying bronchiolitis. The impact of CT on assessing small airways disease is clearly one of the more significant contributions of CT over the past decade (183,229,232, 233,274–284). Of course, accurate interpretation of bronchiolar disease on CT requires thorough familiarity with pertinent lung anatomy (see Chapter 6).

Anatomically, bronchioles are airways that lack cartilage. These include membranous bronchioles, which are purely air conducting, and respiratory bronchioles, which contain alveoli within their walls. Along with their accompanying pulmonary artery branches, bronchioles lie within the center of secondary pulmonary lobules. Although normal intralobular structures cannot be identified, direct and indirect signs of bronchiolar disease have been described (280,278,283). Direct signs result from the presence of bronchiolar secretions, peribronchiolar inflammation, or, less commonly, bronchiolar wall thickening. Most characteristically, these changes result in branching or Y-shaped linear densities, as well as poorly defined centrilobular nodules, or focal small centrilobular lucencies, respectively (183,226,230,233,278). Indirect signs have also been described, the most important of which is the finding of focal air trapping, manifest either as areas of mosaic attenuation on scans obtained in inspiration or as areas of decreased attenuation, focal or global on scans obtained at end-expiration (see Fig. 3-118) (222,285).

Using these signs, one can classify bronchiolitis into one

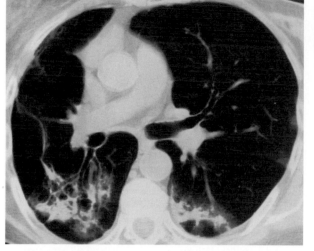

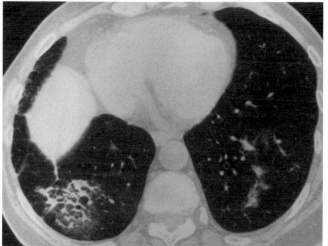

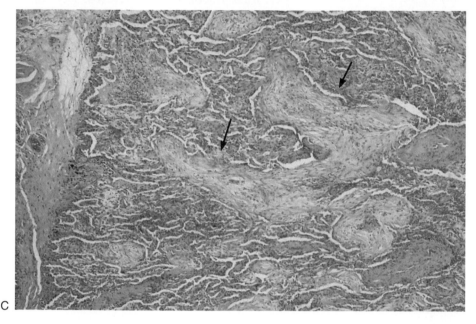

FIG. 3-117. Bronchiolitis obliterans with organizing pneumonia. A,B: Sections through the lower lobes show ill-defined areas of parenchymal consolidation without evidence of underlying parenchymal distortion or honeycombing. This appearance is nonspecific and may be seen as the result of various diseases that cause airspace consolidation. C: Histologic section from open lung biopsy shows characteristic appearance of intraluminal granulation tissue polyps (Masson bodies) (*arrows*) associated with diffuse airspace inflammation.

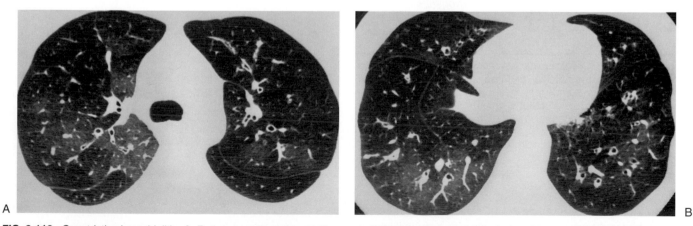

FIG. 3-118. Constrictive bronchiolitis. A, B: 1-mm sections through the upper and lower lobes, respectively, in a 25-year-old woman presenting with increasingly severe dyspnea and a normal chest radiograph (not shown). Evidence of mosaic attenuation is identifiable as geometric areas of apparent ground glass attenuation admixed with areas of relatively low parenchymal attenuation. In this case, the size of the vessels does not vary from region to region; in addition, there is evidence of diffuse bronchiectasis. Open lung biopsy revealed only scant peribronchiolar inflammation without evidence of intraluminal granulation tissue or surrounding airspace or interstitial inflammation. These findings are characteristic of constrictive bronchiolitis.

TABLE 3-12. *Bronchiolar disease: CT classification*

- **Bronchiolar diseases with tree-in-bud pattern**
  Common
  Mycobacterium tuberculosis infection
  Atypical mycobacterial infections (MAC)
  Bacterial infections (especially in patients with cystic fibrosis, and HIV-positive and AIDS patients
  Asian panbronchiolitis
  Uncommon
  Viral and fungal infections, including PCP and CMV
- **Bronchiolar diseases with poorly defined centrilobular nodules**
  Common
  Subacute hypersensitivity pneumonitis
  RB-ILD
  Uncommon
  LIP in AIDS patients
  Follicular bronchiolitis
  Mineral-dust induced bronchiolitis
  Sarcoidosis
- **Bronchiolar disease associated with ground glass attenuation and/or consolidation**
  Common
  Idiopathic BOOP
  BOOP associated with toxic fume inhalation
  Collagen vascular diseases
  Prior infection
  Radiation therapy
  Uncommon
  BOOP associated with unrelated pathologic processes, including neoplasms, infectious granulomas, and vasculitides, or as a component of other diseases, including hypersensitivity pneumonitis and Langerhans cell histiocytosis
- **Bronchiolar disease associated with decreased lung attenuation**
  Common
  Constrictive bronchiolitis after heart-lung and lung and/or bone marrow transplantation
  Uncommon
  Idiopathic
  After childhood infections
  Associated with collagen vascular diseases
  Toxic fume inhalation
  After consumption of *Sauropus androgynus*
  Constrictive bronchiolitis associated with neuroendocrine hyperplasia
  Sarcoidosis

MAC, *M. avuim-intracellulare* complex; HIV, human immunodeficiency virus; AIDS, acquired immunodeficiency syndrome; PCP, *Pneumocystis carinii* pneumonia; CMV, cytomegaloviral infection; RB-ILD, respiratory bronchiolitis with interstitial lung disease; LIP, lymphocytic interstitial pneumonitis; BOOP, bronchiolitis obliterans organizing pneumonia.
Adapted from ref. 278, with permission.

of four basic patterns (Table 3-12). These are as follows: (a) bronchiolar diseases associated with a tree-in-bud appearance; (b) bronchiolar diseases associated with poorly defined centrilobular opacities; (c) bronchiolar diseases associated with focal or diffuse ground glass attenuation or consolidation; and (d) bronchiolar diseases associated with areas of

decreased lung attenuation. As discussed later, this classification is complementary to previously proposed clinicopathologic classifications.

CT Classification

Bronchiolar Diseases Associated with a Tree-in-Bud Pattern

The hallmark of this group of diseases is the finding of dilated, mucus-filled bronchioles resulting in a pattern of centrilobular nodular, branching, or Y-shaped densities that has been aptly referred to as simulating a tree in bud. First described by Akira and colleagues (233) in association with diffuse panbronchiolitis (Fig. 3-119), and Im and associates (183) in patients with endobronchial spread of tuberculosis (Fig. 3-120), this pattern, in fact, is typical of nearly all cases of infectious bronchiolitis (see Fig. 3-104; Fig. 3-121). This includes bacterial, viral, and fungal causes and pertains to both immunocompetent and immunocompromised patients.

As documented by Im and associates (183), the tree-in-bud pattern correlates pathologically with the presence of secretions within dilated terminal and respiratory bronchioles (see Fig. 3-121). These bronchioles characteristically are centrilobular in distribution and are most easily identified in the lung periphery. Less commonly, the buds reflect the presence of peribronchiolar granulomas, a finding especially common in patients with chronic infection due to MAC (286). Of course, other manifestations of acute infection, including areas of ground glass attenuation or consolidation, may be present. Similarly, one can also usually identify poorly defined centrilobular nodules without evidence of branching, the result of sections through distended centrilobular bronchioles seen in cross section. These findings, however, are always ancillary to the main finding of a tree-in-bud pattern. With healing, a distinct tree-in-bud pattern asso-

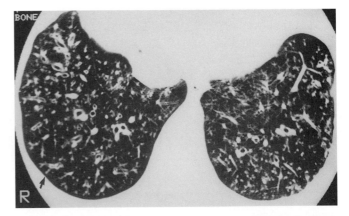

FIG. 3-119. Diffuse panbronchiolitis. A 1-mm section shows diffuse ill-defined nodular and branching or Y-shaped densities throughout both lower lobes in this patient with documented diffuse panbronchiolitis. Most of these fail to reach the pleural surface (*arrow*), consistent with centrilobular versus perilymphatic distribution (see Figs. 6–21 and 6–62B).

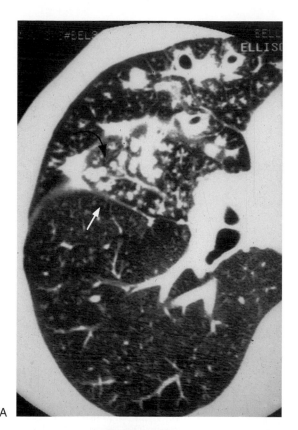

A

FIG. 3-120. Infectious bronchiolitis: endobronchial tuberculosis (TB). **A:** Enlargement of a section through the middle lobe in a patient with documented cavitary TB. Note the typical appearance of a tree-in-bud pattern (*arrow*) resulting from endobronchial spread of TB (see also Fig. 6-23). **B:** Section through the lung bases in a different patient from **A** with documented active cavitary TB again shows characteristic pattern of scattered ill-defined nodules with a tree-in-bud configuration (*white arrow*), as well as Y-shaped branching densities (*black arrow*). These correlate with aspiration of infected secretions with resultant impaction and dilatation of small bronchi and bronchioles. In this case, numerous peripheral cavities can be identified, some of which likely represent foci of cystic bronchiectasis also resulting from endobronchial spread. **C:** A 1-mm section through the right midlung in a patient with long-standing chronic TB resulting in complete atelectasis of the left lung. Small, well-defined nodules are identified adjacent to a peripheral branching vessel around which a distinct zone of hyperlucency can be identified (*arrows*). This appearance correlates with healed endobronchial spread of TB with resulting focal emphysema resulting from prior bronchial and bronchiolar obstruction.

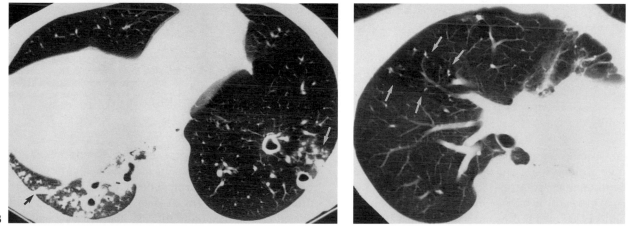

B

C

ciated with secondary lobular emphysema may be identified, presumably the result of bronchial obstruction (see Fig. 3-120).

In the United States, airway infection often results from mycobacterial infections. Of particular importance is the increasingly common finding of airway infection in patients with chronic atypical mycobacterial infections (184,185). Infectious bronchiolitis is also occurring with increasing frequency in HIV-positive and AIDS patients (157,190). The likelihood of diffuse bacterial or viral airway infections occurring in this group of patients appears to be related to decreasing rates of *Pneumocystis carinii* pneumonia as a result of widespread prophylaxis. Probably for similar rea-

sons, the prevalence of fungal airway infections in this same population is also increasing, especially infections with *Aspergillus*.

In Asia, especially in Japan and Korea, a form of diffuse bronchiolitis termed diffuse panbronchiolitis is common (see Fig. 3-119) (233). This disorder has been defined as a clinicopathologic entity characterized by symptoms of chronic cough, sputum, and dyspnea associated with abnormal pulmonary function tests usually indicating mild to moderate airway obstruction and radiographic evidence of ill-defined nodular infiltrates typically basilar in distribution (287). Histologically, diffuse panbronchiolitis is characterized by chronic inflammation with mononuclear cell proliferation

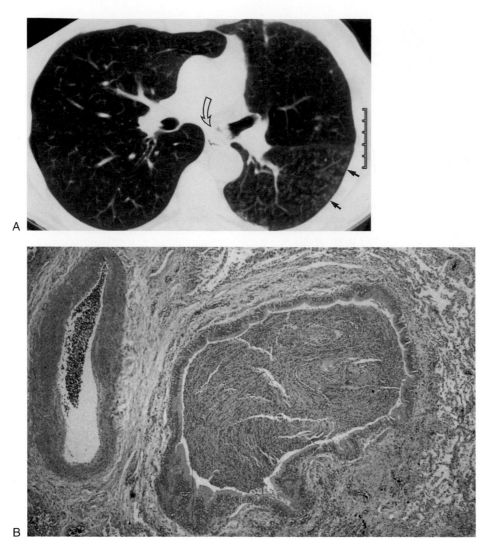

FIG. 3-121. Infectious bronchiolitis: *Chlamydia* pneumonia. **A:** A 5-mm section through the midlung shows a central endobronchial lesion partially obstructing the distal left main stem bronchus (*open arrow*). Throughout the superior segment of the left lower lobe are ill-defined nodules clustered around peripheral vessels (*arrows*), an appearance aptly described as resembling a tree-in-bud. These fail to reach the pleural surface, findings characteristic of a centrilobular as opposed to a perilymphatic distribution (see Figs. 6-21 and 6-62B). Centrilobular nodules with a tree-in-bud appearance are diagnostic of infectious bronchiolitis, in this case pneumonia has resulted from a central carcinoid tumor. **B:** Histologic section obtained in **A** after lobectomy showing inspissated infected secretions within bronchioles.

and foamy macrophages predominantly involving the walls of respiratory bronchioles, adjacent alveolar ducts, and alveoli, constituting the so-called "unit lesion of PB" (287). Inclusion of this entity in the category of infectious causes of bronchiolitis is justified because nearly all patients develop superinfection with *Pseudomonas*. On CT, a characteristic diffuse tree-in-bud pattern is invariably seen, predominately affecting the lung bases, that has been shown to disappear after treatment with erythromycin (see Fig. 3-119) (288). Unfortunately, despite initial improvement, diffuse panbronchiolitis is usually considered a progressive disease, with 5- and 10-year survival rates reported to be in the range of 60% and 30%, respectively (287).

Not surprisingly, the tree-in-bud pattern is frequently found in association with other signs of proximal airway infection. As documented by Acquino and colleagues (286), in a prospective study of 27 cases with a tree-in-bud pattern, 26 had evidence of associated bronchiectasis or proximal airway wall thickening (see Fig. 3-104). Diagnoses in this study included patients with cystic fibrosis, postinfectious bronchiectasis, ABPA, tuberculosis, *Pneumocystis carinii*

pneumonia, and bronchopneumonia, among others (286). Most important, when compared with a control population of 141 studies in patients with other documented airway diseases, including emphysema, respiratory bronchiolitis, constrictive bronchiolitis, BOOP, and extrinsic allergic alveolitis, in none of these cases could a tree-in-bud pattern be identified (see Figs. 3-117 and 3-118). In distinction, in this same control population, 25% of patients with bronchiectasis, and 17% of patients with acute infections bronchitis or pneumonia proved to have this pattern (286). These findings reinforce the concept that a tree-in-bud pattern should be interpreted as a manifestation of infectious bronchiolitis.

Bronchiolar Diseases Associated with Poorly Defined Centrilobular Nodules

In distinction to infectious bronchiolitis, the hallmark of this group of diseases is the finding of ill-defined centilobular nodules in the absence of a tree-in-bud appearance. Pathologically, the finding of centrilobular nodules correlates with the finding of peribronchiolar inflammation with-

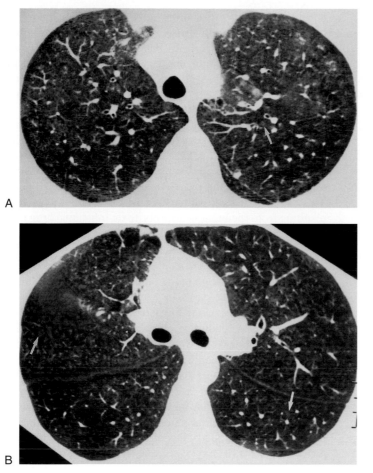

FIG. 3-122. Respiratory bronchiolitis. **A, B:** 1-mm sections through the trachea and carina, respectively, show poorly defined centrilobular nodules (*arrows*) uniformly distributed throughout both lungs. Note the the absence of reticular densities, architectural distortion, or tubular or branching structures (compare with Figs. 3-119–3-121).

out evidence of bronchiolar dilatation or retained secretions. Evidence of proximal bronchial inflammation is also lacking. In our opinion, this pattern is sufficiently distinctive to warrant separate classification.

Within this category are a diverse set of diseases that have in common the finding of peribronchiolar inflammation in the absence of widespread parenchymal consolidation (see Table 3-11). This group includes patients with subacute hypersensitivity pneumonitis, lymphocytic interstitial pneumonitis, follicular bronchiolitis, respiratory bronchiolitis–interstitial lung disease, and mineral dust–induced bronchiolitis (Fig. 3-122), among others. In most cases, differential diagnosis in this group is simplified by detailed clinical correlation, including careful occupational and environmental exposure histories. Characteristic of HRCT findings in this diverse group are those seen in patients with hypersensitivity pneumonitis (see Figs. 6-22, 6-68A,B, and 6-69A). Hypersensitivity pneumonitis is associated with a chronic, nonspecific predominantly lymphocytic interstitial pneumonitis that, early in its course, is primarily distributed around respiratory bronchioles with relative sparing of intervening lung (81). This pattern may persist even later in the course of disease. Additionally, nearly two-thirds of patients also have evidence of nonnecrotizing granulomas, again typically lo-

calized to the peribronchiolar interstitium. Foci of BOOP may also be identified in some cases, with characteristic findings of intraluminal fibrous plugs. Together, these findings result in a pattern of diffuse, poorly defined centrilobular nodular opacities, especially in the subacute phase of disease.

Similar CT findings have been identified in patients with lymphocytic interstitial pneumonitis, especially in AIDS patients (see Chapter 7) (189). Characterized by an interstitial infiltrate of mature lymphocytes, lymphocytic interstitial pneumonitis is part of the spectrum of hyperplasia of bronchus-associated lymphoid tissue that also includes follicular bronchiolitis (81). In this latter disease, lymphoid aggregates containing reactive germinal centers can be identified within the walls of bronchioles representing a localized form of lymphoid hyperplasia. Although characterized by more diffuse interstitial involvement, in fact, histologic differentiation between follicular bronchiolitis and lymphocytic interstitial pneumonitis may be difficult, a finding raising the possibility that the poorly defined centrilobular nodules identified on CT in most cases of lymphocytic interstitial pneumonitis diagnosed by transbronchial biopsy actually represent follicular bronchiolitis. Follicular bronchiolitis has also been described in association with rheumatoid arthritis

(286). In one report in which CT findings showed evidence both of branching or Y-shaped densities and poorly defined centrilobular densities in patients with rheumatoid arthritis with documented follicular bronchiolitis, in all cases the disease was either stabilized or reversed after treatment with erthyromycin, again suggesting that the finding of a tree-in-bud pattern may reflect underlying infection (289).

Also representative of this CT category is the so-called smokers' or respiratory bronchiolitis (see Fig. 3-122). A form of reversible bronchiolitis most often incidentally identified in young smokers, it is characterized histologically by the patchy accumulation of pigmented foamy macrophages predominantly within and around the walls of respiratory bronchioles and alveolar ducts, with or without intraluminal mucus plugs (81,283). When respiratory bronchiolitis is the only cause of disease in patients with clinical evidence of interstitial lung disease, it is then referred to as respiratory bronchiolitis–associated interstitial lung disease. (For a more detailed discussion of respiratory bronchiolitis–interstitial lung disease, see Chapter 6.) Radiographically, up to three-fourths of patients show evidence of reticular or reticulonodular infiltrates (290). CT findings in smokers with respiratory bronchiolitis have been described and include parenchymal and subpleural micronodules, predominately within the upper lobes, associated with areas of ground glass attenuation resulting from filling of airspaces with pigmented macrophages and bronchial dilatation (229,291, 292). The finding of a tree-in-bud pattern is distinctly unusual (286).

Other entities presenting with predominantly ill-defined centrilobular opacities that fit this CT category include mineral dust–induced bronchiolitis, especially due to silicosis, and sarcoidosis (see Figs. 6-21 and 6-62B). In sarcoidosis, centrilobular opacities are almost always associated with other manifestations of perilymphatic disease, including subpleural and perifissural nodules, and peribronchovascular distribution, thereby simplifying the differential diagnosis.

Bronchiolar Diseases Associated with Focal Ground Glass Attenuation or Consolidation

This pattern of presentation is characteristic of BOOP (81,269,273). As previously noted, BOOP is characterized histologically by the presence of granulation tissue polyps within respiratory bronchioles and alveolar ducts (Masson bodies) associated with patchy organizing pneumonia (see Fig. 3-117) (293,294). Investigators have suggested that the term cryptogenic organizing pneumonia is preferable to BOOP because the predominant abnormality clinically, functionally, and radiologically is the organizing pneumonia and because involvement of the bronchioles may be absent in up to 30% of cases (295). However, BOOP is too well established in the literature to be replaced.

Two distinct patterns of intraluminal fibrosis or Masson bodies have been described (296). Type 1 Masson bodies are those that show abundant myxoid matrix, sparse fibrosis,

and little or no fibrin and presumably represent immature mesenchymal cells. In distinction, type 2 Masson bodies contain fibrin and have histochemical properties of myofibroblasts. This distinction may be important because, at least in one study, patients with type 1 disease showed good response to steroid therapy, whereas those with type 2 disease generally failed to respond to treatment (296).

Although most cases of BOOP are idiopathic, similar findings may be seen in association with many different clinical presentations (Fig. 3-123). As described by Katzenstein (81), BOOP may be classified into three separate categories. In the first, BOOP is the primary cause of respiratory illness. This category includes idiopathic BOOP as well as BOOP resulting from rheumatoid arthritis, toxic inhalants, drug toxicity, and collagen vascular diseases, as well as BOOP in response to prior infection, both viral and bacterial (see Fig. 3-123 and Fig. 6-31). Also included in this category is BOOP in association with acute radiation pneumonitis (297). In the second category are cases in which BOOP is found as a nonspecific reaction along the periphery of unrelated pathologic processes, including neoplasms, infectious granulomas, vasculitides, and even infarcts (Fig. 3-124). Finally, BOOP may also be identified as a minor component of other diseases including hypersensitivity pneumonitis, nonspecific interstitial pneumonitis, and Langerhans' cell histiocytosis (81). For this reason, the finding of features consistent with BOOP on transbronchial biopsy is of only limited value in the absence of detailed clinical and radiologic correlation (see Fig. 3-124) (81).

Clinically, patients with idiopathic BOOP usually present with a 1- to 3-month history of nonproductive cough, low-grade fever, and increasing shortness of breath (293,294, 298,299). Various radiographic patterns have been described (300). Most often, radiographs show patchy, nonsegmental, unilateral or bilateral foci of airspace consolidation (294,298,299); however, in a smaller number of cases, both focal nodules as well as irregular predominantly basilar reticular densities have been described. Honeycombing is rare. Infiltrates may be migratory, although as noted by King (297), this rarity may reflect the relative insensitivity of radiographs versus CT scans for detecting subtle areas of parenchymal involvement. Although most patients with ill-defined areas of patchy airspace consolidation respond to treatment with corticosteroids (298), the response in patients with interstitial infiltrates has been noted to be worse (300).

Several studies have reviewed the CT and HRCT findings in patients with BOOP (275,301,302). The most common abnormality consists of patchy bilateral consolidation, seen in approximately 80% of cases, frequently with a predominantly peribronchial and subpleural distribution (see Figs. 3-117, 3-123, and 3-124; see also Fig. 6-31). Bronchial wall thickening and dilatation are commonly present in the areas with consolidation. Although small (1–10 mm), ill-defined, predominately peribronchial or peribronchiolar nodules are seen in 30% to 50% of cases, the finding of a tree-in-bud pattern is distinctly unusual (278). Irregular linear opacities are present in approximately 10% of cases.

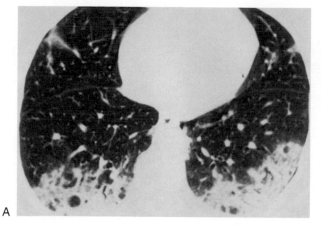

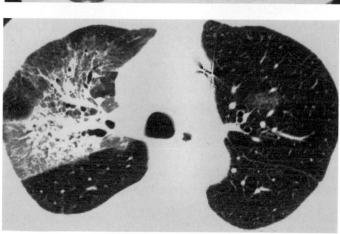

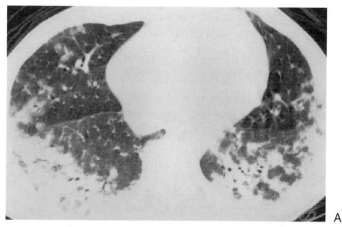

FIG. 3-123. Idiopathic bronchiolitis obliterans organizing pneumonia (BOOP): imaging spectrum. **A–C:** Sections in three different patients with histologically verified BOOP. Most commonly bibasilar and peribronchial in distribution (**A** and **B**), BOOP is frequently associated with mild bronchial wall thickening. BOOP may also appear predominantly unilateral, lobar (**C**), or even nodular (*asterisk* in **B**) (see Fig. 6-31). These findings are nonspecific: identical findings may be seen especially in patients with eosinophilic pneumonia (see Fig. 6-72). However, in distinction to diseases resulting in interstitial fibrosis, evidence of reticulation, architectural distortion, or traction bronchiectasis is unusual.

FIG. 3-124. Bronchiolitis obliterans organizing pneumonia (BOOP): differential diagnosis. **A:** BOOP in polymyositis. High-resolution CT in a 27-year-old man with polymyositis demonstrates peribronchial and subpleural areas of consolidation involving mainly the lower lobes. **B, C:** Selected 1-mm sections in a different patient from **A** show dense areas of ill-defined parenchymal consolidation as well as scattered small, well-defined nodules (*arrows* in **B** and **C**). Although an initial transbronchial biopsy was interpreted as consistent with BOOP, the finding of small, well-defined nodules in a patient with known cervical carcinoma led to open lung biopsy, which confirmed metastatic cervical carcinoma. This case emphasizes that histologic foci of BOOP frequently occur in patients with a wide range of specific disease entities (see text), and consequently, transbronchial biopsy is an unreliable method for establishing this diagnosis.

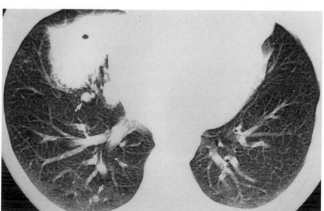

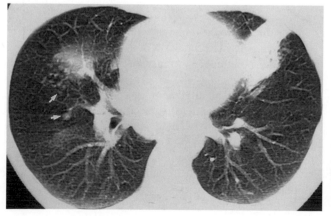

Areas of ground-glass attenuation may be seen in up to 60% of immunocompetent patients with BOOP, but they are seldom the predominant abnormality in these patients (see Fig. 3-123C). Areas of ground glass attenuation are seen more commonly in immunocompromised patients with BOOP and may be the predominant or only abnormality seen in these patients (302). Small nodules are also seen more commonly in immunocompromised patients; nodules 1 to 10 mm in diameter are observed in 6 of 11 (55%) of immuno-compromised patients as compared with 7 of 32 (22%) of immunocompetent patients with idiopathic BOOP reported by Lee and colleagues (302).

In a few cases, BOOP may present as multiple, large (1–5 cm) nodules or masses. In a report by Akira and associates (303), 12 (20%) of 50 patients with BOOP presented with multiple nodules or masses as the predominant finding. Of a total of 60 lesions, 88% proved to have irregular margins, whereas 45% were associated with air bronchograms, and 38% had pleural tags. The finding of an irregular masslike area of consolidation adjacent to pleural surfaces, in particular, proved suggestive. Similar findings have also been reported by Bouchardy and colleagues (275), who also found nodular or masslike opacities to be a frequent finding, occurring in 5 (42%) of 12 patients.

Bronchiolar Diseases Associated with Decreased Lung Attenuation

In this category are patients with obliterative or constrictive bronchiolitis. Constrictive bronchiolitis is defined histologically by the presence of concentric fibrosis involving the submucosal and peribronchial tissues of terminal and respiratory bronchioles exclusively, with resulting bronchial narrowing or obliteration. This process is typically nonuniform, and because the surrounding parenchyma is normal, the condition may be difficult to identify even on open lung biopsy (81,273). Clinically, although these patients may be relatively asymptomatic, in most cases progressive airway obstruction results in severe respiratory compromise that is usually unresponsive to steroid therapy.

Unlike BOOP, which usually proves to be idiopathic, obliterative bronchiolitis is only rarely idiopathic. Conditions associated with constrictive bronchiolitis include heart-lung or lung transplantations, chronic allograft rejection, allogeneic bone marrow transplantation with chronic graft-versus-host disease, and collagen vascular diseases, especially rheumatoid arthritis (see Fig. 3-118; Figs. 3-125–3-127) (81). Also known as the Swyer-James syndrome, constrictive bronchiolitis frequently occurs as the sequela of childhood respiratory tract infections, most often viral, although similar findings may also be seen in children after infection with *Mycoplasma*. Obliterative bronchiolitis has also been linked to consumption of *Sauropus androgynus* (285,304), a small, lowland shrub found in Asia and consumed in the form of an uncooked juice as a means of weight

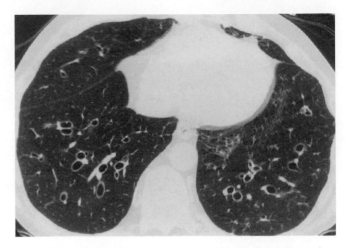

FIG. 3-125. Constrictive bronchiolitis associated with lung transplantation. A 1-mm section in a 48-year-old man with bronchiolitis obliterans after double lung transplantation demonstrates markedly dilated bronchi in both lower lobes and in the right middle lobe. Also note the patchy areas of decreased attenuation and perfusion.

reduction, especially in Taiwan. A CT pattern of mosaic attenuation has also been reported in association with neuroendocrine hyperplasia, especially in patients with carcinoid tumors (305,306).

Obliterative Bronchiolitis Syndrome. Of all causes of constrictive bronchiolitis, most important is the association between constrictive bronchiolitis and heart-lung or lung transplants (see Fig. 3-125). In this setting, constrictive bronchiolitis results from lymphocyte-mediated chronic rejection and is a major cause of both morbidity and mortality. The primary risk factor for posttransplantation constrictive bronchiolitis appears to be the frequency and severity of acute cellular rejection that nearly always occurs in patients in the early postoperative setting (307). Investigators have estimated that as many as 50% of patients receiving heart-lung or lung transplants develop constrictive bronchiolitis, typically within 6 months to a year after organ transplantation, and between 25% and 40% of these patients will die as a direct result. Although the term bronchiolitis obliterans syndrome has been proposed to describe this occurrence, as previously discussed, in our opinion, it is preferable to refer to this entity simply as posttransplantation constrictive bronchiolitis (307).

In distinction to the recipients of heart-lung and lung transplants, constrictive bronchiolitis is far less common in patients after bone marrow transplantation, although it is still problematic (see Fig. 3-126). In this setting, constrictive bronchiolitis is a manifestation of chronic graft-versus-host disease (273,308), and it has been reported in 2% to 13% of patients who underwent allogeneic bone marrow transplantation (309). Clinically, it may develop any time after the third month after bone marrow transplantation (309).

The chest radiograph in patients with constrictive bronchiolitis may be normal, or it may show nonspecific abnormalities, including variable degrees of hyperinflation,

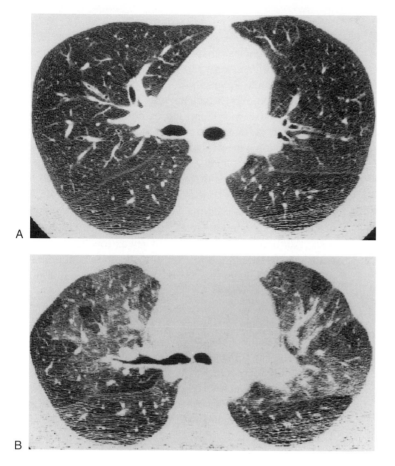

FIG. 3-126. Constrictive bronchiolitis: value of inspiratory/expiratory scanning. **A:** Inspiratory high-resolution CT (HRCT) scan in a 32-year-old woman with bronchiolitis obliterans after bone marrow transplantation is normal. **B:** HRCT performed at end-expiration demonstrates areas of air trapping in the upper and lower lobes.

peripheral attenuation of the vascular markings, and evidence of central airway dilatation (196–198,281). The characteristic HRCT findings consist of mosaic attenuation, air trapping, and bronchial dilatation (see Figs. 3-118 and 3-124–3-126) (197,198,281). Mosaic attenuation results from decreased perfusion of areas distal to bronchiolar obstruction with blood flow redistribution to noninvolved lung. Air trapping resulting from partial airway obstruction is best seen on expiratory HRCT scans (see Fig. 3-126) (198,245,276).

To date, because of the low yield of transbronchial biopsy in the diagnosis of constrictive bronchiolitis, the diagnosis

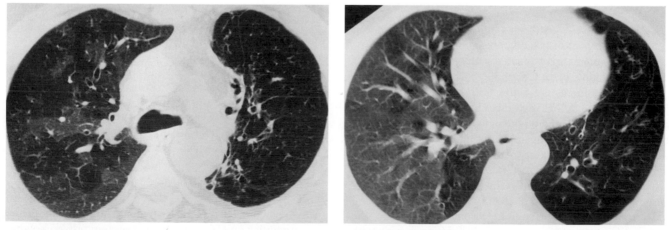

FIG. 3-127. Constrictive bronchiolitis: Swyer-James syndrome. **A, B:** 1-mm sections through the carina and lower lobes, respectively, show hyperlucency of the entire left lung associated with bronchiectasis. Focal areas of hyperlucency are also noted in the right lung, resulting in a pattern of mosaic attenuation. These findings are characteristic of postinfectious constrictive bronchiolitis, which, despite a common misconception, is rarely unilateral.

of posttransplantation constrictive bronchiolitis has been based on a constellation of clinical, radiologic, and primarily physiologic findings, as follows: a decline of 20% in forced expiratory flow at midlung volumes (FEF25–75) from peak values obtained after transplantation and in the absence of definable pathogens on bronchoalveolar lavage in association with a normal radiographic appearance of the transplanted lung (279). Although mosaic perfusion is commonly seen in patients with obliterative bronchiolitis, unfortunately, this feature is of limited value in the diagnosis because it is also common in healthy control subjects and in posttransplant patients without evidence of constrictive bronchiolitis (310). The two most helpful findings in the diagnosis are the presence of bronchial dilatation, particularly in the lower lobes (198,310), and the presence of air trapping on expiratory HRCT (310). Worthy and Flower (310) reviewed the HRCT scans in 15 patients with pathologically proven bronchiolitis obliterans after lung transplantation and 18 control subjects. Findings seen in patients with constrictive bronchiolitis included bronchial dilatation in 80% of cases, mosaic perfusion in 40%, bronchial wall thickening in 27%, and air trapping in 80% of cases, compared with the control subjects who had bronchial dilatation in 22% of cases, mosaic perfusion in 22% of cases, bronchial wall thickening in 0% of cases, and air trapping in 6% of cases (310).

The role of repeated HRCT scans in monitoring the development of bronchiolitis obliterans syndrome after lung transplantation was also assessed by Ikonen and colleagues (311). In a study of 13 lung transplant recipients who underwent a total of 126 HRCT scans during a mean follow-up period of 23 months, 8 of the 13 patients developed bronchiolitis obliterans syndrome. The authors of this study demonstrated that the HRCT findings coincided with the development of the bronchiolitis obliterans syndrome. The overall sensitivity of HRCT for the diagnosis of bronchiolitis obliterans was 93%, and the specificity was 92% (311).

CLINICAL APPLICATIONS: HEMOPTYSIS

Little consensus exists concerning an optimal approach to the management of patients presenting with hemoptysis. At present, patients are evaluated with some combination of chest radiography, chest CT, and FB. The role of FB in the evaluation of patients presenting with hemoptysis has been controversial (312). FB is of proven efficacy in evaluating patients with central endobronchial disease, with definite diagnoses made in more then 95% of endoscopically visible primary malignant diseases (313). In addition to identifying central endobronchial disease, bronchoscopy has also proven valuable in the diagnosis of localizing bleeding sites before surgery, removal of blood clots that may cause obstruction, and removal of foreign bodies. Despite this efficacy, the overall diagnostic accuracy of FB in patients presenting with hemoptysis in most reported series is surprisingly low, especially in patients presenting with normal or nonlocalizing chest radiographs (314–317).

Jackson and associates (316), in a review of 48 consecutive patients presenting with hemoptysis, found that FB resulted in a diagnosis other than endobronchial inflammation in only 4 patients, only 2 of whom proved to have lung cancer. Similarly, Peters and colleagues (315), in a retrospective evaluation of 113 patients with hemoptysis, found that a specific cause was identified in none of the 26 patients with normal radiographs, compared with 35 of 87 patients (40%) in whom corresponding chest radiographs proved localizing. Poe and colleagues (318), in a study of 196 patients with normal or nonlocalizing chest radiographs, found that in only 33 cases (17%) were specific causes established bronchoscopically. Sharma and associates (317) reported normal FB examinations in 81% of 53 patients with hemoptysis. Although the site of bleeding was localized in 5 patients, no specific diagnoses were made, and carcinoma was not detected in any patient during the procedure or at follow-up.

The incidence of bronchogenic carcinoma, in particular, is low in patients presenting with normal or nonlocalizing chest radiographs (314,316–319). Santiago and associates (314) identified cancer in only 4 of 78 patients (5%) presenting with normal radiographs. Similarly, Rath and colleagues (320), in an evaluation of 31 patients presenting with hemoptysis, found that a diagnosis of lung cancer was established in only 1 of 17 patients with normal chest radiographs. In a retrospective study of 196 patients with hemoptysis and nonlocalizing chest radiographs reported by Poe and colleagues (318), only 12 patients (6%) proved to have bronchogenic carcinoma diagnosed endoscopically; furthermore, applying univariate and discriminant analyses using the 3 variables of age older than 50 years, male sex, and a severity of hemoptysis of more than 30 mL per day, the authors of this study concluded that the need to perform bronchoscopy could have been safely reduced by 28%, with the remainder of these patients safely observed. In contrast, bronchoscopy is often diagnostic in patients with localizing radiographs (312,316,319–322). Weaver and associates (321), in their series of 70 patients with hemoptysis, reported that abnormal radiographic findings were identified in all cases of subsequently proved carcinoma.

The accuracy of CT in identifying airway abnormalities has been documented (2,113,115,161). In a retrospective evaluation of 361 abnormal airways, nearly identical sensitivities for both CT and FOB in detecting focal airways lesions were observed (151). Similarly, in an analysis of 50 patients with segmental or lobar atelectasis, obstructive carcinoma was seen on CT in all 27 cases when atelectasis was due to a centrally obstructing tumor (161). CT may disclose tumors, both central and peripheral, otherwise inapparent bronchoscopically (113,151). In 7 of 38 cases reported by Mayr and colleagues (151) as demonstrating focal bronchial abnormalities on CT, initial bronchoscopy proved nondiagnostic: in all 7 cases, tumor was subsequently diagnosed either at surgery or repeat bronchoscopy at the site identified as abnormal at CT. In addition to identifying abnormal air-

TABLE 3-13. *Hemoptysis: CT–flexible bronchoscopy correlations*

	Hirshberg et al. (323)[a] (1997) (n = 208)	McGuinness et al. (114) (1994) (n = 57)	Set et al. (116) (1993) (n = 91)	Naidich et al. (182) (1990) (n = 58)	Millar et al. (181) (1990) (n = 40)	Haponik et al. (203) (1987) (n = 32)
Bronchiectasis (%)	20	25	15	17	18	0
Tuberculosis (%)	1.4	16	0	2	5	0
Lung cancer (%)	19	12	37	33	5	0
Fungal infection (%)	1.4	12	0	2	0	6
Cryptogenic (%)	8	19	34	33	50	37
Bronchitis (%)	18	7	5	0	0	10
Miscellaneous (%)	33	5	9	10	22	3
Multiple causes (%)	0	4	[b]	0	[c]	0

[a] CT performed in 129 (62%) of 208 cases.
[b] Two cases lung cancer and bronchiectasis.
[c] One case peripheral neoplasm and bronchiectasis.
Adapted from ref. 323, with permission.

ways, CT also allows direct visualization of peribronchial tissues. Although bronchoscopic assessment of the extraluminal extent of a lesion and of its relation to bronchi and mediastinal structures in particular is difficult, these features are easily identified with CT.

Various studies have evaluated the role of CT in patients with hemoptysis (Table 3-13) (114,116,181,182,202,323). In an early retrospective study, Haponik and associates (202) compared the contribution of chest radiography, conventional CT, and FB in an evaluation of 32 patients with hemoptysis. CT enabled accurate identification of the source of bleeding in 23 of 26 cases (88%) identified bronchoscopically; furthermore, CT added new diagnostic information in an additional 15 cases (47%), including detection of an unsuspected lung cancer. Nonetheless, these authors found that CT influenced the management of only 6 of 32 cases (19%), a finding that led these investigators to conclude that such limited clinical impact failed to support routine use of CT.

In contrast, all subsequent reports have shown that CT is an accurate method for assessing patients with hemoptysis (181,114–116,323). Millar and colleagues (181) demonstrated that routine CT provided a diagnosis in 20 of 40 patients (50%) with hemoptysis in whom both chest radiographs and FB failed to yield a diagnosis. Set and associates (116) compared the utility of FB and HRCT in 91 patients and found that CT detected all 27 tumors seen bronchoscopically as well as an additional 7, 5 of which were beyond bronchoscopic range. Similarly, McGuinness and associates (114), in a prospective study of 57 consecutive patients presenting with hemoptysis evaluated both with CT and FB, found that CT identified all cancers: furthermore, the overall diagnostic yield of bronchoscopy was documented to be less than that of CT (47% compared with 61%, respectively). CT proved especially valuable in diagnosing bronchiectasis, a diagnosis difficult to establish by FB, present in 25% of cases. CT not only detects abnormalities in patients with normal or nonlocalizing radiographs, but it is also of value

in the presence of localizing findings, even when these findings are suggestive of lung cancer. In this setting, CT may provide information critical to accurate staging in up to 50% of cases (182). As previously discussed, CT is especially valuable in patients for whom TBNA is planned by providing a guide to optimal selection of mediastinal nodes to be evaluated.

Reported causes of hemoptysis have varied during the past 50 years, depending on changing disease prevalence and on the addition of new diagnostic techniques such as FB and chest CT (Table 3-14). Before 1970, tuberculosis, bronchiectasis, and bronchogenic carcinoma were the most common causes of hemoptysis (324–327). With the advent of FB in 1970, most studies concluded that chronic bronchitis and bronchogenic carcinoma had emerged as the predominant causes of hemoptysis (314,321,328). Indeed, by the late 1980s, tuberculosis and bronchiectasis were considered unlikely causes of routine hemoptysis, though they were still significant in the differential diagnosis of massive hemoptysis.

In the late 1980s, HRCT of the chest became the standard radiologic technique for detecting airway disease, particularly bronchiectasis (1,218,243,244). Use of HRCT during this period demonstrated that bronchiectasis again was responsible for a significant portion of cases of otherwise unexplained cases of hemoptysis (114,116,181,182). Millar described 40 patients presenting with hemoptysis and normal chest radiographs and FBs; in 7 cases, bronchiectasis was noted by HRCT (181). Similarly, Set and colleagues (116) and McGuinness and associates (114) found bronchiectasis in 15% and 25% percent of patients presenting with hemoptysis, respectively. These findings are in contrast to previous reports (ranging from 1–3%) that have suggested that bronchiectasis is a rare cause of hemoptysis (314,318,319,322).

These reported differences in the prevalence of bronchiectasis as the cause of hemoptysis likely reflect a lack of bronchographic or CT correlation in most previous reports. In addition, the incidence of bronchiectasis is likely rising,

TABLE 3-14. *Hemoptysis: Etiology*

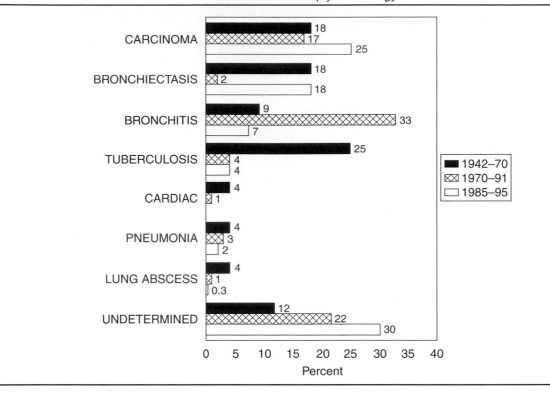

probably as a consequence of the reemergence of tuberculosis. When bronchography was incidently performed in patients with hemoptysis and nonlocalizing chest radiographs, bronchiectasis was diagnosed in 50% of cases (329). In another series, when bronchograms were performed in 13 patients with hemoptysis, bronchiectasis was identified in 8 (62%) (330). Given the accuracy of CT to diagnose both focal and diffuse disease, CT has replaced bronchography as a means of diagnosing bronchiectasis in symptomatic patients.

The relationship between the quantity and duration of hemoptysis and underlying malignancy remains unclear, particularly in patients with normal chest radiographs. Although most reports suggest that mild hemoptysis of protracted duration is typical of malignant disease (244), these findings have been contested (321). Poe and colleagues (318) found that 50% of the cancer patients in their retrospective study had bleeding for less than 1 week, whereas 67% of these patients had mild hemoptysis of less than 30 mL per day. Similarly, definitive correlation is lacking between the size and location of lesions and their propensity to bleed (315,331,332). Adelman and colleagues (333), in an attempt to determine the clinical significance of a negative bronchoscopic examination in patients at risk for lung cancer, reviewed the clinical outcome over a 3-year period of 67 patients with cryptogenic hemoptysis after nondiagnostic bronchoscopy. Eighty-five percent of these patients remained well, whereas 9 died of nonpulmonary conditions.

Only 1 was diagnosed with bronchogenic carcinoma 20 months after bronchoscopy without recurrence of hemoptysis. These results suggest a tenuous relationship between hemoptysis and early carcinoma. Usuda and associates (140), in an evaluation of 105 radiographically occult squamous cell carcinomas in 98 patients, found that only 9 (8%) showed evidence either of bleeding or capillary growth; all these tumors proved larger than 2 mm, a finding suggesting that, at least for central squamous cell carcinomas, lesions must attain a size that should allow identification with CT before they cause hemoptysis (see Fig. 3-71).

The likelihood that small cancers beyond the limits of resolution of HRCT will cause presenting hemoptysis has yet to be determined. Investigators have shown that, in the absence of demonstrable tumor on initial CT evaluation, the likelihood of cancer as the cause of hemoptysis is strikingly low. As reported by Garay and associates (334), in their study of 72 patients initially evaluated in an outpatient setting, in no case was cancer diagnosed despite close monitoring over a minimum period of 2 years if the initial CT study was interpreted as showing no evidence of tumor.

Based on these data, it is apparent that CT and bronchoscopy are not competitive but are complementary modalities. HRCT cannot replace bronchoscopy, especially in its ability to provide biopsy specimens for histologic or cytologic examination. In turn, bronchoscopy is limited in detecting peribronchial abnormalities, as well as in diagnosing parenchymal disease, especially bronchiectasis.

Although current evidence clearly supports a role for CT in evaluating patients with hemoptysis, accurate assessment requires the use of meticulous scan technique. In this regard, despite encouraging results, none of the CT studies published to date have consistently used high-resolution techniques to maximize detection of airway disease (114,116,181,182). It is axiomatic that optimal evaluation of patients presenting with hemoptysis requires that the central airways be closely examined to exclude central endobronchial tumors. With the advent of helical CT technology, the ability to acquire high-quality images consistently through the central airways is now routinely possible. Although some potentially valuable protocols have been proposed, especially in the setting of a normal or nonlocalizing radiograph, we currently recommend a combination of an initial sequence of 5-mm sections reconstructed every 4 mm from the level of the true vocal cords (approximately C5) to just above the carina, followed by a second sequence of 3-mm sections reconstructed every 2 mm from the level of the carina to at the least the level of the inferior pulmonary veins using a pitch of 2. In patients able to maintain a long breath-hold, 3-mm images acquired with a pitch of 2 frequently allow visualization of most of the lower lobes. Finally, to complete the study, 1-mm axial sections are obtained every 10 mm through the lung bases. As outlined, this protocol ensures that the entire length of the central airways is evaluated with overlapping 3- to 5-mm sections, thus ensuring that no central endobronchial lesion is obscured and at the same time allowing for adequate assessment of bronchiectasis. Despite the use of varying collimation, this protocol still allows for the use of both MPRs and virtual bronchoscopic techniques to assess the main, lobar, and segmental airways, regions for which these techniques are of greatest value.

Despite the proven value of HRCT in assessing patients with hemoptysis, whether CT studies should be obtained before or after bronchoscopy remains controversial (114,116,181,335). Colice and colleagues (335), using a statistical model to assess the relative roles of chest radiography, bronchoscopy, sputum cytology, and CT for detecting lung cancer in patients with normal chest radiographs, concluded that a strategy relying on the results of initial sputum cytology as a screen for choosing either immediate bronchoscopy or follow-up chest radiographs results in the lowest number of tests needed to diagnose the condition and hence represents the most cost-effective means of evaluating these patients. Unfortunately, notwithstanding that sputum cytology is not generally relied on in most institutions, this study is based on several assumptions regarding CT that are highly questionable. This includes estimating the sensitivity of CT for detecting endobronchial lesions at 86% based on a single study (114) with a total of only 7 documented endobronchial neoplasms (in which the single false-negative result proved to be due to Kaposi's sarcoma), ignoring other series showing CT sensitivity to be 100% (113,116,151,181), and estimating the specificity of CT at only 61%, again based on findings from this same study (114). Equally disturbing is that such an approach virtually ignores the contribution of CT for establishing other diagnoses in this population, with resultant consequences for patient management. Also ignored are the consequences of delayed diagnosis in patients with peripheral cancers too small to identify on chest radiographs.

In our opinion, CT studies should be routinely obtained in all patients presenting with hemoptysis before bronchoscopy. Even in patients with localizing radiographs, in our experience, CT serves as a guide, allowing precise visualization of the true extent of lesions and more efficacious selection of optimal biopsy sites and procedures. Furthermore, in selected cases, for example nonsmoking patients less than 40 years of age who have a history of questionable or minimal hemoptysis, CT may obviate bronchoscopy altogether by demonstrating the lack of an endobronchial lesion or by identifying bronchiectasis as a probable cause of hemoptysis.

REFERENCES

1. Naidich DP, Harkin TJ. Airways and lung: correlation of CT with fiberoptic bronchoscopy. *Radiology* 1995;197:1–12.
2. Glazer HS, Anderson DJ, Sagel SS. Bronchial impaction in lobar collapse: CT demonstration and pathologic correlation. *AJR Am J Roentgenol* 1989;153:485–488.
3. Perhomaa M, Lahde S, Rossi O, Suramo I. Helical CT in evaluation of the bronchial tree. *Acta Radiol* 1997;38:83–91.
4. Lucidarme O, Grenier P, Coche E, et al. Bronchiectasis: comparative assessment with thin-section CT and helical CT. *Radiology* 1996;200:673–679.
5. Stern EJ, Webb WR. Dynamic imaging of lung morphology with ultrafast high-resolution computed tomography. *J Thorac Imaging* 1993;8:273–282.
6. Stern EJ, Graham CM, Webb WR, Gamsu G. Normal trachea during forced expiration: dynamic CT measurements. *Radiology* 1993;187:27–31.
7. Grenier P, Cordeau M-P, Beigelman C. High-resolution computed tomography of the airways. *J Thorac Imaging* 1993;8:213–239.
8. Remy-Jardin M, Remy J. Comparison of vertical and oblique CT in evaluation of the bronchial tree. *J Comput Assist Tomogr* 1988;12:956–962.
9. Naidich DP, Gruden JF, McGuinness G, McCauley DI, Bhalla M. Volumetric (helical/spiral) CT (VCT) of the airways. *J Thorac Imaging* 1997;12:11–28.
10. Gurney JW. Missed lung cancer at CT: imaging findings in nine patients. *Radiology* 1996;199:117–122.
11. White CS, Romney BM, Mason AC, et al. Primary carcinoma of the lung overlooked at CT: analysis of findings in 14 patients. *Radiology* 1996;199:109–115.
12. Rubin GD, Napel S, Leung AN. Volumetric analysis of volumetric data: achieving a paradigm shift [Editorial]. *Radiology* 1996;200:312–217.
13. Lacrosse M, Trigaux JP, Vanbeers BE, Weynants P. 3D spiral CT of the tracheobronchial tree. *J Comput Assist Tomogr* 1995;19:341–347.
14. Summers RM, Feng DH, Holland SM, Sneller MC, Shelhamer JH. Virtual bronchoscopy: segmentation method for real-time display. *Radiology* 1996;200:857–862.
15. Brink JA. Technical aspects of helical (spiral) CT. *Radiol Clin North Am* 1995;33:825.
16. Napel S, Rubin GD, Jeffrey RB. STS-MIP: a new reconstruction technique for CT of the chest [Technical note]. *J Comput Assist Tomogr* 1993;17:832–838.
17. Fishman EK, Magid D, Ney DR, et al. Three-dimensional imaging. *Radiology* 1991;181:321–337.
18. Kauczor H-U, Wolcke B, Fischer B, et al. Three-dimensional helical CT of the tracheobronchial tree: evaluation of imaging protocols and assessment of suspected stenoses with bronchoscopic correlation. *AJR Am J Roentgenol* 1996;167:419–424.

19. Johnson PT, Heath DG, Bliss DF, Cabral B, Fishman EK. Three-dimensional CT: real-time interactive volume rendering. *Radiology* 1996;200:581–583.

20. Rubin GD, Beaulieu CF, Argiro V, et al. Perspective volume rendering of CT and MR images: applications for endoscopic imaging. *Radiology* 1996;199:321–330.

21. Vining DJ, Ferretti G, Stelt DR, et al. Mediastinal lymph node mapping using spiral CT and three-dimensional reconstructions in patients with lung cancer: preliminary observations. *J Bronchol* 1997;4:18–25.

22. Vining DJ, Liu K, Choplin RH, Haponik EF. Virtual bronchoscopy: relationships of virtual reality endobronchial simulations to actual bronchoscopic findings. *Chest* 1996;109:549–553.

23. Summers RM. Navigational aids for real-time virtual bronchoscopy. *AJR Am J Roentgenol* 1997;168:1165–1170.

24. Quint LE, Whyte RI, Kazerooni EA, et al. Stenosis of the central airways: evaluation by using helical CT with multiplanar reconstructions. *Radiology* 1995;194:871–877.

25. Schlueter FJ, Semenkovich JW, Glazer HS, et al. Bronchial dehiscence after lung transplantation: correlation of CT findings with clinical outcome. *Radiology* 1996;199:849–854.

26. McAdams HP, Murray JG, Erasmus JJ, et al. Telescoping bronchial anastomoses for unilateral or bilateral sequential lung transplantation: CT appearance. *Radiology* 1997;203:202–206.

27. Quint LE, McShan DL, Glazer GM, et al. Three dimensional CT of central lung tumors. *Clin Imaging* 1990;14:323–329.

28. Bhalla M, Naidich DP, McGuinness G, et al. Diffuse lung disease: assessment with helical CT—preliminary observations of the role of maximum and minimum projection images. *Radiology* 1996;200:341–347.

29. Murray JG, Brown AL, Anagnostou EA, Senior R. Widening of the tracheal bifurcation on chest radiographs: value as a sign of left atrial enlargement. *AJR Am J Roentgenol* 1995;164:1089–1092.

30. McGuinness G, Naidich DP, Garay SM, et al. Accessory cardiac bronchus: computed tomographic features and clinical significance. *Radiology* 1993;189:563–566.

31. Katz M, Konen E, Rozenman J, Szeinberg A, Itzchak Y. Spiral CT and 3D image reconstruction of vascular rings and associated tracheobronchial anomalies. *J Comput Assist Tomogr* 1995;19:564–568.

32. Vogel N, Wolcke B, Kauczor HU, Kelbel C, Mildenberger P. Detection of bronchopleural fistula with spiral CT and 3D reconstruction. *Aktuelle Radiol* 1995;5:176–178.

33. Ferretti GR, Knoplioch J, Bricault I, Brambilla C, Coulomb M. Central airway stenoses: preliminary results of spiral-CT–generated virtual bronchoscopy simulations in 29 patients. *Eur Radiol* 1997;7:854–859.

34. Wang K-P. Staging of bronchogenic carcinoma by bronchoscopy. *Chest* 1994;106:588–593.

35. Gamsu G, Webb WR. Computed tomography of the trachea: normal and abnormal. *AJR Am J Roentgenol* 1982;139:3321–3326.

36. Gamsu G, Webb WR. Computed tomography of the trachea and mainstem bronchi. *Semin Roentgenol* 1983;18:51–60.

37. Zwischenberger JB, Sankar AB. Surgery of the thoracic trachea. *J Thorac Imaging* 1995;10:199–205.

38. Kittredge RD. The right posterolateral tracheal band. *J Comput Assist Tomogr* 1979;3:348–354.

39. Breatnach E, Abbott GC, Fraser RC. Dimensions of the normal human trachea. *AJR Am J Roentgenol* 1984;141:903–906.

40. Griscom NT. Computed tomographic determination of tracheal dimensions in children and adolescents. *Radiology* 1982;145:361–364.

41. Effman EL, Fram EK, Vock P, Kirks DR. Tracheal cross-sectional area in children: CT determination. *Radiology* 1983;149:137–140.

42. Greene R. "Saber sheath" trachea: relation to chronic obstructive pulmonary disease. *AJR Am J Roentgenol* 1978;130:441–445.

43. Kwong JS, Müller NL, Miller RR. Diseases of the trachea and mainstem bronchi: correlation of CT with pathologic findings. *Radiographics* 1992;12:647–657.

44. Shepard JO, McLoud TC. Imaging the airways. *Clin Chest Med* 1991;12:151–168.

45. Morrison SC. Case report: demonstration of a tracheal bronchus by computed tomography. *Clin Radiol* 1988;39:208–209.

46. Shipley RT, McLoud TC, Dedrick CG, Shepard JO. Computed tomography of the tracheal bronchus. *J Comput Assist Tomogr* 1985;9:53–55.

47. Siegel MJ, Shackelford GD, Francis RS, McAlister WH. Tracheal bronchus. *Radiology* 1979;130:353–355.

48. O'Sullivan BP, Frassica JJ, Rayder SM. Tracheal bronchus: a cause of prolonged atelectasis in intubated children. *Chest* 1998;113:537–540.

49. Moller GM, ten Berge EJ, Stassen CM. Tracheocele: a rare cause of difficult endotracheal intubation and subsequent pneumomediastinum. *Eur Respir J* 1994;7:1376–1377.

50. Tanaka H, Mori Y, Kurokawa K, Abe S. Paratracheal air cysts communicating with the trachea: CT findings. *J Thorac Imaging* 1997;12:38–40.

51. Berkmen YM. The trachea: the blind spot in the chest. *Radiol Clin North Am* 1984;22:539–562.

52. Stark P. Imaging of tracheobronchial injuries. *J Thorac Imaging* 1995;10:206–219.

53. Devine N, Soyer P, Rebibo G, et al. Bronchial anastomotic complications in lung transplantation: CT assessment. *J Radiol* 1996;77:477–481.

54. Fullerton DA, Campbell DN. Airway problems in lung transplantation. *Semin Respir Crit Care Med* 1996;17:187–196.

55. Herman S, Rappaport D, Weisbrod G, et al. Single-lung transplantation: imaging features. *Radiology* 1989;170:89–93.

56. Murray JG, McAdams HP, Erasmus JJ, Patz EF Jr, Tapson V. Complications of lung transplantation: radiologic findings [Pictorial essay]. *AJR Am J Roentgenol* 1996;166:1405–1411.

57. O'Donovan P. Imaging of complications of lung transplantation. *Radiographics* 1993;13:787–796.

58. Whyte RI, Quint LE, Kazerooni EA, et al. Helical computed tomography for the evaluation of tracheal stenosis. *Ann Thorac Surg* 1995;60:27–31.

59. Rollins RJ, Tocino I. Early radiographic signs of tracheal rupture. *AJR Am J Roentgenol* 1987;148:695–698.

60. Unger JM, Schuchmann GG, Frossman JE, Pellet JR. Tears of the trachea and main bronchi caused by blunt trauma: radiologic findings. *AJR Am J Roentgenol* 1989;153:1175–1180.

61. Weir IH, Müller NL, Connell DG. Case report: CT diagnosis of bronchial rupture. *J Comput Assist Tomogr* 1988;12:1035–1036.

62. Shepard JO. The bronchi: imaging perspective. *J Thorac Imaging* 1995;10:236–254.

63. McCarthy MJ, Rosado-de-Christenson ML. Tumors of the trachea. *J Thorac Imaging* 1995;10:1810–1980.

64. Grillo HC, Mathisen DJ. Primary tracheal tumors: treatment and results. *Ann Thorac Surg* 1990;49:69–77.

65. Kramer SS, Wehunt WD, Stocker JT, Kashima H. Pulmonary manifestations of juvenile laryngotracheal papillomatosis. *AJR Am J Roentgenol* 1985;144:687–694.

66. Kim Y, Lee KS, Yoon JH, et al. Tuberculosis of the trachea and main bronchi: CT findings in 17 patients. *AJR Am J Roentgenol* 1997;168:1051–1056.

67. Moon WK, Im JG, Yeon KM, Han MC. Tuberculosis of the central airways: CT findings of active and fibrotic disease. *AJR Am J Roentgenol* 1997;169:649–653.

68. Choe KO, Jeong HJ, Sohn HY. Tuberculous bronchial stenosis: CT findings in 28 cases. *AJR Am J Roentgenol* 1990;155:971–976.

69. Choplin RH, Wehunt WD, Theros EG. Diffuse lesions of the trachea. *Semin Roentgenol* 1983;18:38–50.

70. Schwartz M, Rossoff L. Tracheobronchomegaly. *Chest* 1994;106:1589–1590.

71. Dunne MG, Reiner B. CT features of tracheobronchomegaly. *J Comput Assist Tomogr* 1988;12:388–391.

72. Roditi GH, Weir J. The association of tracheomegaly and bronchiectasis. *Clin Radiol* 1994;49:608–611.

73. Woodring JH, Barrett PA, Rehm SR, Nurenberg P. Acquired tracheomegaly in adults as a complication of diffuse pulmoary fibrosis. *AJR Am J Roentgenol* 1989;152:743–747.

74. Shin MS, Jackson RM, Ho K-J. Case report. Tracheobronchomegaly (Mounier-Kuhn syndrome): CT diagnosis. *AJR Am J Roentgenol* 1988;150:777–779.

75. Martin CJ. Tracheopathia osteochondroplastica. *Arch Otolaryngol* 1974;64:290–293.

76. Mariotta S, Pallone G, Pedicelli G, Bisetti A. Spiral CT and endoscopic findings in a case of tracheobronchopathia osteochondroplastica. *J Comput Assist Tomogr* 1997;21:418–420.

77. Bottles K, Nyberg DA, Clark M, Hinchcliffe WA. Case report: CT diagnosis of tracheobronchopathia osteochondroplastica. *J Comput Assist Tomogr* 1983;7:324–327.

78. Onitsuka H, Hirose N, Watanabe K, et al. Computed tomography of tracheopathia osteoplastica. *AJR Am J Roentgenol* 1983;140: 268–270.

79. Im J-G, Chung JW, Han SK, Han MC, Kim C-W. CT manifestations of tracheobronchial involvement in relapsing polychondritis. *J Comput Assist Tomogr* 1988;12:792–793.

80. Mendelson DS, Som PA, Crane R, Cohen BA, Spiera H. Relapsing polychondritis studied by computed tomography. *Radiology* 1985; 157:489–490.

81. Katzenstein A-LA. Major problems in pathology. In: *Katzenstien and Askin's surgical pathology of non-neoplastic lung disease,* 3rd ed. Philadelphia: WB Saunders, 1997.

82. Cohen MI, Gore RM, August CZ, Ossoff RH. Case report. Tracheal and bronchial stenosis associated with mediastinal adenopathy in Wegener granulomatosis: CT findings. *J Comput Assist Tomogr* 1984; 8:327–329.

83. Aberle DR, Gamsu G, Lynch D. Thoracic manifestations of Wegener granulomatosis: diagnosis and course. *Radiology* 1990;174:703–709.

84. Stein MG, Gamsu G, Webb WR, Stulbarg MS. Case report: computed tomography of diffuse tracheal stenosis in Wegener granulomatosis. *J Comput Assist Tomogr* 1986;10:868–870.

85. Gross BH, Felson B, Birnberg FA. The respiratory tract in amyoidosis and the plasma cell dyscrasias. *Semin Roentgenol* 1986;21:113–127.

86. Case records of the Massachusetts General Hospital. Weekly clinico-pathological exercises. Case I-1995. An elderly man with a questionable bronchial tumor of long duration and recently increasing tracheal obstructions. *N Engl J Med* 1995;332:110–115.

87. Wilcox P, Miller R, Miller G, et al. Airway involvement in ulcerative colitis. *Chest* 1987;92:18–22.

88. Weibel ER, Taylor CR. Design and structure of the human lung. In: Fishman AP, ed. *Pulmonary diseases and disorders,* 2nd ed, vol 1. New York: McGraw-Hill, 1988:11–60.

89. Murata K, Khan A, Rojas KA, Herman PG. Optimization of computed tomography technique to demonstrate the fine structure of the lung. *Invest Radiol* 1988;23:170–175.

90. Webb WR, Stein MG, Finkbeiner WE, et al. Normal and diseased isolated lungs: high-resolution CT. *Radiology* 1988;166:81–87.

91. Osborne D, Vock P, Godwin J, Silveman P. CT identification of bronchopulmonary segments: 50 normal subjects. *AJR Am J Roentgenol* 1984;142:47–52.

92. Jardin M, Remy J. Segmental bronchovascular anatomy of the lower lobes: CT analysis. *AJR Am J Roentgenol* 1986;147:457–468.

93. Naidich DP, Terry PB, Stitik FP, Siegelman SS. Computed tomography of the bronchi. 1. Normal anatomy. *J Comput Assist Tomogr* 1980;4:746–753.

94. Webb WR, Hirji M, Gamsu G. Posterior wall of the bronchus intermedius: radiographic-CT correlation. *AJR Am J Roentgenol* 1984;142: 907–911.

95. Webb WR, Gamsu G, Glazer G. Computed tomography of the abnormal pulmonary hilum. *J Comput Assist Tomogr* 1981;5:485–90.

96. Naidich SP, Zinn WL, Ettenger NA, McCauley DI, Garay SM. Basilar segmental bronchi: thin-section CT evaluation. *Radiology* 1988;169: 11–16.

97. Lee KS, Im JG, Bae WK, et al. CT anatomy of the lingular segmental bronchi. *J Comput Assist Tomogr* 1991;15:86–91.

98. Lee KS, Bae WK, Lee BH, et al. Bronchovascular anatomy of the upper lobes: evaluation with thin-section CT. *Radiology* 1991;181: 765–772.

99. Jackson CL, Huber JF. Correlated applied anatomy of the bronchial tree and lungs with a system of nomenclature. *Dis Chest* 1943;9: 319–326.

100. Boyden EA. The nomenclature of the bronchopulmonary segments and their blood supply. *Dis Chest* 1961;39:1–6.

101. Boyden EA, Hartmann JF. An analysis of variations in the bronchopulmonary segments of the left upper lobes of fifty lungs. *Am J Anat* 1946;79:321–360.

102. Boyden EA, Scannell JG. An analysis of variations in the bronchovascular pattern of the right upper lobe of fifty lungs. *Am J Anat* 1948; 82:27–73.

103. Ferry RM, Boyden EA. Variations in the bronchosvascular patterns of the right lower lobe in fifty lungs. *J Thorac Cardiovasc Surg* 1951; 22:188–201.

104. Pitel M, Boyden EA. Variations in the bronchovascular patterns of the left lower lobe in fifty lungs. *J Thorac Cardiovasc Surg* 1953;26: 633–653.

105. Yamashita H. *Roentgenologic anatomy of the lung.* Stuttgart: Thieme Medical Publishers, 1978.

106. MacGregor JH, Chiles C, Godwin JD, Ravin CE. Imaging of the axillary subsegment of the right upper lobe. *Chest* 1986;90:763–765.

107. Landay M. Azygos vein abutting the posterior wall of the right main and upper lobe bronchi: a normal CT variant. *AJR Am J Roentgenol* 1983;140:461–462.

108. Jardin MR, Remy J. Comparison of vertical and oblique CT in evaluation of the bronchial tree. *J Comput Assist Tomogr* 1988;12:956–962.

109. Borman N. Broncho-pulmonary segmental anatomy and bronchography. *Minn Med* 1958;41:820–830.

110. Webb WR, Gamsu G. Computed tomography of the left retrobronchial stripe. *J Comput Assist Tomogr* 1983;7:65–9.

111. Mayr B, Heywang SH, Ingrisch H, et al. Comparison of CT with MR imaging of endobronchial tumors. *J Comput Assist Tomogr* 1987;11: 43–48.

112. Davis AL, Salzman SH, eds. *Bronchiectasis.* Philadelphia: WB Saunders, 1991.

113. Henschke CI, Davis SD, Auh PR, et al. Detection of bronchial abnormalities: comparison of CT and bronchoscopy. *J Comput Assist Tomogr* 1987;11:432–435.

114. McGuinness G, Beacher JR, Harkin TJ, et al. Hemoptysis: prospective high-resolution CT/bronchoscopic correlation. *Chest* 1994;105: 1155–1162.

115. Naidich SP, Lee JJ, Garay SM, et al. Comparison of CT and fiberoptic bronchoscopy in the evaluation of bronchial disease. *AJR Am J Roentgenol* 1987;148:1–7.

116. Set PAK, Flower CDR, Smith IE, et al. Hemoptysis: comparative study of the role of CT and fiberoptic bronchoscopy. *Radiology* 1993; 189:677–680.

117. Shure D. Transbronchial biopsy and needle aspiration. *Chest* 1989; 95:1130–1138.

118. Minami H, Ando Y, Nomura F, Sakai S, Shimokata K. Interbronchoscopist variability in the diagnosis of lung cancer by flexible bronchoscopy. *Chest* 1994;105:1658–1662.

119. Colice G, Chappel G, Frenchman S, Solomon D. Comparison of computed tomography with fiberoptic bronchoscopy in identifying endobronchial abnormalities in patients with suspected lung cancer. *Am Rev Respir Dis* 1985;131:397–400.

120. Conces DJ, Tarver RD, Vix VA. Broncholithiasis: CT features in 15 patients. *AJR Am J Roentgenol* 1991;157:249–253.

121. Woodring JH, Reed JC. Radiographic manifestations of lobar atelectasis. *J Thorac Imaging* 1996;11:109–144.

122. Gelb AF, Aberle DR, Schein MJ, Naidich DP, Epstein JD. Computed tomography and bronchoscopy in chest radiographically occult mainstem neoplasm: diagnosis and Nd-YAG laser treatment in 8 patients. *West J Med* 1990;153:385–389.

123. George PJM, Pearson MC, Edwards D, Rudd RM, Hetzel MR. Bronchography in the assessment of patients with lung collapse for endoscopic laser therapy. *Thorax* 1990;45:503–508.

124. Harrow EM, Oldenburg FA. Transbronchial needle aspiration in clinical practice: a five-year experience. *Chest* 1985;96:1268–1272.

125. Mehta A, Kavuru MS, Meeker DP, Gephardt GN, Nunez C. Transbronchial needle aspiration for histology specimens. *Chest* 1989;96: 1228–1232.

126. Schenk DA, Bower JH, Bryan CL. Transbronchial needle aspiration staging of bronchogenic carcinoma. *Am Rev Respir Dis* 1986;134: 146–148.

127. Schenk DA, Strollo PJ, Pickard JS. Utility of the Wang 18-gauge transbronchial histology needle in the staging of bronchogenic carcinoma. *Chest* 1989;96:272–274.

128. Wang KP, Terry PB. Transbronchial needle aspiration in the diagnosis and staging of bronchogenic carcinoma. *Am Rev Respir Dis* 1983; 127:344–347.

129. Wang KP, Brower R, Haponik EF, Siegelmann SS. Flexible transbronchial needle aspiration for staging of bronchogenic carcinoma. *Chest* 1983;84:571–576.

130. Hurter TH, Hanrath P. Endobronchial sonography: feasibility and preliminary results. *Thorax* 1992;47:565–567.

131. Goldberg BB, Steiner RM, Liu JB, et al. US-assisted bronchoscopy with use of miniature transducer-containing catheters. *Radiology* 1994;190:233–237.

132. McAdams HP, Goodman PC, Kussin P. Virtual bronchoscopy for directing transbronchial needle aspiration of hilar and mediastinal

lymph nodes: a pilot study. *AJR Am J Roentgenol* 1998;170: 1361–1364.

133. Jones DF, Chin R, Cappellari JO, Haponik EF. Endobronchial needle aspiration in the diagnosis of small-cell carcinoma. *Chest* 1994;105: 1151–1154.
134. Cropp AJ, DiMarco AF, Lankerani M. False-positive transbronchial needle aspiration in bronchogenic carcinoma. *Chest* 1984;85: 696–697.
135. Morales CF, Patefield AJ, Strollo PJ, Schenk DA. Flexible transbronchial needle aspiration in the diagnosis of sarcoidosis. *Chest* 1994; 709–711.
136. Pastores SM, Naidich DP, Aranda CP, McGuiness G, Rom WN. Intrathoracic adenopathy associated with pulmonary tuberculosis in patients with human immunodeficiency virus infection. *Chest* 1993;103: 1433–1437.
137. Harkin TJ, Karp J, Ciotoli C, et al. Transbronchial needle aspiration in the diagnosis of mediastinal mycobacterial infection [Abstract]. *Am Rev Respir Dis* 1993;147:A801.
138. Webb WR, Gatsonis C, Zerhouni EA, et al. CT and MR imaging in staging non-small cell bronchogenic carcinoma: report of the Radiologic Diagnostic Oncology Group. *Radiology* 1991;178:705–713.
139. Webb WR, Sarin M, Zerhouni EA, et al. Interobserver variability in CT and MR staging of lung cancer. *J Comput Assist Tomogr* 1993; 17:841–846.
140. Usuda K, Saito Y, Nagamoto N, et al. Relation between bronchoscopic findings and tumor size of roentgenographically occult bronchogenic squamous cell carcinoma. *J Thorac Cardiovasc Surg* 1993;106: 1098–1103.
141. Fraser RG, Pare JAP, Pare PD, Fraser RS, Genereux GP. *Diagnosis of disease of the chest*, 3rd ed, vol 1. Philadelphia: WB Saunders, 1988.
142. Proto AV, Tocino I. Radiographic manifestations of lobar collapse. *Semin Roentgenol* 1980;15:117–173.
143. Proto AV. Lobar collapse: basic concepts. *J Eur J Radiol* 1996;23: 9–22.
144. Woodring JH, Reed JC. Types and mechanisms of pulmonary atelectasis. *J Thorac Imaging* 1996;11:92–108.
145. Naidich DP, McCauley DI, Khouri NF, et al. Computed tomography of lobar collapse. 1. Endobronchial obstruction. *J Comput Assist Tomogr* 1983;7:745–57.
146. Naidich DP, McCauley DI, Khouri NF, et al. Computed tomography of lobar collapse. 2. Collapse in the absence of endobronchial obstruction. *J Comput Assist Tomogr* 1983;7:758–67.
147. Naidich DP, Ettinger N, Leitman BS, McCauley DI. CT of lobar collapse. *Semin Roentgenol* 1984;19:222–35.
148. Raasch BN, Heitzman ER, Carsky EW, et al. A computed tomographic study of bronchopulmonary collapse. *Radiographics* 1984;4: 195–232.
149. Khoury MB, Godwin JD, Halvorsen RA, Putman CE. CT of lobar collapse. *Invest Radiol* 1985;20:708–716.
150. Mintzer RA, Sakowicz BA, Blonder JA. Lobar collapse: usual and unusual forms. *Chest* 1988;94:615–620.
151. Mayr B, Ingrisch H, Haussinger K, Huber RM, Sunder-Plassmann L. Tumors of the bronchi: role of evaluation with CT. *Radiology* 1989; 172:647–652.
152. Gurney JW. Atypical manifestations of pulmonary atelectasis. *J Thorac Imaging* 1996;11:165–175.
153. Onitsuka H, Tsukuda M, Araki A, et al. Differentiation of central lung tumor from post obstructive lobar collapse by rapid sequence computed tomography. *J Thorac Imaging* 1991;6:28–31.
154. Heitmiller RF, Marascow WJ, Hruben RH, Marsh BR. Endobronchial metastasis. *J Thorac Cardiovasc Surg* 1993;106:537–542.
155. Zwiebel BR, Austin JHM, Grines MM. Bronchial carcinoid tumors: assessment with CT of location and intratumoral calcification in 31 patients. *Radiology* 1991;179:483–486.
156. Tredaniel J, Peillon I, Ferme C, et al. Endobronchial presentation of Hodgkin's disease: a report of nine cases and review of the literature. *Eur Respir J* 1994;7:1852–1855.
157. McGuinness G, Gruden JF, Bhalla M, et al. AIDS-related airway disease. *AJR Am J Roentgenol* 1997;168:67–77.
158. Shah H, Garbe L, Nussbaum E, et al. Benign tumors of the trcheobronchial tree: endoscopic characteristics and role of laser resection. *Chest* 1995;107:1744–1751.
159. Woodring JH. The computed tomography mucous bronchogram sign. *J Comput Assist Tomogr* 1988;12:165–168.

160. Fishman EK, Freeland HS, Wang KP, Siegelman SS. Case report: intrabronchial lesion on computed tomography secondary to blood clot. *J Comput Assist Tomogr* 1984;8:547–549.
161. Woodring JH. Determining the cause of pulmonary atelectasis: a comparison of plain radiography and CT. *AJR Am J Roentgenol* 1988; 150:757–763.
162. Tobler J, Levitt RG, Glazer HS, et al. Differentiation of proximal bronchogenic carcinoma from post-obstructive lobar collapse by magentic resonance imaging: comparison with computed tomography. *Invest Radiol* 1987;22:538–543.
163. Burke M, Fraser R. Obstructive pneumonitis: a pathologic and pathogenetic reappraisal. *Radiology* 1988;166:699–704.
164. Lee KS, Logan PM, Primack SL, Müller NL. Combined lobar atelectasis of the right lung: imaging findings. *AJR Am J Roentgenol* 1994; 163:43–47.
165. Rosenbloom SE, Ravin CE, Putman CE, et al. Peripheral middle lobe syndrome. *Radiology* 1983;149:17–21.
166. Kwon KY, Myers JL, Swensen SJ, Colby TV. Middle lobe syndrome: a clinicopathological study of 21 patients. *Hum Pathol* 1995;26: 302–307.
167. Gierada DS, Glazer HS, Slone RM. Pseudomass due to atelectasis in patients with severe bullous emphysema. *AJR Am J Roentgenol* 1997; 168:85–92.
168. Felson B. Lung torsion: radiographic findings in nine cases. *Radiology* 1987;162:631–638.
169. Berkman YM. Uncomplicated torsion: case report and literature review. *Chest* 1985;87:695–697.
170. Pinstein ML, Winer-Muram H, Eastridge C, Scott R. Middle lobe torsion following right upper lobectomy. *Radiology* 1985;155:580.
171. Nabawi P, Mantrauaot R, Breyer D, Capek V. Case report: computed tomography of radiation-induced lung injuries. *J Comput Assist Tomogr* 1981;5:568–570.
172. Pagani JJ, Libshitz HI. CT manifestations of radiation-induced change in chest tissue. *J Comput Assist Tomogr* 1982;6:243–248.
173. Mah K, Poon PY, Dyk JV, et al. Assessment of acute radiation-induced pulmonary changes using computed tomography. *J Comput Assist Tomogr* 1986;10:736–743.
174. Huber DJ, Kobzik L, Melasnosn G, Adams DF. The detection of inflammation in collapsed lung by alterations in proton nuclear magnaetic relaxation times. *Invest Radiol* 1985;20:538–543.
175. Shiyoa S, Haida M, Ono Y, Fukuzki M, Yamabayashi H. Lung cancer: differentiation of tumor, necrosis, and atelectasis by means of T1 and T2 values measured in vitro. *Radiology* 1988;167:105–109.
176. Herold CJ, Kuhlman JE, Zerhouni EA. Pulmonary atelectasis: signal patterns with MR imaging. *Radiology* 1991;178:715–720.
177. Glazer HS, Levitt RG, Lee JKT, et al. Differentiation of radiation fibrosis from recurrent pulmonary neoplasms by magnetic resonance imaging. *AJR Am J Roentgenol* 1984;143:729–73.
178. Barker AF, Bardana EJ. Bronchiectasis: update on an orphan disease. *Am Rev Respir Dis* 1988;137:969–978.
179. Stanford W, Galvin JR. The diagnosis of bronchiectasis. *Clin Chest Med* 1988;9:691–699.
180. Currie DC, Goldman JM, Cole PJ, Strickland B. Comparison of narrow section computed tomography and plain chest radiography in chronic allergic bronchopulmonary aspergillosis. *Clin Radiol* 1987; 38:593–6.
181. Millar A, Boothroyd A, Edwards D, Hetzel M. The role of computed tomography (CT) in the investigation of unexplained hemoptysis. *Respir Med* 1992;86:39–44.
182. Naidich DP, Funt S, Ettenger NA, Arranda C. Hemoptysis: CT-bronchoscopic correlations in 58 cases. *Radiology* 1990;177:357–362.
183. Im J-G, Itoh H, Shim Y-S, et al. Pulmonary tuberculosis: CT findings—early active disease and sequential change with antituberculous therapy. *Radiology* 1993;186:653–660.
184. Hartman TE, Swensen SJ, Williams DE. *Mycobacterium avium-intracellulare* complex: evaluation with CT. *Radiology* 1993;187:23–26.
185. Swensen SJ, Hartman TE, Williams DE. Computed tomography in diagnosis of *Mycobacterium avium-intracellulare* complex in patients with bronchiectasis. *Chest* 1994;105:49–52.
186. Moore EH. Atypical mycobacterial infection in the lung: CT appearance. *Radiology* 1993;187:777–782.
187. McGuinness G, Naidich DP, Garay SM, Leitman BS, McCauley DI. AIDS-associated bronchiectasis: CT features. *J Comput Assist Tomogr* 1993;17:260–266.

188. Amorosa JK, Miller RW, Laraya-Cusay L, et al. Bronchiectasis in children with lymphocytic interstitial pneumonia and acquired immune deficiency syndrome: plain film and CT observations. *Pediatr Radiol* 1992;22:603–607.

189. McGuinness G, Scholes JV, Jagirdar JS, et al. Unusual lymphoproliferative disorders in nine adults with HIV or AIDS: CT and pathologic findings. *Radiology* 1995;197:59–65.

190. King MA, Neal DE, St John R, Tsai J, Diaz PT. Bronchial dilatation in patients with HIV infection: CT assessment and correlation with pulmonary function tests and findings at bronchoalveolar lavage. *AJR Am J Roentgenol* 1997;168:1535–1540.

191. King MA, Stone JA, Diaz PT, et al. Alpha(1)-antitrypsin deficiency: evaluation of bronchiectasis with CT. *Radiology* 1996;199:137–141.

192. Kaneko K, Kudo S, Tashiro M, et al. Computed tomography findings in Williams-Campbell syndrome. *J Thorac Imaging* 1991;6:11–13.

193. Watanabe Y, Nishiyama Y, Kanayama H, et al. Congenital bronchiectasis due to cartilage deficiency: CT demonstration. *J Comput Assist Tomogr* 1987;11:701–703.

194. Neeld DA, Goodman LR, Gurney JW, Greenberger PA, Fink JN. Computerized tomography in the evaluation of allergic bronchopulmonary aspergillosis. *Am Rev Respir Dis* 1990;142:1200–1206.

195. Kullnig P, Pongratz M, Kopp W, Ranner G. Computerized tomography in the diagnosis of allergic bronchopulmonary aspergillosis. *Radiology* 1989;29:228–231.

196. Skeens JL, Fuhrman CR, Yousem SA. Bronchiolitis obliterans in heart-lung transplantation patients: radiologic findings in 11 patients. *AJR Am J Roentgenol* 1989;153:253–256.

197. Morrish W, Herman S, Weisbrod G, Chamberlain D. Bronchiolitis obliterans after lung transplantation: findings at chest radiography and high-resolution CT. *Radiology* 1991;179:487–490.

198. Lentz D, Bergin C, Berry G, Stoehr C, Theodore J. Diagnosis of bronchiolitis obliterans in heart-lung transplantation patients: importance of bronchial dilatation on CT. *AJR Am J Roentgenol* 1992;159:463–467.

199. Hruban R, Ren H, Kuhlman J, et al. Inflation-fixed lungs: pathologic-radiologic (CT) correlation of lung transplantation. *J Comput Assist Tomogr* 1990;14:329–335.

200. Graham N, Muller N, Miller R, Shepherd J. Intrathoracic complications following allogeneic bone marrow transplantation: CT findings. *Radiology* 1991;181:153–156.

201. Crawford SW, Clark JG. Bronchiolitis associated with bone marrow transplantation. *Clin Chest Med* 1993;14:741–749.

202. Haponik F, Britt EJ, Smith PL, Bleecker ER. Computed chest tomography in the evaluation of hemoptysis. *Chest* 1987;91:80–85.

203. Gudjberg CE. Roentgenologic diagnosis of bronchiectasis: an analysis of 112 cases. *Acta Radiol* 1955;43:209–226.

204. Reid LM. Reduction in bronchial subdivision in bronchiectasis. *Thorax* 1950;5:233–236.

205. Annest LS, Kratz JM, Crawford FA. Current results of treatment of bronchiectasis. *J Thorac Cardiovasc Surg* 1982;83:546–550.

206. Naidich DP. High-resolution computed tomography of cystic lung disease. *Semin Roentgenol* 1991;26:151–174.

207. Naidich DP, Harkin TJ. Airways and lung: CT versus bronchography through the fiberoptic bronchoscope. *Radiology* 1996;200:613–614.

208. Lynch DA, Tschumper B, Cink TM, Bethel R, Newell JD. Frequency of bronchial dilatation at high-resolution CT in asthmatics and control subjects. Abstract. *Radiology* 1991;181(P):250.

209. Kang EY, Miller RR, Müller NL. Bronchiectasis: comparison of preoperative thin-section CT and pathologic findings in resected specimens. *Radiology* 1995;195:649–654.

210. Smith IE, Jurriaans E, Diederich S, Ali N, Shneerson JM, Flower CDR. Chronic sputum production: correlations between clinical features and findings on high resolution computed tomographic scanning of the chest. *Thorax* 1996;51:914–918.

211. Kim JS, Muller NL, Park CS, et al. Bronchoarterial ratio on thin section CT: comparison between high altitude and sea level. *J Comput Assist Tomogr* 1997;21:306–311.

212. Diederich S, Jurriaans E, Flower CDR. Interobserver variation in the diagnosis of bronchiectasis on high-resolution computed tomography. *Eur Radiol* 1996;6:801–806.

213. Naidich DP, McCauley DI, Khouri NF, Stitik FP, Siegelman SS. Computed tomography of bronchiectasis. *J Comput Assist Tomogr* 1982;6:437–444.

214. Joharjy IA, Bashi SA, Abdullah AK. Value of medium-thickness CT in the diagnosis of bronchiectasis. *AJR Am J Roentgenol* 1987;149:1133–1137.

215. Cooke JC, Currie DC, Morgan MP. Role of computed tomography in the diagnosis of bronchiectasis. *Thorax* 1987;42:272–277.

216. Silverman PM, Godwin JD. CT/bronchographic correlations in bronchiectasis. *J Comput Assist Tomogr* 1987;11:52–56.

217. Young K, Aspestrand F, Kolbenstvedt A. High resolution CT and bronchography in the assessment of bronchiectasis. *Acta Radiol* 1991;32:439–441.

218. McGuinness G, Naidich DP, McAuley DI. Bronchiectasis: CT evaluation [Pictorial essay]. *AJR Am J Roentgenol* 1993;160:253–259.

219. Lynch DA, Brasch RC, Hardy KA, Webb WR. Pediatric pulmonary disease: assessment with high-resolution ultrafast CT. *Radiology* 1990;176:243–248.

220. Kim JS, Müller NL, Park CS, Grenier P, Herold CJ. Cylindrical bronchiectasis: diagnostic findings on thin-section CT. *AJR Am J Roentgenol* 1997;168:751–754.

221. Kim SJ, Im JG, Kim IO. Normal bronchial and pulmonary arterial dimeters measured by thin section CT. *J Comput Assist Tomogr* 1995;19:365–369.

222. Desai SR, Hansell DM. Small airways disease: expiratory computed tomography comes of age. *Clin Radiol* 1997;52:332–337.

223. Seneterre E, Paganin F, Bruel JM, Michel FB, Bousquet J. Measurement of the internal size of bronchi using high resolution computed tomography (HRCT). *Eur Respir J* 1994;7:596–600.

224. Lynch DA, Newell JD, Tschomper BA, Cink TM, Newman LS, Bethel R. Uncomplicated asthma in adults: comparison of CT appearance of the lungs in asthmatic and healthy subjects. *Radiology* 1993;188:829–833.

225. Weibel ER. High resolution computed tomography of the pulmonary parenchyma: anatomical background. Presented at the Fleischner Society Symposium on Chest Disease, Scottsdale, Arizona 1990.

226. Murata K, Itoh H, Todo G, et al. Centrilobular lesions of the lung: demonstration by high-resolution CT and pathologic correlation. *Radiology* 1986;161:641–645.

227. Webb WR, Gamsu G, Wall SD, Cann CE, Proctor E. CT of a bronchial phantom: factors affecting appearance and size measurements. *Invest Radiol* 1984;19:394–398.

228. Bhalla M, Turcios N, Aponte V, et al. Cystic fibrosis: scoring system with thin-section CT. *Radiology* 1991;179:783–788.

229. Remy-Jardin M, Remy J, Boulenguez C, Sobaszek A, Edme J-L, Furon D. Morphologic effects of cigarette smoking on airways and pulmonary parenchyma in healthy adults volunteers: CT evaluation and correlation with pulmonary function tests. *Radiology* 1993;1993:107–115.

230. Gruden JF, Webb WR, Warnock M. Centilobular opacities in the lung on high-resolution CT: diagnostic considerations and pathologic correlation [Pictorial essay]. *AJR Am J Roentgenol* 1994;162:569–574.

231. Murata K, Itoh H, Senda M, et al. Stratified impairment of pulmonary ventilation in "diffuse panbronchiolitis": PET and CT studies. *J Comput Assist Tomogr* 1989;13:48–53.

232. Nishimura K, Kitaichi M, Izumi T, Itoh H. Diffuse panbronchiolitis: correlation of high-resolution CT and pathologic findings. *Radiology* 1992;184:779–785.

233. Akira M, Kitatani F, Lee Y-S, et al. Diffuse panbronchiolitis: evaluation with high-resolution CT. *Radiology* 1988;168:433–438.

234. Hansell DM, Wells AU, Rubens MB, Cole PJ. Bronchiectasis: functional significance of area of decreased attenuation at expiratory CT. *Radiology* 1994;193:369–374.

235. Hansell DM, Strickland B. High-resolution computed tomography in pulmonary cystic fibrosis. *Br J Radiol* 1989;62:1–5.

236. Müller NL, Bergin CJ, Ostrow DN, Nichols DM. Role of computed tomography in the recognition of bronchiectasis. *AJR Am J Roentgenol* 1984;143:971–976.

237. Mootoosamy IM, Reznek RH, Osman J. Assessment of bronchiectasis by computed tomography. *Thorax* 1985;40:920–924.

238. Phillips MS, Williams MP, Flower CDR. How useful is computed tomography in the diagnosis and assessment of bronchiectasis? *Clin Radiol* 1986;37:321–325.

239. Grenier P, Maurice F, Musset D, Menu Y, Nahum H. Bronchiectasis: assessment by thin-section CT. *Radiology* 1986;161:95–9.

240. Giron J, Skaff F, Maubon A. The value of thin-section CT scans in the diagnosis and staging of bronchiectasis: comparison with bronchography in a series of fifty-four patients. *Ann Radiol (Paris)* 1988; 31:25–33.

241. van der Bruggen-Bogaarts BA, van der Bruggen HM, van Waes PF, Lammers JW. Assessment of bronchiectasis: comparison of HRCT and spiral volumetric CT. *J Comput Assist Tomogr* 1996;20:15–19.

242. Engeler CE, Tashjian JH, Engeler CM, et al. Volumetric high-resolution CT in the diagnosis of interstitial lung disease and bronchiectasis: diagnostic accuracy and radiation dose. *AJR Am J Roentgenol* 1993; 163:31–35.

243. Munro NC, Cooke JC, Currie DC, Strickland B, Cole PJ. Comparison of thin section computed tomography with bronchography for identifying bronchiectatic segments in patients with chronic sputum production. *Thorax* 1990;45:135–139.

244. Grenier P, Lenoir S, Brauner M. Computed tomographic assessment of bronchiectasis. *Semin Ultrasound CT MR* 1990;11:430–441.

245. Stern EJ, Webb WR, Gamsu G. Dynamic quantitative computed tomography: a predictor of pulmonary function in obstructive lung diseases. *Invest Radiol* 1994;29:564–569.

246. Zwirewich CV, Mayo JR, Müller NL. Low-dose high-resolution CT of lung parenchyma. *Radiology* 1991;180:413–417.

247. Tarver RD, Conces DJ, Godwin JD. Motion artifacts on CT simulate bronchiectasis. *AJR Am J Roentgenol* 1988;151:1117–1119.

248. Westcott JL, Cole SR. Traction bronchiectasis in end-stage pulmonary fibrosis. *Radiology* 1986;161:665–669.

249. Curtin JJ, Webster ADB, Farrant J, Katz D. Bronchiectasis in hypogammaglobulinemia: a computed tomography assessment. *Clin Radiol* 1991;44:82–84.

250. Patz EF, Swensen SJ, Erasmus J. Pulmonary manifestations of nontuberculous *Mycobacterium*. *Radiol Clin North Am* 1995;33:719–729.

251. Albelda SM, Kern JA, Martinelli DL. Expanding spectrum of pulmonary disease caused by nontuberculous mycobacterial mycobacteria. *Radiology* 1985;157:289–296.

252. Tanaka H, Amitani R, Niimi A, et al. Yield of computed tomography and bronchoscopy for the diagnosis of *Mycobacterium avium* complex pulmonary disease. *Am J Respir Crit Care Med* 1997;155:2041–2046.

253. Friedman PJ. Chest radiographic findings in the adult with cystic fibrosis. *Semin Roentgenol* 1987;22:114–124.

254. Santis G, Hodson ME, Strickland B. High resolution computed tomography in adult cystic fibrosis patients with mild lung disease. *Clin Radiol* 1991;44:20–22.

255. Taccone A, Romano L, Marzoli A, Girosi D. Computerized tomography in pulmonary cystic fibrosis. *Radiol Med (Torino)* 1991;82: 79–83.

256. Nathanson I, Conboy K, Murphy S, Afshani E, Kuhn JP. Ultrafast computerized tomography of the chest in cystic fibrosis: a new scoring system. *Pediatr Pulmonol* 1991;11:81–86.

257. Zhaomking W, Lockey RF. A review of allergic bronchopulmonary aspergillosis. *J Invest Allergol Clin Immunol* 1996;6:144–151.

258. Shah A, Pant CS, Bhagat R, Panchal N. CT in childhood allergic bronchopulmonary aspergillosis. *Pediatr Radiol* 1992;22:227–228.

259. Sandhu M, Mukhopadhyay S, Sharma SK. Allergic bronchopulmonary aspergillosis: a comparative evaluation of computed tomography with plain chest radiography. *Australas Radiol* 1994;38:288–293.

260. Angus RM, Davies ML, Cowan MD, McSharry C, Thompson NC. Computed tomographic scanning of the lung in patients with allergic bronchopulmonary aspergillosis and in asthmatic patients with a positive skin test to *Aspergillus fumigatus*. *Thorax* 1994;49:586–589.

261. Panchal N, Pant C, Bhagat R, Shah A. Central bronchiectasis in allergic bronchopulmonary aspergillosis: comparative evaluation of computed tomography of the thorax with bronchography. *Eur Respir J* 1994;7:1290–1293.

262. Panchal N, Bhagat R, Pant C, Shah A. Allergic bronchopulmonary aspergillosis: the spectrum of computed tomography appearances. *Respir Med* 1997;91:213–219.

263. Webb WR. High-resolution computed tomography of obstructive lung disease. *Radiol Clin North Am* 1994;32:745–757.

264. Reiff DB, Wells AU, Carr DH, Cole PJ, Hansell DM. CT findings in bronchiectasis: limited value in distinguishing between idiopathic and specific types. *AJR Am J Roentgenol* 1995;165:261–267.

265. Goyal R, White CS, Templeton PA, Britt EJ, Rubin LJ. Case report. High attenuation mucous plugs in allergic bronchopulmonary aspergillosis: CT appearance. *J Comput Assist Tomogr* 1992;16:649–650.

266. Logan PM, Müller NL. High-attenuation mucous plugging in allergic bronchopulmonary aspergillosis. *Can Assoc Radiol J* 1996;47: 374–377.

267. Zeinreich SJ, Kennedy SW, Malat M, et al. Fungal sinusitis: diagnosis with CT and MR imaging. *Radiology* 1988;169:439–444.

268. Logan PM, Primack SL, Miller RR, Müller NL. Invasive aspergillosis of the airways: radiographic, CT, and pathologic findings. *Radiology* 1994;193:383–388.

269. King TE. Overview of bronchiolitis. *Clin Chest Med* 1993;14: 607–610.

270. Hogg JC, Macklem PT, Thurlbeck WM. Site and nature of airway obstruction in chronic obstructive lung disease. *N Engl J Med* 1968; 268:1355–1360.

271. Macklem P, Mead J. Resistance of central and peripheral airways measured by a retrograde catheter. *J Appl Physiol* 1967;22:395–401.

272. Colby TV, Myers JL. The clinical and histologic spectrum of bronchiolitis obliterans including bronchiolitis obliterans organizing pneumonia (BOOP). *Semin Respir Dis* 1992;13:119–133.

273. Myers JL, Colby TV. Pathologic manifestations of bronchiolitis, constrictive bronchiolitis, cryptogenic organizing pneumonia and diffuse panbronchiolitis. *Clin Chest Med* 1993;14:611–623.

274. Bartter T, Irwin RS, Nash G, Balikian JP, Hollingsworth HH. Idiopathic bronchiolitis obliterans organizing pneumonia with peripheral infiltrates on chest roentgenogram. *Arch Intern Med* 1989;149: 273–279.

275. Bouchardy LM, Kuhlman JE, Ball WC, et al. CT findings in bronchiolitis obliterans organizing pneumonia (BOOP) with radiographic, clinical, and histologic correlation. *J Comput Assist Tomogr* 1993;17: 352–357.

276. Garg K, Lynch DA, Newell JD, King TE Jr. Proliferative and constrictive bronchiolitis: classification and radiologic features. *AJR Am J Roentgenol* 1994;162:803–808.

277. Hansell DM. What are bronchiolitis obliterans organizing pneumonia (BOOP) and cryptogenic organizing pneumonia (COP)? *Clin Radiol* 1992;45:369–370.

278. Hartman TE, Primack SL, Lee KS, Swensen SJ, Müller NL. CT of bronchial and bronchiolar diseases. *Radiographics* 1994;14: 991–1003.

279. Keller CA, Cagle PT, Brown RW, Noon G, Frost AE. Bronchiolitis obliterans in recipients of single, double, and heart-lung transplantation. *Chest* 1995;107:973–980.

280. Lynch D. Imaging of small airways diseases. *Clin Chest Med* 1993; 14:623–634.

281. Müller NL, Miller RR. Diseases of the bronchioles: CT and histopathologic findings. *Radiology* 1995;196:3–12.

282. Padley SPG, Adler BD, Hansell DM, Müller NL. Bronchiolitis obliterans: high-resolution CT findings and correlation with pulmonary function tests. *Clin Radiol* 1993;47:236–240.

283. Teel GS, Engeler CE, Tshijian JH, duCret RP. Imaging of small airways disease. *Radiographics* 1996;16:27–41.

284. Wells AU, duBois RM. Bronchiolitis in association with connective tissue diseases. *Clin Chest Med* 1993;14:655–666.

285. Yang CF, Wu MT, Chiang AA, et al. Correlation of high-resolution CT and pulmonary function in bronchiolitis obliterans: a study based on 24 patients associated with consumption of *Sauropus androgynus*. *AJR Am J Roentgenol* 1997;168:1045–1050.

286. Aquino SL, Gamsu G, Webb WR, Kee ST. Tree-in-bud pattern: frequency and significance on thin section CT. *J Comput Assist Tomogr* 1996;20:594–599.

287. Iwata M, Colby TV, Kitaichi M. Diffuse panbronchiolitis: diagnosis and distinction from various pulmonary diseases with centrilobular interstitial foam cell accumulations. *Hum Pathol* 1994;25:357–363.

288. Ichikawa Y, Hotta M, Sumita S, Fujimoto K, Oizumi K. Reversible airway lesions in diffuse panbronchiolitis: detection by high-resolution computed tomography. *Chest* 1995;107:120–125.

289. Hayakawa H, Sato A, Imokawa S, Toyoshima M, Chida K, Iwata M. Bronchiolar disease in rheumatoid arthritis. *Am Rev Respir Crit Care Med* 1996;154:1531–1536.

290. Yousem SA, Colby TV, Gaensler EA. Respiratory bronchiolitis–associated interstitial lung disease and its relationship to desquamative interstitial pneumonia. *Mayo Clin Proc* 1989;64:1373–1380.

291. Holt RM, Schmidt RA, Godwin JD, Rghu G. HRCT in respiratory bronchiolitis–associated interstitial lung disease. *J Comput Assist Tomogr* 1993;17:46–50.

292. Gruden J, Webb WR. Case report: CT findings in a proved case of respiratory bronchiolitis. *AJR Am J Roentgenol* 1993;161:44–46.

293. Davidson AG, Heard BE, McAllister WC, Turner-Warwick MEH. Cryptogenic organizing pneumonitis. *Q J Med* 1983;52:382–393.

294. Epler GR, Colby TV, McLoud TC, Carrington CG, Gaensler EA. Idiopathic bronchiolitis obliterans with organizing pneumonia. *N Engl J Med* 1985;312:152–159.

295. Thurlbeck WM, Miller RR, Müller NL, Rosenow ECI. *Diffuse diseases of the lung: a team approach.* Philadelphia: BC Decker, 1991.

296. Yoshinouchi T, Ohtsuki Y, Kubo K, Shikata Y. Clinicopathological study on two types of cryptogenic organizing pneumonitis. *Respir Med* 1995;89:271–278.

297. King TE. BOOP: An important cause of migratory pulmonary infiltrates? *Eur Respir J* 1995;8:193–195.

298. Epler GR, Colby TV, McLoud TC, et al. Bronchiolitis obliterans organizing pneumonia. *N Engl J Med* 1985;312:152–158.

299. Müller NL, Guerry-Force ML, Staples CA, et al. Differential diagnosis of bronchiolitis oliterans with organizing pneumonia and usual interstitial pneumonia: clinical, functional, and radiologic findings. *Radiology* 1987;162:151–156.

300. Cordier JF, Loire R, Brune J. Idiopathic bronchiolitis obliterans organizing pneumonia. *Chest* 1989;96:999–1005.

301. Müller NL, Staples C, Miller R. Bronchiolitis obliterans organizing pneumonia: CT features in 14 patients. *AJR Am J Roentgenol* 1990;154:983–987.

302. Lee KS, Kullnig P, Hartman TE, Müller NL. Cryptogenic organizing pneumonia: CT findings in 43 patients. *AJR Am J Roentgenol* 1994;162:543–546.

303. Akira M, Yamamoto S, Sakatani M. Bronchiolitis obliterans organizing pneumonia manifesting as multiple large nodules or masses. *AJR Am J Roentgenol* 1998;170:291–295.

304. Chang H, Wang J-S, Tseng H-H, Lai R-S, Su J-M. Histopathological study of *Sauropus androgynus*–associated constrictive bronchiolitis obliterans. *Am J Surg Pathol* 1997;21:35–42.

305. Miller RR, Müller NL. Neuroendocrine cell hyperplasia and obliterative bronchiolitis in patients with peripheral carcinoid tumors. *Am J Surg Pathol* 1995;19:653–658.

306. Brown MJ, English J, Müller NL. Case report. Bronchiolitis obliterans due to neuroendocrine hyperplasia: high-resolution CT–pathologic correlation. *AJR Am J Roentgenol* 1997;168:1561–2.

307. Dauber JH. Posttransplant bronchiolitis obliterans syndrome: where have we been and where are we going? [Editorial] *Chest* 1996;109:857–859.

308. Wright JL, Cagle P, Churg A, Colby TV, Myers J. Diseases of the small airways. *Am Rev Respir Dis* 1992;146:240–262.

309. Soubani AO, Miller KB, Hassoun PM. Pulmonary complications of bone marrow transplantation. *Chest* 1996;109:1066–1077.

310. Worthy SA, Flower CDR. Computed tomography of the airways. *Eur Radiol* 1996;6:717–729.

311. Ikonen T, Kivisaari L, Harjula ALJ, et al. Lung and heart-lung transplantation: value of high-resolution computed tomography in routine evaluation of lung transplantation recipients during development of bronchiolitis obliterans syndrome. *J Heart Lung Transplant* 1996;15:587–595.

312. Rohwedder JJ. Enticements for fruitless bronchoscopy [Editorial]. *Chest* 1989;96:708–710.

313. Dierkesman R. The diagnostic yield of bronchoscopy. *Cardiovasc Intervent Radiol* 1991;14:24–28.

314. Santiago S, Tobias J, Williams AJ. A reappraisal of the causes of hemoptysis. *Arch Intern Med* 1991;151:2449–2451.

315. Peters J, McClung HC, Teague RB. Evaluation of hemoptysis in patients with a normal chest roentgenogram. *West J Med* 1984;141:624–626.

316. Jackson CV, Savage PJ, Quinn DL. Role of fiberoptic bronchoscopy in patients with hemoptysis and normal chest roentgenograms. *Chest* 1985;87:142–144.

317. Sharma SK, Dey AB, Pande JN, Verma K. Fiberoptic bronchoscopy in patients with haemoptysis and normal chest roentgenograms. *Indian J Chest Dis Allied Sci* 1991;33:15–18.

318. Poe RH, Israel RH, Marin MG, et al. Utility of fiberoptic bronchoscopy in patients with hemoptysis and a nonlocalizing chest roentgenogram. *Chest* 1988;92:70–75.

319. Lederle FA, Nichol KL, Parenti CM. Bronchoscopy to evaluate hemoptysis in older men with nonsuspicious chest roentgenograms. *Chest* 1989;95:1043–1047.

320. Rath GS, Schaff JT, Snider GL. Flexible fiberoptic bronchoscopy: techniques and review of 100 bronchoscopies. *Chest* 1973;63:689–693.

321. Weaver LJ, Sollioday N, Cugell DW. Selection of patients with hemoptysis for fiberoptic bronchoscopy. *Chest* 1979;76:7–10.

322. Suri JC, Singla R. Cryptogenic hemoptysis: role of fiberoptic bronchoscopy. *Indian J Chest Dis Allied Sci* 1990;32:149–152.

323. Hirshberg B, Biran I, Glazer M, Kramer MR. Hemoptysis: etiology, evaluation, and outcome in a tertiary referral hospital. *Chest* 1997;112:440–444.

324. Jackson CL, Diamond S. Hemorrhage from the trachea, bronchi, and lungs of non-tuberculous origin. *Am Rev Tuberc* 1942;46:126–138.

325. Abbott GA. The clinical significance of pulmonary hemorrhage: a study of 1316 patients with chest disease. *Dis Chest* 1948;14:824–842.

326. Moersch HJ. Clinical significance of hemoptysis. *JAMA* 1952;148:1461–1465.

327. Pursel SE, Lindskog GE. Hemoptysis: a clinical evaluation of 105 patients examined consecutively on a thoracic surgical service. *Am Rev Respir Dis* 1961;84:329–336.

328. Johnston H, Reisz G. Changing spectrum of hemoptysis: underlying causes in 148 patients undergoing diagnostic flexible bronchoscopy. *Arch Intern Med* 1989;149:1666–1668.

329. Heimer D, Bar-Ziv J, Scharf SM. Fiberoptic bronchoscopy in patients with hemoptysis and nonlocalizing chest roentgenograms. *Arch Intern Med* 1985;145:1427–1428.

330. Gong H, Salvatierra C. Clinical efficacy of early and delayed fiberoptic bronchoscopy in patients with hemoptysis. *Am Rev Respir Dis* 1981;124:221–225.

331. Colletti PM, Peck S, Boswell WD, et al. Computed tomography in endobronchial neoplasms. *Comput Med Imaging Graph* 1990;14:257–262.

332. Snider GL. When not to use the bronchoscope for hemoptysis [Editorial]. *Chest* 1979;76:1–2.

333. Adelman M, Haponik EF, Bleeker ER, Britt EJ. Cryptogenic hemoptysis: clinical features, bronchoscopic findings, and natural history in 67 patients. *Ann Intern Med* 1985;102:829–834.

334. Garay SM, Naidich DP, Lin WC, et al. Hemoptysis: CT/fiberoptic bronchoscopic correlations in an outpatient population (abstract). *Chest* 1995;175(Suppl.):108.

335. Colice GL. Detecting lung cancer as a cause of hemoptysis in patients with a normal chest radiograph: bronchoscopy vs CT. *Chest* 1997;111:877–884.

336. McGuinness G, Naidich DP. Bronchiectasis: CT/clinical correlations. *Semin Ultrasound CT MRI* 1995;16:395–419.

CHAPTER 4

Focal Lung Disease

Assessment of patients with focal lung abnormalities presents an important problem in pulmonary diagnosis (1). Despite considerable advances in both imaging and biopsy techniques, controversy persists concerning the optimal evaluation and management of these cases, with little consensus on the definition of standard of care. Even the definition of a solitary nodule varies, leading us to favor, wherever applicable, the more inclusive term focal lung disease to solitary pulmonary nodule.

When assessing the role of CT in the evaluation of focal lung disease, it is appropriate to consider three separate albeit overlapping categories: detection, characterization, and management.

DETECTION

Pulmonary Metastases

Evaluation of patients with known or suspected pulmonary metastases serves as an ideal model for assessing both the strengths and limitations of computed tomography (CT) for detecting focal lung disease (2).

The superior sensitivity of CT compared with both routine chest radiography and conventional lung tomography for the detection of metastatic pulmonary nodules was documented soon after its introduction. Muhm et al., in a series of 91 patients, found more nodules with CT (35%) than with lung tomography (3). In 14% of cases, bilateral nodules were detected when conventional tomography showed only unilateral disease and nodules were detected in 6% of cases where none were seen with conventional techniques. Eighty-three percent of the additional nodules detected with CT were found at surgery to represent metastatic tumor. Similarly, in another early study Crow et al. found 59% of metastatic lesions measured 5 mm or less, a size rarely detected with standard radiography (4).

Despite these reports and numerous others confirming the value of CT to detect pulmonary metastases (5), from the outset the clinical value of CT for assessing metastatic tumor has been controversial. Schaner et al., in a prospective radiologic pathologic study in 1978, confirmed that CT defined more nodules than did conventional tomography (6). CT was much more effective for nodules in the 3 to 6 mm range. Nonetheless, 60% of the additional nodules detected by CT proved to be granulomas and pleural-based lymph nodes at resection. In addition, nearly one-third of the nodules discovered by CT could not be found by the surgeon. Similar limitations have been documented in a more recent investigation by Chalmers et al. (7). In their study of 146 patients with documented extrathoracic primary tumors, 16 (13%) of CT scans showed a total of 23 pulmonary nodules in patients with normal chest radiographs including 19 with nodules 5 mm or less in size: in over 80% of these cases, however, nodules proved to be benign. It should be noted, however, that assessment of most nodules in this study was clinical and that histologic confirmation was generally unavailable.

In a study involving radiologic-surgical correlation Peuchot and Libshitz evaluated 84 patients with previously documented extrathoracic malignancies and newly identified pulmonary nodules (8). These authors noted important limitations both in the sensitivity and specificity of CT. Of a total of 237 nodules resected, CT was able to identify only 173 (73%): 207 (87%) proved to be metastatic in etiology whereas 21 (9%) proved to be benign and nine (4%) were bronchogenic carcinomas. Of 65 nodules interpreted as solitary on chest radiographs, 46% were shown to have multiple nodules on CT. However, of those only 84% proved to be metastases (8).

In our experience specificity has proven to be related to patient status. The best specificity (a very high percentage of small nodules truly representing metastatic disease) is encountered in the initial staging of previously untreated younger patients. Positive findings on CT are less apt to be reliable when patients are examined months or years after a course of chemotherapy because of false positive results from nonneoplastic inflammatory changes.

In addition to limitations in both sensitivity and specificity, problems with interobservor variability have also been noted. In one study the value of CT in staging 202 patients with Wilm's tumors and normal chest radiographs was assessed by three independent observers (9). Although the three observers identified a total of 78 nodules, only 19 (24%) of these nodules were identified by all three readers. Of still greater concern, only 14 of the 202 patients actually developed documented pulmonary disease. Of these 14, only five had nodules identified by all three readers; furthermore, in five other cases, CT studies were interpreted as normal by all three readers. Although these data support a limited role for the use of CT in assessment of pulmonary metastases it should be noted that this study, extended from 1978 to 1995, raised issues both of reader experience, especially early in the study, as well as technique as a consequence of well documented limitations of early CT scanners.

Lung Cancer

Limitations in the ability of CT to identify patients with bronchogenic carcinoma also have been documented although to a far lesser degree than in studies assessing lung metastases. On occasion lung cancer may be diagnosed in a patient with a prior CT examination in which an abnormality was detectable but not reported. In a retrospective review of 35,000 CT studies reported by White et al., missed lung cancers were identifiable in 14 cases (10). Of these the majority were endobronchial (n = 10). In two cases each, solitary parenchymal nodules and focal peripheral air-space disease was retrospectively identified. Similar findings have been noted by Gurney et al., who reported on imaging findings in nine patients with missed lung cancers (11). Based on these studies it would appear that the lower limit of visibility of most parenchymal lesions is approximately 3 mm (12).

That missed lung cancers may represent a far larger group than previously appreciated has recently come to light as a result of the increasing frequency with which lung reduction surgery is being performed (13). Hazelrigg et al., in a study of 281 patients undergoing lung reduction surgery for emphysema found that a total of 110 (39.5%) patients had at least one nodule (14). Excluding calcified granulomas, there were 98 nodules further evaluated either surgically (n = 78) or with clinical follow-up (n = 20). Seventeen (22%) of those resected proved to be malignant. Of these, 14 proved retrospectively to have false negative CT studies.

Computer Simulation of Lung Nodules

Given the limitations noted above, efforts to further define variables affecting pulmonary nodule detection with CT have led investigators to explore the use of three-dimensional computer simulation (12). In one study 804 simulated nodules randomly distributed on 1.5-, 5-, and 10-mm thick sections, respectively, were evaluated by three experienced thoracic radiologists. The overall sensitivity in identifying nodules was only 62% whereas the corresponding specificity was 80% (12). Major determinants of lesion detectability included size (with observers identifying 1%, 48%, 82%, and 91% of nodules less than 1.5, 3, 4.5, and 7 mm, respectively), as well as location (with peripheral nodules easier to identify than central, perihilar nodules). Angiocentric nodules were more difficult to detect (Fig. 4-1). Results have also been recently reported using computer simulation to evaluate nodule detection comparing standard (200 mAs) with low-dose (20 mAs) scans (15). Interestingly, in this study no significant difference could be identified between low-dose and standard techniques, with sensitivities of 60% and 63%, and specificities of 88% versus 91% noted, respectively.

Conventional Versus Volumetric CT

From the outset it has been appreciated that an important use of spiral or helical CT is detecting pulmonary nodules (16–18). As reviewed in Chapter 1, a number of important advantages result from volumetric (helical/spiral) data acquisition. These include reduction in the time of examination, allowing the entire thorax to be imaged in a single breath hold, and the ability to obtain overlapping reconstructions without the need to obtain additional scans (19).

Helical CT has clearly improved the sensitivity of detecting small nodules (Fig. 4-2). Heywang-Köbrunner et al., in an early study of 40 patients evaluated both with conven-

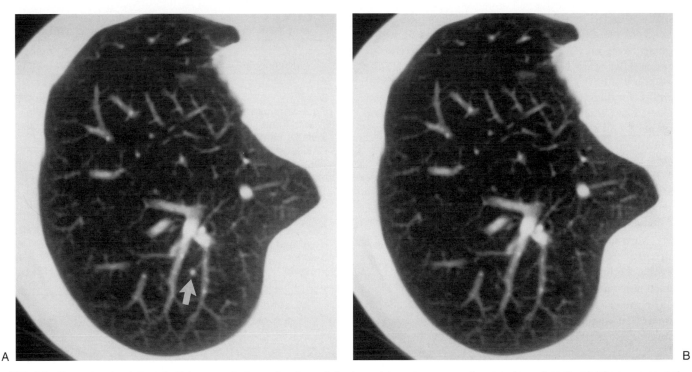

FIG. 4-1. Computer simulation. **A:** Enlargement of a section through the lower lobes shows a small nodule (*arrow*) easily mistaken as a normal vessel. **B:** Identical section to **A**, prior to computer simulation of the nodule seen in **A**. As shown here, nodules less than 3 mm are usually impossible to identify unless they are subpleural in location.

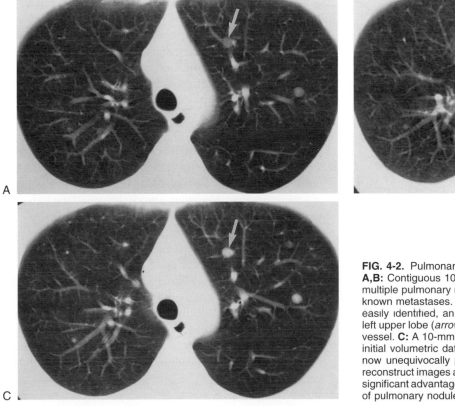

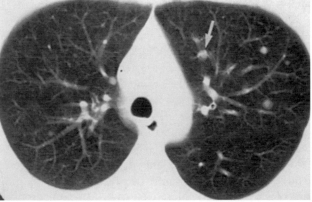

FIG. 4-2. Pulmonary nodule detection: volumetric CT evaluation. **A,B:** Contiguous 10-mm sections obtained with a pitch of 1 show multiple pulmonary nodules present in both lungs in a patient with known metastases. Note that although most of these nodules are easily identified, an apparent nodule in the medial portion of the left upper lobe (*arrows*) could be confused with a prominent central vessel. **C:** A 10-mm section retrospectively reconstructed from the initial volumetric data centered 5 mm below **A**. Central nodule is now unequivocally present (*arrow*). The ability to retrospectively reconstruct images at any arbitrary level represents one of the most significant advantages of spiral scanning, especially in the detection of pulmonary nodules. (From ref. 197, with permission.)

tional CT and volumetric CT found that although 245 nodules were identified by both techniques, an additional 22 nodules were only identified with spiral CT whereas only four nodules were identified with conventional CT (20). Costello et al., documented in a study of 19 patients that spiral CT using 10-mm slice thickness with a pitch of one detected 22% more nodules than conventional CT using contiguous 8 mm sections (17). Remy-Jardin et al., compared standard CT using sequential 10-mm sections to spiral CT using 10-mm sections with a pitch of one (21). In a series of 39 patients, the mean number of nodules detected per patient was significantly higher with spiral versus conventional CT (18 ± 4.5 versus 12.6 ± 3.2), as were the number of nodules less than 5 mm (12.7 ± 3.7 versus 8.4 ± 2.3) (21). Most importantly, multiple nodules were identified in three patients in whom conventional CT identified only one, whereas solitary nodules were identified in two cases in which conventional CT was interpreted as normal (21).

The greater accuracy of spiral CT compared to conventional CT in demonstrating lung nodules is due to its greater average contrast and spatial resolution provided that overlapping sections are obtained (22). Although, because of differences in slice sensitivity profiles, each individual spiral CT section is inferior to the corresponding conventional CT, optimal contrast and spatial resolution on conventional CT studies requires that nodules be precisely centered in the plane of section. For those nodules that lie between contiguous axial images, contrast and spatial resolution may decline by as much as 50%. Volumetrically acquired images reconstructed with overlapping reconstructions improve small lesion contrast by a factor of up to 1.8 (see Fig. 4-1).

Validation of an advantage to obtaining overlapping reconstructions has been documented. Buckley et al., in a retrospective evaluation of 67 spiral CT studies with a total of 116 nodules using four reviewers of varying interpretative skill compared contiguous 8-mm sections with 8-mm sections reconstructed every 4 or 5 mm (23). These authors documented a significant effect on interpreter's degree of confidence with more definite nodules and fewer indeterminate nodules identified (482 versus 431 and 101 versus 135, respectively; $p < .055$). As important, the number of false positive diagnoses significantly decreased with nearly one-third of scans initially interpreted as positive reinterpreted as normal with the advantage of overlapping sections. Nonetheless, it should be emphasized that despite these advantages, a total of 58 false positive studies were still recorded by even the most experienced interpreters. In this regard it should be noted that use of even thinner slice collimation (4 or 5 mm) would likely increase sensitivity still further, as many 2 or 3 mm peripheral subpleural metastases are apt to be missed with thicker sections.

Unfortunately, the use of overlapping reconstructions results in a considerable increase in the number of images to be evaluated, an effect that is clearly accentuated by use of thinner sections. As overlapping reconstructions are time-consuming both to generate as well as to interpret, our pres-

TABLE 4-1. *Incidence of pulmonary metastases from extrathoracic primaries (at presentation and autopsy)[a]*

Primary lesion	Presentation (%)	Autopsy (%)
Choriocarcinoma (female)	60	70–100
Kidney	5–30	50–75
Rhabdomyosarcoma	21	25
Wilm's tumor	20	60
Ewing's sarcoma	18	77
Osteosarcoma	15	75
Testicular (germinal)	12	70–80
Melanoma	5	66–80
Thyroid	5–10	65
Breast	5	60
Hodgkin's lymphoma	5	50–70
Colon/rectum	5	25–40
Head and neck	5	13–40
Bladder	5–10	25–30
Prostate	5	13–53
Non-Hodgkin's lymphoma	1–10	30–40

[a] Modified from ref. 38.

ent approach is to use minimum overlap in routine cases (i.e., 7- to 8-mm. sections reconstructed every 6 to 7 mm, respectively), reserving greater degrees of overlap only in those cases in which there is an especially high clinical index of suspicion that a nodule is present. This includes, in particular, patients with extrapulmonary malignancies with a known predilection for metastasizing to the lungs in whom detection of solitary and/or additional nodules may lead to a change in clinical management. As reviewed by Davis, the malignancies of concern are those with venous drainage to the lung. These include: carcinomas of the head and neck, kidneys, testes, choriocarcinomas, melanomas, bone and soft tissue sarcomas, endocrine tumors, and the major pediatric tumors with the exception of neuroblastoma (Table 4-1) (2).

Newer Approaches

Despite the advantages of volumetric scanning compared with conventional CT to identify pulmonary nodules, as noted above, significant limitations remain. It is not surprising therefore that alternative approaches continue to be explored. One relatively simple method has been to use cine viewing at a computer workstation in place of film. As proposed by Seltzer et al., the potential advantage of this approach is improvement in one's ability to trace vessels as they course three-dimensionally through the scan volume (24). Not surprisingly, in a preliminary study of 10-mm collimated spiral images evaluated at 2 mm intervals at frame rates as fast as 10 frames per second, these authors showed that a greater number of simulated nodules could be identified with the cine presentation than with film (mean of 0.69 versus 0.58 nodules per case, respectively, $p = .006$) (24). More recently, Tillich et al., in a similarly designed study,

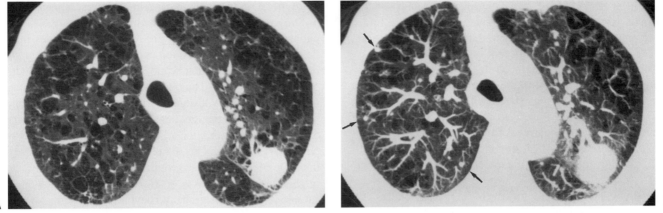

FIG. 4-3. Pulmonary nodule detection: use of maximum intensity projection images. **A:** One-millimeter section through a mass in the left upper lobe shows evidence of diffuse emphysema. Although subtle nodularity can be appreciated along the lateral pleural surface on the right side, no definite nodules can be identified. **B:** Maximum projection image obtained using five contiguous helical 1-mm sections using a pitch of 1 through the nodule shown in **A**. Note that the most dramatic effect of maximum projection images through the lungs is to accentuate vascular structures, allowing easier identification of pulmonary nodules (*arrows*). In this case, note that the nodules appear related to adjacent vessels, the so called feeding vessel sign.

also found an advantage to cine versus film-based viewing for identifying nodules (25). However, as noted by these authors, the major difference was in identifying small nodules less than 5 mm in size: larger nodules were identified with equal accuracy using both viewing techniques. With increasing focus on the advantages of filmless radiology, it may be anticipated that reliance on cine viewing will gain increasing acceptance.

Employing a technically more sophisticated approach, Napel et al., have shown that high resolution CT images of the lung can be obtained using sliding thin-slab maximum intensity projection (STS-MIP) as a technique for enhanced visualization of pulmonary vascular anatomy (Fig. 4-3) (26). Using 1- to 3-mm sections, these authors devised a method for rapidly computing a series of either overlapping maximum (MIP) or minimum (MINIP) intensity projection images through a thin slab of lung retaining a normal superoinferior or axial orientation. This results in images of high contrast resolution allowing enhanced visualization of peripheral blood vessels in particular using MIP reconstructions. This approach already has proved of some value for detecting micronodules in patients with diffuse infiltrative lung disease (27). Still considered to be experimental, this technique offers considerable promise in further improving nodule evaluation with volumetric CT.

More speculative is the use of automated segmentation to improve detection of pulmonary nodules (Fig. 4-4). As demonstrated by Croisille et al., using a three-dimensionally seeded region-growing algorithm to identify computer generated lung nodules, it is possible to connect and thus extract vessels from lung images increasing the conspicuity of lung nodules not attached to vessels (28). In an analysis of eight patients referred for possible nodules, these authors documented improved sensitivity ranging between 58% to 78% for three experienced radiologists using automated vessel

subtraction for detecting pulmonary nodules. As important, the proportion of false-positive interpretations decreased from 55% to 12%.

Although these preliminary results are promising, further studies need to be performed to determine the diagnostic accuracy and clinical utility of these techniques.

MR Imaging

The potential for magnetic resonance (MR) to detect pulmonary nodules is limited because of inferior spatial resolution as compared with CT. Nonetheless, MR does present some advantages that in select cases may allow identification of lesions with more certainty than CT. As noted by Müller

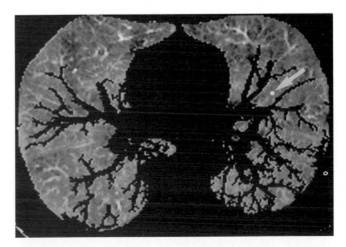

FIG. 4-4. Nodule detection: automated segmentation. CT image demonstrates the use of an automated three-dimensional seeded region growing algorithm to outline pulmonary vessels in black, facilitating identification of nodules separate from blood vessels (*arrow*).

et al., in an early study of 25 patients evaluated with both CT and MR using T2-weighted sequences, whereas CT allowed more precise identification of small nodules, MR was superior for detecting lesions adjacent to blood vessels (29).

More recently, Feuerstein et al., in a prospective study comparing CT with MRI in the evaluation of 12 cases with suspected pulmonary metastases with surgical correlation, found that MR and CT were equivalent for classifying patients as positive or negative for metastatic disease: surprisingly, this also proved true for individual nodules as well (30). Among the various pulse sequences employed, the most sensitive proved to be short inversion time inversion-recovery (STIR) images, identifying 82% of nodules. By comparison, gadolinium enhanced T1-weighted, and T2-weighted sequences proved less sensitive. Given the greater contrast resolution of MR, it is perhaps not surprising that MR would perform so well, especially in the detection of central or perihilar nodules (31). As reported by Doppman et al., MR has already been shown to be of value in detecting small, centrally located adrenocorticotrophic hormone producing bronchial carcinoid tumors (32). Nonetheless, given the advantages of greater spatial resolution and the ability to detect calcification, it is likely that helical CT will remain the method of choice for detecting pulmonary nodules for the foreseeable future.

CHARACTERIZATION

Definition

Various authors have applied a wide range of restrictions on what constitutes a solitary nodule. However, any patient whose chest roentgenogram shows a single rounded or ovoid lesion in the lung parenchyma, which is not associated with atelectasis or pneumonia, must be considered to have a solitary pulmonary nodule. The term *coin lesion* was suggested by O'Brien et al., to describe a focal mass (33). The term enjoyed a short-lived popularity but has since been disparaged since the description implies a flattened object instead of a spherical mass. Solitary pulmonary nodule (SPN) has been the most appropriate designated name for such lesions (34,35).

Clinical Evaluation

In the evaluation of pulmonary nodules a number of clinical and historical data should be considered. In addition to age and smoking history, these include: risk factors for cancer other than smoking, especially occupational exposure as well as the presence of coexisting parenchymal disease; history of a known prior malignancy; geographic considerations, including travel history; and results of diagnostic tests, especially skin testing (1).

Of these, probably the most reliable is assessment of age. Solitary pulmonary nodules are almost invariably benign in patients under 30. Taylor et al., resected 81 nodules in patients aged 20 to 29 and found one bronchogenic carcinoma, one "bronchial adenoma," and 79 benign lesions including 67 granulomas (36). Thus, unless there is a known primary malignancy, solitary lesions in patients younger than 30 may be presumed to be benign, but should be followed with serial chest roentgenograms for at least two years. In distinction, pulmonary malignancies should not be considered rare in the 30 to 39 year-old age group. Among 39 lesions resected in this age group, Davis et al., found nine bronchogenic carcinomas (37). At age 40 and beyond, there is greater probability of malignancy in any newly discovered solitary pulmonary nodule. Given that nearly 90% of these lesions may prove resectable, early diagnosis remains essential.

Patients with a history of extrathoracic malignancies pose a particular diagnostic problem, especially in the presence of small, less than 5 mm, sized nodules. Furthermore, these are difficult to biopsy percutaneously and may be difficult to palpate at surgery. In this context, clinical correlation can be of value. The propensity of certain tumors to metastasize to the lungs, in particular, varies and should be taken into account. Gilbert and Kagan, for example, have studied the estimated incidence of lung metastases for various primary neoplasms at presentation and autopsy (38). In their study, those tumors most likely to metastasize to the lung included choriocarcinoma, renal cell carcinoma, and bone and soft tissue sarcomas, in particular (see Table 4-1). A similar propensity for sarcomas as compared to carcinomas to metastasize to the lungs has been documented by Peuchot and Libshitz (8).

Solitary pulmonary nodules are a common finding on routine screening chest roentgenograms in adults. The vast majority of such incidentally detected lesions are benign. In two mass screening studies of the general population, only 3% to 6% of solitary nodules proved to be malignant (39, 40). This is in marked distinction to the prevalence of malignant nodules in clinical studies of patients referred for nodule evaluation. In this setting, estimates of the prevalence of cancer vary from 10% to 70%, presumably reflecting differences due to referral bias (41). Lung cancer, particularly early treatable malignancies, often manifests as a peripheral pulmonary nodule. In the early 1950s, Steele summarized the results of nine separate series that included a minimum of 100 resected solitary nodules (34): Although the incidence of malignant disease ranged from 10% to 68%, in two-thirds of these studies it exceeded 40%. In a more recent review of 1,267 lung cancers by Theros, 507 or 40% of cases initially presented as peripheral lung masses (42). Solitary lung nodule is the most common radiologic manifestation in patients with asymptomatic lung cancer. Stitik and Tockman in a surveillance study of male smokers found that 72% of the cancers detected in asymptomatic subjects were peripheral nodules (43).

Morphologic Evaluation

Unfortunately, clinical data rarely allow definitive evaluation. As a consequence, attention has necessarily been focused on radiographic characterization. Prior to the advent of CT, the radiologic factors most often considered useful in determining the nature of a pulmonary nodule included: (a) the presence of calcification; (b) the growth rate of the lesion; (c) lesion size; and (d) lesion contour. With the introduction of CT, the degree of accuracy with which these features may be assessed has improved. Furthermore a number of newer features, both morphologic and densitometric, may now be evaluated further expanding our ability to characterize focal parenchymal abnormalities.

Size

The likelihood of malignancy in an indeterminate pulmonary nodule detected by chest roentgenography is a direct function of the size of the lesion. This principle was well established in the years preceding the advent of CT. Thus, Steele et al., in a study of 756 resected asymptomatic solitary pulmonary nodules, noted a benign/malignant ratio of 13:1 in a group of 112 lesions 1 cm or less in size versus a ratio 1:4 in the 144 lesions greater than 3.0 cm in diameter (34). Experience with CT further documented that smaller lesions are more apt to be benign. Thus, in three published series of solitary nodules assessed by CT, the authors found that among all 1,000 nodules studied 67.5% of the 246 lesions from 0.5 to 1.0 cm in diameter proved to be benign, the 481 lesions from 1.0 to 2.0 cm were equally divided between benign and malignant, whereas over 85% of 322 lesions greater than 2.0 cm in diameter were malignant (44–46).

Despite these data it is apparent that lesion size, although a statistically significant discriminator between groups of benign and malignant lesions, is of only limited value in individual cases. In fact, even very small lesions may be malignant (Fig. 4-5). In a retrospective study of 64 patients with nodules less than one centimeter in size subsequently evaluated by video-assisted thoracoscopy reported by Munden et al., 38 (57%) proved to be neoplastic, including 37 nodules in patients without prior history of malignancy (47). Strikingly, in eight cases with nodules less than 5 mm in size (so-called ditzels), six of eight proved malignant whereas two proved to be due to intrapulmonary lymph nodes.

Location

It has long been established that primary lung cancers are more commonly found in the upper lobes, especially on the right side. This remains true to the present. In a recent review of 40 solitary nodules identified in an outpatient department, SPNs were identified in the right lung in 70% of cases and in the upper lobes in 65% (48). Not surprisingly, radiographically SPNs were most often identified in the lung periphery seen in 60% of cases, compared with the medial third and middle third of the lung in 10% and 30%, respectively (48). Similarly, metastatic lesions tend to be subpleural in location. In a study of serial sections of resected lungs containing metastatic nodules, Scholten and Kreel found that 60% of the lesions were in an immediate pleural or subpleural location and an additional 25% were located in the outer third of the lung (49). Furthermore, two-thirds of metastatic lesions occur in the lower lobes. Unfortunately, a number of other lesions also have a predilection for subpleural portions of the lungs. As documented by Bankoff et al., in a study including 96 patients with well-circumscribed peripheral pulmonary nodules undergoing minithoracotomies, 17 (18%)

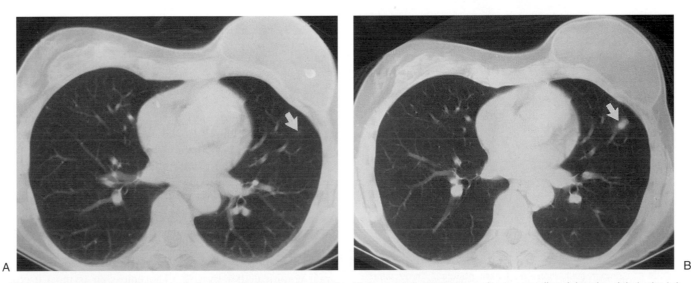

FIG. 4-5. Metastatic breast cancer. **A:** Seven-millimeter section obtained following left mastectomy shows a small peripheral nodule in the left upper lobe (*arrow*). Given the small size of this lesion it was elected to follow this radiographically. **B:** Follow-up CT study 4 months later at the same level confirms substantial interval growth (*arrow*) because of biopsy-proved metastatic breast cancer.

proved to have intrapulmonary lymph nodes (50). It should be noted that most of these proved to be solitary with 12 located within the lower lobes.

Contour and Edge

Malignant nodules are much more apt to have an irregular contour and an ill-defined, irregular, or spiculated margin (Fig. 4-6) (51) and this pertains even to calcified lesions. Benign lesions, on the other hand, much more commonly exhibit a round or oval contour and a sharply defined edge. This has proved true both for primary and metastatic nodules. In patients with known neoplasms and multiple pulmonary nodules, Gross et al. found that metastatic lesions on CT are more likely to be spherical or ovoid in shape (52) whereas linear, triangular, irregularly shaped, or multiple ill-defined lesions, especially when centrally located, are less likely to represent metastases. These authors also found that if noncalcified round lesions, larger than 2.5 cm, were present or if more than 10 lesions were visualized in any one patient, the likelihood of metastatic disease was very high.

Nonetheless, although the contour and shape of lesions may provide some indication as to the likelihood of malignancy, it is not unusual both for primary lung neoplasms and, in particular, solitary metastases to present with smooth, sharply marginated contours. Hirakata et al., in a study of 87 metastatic lesions identified at autopsy, including 43 nodules less than 5 mm in size (53), found 38% of nodules to be well-defined with smooth margins using high resolution

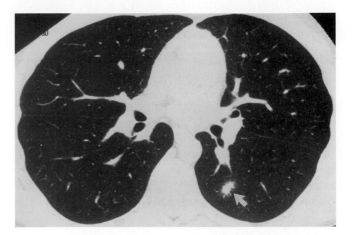

FIG. 4-7. Contour evaluation—tuberculosis. One millimeter CT section through the superior segment of the left lower lobe shows an approximately 1 cm spiculated lesion without CT evidence of calcification. Despite irregular margins and an associated subtle halo sign this lesion proved on resection to be caused by tuberculosis.

computed tomography (HRCT), whereas 16% had poorly defined smooth margins and 30% had poorly defined, irregular margins. Well-defined lesions correlated with the presence of tumor displacing surrounding normal structures by uniform expansion, whereas irregular margins correlated with proliferation of tumor into the adjacent interstitium. Less well appreciated is the fact that benign lesions may also have spiculated margins, further limiting the usefulness of this sign (Fig. 4-7).

Surprisingly, given the importance usually attributed to the edges of lesions, significant interobserver variability in the assessment of this sign has also been reported. In a study characterizing nodules in 66 patients, the largest discrepancy between four board certified readers was in classification of nodule contour (54). This suggests that accurate evaluation of this sign may require a more precise definition of this sign, perhaps even the potential use of a more quantitative assessment (55,56).

Halo Sign

The halo sign by definition is a discrete nodule surrounded by a circular margin of ground glass attenuation (Fig. 4-8). Usually representing edema or hemorrhage, this sign has proved useful in the proper clinical situation as an early indication of invasive pulmonary aspergillosis (IPA) (see Fig. 4-8A) (57–61). When identified in immunocompromised patients, particularly those with acute leukemia, following aggressive therapeutic marrow suppression accompanied by severe leukopenia, detection of the halo sign has proved sufficiently characteristic of fungal infection to warrant empirical therapy (62). The halo sign is most useful early in the course of infection. As noted by Blum et al., in their prospective study of 38 neutropenic patients presenting

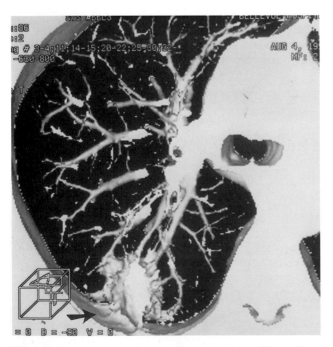

FIG. 4-6. Contour evaluation—malignant nodules. Three dimensional surface reconstruction showing to good effect the spiculated nature of this peripheral lung cancer. Note the presence of parietal pleural invasion (*arrow*). (From ref. 198, with permission.)

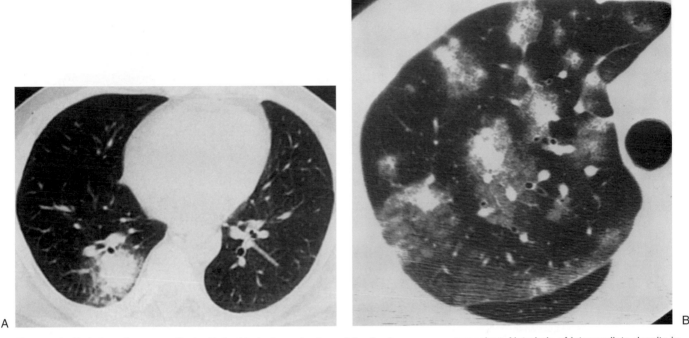

FIG. 4-8. A: Early invasive aspergillosis. Patient in leukopenic phase following bone marrow transplant. Note halo of intermediate density in the transition zone between the nodule and the normal lung. This sign is suggestive of infection by angiotropic organisms, the most common of which is *Aspergillus fumigatus*. **B:** One-millimeter target reconstructed image through the right upper lobe shows multiple ill-defined nodules all associated with adjacent areas of ground glass attenuation. In this case with documented pulmonary Kaposi's sarcoma, areas of ground glass attenuation represent associated lung hemorrhage. Based on these cases it may be concluded that the finding of a halo sign, per se, is nonspecific (see Fig. 4-7).

with radiographic evidence of nodular lung disease, a halo sign was noted in 16 of 22 patients evaluated within the first seven days with documented IPA, with no false positive studies: in distinction, a halo sign could be identified in only 3 of 13 patients with proved invasive aspergillosis evaluated only after 10 days (61). As most of these patients also have extremely low platelet counts making biopsy infeasible, CT findings play a critical role in the management of these patients (58). It is only later following successful therapy when granulocytes begin to return to the blood stream and patients begin to recover, that the characteristic air crescent sign traditionally identified on plain radiographs as diagnostic of fungal infection is seen as the central infarcted portion of the lesion becomes demarcated.

Mori et al., in a study of 33 febrile bone marrow recipients found that CT showed nodules in 20 of 21 episodes of documented fungal infection but none in nine bacteremic episodes (62). Based on these data, these authors concluded that CT studies documenting the presence of nodules in this population could be taken as presumptive evidence of fungal infection warranting empiric therapy without the need for bronchoscopy. It should be emphasized, however, that the halo sign is nonspecific and has been reported in a variety of other lesions in which both inflammatory and neoplastic processes compromise blood vessels or nodules are surrounded by hemorrhage. Primack et al., have described this

sign in patients with other infections including candidiasis, cytomegalovirus infection, and herpes pneumonia, as well as in patients with Kaposi's sarcoma and metastatic angiosarcoma (see Fig. 4-8B) (63). The halo sign has also been reported to occur in patients with tuberculomas (64).

Recently, a potential role for MRI has been suggested for assessing patients with suspected IPA (Fig. 4-9) (61,65). In particular, it has been noted that the finding of lower signal intensity in the center of a lesion with higher signal intensity along the rim (so-called target sign) on T2-weighted sequences in the appropriate setting should suggest IPA, especially early in the course of infection (65). Presumably, the finding of rim enhancement on T2-weighted sequences is a reflection of either subacute hemorrhage or peripheral inflammation or edema. However, the value of this sign has been questioned, especially early in the course of infection. Contrary to prior reports, Blum et al., in a study of 38 patients evaluated with contrast-enhanced MRI, found no evidence of rim enhancement in any patient imaged less than 10 days following the appearance of nodules on corresponding chest radiographs (61). However, a target sign was noted in 13 patients late in the course of infection (greater than 10 days) in patients with fully developed infection as well as those with resolving IPA. Given these contradictory results, it is apparent that MRI should at present be deemed of only limited value in assessing patients with suspected IPA.

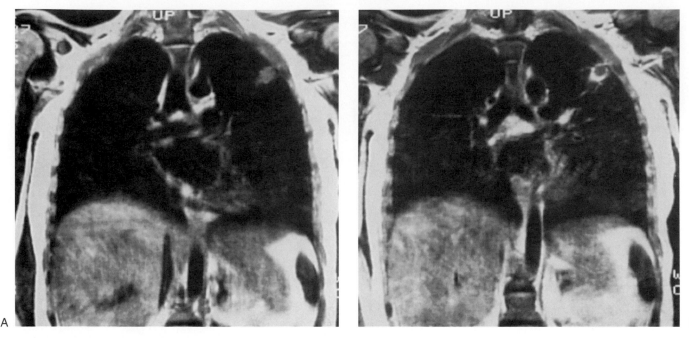

FIG. 4-9. Focal invasive pulmonary aspergillosis in an immunocompromised patient. **A:** T1-weighted coronal scan. **B:** T1-weighted scan post GdDTPA enhancement. Note target-like appearance of lesion with high signal intensity rim and nonenhancing center. (From Herold CJ, Karmer J, Sertl K, et al. Invasive pulmonary aspergillosis: evaluation with MR imaging. *Radiology* 1989;173:717–721, with permission.)

Positive Bronchus Sign

The presence of a positive bronchus sign or air-bronchogram is an important and common finding with thin-section CT (Figs. 4-10 and 4-11). Gaeta et al., reported a prevalence of a positive bronchus sign in 66.7% of solitary pulmonary nodules evaluated by thin-section CT whereas Kuriyama et al., reported a prevalence of 35.0% (14 out of 40 cases) in patients with documented malignant nodules (66,67). Although nonspecific, pulmonary lesions that directly abut, displace, or narrow a visible bronchial lumen should not be assessed as benign (44, 67–69). In a retrospective study of 132 patients with solitary nodules evaluated with CT, Kui et al. identified a total of 34 lesions with air-bronchograms: altogether 33 (28.7%) of 115 proved lung cancers but only 1 (5.9%) of 17 benign lesions had air-bronchograms identified (69). When assessed morphologically, airways seen in relation to lung cancers were invariably abnormal, being either tortuous, ectatic, or cut-off, confirming earlier descriptions by Gaeta et al. (70).

Cystic/Cavitary Disease

A number of mechanisms have been proposed to account for parenchymal cysts and cavities. These include: (a) vascular occlusion with ischemic necrosis, as occurs in patients with infections, including septic emboli and IPA, vasculitidies, and tumors; (b) airway dilatation, resulting from bron-chial occlusion and/or peribronchial fibrosis; (c) disruption of the elastic fiber network of the lung resulting in pulmonary emphysema; (d) remodeling of the lung parenchyma as occurs in patients with extensive fibrosis; and (e) multifactorial or unknown mechanisms (71). Although most of these result in diffuse cystic change or cavitation, most may occasionally present with isolated or focal disease.

CT improves both the detection and characterization of lung cysts and cavities (Figs. 4-12–4-14). In addition to assessing the relationship between cavities and airways and surrounding parenchyma, CT allows precise evaluation of the thickness of cavity walls as well as the presence of intracavitary filling defects and/or air-fluid levels. As reported by Woodring et al., the most important of these is assessment of cavity wall thickness (72). Of 65 solitary lung cavities initially assessed by these authors using plain radiographs, all lesions in which the thickest part of the cavity wall was 1 mm were benign: in distinction, of those with greatest wall thickness measuring between 5 to 15 mm, 51% were benign, whereas of those over 15 mm, 95% were malignant. In a follow-up prospective study of 61 additional patients reported by these same authors, 19 (95%) of 20 cavities with a maximum wall thickness of 4 mm again proved benign, whereas 16 (84.2%) of 19 cavities with maximum wall thickness of 16 mm proved malignant (73). In our experience, although thin-walled cavities are almost always benign, thick-walled cavities are usually of indeterminate etiology (see Fig. 4-13).

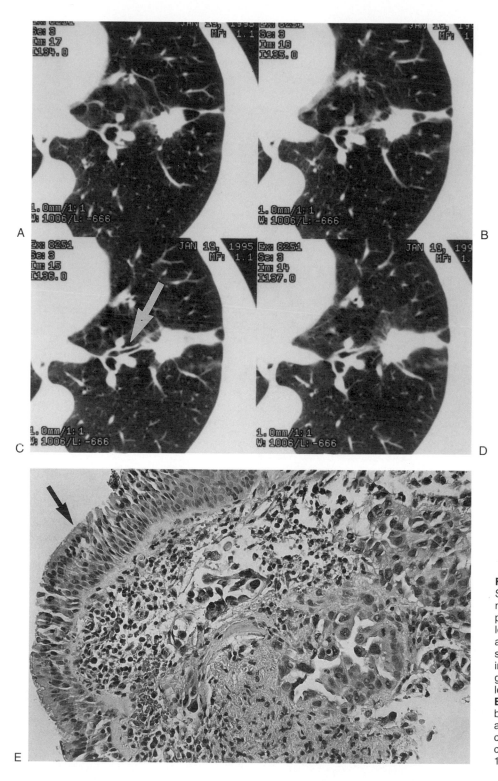

FIG. 4-10. Positive bronchus sign. **A–D:** Sequential 1-mm sections obtained volumetrically through the left midlung show presence of a poorly defined lesion in the left lower lobe. Note that in this case the anterobasilar bronchus can be traced on sequential images into this lesion (*arrow* in C). This appearance correlates with a greater likelihood of obtaining a histologic diagnosis on transbronchial biopsy. **E:** Histologic section obtained by transbronchial biopsy identifying this lesion as a nonsmall cell lung cancer. Note the close proximity of tumor cells to the adjacent bronchial mucosa (*arrow*). (From ref. 198, with permission.)

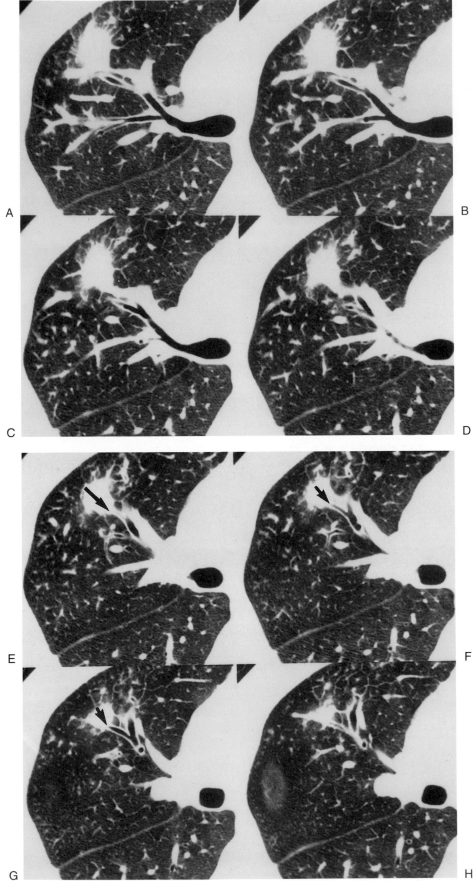

FIG. 4-11. Positive bronchus sign. **A–H:** Sequential 1-mm helical CT sections from above-downward in a patient with a spiculated right upper lobe nodule first through the right upper lobe bronchus (**A–D**) and then the bronchus intermedius (**E–H**) allow central airway branches to be traced sequentially. Note that in this case, a lateral sub-subsegmental branch of the anterior segmental bronchus can be traced to this lesion (*arrows* in **E–G**). The ability to identify a relationship between airways and nodules has clear implications for the likely success of transbronchial biopsy in establishing a definitive histologic diagnosis. Bronchoscopically verified nonsmall cell lung cancer.

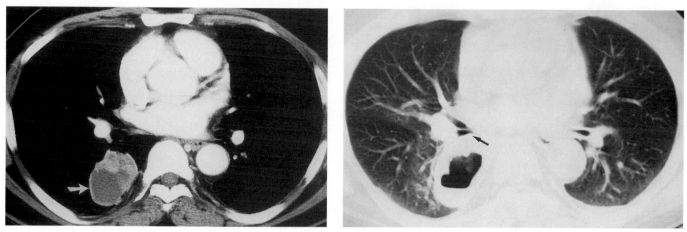

FIG. 4-12. Cavitation—lung cancer. **A:** Contrast enhanced CT section shows a heterogeneous mass in the superior segment of the right lower lobe in which low density is easily identified consistent with necrosis (*arrow*). **B:** Follow-up CT section at the same level through the middle lobe bronchus shows that this neoplasm has enlarged and cavitated and now contains an air-fluid level. Note that there is narrowing of the right lower lobe bronchus (*arrow*), suggesting bronchial communication to account for the presence of air within the tumor.

Feeding Vessel Sign

Focal disease in which identification of the relationship between nodules and adjacent or feeding vessels have been described include metastases, infarcts, and arteriovenous malformations. Particularly intriguing has been the observations made by some investigators of a connection between pulmonary metastases and adjacent pulmonary arteries, the so-called feeding vessels sign (Fig. 4-15). Meziane et al., in a radiologic-pathologic correlative study, noted frequent identification of pulmonary vessels leading to the center of metastatic lesions (74). These results have received further confirmation using microangiographic techniques (75). However, in a more recent study comparing the thin section CT appearance of metastases with histopathologic findings, Hirakata et al. studied 87 metastatic lesions identified at autopsy, including 43 nodules less than 5 mm in size (53). Contrary to previous reports, these investigators found that in the majority of lesions no discernible relationship could be identified between metastases and adjacent pulmonary vessels. It is worth noting that this latter study was based on careful analysis of high resolution CT images. It is likely that the higher prevalence of the feeding vessel sign in previous investigations was in part artifactual because of volume averaging of thicker CT sections.

Although a vascular connection is not commonly seen, when present it is helpful for distinguishing hematogenous metastases from either primary carcinomas or granulomatous lesions (see Fig. 4-15). The finding of a feeding vessel sign has also proven reliable in diagnosing patients with septic emboli and in the appropriate clinical setting may suggest a diagnosis of pulmonary vasculitis: in these cases, however, multiple nodules are almost always present (Fig. 4-16). A major potential pitfall in using this mass-vessel sign is the possibility of partial volume effects making a lesion appear connected to an adjacent but unrelated vessel, especially one coursing obliquely through the scan plane. To obviate this pitfall it should be emphasized that thin sections are necessary in order to properly assess this sign.

Other indirect signs suggesting a hematogenous or vascular etiology have been described. One is the finding of a zone of hypodensity distal to nodules. Presumably, this represents hypoperfusion distal to a pulmonary artery occluded by metastases. Even after successful chemotherapy in patients with documented metastatic lung disease, a mass-vessel connection can still be seen. Other indirect but suggestive findings indicative of vascular disease have been described in patients with documented pulmonary infarction (76).

Morphologic Characteristics: Specific Etiologies

In a number of instances, morphologic characteristics, alone or in combination with other findings, including calcification and/or patterns of contrast enhancement, are sufficiently specific to suggest definitive diagnoses. In our experience these include carcinoid tumors (see also Chapter 3), bronchoalveolar cell carcinomas, arteriovenous malformations, pulmonary infarcts, and round atelectasis (see also Chapter 9).

Carcinoid Tumors

Classified as part of the spectrum of neuroendocrine lung neoplasms, carcinoids are further characterized as either typical or atypical (77). These tumors tend to exhibit variable growth patterns. Most arise as endobronchial obstructing lesions, resulting on occasion in an appearance of focal mucoid impaction; alternatively they may extend extraluminally, resulting in so-called iceberg lesions. Unlike typical carci-

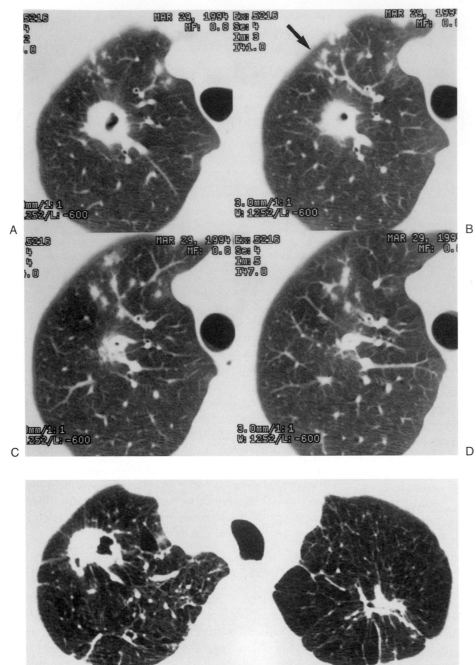

FIG. 4-13. Thick-walled cavities: differential diagnosis. **A–D:** Sequential high resolution sections through the right upper lobe show a thick walled cavity associated with adjacent nodules with a tree-in-bud configuration (*arrow* in **B**). This constellation of findings is strongly suggestive of active tuberculosis, subsequently verified at bronchoscopy. **E:** CT section in a different patient than **A–D**, also shows bilateral irregular thick-walled cavities. In this case, the lesion in the right upper lobe proved to be a cavitary lung cancer whereas the lesion in the left upper lobe proved to be caused by tuberculosis (biopsy proved). As shown in these cases, the presence of a thick-walled cavity in itself is nonspecific.

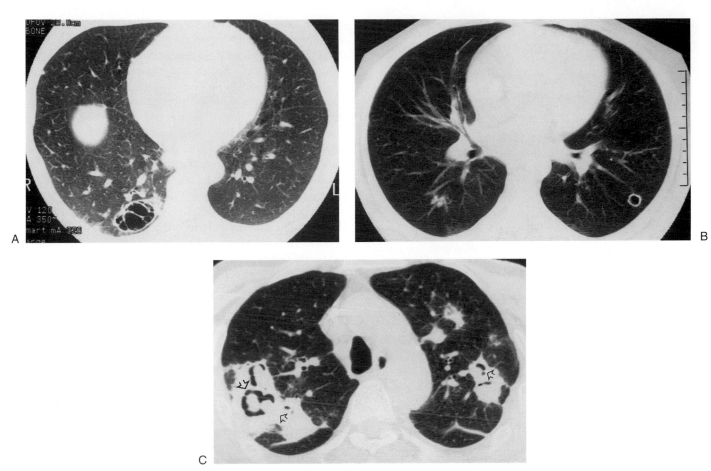

FIG. 4-14. Cavitation: benign disease. **A:** High resolution CT section shows a multiseptated, thin-walled cavity in the posterobasilar segment of the right lower lobe, associated with minimal eccentric consolidation and ground glass attenuation. Findings consistent with clinically documented cryptococcal infection. **B:** High resolution CT section shows sharply defined, thin walled cavity in the left lower lobe in an acquired immune deficiency syndrome (AIDS) patient, subsequently documented to have atypical mycobacterial infection (MAI). Note as well the presence in the right lower lobe of a focal area of mucoid impaction. The finding of thin-walled cavities, with or without septations is a reliable sign of benignancy. **C:** CT section through the distal trachea shows multiple thick-walled cavities in this patient with prior treated tuberculosis within which are nodular filling defects (*arrows*), findings consistent with superimposed fungal infection, in this case caused by Aspergillus species.

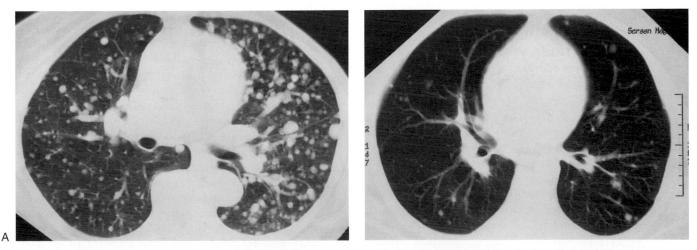

FIG. 4-15. Feeding vessel sign: metastatic disease. **A:** Seven-millimeter section in a patient with documented metastatic disease shows numerous nodules, many in close proximity to small vessels. **B:** Seven-millimeter section in a different patient with distinctly fewer nodules than in **A** again shows many with apparent feeding vessels. This sign is more likely to occur in patients with multiple nodules, suggesting that this sign is partly coincidental.

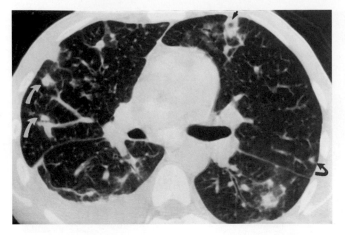

FIG. 4-16. Feeding vessel sign: septic pulmonary emboli. One-millimeter section shows scattered nodules in both lungs, some clearly cavitary (*straight arrow*), many of which are either associated with peripheral vessels (*curved arrows*), or are subpleural in location associated with a moderate-sized right pleural effusion. This constellation of findings is suggestive of septic pulmonary emboli, in this case confirmed by blood cultures as caused by staphylococcal infection. (From ref. 198, with permission.)

noids, atypical carcinoids show a marked propensity to metastasize early, especially to regional lymph nodes.

A typical triad of features has been described for central carcinoid tumors and includes: (a) a well defined round or slightly lobulated lesion that; (b) abuts or narrows a central airway; (c) in which eccentric calcifications can be identified (Fig. 4-17). As will be discussed in greater detail below, eccentric calcification is common, especially in central tumors, with foci of calcification or even ossification shown histologically in up to 30% of cases (78). In addition, these lesions are characteristically extremely vascular and therefore show marked contrast enhancement following intravenous contrast administration (Fig. 4-18). Although accurate preoperative evaluation requires precise definition of both the intraluminal and the extraluminal components of these tumors, recognition of the vascular nature of these lesions is also of obvious value especially prior to bronchoscopy given the propensity of these lesions to hemorrhage, sometimes massively, when biopsied.

Bronchoalveolar Cell Carcinoma

Of all tumors, the relationship between airways and lesions has been most carefully assessed in patients with bronchoalveolar cell carcinomas (BAC) (Fig. 4-19) (51,66,79,80). Gaeta et al., in a review of thin-section CT in 11 patients with nodular BAC, showed a positive bronchus sign in 36%: in two lesions these authors further observed serpentine radiolucencies that subsequently were shown histologically to represent air-containing glandular spaces within the tumor (81). Kuhlman et al., in a study of 30 patients with documented focal bronchoalveolar cell carcinomas, similarly described a pattern they interpreted as sugges-

tive of pseudocavitation in 18 cases (80). Defined as small, oval areas of lucency appearing in or around pulmonary masses, this appearance was interpreted as consistent with residual dilated bronchioles and expanded air spaces, the result of the distinctive propensity of these tumors to extend along alveolar walls without distortion of the underlying architecture.

It should be noted that the finding of an air-bronchogram leading to or within a nodule, per se, is less characteristic than so-called pseudocavitation (see Fig. 4-19A–C). As noted by Zwirewich et al., bubble-like lucencies are seen more commonly in bronchoalveolar cell carcinoma (50%) than in acinar adenocarcinomas (31%) or other lung tumors (11%) making this sign highly suggestive of BAC (see Fig. 19) (51). In distinction, although highly suggestive of malignancy, the appearance of a positive bronchus sign in itself is not predictive of cell type (69).

It cannot be overemphasized that solitary bronchoalveolar carcinomas may have a wide range of radiologic manifestations (see Fig. 4-19). In addition to air-bronchograms and pseudocavitation, these include: focal ill-defined areas of poorly marginated ground glass attenuation (see Fig. 4-19E) (79,82); denser lesions with markedly irregular contours; a propensity towards subpleural localization, often in association with pleural retraction (a so-called pleural tag); a cystic or cavitary appearance (83); and even a positive halo sign (81). A pattern of lobar consolidation has also been described, including the finding of a so-called angiogram sign (84): Unfortunately, this is nonspecific, as it is frequently identified in patients with simple lobar consolidation and even lymphoma. As reported by Gaeta et al., although 36% of lesions showed air-bronchograms, an equal number had spiculated margins and evidence of pleural retraction, and 18% demonstrated surrounding ground glass attenuation (81). Similar findings have been reported by Kuhlman et al. (80).

Arteriovenous Malformations

Not surprisingly, the most compelling evidence substantiating the value of the feeding vessel sign comes from patients with known or suspected arteriovenous malformations (see Fig 4-6; Figs. 4-20 and 4-21). The presence of pulmonary vascular malformations is often suspected based on a clinical history and findings on plain chest radiography. A high percentage of patients with lung lesions are affected with Osler-Weber-Rendu disease. Chest roentgenography often shows a complex lesion consisting of a lobulated or serpiginous mass associated with tortuous feeding arteries and draining veins. However, for smaller lesions the vasculature may be subtle or inapparent and the lesion may be manifest as a solitary pulmonary nodule: associated vasculature may be visualized only on CT.

Remy et al., have demonstrated that spiral CT allows accurate assessment of the presence and number of arteriovenous pleural malformations, being superior to angiography for demonstrating small lesions (85,86). As important, unen-

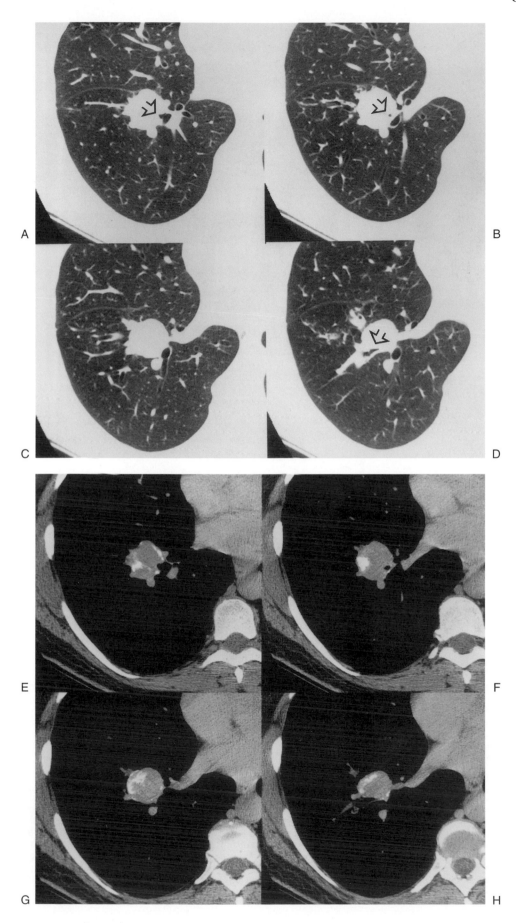

FIG. 4-17. Carcinoid tumor. **A–D:** Sequential 1-mm sections show well-defined central mass in the lower portion of the right hilum causing marked compression of the basilar segmental airways (*arrows* in **A, B** and **D**). **E–H:** Identical sections as shown in **A–D**, imaged with mediastinal windows shows the presence of peripheral calcification. This constellation of findings is characteristic of a carcinoid tumor, subsequently verified surgically.

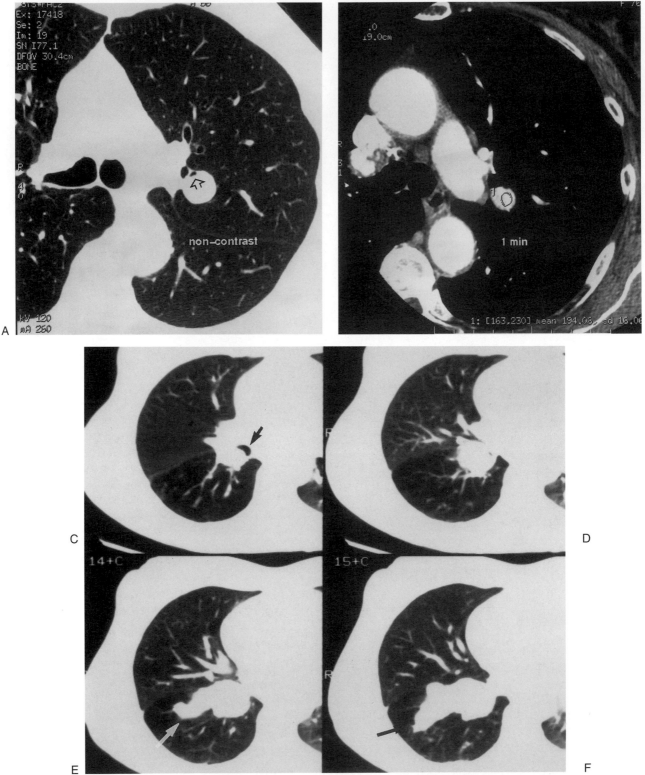

FIG. 4-18. Hilar carcinoid: evaluation with contrast enhancement. **A,B:** Enlargement of 3-mm section acquired helically through the left hilum, imaged with wide and narrow windows, respectively, 1 minute after the administration of intravenous contrast media shows a left hilar mass causing slight compression of the adjacent bronchus (*arrow* in **A**). Note that with mediastinal windowing this mass has the same density as the adjacent left pulmonary artery and aorta, measuring 163 HU, indicative of an extremely vascular lesion. This degree of enhancement within a central mass abutting a bronchus is characteristic of a carcinoid tumor, subsequently verified at surgery. (From ref. 199, with permission.) **C–F:** Sequential images through the distal bronchus intermedius and proximal middle and lower lobe airways imaged with lung windows in a different patient than in **A** and **B** shows marked distortion of the bronchus intermedius (*arrow* in **C**) with complete obstruction of the basilar airways. Note the presence of a serpiginous density extending laterally (*arrows* in **E** and **F**) consistent with mucoid impaction.

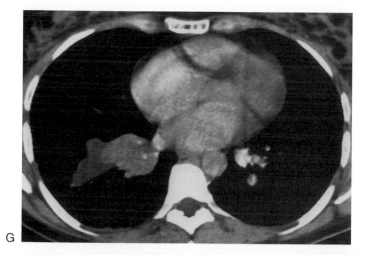

G

FIG. 4-18. *Continued.* **G:** Delayed image following contrast enhancement at the same level as shown in **E** confirms the presence of a hilar mass easily differentiated from peripheral mucoid impaction (*arrow*) because of considerable neovascularity (compare visually with corresponding density within the left atrium). Use of contrast enhancement may be invaluable in identifying central lesions in patients with peripheral airway obstruction and/or atelectasis. **H–K:** Sequential gadolinium-enhanced MR images through the lower portion of the right hilum also show evidence of a centrally enhancing mass with peripheral mucoid impaction. In this case, identification of central tumor is equally well-established using either CT or MR.

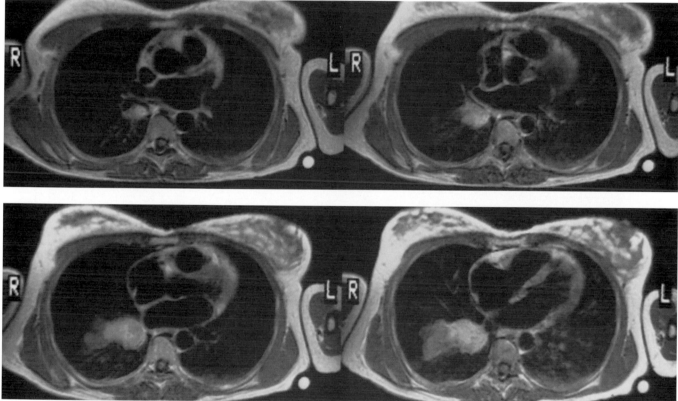

H   I

J   K

hanced three dimensional CT can provide a reliable analysis of the angioarchitecture of lesions and is therefore useful in follow-up both of treated and untreated patients.

Pulmonary Infarction

Pulmonary infarcts characteristically present as focal masses with a broad pleural base, convex margins (representing Hampton's hump), strands leading from the apex of the lesion toward the pulmonary hilus, and scattered lucencies

(Fig. 4-22) (76). An apparent feeding vessel also may be identified. This may be especially easy to identify with use of multiplanar reconstructions (Fig. 4-23). Following intravenous contrast administration, peripheral enhancement is frequently seen along the margins of the infarct including the pleural surface: Presumably this is the result of collateral perfusion from the bronchial arterial circulation. In our judgment this constellation of findings allows a correct diagnosis in most patients, even in the absence of a clinical diagnosis of pulmonary embolism.

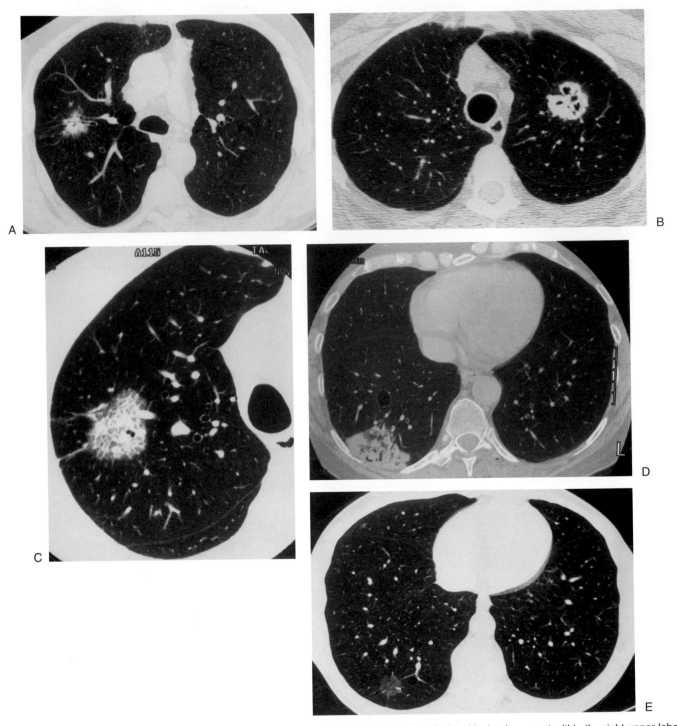

FIG. 4-19. The many faces of bronchoalveolar cell carcinoma (BAC). **A:** An ill-defined, spiculated lesion is present within the right upper lobe through which a peripheral bronchus clearly traverses. **B:** An irregular, slightly lobulated mass can be seen in the left upper lobe within which multiple dilated cystic spaces can be identified, an appearance that has been described as pseudocavitation. **C:** Within the right upper lobe there is a focal lesion within which distinct reticular elements can be identified on a background of ground glass attenuation. Focally dilated airways can also be identified within this lesion as well. Note the presence of linear strands extending to the pleural surface, indicative in this case of cicatricial changes around this tumor. **D:** There is a focal area of apparent parenchymal consolidation in the peripheral portion of the right lower lobe associated with dilated airways and a suggestion of mild cavitation. Although superficially mimicking the appearance of a focal pneumonia, this lesion remained unchanged despite aggressive antibiotic therapy. Surgically verified bronchoalveolar cell carcinoma. **E:** There is a focal area of ground glass attenuation noted in the posterior portion of the right lower lobe through which normal vessels can be identified. A few thin linear strands can be identified extending from this lesion to the pleural surface. Subsequently surgery verified BAC. Despite a wide range of presentations, this tumor should be identifiable in most cases, especially in the appropriate clinical setting.

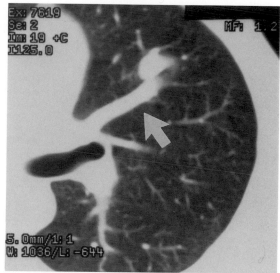

FIG. 4-20. Posttraumatic AV fistula. **A–C:** Sequential 5-mm helical sections through the left upper lobe show a well-defined nodular density closely related to an enlarged left superior pulmonary vein (*arrow* in **A**). **D:** Coned-down early radiograph from a selective left pulmonary artery injection confirms the presence of an AV fistula in the left upper lobe with rapid filling of the left upper lobe pulmonary vein. Note the presence of suture material, the result of a previous knife wound several months prior to this admission. **E:** Three dimensional surface rendering derived from 5-mm sections reconstructed every 3 mm obtained following a bolus of 100 cc of nonionic intravenous contrast material injected at a rate of 3 cc clearly depicts the enlarged draining pulmonary vein extending to the hilum. (From ref. 198, with permission.)

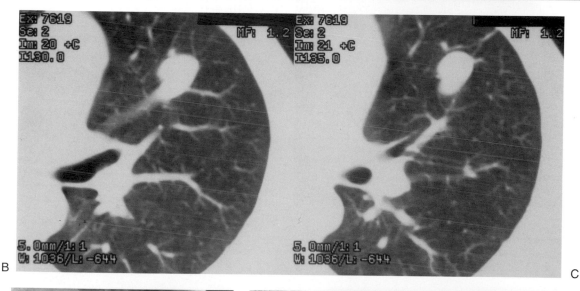

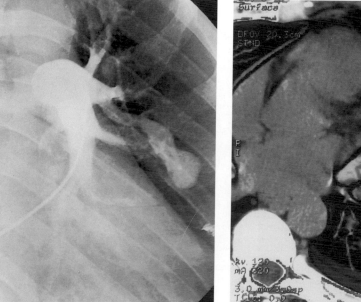

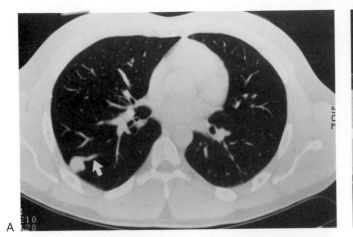

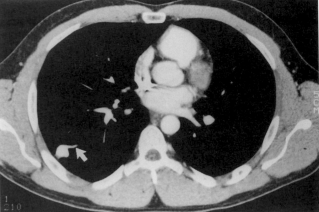

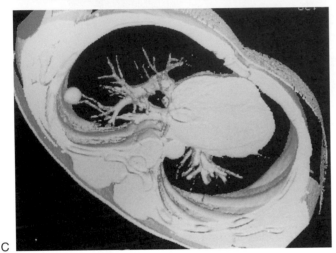

FIG. 4-21. Arteriovenous malformation. **A,B:** Section through the lower lobes following a bolus of intravenous contrast media imaged with wide and narrow windows, respectively, show a peripheral nodule interpreted as likely representing a vascular malformation because of markedly enhancing vessel-like strand extending medially (*arrows* in **A** and **B**). **C:** Three dimensional reconstruction shows to better advantage the feeding artery and draining vein.

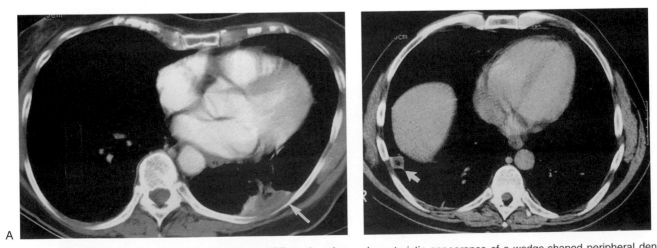

FIG. 4-22. Pulmonary infarction. **A:** Contrast enhanced CT section shows characteristic appearance of a wedge-shaped peripheral density abutting the pleura with subtle enhancement noted along the base of the triangle (*arrow*). **B:** Contrast enhanced CT scan in a different patient than in **A** again shows characteristic findings of a small pulmonary infarct with a slightly more rectangular density abutting the pleura surface with enhancement along the base (*arrow*). Note that in both **A** and **B**, subtle cavitation may be identified within the area of infarction.

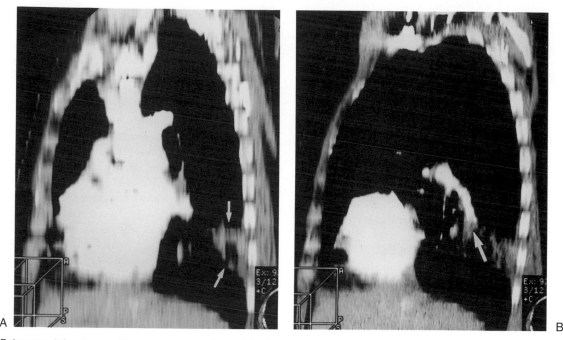

FIG. 4-23. Pulmonary infarction: multiplanar reconstructions. **A,B:** Contiguous sagittal reconstructions through the left lower lobe in a patient with documented pulmonary emboli show characteristic peripheral wedge-shaped or triangular density abutting the pleural surface *(arrows in* **A**), seen to better advantage in this plane. Note the presence of a discrete filling defect within the left lower lobe pulmonary artery *(arrow in* **B**). (From ref. 198, with permission.)

Growth Characteristics

Growth Rate

The absence of detectable growth over a two-year period of observation is a reliable criterion for establishing that a pulmonary nodule is benign. It is for this reason that review of prior chest roentgenograms is a critical factor in the evaluation of a patient with a solitary nodule. If a lesion is unchanged in size and appearance over a two-year period, the likelihood of benignancy is close to 100% (87).

Despite widespread acceptance, the value of two year stability recently has been questioned (88). Yankelevitz et al., citing earlier works by Good et al., have indicated that the actual published data do not support the reliability of absence of growth as a criterion for benignancy (89). Key to this reinterpretation is a previously published table that provided information on a group of patients with pulmonary resections performed between 1940 and 1951 (89). Of nine patients with lung cancers evaluated with serial chest roentgenograms prior to surgery (see Table 4-1), four lesions showed evidence of growth with the implication that five of nine carcinomas showed no growth (89). However, there is no indication of the interval between studies, no illustrations of a case of malignancy without growth, and no specific mention of the data in the body of the paper. In our judgment, this report simply does not provide sufficient information to draw definitive conclusions. Moreover, in a subsequent paper on patients seen at the Mayo Clinic from 1951 to 1954 reported by this same author, 35 of 37 cases with nodules unchanged over a two-year period were not sent to surgery

because the lesions were stable (90). Despite these limitations, we concur with the statement of Good in 1963 that, "we believe we are on safe ground to recommend repeated periodic roentgenologic examination rather than excision if the mass has not enlarged in two years. So far we have not had reason to reject this advice" (91).

In distinction to absence of growth over a two year period, the reliability of slow growth as an indicator of benign disease is difficult to document. This is because to date there is no prospective study of serial growth of focal lung lesions in an unselected group of patients: To knowingly follow a group of suspicious lesions would be contrary to accepted medical practice. Measuring the diameter of lesions, and determining the period in which a nodule doubled in volume, Collins and Nathan in a series of seminal papers studied the growth rate of 177 malignant nodules and 41 benign nodules in patients with available serial chest roentgenograms (87, 92). Since the volume of a sphere is equal to $4/3 \pi r^3$, a 26% increase in diameter yields a doubling in volume. They concluded among patients of all age groups, pulmonary nodules enlarging more slowly than one doubling every 18 months were invariably benign. It should be noted that although the study ostensibly included 21 benign nodules with doubling times in excess of three years, including 13 patients with proved hamartomas (two of which showed no growth) and 7 with granulomas, one of these lesions was mistakenly labeled as a benign carcinoid tumor. At the time, the authors noted only one exception—an adenocarcinoma that showed no growth in three months (87). Similar results have been retrospectively reported by Weiss et al., who obtained serial chest radiographs in a group of men with lung lesions and confirmed that the doubling time for malignancies was 1.8 to 10 months (93).

Despite these data supporting slow growth as indicative of a likely benign etiology, opinions have varied from the beginning on whether growth rate is a sufficiently reliable parameter to be useful in the management of patients. Good, for example, expressing greater confidence in the presence of calcification as a sign of benign disease noted that although a two-year period of stability "greatly lengthens the odds against lesions being malignant... (it) is not incontrovertible evidence that a lesion is benign" (89). Rigler similarly was cautious about endorsing lack of growth, stating that he had personally observed two startling exceptions of slowly growing carcinomas (94).

At the other end of the spectrum, Nathan authored a proposal that growth rate be used prospectively to evaluate small nodules in patients 30 to 45 years old in areas with a high incidence of granulomatous disease (95). Rather than an immediate thoracotomy, Nathan advised a 2-week delay to obtain a follow-up chest roentgenogram. If no growth of the nodule could be detected, a second delay of 4 weeks was proposed: If again no growth could be detected, chest radiographs were advised at continually increasing intervals up to 2 years, at which point the nodule could safely be deemed benign. If any definite growth of the nodule was observed at any point in this sequence, surgery was then deemed advisable (95). Although it is now common, based largely on these observations, to routinely follow a wait-and-see policy in all patients in whom initial clinical and radiographic findings are deemed equivocal, with initial follow-up radiographs generally obtained between 6 weeks and 3 months, it is apparent that reliance on slow-growth in itself cannot be deemed definitive proof of benignancy.

The Dormant Scar Carcinoma

Many clinical investigators have suggested that cancer may arise from a previously stable scar (87,96). Bennett et al. found that almost half of adenocarcinomas of the lung in men were associated with preexistent pulmonary scars (96). Scars were documented by the detection of increased elastica and abundant anthracotic pigment as thin dense hyalinized connective tissue. Cancers frequently occur at the periphery of old scars. The nature of the premalignant process of fibrosis is due to prior tuberculosis, old infarcts, or nonspecific granulomas. Active scars, presumably with increased metabolic activity may display peripheral areas of epithelial hyperplasia, atypical metaplasia, and finally adenocarcinoma (96). A modern hypothesis to explain this phenomenon is that, in association with the increased metabolic activity of areas of scarring, a mutation in the p53 gene (a cancer suppressing gene) leads to focal development of malignancy (97). It appears that during mitosis p53 directs a series of processes whereby damaged DNA is repaired. With mutations of the p53 gene the structure of the molecule is altered leading to the production and survival of cells with abnormal tumorigenic DNA. Recently, smoking has been shown to produce mutations in the p53 gene (98).

Despite these reports, although focal fibrosis and carcinoma are frequently associated histologically, a causal relationship between a scar and carcinoma is difficult to prove (Fig. 4-24). Furthermore, it is well known that carcinoma can lead to active production of collagen and focal desmoplastic reaction (99,100). Therefore, although focal areas of fibrosis may indeed be pathogenetically important in the development of bronchogenic carcinomas in some patients, the incidence of true scar carcinoma has probably been overestimated in the past. An increase in the incidence of bronchogenic carcinoma has been clearly shown, however, in patients who have interstitial pulmonary fibrosis, particularly in patients with asbestosis and, less commonly, progressive systemic sclerosis, rheumatoid disease, dermatomyositis, idiopathic pulmonary fibrosis, and sarcoidosis (101–105).

Calcification

It is well documented that the radiographic presence of calcification within a pulmonary lesion is generally a reliable sign that the lesion is benign (39,40). The best documentation of the nature of calcification within pulmonary nodules was carried out at the Mayo Clinic and reported in a series of articles in the 1950s (89,90,106). In addition to confirming a strong correlation between radiographic and/or tomographic evidence of calcification and benign disease, these authors also defined characteristic patterns of calcification. Based on specimen radiography obtained on a total of 207 solitary pulmonary masses four different patterns of benign calcification were identified (Fig. 4-25):

1. A laminated pattern with calcium deposited in concentric layers, between rings of fibrous tissue.
2. A dense central nidus.
3. Diffuse and/or irregular or nodular (so-called popcorn) calcification.
4. Punctate calcification.

With minor variation, these guidelines for pattern recognition remain in effect. Although the four patterns cited adequately categorize the range of heterogeneous calcifications encountered, it should be emphasized that for small nodules, particularly those that are 1 cm or less in size, the commonest finding is diffuse homogeneous calcification.

CT Densitometry

The concept of using CT to evaluate the solitary pulmonary nodule was first published by Siegelman et al., in 1980 (107). In this initial series, 91 patients without radiographic or tomographic evidence of calcification were evaluated with thin-section CT and assigned a representative CT number based on average of continuous pixels measured within the estimated center of the lesion. These authors reported that although all 45 primary neoplasms and 13 metastases had representative CT less than 164 Hounsfield units (HU),

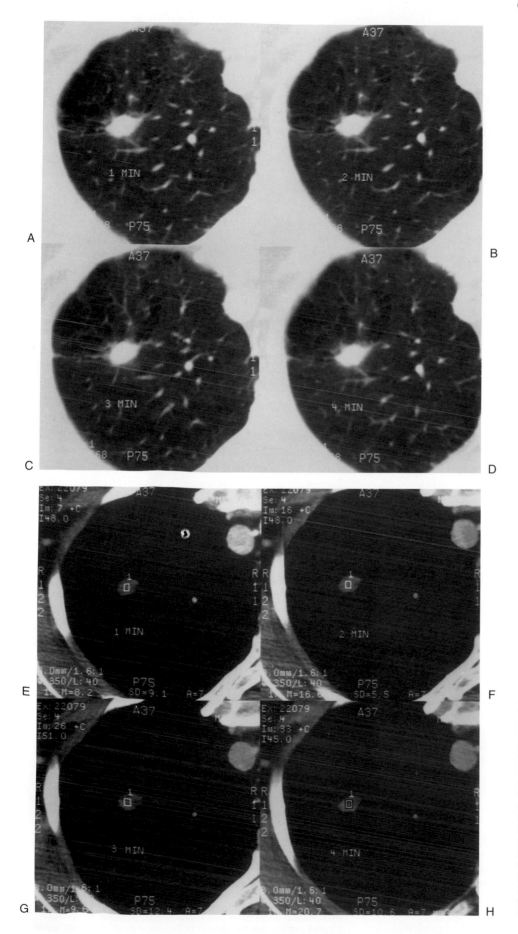

FIG. 4-24. Nonenhancing lung cancer related to a scar. **A–D:** Three-millimeter section obtained at the same level 1, 2, 3, and 4 minutes following a bolus of intravenous contrast imaged with lung windows shows the presence of a slightly irregular, oblong nodule adjacent to an area of focal pulmonary emphysema anteriorly. **E–H:** Identical images as shown in **A–D,** imaged with narrow widows. In this case the mean density within this lesion (shown on the bottom of each image) measured 8.2, 16.6, 9.6 and 20.7 HU, respectively, never exceeding 15 HU above the baseline noncontrast section (not shown). Histologic section through this lesion confirming the presence of foci of adenocarcinoma. By visual inspection, greater than 90% of this lesion proved to be fibrotic tissue, accounting for the lack of contrast enhancement note in **D–G:** Extensive fibrosis within pulmonary nodules, whether or not this constitutes a scar carcinoma, represents a potential pitfall in the use of contrast enhancement to identify benign pulmonary nodules.

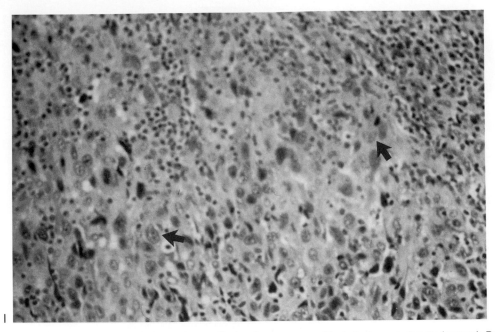

FIG. 4-24. *Continued.* **I:** Histologic section through this lesion confirming the presence of foci of adenocarcinoma (*arrows*). By visual inspection, greater than 90% of this lesion proved to be fibrotic tissue, accounting for the lack of contrast enhancement noted in **D–G**. Extensive fibrosis within pulmonary nodules, whether or not this constitutes a "scar" carcinoma, represents a potential pitfall in the use of contrast enhancement to identify benign pulmonary nodules.

20 of 33 benign lesions proved to have representative CT numbers greater than 164 HU. If the correct diagnosis of a benign lesion is considered a true positive and the designation of a malignancy as benign is considered a false positive, then the overall sensitivity of CT in this initial study proved to be 59%, with a sensitivity of 73% for lesions 1 cm or less in diameter, and a specificity of 100% (107).

In 1986, a follow-up study presented the results of 634 solitary pulmonary nodules found that 44% proved to be benign: of these, 176 (63%) were correctly assessed as benign by CT criteria, including 90 lesions identified as indeterminate on conventional tomography (44).

Despite these encouraging results, difficulties remained in extrapolating these data to other scanners in other locales. The density of a lesion, as measured by the degree to which it attenuates a collimated beam of x-rays, is an innate property of its tissue content. However, the determination of a reliable measurement in Hounsfield units is subject to extensive variation. Measurements vary as a function of partial volume averaging, the reconstruction algorithm, true slice thickness, the size of the lesion, kilovoltage, and beam hardening artifacts (108). In an attempt to solve problems related to scanner variability, Zerhouni et al., showed that these variations could be eliminated by use of a standardized anthropomorphic reference phantom (108). By simulating the size and position of nodules within the patient's lung with cylinders of various diameters made to correspond to the density of a calcified nodule, thin sections through patient's nodules could be compared with similar sections obtained in the same location using the phantom. The value of this approach was quickly verified in a multi-institutional cooperative study (46). Of 284 nodules evaluated, 118 (31%) proved to be benign: among these, unsuspected calcification was detected in 65 (55%). Interestingly, approximately 5% of patients referred for evaluation of solitary pulmonary nodules identified on chest radiographs had extrapulmonary lesions such as pleural plaques or rib abnormalities. Of the 229 lesions interpreted as indeterminate, 176 proved to be malignant, 53 benign. Significantly, in only one case was a lesion that was interpreted as benign by CT criteria shown to be malignant. Similar data have been reported by Jones et al. (109). In their study 31 nodules in 29 patients were evaluated using a reference phantom: 10 of 11 nodules interpreted as benign were later confirmed with one lesion, an adenocarcinoma, representing the sole false positive.

The use of CT to evaluate nodules is now well established. As problems related to standardization of tissue attenuation

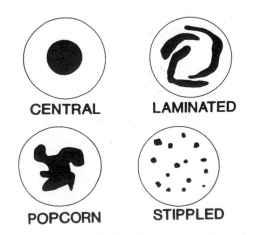

FIG. 4-25. Patterns of calcification. Central, laminated, and popcorn-like calcification patterns are characteristic of benign nodules. The stippled pattern can be seen in both benign and malignant lesions.

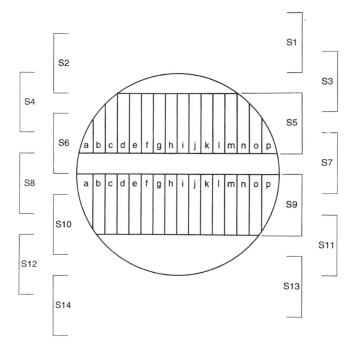

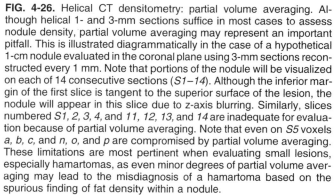

FIG. 4-26. Helical CT densitometry: partial volume averaging. Although helical 1- and 3-mm sections suffice in most cases to assess nodule density, partial volume averaging may represent an important pitfall. This is illustrated diagrammatically in the case of a hypothetical 1-cm nodule evaluated in the coronal plane using 3-mm sections reconstructed every 1 mm. Note that portions of the nodule will be visualized on each of 14 consecutive sections (*S1–14*). Although the inferior margin of the first slice is tangent to the superior surface of the lesion, the nodule will appear in this slice due to z-axis blurring. Similarly, slices numbered *S1, 2, 3, 4,* and *11, 12, 13,* and *14* are inadequate for evaluation because of partial volume averaging. Note that even on *S5* voxels *a, b, c,* and *n, o,* and *p* are compromised by partial volume averaging. These limitations are most pertinent when evaluating small lesions, especially hamartomas, as even minor degrees of partial volume averaging may lead to the misdiagnosis of a hamartoma based on the spurious finding of fat density within a nodule.

measurements have been notably lessened, in particular, by algorithms to correct beam hardening artifacts, the need for a reference phantom has declined (110). Reliance on the use of a phantom has been further diminished with the introduction of spiral scanning, which minimizes partial volume averaging. As a consequence, it is generally held that in the majority of cases, calcified lesions are readily recognized by obvious high attenuation values without the need for a reference phantom. In fact, even with modern scanners, the superiority of phantoms as a means for performing CT densitometry has yet to be challenged. Khan et al., in an study of 62 nodules in 59 patients, compared noncontrast, thin-section CT with CT densitometry using a phantom (111). Although 21 lesions were assessed as benign using noncontrast thin section CT, 33 were assessed as benign with use of the reference phantom, an increase in sensitivity of 22%. Only two lesions classified as benign subsequently proved to be malignant: both were assessed as calcified using thin-section and reference phantom CT. Supporting data have been published by Swensen et al., who found in a retrospective study of 296 cases of solitary nodules evaluated with a reference phantom, 85 patients in whom nodules were interpreted as calcified using the phantom only (112). In distinction to the data reported by Khan et al., in this study, 10 of these lesions subsequently proved to be malignant, clearly representing an important limitation to this technique.

It should be noted that reported variations in the accuracy of CT phantom densitometry in part is a reflection of differences between studies in phantom design. Initial reports were based on use of reference nodules standardized to 264 HU: in distinction, more recent studies, including that of Swensen et al., have made use of 185 HU reference nodules (54,112). Although use of the lower density reference nodules increases the sensitivity of this technique, a mean difference of 79 HU undoubtedly accounts, at least in part, for the greater number of false negative studies reported for 185 HU reference nodules.

Despite these findings documenting increased sensitivity, the use of a reference phantom has all but been abandoned in most institutions. As a consequence, it is mandatory that studies be performed with close attention to scan technique. Although thin-section CT suffices in the majority of cases, an adequate study should consist of a series of narrowly collimated scans through the lesion (Fig. 4-26). With conventional scanners, patients should be told to breathe in exactly the same fashion for each scan, preferably at end-expiratory lung volume to maximize reproducibility. Slice collimation should be less than half the diameter of the nodule to eliminate partial volume averaging. The table should be advanced by small increments so that at least three sections close to the center of the lesion are obtained, with measurements most appropriately obtained from the section in which the nodule has the maximum diameter. Although many of these problems may be obviated with use of helical CT, it should be emphasized that even in this setting only a few sections will truly be representative (see Fig. 4-26).

For small lesions, attenuation values will be overestimated by an edge-enhancing (sharp) algorithm and underestimated by a smoothing algorithm (108). Selection of a high-spatial-frequency reconstruction algorithm, in particular, may artificially create the erroneous impression of calcification within lesions, especially along their edge (113). This technical fact should not obscure the fact that 1-mm sections frequently disclose the presence of calcification when thicker 7- to 10-mm sections do not (Fig. 4-27).

Parenthetically, it is worth noting that some have advocated the use of dual kVp to analyze nodules as an alternate method for detecting calcium (Fig. 4-28) (114). This may

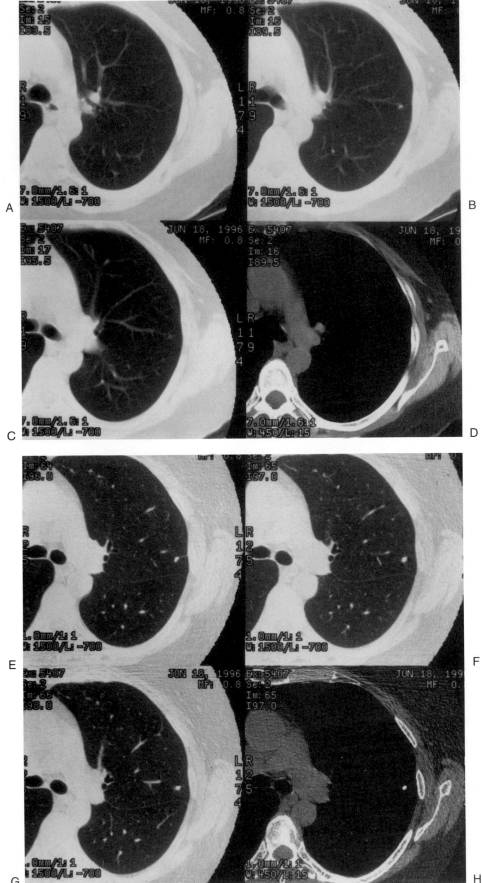

FIG. 4-27. CT densitometry: 1- versus 7-mm section. **A–C:** Sequential 7-mm helical sections through the left upper lobe reconstructed every 6 mm show a small nodule in the left upper lobe. **D:** Identical section as **B**, imaged with narrow windows, shows no obvious calcifications within the nodule. **E–G:** Sequential 1-mm helical images through the same portion of the left upper lobe as in **A–C** again show small peripheral lung nodule. **H:** Identical image as in **F**, imaged with narrow windows clearly shows this lesion to be densely calcified. This case illustrates that 1-mm sections are often necessary to perform adequate CT densitometry. Helical acquisition is especially helpful for evaluating very small nodules as it markedly simplifies acquisition of sections through the center of lesions (see Figure 4-25).

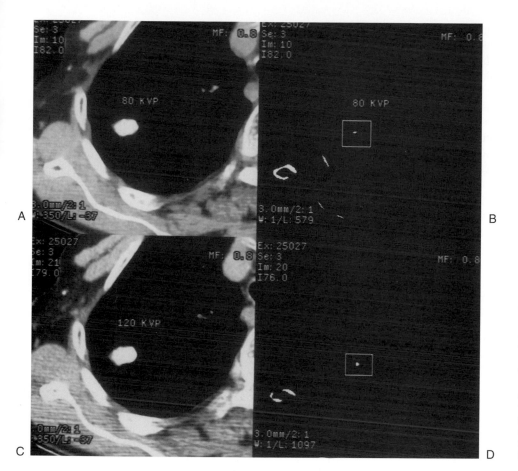

A
B
C
D

FIG. 4-28. CT densitometry: dual kVp technique. **A,B:** Three-millimeter section obtained using 80 kVp imaged with window widths of 350 and 1, and corresponding window levels of −87 and 579, respectively, show a densely calcified nodule in the right upper lobe. Using a window of 1 (as shown in **B**) effectively renders the CT scanner a densitometer. Only a few remaining pixels may be identified within the nodule in **B** that is now outlined by a square. These few pixels represent the highest HU within this nodule using 80 kVp. **C,D:** Identical images as shown in **A** and **B**, except for the fact that these were obtained with 120 kVp. Note that in this case, when the window width is reduced to 1 as shown in **D**, the same pixels shown in **B** now measure 1097 HU. This change is caused by the presence of calcification within the lesion. It should be emphasized that use of a dual kVp technique is limited because of the requirement that images be acquired at the exact same level.

be performed by first obtaining 3-mm sections with 140 kVp, 280 mA, using a standard algorithm with images reconstructed every 2 mm if helical CT is employed, followed by a second set of images using 80 kVp. If the 80 kVp image density measures greater than that measured on the corresponding 140 kVp images, the lesion likely contains sufficient calcification to qualify as benign. The necessity for images to be obtained at precisely the same level for comparison purposes has, to date, proved a major limitation to this technique. It is possible that helical scanning may sufficiently address this limitation to warrant further consideration.

Calcification in Malignancy

Primary lung malignancies may contain areas of calcification or ossification. Theros, for example, found seven examples of radiologically detected calcification in 1,267 lung cancers, a prevalence of approximately 1% (42). O'Keefe et al., using radiographs of resected lung specimens, found calcification in 8 (15%) of 52 resected primary lung cancers (106). With the addition of CT the likelihood of detecting calcification within tumors has increased (Fig. 4-29) (46,109,111,115,116). As documented by Grewal and Austin, 53 (10.6%) of 500 consecutive patients with provisional diagnoses of lung cancer were found to have calcification on CT (116).

Calcification within tumors may result for a number of reasons. These include: (a) tumor engulfing previous calcification, as may occur with a preexisting granuloma; (b) dystrophic calcification, occurring in areas of tumor necrosis; and (c) primary tumor calcification, as may be seen in particular within mucinous adenocarcinomas.

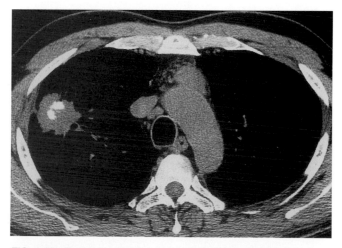

FIG. 4-29. Tumor calcification. One-millimeter section shows eccentric foci of dense calcification within a spiculated right upper lobe mass. With the addition of CT the likelihood of identifying calcification within tumors has increased. Note presence of extensive mediastinal adenopathy.

Radiographically, calcification within lung neoplasms typically appears stippled or eccentric and usually occurs in large central lesions (see Fig. 4-29) (106). In their study of 53 patients with histologically verified calcification compared to a control group of 15 patients, Grewal and Austin recorded a mean diameter of 6.2 ± 3 cm for calcified neoplasms versus 4.4 ± 2.3 cm for noncalcified tumors, with 33 (85%) of the calcified tumors measuring more than 3 cm (116). In a smaller study, Mahoney et al., also noted a propensity for calcification to occur in larger lesions: of 20 lesions, 15 (75%) were 5 cm or greater in size, whereas only three were 2 cm or smaller (115). Although a number of different patterns of calcification have been noted in these studies, including peripheral, central, diffuse, and amorphous, to date no study has shown any consistent correlation between patterns of calcification and histologic subtype. Indeed, virtually all primary lung cancers, including small cell carcinoma, may have areas of calcification identified on CT scans (46,109,111,115,116).

In addition to bronchogenic carcinoma, calcification has been identified in other primary lung tumors (117). By far the commonest of these are central carcinoid tumors (see Fig. 4-17) (78,111,116,118). In a retrospective study of 31 patients with documented carcinoids (27 typical, 4 atypical) Zweibel et al. found that 18 (58%) were central whereas 13 (42%) were peripheral in location: of these calcification was identified in 7 (39%) of central lesions, but seen in only 1 (8%) of peripheral lesions (78). In a similar study of 12 pulmonary carcinoids, Magid et al., also noted a propensity for central tumors to preferentially calcify (119). In our judg-

ment, the triad of a well-defined central lesion abutting or narrowing an adjacent bronchus with eccentric areas of calcification are all but pathognomonic of this diagnosis (120). The one exception is the rare case of a central, endobronchial hamartoma.

Despite the fact that most calcified parenchymal neoplasms are identifiable as such with CT, it should be emphasized that malignant lesions may still mimic the appearance of benign calcified granulomas. In addition to the well described finding of calcified metastases from osteogenic and chondrosarcomas, adenocarcinomas, both primary and metastatic, not infrequently are calcified. In a retrospective study of 296 cases of solitary nodules evaluated with a reference phantom, Swenson et al., identified 85 patients in whom nodules appeared calcified with use of the phantom only (112). Ten of these (including eight interpreted as having a high probability of being benign) subsequently proved to be malignant: four proved to be metastases (including three patients with metastatic adenocarcinomas of the breast) whereas the remainder included three primary adenocarcinomas of the lung (112). Review of previous published studies also confirm that primary and metastatic adenocarcinoma remains the lesion most likely to be misinterpreted as benign (46,54,109,111). We have additionally noted several compound lesions in which an adenocarcinoma lies adjacent to a dense scar. Thus, although a single thin section through the center of a 5- to 9-mm spherical nodule usually constitutes an adequate examination, larger nodules and complex lesions require more extensive detailed study (Fig. 4-30). Based on

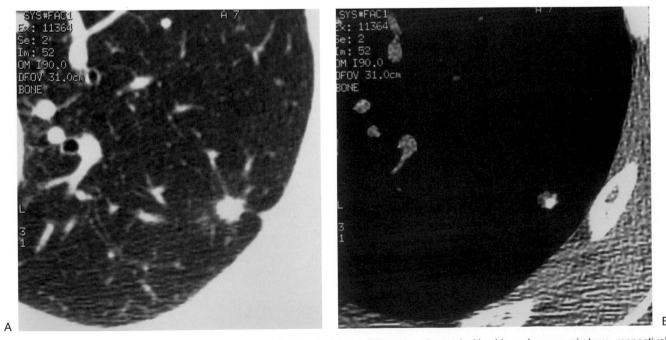

FIG. 4-30. CT densitometry: indeterminate appearance. **A,B:** Identical 1 mm CT sections imaged with wide and narrow windows, respectively show a slightly spiculated nodule with a linear density extending to the pleural surface associated with a faint halo sign. Note that although a portion of this lesion is densely calcified, there is an eccentric rim of soft tissue density along the medial border of this nodule. This case illustrates that in any given case features suggestive of both benign and malignant disease may coexist, and that, necessarily, these lesions are indeterminate in nature. In this case, follow-up CT studies have revealed no interval growth for over 1 year following treatment for tuberculosis.

these findings, even when a calcified lesion is identified on CT it is suggested that continued surveillance with follow-up radiographs be obtained for at least 1 year following initial evaluation, especially in patients with known extrathoracic malignancies, as discussed.

Fat

The presence of fat within the parenchyma is indicative of one of two diagnoses: hamartoma (Figs. 4-31–4-33), or exogenous lipoid pneumonia (Figs. 4-34 and 4-35) (see also Chapter 6).

Hamartoma

Hamartomas, the third commonest cause of a solitary pulmonary nodule, are considered benign neoplasms that originate in fibrous connective tissue beneath the mucous membrane of the bronchial wall (121,122). These lesions contain mixtures of myxomatous connective tissue, cartilage, epithelial-lined clefts, and variable amounts of fat, smooth muscle, marrow, and bone (123). Fat is a key element; if one combines three reported series with data on histology, 37/68 (54%) of the lesions contain fat (124–126). Calcification is more common in large lesions occurring in less than 10% of lesions smaller than two cm, one-third of tumors 3 to 4 cm in diameter and 75% of lesions larger than 5 cm (127). Cartilage usually predominates but occasionally fat or myxomatous connective tissue may be most prominent.

Although the initial basis for using CT for nodules was to detect diffuse calcification in granulomas, an additional function became apparent when it was appreciated that hamartomas containing fat or calcium may have a distinctive appearance (121). Hamartomas may be diagnosed when they are manifest on CT as lesions that contain fat, or fat plus calcium, and have a smooth contour and sharp outline (see

Figs. 4-31–4-33) (111,121). In a report of 47 lesions studied by CT, 30 (63.8%) contained fat only (n = 18), calcium and fat (n = 10) or calcium alone (n = 2) (121). The remaining lesions were diagnosed as indeterminate and managed with surgery or lung biopsy (121). In our experience, lung cancers never manifest as smoothly marginated lesions containing fat.

Thin sections must be used to identify fat with certainty (see Fig. 4-32). On thicker sections, a small cavity may be confused with fat because of partial volume averaging (see Fig. 4-26). The incorporation of a solid portion of the lesion adjacent to a cavity may raise the CT attenuation values into the range of fat (e.g., assuming that a lesion with a CT attenuation of 100 HU has a 2-mm cavity with a CT attenuation of (−) 1000 HU. A 10-mm section through the lesion will have a CT measurement of $(8 \times 100) - (2 \times 1000) = (-)120$ HU.

Pulmonary hamartoma is a lesion of adults. Three-quarters of the 47 patients diagnosed by CT were in their fifth or sixth decades and we have personally encountered more than a dozen patients over the age of 65. It should be emphasized that despite their benign nature, hamartomas grow, albeit slowly. Bateson and Abbott noted slow growth in 40 of 45 patients with available serial chest roentgenograms (127). In one study of 11 cases that exhibited enlargement, recognizable changes were present only in those studied for at least 3 years (128). We, too, have demonstrated fat in a number of pulmonary lesions with documented slow growth enlarging between 1.4 to 1.7 cm over a 4-year period subsequently confirmed to be hamartomas.

Fluid

In select cases, CT identification of characteristic tissue densities (especially when coupled with morphologic evalu-

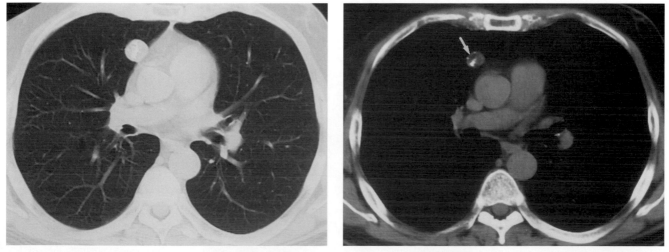

FIG. 4-31. Hamartoma. **A,B:** Identical sections imaged with wide and narrow windows, respectively, show a well defined lesion in the medial portion of the right upper lobe. Note the presence of both dense foci of calcification as well as a small quantity of fat (*arrow* in **B**). In fact, many hamartomas appear to be of soft-tissue density and are otherwise nonspecific in appearance.

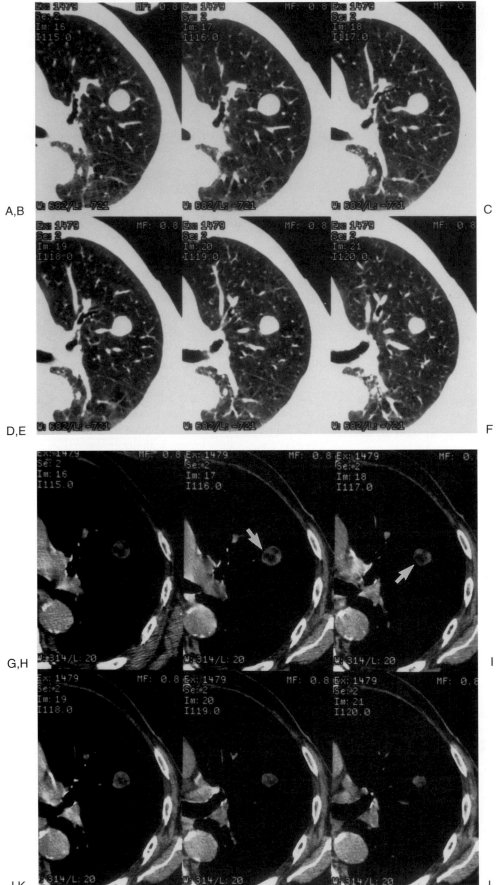

FIG. 4-32. Hamartoma. **A–F:** Sequential 1-mm sections show a well defined left upper lobe nodule. In this case the presence of an apparent feeding vessel in **C** and **D** is caused by incidental proximity. **G-L:** Identical 1-mm sections as shown in **A–F** imaged with narrow windows again show a well defined lesion within which fat is clearly present (*arrows* in **H** and **I**). As diagrammatically shown in Figure 4-26, when assessing small lesions such as this the use of helical acquisition insures that at least some sections are truly representative of the lesions density without partial volume averaging.

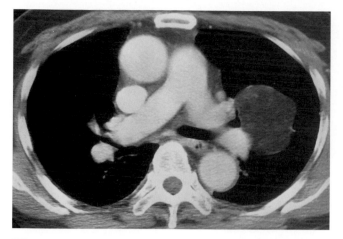

FIG. 4-33. Hamartoma. Contrast-enhanced CT section shows a giant fat containing hamartoma within the left upper lobe. In this case partial volume averaging is not a significant concern.

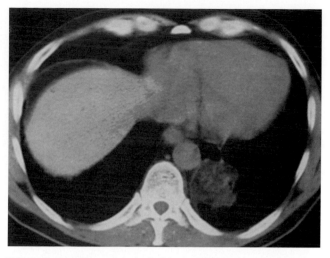

FIG. 4-35. Lipoid pneumonia. Left lower lobe mass in an elderly patient using oily drops for nasal dryness. Note focal infiltrate with large areas of low attenuation in the range of fatty tissues typical of this entity. (Case courtesy of Dr. Norman Ettenger, Manhattan V.A. Hospital, NY.)

ation) allows specific diagnoses to be suggested even in the absence of demonstrable calcification or fat (Table 4-2). Included in this group are patients with lung abscesses (Figs. 4-36 and 4-37), mucoid impaction of the airways (Fig. 4-38), and cysts, including, rarely, intrapulmonary bronchogenic cysts (129) (see Table 4-2) (Fig. 4-39). By establishing the presence of fluid within lesions, following the bolus administration of intravenous contrast media, lung abscesses characteristically appear well-defined and smooth walled prior to the development of bronchial or pleural communications, and consequently are easily differentiated from tumors with CT. Similarly, mucoid impaction of the airways is easily identifiable by the presence of characteristic focal fluid-filled, nonenhancing, branching structures, frequently asso-

ciated with peripheral areas of emphysema (see Fig. 4-36). Less commonly, central endobronchial tumors may present with focal mucoid impaction: In these cases, the use of a bolus of intravenous contrast may be of help in differentiating the central enhancing tumor from peripheral fluid-filled

TABLE 4-2. *CT densitometry in evaluation of focal lung disease*[a]

Calcification
Common
   Calcified granulomas (central or diffuse)
   Hamartomas (central, diffuse, popcorn)
   Carcinoid tumors (punctate, eccentric)
Uncommon
   Bronchogenic carcinomas (punctate, eccentric)
   Metastases (diffuse, punctate)
Rare
   Mucoid impaction (branching)
   Sclerosing hemangiomas (punctate, eccentric)
Fat
Common
   Hamartomas ($\pm$) calcification
Uncommon
   Exogenous lipoid pneumonia
Contrast Enhancement
Common
   Bronchogenic carcinomas
   Carcinoid tumors
   Arteriovenous malformations
Fluid
Common
   Lung abscesses (bacterial and fungal)
   Mucoid impaction
Rare
   Intrapulmonary bronchogenic cyst
Iodine
Amiodarone toxicity

[a] From ref. 120, with permission.

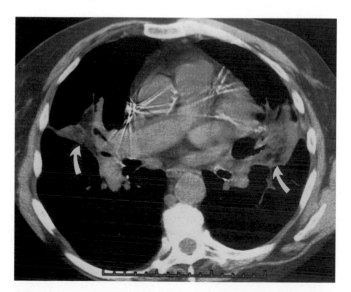

FIG. 4-34. Lipoid pneumonia. CT section through the mid portions of both lungs show bilateral ill-defined areas of parenchymal consolidation within which there is unmistakable evidence of fat density (*arrows*).

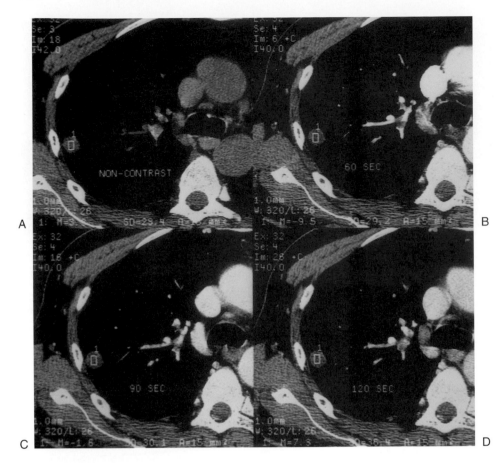

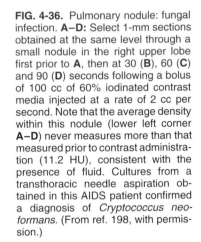

FIG. 4-36. Pulmonary nodule: fungal infection. A–D: Select 1-mm sections obtained at the same level through a small nodule in the right upper lobe first prior to A, then at 30 (B), 60 (C) and 90 (D) seconds following a bolus of 100 cc of 60% iodinated contrast media injected at a rate of 2 cc per second. Note that the average density within this nodule (lower left corner A–D) never measures more than that measured prior to contrast administration (11.2 HU), consistent with the presence of fluid. Cultures from a transthoracic needle aspiration obtained in this AIDS patient confirmed a diagnosis of *Cryptococcus neoformans*. (From ref. 198, with permission.)

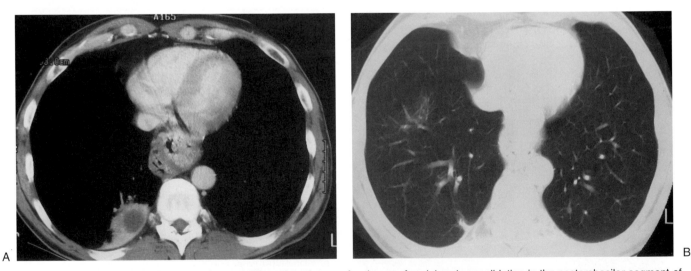

FIG. 4-37. Lung Abscess. A: Contrast enhanced CT section shows a focal area of peripheral consolidation in the posterobasilar segment of the right lower lobe within which there is a sharply defined rounded area of lucency measuring within the range of fluid (HU not shown). This appearance is suggestive of a lung abscess, in this case possibly caused by aspiration in a patient with a moderate sized hiatal hernia. B: Section at the same level as A following a 6 week course of antibiotic therapy shows that the previous abscess has near completely resolved leaving behind only an ill-defined linear density to mark the spot.

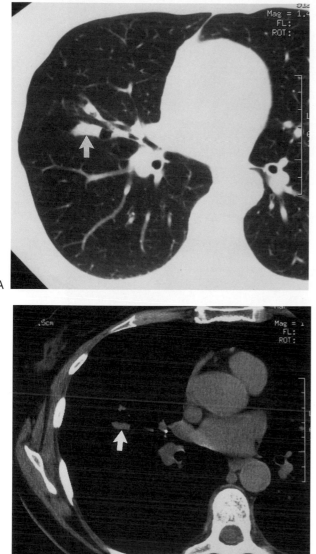

A

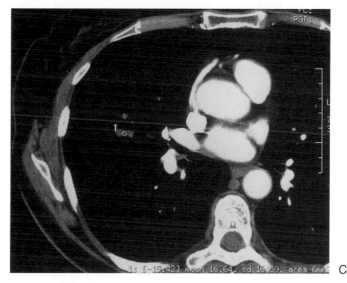

B

C

FIG. 4-38. Mucoid impaction. **A,B:** Identical 3-mm sections through the right upper lobe imaged with wide and narrow windows, respectively, prior to the IV injection of contrast media show a tubular structure (*arrows* in **A** and **B**) most likely representing fluid within a distended bronchus. **C:** Section at the same level as in **A** and **B**, following a bolus of 120 cc 60% iodinated contrast media injected at a rate of 2 cc/second confirms that this is a dilated, fluid-filled bronchus. There is no evidence of a central obstructing mass or evidence of abnormal vessels to account for this focal area of bronchiectasis. Although in this case the density within this bronchus measured within the range of fluid, frequently inspissated secretions, especially when long standing, may measure well above the density of water. In this setting, the use of contrast is critical as, regardless of the baseline density, no enhancement will occur (compare with Fig. 4-18 C–G).

airways. Care should be taken to insure that tumor has not invaded the airways directly by measuring attenuation values within these areas both prior to and following the injection of contrast media. Alternatively, differentiation of tumor from fluid-filled airways may be obtained with T2-weighted MR images (see Fig. 4-18) (130,131).

Contrast Enhancement

CT Evaluation

The determination of distinctive enhancement patterns as a means of differential diagnosis of lesions throughout the body has been the basis for various CT studies. Enhancement of focal malignant breast lesions was demonstrated as early as 1978 (132,133). Increasingly sophisticated analyses of enhancement properties of liver lesions have been used for a number of years. More recently CT studies have been di-

rected at adrenal nodules in an attempt to distinguish metastases (which show delayed enhancement) from incidental nonhyperfunctioning adenomas (significantly less enhancement) (134). The phenomenon of enhancement of pulmonary malignancies by intravenous injection of contrast media was first documented by Littleton et al., using trispiral tomography of lung masses (135). This author showed that there is a fundamental difference in vascularity between focal malignant and benign lesions: Malignant lesions (Figs. 4-40 and 4-41) contain neovascularity and hence are much more apt to enhance following injections of contrast media. This distinctive feature has been exploited using CT first by Swensen et al. (136,137), and subsequently by Yamashita and associates (see Figs. 4-12, 4-18, 4-24, 4-40, 4-41) (138).

In an initial study of 163 patients, Swenson et al., found the median enhancement of malignant nodules (n = 111) to be 40 HU (range = 20 to 108 HU) compared to 12 HU (range = 4 to 58 HU) for benign lesions (n = 52). Using 20

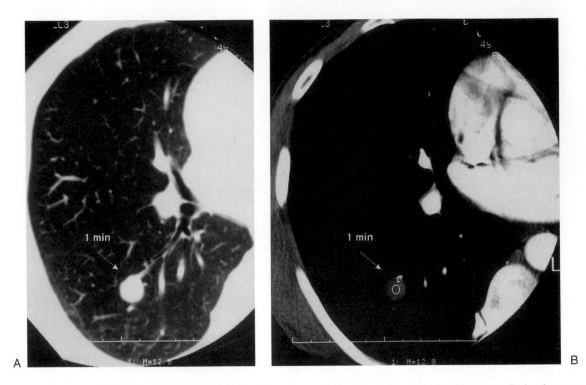

FIG. 4-39. Intrapulmonary bronchogenic cyst. **A,B:** Identical sections imaged with wide and narrow windows, respectively, show a well-defined peripheral nodule in the superior segment of the right lower lobe in close proximity to a subsegmental bronchus. Note that one minute following a bolus of intravenous contrast media this lesion is uniform in appearance and measures 12 HU, indicating that it is within the range of fluid. Subsequent images obtained at 2, 3, and 4 minutes failed to show any significant enhancement suggesting the possibility of an intraparenchymal cyst or abscess. At transthoracic needle biopsy approximately 2 cc of clear sterile fluid were aspirated. At thoracotomy this lesion proved to have cartilage in the wall, confirming the diagnosis of an intrapulmonary bronchogenic cyst. (From ref. 199, with permission.)

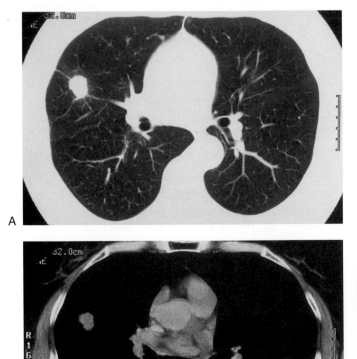

FIG. 4-40. Malignant nodule: contrast enhancement. **A:** Five-millimeter section through the right midlung shows a spiculated nodule in the right upper lobe with a positive tail sign extending to the pleural surface. **B,C:** Select 5-mm sections obtained through this nodule obtained first prior to (**B**) and then 90 seconds (**C**) following injection of 100 cc of 60% iodinated contrast media at a rate of 2 cc per second. The density measured within the nodule changed from a precontrast level of 15 to 69.5 HU, indicating considerable vascularity. Surgically proved adenocarcinoma. (From ref. 198, with permission.)

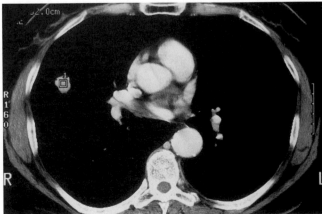

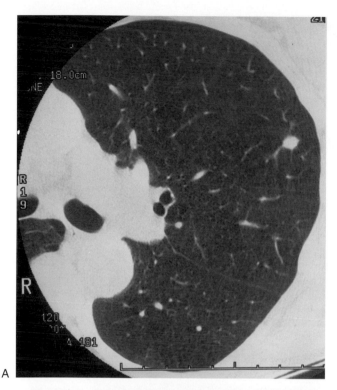

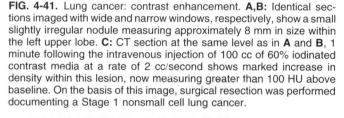

FIG. 4-41. Lung cancer: contrast enhancement. **A,B:** Identical sections imaged with wide and narrow windows, respectively, show a small slightly irregular nodule measuring approximately 8 mm in size within the left upper lobe. **C:** CT section at the same level as in **A** and **B**, 1 minute following the intravenous injection of 100 cc of 60% iodinated contrast media at a rate of 2 cc/second shows marked increase in density within this lesion, now measuring greater than 100 HU above baseline. On the basis of this image, surgical resection was performed documenting a Stage 1 nonsmall cell lung cancer.

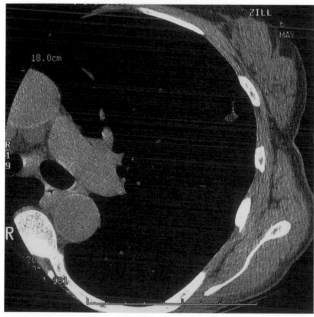

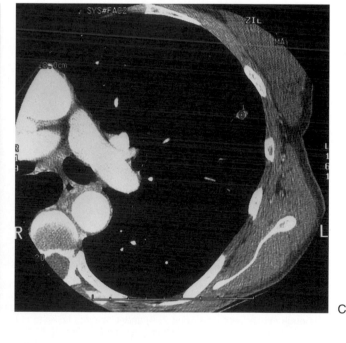

HU as a threshold separating malignant from benign lesions, these authors reported sensitivity of 100%, specificity of 76.9% and accuracy of 92.6% (136). Again using 20 HU as a threshold, Yamashita et al. have reported nearly identical results (138). In a follow-up to their original report, Swenson et al., reported findings in an additional 107 patients. Again using 20 HU as a threshold, median enhancement in malignant lesions (n = 52) proved significantly higher than benign lesions with sensitivity = 98%, specificity = 73%, and accuracy = 85%, with positive and negative predicative

values measuring 77% and 98%, respectively (137). Only one false negative study was reported (see Fig. 4-24). Eight nodules were identified that measured between 16 and 24 HU: four of these proved malignant, leading the authors to define this range as inconclusive (137).

The value of contrast enhancement for evaluating nodules has recently been confirmed in a multi-center prospective study of 356 nodules involving seven centers (139). Using 15 HU as a threshold for a positive test result, the sensitivity was 98%, specificity was 58% and accuracy was 77%. Con-

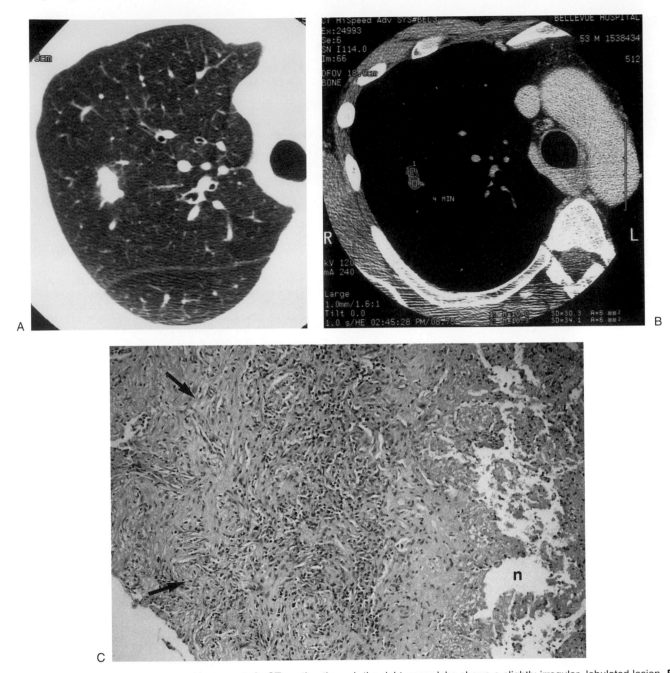

FIG. 4-42. Benign disease: contrast enhancement. **A:** CT section through the right upper lobe shows a slightly irregular, lobulated lesion. **B:** CT section at the same level as in **A** obtained 1 minute following the intravenous injection of 100 cc of 60% iodinated contrast media at a rate of 2 cc/second. In this case, two regions of interest were employed reflecting the lobulated nature of this lesion. Note that both measure 10 HU. Although subsequent images at 2, 3, and 4 minutes failed to show significant contrast enhancement this lesion was surgically removed because of its unusual shape. **C:** Histologic section confirming that this lesion in fact represented a chronic lung abscess. Note the presence of a dense fibrotic wall (*arrows*) outlining central necrosis (*n*). Subsequent cultures proved negative, likely the result of prior antibiotic therapy.

firming previous results, median enhancement within malignant nodules (median, 38 HU; range, 14 to 165) was significantly greater than benign nodules (median, 10 HU; range 20 to 96) ($p < 0.0001$). Based on these data it is now possible to conclude that lack of enhancement within a nodule is strongly suggestive of a benign etiology and that this data should be incorporated into any CT algorithm for nodule assessment (Fig. 4-42).

It cannot be overemphasized that use of contrast enhancement for evaluating nodules necessitates meticulous technique. This has been outlined by Swensen et al. as follows: Following initial unenhanced scans a total of 420 mg I/kg, 300 mg I/mL (100 mL for a 70 kg subject) is injected at a rate of 2 mL/second. Three-millimeter thick sections are obtained using a standard algorithm employing a 19 cm field-of-view. Images are then obtained at 1, 2, 3, and 4 minute intervals using identical technique. Although conventional scanners may be employed (136), the advantages of helical scanning are obvious. In addition to allowing data acquisition in a single breath-hold period, the ability to both prospectively and if necessary retrospectively reconstruct images both insures that at least one image will be reconstructed through the center of the nodule (thus minimizing partial volume artifact) as well as allow more precise comparison of scans obtained at different times by insuring that scans are evaluated at the same exact level. Using 3-mm collimation, images should be reconstructed every 2 mm, with the section most clearly through the center of the nodule selected for analysis using an ROI occupying 60% of the total diameter of the nodule (137).

Despite apparently compelling data, numerous questions remain regarding this technique. In particular, it is yet unclear how to interpret nodules with heterogeneous density (Fig. 4-43). Also unclear is the use of this technique for extremely small nodules, especially those less than 5 mm in size for which 1 mm collimation would be necessary (see Fig. 4-41). Also unclear is the optimum number of data acquisitions to properly assess nodules while minimizing radiation dose. As noted by Swensen et al., in their initial study of 163 patients, 50 (31%) had peak nodule enhancement at either 3 or 4 minutes: in six of these studies, failure to obtain delayed images would have resulted in false negative diagnoses (140). Finally, it is likely that some means for determining the adequacy of contrast administration will be necessary. Appropriately, Swensen et al., excluded eight subjects (two examined with spiral CT) because of technical difficulties (137).

Recently, Zhang and Kono et al. have attempted to address many of these issues by emphasizing the need to assess blood flow patterns (141). Utilizing rapid contrast infusion (4 mm/second) with single level dynamic CT to acquire clusters of images at 15 and 65 seconds, these authors were able to assess the following parameters: peak levels of nodule enhancement (including the ratio of peak enhancement within nodules versus the aorta), time-attenuation curves, and nodule perfusion as well as patterns of contrast enhancement. Defining nodules as either malignant (n = 42), benign (n = 16), or inflammatory, defined as foci of active inflammation (n = 7), these authors showed that significant differences could be measured in the peak height of enhancement within malignant (41.9 HU) and inflammatory nodules (43.6 HU) nodules compared with benign nodules (13.4) HU, respectively ($p < .001$) (141). Similarly, significant differences could be identified between these groups calculating both the ratio of peak enhancement within nodules to the aorta as well as nodule perfusion (141). Using an absolute peak enhancement of 20 HU (in place of an incremental change in density of 20 HU as proposed by Swensen et al.) 2 of 42 malignant nodules were interpreted as benign. Interestingly, significant differences were also identified in this study when patterns of nodule enhancement were assessed. In addition to absence of enhancement, specific patterns evaluated included homogeneous versus heterogeneous enhancement, and central versus peripheral or rim enhancement. Significantly, although benign nodules characteristically showed either no enhancement (56%) or less commonly peripheral enhancement (31%), there were no cases of heterogeneous enhancement within this group. In distinction, malignant nodules most commonly showed homogeneous enhancement (55%) with heterogeneous enhancement next most commonly seen (30%): in no case did a malignant nodule show no measurable enhancement. Changes in patterns of enhancement in time also were evaluated, specifically the finding of heterogeneous enhancement converting to homogenous enhancement exclusively in patients with malignant nodules.

Although these data clearly represent an intriguing addition to the work of Swensen et al., and Yamashita, it should be stressed that many of these observations are preliminary, based on a total of only 65 patients. Furthermore, an important limitation of this approach, acknowledged by the author's themselves, is that this technique allows only a single level through nodules to be evaluated. This may be problematic both for nonspherical nodules as well as, more importantly, small nodules in which minor variations in respiratory excursion may result in questionably usable data.

Allowing for differences in technique, contrast enhanced CT clearly has the potential to serve as an additional means to reach an informed decision on the management of select

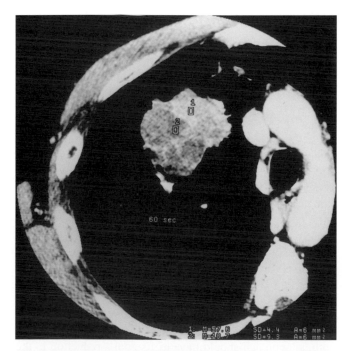

FIG. 4-43. Lung cancer: heterogeneous enhancement. Contrast enhanced CT section shows a heterogeneous mass in the right upper lobe. Note that density within this lesion varies markedly depending on the location of the cursor, in this example varying between 57 and −18 HU. It is apparent that for lesions such as this one region of interest is insufficient for accurate assessment following contrast enhancement. Biopsy proved nonsmall cell lung cancer.

patients with pulmonary nodules. Undoubtedly, the greatest potential use will be its role in providing support for conservative follow-up of noncalcified lesions, which are considered likely benign clinically and morphologically. The use of contrast enhancement clearly will be less helpful in patients with features suggestive of malignancy such as large nodules or those with spiculated borders. Such lesions usually demand tissue diagnosis. Enhancement of a lesion, per se, is of less value, given the significant number of false positive examinations (137).

MRI

Based on the same principle of increased vascularity of malignancies, success has been achieved using MRI to better visualize and assess focal lesions (142,143). MRI contrast agents change T1 and T2 relaxation values leading to detectable alterations (generally an increase) in signal intensity. After intravenous injection, more contrast is delivered to tissues with greater vascularity distinguishing them from less vascular benign processes. As shown by Kono et al., significant differences can be demonstrated in the percent change in signal intensity (SI) measured within malignant (n = 13) compared to benign (n = 5) nodules ($p < .001$) (142). It should be emphasized, however, that simply measuring percent change in SI following contrast administration may not be sufficiently accurate to consistently differentiate benign from malignant nodules, such evaluation requiring more sophisticated data analysis. In a prospective study of 28 SPN (20 malignant, 8 benign) between 10 and 30 mm, Guckel et al., found no significant difference between malignant and benign nodules measuring percent change in signal intensity (%SI) using pre and postcontrast 10-mm axial, ECG-gated, T1-weighted spin-echo (SE) sequences (143). However, in this same population, significantly higher SIs were demonstrated in malignant lesions when enhancement curves (%SI/second) were evaluated during the first transit of a bolus of contrast media using dynamic snapshot sagittal GRE images ($p < .0001\%$). Similar to recent CT findings reported by Zhang and Kono (141), these data suggest that optimal measurement of MR signal intensity may require data acquisition as early as possible following injection of contrast prior to a later stage during equilibrium of intravascular and interstitial contrast media.

It should be emphasized that the use of MR to evaluate contrast enhancement within nodules is still preliminary. Given the additional cost and relative greater inaccessibility of MRI, coupled with decreased spatial resolution, and most importantly, the inability of MR to reliably identify the presence of calcium, it is unlikely that this technique will replace standard CT anytime soon.

Positron Emission Tomography

In distinction to MRI, considerable interest has focused on the potential use of positron emission tomography (PET), especially with 2-[fluorine-18]-fluoro-2-deoxy-D-glucose (FDG) to characterize pulmonary nodules (144–149). Briefly, FDG is a D-glucose analog radiopharmaceutical labeled with a positron emitter ^{18}F that is transported through the cell membrane and phosphorylated using normal glycolytic pathways. Increased uptake and accumulation of FDG has been shown to occur in tumor cells, although the effect is nonspecific and may be seen as well in foci of inflammation. Once inside tumor cells, FDG is only slowly metabolized allowing identification with PET (Fig. 4-44) (146).

To date, a number of studies have evaluated the efficacy of FDG-PET for differentiating between malignant and benign SPN (146,148,150,151) with reported sensitivities ranging between 93% and 100% and specificities between 82% and 88%. As reported by Gupta et al., in a prospective evaluation of 61 patients with radiographically indeterminate nodules, the probability of malignancy in a patient with a positive study is 83%, which increases with increasing age (greater than 90%) and lesion size (146): in distinction, the probability of malignancy in a patient with a negative study is only 4.7%. It should be noted that the accuracy of PET scanning improves with semiquantitative methods instead of simple visual interpretation, including standardized uptake values as well as calculation of the rate of radiotracer accumulation (150). Coupled with the apparent increased sensitivity and specificity of this technique for evaluating hilar and mediastinal nodes (146,148,152,153), it is possible that PET scanning will become the method of choice for evaluating solitary nodules as well as staging lung cancer, pending greater accessibility.

MANAGEMENT

It is estimated that nearly 130,000 individuals or 52 of every 100,000 people present each year with radiographic evidence of focal parenchymal disease (146). Unfortunately, to date, there is still little consensus concerning optimum management of these patients (1,120,154). Patients with indeterminate nodules are particularly problematic as nearly 60% of these subsequently prove benign. In an evaluation of pulmonary resections performed over a 20-year period in patients with solitary lung nodules, Ray et al., found that only 27 of 179 lesions (15%) were malignant (155). Only slightly better results have been reported by Keagy et al., who found that 79 of 122 patients (65%) undergoing minor resections (biopsy, wedge resections, or segmentectomies) and 33 of 102 patients (32%) undergoing major resections (lobectomies or pneumonectomies) proved to have benign disease (156). In distinction, more recent data has shown a larger proportion of malignant nodules (51). Clearly, an optimal approach should have as its goal a reduction in the number of thoracotomies performed for benign disease.

Available methods for evaluating pulmonary nodules include clinical assessment of the likelihood of malignancy (including the use of statistical methodologies such as Bayesian analysis) and/or lung biopsy, either via fiberoptic bron-

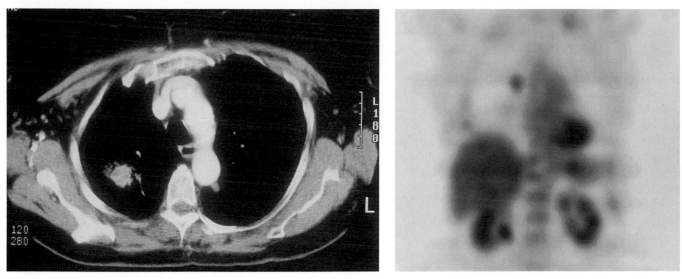

FIG. 4-44. Pulmonary nodule: evaluation with 2-[fluorine-18]-fluoro-2-deoxy-D-glucose-positron emission tomography (FDG-PET) scanning. **A:** CT section through the upper lobes shows an irregular nodule in the right upper lobe. Note that a smaller nodule is also present immediately posterior to the aortic arch. **B:** Coronal FDG-PET image shows intense accumulation of FDG within the right upper lobe nodule, subsequently surgically proved to be a nonsmall cell lung cancer. Note the absence of accumulation within the left upper lobe lesion, which has remained stable on subsequent follow-up CT examinations. The value of FDG-PET scans is similar to that of contrast-enhanced CT scans in that whereas a positive nodule study is relatively nonspecific, absence of uptake within a nodule is strong evidence of benign disease.

choscopy (FB), transthoracic needle biopsy (TTNB), or surgery, including video-assisted thoracotomy (VATS).

Use of Bayesian Analysis in Asessing CT Characteristics

Clinical correlation continues to play a critical role in the assessment of patients with pulmonary nodules. For example, a lung nodule in a patient over the age of 40, especially a smoker, is much more likely to be a bronchogenic carcinoma than a nodule seen in a younger patient or an immunocompromised patient presenting with fever (157,158).

In an attempt to more precisely define various known risk factors, both clinical and radiologic, an increasing number of investigators have made use of Bayesian analysis. Briefly, the odds-likelihood ratio form of the Bayes theorem allows calculation of the probability of malignancy by estimating likelihood ratios for various individual radiographic and clinical characteristics derived from previous literature. The likelihood ratio is a measure of the probability of a positive test result or finding in a patient with disease (i.e., sensitivity or true positive fraction) divided by the probability of a positive result or finding in a patient without disease (i.e., 1—specificity, or false positive fraction). Likelihood ratios range from zero to infinity: tests strongly suggestive of malignancy, for example, have a likelihood ratio much greater than one, whereas those strongly suggestive of benignancy approximate zero. A likelihood ratio equal to one contains no diagnostic information. Using these calculations, it is possible to combine individual probabilities into an overall estimate of the odds favoring malignancy in solitary nodules, for example, by multiplying the prior probability (or preva

lence) of cancer in the population studied by the likelihood ratios of a variety of clinical or radiographic characteristics, as long as these are conditionally independent from each other (41,159,160).

To date, investigators have reported accuracies ranging between 53% and 96% for predicting the likelihood of malignancy (41). The highest accuracy, reported by Edwards et al., made use of 27 characteristics derived from a retrospective review of their own case material (161). Unfortunately, this included characteristics otherwise unrelated to nodule characterization, such as mediastinal, hilar, and pleural abnormalities. Nonetheless, of 15 benign lesions 13 (87%) were correctly predicted.

It has been suggested that as few as four characteristics only need be assessed, including the nodule diameter, the patient's age and smoking history, and data on overall prevalence of malignancy (159); however, most studies have relied on evaluation of a far greater number of factors. In the most thorough study to date, Gurney et al., derived likelihood ratios for six radiographic and four clinical characteristics including: radiographic findings of size (subdivided in centimeter intervals), edge characteristics (including smooth, lobulated, irregular, and spiculated), the presence or absence of calcification (both radiographically and using CT phantom densitometry), growth rate (malignant versus benign), cavitation (thin versus thick-walled), and location (upper/middle versus lower lung zone); and clinical findings, including age (subdivided by decade), smoking history (subdivided by type and duration) as well as a history either of hemoptysis or prior malignancy (41). From these data a total of 15 malignant and 19 benign indicators could be identified on the basis of likelihood ratios. For malignancy, the most important radiographic findings were thickness of cavity walls, spiculation, and nodule diameter greater than 3 cm. Not surprisingly, for benignancy the most important radiographic findings included benign growth rates and calcification. It should be noted that part of the evaluation in this study included findings derived from routine tomography, a methodology only rarely employed currently in most institutions.

Using these data, these same authors then applied these estimates to a study of 66 cases of solitary pulmonary nodules (44 malignant, 22 benign, of which 10 had histologic verification) (54). Four interpreters first estimated the probability of malignancy by assessing radiographs alone and then in conjunction with all other available clinical and imaging studies: this included CT studies in 57 patients, with phantom densitometry performed in seven. Two other readers then evaluated the same material independently, with their findings used to estimate the probability of malignancy using previously derived likelihood ratios (41). Using a probability of 20% or less as indicative of benignancy, and 50% or greater as indicative of malignancy, overall, readers using Bayesian analysis performed significantly better ($p < .05$) than those only interpreting radiographs by visible inspection alone. Not surprisingly, there was considerable interobserver variation in the number of false negative interpretations recorded for the group visually assessing nodules, ranging between 14% and 41%. Inexplicably, however, for this same group of readers, the availability of ancillary studies, including prior radiographs and CT examinations, did not make a significant difference in readers interpretations. In comparison, there were far fewer false negative studies using Bayesian analysis (n = 8) when compared to routine evaluation (n = 27). Of eight false negative studies, five proved to be misinterpreted because of the presence of diffuse calcification within adenocarcinomas, including four metastases and one primary lung cancer. Nonetheless, employing Bayesian analysis the overall accuracy for interpreting nodules only proved to be 77.5%, even using all available information, compared with an accuracy of 62.5% when nodules were assessed only visually. These data suggest that although of potential value, the use of quantitative methods relying on standard radiologic and clinical criteria remains to be established.

More recently, Dewan et al., have compared the utility of PET scanning with standard criteria using Bayesian analysis in a retrospective study of 52 patients also undergoing CT evaluation (162). These investigators found that the likelihood ratios for malignancy in SPN with abnormal FDG-PET scans was 7.11 (indicative of a very high probability of malignancy for positive studies) and 0.06 for benignancy (indicative of a very high probability of benignancy for negative studies). FDG-PET proved to be a better predictor of malignancy as a stand-alone test than standard radiographic and clinical criteria either alone or surprisingly even in conjunction with FDG-PET results (162). Although these results are based on retrospective analysis they again point out the limitations of Bayesian analysis based on routine clinical and radiologic data.

Biopsy

Because of the limitations of currently available noninvasive methods for assessing nodules, biopsy is often required for a definitive diagnosis. It is also not surprising that as with other aspects of SPN evaluation there is little unanimity of opinion regarding the best method for performing nodule biopsies. In addition to sputum cytology, currently available methods include fiberoptic bronchoscopy (FB), TTNB, and surgery, including VATS.

Fiberoptic Bronchoscopy

Fiberoptic bronchoscopy is of limited value in the assessment of lung nodules. Although transbronchial biopsy is extremely accurate for assessing focal endobronchial lesions within the visual range of the bronchoscope, including those within lobar and segmental airways, the yield of FB for peripheral nodules, especially when these are less than 2 cm in size is disappointing, ranging between 20% and 83%. As recently summarized by Westcott, in a review of 15 large studies including 680 peripheral cancers, overall FB proved diagnostic in only 389 (sensitivity = 57%) (163). When assessed by nodule size, FB proved diagnostic in only 25% to 30% of nodules less than 2 cm in size. Although the yield of FB increases when only those cases in which nodules are associated with airways are selected when evaluated by CT, even in this setting, the sensitivity of FB increases only to approximately two-thirds of cases (67,164). FB has also proved of only limited value in diagnosing benign disease, even in situations in which the prevalence of benign disease is high, as in select populations with suspected tuberculosis (165). Given the accuracy of CT to evaluate the central airways, little additional benefit is derived by FB in assessing SPNs. It should be emphasized, however, that an important exception is the case in which a parenchymal nodule(s) is associated with either hilar or more importantly mediastinal adenopathy. In these cases the ability to perform transbronchial needle aspirations and biopsies (TBNA or Wang needle biopsies) using CT as a road map, in the appropriate hands, may allow definitive staging of lung cancer in a significant proportion of cases (166,167).

Transthoracic Needle Biopsy

The use of transthoracic needle aspirate (TTNA) and/or transthoracic needle biopsy (TTNB) for assessing solitary nodules is well established (Fig. 4-45). To date, numerous studies have shown that the accuracy of needle aspiration for diagnosing malignancy is uniformly greater than 90% (168). Recent advances in this technique, including the use of CT guidance, immediate cytopathology, the introduction of core biopsy techniques, and postbiopsy positional restric-

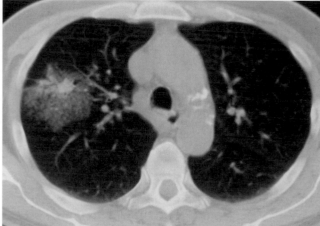

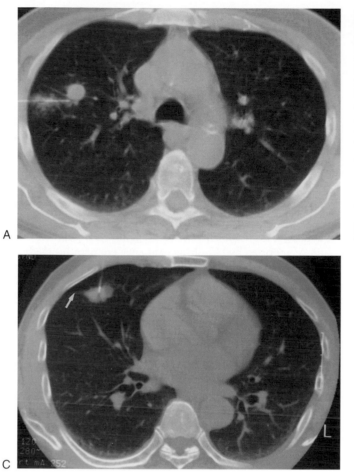

FIG. 4-45. Transthoracic needle biopsy: complications. **A:** CT section through the right upper lobe shows presence of a 21-gauge aspiration needle in close proximity to a right upper lobe nodule. **B:** Section obtained at approximately the same level as **A** following withdrawal of the needle shows ill defined airspace consolidation appearing adjacent to the nodule resulting from hemorrhage. Despite this finding the patient reported no undue discomfort, nor was there evidence of subsequent hemoptysis. Cytologically verified nonsmall cell lung cancer. **C:** CT section through the middle lobe in a different patient than **A** and **B** shows a 21-gauge cytology needle anteriorly with the tip within a right upper lobe nodule. In this case, transthoracic biopsy resulted in a small pneumothorax (*arrow*) incidentally confirming that the lesion is separate from the adjacent parietal pleura. Despite this complication, aspiration was successful, confirming this lesion as a nonsmall cell lung cancer, subsequently resected.

tions to limit the incidence of pneumothoraces have made this option still more attractive (see Fig. 4-45).

In our judgment, in most cases the true utility of TTNB is in diagnosing benign disease (169). Unfortunately, despite some reports suggesting that a benign diagnosis could be established in as many as 64% of lesions (170) in most series the accuracy of TTNA for definitive diagnosis of benign disease has proved limited, typically below 50% (171,172). Calhoun et al., in an early study using fine needle aspiration under fluoroscopic guidance, for example, were able to definitively diagnose only 16 (12%) of 132 cases interpreted as showing no evidence of malignancy on initial aspiration biopsy, and one of these 16 subsequently proved malignant (173). Furthermore, in the same group of 132 patients, 38 (29%) subsequently proved malignant.

These data emphasize the need to clearly distinguish between a true benign versus a nonspecific diagnosis at TTNA and biopsy. Included in the former category are hamartomas, granulomas, infectious etiologies in which microorganisms can be demonstrated, including lung abscesses, and cores of fibrous tissue; included in the latter category are the findings of blood, histiocytes, necrosis, inflammatory cells, alveolar lining cells, and bronchial epithelium (168,172).

A number of reasons have been cited to explain the low yield of TTNB for establishing a benign diagnosis. These include an insufficient number of biopsies, lack of on-site cytology, technical inexperience, and small lesion size, among others. Use of repeated biopsies has been shown to increase the likelihood of a benign diagnosis by biopsies as much as 30% (163). Similarly, the presence of on-site cytological evaluation has been shown to reduce the number of false-negative studies in at least some studies. The effect of small lesion size (less than 1.5 cm) is somewhat more controversial (168,174,175). Li et al., have reported a significant difference in the diagnostic accuracy of TTNB between small and large lesions (74% versus 96%, respectively) (174). More recently, however, Wescott et al., in a study of 74 biopsies of 64 small (less than 1.5 cm) lesions, including 21 benign lesions and 43 malignant lesions, reported a sensitivity of 93%, a specificity of 100% with an accuracy of 95% (168). As noted by these authors, discrepancies in the diagnostic accuracy of TTNB for small lesions likely reflect a combination of experience and the number of attempted biopsies. With these issues in mind, in most centers cases that meet truly benign criteria can now safely be managed conservatively.

Recently, it has been shown that the ability to establish a definitive benign diagnosis may be improved significantly by use of coaxial core needle biopsy using an automated cutting biopsy needle (176). The advantage of this approach is inherent in the ability to acquire histologic sections. Klein et al., in a retrospective study comparing the accuracy of routine cytology versus core needle biopsy, found that although no difference could be seen for diagnosing malignancy, fine needle aspiration yielded a benign diagnosis in only 44% of cases as compared with 100% using core biopsy (169). It should be noted that in this series, originating from the American Southwest, 30% of benign lesions were caused by *Coccidiomycosis* infection, an unusual distribution compared with most other series.

The use of an automated spring-loaded gun allows better penetration of firm lesions less amenable to fine aspirating needles. Another advantage of core needle biopsy is the ability to more precisely characterize malignant lesions, including pulmonary metastases and especially parenchymal lymphoma. Unfortunately, the incidence of pneumothoraces does increase to as high as 54% with use of a core needle-biopsy gun (169): in distinction, although the incidence of pneumothoraces resulting from transthoracic needle aspiration has been reported to be as high as 50%, in most series, the incidence averages around 20 to 25%, with the need for chest tube placement occurring in less than 5% (163). As noted by Kazerooni et al., the risk of complications does increase with smaller lesion, especially when centrally located (177). Given these data, the use of core needle biopsy is advocated in patients in whom the suspicion of malignancy is low, or for whom initial cytologic evaluation has proved nonspecific.

Video-Assisted Thoracic Surgery

Recent advances in video technology have led to considerable interest in the use of video-assisted thoracic surgery (VATS) to assess indeterminate pulmonary nodules (105,178,179). VATS is performed using a double-lumen endobronchial tube to allow ventilation of the contralateral lung, usually under general anesthesia. Following collapse of the ipsilateral lung, three incisions are typically made with introduction of a telescope coupled to a video camera: if necessary these incisions also allow insertion of a palpating finger in those cases in which peripheral abnormalities are not apparent by inspection. Wedge and less commonly lobar resections are performed either using an endoscopic stapler, or less commonly, neodymium:yttrium-aluminum garnet (YAG) laser resection (180). Following the procedure, a chest tube is always inserted.

Initial results using video-assisted thoracoscopic excisional biopsy has confirmed that this is a viable approach for diagnosing peripheral pulmonary nodules. Mack et al., in a study of 242 indeterminate pulmonary nodules were able to establish definitive diagnoses in all patients, including benign diagnoses in 127 patients who otherwise may have required thoracotomies (52%) (181). Viewed from a different perspective, of course, it is unclear how many of these lesions may have been successfully diagnosed with modern transthoracic needle biopsy techniques. Of the 127 patients with benign diagnoses, 12 had pulmonary hamartomas, and 34 had granulomas, diagnoses that may have been established definitively using transthoracic needle biopsy for which resection is unnecessary (181). Furthermore, of the 115 patients diagnosed with malignant nodules, 64 (56%) proved to be metastatic in origin, a diagnosis again that preferentially should be made prior to thoracoscopy.

It should be emphasized that in most large series as many as 25% of cases require conversion to thoracotomy, either because of the need for more extensive or definitive resection in patients with resectable lung cancers, inability to detect pathology, prior adhesions, bleeding, and/or equipment failure. As reported by Hazelrigg et al., in a cooperative study of 1,820 cases, 865 of which were performed for indeterminate pulmonary nodules, there were 65 cases (7.5%) in which nodules could not be detected (179). Especially problematic are central lesions variously defined as greater than one to three centimeters from adjacent visceral pleura or adjacent to segmental or subsegmental pulmonary vasculature (182). In this setting, the diagnostic accuracy of VATS may be as low as 67%. As a result, a number of investigators have suggested use of CT-guided wire placement using a variety of needles with or without injection of methylene blue dye prior to VATS (Fig. 4-46) (183–185). Using a Kopans wire, Shah et al., were able to successfully place hook wires in 16 of 17 nodules prior to VATS with only one of these dislodging (183). Similarly, Shepard et al., also using a Kopans hook wire reported successfully positioning 8 of 10 wires with only two dislodging prior to surgery (184). More recently, Asamura et al., have suggested use of CT-guided injection of a metallic coil with subsequent thoracoscopic resection under fluoroscopic guidance as a method to improve thoracoscopic localization (186).

Despite these reports, recent reviews have suggested that in most cases, prethoracoscopic nodule localization may not be necessary provided surgeons make adequate use of finger palpation at the time of thoracoscopy (105). As pointed out by Westcott, it is difficult to follow the logic of performing wire localization without first attempting needle aspiration or biopsy given that the procedure requires identical skills, equipment, and expense as routine CT-guided transthoracic needle biopsy (168). It should be noted that alternative approaches, in particular intraoperative sonography, have been advocated by some as a more definitive means for more precise localization of nodules again obviating prethoracoscopic needle localization (187).

Current Strategy

It is apparent that despite considerable technical advances, both radiographic and surgical, optimal management of patients with solitary nodules still requires considerable clinical acumen. No single algorithm applies in all cases making

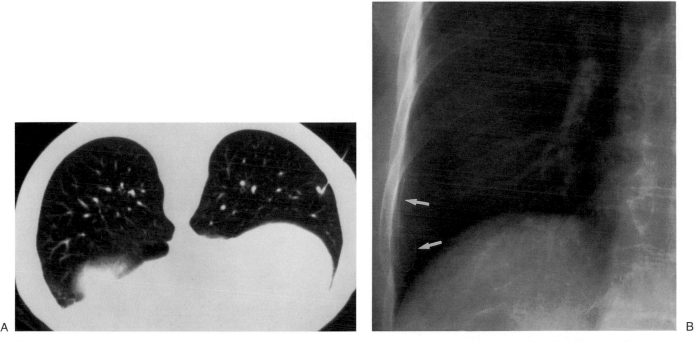

FIG. 4-46. CT-guided needle localization. **A:** Prone CT section through the lung bases shows a localization needle adjacent to a small peripheral lung nodule. **B:** Coned down radiograph of the right costophrenic angle following placement of needle localization wire shows the wire still in place prior to surgery (*arrows*). Although CT may be used for this purpose, in our experience it is preferable to simply attempt an aspiration/biopsy instead.

clinical judgment an absolute prerequisite for proper care (1,154).

In general, one of three broad strategies are usually employed. These include: (a) observation, followed by biopsy if interval change is noted; (b) bronchoscopic and/or transthoracic needle aspiration or biopsy, followed by continued observation or surgery as indicated; and (c) immediate surgery. As noted by Cummings et al., the choice between these strategies may indeed be a close call (159). Using decision analysis these authors showed that immediate surgery produced a slightly longer life expectancy provided the probability of cancer clinically was high, whereas observation produced a slightly longer life expectancy in patients with a low probability of malignancy (159). These differences, however, were extremely small. Unfortunately, many studies purporting to evaluate optimal strategies based on either decision analysis, or cost-effectiveness have been reported prior to the introduction of video-assisted tomography, PET scanning and/or contrast enhanced CT densitometry, limiting their value (159,188).

Our present approach centers on the use of CT as an initial means for assessing nodules (see Tables 4-3 and 4-4). CT represents the most practical method available to confirm the presence and location of nodules, insure that they are solitary, and allow initial characterization based on size, shape, position, configuration, and density. Unfortunately, it may be anticipated that following routine CT evaluation 30% to 40% of nodules will remain indeterminate. Although surgery has been advocated by some in all such cases, in our opinion this would lead to a large number of unnecessary thoracotomies. Instead, the following guidelines for management are recommended:

1. Nodules greater than 3 cm in size especially in patients over the age of 30 are likely malignant (greater than 90%). In these cases, especially when otherwise deemed potentially resectable, these patients should proceed directly to surgery. Immediate surgery may also be applicable in patients for whom reliable follow-up assessment may not be possible.

TABLE 4-3. *Diagnostic algorithm: SPNs < 3 cm*

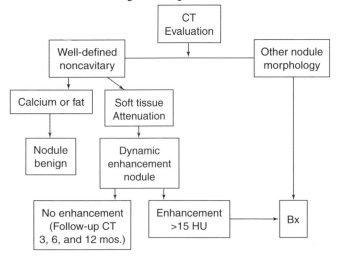

TABLE 4-4. *Diagnostic algorithm: SPNs < 5 mm*

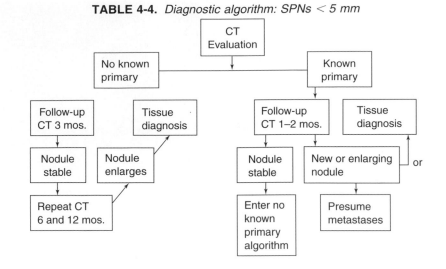

2. In distinction, nodules that are unchanged in size for two years, or show benign patterns of calcification or fat may be safely observed. It should be emphasized, however, given numerous reports documenting the propensity for some adenocarcinomas to calcify that follow-up radiologic or CT surveillance should be mandatory for a period of no less than 1 year especially in patients with known extrathoracic malignancies.

3. In patients with indeterminate CT studies, the use of contrast-enhanced CT densitometry may prove invaluable by increasing the degree of certainty that a lesion is benign in the absence of significant contrast enhancement. This may be especially helpful in patients in whom the suspicion of malignancy is low, as for example, patients under the age of 30, or those living in regions in which granulomas are endemic. PET scanning, although potentially more accurate, remains at present more investigational. It may be anticipated, however, that with increasing availability, the role of PET scanning for characterizing nodules will expand.

4. Fiberoptic bronchoscopy should be reserved only for those patients in whom lesions either are clearly endobronchial on CT, or for whom transbronchial needle aspiration or biopsy (TBNA) is deemed appropriate for definitive staging of mediastinal nodes.

5. Transthoracic needle aspiration or biopsy should be performed preferentially on indeterminate nodules, especially those deemed likely benign or in patients with known extrathoracic malignancies in whom metastatic disease is likely. In these cases, core needle biopsies should be performed either if the initial cytology proves non-specific, or when more definitive characterization of malignancy is indicated, especially in patients with suspected lymphoma. Although core needle biopsies result in greater morbidity, this is more than offset by the higher yield of true benign diagnoses. CT guidance is recommended particularly for those cases in which nodules are small, central in location, or difficult to identify on biplane fluoroscopy.

6. Video-assisted thoracostomy should be considered at present primarily a diagnostic modality, and should be reserved for those cases in which alternate methods prove nondiagnostic. Routine use of video-assisted thoracoscopy entails considerably greater cost given the need for general anesthesia in most cases coupled with the fact that between 30% to 40% of cases require conversion to thoracotomy either for definitive resection of lung cancer, or because of inability to localize disease. Therapeutic indications yet to be validated include video-assisted lobectomies, and metastasectomies. The use of CT-guided wire localization may be of value in select cases, especially when nodules are central in location.

It should be emphasized that these recommendations pertain primarily to lesions greater than 5 mm in size. To date, most reported series, including those emphasizing a role for contrast enhancement as well as transthoracic needle biopsies have almost exclusively focused on nodules greater than 5 mm in size. What to do with so-called ditzels remains extremely controversial. As documented by Munden et al., in their retrospective study of 64 nodules less than 1 cm in size evaluated with video-assisted thoracostomy, 37 proved to be malignant in patients without a known primary or prior history of malignancy (47). Importantly, six of eight nodules less than 5 mm in size proved to be malignant. Although this study is likely biased by patient selection, the problem of managing incidentally noted small nodules remains problematic (see Fig. 4-44).

In this regard, recent attention has focused on the potential for more precise computer evaluations of nodule contour and especially growth. Anyone who has attempted to sequentially follow small nodules knows of limitations using currently available scan technology for precisely measuring the size of nodules. In addition to technical factors such as those related to optimal windowing and variable field-of-view, serious limitations also result from minor variations in scan location that occur between studies. It should be remembered that a nodule measuring 4 mm in diameter need

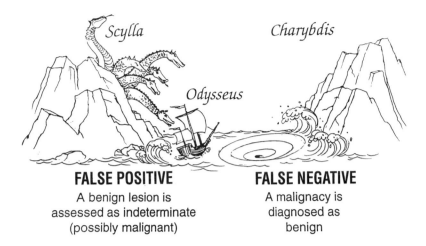

FALSE POSITIVE
A benign lesion is assessed as indeterminate (possibly malignant)

FALSE NEGATIVE
A malignancy is diagnosed as benign

FIG. 4-47. Illustration denoting conservative approach to diagnosis of a solitary pulmonary nodule. Given a choice between the two evils, the Scylla of false positive (a benign lesion assessed as indeterminate) and the Charybdis of false negative (a malignancy diagnosed as benign), Odysseus steers his ship closer to Scylla, the lesser of two evils. For indeterminate lesions, additional studies, such as needle biopsy, are indicated.

only grow to 5 mm for the nodule to have doubled in volume. Using currently available computer calipers is rarely sufficient for reliable measurements of such small increments. As preliminarily reported by Reeves et al., using automatic three dimensional evaluation of nodule shape and size, quantitative measurement of even small changes in nodules may be possible allowing for far more precise characterization of nodule growth in considerably shorter time frames than currently available (189). Clearly, the clinical utility of such assessment must await further prospective validation.

It remains only to emphasize that the choice of strategy for managing patients with pulmonary nodules also entails considerations of the various levels of expertise (including those of the interventional radiologist, bronchoscopist, cytologist, and surgeon) as well as patient factors, in particular the effect of patient's risk-taking attitude towards testing strategies (190). The proper approach to the assessment of a focal pulmonary lesion is conservative. Patients with nodules diagnosed as benign by CT should have follow-up chest roentgenograms. No lesion with a questionable or disturbing morphologic feature should be certified as benign. In a difficult situation it is preferable to designate a benign mass as indeterminate (false positive) with a goal of never diagnosing a malignant lesion as benign (false negative). This philosophy is illustrated in Figure 4-47. The radiologist must steer carefully between the perils of Scylla and Charybdis, favoring a cautious course as far as possible from the whirlpool of a false positive diagnosis.

CT Screening

As is well known, routine radiographic screening of lung cancer has failed to gain general acceptance. The results of four randomized controlled studies including 37,724 individuals performed in the early 1980s failed to show evidence of improved disease-specific mortality (191), leading most critics to conclude that there is no indication for routine radiographic screening (192,193). Less well appreciated is the fact that despite this consensus, controversy persists over the true significance of these studies (194,195). Although a detailed evaluation of this topic is outside the intended scope of the present review, recent interest has focused on the potential use of CT as a method for early detection of lung cancer (Fig. 4-48). As reported by Kaneko et al., in a combined prevalence and incidence study of 1,369 patients evaluated using low-dose volumetric CT over a three year interval, a total of 701 nodules greater than 5 mm in size were identified either by chest radiography (n = 57), CT (n = 588) or both (N = 56) (196). Two hundred and twenty nine nodules were further evaluated using high-resolution CT scans of which 19 (8.3%) were ultimately biopsied. Of these, 16 of 19 proved to be malignant including 15 patients with primary lung cancer and one patient with metastatic disease. Of 15 primary lung cancers, 14 (93%) proved to be stage 1 neoplasms with mean diameters of 16 mm ($\pm$ 7 mm) with a range of eight to 35 mm: not surprisingly, of these 11 were identified by CT only (196). Further analysis showed that 10 nodules were first identified on prevalence CT examinations, with the remaining five nodules detected on follow-up of true incidence CT examinations. Of note in this study is the fact that in Japan, within a single for-profit program, thousands of individuals with a history of 20 pack-years of smoking or more, regarded conventional radiographic-cytologic screening worth the out-of-pocket expense of $350 per year.

Although intriguing, these results raise more questions than they answer. It is unclear, for example, by what criteria it was determined that of the 701 nodules identified only 229 cases (6.6%) were subsequently evaluated by HRCT. Furthermore, it is unclear why of these 229 cases only 19 were subsequently biopsied. As any screening protocol relying on CT is likely to identify a large number of small parenchymal nodules, decisions concerning the efficacy of screening will necessarily have to contend with the issue of how to manage these cases. Of equal importance is the issue of cost as well as the frequency with which patients will have

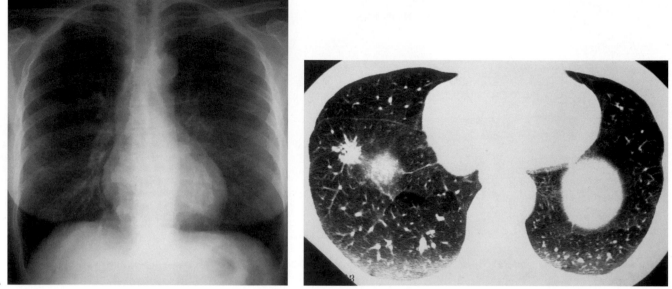

FIG. 4-48. CT screening. **A:** Posteroanterior radiograph shows no apparent parenchymal abnormality. **B:** One-millimeter CT section obtained following a preliminary low-dose CT scan through the lungs confirms the presence of a spiculated lesion just above the right hemidiaphragm, not visible on the accompanying chest radiograph including the lateral view (not shown), even in retrospect.

to be scanned for screening to be efficacious. These caveats notwithstanding, a potential role for CT as a screening modality for lung cancer is currently being assessed in a number of institutions around the world, and may well shortly be established.

REFERENCES

1. Webb WR. Radiologic evaluation of the solitary pulmonary nodule. *AJR Am J Roentgenol* 1990;154:701–708.
2. Davis SD. CT evaluation for pulmonary metastases in patients with extrathoracic malignancy. *Radiology* 1991;180:1–12.
3. Muhm JR, Brown LR, Crowe JK, et al. Comparison of whole lung tomography and computed tomography for detecting pulmonary nodules. *AJR Am J Roentgenol* 1978;131:981–984.
4. Crow J, Slavin G, Kreel L. Pulmonary metastases: a pathologic and radiologic study. *Cancer* 1981;47:2595–2602.
5. Reiner B, Siegel E, Sawyer R, et al. The impact of routine CT of the chest on the diagnosis and management of newly diagnosed squamous cell carcinoma of the head and neck. *AJR Am J Roentgenol* 1997; 169:667–671.
6. Schaner EG, Chang AE, Doppman JL, et al. Comparison of computed and conventional whole lung tomography in detecting pulmonary nodules: a prospective radiologic-pathologic study. *AJR Am J Roentgenol* 1978;131:51–54.
7. Chalmers N, Best JJK. The significance of pulmonary nodules detected by CT but not by chest radiography in tumor staging. *Clin Radiol* 1991;44:410–412.
8. Peuchot M, Libshitz HI. Pulmonary metastatic disease: radiologic-surgical correlation. *Radiology* 1987;164:719–722.
9. Wilimas JA, Kaste SC, Kauffman WM, et al. Use of chest computed tomography in the staging of pediatric Wilms tumor: interobserver variability and prognostic significance. *J Clin Oncol* 1997;15: 2631–2635.
10. White CS, Romney BM, Mason AC, et al. Primary carcinoma of the lung overlooked at CT: analysis of findings in 14 patients. *Radiology* 1996;199:109–115.
11. Gurney JW. Missed lung cancer at CT: imaging findings in nine patients. *Radiology* 1996;199:117–122.
12. Naidich DP, Rusinek H, McGuinness G, et al. Variables affecting pulmonary nodule detection with computed tomography: evaluation with three-dimensional computer simulation. *J Thorac Imaging* 1993; 8:291–299.
13. Venuta F, Rendina EA, Pescarmona EO, et al. Occult lung cancer in patients with bullous emphysema. *Thorax* 1996;52:289–290.
14. Hazelrigg SR, Boley TM, Weber D, Magee MJ, Naunheim KS. Incidence of lung nodules found in patients undergoing lung volume reduction. *Ann Thorac Surg* 1997;64:303–306.
15. Rusinek H, Naidich DP, McGuinness G, et al. Pulmonary nodule detection: low-dose versus conventional CT. *Radiology* 1998 *(in press)*.
16. Kalender WA, Seissler W, Klotz E, Vock P. Spiral volumetric CT with single-breath-hold technique, continuous transport, and continuous scanner rotation. *Radiology* 1990;176:181–183.
17. Costello P, Anderson W, Blume D. Pulmonary nodule: evaluation with spiral volumetric CT. *Radiology* 1991;179:875–876.
18. Vock P, Soucek M, Daepp M, Kalender WA. Lung: spiral volumetric CT with single-breath-hold technique. *Radiology* 1990;176:864–867.
19. Brink JA. Technical aspects of helical (spiral) CT. *Radiol Clin North Am* 1995;33:825.
20. Heywang-Koebrunner S, Lommatzsch B, Fink U, Maayr B. Comparison of spiral and conventional CT in the detection of pulmonary nodules [abstr]. *Radiology* 1992;185(P):131.
21. Remy-Jardin M, Remy J, Giraud F, Marquette CH. Pulmonary nodules: detection with thick-section spiral CT versus conventional CT. *Radiology* 1993;187:513–520.
22. Kalender WA, Polacin A, Suss C. A comparison of conventional and spiral CT: an experimental study on the detection of spherical lesions. *J Comput Assist Tomogr* 1994;18:167–176.
23. Buckley JA, Scott WW, Siegelman SS, et al. Pulmonary nodules: effect of increased data sampling on detection with spiral CT and confidence in diagnosis. *Radiology* 1995;196:395–400.
24. Seltzer SE, Judy PF, Adams DF, et al. Spiral CT of the chest: comparison of cine and film-based viewing. *Radiology* 1995;197:73–78.
25. Tillich M, Kammerhuber F, Reittner P, et al. Detection of pulmonary nodules with helical CT: comparison of cine and film-based viewing. *AJR Am J Roentgenol* 1997;169:1611–1614.
26. Napel S, Rubin GD, Jeffrey RB. Technical note. STS-MIP: a new reconstruction technique for CT of the chest. *J Comput Assist Tomogr* 1993;17:832–838.
27. Remy-Jardin M, Remy J, Artaud D, Deschildre F, Duhamel A. Diffuse infiltrative lung disease: clinical value of sliding-thin-slab maximum intensity projection CT scans in the detection of mild micronodular patterns. *Radiology* 1996;200:333–339.

28. Croisille P, Souto M, Cova M, et al. Pulmonary nodules: improved detection with vascular segmentation and extraction with spiral CT. *Radiology* 1995;197:397–401.

29. Müller NL, Gamsu G, Webb WR. Pulmonary nodules: detection using magnetic resonance and computed tomography. *Radiology* 1985;155:687–690.

30. Feuerstein IM, Jicha DL, Pass HI, et al. Pulmonary metastases: MR imaging with surgical correlation—a prospective study. *Radiology* 1992;182:123–129.

31. Panicek DM. Editorial. MR imaging for pulmonary metastases? *Radiology* 1992;182:10–11.

32. Doppman JL, Pass HI, Niemen L, et al. Detection of ACTH-producing bronchial carcinoid tumors: MR imaging vs CT. *AJR Am J Roentgenol* 1991;156:39–43.

33. O'Brien EJ, Tuttle WM, Ferkaney JE. The management of the pulmonary "coin" lesion. *S Clin North Am* 1948;28:1313–1322.

34. Steele JD. The solitary pulmonary nodule. Report of a cooperative study of resected asymptomatic solitary pulmonary nodules in males. *J Thoracic Cardiovasc Surg* 1963;46:21–39.

35. Walske BR. The solitary pulmonary nodule. *Dis Chest* 1966;49:302–304.

36. Taylor RR, Rivkin LN, Salyer JM. The solitary pulmonary nodule. *Ann Surg* 1958;147:197–202.

37. Davis EW, Peabody JE, Katz S. The solitary pulmonary nodule. *J Thoracic Surg* 1956;32:728–770.

38. Gilbert HA, Kagan AR. Metastases: incidence, detection and evaluation without histologic confirmation. In: *Fundamental aspects of metastases.* Amsterdam: North-Holland Publishing, 1976.

39. Holin SM, Dwork RE, Glaser S, Rikli AE, Stocklen JB. Solitary pulmonary nodules found in a community-wide chest roentgenographic survey: a five year follow-up study. *Am Rev Tuberc* 1959;79:427–439.

40. McClure CD, Boucot KF, Shipman GA, et al. The solitary pulmonary nodule and primary lung malignancy. *Arch Environ Health* 1961;3:127–139.

41. Gurney JW. Determining the likelihood of malignancy in solitary pulmonary nodules with Bayesian analysis. Part 1. Theory. *Radiology* 1993;186:405–413.

42. Theros EG. Varying manifestations of peripheral pulmonary neoplasms: a radiologic-pathologic correlative study. *Am J Roentgenol* 1977;128:893.

43. Stitik FP, Tockman MS. Radiographic screening in the early detection of lung cancer. *Radiol Clin North Am* 1978;16(3):347–366.

44. Siegelman SS, Khouri NF, Leo FP, et al. Solitary pulmonary nodules: CT assessment. *Radiology* 1986;160:307–312.

45. Proto AV, Thomas SP. Pulmonary nodules studied by computed tomography. *Radiology* 1985;156:149–153.

46. Zerhouni EA, Stitik FP, Siegelman SS, et al. CT of the pulmonary nodule: a cooperative study. *Radiology* 1986;160:319–327.

47. Munden RF, Pugatch RD, Liptay MJ, Sugarbaker DJ, Le LU. Small pulmonary lesions detected at CT: clinical importance. *Radiology* 1997;202:105–110.

48. Libby DM, Henschke CI, Yankelevitz DF. The solitary pulmonary nodule: update 1995. *Am J Med* 1995;99:491–496.

49. Scholten ET, Kreel L. Distribution of lung metastases in the axial plane: a radiological-pathological study. *Radiol Clin (Basel)* 1977;46:248–265.

50. Bankoff MS, McEniff NJ, Bhadelia RA, Garacia-Moliner M, Daly BDT. Prevalence of pathologically proven intrapulmonary lymph nodes and their appearance on CT. *AJR Am J Roentgenol* 1996;167:629–630.

51. Zwirewich CV, Vedal S, Miller RR, Müller NL. Solitary pulmonary nodule: high-resolution CT and radiologic-pathologic correlation. *Radiology* 1991;179:469–476.

52. Gross BH, Glazer GM, Bookstein FL. Multiple pulmonary nodules detected by computed tomography: diagnostic implications. *J Comput Assist Tomogr* 1985;9:880–885.

53. Hirakata K, Nakata H, Haratake J. Appearance of pulmonary metastases on high-resolution CT scans: comparison with histopathologic findings from autopsy specimens. *AJR Am J Roentgenol* 1993;161:37–43.

54. Gurney JW, Lyddon DM, McKay JA. Determining the likelihood of malignancy in solitary pulmonary nodules with Bayesian analysis: part II. Application. *Radiology* 1993;186:415–422.

55. Kido S, Kuriyama K, Kumatani Y, et al. Fractal analysis of internal texture of small peripheral pulmonary adenocarcinomas in thin-section computed tomography: radiologic-pathologic correlation. *Radiology* 1997;205(P):396.

56. McNitt-Gray MF, Hart EM, Wycoff N, et al. Characterization of solitary pulmonary nodules using measures extracted from high resolution CT images. *Radiology* 1997;205(P):395.

57. Kuhlman JE, Fishman EK, Siegelman SS. Invasive pulmonary aspergillosis in acute leukemia: characteristic findings on CT, the CT halo sign, and the role of CT in early diagnosis. *Radiology* 1985;157:611–614.

58. Kuhlman JE, Fishman EK, Burch PA, et al. Invasive pulmonary aspergillosis in acute leukemia: the contribution of CT to early diagnosis and aggressive management. *Chest* 1987;92:95–99.

59. Kuhlman JE, Fishman EK, Burch PA, et al. CT of invasive pulmonary aspergillosis. *AJR Am J Roentgenol* 1988;150:1015–1020.

60. Barloon TJ, Galvin JR, Mori M, Stanford W, Gingrich RD. High-resolution ultrafast chest CT in the clinical management of febrile bone marrow transplant patients with normal or nonspecific chest roentgenograms [see comments]. *Chest* 1991;99:928–933.

61. Blum U, Windfuhr M, Buitrago-Tellez C, et al. Invasive pulmonary aspergillosis. MRI, CT and plain radiographic findings and their contribution for early diagnosis. *Chest* 1994;106:1156–1161.

62. Mori M, Galvin JR, Barloon TJ, Gingrich RD, Stanford W. Fungal pulmonary infections after bone marrow transplantation: evaluation with radiography and CT. *Radiology* 1991;178:721–726.

63. Primack SL, Hartman TE, Lee KS, Müller NL. Pulmonary nodules and the CT halo sign. *Radiology* 1994;190:513–515.

64. Gaeta M, Volta S, Stroscio S, Romeo P, Pandolfo I. CT "halo sign" in pulmonary tuberculoma. *J Comput Assist Tomogr* 1992;16:827–828.

65. Herold CJ, Kramer J, Sertl K, et al. Invasive pulmonary aspergillosis: evaluation with MR imaging. *Radiology* 1989;173:717–723.

66. Kuriyama K, Tateishi R, Doi O. Prevalence of air bronchograms in small peripheral carcinomas of the lung on thin-section CT: comparison with benign tumors. *AJR Am J Roentgenol* 1991;156:921–924.

67. Gaeta M, Pandolfo I, Volta S, et al. Bronchus sign on CT in peripheral carcinoma of the lung: value in predicting results of transbronchial biopsy. *AJR Am J Roentgenol* 1991;157:1181–1185.

68. Kuriyama K, Tateishi R, Doi O, et al. CT-pathologic correlation in small peripheral lung cancers. *AJR Am J Roentgenol* 1987;149:1139–1143.

69. Kui M, Templeton PA, White CS, et al. Evaluation of the air bronchogram sign on CT in solitary pulmonary lesions. *J Comput Assist Tomogr* 1996;20:983–986.

70. Gaeta M, Barone M, Russi EG, et al. Carcinomatous solitary pulmonary nodules: evaluation of the tumor-bronchi relationship with thin-section CT. *Radiology* 1993;187:535–539.

71. Kuhlman JE, Reyes BL, Hruban RH, et al. Abnormal air-filled spaces in the lung. *Radiographics* 1993;13:47–75.

72. Woodring HH, Fried AM, Chung VP. Solitary cavities of the lung: diagnostic implications of cavity wall thickness. *AJR Am J Roentgenol* 1980;135:1269–1271.

73. Woodring JH, Fried AM. Significance of wall thickness in solitary cavities of the lung: a follow-up study. *AJR Am J Roentgenol* 1983;140:473–474.

74. Meziane MA, Hruban RH, Zerhouni EA, et al. High resolution CT of the lung parenchyma with pathologic correlation. *Radiographics* 1988;8:27–54.

75. Milne ENC, Zerhouni EA. Blood supply of pulmonary metastases. *J Thorac Imag* 1987;2:15–23.

76. Balakrishnan J, Meziane MA, Siegelmn SS. Pulmonary infarction: CT appearance with pathologic correlation. *J Comput Assist Tomogr* 1989;13:941–945.

77. Forster BB, Müller NL, Miller RR, Nelems B, Evans KG. Neuroendocrine carcinomas of the lung: clinical, radiologic, and pathologic correlation. *Radiology* 1989;170:441–445.

78. Zweibel BR, Austin JHH. Carcinoid tumors: CT evaluation. *Radiology* 1991;178:473–486.

79. Kushihashi T, Munechika H, Ri K, et al. Bronchoalveolar adenoma of the lung: CT-pathologic correlation. *Radiology* 1994;193:789–793.

80. Kuhlman JE, Fishman EK, Kuhajda FP, et al. Solitary bronchoalveolar carcinoma: CT criteria. *Radiology* 1988;167:379–382.

81. Gaeta M, Barone M, Caruso R, Bartiromo G, Pandolfo P. CT-pathologic correlation in nodular bronchoalveolar carcinoma. *J Comput Assist Tomogr* 1994;18:229–232.

82. Jang HJ, Lee KS, Kwon OJ, et al. Bronchioloalveolar carcinoma: focal area of ground-glass attenuation at thin-section CT as an early sign. *Radiology* 1996;199:485–488.

83. Weisbrod GL, Towers MJ, Chamberlain DW, Herman SJ, Matzinger

FR. Thin-walled cystic lesions in bronchioalveolar carcinoma. *Radiology* 1992;185:401–405.

84. Im JG, Han MC, Yu EJ, et al. Lobar bronchioloalveolar carcinoma: angiogram sign on CT scans. *Radiology* 1990;176:749–753.

85. Remy J, Remy-Jardin M, Wattinne L, Deffontaines C. Pulmonary arteriovenous malformations: evaluation with CT of the chest before and after treatment. *Radiology* 1992;182:809–816.

86. Remy J, Remy-Jardin M, Giraud F, Wattinne L. Angioarchitecture of pulmonary arteriovenous malformations: clinical utility of three-dimensional helical CT. *Radiology* 1994;191:657–664.

87. Nathan MH, Collins VP, Adams RA. Differentiation of benign and malignant pulmonary nodules by growth rate. *Radiology* 1962;79:221–231.

88. Yankelevitz DF, Henschke C. Does 2-year stability imply that pulmonary nodules are benign? *AJR Am J Roentgenol* 1997;168:325–328.

89. Good CA, Hood Jr RT, McDonald JE. Significance of a solitary mass in the lung. *Am J Roentgenol* 1953;70:543–554.

90. Good CA, Wilson TW. The solitary circumscribed pulmonary nodule. *JAMA* 1958;166:210–215.

91. Good CA. The solitary pulmonary nodule: a problem of management. *Radiol Clin North Am* 1963;1:429–438.

92. Collins VP, Loeffler RK, Tivey H. Observations on growth rates of human tumors. *AJR Am J Roentgenol* 1956;76:988–1000.

93. Weiss W, Boucot KE, Cooper DA. Survival of men with peripheral lung cancer in relation to histologic characteristics and growth rate. *Am Rev Resp Dis* 1968;98:75–92.

94. Rigler L. The roentgen signs of carcinoma of the lung. *AJR Am J Roentgenol* 1955;74:415–428.

95. Nathan MH. Management of solitary pulmonary nodules. An organized approach based on growth rate and statistics. *JAMA* 1974;227:1141–1144.

96. Bennett DE, Sasser WF, Ferguson TB. Adenocarcinoma of the lung in men. *Cancer* 1969;23:431–439.

97. Ireland AP, Clark WWB, DeMeester TR. Barrett's esophagus: the significance of p53 in clinical practice. *Annals Surg* 1997;225:17–30.

98. Denissenko MF, Pao A, Tang M-S, Pfeifer GP. Preferential formation of benzo[a]pyrene adducts at lung cancer mutational hotspots in p53. *Science* 1996;274:430–432.

99. El-Torky M, Giltman LI, Dabbous M. Collagens in scar carcinoma of the lung. *Am J Pathol* 1985;171:322.

100. Barsky SH, Huang SJ, Bhuta S. The extracellular matrix of pulmonary scar carcinoma is suggestive of a desmoplastic origin. *Am J Pathol* 1986;124:412–419.

101. Kawai T, Yakumaaru K, Suzuki Mea. Diffuse interstitial pulmonary fibrosis and lung cancer. *Acta Pathol Jpn* 1987;37:11.

102. Hughes JM, Weil H. Asbestosis as a precursor of asbestos related lung cancer: results of a prospective mortality study. *Br J Ind Med* 1991;48:229.

103. Mellemkjaer L, Linet MS, Gridley Gea. Rheumatoid arthritis and cancer risk. *Eur J Cancer* 1996;32A:1753–1757.

104. Roumm AD, Medsger TA Jr. Cancer and systemic sclerosis: an epidemiologic study. *Arthritis Rheum* 1985;28:1336–1340.

105. Kaiser LR, Shrager JB. Video-assisted thoracic surgery: the current state of the art. *AJR Am J Roentgenol* 1995;165:1111–1117.

106. O'Keefe Jr ME, Good CA, McDonald JE. Calcification in solitary nodules in the lung. *Am J Roentgenol* 1957;77:1023–1033.

107. Siegelman SS, Zerhouni EA, Leo FP, Khouri NF, Stitik FP. CT of the solitary pulmonary nodule. *AJR Am J Roentgenol* 1980;135:1–13.

108. Zerhouni EA, Spivey JF, Morgan RH, et al. Factors influencing quantitative CT measurements of solitary pulmonary nodules. *J Comput Assist Tomogr* 1982;6:1075–1087.

109. Jones FA, Wiedemann HP, O'Donovan PB, Stoller JK. Computerized tomographic densitometry of the solitary pulmonary nodule using a nodule phantom. *Chest* 1989;96:779–783.

110. Im J-G, Gamsu G, Gordon D. CT densitometry of pulmonary nodules in a frozen human phantom. *AJR* 1988;150:61–66.

111. Khan A, Heerman PG, Vorwerk PS, et al. Solitary pulmonary nodules: comparison of classification with standard, thin-section, and reference phantom CT. *Radiology* 1991;179:477–481.

112. Swensen SJ, Harms GF, Morin RL, Myers JL. CT evaluation of solitary pulmonary nodules: value of 185-H reference phantom. *AJR Am J Roentgenol* 1991;156:925–929.

113. Swensen SJ, Morin RL, Aughenbaugh GL, Leimer DW. CT reconstruction algorithm selection in the evaluation of solitary pulmonary nodules. *J Comput Assist Tomogr* 1995;19:932–935.

114. Bhalla M. Use of dual kVp to assess solitary pulmonary nodules. *J Comput Assist Tomogr* 1995;19:44–47.

115. Mahoney MC, Shipley RT, Cocoran HL, Dickson BA. CT demonstration of calcification in carcinoma of the lung. *AJR* 1990;154:255–258.

116. Grewal RG, Austin JHM. CT demonstration of calcification in carcinoma of the lung. *J Comput Assist Tomogr* 1994;18:867–871.

117. Im J-G, Kin WH, Han MC, et al. Sclerosing hemangiomas of the lung and interlobar fissures: CT findings. *J Comput Assist Tomogr* 1994;18:34–38.

118. Naidich DP, McCauley DI, Siegelman SS. Computed tomography of bronchial adenomas. *J Comput Assist Tomogr* 1982;6:725–732.

119. Magid D, Siegelman SS, Eggleston JC. Pulmonary carcinoid tumors: CT assessment. *J Comput Assist Tomogr* 1989;13:244–247.

120. Naidich DP, Garay SM. Radiographic evaluation of focal lung disease. *Clin Chest Med* 1991;12:77–95.

121. Siegelman SS, Khouri NF, Scott WW, et al. Pulmonary hamartoma: CT findings. *Radiology* 1986;160:313–317.

122. Bateson EM. So-called hamartoma of the lung—a true neoplasm of fibrous connective-tissue of the bronchi. *Cancer* 1973;31:1458–1467.

123. Bateson EM. Relationship between intrapulmonary and endobronchial cartilage-containing tumors (so-called hamartomata). *Thorax* 1965;20:447.

124. Hickey PM, Simpson WM. Primary chondroma of the lung. *Acta Radiol* 1926;5:475–500.

125. McDonald JR, Harrington SW, Clagett OT. Hamartoma (often called chondroma) of the lung. *J Thoracic Surg* 1945;14:128–143.

126. Benninghoven CD, Pierce CB. Primary chondroma of the lung. *AJR Am J Roentgenol* 1933;29:805–812.

127. Bateson EM, Abbott EK. Mixed tumors of the lung, or hamarto-chondromas: a review of the radiological appearances of cases published in the literature and a report of fifteen new cases. *Clin Radiol* 1960;11:232–247.

128. Jensen KG, Schiodt T. Growth conditions of hamartoma of the lung. *Thorax* 1958;13:233–237.

129. Ribet ME, Copin M-C, Gosselin BH. Bronchogenic cysts of the lung. *Ann Thorac Surg* 1996;61:1636–1640.

130. Naidich DP, Rumanick WM, Ettenger NA. Congenital anomalies of the lung in adults: MR diagnosis. *AJR Am J Roentgenol* 1988;151:13–19.

131. Weinreb JC, Naidich SP. Thoracic magnetic resonance imaging. *Clin Chest Med* 1991;12:33–54.

132. Chang CHJ, Sibala JL, Lin F, Jewell WR, Templeton AW. Preoperative diagnosis of potentially precancerous breast lesions by computed tomography breast scanner: preliminary study. *Radiology* 1978;129:209–210.

133. Chang CHJ, Nesbit DE, Fisher DR, et al. Computed tomographic mammography using a conventional body scanner. *AJR Am J Roentgenol* 1982;138:553–558.

134. Korobkin M, Brodeur FJ, Francis IR, et al. Delayed enhanced CT for differentiation of benign from malignant adrenal masses. *Radiology* 1996;200:737–742.

135. Littleton JT, Durizch ML, Moeller G, Herbert DE. Pulmonary masses: contrast enhancement. *Radiology* 1990;177:861–871.

136. Swensen SJ, Brown LR, Colby TV, Weaver AL. Pulmonary nodules: CT evaluation of enhancement with iodinated contrast material. *Radiology* 1995;194:393–398.

137. Swensen SJ, Brown LR, Colby TV, Weaver AL, Midthun DE. Lung nodule enhancement at CT: prospective findings. *Radiology* 1996;201:447–455.

138. Yamashita K, Matsunobe S, Takahashi R, et al. Small peripheral lung carcinoma evaluated with incremental dynamic CT: radiologic-pathologic correlation. *New Engl J Med* 1995;196:401–408.

139. Swensen SJ, Viggiano RW, Midthun DE, et al. Lung nodule enhancement at CT: multicenter study. Abstract. *Radiology* 1998 (submitted).

140. Swensen SJ. Lung nodule enhancement at CT—Response. *Radiology* 1997;204:283.

141. Zhang M, Kono M. Solitary pulmonary nodules: evaluation of blood flow patterns with dynamic CT. *Radiology* 1997;205:471–478.

142. Kono M, Adachi S, Kusumoto M, Sakai E. Clinical utility of Gd-DTPA-enhanced magnetic resonance imaging in lung cancer. *J Thorac Imag* 1993;8:1:18–26.

143. Guckel C, Schnabel K, Deimling M, Steinbrich W. Solitary pulmonary nodules: MR evaluation of enhancement patterns with contrast-enhanced dynamic snapshot gradient-echo imaging. *Radiology* 1996;200:681–686.

144. Gambhir SS, Hoh EK, Phelps ME, Madar I, Maddahi J. Decision tree sensitivity analysis for cost-effectiveness of FDG-PET in the staging

and management of non-small-cell lung carcinoma. *J Nucl Med* 1996; 37:1428–1436.

145. Gupta NC, Frank AR, Dewan NA, et al. Solitary pulmonary nodules: detection of malignancy with PET with 2-[F-18]-fluoro-2-deoxy-D-glucose. *Radiology* 1992;184:441–444.

146. Gupta NC, Maloof J, Gunel E. Probability of malignancy in solitary pulmonary nodules using fluorin-18-FDG and PET. *J Nucl Med* 1996; 37:943–948.

147. Cook GJR, Maisey MN. Review. The current status of clinical PET imaging. *Clin Radiol* 1996;51:603–613.

148. Duhaylongsod FG, Lowe VJ, Patz EF, et al. Detection of primary and recurrent lung cancer by means of F-18 fluorodeoxyglucose positron emission tomography (FDG PET). *J Thorac Cardiovas Surg* 1995; 110:130–140.

149. Patz EF, Lowe VJ, Hoffman JM. Focal pulmonary abnormalities; evaluation with F-18 fluorodeoxyglucose PET scanning. *Radiology* 1993;188:487–490.

150. Hubner KF, Buonocore E, Gould HR, et al. Differentiating benign from malignant lung lesions using "quantitative" parameters of FDG PET images. *Clin Nucl Med* 1996;21:941–949.

151. Bury T, Dowlati A, Paulus P, et al. Evaluation of the solitary pulmonary nodule by positron emission tomography imaging. *Eur Resp J* 1996;9:410–414.

152. Sazon DAD, Santiago SM, Soo Hoo GW, et al. Fluorodeoxyglucose-positron emission tomography in the detection and staging of lung cancer. *Am J Respir Crit Care Med* 1996;153:417–421.

153. Patz Jr EF, Lowe VJ, Goodman PC, Herndon J. Thoracic nodal staging with PET imaging with 18FDG in patients with bronchogenic carcinoma. *Chest* 1995;108:1617–1621.

154. Swensen SJ, Jett JR, Payne WS, et al. An integrated approach to evaluation of the solitary pulmonary nodule. *Mayo Clin Proc* 1990; 65:173–186.

155. Ray JF, Lawton BR, Magnin GE, et al. The coin lesion story: update 1976. Twenty years experience with early thoracotomy for 179 suspected malignant coin lesions. *Chest* 1976;70:332–336.

156. Keagy BA, Starek PJ, Murray GF, et al. Major pulmonary resection for suspected but unconfirmed malignancy. *Ann Thorac Surg* 1984; 38:314–316.

157. Scott WW, Kuhlman JE. Focal pulmonary lesions in patients with AIDS: percutaneous transthoracic needle biopsy. *Radiology* 1991; 180:419–421.

158. End A, Helbich T, Wisser W, Dekan G, Klepetko W. The pulmonary nodule after lung transplantation: cause and outcome. *Chest* 1995; 107:1317–1322.

159. Cummings SR, Lillington GA, Richard RJ. Estimating the probability of malignancy in solitary pulmonary nodules: a Bayesian approach. *Am Rev Respir Dis* 1986;134:449–452.

160. Edwards FH, Schaefer PS, Callahan S, Graeber GM, Albus RA. Bayesian statistical theory in the preoperative diagnosis of pulmonary lesions. *Chest* 1987;92:888–891.

161. Edwards FH, Schaefer PS, Cohen AJ, et al. Use of artificial intelligence for the preoperative diagnosis of pulmonary lesions. *Ann Thor Surg* 1989;48:556–559.

162. Dewan NA, Shehan CJ, Reeb SD, et al. Likelihood of malignancy in a solitary pulmonary nodule: comparison of Bayesian analysis and results of FDG-PET scan. *Chest* 1997;112:416–422.

163. Westcott JL. Diagnostic approach to solitary pulmonary nodule. *J Bronchol* 1996;3:316–323.

164. Naidich DP, Sussman R, Kutcher WL, et al. Solitary pulmonary nodules: CT-bronchoscopic correlation. *Chest* 1988;93:595–598.

165. Lai RS, Lee SSJ, Ting YM, Wang HC, Lin CC. Diagnostic value of transbronchial lung biopsy under fluoroscopic guidance in solitary pulmonary nodule in an endemic area of tuberculosis. *Resp Med* 1996; 90:139–143.

166. Wang K-P. Staging of bronchogenic carcinoma by bronchoscopy. *Chest* 1994;106:588–593.

167. Shure D. Transbronchial biopsy and needle aspiration. *Chest* 1989; 95:1130–1138.

168. Westcott JL, Rao N, Colley DP. Transthoracic needle biopsy of small pulmonary nodules. *Radiology* 1997;202:97–103.

169. Klein JS, Salomon G, Stewart EA. Transthoracic needle biopsy with a coaxially placed 20-gauge automated cutting needle: results in 122 patients. *Radiology* 1996;198:715–720.

170. Khouri NF, Stitik FP, Erozan YS, et al. Transthoracic needle aspiration biopsy of benign and malignant lung lesions. *AJR* 1985;144:281–288.

171. Stanley JH, Fish GD, Andiole JG, et al. Lung lesions: cytologic diagnosis by fine-needle biopsy. *Radiology* 1987;162:389–391.

172. Fraser RS. Transthoracic needle aspiration. The benign diagnosis. *Arch Pathol Lab Med* 1991;115:751–761.

173. Calhoun P, Feldman PS, Armstrong P, et al. The clinical outcome of needle aspirations of the lung when cancer is not diagnosed. *Ann Thorac Surg* 1986;41:592–596.

174. Li HQ, Boiselle PM, Shepard JAO, Trotmandickenson B, McLoud TC. Diagnostic accuracy and safety of CT-guided percutaneous needle aspiration biopsy of the lung: comparison of small and large pulmonary nodules. *Am J Roentgenol* 1996;167:105–109.

175. Yankelevitz DF, Henschke CI, Koizumi JH, Altorki NK, Libby D. CT-guided transthoracic needle biopsy of small solitary pulmonary nodules. *Clin Imag* 1997;21:107–110.

176. Moulton JS, Moore PT. Coaxial percutaneous biopsy technique with automated biopsy devices: value in improving accuracy and negative predictive value. *Radiology* 1993;186:515–522.

177. Kazerooni EA, Lim FT, Mikhail A, Martinez FJ. Risk of pneumothorax in CT-guided transthoracic needle aspiration biopsy of the lung. *Radiology* 1996;198:371–375.

178. Bernard A, Azorin J, Bellenot F, et al. Resection of pulmonary nodules using video-assisted thoracic surgery. *Ann Thorac Surg* 1996;61: 202–204.

179. Hazelrigg SR, Nunchuck SK, LoCicero III J. Video Assisted Thoracic Surgery Study Group Data. *Ann Thorac Surg* 1993;56:1039–1044.

180. Kirby TJ, Mack MJ, Landreneau RJ, Rice TW. Initial experience with video-assisted thoracoscopic lobectomy. *Ann Thorac Surg* 1993;56: 1248–1253.

181. Mack MJ, Haellrigg SR, Landreneau RJ, Acuff TE. Thoracoscopy for the diagnosis of the indeterminate solitary pulmonary nodule. *Ann Thorac Surg* 1993;56:825–832.

182. Schwarz CD, Lengliner F, Eckmayr J, et al. VATS (video-assisted throacic surgery) of undefined pulmonary nodules. Preoperative evaluation of videoendoscopic resectability. *Chest* 1994;106:1570–1574.

183. Shah RM, Spirn PW, Salazar AM, et al. Localization of peripheral pulmonary nodules for thoracoscopic excision: value of CT-guided wire placement. *AJR Am J Roentgenol* 1993;161:279–283.

184. Shepard J-AO, Mathisen DJ, Muse VV, Bhalla M, McLoud TC. Needle localization of peripheral lung nodules for video-assisted thoracoscopic surgery. *Chest* 1994;105:1559–1563.

185. Shennib H. Intraoperative localization techniques for pulmonary nodules. *Ann Thorac Surg* 1993;56:745–748.

186. Asamura H, Kondo H, Narike T, et al. Computed tomography-guided coil injection and thoracoscopic pulmonary resection under roentgenographic fluoroscopy. *Ann Thorac Surg* 1994;58:1542–1544.

187. Greenfield AL, Steiner RM, Liu JB, et al. Sonographic guidance for the localization of peripheral pulmonary nodules during thoracoscopy. *Am J Roentgenol* 1997;168:1057–1060.

188. Goldberg-Kahn B, Healy JC, Bishop JW. The cost of diagnosis: a comparison of four different strategies in the workup of solitary radiographic lung lesions. *Chest* 1997;111:870–876.

189. Reeves AP, Zhao B, Yankelevitz DF, Henschke CI. Characterization of three-dimensional shape and size changes of pulmonary nodules over time from helical CT images. *Radiology* 1997;205(P):396.

190. Raab SS, Hornberger J. The effect of a patient's risk taking attitude on the cost effectiveness of testing strategies in the evaluation of pulmonary lesions. *Chest* 1997;111:1583–1590.

191. Berlin NI, Buncher CR, Fonatana RS, Frost JK, Melamed MR. The National Cancer Institute cooperative early lung cancer detection program. Results of the initial screen (prevalence). Early lung cancer detection: Introduction. *Am Rev Resp Dis* 1984;130:545–549.

192. Eddy D. Screening for lung cancer. *Ann Int Med* 1989;111:232–237.

193. Black WC, Welch HG. Screening for disease. *AJR* 1997;168:3–11.

194. Fontana R, Sanderson DR, Woolner LB. Lung cancer screening: the Mayo Program. *J Occup Med* 1986;28:746–750.

195. Strauss GM, Gleason RE, Sugarbaker DJ. Screening for lung cancer—another look; a different view. *Chest* 1997;111:754–768.

196. Kaneko M, Eguchi K, Ohmatsu H, et al. Peripheral lung cancer: screening and detection with low-dose spiral CT versus radiography. *Radiology* 1996;201:798–802.

197. Naidich DP. Helical computed tomography of the thorax. Clinical applications. *Radiol Clin N Am* 1994;32:759–774.

198. Naidich DP. Volumetric CT in the evaluation of focal pulmonary disease. In: Remy-Jardin M, Remy J, eds. *Spiral CT of the chest.* Berlin: Springer-Verlag, 1997:129–151.

199. Costello P, Naidich DP. Protocols for helical CT of the chest. In: Silverman PM, ed. *Helical (spiral) computed tomography. A practical approach to clinical protocols.* Philadelphia: Lippincott–Raven, 1998:65–101.

CHAPTER 5

Lung Cancer

Lung cancer is the leading cause of cancer death in the world. In the United States, 96,000 men and 73,900 women died of this disease in 1995 (1). It currently accounts for 33% of deaths from cancer in males, compared to carcinoma of the prostate, the second most common cause, which accounts for 14%. Lung cancer accounts for 24% of cancer deaths in women in the United States compared to 18% caused by breast carcinoma, now the second most common cause of death from cancer in women (1). The five year survival of lung cancer is only 10% to 15% because most bronchogenic carcinomas are unresectable when first diagnosed. Complete surgical excision of carcinoma remains the most effective form of therapy and offers the patient the only reasonable hope for cure.

Accurate staging is critical in the selection of treatment and in the evaluation of prognosis of patients with bronchogenic carcinoma. The responsibility for accurate staging is shared by the surgeon, pulmonologist, radiologist, and pathologist. A uniform staging system enables every participant in the management of the patient to communicate results unambiguously. Recently, new revisions in the international system for staging lung cancer and regional lymph node classification have been proposed (Tables 5-1 and 5-2) (2–4). Familiarity with these modifications in the current staging system for lung cancer is essential to an understanding of the role of imaging in the assessment of these patients.

Although this is especially true of computed tomography (CT) and magnetic resonance (MR), familiarity with the current staging system for nonsmall cell lung cancer also is of importance in assessing the potential role of positron emission tomography (PET) scanning in assessing lung cancer. Presently, CT remains the main imaging modality used for the intrathoracic staging of lung cancer, with magnetic resonance imaging (MRI) and PET scanning ancillary techniques which complement CT in a relatively small but important percentage of cases (4). As will be discussed, this is likely to change.

The staging system devised for lung cancer has evolved over the years, following the establishment of the American Joint Committee on Cancer and End Results Reporting (AJCC) in 1959. In 1970, the task force on lung cancer of the AJCC adopted the T, N, M system originally proposed by Pierre Denoix (5). The initial classification scheme was published in 1973 and a modified version appeared in 1979 (6,7). At the World Conference on Lung Cancer in 1985, a new uniform international staging system was adopted (8). This system, based largely on the prior AJCC formulation, has successively been modified to reflect changes in the therapeutic approach to lung cancer. The present International Staging System again has two major components: anatomic extent of disease (TNM) and cell type (2,3). Lung cancer stage is determined by the extent of the primary tumor (T),

TABLE 5-1. Definition of primary tumor, nodal involvement, and distal metastases (TNM) characteristics in lung cancer

Primary tumor (T)

TX	Primary tumor cannot be assessed, or tumor proven by the presence of malignant cells in sputum or bronchial washings but not visualized by imaging or bronchoscopy
T0	No evidence of primary tumor
Tis	Carcinoma *in situ*
T1	Tumor ≤ 3 cm in greatest dimension, surrounded by lung or visceral pleura, without bronchoscopic evidence of invasion more proximal than the lobar bronchus[a] (i.e., not in the main bronchus)
T2	Tumor with any of the following features of size or extent: >3 cm in greatest dimension Involves main bronchus, ≥ 2 cm distal to the carina Invades the visceral pleura Associated with atelectasis or obstructive pneumonitis that extends to the hilar region but does not involve the entire lung
T3	Tumor of any size that directly invades any of the following: chest wall (including superior sulcus tumors), diaphragm, mediastinal pleura, parietal pericardium; or tumor in the main bronchus <2 cm distal to the carina, but without involvement of the carina; or associated atelectasis or obstructive pneumonitis of the entire lung
T4	Tumor of any size that invades any of the following: mediastinum, heart, great vessels, trachea, esophagus, vertebral body, carina; or tumor with a malignant pleural or pericardial effusion,[b] or with satellite tumor nodule(s) within the ipsilateral primary-tumor lobe of the lung

Regional lymph nodes (N)

NX	Regional lymph nodes cannot be assessed
N0	No regional lymph node metastasis
N1	Metastasis to ipsilateral peribronchial and/or ipsilateral hilar lymph nodes, and intrapulmonary nodes involved by direct extension of the primary tumor
N2	Metastasis to ipsilateral mediastinal and/or subcarinal lymph node(s)
N3	Metastasis to contralateral mediastinal, contralateral hilar, ipsilateral or contralateral scalene, or supraclavicular lymph node(s)

Distant metastasis (M)

MX	Presence of distant metastasis cannot be assessed
M0	No distant metastasis
M1	Distant metastasis present[c]

[a] The uncommon superficial tumor of any size with its invasive component limited to the bronchial wall, which may extend proximal to the main bronchus, is also classified T1.

[b] Most pleural effusions associated with lung cancer are due to tumor. However, there are a few patients in whom multiple cytopathologic examinations of pleural fluid show no tumor. In these cases, the fluid is nonbloody and is not an exudate. When these elements and clinical judgment dictate that the effusion is not related to the tumor, the effusion should be excluded as a staging element and the patient's disease should be staged T1, T2, or T3. Pericardial effusion is classified according to the same rules.

[c] Separate metastatic tumor nodule(s) in the ipsilateral nonprimary-tumor lobe(s) of the lung also are classified M1.

From ref. 2, with permission.

TABLE 5-2. New international revised stage grouping

Classification stages	TNM classification
Stage 0	TIS
Stage IA	T1, N0, M0
Stage IB	T2, N0, M0
Stage IIA	T1, N1, M0
Stage IIB	T2, N1, M0; T3, N0, M0
Stage IIIA	T1-3, N2, M0; T3, N1, M0
Stage IIIB	T4, any N, M0; any T, N3, M0
Stage IV	any T, any N, M1

TIS, tumor *in situ*; T, tumor; N, node; M, metastasis.
From ref. 2, with permission.

presence of intrapulmonary, hilar, or mediastinal lymph node metastases (N) and presence of extrathoracic metastases (M). Small cell carcinoma is still staged as either limited or extensive disease, and consequently will be considered separately (9).

STAGING OF THE PRIMARY TUMOR EXTENT

T is the descriptor given to the primary tumor and its local extent. The precise definitions are given in Table 5-1. As pertains to radiologic interpretation, T staging is subdivided in four groups: T1 to T4. T1 lung cancer is a tumor that is 3 cm or less in greatest dimension, is surrounded by lung or visceral pleura, and has no evidence of invasion proximal to a lobar bronchus at bronchoscopy. Patients with surgical-pathological T1 (pT1) lesions without associated lymph node involvement have a 5 year survival of between 65 to 80% following lobectomy (2,3,10). These lesions are usually treated by lobectomy because of the increased local recurrence rate and decreased 5 year survival in patients following segmentectomy or wedge resection (10). Wedge resection is therefore only recommended for patients with limited cardiopulmonary reserve.

T2 lung cancer is a tumor more than 3.0 cm in greatest diameter, or a tumor of any size that invades the visceral pleura or has associated atelectasis or obstructive pneumonitis extending to the hilar region. Patients with pT2 lesions without associated nodal involvement have a 5 year survival of approximately 65% following lobectomy (2,3,10). In distinction, patients with pT2 lesions associated with nodal disease have a 5 year survival of approximately 40%.

Although T1 and T2 lesions have different prognoses, in clinical practice distinction between these tumors is usually not necessary because they are treated in a similar fashion. Of considerable importance, however, is the recognition of T3 lesions and their distinction from T4 tumors. This is because T3 lesions have extended beyond the lung but are potentially resectable and T4 lesions are, by definition, unresectable. A T3 cancer is defined as a tumor of any size with direct extension into the chest wall (including superior sulcus tumors), diaphragm, or the mediastinal pleura or pericardium without involving the heart, great vessels, trachea, esophagus, or vertebral body, or a tumor in the main bronchus within 2 cm of the tracheal carina without involvement of the carina (see Table 5-1). This may be associated with either atelectasis or obstructive pneumonitis involving the entire lung. Patients with T3 lung lesions without associated nodal involvement have a 5 year survival ranging from 30% to 50% following complete resection (10–16). Many of the patients receive adjuvant radiotherapy.

Direct invasion of the pleura and chest wall by a peripheral bronchogenic carcinoma is potentially resectable (T3) provided vertebral bodies and major structures such as the brachial plexus are not involved (8). Surgery consists of lobectomy, bilobectomy or pneumonectomy usually with extrapleural resection if the tumor is limited to the parietal pleura and full-thickness chest wall resection when the tumor is invading the ribs or the chest wall muscles (10). Preoperative radiation is usually used in patients who have superior sulcus tumors with chest wall invasion (10).

The only CT findings that allow a reliable diagnosis of chest wall invasion are presence of rib destruction (17) or an obvious chest wall mass (18). These findings, however, have a low sensitivity being present in only 20% to 40% of patients with surgically proven chest wall invasion (19,20). A number of other CT findings have also been assessed but are considerably less accurate. Glazer et al., in a study of 47 patients with peripheral tumors contacting the chest wall or pleural surface, found that the presence of an obtuse angle between the mass and pleura, pleural contact over a distance greater than 3 cm, and associated pleural thickening yielded a sensitivity of 87% for chest wall invasion with a specificity of only 59%, and a diagnostic accuracy of 68% (21). In this study, the presence of focal chest pain, although not as sensitive as CT, was more specific (94%) and accurate (85%) in making the diagnosis of chest wall invasion (21). Thus, tumors abutting the pleura, even when associated with local pleural thickening, may not be invasive (19–21).

Two preliminary studies have suggested that the accuracy of CT in the detection of parietal pleural and chest wall invasion can be improved by assessing tumoral movement along the chest wall during expiration (22,23). In the first, Shirrakawa et al. used spiral CT performed during deep inspiration and at end-expiration to evaluate 17 patients with peripheral lung cancers in contact with the chest wall (22). Six of 10 lesions in the middle and lower lobes showed considerable respiratory phase shift; all were proved at surgery not to have invaded the parietal pleura. Three lesions showed no respiratory phase shift and had parietal pleural invasion at surgery. The remaining lesion showed no respiratory phase shift and no invasion at surgery. In this case, benign pleural adhesion caused by previous pleuritis was identified at surgery (22). CT findings for tumors in the upper lobe did not correlate with the surgical findings. In a second study, Murata et al. evaluated the use of multisection dynamic expiratory CT scans obtained during a single expiratory maneuver evaluated in cine mode to assess tumoral movement along the chest wall or mediastinum (23). Free movement of tumor along the peripheral or mediastinal pleura was shown on dynamic CT in 10 patients, whereas in five patients dynamic CT showed the tumors to be fixed to the chest wall or mediastinum: In all 15 cases the findings on multisection expiratory dynamic CT were proved to be correct at surgery. Although these results are preliminary, they are encouraging and therefore it is recommended that spiral CT scans at end-expiration be obtained in patients with questionable chest wall invasion on inspiratory scans. Although it has been shown that the use of induced pneumothorax results in a sensitivity of 100% in the detection of chest wall and mediastinal pleural invasion on CT with specificities ranging from 57% to 80% (24,25), this technique has not gained widespread acceptance and is unlikely to ever be used in routine clinical practice.

With the advent of bronchial reconstruction procedures, select patients whose tumors are within 2 cm of the tracheal carina (T3) can undergo curative resection (26,27). Determination of the proximity of lesions to the carina, however, may be problematic (Fig. 5-1). Bronchoplastic procedures are relatively safe, with a mortality of 2% to 9% (10). The tumor may be resectable with "sleeve lobectomy" rather than pneumonectomy, thus conserving the lung and providing improved quality of survival (10).

Mediastinal invasion which may be technically resectable (T3) includes limited invasion of the pericardium, mediastinal pleura or fat, and vagus and phrenic nerves (8,28). A lesion that abuts or makes only limited contact with the mediastinum, even if adjacent to areas of pleural or pericardial thickening, cannot confidently be diagnosed as being invasive because associated desmoplastic reaction and inflammation can simulate tumor extension into an adjacent structure (19,29) (Fig. 5-2). Likewise, microscopic invasion may be completely missed. The low reliability of CT in this context has been documented by several authors (28–30).

Glazer et al. have described three criteria that help identify patients with indeterminate mediastinal or pleural invasion whose lesions are likely to be technically resectable (28). These criteria include: (a) less than 3 cm of contact between the tumor and the adjacent mediastinum; (b) less than 90 degrees circumferential contact between the tumor and the aorta; and the presence of mediastinal fat between the mass and adjacent mediastinal structures. In their study, 36 out of 37 masses with one or more of these CT findings were technically resectable (28).

T4 lung cancer is a tumor of any size with invasion of the mediastinum or involving heart, great vessels, trachea, esophagus, vertebral body or tracheal carina or associated with malignant pleural effusion (Fig. 5-3). As recently modified, T4 also now includes evidence of satellite tumor nodule(s) within the ipsilateral primary-tumor lobe of the lung (Fig. 5-4). Patients with T4 tumors are considered to have surgically unresectable disease and have a five year survival of less than 10% (2,3,8).

The most important role of the radiologist in T staging is

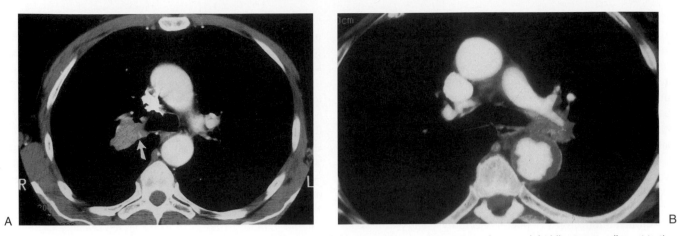

FIG. 5-1. Endobronchial (T3) disease. **A:** Section through the carina following contrast enhancement shows a right hilar tumor adjacent to the lateral wall of the right main-stem bronchus (*arrow*) consistent with a T3 lesion. **B:** CT section in different patient than **A** shows a left hilar mass encasing the left main pulmonary artery, adjacent to the left main bronchus. In these two cases, identification of tumor near the carina is of limited value in predicting resectability, partially because of the oblique course of the proximal right and left main bronchi, partly because CT is of limited value in predicting submucosal extension of disease especially compared with fiberoptic bronchoscopy. Although surgical resection was successfully performed in the patient illustrated in **A**, in the second case, surgical resection was not considered because of encasement of the left pulmonary artery.

to assess whether a T4 classification is warranted on the basis of unequivocal CT findings. Indeed, CT staging should support curative surgery in potentially resectable tumors. CT can reliably determine the presence of mediastinal soft-tissue invasion or involvement of major mediastinal structures, such as the heart, great vessels, trachea, esophagus, and vertebral bodies. However, definite involvement should only be considered if clear-cut destruction and interdigitation of the tumor with the given structure is demonstrated. A CT diagnosis of T4 status applies to the following situations:

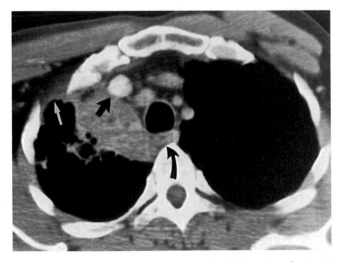

FIG. 5-2. Stage 3A disease: mediastinal pleural invasion. Contrast-enhanced CT scan shows a tumor (T3) in the right upper lobe that abuts the entire length of the mediastinum. Note that mediastinal fat planes are well preserved except anteriorly adjacent to the lateral aspect of the superior vena cava (*black arrow*), and posteriorly in the region of the posterior wall of the trachea (*curved arrow*). This appearance is nonspecific, as is evidence of subtle pleural thickening along the anterolateral pleural surface (*white arrow*). At surgery there was no evidence of mediastinal invasion.

1. Tumors involving the trachea or narrowing the carina, usually involving both sides of the carina (Fig. 5-5).
2. Tumors surrounding, encasing, or abutting for more than 180 degrees the superior vena cava, the aorta, main pulmonary artery, right or left pulmonary artery beyond the mediastinal pleural reflection, or a major branch of any vessel within the mediastinal fat (see Figs. 5-1B and 5-3).
3. Erosion of a vertebral body (Fig. 5-6) or involvement of the brachial plexus (Fig. 5-7).
4. Pleural masses or pleural effusion (Fig. 5-8). A pleural effusion generally predicts a poor prognosis for patients with lung cancer, justifying a T4 classification. However, the possibility that a pleural effusion is only reactive (as may occur in patients with obstructive atelectasis, underlying pneumonia, or possible obstruction of the lymphatics) requires that the malignant nature of any effusion be proven before considering a patient unresectable. In particular, otherwise unsuspected small pleural effusions may be seen on thoracic CT; these should not be considered prima facie evidence of unresectability until malignant cells have been documented within the effusion.

The interpretation of a CT examination in patients with T4 lesions is generally not difficult. Often, multiple findings that would indicate a T4 status co-exist. Tumors surrounding blood vessels also implicate the soft tissues of the mediastinum. Patients with T4 lesions are also more apt to demonstrate advanced nodal disease, as well as distant metastases. It cannot be overemphasized, however, that when interpreting CT scans for staging, difficulties may be encountered if findings prove less than unequivocal. This is especially true in anatomic areas where partial volume effects may blur boundaries, such as superior sulcus tumors or central masses, including medially located lower lobe masses. In select cases, many of these difficulties may be obviated by the use

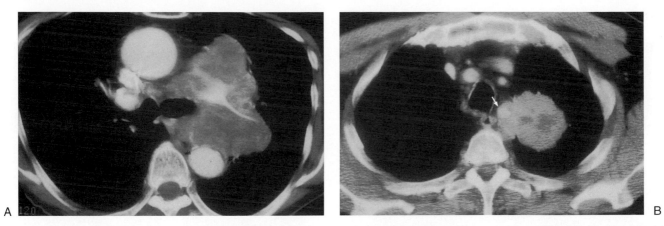

FIG. 5-3. T4 disease. **A:** CT section at the level of the carina shows extensive tumor infiltration with encasement of the entire length of the left pulmonary artery as well as the entire left main bronchus (compare with Fig. 5-1B). These findings are reliable signs of unresectability. **B:** CT section in a different patient than in **A**, shows a focal tumor mass in the left upper lobe that is invading the mediastinum with resultant encasement of the left subclavian artery (*arrow*).

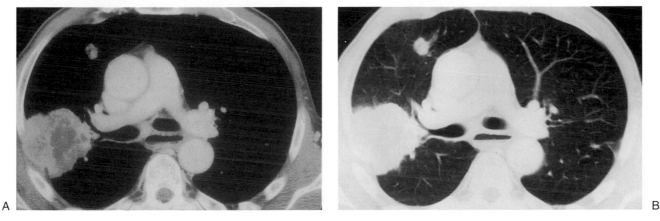

FIG. 5-4. T4 disease. **A,B:** CT sections through the right upper lobe, imaged with lung and mediastinal windows, respectively, show a necrotic tumor extending from the hilum to the chest wall. Although this appearance is consistent with a T3 lesion, an additional lesion in the same lobe makes this technically a T4 lesion and hence unresectable (see Table 5-1).

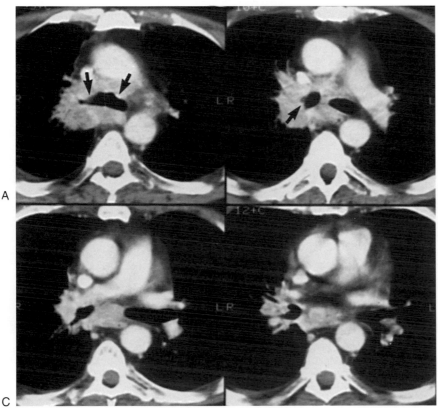

FIG. 5-5. Stage 3B disease: mediastinal invasion. **A–D:** Enlargements of contrast-enhanced CT sections through the mediastinum show the presence of extensive tumor (T4) encasing the carina and main-stem bronchi, associated with enlarged subcarinal lymph nodes. Note that the contours of both main-stem bronchi are nodular, indicating invasion and fixation of the central airways (*arrows* in **A** and **B**).

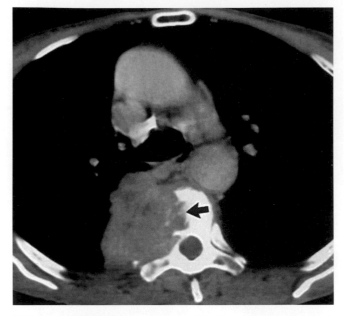

FIG. 5-6. Stage 3B disease: invasion of the thoracic spine. Contrast-enhanced CT section shows a large tumor (T4) in the right lower lobe directly invading the adjacent vertebral body (*arrow*).

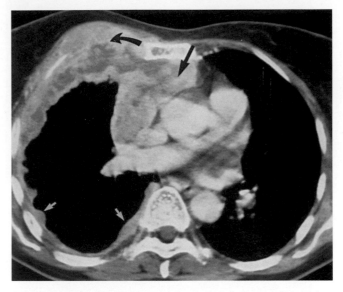

FIG. 5-8. Stage 3B disease: mediastinal and chest wall invasion. Contrast-enhanced CT section at the level of the right main pulmonary artery shows extensive tumor (T4) infiltrating the mediastinum (*black arrow*) as well as the chest wall (*curved arrow*). Note that the pleura circumferentially on the right side is thickened, nodular, and irregular caused by extensive infiltration by tumor (*white arrows*).

of thin-section CT scans to define better the relationship of the tumor to the surrounding structures. Contrast enhancement is also critical in all cases where the relationship of major vessels to tumor is questioned (Fig. 5-9). Although difficulties may be encountered when tumors are associated with pneumonitis or obstructive atelectasis, caused by blurring of the boundaries between the tumor and surrounding inflamed parenchyma, contrast-enhanced studies often can resolve the uncertainty (see Fig. 5-9 and Fig. 5-10).

The diagnosis of T4 status is perhaps the most valuable contribution of CT to the management of patients with advanced lung cancers. This contribution has not been stressed

in the literature because such patients rarely undergo surgery. However, it is one of the main reasons stated by surgeons to justify the use of CT in lung cancer staging (31). In a study of 275 patients with bronchogenic carcinoma by Primack et al., CT scans demonstrated surgically unresectable tumors (T4) in 34 patients (12%) caused by extensive mediastinal invasion, destruction of a vertebral body, or findings suggestive of malignant pleural involvement that was confirmed by thoracentesis or pleural biopsy (32). Similarly, in a prospective cooperative trial involving 250 patients, only two patients underwent a thoracotomy and were found to harbor T4 disease undetected by CT (30). CT therefore

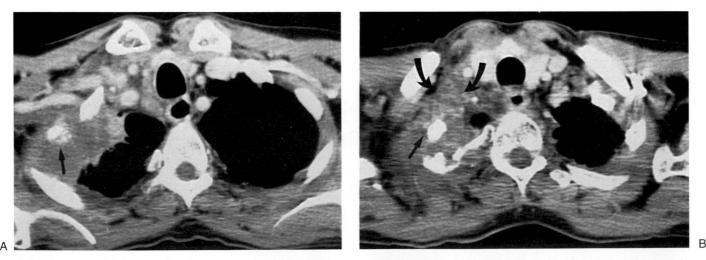

FIG. 5-7. Stage 3B disease: invasion of the chest wall and brachial plexus. **A,B:** Sequential contrast-enhanced CT scans through the thoracic inlet. An irregular, heterogeneous low-density mass is present in the right upper lobe, clearly invading the chest wall associated with lytic destruction of the first three ribs (*arrows* in **A** and **B**). Note that superiorly the tumor (T4) has extended into the base of the neck where it has obliterated all normal landmarks (*curved arrows* in **B**). Clinically this patient had evidence of brachial plexus involvement.

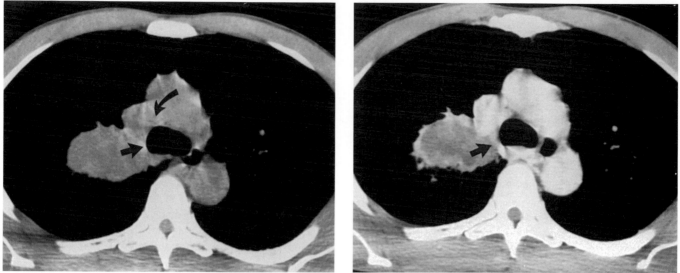

FIG. 5-9. The role of contrast enhancement in CT staging. **A,B:** CT sections through the carina, obtained pre and postadministration of intravenous contrast media, respectively. Note that without contrast enhancement, the tumor appears to abut the lateral wall of the right main-stem bronchus (*arrow* in **A**); furthermore, delineation of mediastinal facial planes is limited and adenopathy cannot be excluded (*curved arrow* in **A**). Following contrast enhancement, the tumor clearly lies lateral to the azygos vein (*arrow* in **B**). No mediastinal adenopathy is identified. Surgery documented T2N1 disease.

appears to be an effective method for preventing unnecessary thoracotomies in unequivocal T4 disease.

It is clear that in many patients with bronchogenic carcinoma, CT allows accurate distinction of potentially resectable T1-T3 lesions from unresectable T4 tumors. Unfortunately in some cases the presence of mediastinal invasion and the distinction of resectable from unresectable tumors cannot be reliably made based on the CT findings. This is particularly the case when there is extensive contact between the tumor and the mediastinum with loss of the fat plane between the tumor and mediastinal structures or evidence of mass effect on the mediastinal structures but no obvious encasement (33). These findings are not reliable in the diagnosis of mediastinal invasion or unresectability. Herman et al. assessed the diagnostic accuracy of CT in the assessment of direct mediastinal invasion in 90 patients who underwent

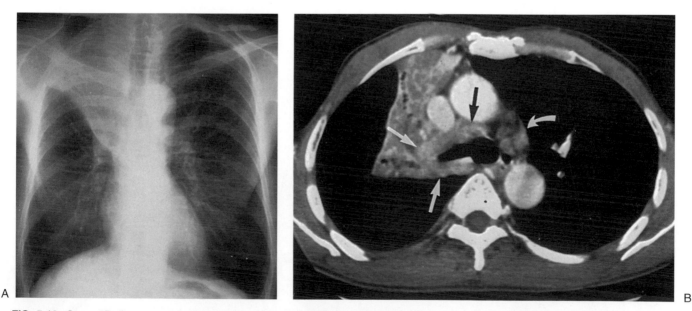

FIG. 5-10. Stage 3B disease: encasement of the carina; contralateral mediastinal adenopathy. **A:** Posteroanterior radiograph shows classic appearance of right upper lobe atelectasis, limiting evaluation of the hilum and mediastinum. There is no radiographic evidence to suggest this lesion is unresectable. **B:** Contrast-enhanced CT section through the carina shows classic CT appearance of right upper lobe atelectasis. In addition to evidence of tumor (T4) encasing the right main-stem bronchus (*straight arrows*), there are enlarged contralateral mediastinal lymph nodes easily identified within the aorticopulmonary window (*curved arrow*). Involvement of the carina and right main-stem bronchus was confirmed bronchoscopically.

CT and thoracotomy (33). A total of 785 mediastinal structures (25 with tumor invasion) were analyzed. Only 11 of 17 mediastinal structures distorted by adjacent tumor (65%) and five of seven structures with apparent intraluminal tumor on CT (71%) were shown to be involved at thoracotomy (T4). Greater than 90 degrees contact of tumor with a mediastinal structure had a sensitivity of 40% (10 of 25 structures), and a specificity of 99% (752 of 760 structures) in the detection of mediastinal tumor invasion. All seven structures with more than 180 degrees of contact with the tumor were involved (specificity 100%), but the sensitivity was only 28%. Although the authors concluded that CT is insensitive in the detection of mediastinal invasion by bronchogenic carcinoma, this conclusion is unwarranted because they excluded from the study 48 patients who had clearly unresectable disease because of advanced local extension (T4 lesions) or presence of extrathoracic disease as well as 60 patients with positive mediastinoscopy.

White et al. assessed the ability of CT in distinguishing the various T stages in 97 patients who underwent thoracotomy for resection of lung cancer (34). CT findings interpreted as indicating resectable mediastinal invasion (T3) included focal involvement of fat or pericardium with no evidence of involvement of heart, great vessels, trachea, or esophagus. Findings interpreted as indicating unresectable disease (T4) included the presence of infiltration of mediastinal fat planes or encasement of mediastinal structures. Of 82 cases considered to have T1 or T2 tumors on CT, 93% had no mediastinal invasion at thoracotomy, 2% had resectable T3 lesions, and 5% had unresectable T4 tumors. Of 13 patients considered to have potentially resectable T3 tumors, 54% had no mediastinal invasion (T1, T2), 2% had T3 tumors, and 2% had unresectable T4 tumors. The study only included two patients with CT findings suggesting unresectable T4 tumors, presumably because the study included only patients "undergoing thoracotomy for intended resection" and therefore presumably excluded patients with obviously unresectable disease. Another major limitation of this study is that only 50% of patients received intravenous contrast. We believe that the use of intravenous contrast is essential for the assessment of mediastinal invasion by lung cancer. The authors concluded correctly that "patients should not be denied the opportunity for curative surgery on the basis of equivocal CT findings."

NODAL STAGING

The descriptor *N* refers to the presence or absence of regional lymph node metastases (Fig. 5-11). The definitions used in the new international system are listed in Table 5-3 and include anatomic landmarks for 14 hilar, intrapulmonary, and mediastinal lymph node stations. It should be emphasized that although prognosis is affected by the number and size of involved nodes, as well as the levels of involve-

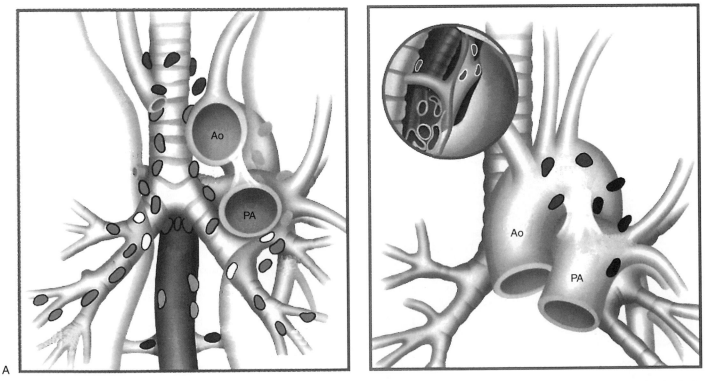

FIG. 5-11. A,B: Regional nodal stations for lung cancer staging. Superior mediastinal nodes: *1*, highest mediastinal; *2*, upper paratracheal; *3*, prevascular and retrotracheal; *4*, lower paratracheal. Aortic nodes: *5*, subaortic (A–P window); *6*, paraaortic (ascending aorta or phrenic). Inferior mediastinal nodes: *7*, subcarinal; *8*, paraesophogeal (below carina); *9*, pulmonary ligament. N¹ nodes: *10*, hilar; *11*, interlobar; *12*, lobar; *13*, segmental; *14*, subsegmental. *PA*, pumonary artery; *Ao*, aorta.

TABLE 5-3. *Lymph node map definitions*

Nodal station	Anatomic landmarks
N2 nodes—All N2 nodes lie within the mediastinal pleural envelope	
1 Highest mediastinal nodes	Nodes lying above a horizontal line at the upper rim of the brachiocephalic (left innominate) vein where it ascends to the left, crossing in front of the trachea at its midline
2 Upper paratracheal nodes	Nodes lying above a horizontal line drawn tangential to the upper margin of the aortic arch and below the inferior boundary of No. 1 nodes
3 Prevascular and retrotracheal nodes	Prevascular and retrotracheal nodes may be designated 3A and 3P; midline nodes are considered to be ipsilateral
4 Lower paratracheal nodes	The lower paratracheal nodes on the right lie to the right of the midline of the trachea between a horizontal line drawn tangential to the upper margin of the aortic arch and a line extending across the right main bronchus at the upper margin of the upper lobe bronchus, and contained within the mediastinal pleural envelope; the lower paratracheal nodes on the left lie to the left of the midline of the trachea between a horizontal line drawn tangential to the upper margin of the aortic arch and a line extending across the left main bronchus at the level of the upper margin of the left upper lobe bronchus, medial to the ligamentum arteriosum and contained within the mediastinal pleural envelope
	Researchers may wish to designate the lower paratracheal nodes as No. 4s (superior) and No. 4i (inferior) subsets for study purposes; the No. 4s nodes may be defined by a horizontal line extending across the trachea and drawn tangential to the cephalic border of the azygos vein; the No. 4i nodes may be defined by the lower boundary of No. 4s and the lower boundary of No. 4, as described above.
5 Subaortic (aorto-pulmonary window)	Subaortic nodes are lateral to the ligamentum arteriosum or the aorta or left pulmonary artery and proximal to the first branch of the left pulmonary artery and lie within the mediastinal pleural envelope
6 Para-aortic nodes (ascending aorta or phrenic)	Nodes lying anterior and lateral to the ascending aorta and the aortic arch or the innominate artery, beneath a line tangential to the upper margin of the aortic arch
7 Subcarinal nodes	Nodes lying caudal to the carina of the trachea, but not associated with the lower lobe bronchi or arteries within the lung
8 Paraesophageal nodes (below carina)	Nodes lying adjacent to the wall of the esophagus and to the right or left of the midline, excluding subcarinal nodes
9 Pulmonary ligament nodes	Nodes lying within the pulmonary ligament, including those in the posterior wall and lower part of the inferior pulmonary vein
N1 nodes—All N1 nodes lie distal to the mediastinal pleural reflection and within the visceral pleura	
10 Hilar nodes	The proximal lobar nodes, distal to the mediastinal pleural reflection and the nodes adjacent to the bronchus intermedius on the right; radiographically, the hilar shadow may be created by enlargement of both hilar and interlobar nodes
11 Interlobar nodes	Nodes lying between the lobar bronchi
12 Lobar nodes	Nodes adjacent to the distal lobar bronchi
13 Segmental nodes	Nodes adjacent to the segmental bronchi
14 Subsegmental nodes	Nodes around the subsegmental bronchi

From ref. 3, with permission.

ment, and intracapsular versus extracapsular, or microscopic versus macroscopic nodal disease, these characteristics are not considered in the current TNM staging system.

N0 indicates no demonstrable metastases to regional lymph nodes. Only 10% to 15% of patients have N0 status at diagnosis. N1 status is characterized by direct tumor extension or metastases to ipsilateral peribronchial or hilar nodes. These nodes are all within the lung and are completely covered by pleura. Although the presence of N1 disease adversely affects prognosis, it usually does not affect resectability. However, N1 status may necessitate a pneumonec-

tomy (rather than a lobectomy) for total removal of disease (Fig. 5-12).

N2 status refers to the presence of metastases to ipsilateral mediastinal lymph nodes and subcarinal lymph nodes. Several studies have shown that complete resection of the primary tumor and ipsilateral mediastinal lymph nodes, with or without adjuvant radiotherapy, results in improved prognosis (Fig. 5-13) (12,35,36). Five-year survival rates ranging from 14% to 42% have been reported. The best prognosis appears to be in the group of patients in whom only low ipsilateral lymph nodes are involved and in patients with

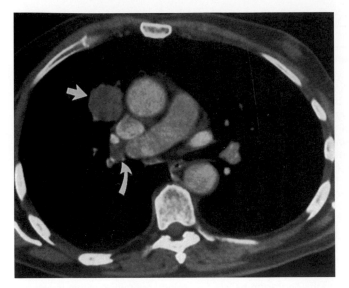

FIG. 5-12. Stage 2 disease: ipsilateral hilar adenopathy. Contrast-enhanced CT scan shows a well-defined right upper lobe mass abutting the mediastinum without evidence of invasion (*arrow*), associated with enlarged right hilar (11R) node (N1) (*curved arrow*).

squamous cell carcinoma. Other authors do not find a significant dependence on cell type (37,38). The extent of nodal involvement by tumor has an impact on prognosis. Patients with a single involved N2 node have a five-year survival of approximately 40% compared to a 20% five-year survival for patients with multiple nodal involvement (39). It should be noted that in the majority of studies only 10% to 20% of patients with N2 disease discovered by routine surgical exploration have completely resectable lung cancer (10,40,41). The prognosis and chance of complete surgical resection are better when N2 nodes are detected only at thoracotomy after a negative mediastinoscopy than when metastases to mediastinal lymph nodes are identified at mediastinoscopy (40). Pearson has shown that among patients in whom N2 disease was identified at mediastinoscopy, the five-year survival following surgery was 9%, whereas patients with N2 disease discovered at thoracotomy following a negative mediastinoscopy had a five-year survival rate of 24% (40).

The prognosis of N2 nodes is considerably worsened when there is permeation of the node and extension through the capsule. Capsular penetration appears to be an indication that the tumor has spread to other nodes or entered the systemic circulation. In one study, the five year survival following resection was 43% in 35 patients with entirely intranodal

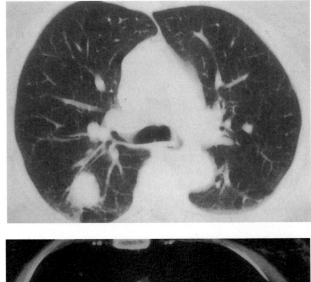

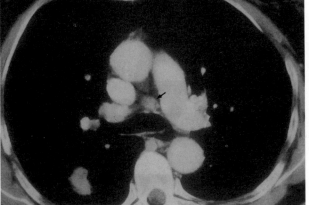

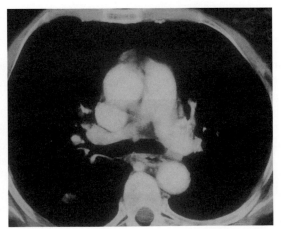

FIG. 5-13. N2 disease: role of neoadjuvant chemotherapy. **A,B:** CT section through the right upper lobe imaged with lung and mediastinal windows, respectively, shows an irregular mass less than 3 cm in size (T2) in the right upper lobe with an enlarged lower paratracheal node (*arrow* in **B**). Although this is slightly to the left of midline, this was still interpreted as N2 disease. **C:** Follow-up CT section at approximately the same level as **A** and **B**, three months later following neoadjuvant chemotherapy shows complete regression of nodal enlargement and marked decrease in size of the primary tumor. This patient subsequently underwent successful resection.

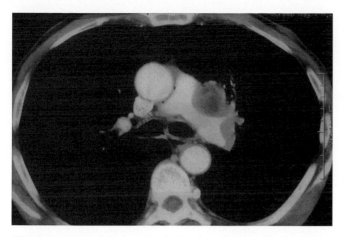

FIG. 5-14. N2 disease: low-density lymph nodes. Section through the carina shows markedly enlarged low density left hilar and subaortic (aortopulmonary window) nodes causing marked compression of the adjacent left main pulmonary artery. In our experience, necrotic nodes carry a worse prognosis.

cancer as opposed to 4.3% survival in 47 patients with malignancy extending through the capsule (42). Other investigators have cited similar statistics (43). The size of the involved nodes seems to have no impact on survival as long as the nodes are encapsulated and completely removed (39). Although less well established, in our experience the prognosis is also worse in patients with necrotic or low-density lymph nodes (Fig. 5-14).

As recently defined, the N2 category includes all patients with ipsilateral mediastinal lymph node or subcarinal lymph node involvement (Fig. 5-15). In particular, subcarinal nodes remain, by definition, N2 despite the fact that in a few series,

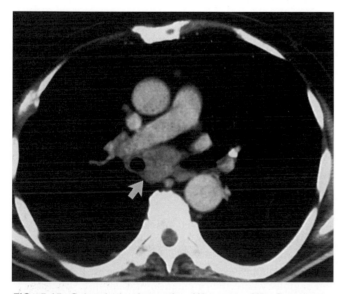

FIG. 5-15. Subcarinal adenopathy: N2 versus N3. Contrast-enhanced CT scan shows extensive subcarinal adenopathy (*arrow*). Although technically not considered evidence of contralateral disease (see Table 5-2), the significance of subcarinal adenopathy in staging lung cancer is controversial.

when careful nodal analysis was undertaken, metastases to the subcarinal lymph nodes carried a poor prognosis (36,38,44). There is also some disagreement about the significance of uppermost ipsilateral mediastinal lymph node involvement, which is listed as a contraindication for surgical resection by some authors (40,45) but not by others (38).

Although some residual controversy surrounds the interpretation of N2 disease, there is general agreement that N3 status implies nonresectability. It should be emphasized that in select cases, N3 status may be conferred as the result of clinical sequelae, as in patients with signs of recurrent laryngeal nerve involvement. It should also be noted that in the current staging system, both ipsilateral and contralateral supraclavicular and scalene nodes are included as "regional" nodes because radiotherapists can include them in the radiation therapy portal. Consequently, metastases to the scalene and supraclavicular nodes are classified as N3.

The significance of mediastinal nodal disease is being actively reassessed. With the changing surgical attitude toward the management of mediastinal nodes, interpretation of nodal staging by CT requires adaptability to the predominant philosophy at a given institution (46). The current system for interpreting nodal disease is based on the concept that thoracic nodes are better defined if their relationship to fixed anatomic structures (such as the azygos vein, bronchi, or aortic arch) can be described (see Table 5-3 and Fig. 5-11). Such anatomic structures are easily recognizable at surgery, mediastinoscopy, and for the most part on CT scans. A major goal of the American Thoracic Society (ATS) system is to improve the separation of so-called hilar (N1) nodes, designated by double digits, from mediastinal (N2) nodes, designated by a single digit. The AJCC definition for N1 nodes includes all nodes within the pleural reflection at surgery. This definition is somewhat arbitrary since the visceral pleura cannot always be visualized and some nodes may be partially covered by visceral pleura even though they are anatomically within the hilum. In this regard, separation between these groups with current imaging methods—both CT and MR—may be problematic, especially, in our experience, between 4R (lower paratracheal) and 10R (right hilar) nodes. To facilitate interpretation, it has been proposed that nodes lying between the cephalic border of the azygos vein and a line extending across the right main bronchus at the upper margin of the right upper lobe bronchus are designated 4i (for inferior) and should be interpreted as lying within the mediastinal pleural envelope (3).

Critical for interpretation of CT studies in patients being assessed for lung cancer staging is familiarity with the accessibility of nodes via both mediastinoscopy as well as transbronchial needle aspiration and biopsy (TBNA) (47). After polling thoracic surgeons at major university hospitals, it has been determined that the mediastinoscopist should be able to characterize nodes in the upper paratracheal (2R, 2L), lower paratracheal (4R, 4L), right tracheobronchial (10R), left peribronchial (10L), and subcarinal (7) nodal stations. Aortopulmonary window and anterior mediastinal nodes

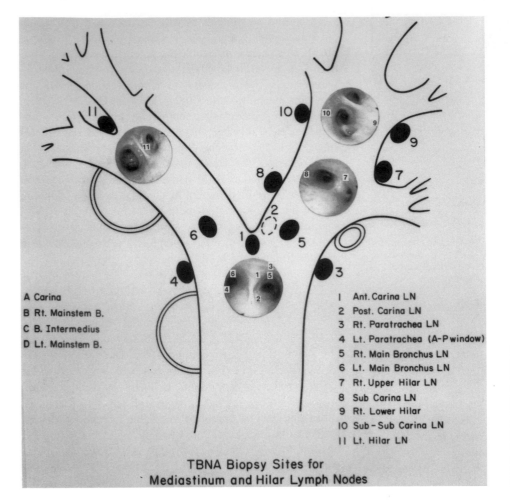

A Carina
B Rt. Mainstem B.
C B. Intermedius
D Lt. Mainstem B.

I   Ant. Carina LN
2   Post. Carina LN
3   Rt. Paratrachea LN
4   Lt. Paratrachea (A-P window)
5   Rt. Main Bronchus LN
6   Lt. Main Bronchus LN
7   Rt. Upper Hilar LN
8   Sub Carina LN
9   Rt. Lower Hilar
10 Sub-Sub Carina LN
11 Lt. Hilar LN

TBNA Biopsy Sites for
Mediastinum and Hilar Lymph Nodes

FIG. 5-16. Endobronchial map of transbronchial needle aspiration biopsy sites for mediastinal and hilar lymph nodes as visualized bronchoscopically. By convention, the airways are oriented from above-downwards, with right-sided airways on the right side. Unfortunately, although widely accepted, the numbering system employed in this map is different than that recently proposed by the American Thoracic Society.

(stations 5 and 6) are not accessible to the mediastinoscope.

It should be emphasized that not all mediastinal or hilar nodes are equally accessible to transbronchial needle aspiration/biopsy. This has led to the development by Wang of a correlative CT-bronchoscopic nodal map meant to improve the yield of TBNA (Fig. 5-16) (47). Unfortunately, this map uses a numbering system to designate lymph node groups different than that proposed by the ATS (see Fig. 5-11). Despite this, familiarity with this approach is essential for predicting the likely yield of TBNA. It cannot be overemphasized that just because a node can be identified adjacent to an airway on CT that node is therefore easily accessible to bronchoscopists performing TBNA.

Role of CT

CT Technique

The detectability of mediastinal nodes correlates directly with the amount of mediastinal fat that provides a natural contrasting background (see Fig. 5-12). With reduced amounts of mediastinal fat, interpretation may be difficult. An easy method to gain familiarity with the ATS classifica-

tion is by referring to the pictorial essay by Glazer et al. that illustrates examples of calcified nodes in various nodal stations (48).

Another problem is related to the partial volume effect in anatomic areas oriented obliquely relative to the plane of scanning (see Chapter 1). Comparison of lymph node size and number in cadavers imaged by CT and followed by lymph node dissection has shown excellent correlation between CT and pathology for right-sided mediastinal lymph nodes (49,50). However, CT has been shown to be less accurate on the left side failing to demonstrate several normal nodes in the left tracheobronchial region (10L), aortopulmonary window (station 5), and subcarinal region (station 7) (49,50). There is, therefore, a risk of understaging lymph nodes on the left side of the mediastinum. In addition, it is often difficult to distinguish lymph nodes from hilar vessels without the use of contrast media. These considerations have led to a change in the imaging strategy for the mediastinum. For regions where the orientation of anatomic structures is essentially perpendicular to the plane of scanning, 7- to 10-mm sections are adequate. However, thinner 5-mm sections may need to be obtained from the top of the aortic arch through the subcarinal regions. In addition, contrast enhancement is recommended for better definition of low mediastinal and aorticopulmonary window nodes. Critical areas where contrast enhancement is most often useful are:

1. The region of the aorticopulmonary window where the inferior margin of a prominent distal aortic arch or the superior aspect of the main pulmonary artery may be misinterpreted as a nodal mass;
2. The right pulmonary artery as it passes around the bronchus intermedius, and the left pulmonary artery as it arches over the left upper lobe bronchus, where nodes adjacent to the vessels may be misinterpreted as nodular portions of the pulmonary artery (see Fig. 5-12);
3. The truncus anterior, the first branch of the right pulmonary artery, as it courses through the mediastinum en route to the right upper lobe. It may be confused with a node when it is seen in cross-section. Small collections of connective tissue near the truncus anterior may mimic nodes; however, the fatty density of these collections should be a clue to the true nature of this normal variant (51).

Blood vessels, such as a tortuous innominate artery or a persistent left superior vena cava, are most apt to be mistaken for mediastinal nodes. The recesses of the pericardium also present an additional potential source of confusion (see Chapter 2, Fig. 2-11B). The superior sinus, the most prominent of the pericardial recesses, may be visualized as a soft-tissue structure in the mediastinum anterior to the tracheal bifurcation and directly posterior to the ascending aorta (52). The key feature that distinguishes the superior sinus from a lymph node is the near-water density of this structure.

It cannot be overemphasized that proper evaluation of mediastinal lymph nodes requires detailed knowledge of mediastinal vascular anatomy. Although the use of intravenous contrast medium facilitates the distinction of nodes from other mediastinal structures, it is probably not required in the routine assessment of patients with lung cancer, particularly when using spiral CT with 5 to 7 collimation. In a study of 79 adult patients, 5-mm thick sections without intravenous contrast allowed identification of more mediastinal nodes than 10-mm thick sections with intravenous contrast and tended to show slightly (1 to 2 mm) larger nodes than the 10-mm contrast enhanced CT scans (53). Optimal assessment of nodal disease is facilitated by awareness of the pattern of tumor spread to regional lymph nodes.

Patterns of Nodal Spread

A knowledge of the patterns of metastatic spread to regional lymph nodes is valuable when interpreting CT findings. Rouviere was the first to systematically study the lymphatic drainage of the lung (54). Typically, lymph flows into intrapulmonary nodes around segmental bronchi, then to lobar or interlobar nodes, and then to lymph nodes at the hilar areas. The spread of lung cancer generally follows the same pathway. The lymphatic pathways from the individual lobes to the mediastinum are constant.

In 1952, Borrie described more precisely the mechanisms of lymph drainage (55). In the right lung, a collection of intrapulmonary lymph nodes that lie between the upper lobe bronchus and the superior segmental or middle lobe bronchi appeared to be the common drainage pathway for all three lobes. In addition, the right upper lobe drains to nodes in the region of the azygos vein, also called the right tracheobronchial nodes, contiguous with nodes in the lower paratracheal area. The middle and lower lobes also drain to the subcarinal nodes and to nodes in the pulmonary ligament and adjacent to the esophagus (56). A group of lymph nodes located between the left upper lobe bronchus and the left superior segmental bronchus drains both the left upper and left lower lobes. In addition, the left upper lobe drains to nodes in the aorticopulmonary window, the anterior mediastinum, the left paratracheal area, and the subcarinal nodes. As on the right side, the left lower lobe exhibits preferential drainage to the subcarinal nodes, para-esophageal nodes, and nodes of the pulmonary ligament.

An important consideration is the pattern of lymphatic spread. Does it occur in an orderly manner or can some proximal nodes be spared while more distal nodes are involved by disease? Two studies suggest that the latter is true. Nearly 30% of patients with lung cancer had "skipped" metastases to mediastinal lymph nodes with no involvement of lobar or hilar nodes (38,57). Thus, one should not assume that absence of hilar nodes indicates the absence of disease in the mediastinal nodes. Likewise, it is important to understand differences in the patterns of tumor spread throughout the various pulmonary lobes. Although as a rule bronchogenic carcinoma tends to spread to ipsilateral mediastinal lymph nodes, significant exceptions occur.

Although right lung cancers initially spread almost exclusively to ipsilateral mediastinal nodes, left lung tumors have a higher propensity for contralateral spread (Fig. 5-17). In one study, contralateral spread was observed in 3.6% of patients with right upper lobe tumors, 3.7% in those with right lower lobe tumors, 11% in patients with left upper lobe tumors, and 25% in patients with left lower lobe tumors (58). Right lung cancers tend to involve mainly stations 10R and 4R and extend to the higher paratracheal node stations (2R) and finally to the scalene or inferior deep cervical nodes. Tumors in the right lower and middle lobe frequently spread to subcarinal (station 7), tracheobronchial (10R) and paratracheal nodal stations (4R and 2R). It should be noted that subcarinal nodes are midline nodes connected to both right and left lymphatic systems and from which contralateral spread can occur. Once again the new staging system classifies subcarinal nodes as ipsilateral and resectable (3).

Contralateral lymphatic spread is more common with left lung tumors, especially those in the left lower lobe (see Fig. 5-17). Regional lymph node stations 4L and 10L are commonly involved. Left upper lobe tumors often metastasize to subcarinal (station 7), the aorticopulmonary window (station 5), and anterior mediastinal nodes (station 6). The left

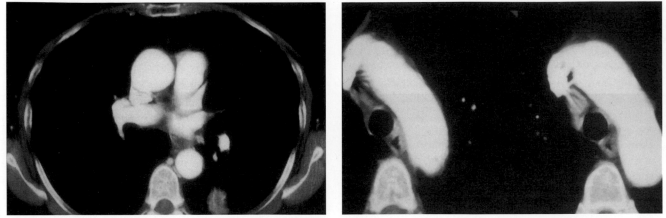

FIG. 5-17. Patterns of spread: N3 disease. **A:** CT section shows tumor in the left lower lobe in the absence of obvious hilar adenopathy. **B:** Contiguous CT sections through the mediastinum in the same patient show evidence of enlarged contralateral right paratracheal (N3) nodes. These were subsequently confirmed to be malignant by mediastinoscopy. Left lower lobe tumors in particular have a tendency to involve contralateral right paratracheal nodes.

lower lobe lesions are the ones most likely to spread contra-laterally via the subcarinal node (station 7) to the right paratracheal regions (4R) and to the pulmonary ligament and para-esophageal stations.

Accuracy of Lymph Node Staging by CT

A large number of studies has assessed accuracy of CT in staging nodal disease in lung cancer patients. The majority of studies have used nodal size alone as the diagnostic criterion. To date, there is no definite evidence that characteristics other than size (such as shape or appearance of borders) are of value in staging lung cancer. Although correlating lymph node size with presence or absence of metastatic disease would seem to constitute a straightforward study design, the reported accuracies of CT in assessing metastatic nodal disease cover a bewildering range of values, ranging from the low 40% to the high 90% (30,32,59–72). This wide range

of findings is related to a number of factors including different size criteria to distinguish normal from enlarged nodes, different CT scanners, different collimation and scan intervals, and thoroughness of mediastinal dissection at surgery.

Normal Mediastinal Nodes

Because the primary goal of nodal staging is to determine the presence or absence of metastatic lymphadenopathy, knowledge of normal nodal anatomy is important. Although several studies have assessed the size and number of nodes in normal subjects or in cadavers (49,50,73,74), we will limit our discussion to the most relevant studies using the ATS nodal map.

Glazer et al. performed a thorough investigation of lymph node size by CT in 56 normal subjects (Table 5-4) (74). They measured the longest and shortest axes in the transverse plane. Short axis was the most reliable parameter of nodal

TABLE 5-4. *Lymph node size by American Thoracic Society lymph node station, measured using CT in 56 normal subjects*

ATS station	Patients with nodes (%)	Number of nodes ± SD	Maximum number of nodes	Short axis diameter ± SD (mm)	Upper limits of normal (mm) (mean + 2 SD)
2R	95	2.1 ± 1.3	6	3.5 ± 1.3	6.1
2L	75	1.9 ± 1.6	6	3.3 ± 1.6	6.5
4R	100	3.2 ± 2.0	10	5.0 ± 2.0	9.0
4L	84	2.1 ± 1.6	7	4.7 ± 1.9	8.5
5	59	1.2 ± 1.1	3	4.7 ± 2.1	8.9
6	86	4.8 ± 3.5	12	4.1 ± 1.7	7.5
7	95	1.7 ± 1.1	6	6.2 ± 2.2	10.6
8R	57	1.0 ± 1.1	4	4.4 ± 2.6	9.6
8L	45	0.8 ± 1.2	6	3.8 ± 1.7	7.2
10R	100	2.8 ± 1.3	7	5.9 ± 2.1	10.1
10L	70	1.0 ± 0.8	3	4.0 ± 1.2	6.4

ATS, American Thoracic Society; SD, standard deviation.
From ref. 74, with permission.

TABLE 5-5. *Lymph node size by American Thoracic Society lymph node station, measured in 40 cadavers*

ATS station	Patients with nodes (%)	Number of nodes ± SD	Maximum number of nodes	Short axis diameter (mm)	Upper limits of normal (mm) (mean + 2 SD)
2R	80	2.5 ± 2.2	11	3.4	7.8
2L	68	2.1 ± 2.2	7	2.8	5.6
4R	98	4.8 ± 2.8	11	3.4	9.2
4L	98	4.5 ± 2.9	16	3.6	9.2
5	58	1.1 ± 1.4	6	3.3	8.5
6	85	4.7 ± 3.9	15	3.0	7.2
7	100	2.9 ± 1.4	6	5.5	12.3
8R	58	1.2 ± 1.4	6	3.6	8.2
8L	50	1.1 ± 1.4	5	2.4	6.1
9R	10	0.1 ± 0.4	2	2.3	3.9
9L	35	0.5 ± 0.8	3	3.1	6.5
10R	95	3.5 ± 2.3	10	4.0	10.8
10L	90	2.4 ± 1.9	7	3.2	6.8

ATS, American Thoracic Society; SD, standard deviation.
From ref. 75, with permission.

size because it is less dependent on the spatial orientation of the node relative to the transaxial scan. They found that the largest nodes in normal individuals were subcarinal (region 7), where the mean short axis was 6.2 mm ± 2.2 and right tracheobronchial (region 10R), and where the mean short axis was 5.9 ± 2.1. Based on their data, they concluded that 10 mm is the short axis measurement above which a node should be considered enlarged (74).

A study on 40 adult cadavers by Kiyono et al., confirmed the greater variation in the size of normal long axis diameters compared to maximum short axis measurements of lymph node size (Table 5-5) (75). These authors also observed that nodes are seen most frequently in the lower paratracheal (station 4), right tracheobronchial (10R), and subcarinal regions (station 7), where they can be demonstrated in 90% to 100% of subjects. The mean short diameter of nodes in their transverse plane ranged from 2.4 to 5.6 mm. The largest nodes were subcarinal (region 7), with 25% of cadavers demonstrating nodes larger than 10 mm in short axis in that region. For the subcarinal region, using mean − 2 standard deviations, these authors found a value of 12.3 mm as the upper limit of normal. In region 10R the upper limit of normal was 10.8 mm. For all other regions, the mean plus two standard deviations did not exceed 10 mm. They also found that upper paratracheal nodes are smaller than lower paratracheal nodes and left paratracheal nodes are smaller and less numerous than right paratracheal nodes. The main findings of these studies have been summarized in Tables 5-4 and 5-5.

Existing data indicate that the short axis measurement of lymph nodes is the least variable measure of enlargement. The normal size of lymph nodes varies depending on its location in the mediastinum. A threshold value of 10 mm appears to represent two standard deviations for the population studied, except in the subcarinal region where a 12-mm value can be used. However, these findings should not be interpreted too rigidly. First, the sample size is small. Also,

age-related and environmentally related variations may exist. Thus, threshold values should be considered only as guidelines. Further, it has been suggested that defining node size in a given region relative to other regions may be a more reliable parameter for detecting nodal disease. This method was suggested by Buy et al., who demonstrated increased accuracy in detecting nodal pathology when nodes were defined as abnormal only when larger than 10 mm in the short axis, and if a difference could be documented between these same nodes and the largest node identifiable in other territories (76). Their working hypothesis was that size comparison between regions may decrease false positive diagnoses caused by underlying inflammatory disease.

A review of the literature indicates that variations in accuracy of CT in the staging of mediastinal lymph nodes can be attributed to some extent to the different methodologies used by the investigators. First, numerous size criteria have been used to define enlarged nodes. Most authors agree that lymph nodes less than 1 cm in diameter are normal in size even though they may still harbor microscopic metastases; however, there has been considerable variation in the size criteria used to identify abnormal nodes. Whereas lymph nodes greater than 15 mm were generally considered abnormal, lymph nodes between 11 to 15 mm were variably categorized. Second, the problem of defining abnormal size criteria has been further compounded by the use of different criteria for measuring lymph node size. Although Glazer et al. (77) and Kiyono et al. (75) advocate the use of the short axis measurement, a study by Staples et al. suggested that a long axis measurement greater than 10 mm was the best criterion on CT (71). These differences in size criteria result in considerable changes in the sensitivity and specificity of CT (32,71).

The absence of a uniform size criterion among studies only partially explains the wide disparity in results. Most studies involved small series of patients—usually 50 or less—leading to considerable statistical variation. Also, populations within reported series have not been homogeneous in terms of disease severity. Indeed, the prevalence of nodal metastases is known to vary depending on the T stage of the tumor, with the likelihood of negative nodes being higher in patients with stage T1 disease. Thus a negative test is more likely to be correct in that group of patients than in patients with more advanced disease. In the study by Primack et al. (32), the prevalence of mediastinal nodal metastases was 22% in patients with T1 tumors, 42% in patients with T2 disease, and 50% in patients with T3 disease. On a per patient basis, the sensitivity of CT in the detection of mediastinal nodal metastases was 40% in patients with T1 lesions, 56% in T2 lesions, and 87% in T3 lesions. However, the specificity decreased from 97% in T1 lesions to 83% in T2 lesions and 69% in T3 lesions. The decreased specificity of CT in T2 and T3 lesions is caused by the increased likelihood of finding enlarged reactive inflammatory nodes related to the postobstructive pneumonitis and atelectasis (63,78).

Another confounding variable has been the lack of uniformity in the measure of truth used by investigators. Some studies have relied on surgical as well as pathologic correlation to establish the accuracy of CT interpretations. Many early studies, however, did not include a thorough exploration of the mediastinum at the time of thoracotomy. As a result, small lymph nodes that appeared normal macroscopically and at palpation could easily have been overlooked at the time of surgery, and consequently, be called negative even though they harbored microscopic disease. Obviously, this would tend to reduce the number of false negative studies and improve the apparent sensitivity of the test. Moreover, surgeons cannot sample contralateral nodes at the time of surgery. In some studies, mediastinoscopy was used to verify the status of contralateral nodes. In others, however, a negative CT scan was considered sufficient to avoid preoperative mediastinoscopy.

These problems were appreciated early on by a few investigators. In 1984, Libshitz and McKenna studied 86 patients with bronchogenic carcinoma who had mediastinal CT and full nodal sampling (63). In 33% of cases, metastases involved nodes less than 1 cm in diameter. These nodes were either missed or classified as normal using CT. In an extension of this study (79), the same authors found a 10% incidence of metastatic disease in lymph nodes smaller than 1 cm. In the group of patients with metastatic disease (25 of 102 patients), CT detected only 60% of lesions using 1 cm as a threshold value. Similarly, in 1988, Staples et al. reported results from a series of patients who underwent preoperative mediastinoscopy and thorough mediastinal exploration (71). In this study, the authors tried to match nodal stations examined by CT with nodal stations examined by mediastinoscopy or surgery. They documented a sensitivity of 79% and a specificity of 65%. Additionally, these authors found that in 7 of 44 patients, tumor was absent in the enlarged nodes seen on CT but was present in normal-sized lymph nodes located in a different nodal station. Thus the overall sensitivity of CT in predicting the number of patients with mediastinal metastasis was 79%, whereas the sensitivity for individual lymph node stations was only 66%. This study and a subsequent study by Seely et al. (80), point out that it may be difficult at CT and at surgery to determine precisely the boundaries between adjacent nodal stations. In the study by Seely et al., a total of 362 mediastinal lymph nodal stations were sampled at mediastinoscopy or thoracotomy in 104 patients with T1 bronchogenic carcinomas. The overall sensitivity of CT (short axis measurements) in the detection of metastases to mediastinal lymph nodes on a per node basis was 41%. When adjacent nodal stations were included in the analysis, that is, when it was assumed that the CT findings were positive whenever a node was identified at surgery in the same or in adjacent nodal stations, the sensitivity increased to 59%, which corresponded exactly to the sensitivity on a per patient basis. Prospective studies that reported a very low accuracy of CT made no allowance for this potential pitfall (30,72). McLoud et al. reported a CT sensitivity of 41% and a specificity of 84% (72). In a multi-center cooperative study of the Radiology Diagnostic Oncology Group that included prospective blinded readings and systematic surgical sampling, the sensitivity of CT was 52% and specificity was 69% (30). It is probable that the lower accuracy in these two studies is in part caused by the analysis on a per node basis rather than on a per patient basis. Meta-analysis of 42 studies published between 1980 and 1988 demonstrated that the sensitivity of CT is 83%, the specificity 81%, and the accuracy 81%, on a per patient basis (81). This is similar to the recent prospective multicenter Canadian Lung Oncology Group study which showed CT to have a sensitivity of 78% and a specificity of 69% in the detection of mediastinal N2 disease (82).

The relatively low specificity of CT is directly related to the number of enlarged nodes that do not harbor disease. As mentioned previously, Libshitz and McKenna examined this problem in patients with lung cancer and concomitant atelectasis, pneumonitis, or evidence of granulomatous disease (57). Of their 86 patients, 39 had associated pneumonia or atelectasis; of these 39, 54% had lymph nodes larger than 1 cm. Ten of these patients harbored metastatic disease, but 11 had reactive enlarged lymph nodes. Likewise, Hirleman et al. found that five of seven patients with a false positive reading from CT images had evidence of postobstructive atelectasis or pneumonia (78). The specificity of CT decreases with increasing T stage. In the study by Primack et al., the specificity of CT decreased from 97% for T1 lesions to 69% in T3 lesions (32).

What conclusions can be drawn about the role of CT in mediastinal nodal staging? Clearly, there are serious limitations in the use of CT for assessing mediastinal nodal involvement by tumor. Nonetheless, CT currently remains the primary noninvasive modality for staging local invasion and nodal status (Fig. 5-18) (4).

One should be keenly aware that staging issues constantly evolve as results of different therapeutic approaches become

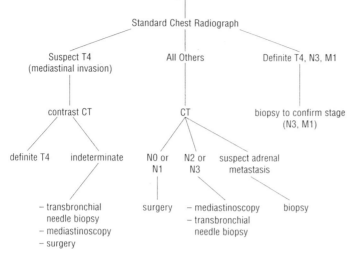

Lung Cancer

Standard Chest Radiograph

Suspect T4 (mediastinal invasion) — All Others — Definite T4, N3, M1

contrast CT — CT — biopsy to confirm stage (N3, M1)

definite T4 — indeterminate — N0 or N1 — N2 or N3 — suspect adrenal metastasis

– transbronchial needle biopsy
– mediastinoscopy
– surgery

surgery

– mediastinoscopy
– transbronchial needle biopsy

biopsy

FIG. 5-18. Imaging schematic for clinical evaluation of nonsmall cell lung cancer.

known. For example, the evidence that patients with N2 disease have a better prognosis following extensive lymph node dissection is still being evaluated. Clinical data now support the hypothesis that survival of such patients depends on the underlying character of the nodal involvement. Bergh and Schersten reported a 43% survival rate when resected cancer was entirely intranodal, as opposed to a 4.3% survival rate when malignancy extended through the capsule (42). Simi-

larly, it has been shown that patients in whom nodal disease is not detected during mediastinoscopy but only at thoracotomy have a better prospect of survival (83,84). Such findings suggest that normal-sized lymph nodes harboring metastatic disease may not have the same prognostic significance as larger positive nodes with penetration of tumor through the capsule (Fig. 5-19). In this context, false negative CT examinations in normal-sized lymph nodes may not be a limiting

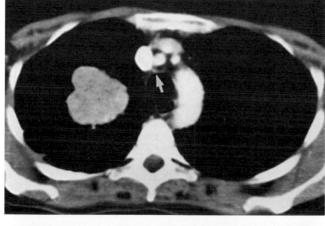

A

FIG. 5-19. Stage 3A disease: ipsilateral mediastinal metastases. **A:** Contrast-enhanced CT shows a lobulated mass in the right upper lobe. A very small paratracheal lymph node (*arrow*) corresponding to region 2R can just be identified. Similar-sized mediastinal nodes were seen throughout the mediastinum and right hilum (not shown). **B,C:** T1- and T2-weighted MR images at approximately the same level as **A**, respectively. Paratracheal lymph nodes are shown to good advantage, embedded in mediastinal fat (*arrow* in **B**). Note that the T2-weighted image shows bright signal within nodes identified on the T1-weighted scan (*arrow* in **C**). At surgery, these nodes proved positive. Unfortunately, signal intensity within nodes is nonspecific; a similar appearance may be seen as well in hyperplastic lymph nodes.

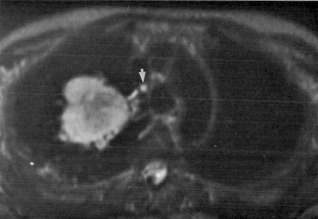

B

C

factor since these patients are now considered candidates for surgery. As removal of all nodes becomes important, CT is valuable for its ability to visualize all nodes, whether normal or abnormal. In addition, if patients with varied prognoses can be segregated according to the degree of abnormal node involvement, detailed CT analysis of the morphologic features of lymph nodes may become important (Fig. 5-20). If CT scans show no enlarged lymph nodes and no evidence of capsular penetration, it would seem reasonable to bypass surgical staging procedures (such as mediastinoscopy) and proceed directly to thoracotomy.

The main role of CT in the assessment of mediastinal nodes is to exclude disease. A negative CT study is of value by obviating mediastinoscopy or transbronchial needle aspiration prior to thoracotomy. Evidence for the value of a negative CT study was published by Daly et al. (85). Of 501 patients with normal size mediastinal nodes on CT, a total of 37 proved to have N2 disease either at thoracotomy or mediastinoscopy. Surgical resection was performed in 33 (92%) of these 37 patients with projected five year survival

of 31%. These data support the role of thoracotomy without mediastinoscopy in most patients with a normal CT. It has also been demonstrated that in patients with a normal CT, the yield of transthoracic needle biopsy is limited (86). The utility and cost effectiveness of CT in the assessment of mediastinal nodal disease were recently confirmed in a prospective study performed by the Canadian Lung Oncology Group (82). This prospective multicenter study included 685 patients, 342 of which were randomized to have mediastinoscopy for preoperative staging of mediastinal nodes and 343 were randomized to have CT. Patients who underwent CT proceeded to mediastinoscopy if they had any mediastinal nodes greater than 10 mm in short axis diameter, or directly to thoracotomy if all nodes were 10 mm or less in diameter. The primary end point, chosen before the study began, was thoracotomy without cure. This was defined as including patients who had unresectable disease at the time of thoracotomy, patients who underwent incomplete resections, or in whom recurrent disease developed within three years. The sensitivity of CT in detecting mediastinal nodal

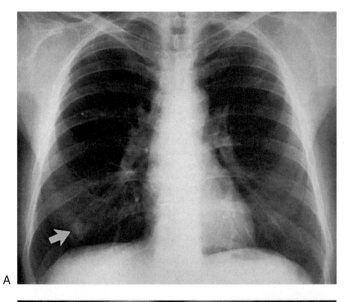

A

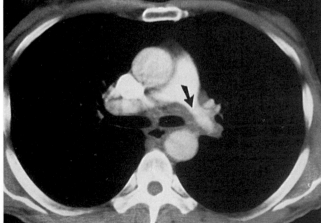

B

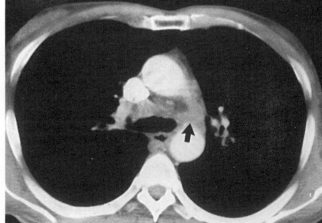

C

FIG. 5-20. Radiographic T1N0M0 disease: the role of CT. **A:** Posteroanterior radiograph shows a nodule in the right lower lobe (*arrow*). The hilar and mediastinal contours are normal. **B,C:** Sequential contrast-enhanced CT scans show extensive tumor throughout the mediastinum. This appearance is consistent with extranodal spread of disease (*arrow* in **C**). Note that the left main pulmonary artery is encased (*arrow* in **B**). This case shows the value of CT in more precisely defining the extent of disease prior to attempting surgical resection.

involvement on a per patient basis was 78% and the specificity 69%. The percentage of patients with positive N2 nodes at thoracotomy was similar in the CT group as in the mediastinoscopy group (23%). Overall, the number of thoracotomies without cure was slightly lower in the CT group (103 of 343, 30%) than in the mediastinoscopy group (109 of 342, 32%). The number of thoracotomies in patients with benign disease was also lower in the CT group (4 of 20, 20%) than in the mediastinoscopy group (12 of 25, 48%). The CT strategy therefore produced the same number of or fewer unnecessary thoracotomies than doing mediastinoscopy on all patients, and also was less expensive. The authors recommended that CT rather than mediastinoscopy be performed in all patients with nonsmall cell bronchogenic carcinoma (82). Patients with normal sized nodes may proceed directly to thoracotomy.

Unfortunately, CT does not provide histologic specificity. Therefore patients with enlarged nodes need to have further evaluation by mediastinoscopy or needle biopsy because the enlarged nodes may simply be the result of benign reactive changes. In the context of advanced disease with associated pneumonitis, atelectasis, or inflammation, preoperative sampling of these nodes becomes essential for two reasons: (a) to prove the presence of disease; and (b) to evaluate the presence of nodal disease in the contralateral mediastinum rather than in the ipsilateral nodes that are all accessible during thoracotomy. This last point is especially important in the context of the new staging system. A valid question would be to determine the accuracy of CT in assessing the contralateral mediastinum. This could prove especially important in the management of left-sided lung tumors, particularly left lower lobe lesions, which have a higher propensity for contralateral spread. It is possible that contralateral disease distant from the primary site may be less affected by the problem of false positive diagnoses related to associated inflammation.

STAGING OF DISTANT METASTASES

The descriptor *M* relates to the presence of distant metastases (M1) or their absence (M0) (see Table 5-1). Now included in the category M1 as well are patients with separate metastatic tumor nodules in the ipsilateral nonprimary-tumor lobe(s) of the lung (2).

Extrathoracic metastases are present in approximately 40% of patients with newly diagnosed bronchogenic carcinoma (87). Patients with distant metastases carry a very poor prognosis and are generally treated with chemotherapy, radiotherapy, or both. For didactic purposes, the TNM system is described in an orderly pathophysiologic progression from local extension T to distant metastasis M. In fact, the clinical work-up of a patient with lung cancer generally proceeds in the opposite direction, that is, from M to T (4). Initial clinical evaluation and laboratory tests strive to detect M1 disease, which will preclude more aggressive and expensive work-up and therapy. Biopsies are performed for suspicious skin lesions or palpable lymph nodes. Abnormal biochemical tests may indicate the necessity for imaging of the liver or bones to detect distant metastases. Neurologic findings may indicate central nervous system disease, to be confirmed by CT or MRI. Thoracic CT becomes important in the staging process only when these initial steps are negative. Often, clinically silent sites of distant metastatic disease can be discovered. Mathews et al. studied 200 patients who died within 30 days of presumed curative surgery. At autopsy, 48 of these patients (23.4%) had metastases, 18 of them to the adrenal gland and 16 to the liver (88). In a comparable population, a 26% incidence of extrathoracic metastases was found at autopsy (89). In a study of 95 patients with bronchogenic carcinoma in whom preoperative CT scan showed a solitary lung mass without evidence of hilar or mediastinal lymphadenopathy, 25% had extrathoracic metastases (90). The majority of these patients (67%) had adenocarcinoma. It is therefore common practice to obtain scans of the upper abdomen at the same time as the examination of the thorax to evaluate the liver and adrenal glands for clinically silent metastatic disease.

Salvatierra et al. assessed the value of systematic evaluation of extrathoracic metastases in a prospective study of 146 patients with potentially resectable nonsmall cell bronchogenic carcinoma (91). The study protocol included CT of the brain and upper abdomen, abdominal ultrasonography, and whole-body bone scanning. They demonstrated that in 61% (11/18) of patients with hepatic metastases, there were no organ-specific indicators. The series showed a 7.5% incidence of adrenal metastases. Twenty-one percent (4/19) of brain metastases were asymptomatic. Bone scanning detected metastases in 3.4% (4/116) of the asymptomatic patients. The rate of metastases for adenocarcinoma was significantly larger than other cell types and it did not correlate with the TN staging (91). They therefore recommended that upper abdominal CT scan or ultrasonography be performed in all patients except for those with asymptomatic stage 1 squamous cell carcinoma. Other studies have also suggested that cranial CT be performed in all patients with nonsmall cell lung cancer prior to surgical resection (92) or at least in patients in whom mediastinal disease is suspected before proceeding to surgery (93). However, meta-analysis of 25 studies assessing the performance of the clinical evaluation compared with brain and abdomen CT and radionuclide bone scans in detecting extrathoracic metastases in patients with newly diagnosed bronchogenic carcinoma has questioned the need for performing CT or bone scan in asymptomatic patients (94). The meta-analysis included 25 studies published between 1977 and 1992, with a total of 3,089 imaging scans obtained in the patients after a clinical evaluation. The mean negative predicted value of the clinical evaluation for CT of the brain, abdomen, and radionuclide bone scan was 95%, 94%, and 89%, respectively. The use of CT in the assessment of extrathoracic metastases in asymptomatic patients with normal biochemistry is therefore controversial.

We believe that CT of the upper abdomen is probably warranted in the following settings:

1. In patients with adenocarcinoma or poorly differentiated carcinomas, because the risk of distant metastases in this population is generally higher.
2. In patients with T3 lesions, because justification for thoracotomy may be borderline, and in these cases, again, there is a higher likelihood of distant metastases. This is true even in patients who demonstrate no evidence of mediastinal adenopathy since only 70% of patients with distant metastatic disease demonstrate lymph node involvement in the mediastinum.
3. In patients with N2 disease, particularly when the histology is other than squamous cell carcinoma.
4. In patients with questionable physiologic status who may not withstand surgical resection.

It cannot be overemphasized that the accuracy of CT in detecting upper abdominal pathology directly correlates with scan technique, especially when evaluating the liver. Proper examination of the liver by CT is in itself an exacting task. In the thorax, parenchymal lesions and lymph nodes are accentuated either by surrounding aerated lung or mediastinal fat. Liver metastases can be detected only by virtue of a difference in attenuation between tumor and adjacent normal liver. A bolus of intravenous contrast medium increases the ability to identify metastases, which typically exhibit less enhancement than normal liver. The accuracy of CT in detecting liver metastases is a function of the quality of the CT examination. In patients in whom there is a strong suspicion of hepatic disease (based on clinical evidence either of hepatomegaly or abnormal liver function), it is our practice to use a combined thoracic-upper abdominal oncologic survey protocol (see Chapter 2, Table 2-1) (95). This entails obtaining images through the upper abdomen (7 to 8 mm slice thickness; pitch = 1.6; reconstruction interval = 3.5 to 4 mm) following an initial bolus of 125–150 cc 60% iodine solution injected at a rate of 2 to 3 cc/second, starting at the thoracic inlet and scanning caudally, allowing a 15 second interval between thoracic and abdominal sequences to provide time for patients to catch their breath. Typically this results in sections being obtained through the liver 60 to 75 seconds following the initial administration of intravenous contrast medium—coinciding with the portal venous phase of contrast enhancement, optimal for identifying most liver metastases originating from the lung. As with thoracic lesions, in most cases the nature of hepatic masses must be histologically confirmed before a patient is declared unresectable.

Although histologic confirmation of adrenal lesions is also often sought, a confident diagnosis of a benign adrenal adenoma may now be reliably obtained using both CT and MRI. A fair proportion of cases of nodular adrenal enlargement will be found to represent benign adrenal adenomas or adrenal hyperplasia (96). Although optimal assessment of the liver on CT requires use of intravenous contrast, differentiation of adrenal adenomas from metastatic bronchogenic carcinoma on CT is facilitated by measurement of attenuation values in scans performed either prior to injection (Fig. 5-21) (97,98), or following delay (99). As documented by Korobkin et al., the mean attenuation value of adenomas is significantly lower than nonadenomas (2.5 Hounsfield units [HU] $\pm$ 14 compared with 32 HU $\pm$ 6.4) (97). In this study, the lowest unenhanced CT attenuation value of metastatic bronchogenic carcinoma and other nonadenomas was 18 HU; therefore, the sensitivity:specificity ratio for the diagnosis of adenomas was 85%–100% at a threshold value of 18 HU. At this threshold, the positive predictive value was 100% and the negative predictive value was 77%. As recently shown by Macari, initial noncontrast scans through the adrenals are easily obtained in those cases in which there is heightened suspicion for extrathoracic metastases without the need for routine physician monitoring (98).

STAGE GROUPINGS

Based on comparable extent of disease, anticipated treatment, and prognosis, TNM subsets have been defined corresponding to 4 stages of disease, not including carcinoma in situ (see Table 5-2). Initially formulated on the basis of result of careful studies by Mountain (8) of the prognostic factors and treatment outcomes in 3,753 patients, recently modifications have been adopted (2). These primarily involve dividing previous stage 1 and 2 disease into 1A, 1B, 2A, and 2B categories.

As noted, compared to the previous staging system, Stage 1 has now been subdivided into 1A (T1N0M0) and 1B (T2N0M0) categories to reflect differences in survival between these two groups: 67% of patients with surgical-pathological stage 1A disease survive 5 years compared to 57% with stage 1B disease (2).

Similarly, the new classification calls for subdividing previous Stage 2 disease into 2A (T1N1M0) and 2B (including both T2N1M0 and T3N0M0) reflecting the prognostic implications of hilar nodal status, tumor size and location (including extrapulmonary extension in the absence of adenopathy): 55% of patients with stage 2A survive 5 years compared with 38% and 39% of patients with T2N1M0 and T3N0M0 tumors, respectively (2). It should be noted that as part of this revision, T3N0M0, previously classified as stage 3A is now considered Stage 2B (see Table 5-2).

Modifications in the stage 3 classification include reclassifying T3N0M0 as stage 2B, as noted above. Otherwise, stage 3 remains unchanged, subdivided into two subgroups. Stage 3A (T3N1M0, or T1-T3N2M0) represents patients with advanced disease in whom extensive surgery (including resection of all ipsilateral and subcarinal lymph nodes) may be of value, especially if adjuvant radiotherapy or chemotherapy is used. Stage 3B includes all cases of more advanced disease without distant metastases. Stage 4 represents any patient with evidence of distant metastases.

Patients with stage 3B disease may benefit from radiation

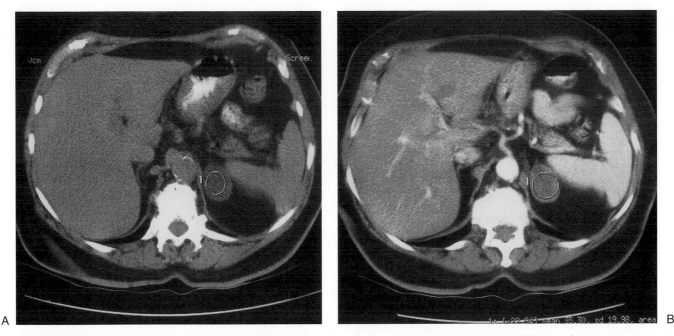

FIG. 5-21. Benign adrenal adenoma: CT evaluation. **A:** CT section through the upper abdomen prior to the injection of intravenous contrast media shows a well-defined left adrenal lesion (*round cursor* in **A** and **B**) with a mean density of −18 Hounsfield units (HU). **B:** Section at the same level following a bolus of intravenous contrast medium shows that there is heterogeneous enhancement within this mass with a mean density measuring 35 HU. The mean attenuation of adrenal adenomas on noncontrast enhanced CT is significantly lower than nonadenomas and may be reliably diagnosed when the mean density is less than 15 HU. Although the appearance of adenomas is less characteristic on a single contrast enhanced image, delayed contrast enhanced images through the adrenal glands may be equally diagnostic (see text).

therapy, often in conjunction with chemotherapy. This group is often referred to as the extensive radiotherapy group. Patients with stage 4 disease are generally treated with chemotherapy with limited use of palliative radiotherapy. This group is referred to as the chemotherapy group. The radiologist interpreting CT scans needs to be familiar with the staging groups and their implications to enhance both the technical quality of studies and the quality of interpretation.

It is worth noting that there is no optimal CT technique to stage lung cancer. Instead, each study should reflect an initial estimate of the probable stage of disease based on routine chest radiographs, as well as an estimate of the patient's clinical status. For example, in patients suspected of stage 1A disease in whom a diagnosis of malignancy has not yet been established, initial scans should be obtained prior to the administration of intravenous contrast, utilizing thin (1.5 to 2 mm) sections in order to accurately measure tissue density (see Chapter 4). In select cases, further evaluation using contrast enhancement to evaluate tissue vascularity may be indicated, especially for well-defined rounded lesions. As already discussed, this approach differs fundamentally from patients in whom a diagnosis of lung cancer has already been established and in whom distant metastases are suspected, especially within the liver. In cases in which tumor appears primarily central, especially when associated with peripheral atelectasis, initial attention should be paid to the region of the pulmonary hilum. As discussed in detail in Chapter 3, evaluation of the central airways and hilum is best achieved using volumetric acquisition following a bolus administration of intravenous contrast media to allow optimal differentiation between central lesions and postobstructive pneumonitis. In patients in whom evaluation centers on differentiating stage 3A from 3B disease, a similar technique as described for the hilum also can be used, with scans initially obtained either through the center of lesions suspected of invading either the chest wall or mediastinum, or from the level of the thoracic inlet to the carina in patients for whom the critical question is evaluation of mediastinal nodal disease. In patients with possible chest wall invasion, further evaluation using expiratory scans may also be of value as discussed previously. In each case scan technique optimization is based on an initial assessment of the probable disease stage based largely on radiographic appearances. It should be emphasized that regardless of technique, all patients in whom lung cancer is suspected should have additional images obtained through the upper abdomen to include the adrenal glands as part of a routine chest CT study (4). This requires very little extra time and is of sufficient benefit to warrant routine acquisition of these few extra images.

SMALL CELL LUNG CANCER

Small cell lung cancer is a tumor with a very high biologic malignancy, which tends to be widespread at the time of diagnosis. Small cell carcinoma account for 20% to 25% of bronchogenic carcinomas. Although the AJCC recommended that patients with small cell carcinoma be staged identically to those with nonsmall cell carcinomas, in practice the majority of oncologists use a 2-stage system based on studies of the Veterans Administration Lung Study Group. In this system, patients with small cell carcinoma are classified as having either limited or extensive disease (9). Limited disease refers to tumor that can be treated within a tolerable single radiation port (100). It includes tumor confined to one hemithorax and to the regional lymph nodes, including regional hilar, ipsilateral and contralateral mediastinal nodes, ipsilateral and contralateral scalene nodes, and with ipsilateral pleural effusion independent of whether the pleural fluid is benign or malignant (101). Extensive disease refers to any tumor burden more than limited disease. Extensive disease is present in 60% to 80% of patients with newly diagnosed small cell lung cancers.

Untreated patients with small cell carcinoma have a median survival of only 6 to 17 weeks, but even with treatment the five year survival is usually less than 10% (101). Treatment usually consists of radiotherapy and chemotherapy. However, in patients with small cell carcinoma presenting with a single lung nodule or mass (T1 or T2 lesions) without associated lymphadenopathy (stage I disease) surgical resection followed by chemotherapy results in a five year survival of 30% to 50% (102–104). Review of long term survivors with small cell carcinoma demonstrated that only patients who underwent surgery for either stage I or II disease had survival beyond two years (105). Currently, the recommended treatment for stage I and II small cell carcinoma is surgical resection followed by postoperative chemotherapy with additional mediastinal radiation therapy for nodal disease (10). Therefore it seems reasonable to use the new International Staging System for Bronchogenic Carcinoma rather than the 2-tier system to classify small cell carcinoma. It would also seem reasonable to stage patients with small cell carcinoma with CT of the chest and abdomen except perhaps in patients with obviously extensive disease on the chest radiograph. CT is also of value as a monitoring tool to assess the response of the disease to radiotherapy or chemotherapy (Fig. 5-22).

ROLE OF MR IN STAGING LUNG CANCER

Since the advent of MRI, several studies have been performed to assess its value relative to CT in the management of patients with lung cancer (69,106–111). MRI offers inherent advantages that may be of use in lung cancer staging. First, the delineation of mediastinal and hilar vessels does not require the administration of intravenous contrast medium. Second, direct coronal, sagittal, and oblique imaging provides superb anatomic detail in regions difficult to study with CT, such as the lung apex, the aortopulmonary window, and the supradiaphragmatic regions. Third, the increased soft-tissue differentiation achievable with MRI may also be helpful in differentiating tumor from other processes.

It should be emphasized that MRI also exhibits significant disadvantages relative to CT. It is costly and time-consuming, and the spatial resolution is less than that achievable with CT. Artifacts and blurring of structures related to respiratory and cardiac motion are a potential problem, although this has been greatly reduced by the advent of motion compensation techniques and the systematic use of cardiac gating. The general consensus at present is that MRI and CT have similar accuracies, therefore in our opinion, CT remains the imaging modality of choice both for assessing patients with abnormal chest radiographs suspected of having lung cancer, and staging patients with documented bronchogenic carcinoma (4). Nonetheless, as will be discussed in detail, in select cases MRI can play a significant complementary role in the evaluation and staging of lung cancer.

Assessment of Chest Wall and Mediastinal Invasion

Chest wall invasion adjacent to a lung tumor may be better demonstrated by MRI than by CT. This is because MRI provides better tissue contrast, particularly on T2-weighted images, between tumor, chest wall, fat, and muscles (69,111,112). A thin layer of extrapleural fat separating the tumor mass from the chest wall can almost always be seen on high quality MR images. This thin layer of extrapleural fat, located beneath the parietal pleura, may be effaced in the presence of early invasion (Fig. 5-23). Using conventional CT, this fat layer is more difficult to see. Although plain radiographs generally demonstrate rib destruction better than MRI, MRI most clearly demonstrates the mass within the chest wall. It should be noted that although MRI is helpful in the assessment of chest wall invasion in select cases, in the report of the Radiology Diagnostic Oncology Group (RDOG) trial involving 23 patients with surgical and pathologic correlation, CT and MRI were equivalent in the assessment of chest wall invasion (30). In the study by Haggar et al., however, MRI allowed accurate diagnosis of presence or absence of chest wall invasion in nine cases in which CT findings were equivocal (111). In a more recent study by Padovani et al. in 34 patients MRI had a sensitivity of 90% and a specificity of 86% in the detection of chest wall invasion (112). Several studies have demonstrated that MRI is of relatively limited value in the assessment of invasion of the lateral chest wall but that MRI images in the sagittal or coronal planes are particularly advantageous in imaging superior sulcus tumors (Figs. 5-24 and 5-25) (30,72,113–115). Sagittal or coronal plane images often show the extent of chest wall invasion and involvement of the subclavian artery or brachial plexus better than either transaxial CT or MR images (116,117). Therefore MRI is strongly recommended when superior sulcus invasion is suspected.

A significant advantage of MRI is its ability to demonstrate the relationship between tumor and major mediastinal vascular structures without the need for administration of intravenous contrast media. Indeed, with MRI, good contrast is generally observed between the flow void within blood vessels and the high signal intensity mediastinal fat and the

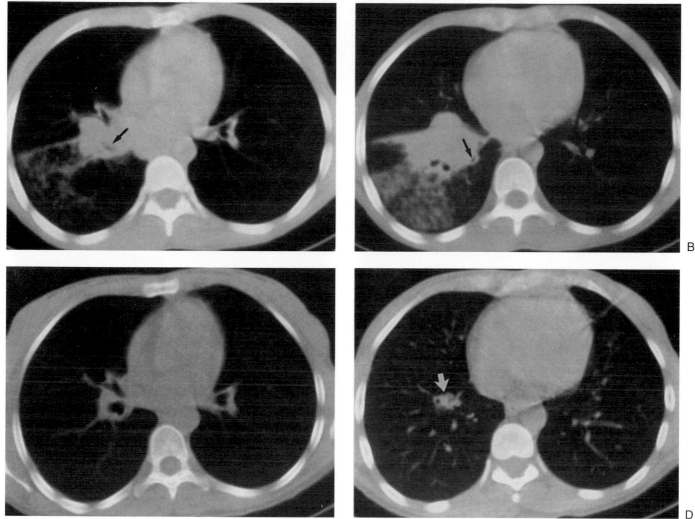

FIG. 5-22. Small-cell lung cancer: CT evaluation. **A,B:** Sequential CT sections through the right hilum show extensive tumor deforming both the middle lobe and right lower lobe bronchi (*arrows* in **A** and **B**), causing distal consolidation and atelectasis. Diagnosis established by transbronchial biopsy. **C,D:** CT scans through the same levels as shown in **A** and **B**, following 6 months of chemotherapy. Note that there has been near complete regression of tumor, although there is a small, residual, soft-tissue density adjacent to the basilar bronchi (*arrow* in **D**). CT allows precise evaluation of response to therapy in these cases, allowing for close monitoring and potentially early detection of tumor recurrence.

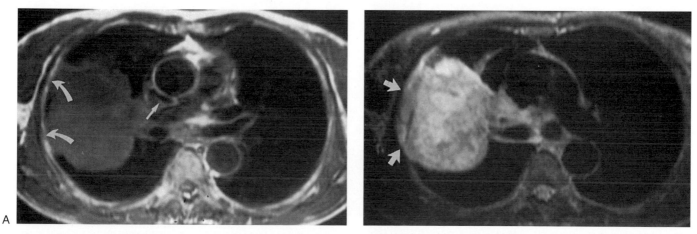

FIG. 5-23. Stage 3A disease: ipsilateral mediastinal adenopathy/chest wall invasion. **A:** T1-weighted MRI scan shows a right hilar mass with apparent extension into the mediastinum, causing compression of the superior vena cava (*straight arrow*). Laterally, there is a suggestion that tumor has infiltrated extrapleural fat, identifiable as focal areas of decreased signal intensity (*curved arrows*). **B:** T2-weighted MRI scan, at the level slightly higher than **A**. Tumor clearly extends into the chest wall (*arrows*). At surgery, the vena cava was found not to be invaded. Hilar and mediastinal nodes proved positive, without evidence of mediastinal invasion. The tumor was successfully resected despite chest wall invasion.

mediastinal pleural margins. In addition, the pericardium is routinely demonstrated, identifiable as a line of hypointensity surrounding the heart and the base of the major vessels. Although neither MRI nor CT are capable of demonstrating minimal invasion of either the mediastinal pleura or mediastinal fat, significant obliteration of mediastinal fat planes or compression or encasement of mediastinal vessels appear better demonstrated by MRI than CT. In a prospective study by the RDOG, no statistically significant differences were observed in the relative accuracies of CT and MRI in staging lung cancer, except for significantly better delineation of mediastinal and superior sulcus invasion by MRI (30). The specific instances in which we believe MRI to be useful are as follows:

1. Superior sulcus tumors (chest wall invasion). MRI shows extent of chest wall invasion and proximity to spine, spinal canal, nerves (including the recurrent laryngeal nerves as well as the brachial plexus), and the spinal cord in an exquisite fashion (see Figs. 5-24 and 5-25).

2. Tumor in contact with the heart, in particular the left atrium. MRI is helpful in determining pericardial involvement (T3 disease) versus pericardial and cardiac muscle involvement (T4 disease).

3. Central tumor with direct extension in the subcarinal region. In this setting, coronal images in particular are extremely valuable in determining the precise extent of tumor, especially in relation to the carina (Fig. 5-26).

4. Tumor extension into the aorticopulmonary window. Again, coronal images may be extremely helpful in determining encasement of the pulmonary artery and aorta (Fig. 5-27).

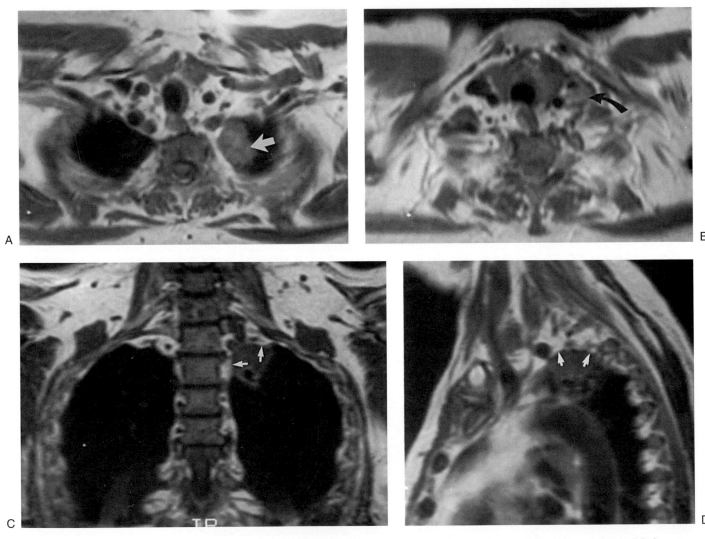

FIG. 5-24. Stage 3A disease: Pancoast tumor. **A,B:** Sequential MR images through the thoracic inlet from below-upward show a lobular mass in the left lung apex (*arrow* in **A**). Note that the medial border of the tumor is well delineated by fat. A large supraclavicular lymph node is present on the left, as well, just posterior to the left jugular vein and lateral to the left carotid artery (*arrow* in **B**). **C,D:** Coronal and sagittal images through the lung apex, respectively, show sharp demarcation between the tumor and adjacent mediastinal and extrapleural fat along most of the course of the tumor-pleural interface (*arrows* in **C** and **D**). No contact is seen with the spine. Although these findings suggested a lack of gross chest wall invasion, at surgery microscopic invasion was documented with minimal tumor extension into the extrapleural fat. The supraclavicular node shown in **A** proved to be positive.

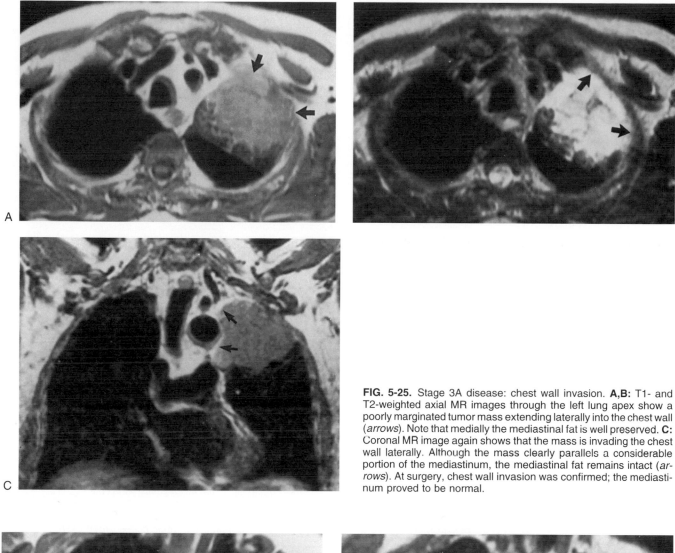

FIG. 5-25. Stage 3A disease: chest wall invasion. **A,B:** T1- and T2-weighted axial MR images through the left lung apex show a poorly marginated tumor mass extending laterally into the chest wall (*arrows*). Note that medially the mediastinal fat is well preserved. **C:** Coronal MR image again shows that the mass is invading the chest wall laterally. Although the mass clearly parallels a considerable portion of the mediastinum, the mediastinal fat remains intact (*arrows*). At surgery, chest wall invasion was confirmed; the mediastinum proved to be normal.

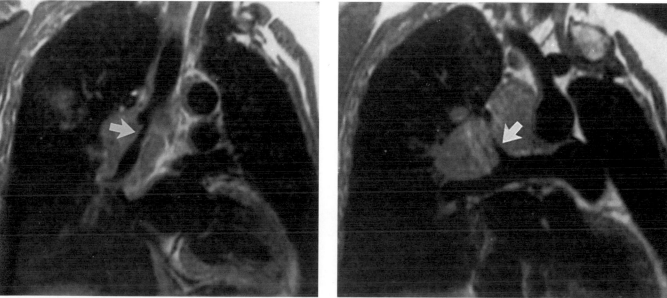

FIG. 5-26. Stage 3B disease: mediastinal adenopathy coronal images. **A,B:** Sequential coronal MR images through the mediastinum show extensive adenopathy surrounding and narrowing the bronchus intermedius (*arrow* in **A**), as well as encasing the truncus anterior (*arrow* in **B**). Note the extensive paratracheal adenopathy, especially well seen in **B**. In select cases, coronal images may be of particular value in determining the true extent of disease.

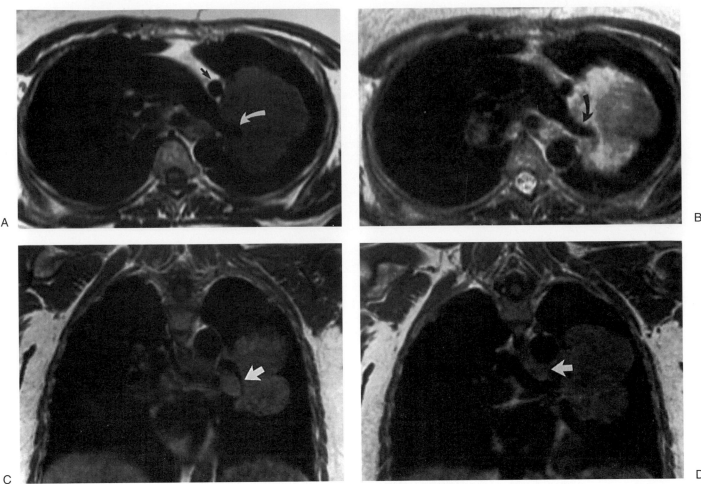

FIG. 5-27. Stage 3B disease: mediastinal invasion. **A,B:** Axial T1- and T2-weighted MR images at the same level through the carina in a patient with squamous cell carcinoma. Tumor clearly encases the left pulmonary artery (*curved arrows* in **A** and **B**). Note the presence of a persistent left superior vena cava, a normal variant (*straight arrow* in **A**). **C,D:** Coronal T1-weighted images show encasement of the left pulmonary artery to better advantage (*arrow* in **C**). Note the presence of enlarged aorticopulmonary and left paratracheal lymph nodes (*arrow* in **D**).

5. Invasion of the superior vena cava and adjacent mediastinal soft tissues in patients with otherwise radiographically resectable right hilar disease (Fig. 5-28).

6. Tumor located in the cardiophrenic angles and in the medial aspect of the lower lobes. MRI is helpful in determining invasion of the aorta and paraesophageal tissues as well as determining pericardial versus cardiac involvement.

Recently, it has been suggested MRI using gadolinium enhancement may be of value in the initial assessment of solitary lung nodules (see Chapter 3). Similar to contrast enhanced CT nodule evaluation, a lack of enhancement on MRI has been cited as evidence of a likely benign etiology. At present, this application remains speculative.

Role of MR in the Evaluation of the Hila

Contrast-enhanced CT and MRI are both accurate in detecting hilar masses and adenopathy. However, in patients in whom there is a contraindication to the intravenous administration of contrast media or with poor vascular opacification, MRI may allow a more confident diagnosis, especially of hilar invasion. On occasion, MRI can demonstrate node enlargement not visible on CT, especially when partial volume effects between adjacent vessels and nodes prevent identification. Because blood vessels usually have a low signal and nodes have a relatively higher signal, such a confusion is less likely with MRI (Fig. 5-29). It should be noted, however, that slow flow in hilar vessels may be associated with significant signal, even in normal individuals. Additionally, MRI is unable to detect nodal calcifications. These drawbacks render MRI unsuitable as a routine imaging modality for evaluating the pulmonary hila. In select cases, MRI may aid surgical planning by determining the extent of invasion of both central pulmonary arteries or veins. This may be of particular value in deciding whether a patient requires a pneumonectomy or, instead, special reconstructive techniques. In select cases, especially those in which detailed

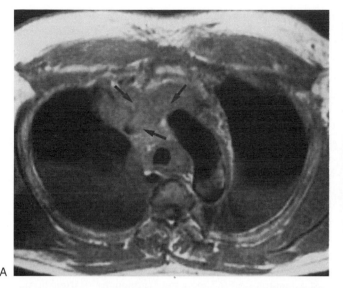

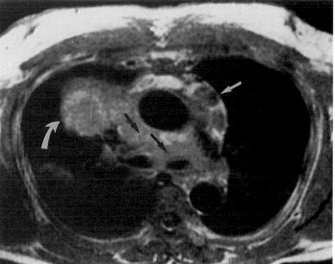

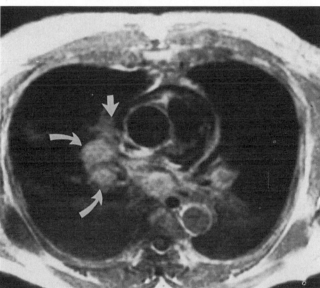

FIG. 5-28. Stage 3B disease: superior vena caval obstruction; contralateral lymphadenopathy, extranodal extension. A–C: Sequential MR images show extensive metastatic lymphadenopathy in a patient with a primary right upper lobe lung cancer (*curved arrow* in **B**). Note transcapular extension of disease from the nodes into surrounding fat, as well as encasement of the superior vena cava (*black arrows* in **A** and **B**). In addition, contralateral mediastinal lymph nodes are identifiable in **B**, just anterior to the left main pulmonary artery (*straight white arrow*), as well as enlarged subcarinal node and right hilar nodes surrounding the bronchus intermedius (*curved arrows* in **C**). Note that there are bilateral pleural effusions as well as pericardial effusion, the latter probably secondary to direct extension of tumor (*straight arrow* in **C**).

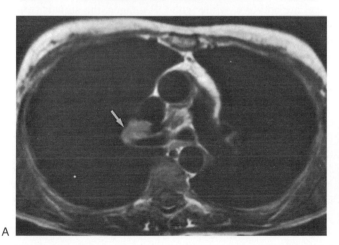

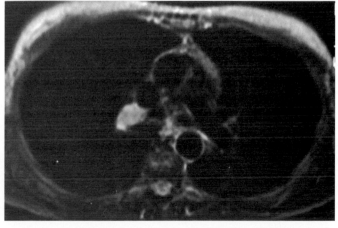

FIG. 5-29. Hilar lymphadenopathy: MRI evaluation. **A:** T1-weighted MR image through the right hilum shows evidence of moderately enlarged right hilar nodes just anterior to the right upper lobe bronchus (*arrow*), identifiable as a focal area of intermediate signal intensity (compare with the normal appearing left hilum). **B:** T2-weighted MRI scan at approximately the same level as in **A** shows considerably enhanced signal within the right hilum, again confirming the presence of enlarged nodes. Unfortunately, there is nothing in the appearance of these nodes that allows differentiation between benign and malignant lymphadenopathy. Surgically proven metastatic lymph nodes in a patient with a right upper lobe tumor (not shown).

evaluation of the pulmonary arteries or veins is requisite, gadolinium-enhanced MRI may be preferential.

Because of its better spatial resolution, CT is superior to MRI in determining the presence or extent of endobronchial tumors (106). As discussed in Chapter 3, in select cases in which proximal bronchial obstruction is associated with postobstructive pneumonitis, MRI can help by differentiating the obstructing carcinoma from surrounding atelectatic lung, especially on T2-weighted or gadolinium-enhanced images (see Chapter 3). In such patients, the consolidated lung typically exhibits a higher signal intensity than the central hilar mass (118–120).

Role of MR in Nodal Staging

Differentiation between mediastinal lymph nodes and mediastinal fat is easily accomplished on T1-weighted MRI sequences. In general, MRI is similar to CT in its ability to detect and define mediastinal lymph nodes (113). However, with the limited spatial resolution of MRI and its inability to obtain scans at suspended respiration, blurring of structures may occur. On occasion, several small lymph nodes have been mistaken by MRI for a single, large, abnormal node mass (106). As already noted, MRI is significantly disadvantaged because of its inability to detect calcification within mediastinal or hilar nodes. Although coronal or sagittal MRI may be helpful in studying aorticopulmonary window or subcarinal nodes, this is only occasionally indicated and clearly does not justify the routine use of MRI.

With the advent of MRI, it was hoped that malignant and benign nodes could be differentiated based on differences in relaxation times. In a study by De Geer et al., a difference was found in the T1 values of nodes enlarged because of sarcoidosis (mean, 544 ms) compared with nodes enlarged because of metastatic tumor (mean, 769 ms); unfortunately, however, considerable overlap between these groups existed (121). Glazer et al. performed an *in vitro* study of freshly resected nodes in patients with lung cancer (122). They found that although groups of involved and uninvolved nodes differed in average T1 values, with metastatic nodes exhibiting a longer T1 (mean, 640 ms versus 566 ms), there was too much overlap between the groups to allow differentiation. A preliminary report by Laissy et al. suggests that contrast-enhanced MR imaging may be helpful in distinguishing malignant from benign mediastinal lymph nodes (123). In this study, nine patients with bronchogenic carcinoma underwent dynamic MR imaging following intravenous bolus of gadoterate meglumine. Malignant mediastinal lymph nodes demonstrated marked enhancement whereas granulomatous and anthracotic lymph nodes displayed only minimal enhancement (123).

The Role of MR in the Assessment of Distant Metastases

Because of the examination length and the cost, MRI is not recommended for routine staging of distant metastases in the upper abdomen. However, it may be used to further characterize adrenal masses seen on CT (Figs. 5-30 and 5-31). It has been recently shown that adrenal masses with CT attenuation values of 18 HU or less can be confidently diagnosed as representing adenomas (see Fig. 5-21) (97,98). The positive predictive value for the diagnosis of adenomas using this threshold value was 100% and the negative predictive value 77%. The discrimination between adenomas and metastatic bronchogenic carcinomas or other adrenal tumors on CT is better without the use of intravenous contrast (97). MRI may be helpful in further characterizing adrenal lesions that have attenuation values greater than 18 HU. Features that suggest a malignant lesion include large size (greater than 3 cm); irregular margins, with or without invasion of adjacent structures; inhomogeneous CT density; and a thick, irregular, enhancing rim (124).

On MR, metastases have a higher signal intensity than most adenomas on T2-weighted sequences. Ratios of the intensity of the adrenal tumor to adjacent liver, muscle, or fat have been used (125–128). Metastatic lesions tend to have a higher signal intensity than that of liver or muscle and near or higher than that of fat, whereas benign adenomas have signal intensities similar to or less than that of liver. Pheochromocytomas characteristically exhibit very high T2-weighted signal intensity. Unfortunately, some overlap can be observed in the relaxation times of benign and malignant masses (128). The efficacy of various MRI sequences for the differentiation of adrenal masses was assessed in 46 patients with a total of 53 adrenal masses (129). Gradient-recalled echo (GRE) sequences with chemical-shift induced signal change (see Fig. 5-31) and T2-weighted imaging allowed the best differentiation of adenomas, metastases, and pheochromyocytomas. With GRE sequences, echo times can be varied to produce fat and water signals that are either in-phase (IP) or out-of-phase (or opposed phase) (OP). On IP images, the signals from water and lipids within the same voxel are additive, while with OP images, the signals from water and fat within the same voxel are destructive. The resultant signal is equal to the absolute value of the vector sum of the two. Loss of signal in a voxel containing both water and fat protons allows confident identification of fat within adrenal adenomas (see Fig. 5-31). Use of a short TE is particularly important, as this not only maximizes anatomic coverage in a given TR, but also improves T1 contrast as there is less T2 decay allowing improved signal to noise (S/N).

Although these techniques allowed accurate differentiation of groups of lesions, significant overlap has been noted in individual patients. This has led some authors to conclude that MR is not accurate enough to allow a confident diagnosis (129). In our experience, one-third of cases with positive adrenal findings present with small (less than 1.5 cm) adrenal masses with low signal intensity on T2-weighted scans, a typical presentation of nonfunctioning cortical adenomas. In another one-third of cases, lesions demonstrate a combination of features including large size, irregular margins, and

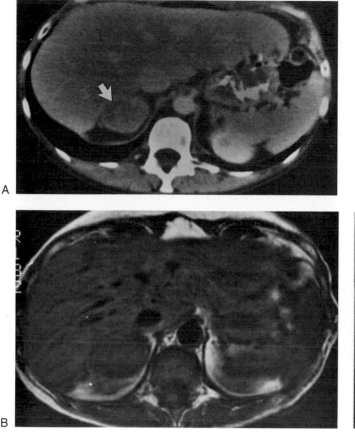

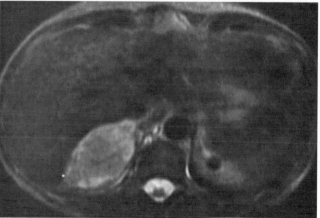

FIG. 5-30. Stage 4 disease: adrenal metastases. **A:** Contrast-enhanced CT scan through the adrenals shows an approximately 3 × 3 cm mass in the right adrenal gland (*arrow*) in a patient with known adenocarcinoma of the lung metastatic to mediastinal lymph nodes. **B,C:** T1- and T2-weighted MR images at the same level as in **A**, respectively. The right adrenal mass appears moderately hyperintense on the T2-weighted image relative to liver with slight heterogeneity, features suggestive of metastatic disease (histologically confirmed adrenal metastases).

heterogeneity, although predominantly high intensity, on T2-weighted scans; these findings all suggest metastatic disease. In the majority of these cases, intrathoracic disease is almost always advanced, generally involving T2 or T3 lesions associated with evidence of enlarged mediastinal nodes. Finally, in one-third of cases, lesions measure be-

tween 1.5 and 2.5 cm in size, morphologic or signal features are not characteristic, and needle biopsies are required for further diagnosis.

Although MRI is of only limited value in the assessment of adrenal and liver metastases, gadolinium-enhanced MR imaging is far superior to CT in the detection of cerebral

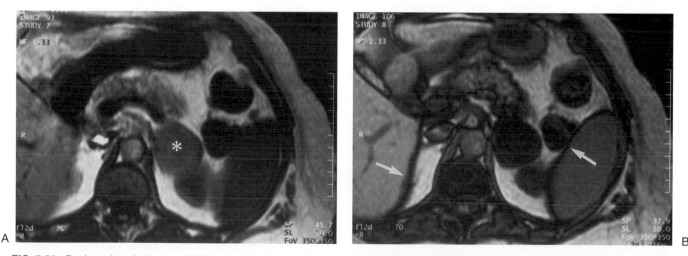

FIG. 5-31. Benign adrenal adenoma: MR evaluation. **A:** In-phase breathhold gradient-recalled echo (GRE) image at 1.0T (160/6/70, TR/TE/Flip angle) demonstrates a left adrenal mass (*asterisk*) brighter in signal intensity than the adjacent spleen. **B:** Opposed-phase (OP) GRE image (160/4/70) shows that the signal intensity of the mass is now hypointense compared to the spleen. This decrease in signal intensity is due to destructive interference between the signals from cytoplasmic fat and water within the adrenal lesion. Increased fat within the cytoplasm leading to signal decrease on this OP image is the histologic substrate used for making the diagnosis of an adrenal adenoma. Note the characteristic "India ink" artifact where the liver and spleen interface with adjacent fat (*arrows*). (Case courtesy of Neil Rofsky, M.D., New York University Medical Center, New York, NY.)

metastases. It is likely that the prevalence of asymptomatic brain metastases in asymptomatic patients is higher than the approximately 5% suggested on meta-analysis of CT data (94). Because the prevalence of metastases is higher in patients with T3 lesions and in patients with adenocarcinoma, it would seem reasonable to perform MRI of the brain in these patients even if they are asymptomatic.

ROLE OF MR AND CT IN THE FOLLOW-UP OF TREATED LUNG CANCER

In select cases, MRI seems to be able to differentiate tumor from fibrosis. In patients who have undergone radiation therapy for treatment of carcinoma, radiation-induced fibrosis in a recurrent tumor can be difficult to differentiate with CT. It has been reported that recurrent tumor can be distinguished from posttreatment radiation fibrosis by using T2-weighted MRI pulse sequences (130). In a study of 12 patients, posttreatment fibrosis had a low signal intensity on both T1- and T2-weighted images, whereas tumor showed relatively increased intensity on T2-weighted sequences. Unfortunately, such differentiation is difficult in patients who have recently completed treatment because inflammatory reaction secondary to radiation therapy may also lead to high signal intensity on T2-weighted sequences. In addition, associated inflammatory disease from other causes cannot

be differentiated from recurrent tumor. Another problem encountered in attempting to differentiate postradiation fibrosis from tumor recurrence within the lung is that retained secretions within airways can simulate recurrent tumor. It is presumed that destruction of the ciliated epithelium in the paramediastinal regions of the lung following radiation therapy prevents effective clearance of secretions. These secretions generate high T2-weighted signal because of their high free-water content.

A far more prosaic use of MRI is in the evaluation of patients following lobectomy or pneumonectomy. In this regard, CT is generally more useful to evaluate recurrent disease (Figs. 5-32 and 5-33). MRI may be especially valuable (a) in patients in whom extensive surgical clips limit CT interpretation, and (b) in patients unable to receive intravenous contrast (Fig. 5-34). In the setting of patients who require multiple follow-up examinations, MRI can replace CT as the imaging method of choice.

SUMMARY: CT/MR CORRELATIONS

It is apparent that the use of CT in staging patients with lung cancer has gained wide acceptance (see Fig. 5-18) (4). In 1986, Pearson reported on the lung cancer incidences in Toronto over the past 25 years (131). In his experience, the number of thoracotomies for unresectable disease had de-

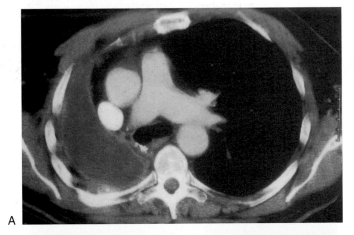

A

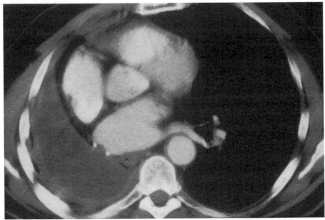

B

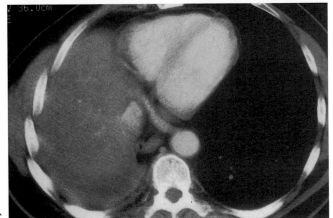

C

FIG. 5-32. Postpneumonectomy space: CT evaluation. **A–C:** Sequential contrast enhanced CT images show characteristic appearance of a normal postpneumonectomy space. Note that fluid fills the pneumonectomy space: pleural surfaces remain smooth except at the base of the right hemithorax. This appearance is typical and should not be misconstrued as evidence of pleural malignancy. Note the presence of surgical clips at the level of the right main bronchus. Use of contrast is recommended in these cases to facilitate identification of normal mediastinal, pleural and chest wall structures.

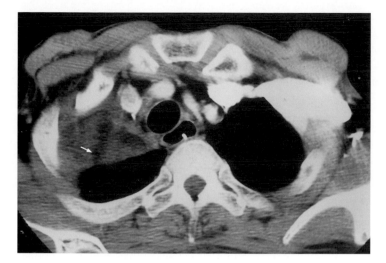

FIG. 5-33. Postlobectomy space: CT evaluation. Contrast-enhanced CT section following resection of the right upper lobe shows heterogeneous density in the anterior portion of the hemithorax. Although this superficially mimics tumor, the presence of fat (*arrow*) in this case is the clue that this appearance is caused by the use of a pectoral flap to occupy the postlobectomy space. In general the key to interpreting scans following lobectomy is to match surgical clips with the appropriate corresponding airway(s).

creased from 25% to 5%, with operative mortality decreasing from 10% to 3%, and 5-year survival increasing from 23% to 40%. Pearson cited better selection of surgical candidates owing to both invasive and noninvasive techniques as the major factor for these improved statistics. That CT has had a significant impact on lung cancer staging has also been documented by Epstein et al. (31). In a survey of over 500 thoracic surgeons, 98% of the responding surgeons advocated the use of CT, and more than one-third said they used it routinely. Surgeons cited the determination of resectability in patients with a central mass, with or without associated atelectasis, a prominent hilum, or an abnormal mediastinum on plain chest radiography as the most important indications. These results appear to indicate that for most surgeons, the major contribution of CT staging lies in its use as a diagnostic tool preventing unnecessary thoracotomies, excluding ad-

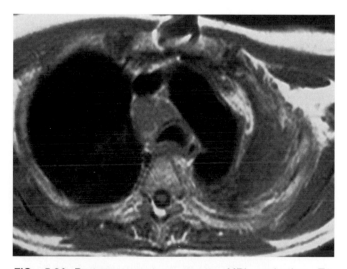

FIG. 5-34. Postpneumonectomy space: MRI evaluation. T1-weighted MR image through the mediastinum shows enlarged pretracheal nodes following a left-sided pneumonectomy. MR should replace CT in patients with extensive surgical clips, or in whom intravenous contrast is contraindicated.

vanced cases of lung cancer from surgical consideration. Significantly, only 57% of surgeons agreed that a negative CT examination of the mediastinum obviated the need for mediastinoscopy.

It is our belief, too, that the first and foremost contribution of CT staging is to exclude patients with clear-cut invasion of major structures or evidence of otherwise unsuspected metastatic disease from surgical consideration. New prospective studies with carefully controlled patient populations and pathologic correlation indicate a lower accuracy for CT in the staging of nodal metastases. This lower accuracy, foreseen by earlier investigators, has been confirmed by several independent groups. As the role of CT has been assessed, the staging system itself has been revised. This revision was prompted by new evidence indicating that aggressive surgery, with or without adjuvant forms of therapy, may offer improved prospects for patients with lung cancer. Resection of ipsilateral lymph node metastases, when confined to normal-sized nodes in particular, appears to enhance survival. As a consequence, in our opinion, a negative CT examination (with normal-sized nodes less than 10 mm in diameter) can be construed as justification to bypass preoperative staging procedures including mediastinoscopy. However, this statement should be tempered by the fact that left-sided lung lesions have a higher propensity for contralateral nodal metastases. Furthermore, because of partial volume effects in the region of the aorticopulmonary window and subcarinal space, these lesions may be more difficult to stage with conventional CT. Careful examination of the contralateral mediastinum, especially in left-sided lesions, is mandatory. Significantly, the accuracy of CT in staging distant sites, such as contralateral nodal stations, has not been addressed by prospective studies. For now, a reasonable solution to this problem would be to initiate preoperative mediastinal exploration whenever enlarged nodes are found in the mediastinum contralateral to a known tumor.

Although small-sized positive nodes should not influence management, enlarged lymph nodes should always be aggressively pursued. Patients should never be denied a potentially curative resection based solely on the radiographic appearance of lymph nodes. Because they may represent benign disease, enlarged nodes should always be assessed histologically. This policy will provide a firm rationale for decisions about curative resection. Although evidence suggests that grossly enlarged nodes are more likely to exhibit capsular penetration, a poor prognostic indicator, until more data is accumulated concerning the accuracy of CT in predicting capsular invasion, in most cases histologic proof is still strongly recommended for any enlarged mediastinal nodes, especially those in regions 4R, 2R, 10L, 4L, and 2L.

It should be emphasized that in the report by Epstein et al., only 10% of surgeons indicated that CT was useful in patients with small peripheral nodules (31). Indeed, there is some controversy about the utility of CT in patients with small peripheral nodules and an apparently normal mediastinum on plain chest radiographs (132–134). Pearlberg et al. found that CT contributed useful information in only 1 of 23 patients with T1N0M0 lesions (132). On the other hand, Heavey et al. found significant findings in 5 of 31 patients with peripheral nodules (133). Seely et al. assessed the prevalence of mediastinal nodal metastases and diagnostic accuracy of CT in 104 patient with T1 lesions (80). Nodal metastases were present in 22 patients (21%). Although CT had a sensitivity of only 59% for the detection of nodal metastases, the specificity was 91%. The authors therefore recommended that CT be performed in all patients with lung cancer (80).

It should be emphasized that the role of CT in evaluating patients with solitary pulmonary nodules depends on whether or not a diagnosis of cancer has or has not been established. In patients in whom a diagnosis of cancer has not been established, CT may be of considerable value by detecting the presence of either significant calcification or fat, findings indicative of benign disease. CT may also help in determining the best approach to obtaining histology by predicting the likely results of transbronchial biopsy versus transthoracic needle aspiration or biopsy. In patients with undiagnosed disease, CT should always be obtained prior to surgical resection. In patients in whom a diagnosis of cancer has already been established, as already indicated, the role of CT is more controversial. Although no dogmatic advice can be offered, in our experience, patients with peripheral adenocarcinomas and small cell undifferentiated carcinomas exhibit a higher incidence of mediastinal nodal disease than patients with squamous cell cancers. Consequently, we recommend that CT scans be obtained when tumors of these cell types are identified. In addition, given the propensity for contralateral metastases in left-sided lesions, it may be prudent to scan all left-sided T1N0M0 lesions regardless of cell type.

The main role of MRI at this time is as a problem-solving tool. Limited and focused MRI examinations should be used to evaluate or to resolve specific questions related to invasion of the chest wall or mediastinum, especially in the evaluation of vascular or neural invasion. MRI may also be valuable, albeit to a lesser extent, in adrenal mass characterization. Finally, MRI should be considered an alternative for all patients who cannot tolerate the administration of intravenous contrast media.

^{18}FDG-POSITRON EMISSION TOMOGRAPHY

Given the relatively poor sensitivity and specificity of both CT and MRI for staging lung cancer, it is not surprising that considerable interest has focused on the potential role of positron emission tomography (PET), especially with 2-(fluorine-18)-fluoro-2-deoxy-D-glucose (FDG) (135–139). FDG is a D-glucose analog radiopharmaceutical labeled with a positron emitter ^{18}F that is facilitatively transported through the cell membrane and phosphorylated using normal glycolytic pathways, especially by primitive fermenting cells with a high anaerobic:aerobic metabolic ratio (137). This includes neoplastic cells, irrespective of cell type, as well as inflammatory cells. Failure of further metabolism results in intracellular trapping of the tracer.

The efficacy of FDG-PET for lung cancer staging has been evaluated for both the intra and extrathoracic spread of disease. The role of ^{18}FDG-PET scans in the evaluation of solitary pulmonary nodules is discussed in detail in Chapter 4. To date, despite considerable variability, the reported sensitivities and specificities of ^{18}FDG-PET scans for identifying mediastinal nodal (N2) metastases have consistently outperformed both CT and MRI (Fig. 5-35). Valk et al., for example, in a prospective study of 76 patients with nonsmall cell lung cancer (NSCLC) with histologically or clinically documented mediastinal disease reported a sensitivity and specificity for the diagnosis of N2 disease of 83% and 94% with ^{18}FDG-PET compared with 63% and 73% for CT, respectively (136). Similar results have been reported by others (135,137,140–143). Comparing blinded prospective interpretations of CT scans alone, PET alone, CT and PET together and fusion images in 23 patients with either newly diagnosed or suspected NSCLC, Wahl et al. found both PET alone and fusion images to have a sensitivity of 82%, specificity of 81% and an accuracy of 81% compared to CT alone, which proved only 64% sensitive, 44% specific and 52% accurate (142). Although less impressive results have been noted for evaluating N1 disease, presumably because of a greater prevalence of hyperplastic intrapulmonary or hilar nodes, ^{18}FDG-PET has also been noted to be more accurate in this group as well (135,136).

More impressive still have been the results of studies employing total body ^{18}FDG-PET scanning for staging lung cancer. Bury et al., in a prospective study of comparing the efficacy of whole body ^{18}FDG-PET to conventional imaging in 109 patients found distant metastatic foci (n = 59) in 39 patients: of these, ^{18}FDG-PET correctly changed the M status in 15 (14%) (138). Although there were five false-positive sites, including moderate ^{18}FDG uptake in two patients with enlarged axillary nodes as well as on patient with a

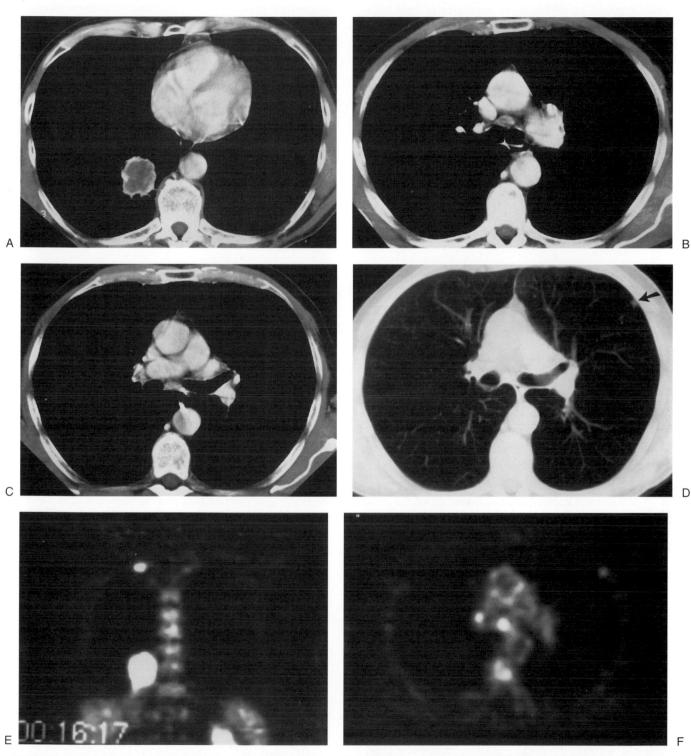

FIG. 5-35. 18FDG-PET: Lung cancer staging. **A:** Contrast-enhanced CT section shows an irregular mass in the right lower lobe. **B,C:** Sequential sections through the carina and subcarinal space, respectively, show enlarged precarinal nodes on **B**; subcarinal nodes are within the upper limits of normal in size. **D:** Identical section as in **C**, imaged with lung windows shows a small subpleural nodule present in the left upper lobe (*arrow*). **E:** Coronal image from 2-[fluorine-18]-fluoro-2-deoxy-D-glucose (FDG)-positron emission tomography (PET) scan shows marked tracer uptake in the primary lesion in the right lower lobe as well as within a right supraclavicular node, not appreciated on the corresponding CT (not shown). Note that moderate uptake is also present in the marrow, liver and spleen and upper pole of the left kidney. **F:** Axial image from the same study shows marked uptake within both subcarinal and right hilar nodes. There is also uptake noted in the subpleural nodule identified on the CT scan in the left upper lobe. This lesion was subsequently confirmed to represent a contralateral pulmonary metastasis. This case clearly illustrates the potential role of PET as a method for more definitive lung cancer staging compared to CT. (Case courtesy of Edward Patz, M.D., Duke University, Durham, NC.)

substernal goiter, by comparison, there were at total of 14 false positive CT examinations. There were no false negative studies. Similar results have been reported by others (135,144). Valk et al. found unsuspected distant metastases in 11 (11%) of 99 patients (136). Normal PET scans were obtained in 19 patients with abnormal CT studies only one of which proved to be falsely negative.

PET scanning has also proved of value for assessing disease recurrence (145–148). As summarized by Hughes, in a review of recent studies including total of 219 patients, recurrent cancer was missed in only four (3%) of 139 cases

of recurrent tumor (137). At the same time, the corresponding false positive rate was 15 (81%) of 80 cases reported, giving an overall accuracy of 91%.

Despite these consistently positive reports, it should be emphasized that there are a number of important limitations to the use of ^{18}FDG-PET. As noted by Heelan, given its limited spatial resolution, ^{18}FDG PET is of little value for assessing local tumor extent (T disease) especially for evaluating invasion of contiguous structures such as the chest wall, bronchi, or mediastinal structures (Fig. 5-36) (149). Although this has led some to investigate the use of fusion

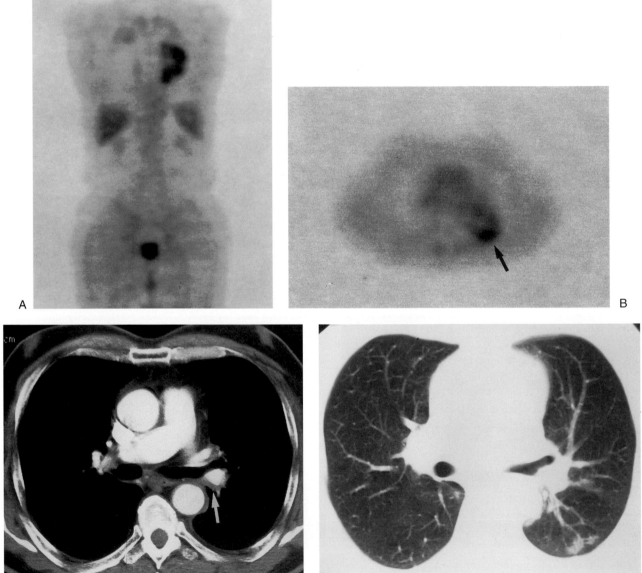

FIG. 5-36. ^{18}FDG PET: Evaluation of tumor recurrence. **A,B:** Coronal and axial views, respectively, from a positron-emission tomography (PET) scan obtained from a patient 6 months after radiation therapy for nonsmall cell lung cancer initially involving the left hilum. While marked uptake is present on both the coronal and axial views, precise anatomic localization is difficult: The appearance on the coronal view is consistent with nodal disease, while localization on the axial view appears to be predominantly posterior (*arrow* in **B**). **C:** Contrast-enchanced CT section shows only minimal residual soft tissue density in the left hilum posterior to the interlobar pulmonary artery (*arrow*) as well as adjacent to the descending aorta. **D:** Section at a slightly lower level than in **C** shows ill-defined, patchy consolidation in the superior segment of the left lower lobe. These findings on CT are compatible with prior radiation therapy with mild radiation pneumonitis and minimal residual fibrosis in the left hilum, accounting for the changes seen on the corresponding PET images. Lack of anatomic detail is an important potential limitation of PET scanning and is one rationale for CT–PET correlation.

images, in fact these are likely to prove of little additional value as compared to simply combining the physiologic data inherent in PET scanning with the superior spatial resolution of CT by themselves (142). In this regard, as noted by Hughes, although the sensitivity, specificity, and accuracy of PET versus CT for assessing mediastinal metastases in 30 patients with NSCLC proved to be 78%, 81%, and 80% for PET compared with 56%, 86%, and 77% respectively, the diagnostic accuracy of combined CT and PET imaging equaled 90% (137).

[18]FDG normally accumulates in a number of sites, including especially the brain, heart, renal collecting system, and bladder. This limits evaluation of tumor in these locations, especially within the brain. In order to enhance evaluation of the pelvis, some routinely catheterize patients prior to evaluation. Moderate activity is also commonly noted in the liver, spleen, bone marrow, breast and gastrointestinal tract. Within the thorax, 18FDG also accumulates in both residual thymic tissue as well as thyroid tissue, including nodular goiters, sites easily mistaken for mediastinal metastases (138). It should also be noted that [18]FDG PET may be of limited value in diabetics: This is because elevations of blood glucose (or insulin levels) leads to increased accumulation of FDG in muscle and decreased accumulation of uptake within malignant tissue (139).

Perhaps most important, PET scanners are still not generally available even though the price of these is now comparable to spiral CT or magnetic resonance scanners. As a consequence, recent interest has focused on the potential of either 511-keV SPECT or coincidence imaging with dual-detector single photon emission computed tomographic (SPECT) cameras as an alternate method for emission scanning. Unfortunately, to date, neither of these methods provides equivalent spatial resolution compared to dedicated PET scanners. In a recent study, Shreve et al. compared a dual-head SPECT scanner with a dedicated PET scanner in 31 patients with known or suspected malignant neoplasms undergoing total body PET scans (150). Although SPECT identified 13 (93%) of 14 lung nodules or masses, only 20 (65%) of 31 mediastinal nodes were correctly identified compared with PET. Furthermore, only 11 (50%) of 22 bone metastases and six (23%) of 26 abdominal tumor deposits were correctly identified by the coincidence gamma camera (150). These data suggest that pending further technologic improvements, SPECT imaging will remain of only limited value for lung cancer staging.

Despite these limitations, it is apparent that the impact of [18]FDG PET scanning in oncologic imaging is likely to increase especially with increasing availability of both PET scanners and isotopes. It is likely that in the near future, optimal lung cancer diagnosis and staging will require some combination of both PET and CT.

REFERENCES

1. Wingo P, Tong T, Bolden S. Cancer Statistics 1995. *Cancer J Clin* 1995;45:8–31.
2. Mountain CF. Revisions in the International System for Staging Lung Cancer. *Chest* 1997;111:1710–1717.
3. Mountain CF, Dresler CM. Regional lymph node classification for lung cancer staging. *Chest* 1997;111:1718–1723.
4. Society ATSER. Pretreatment evaluation of non-small-cell lung cancer. *Am J Resp Crit Care Med* 1997;156:320–332.
5. Denoix PF. Enquete permanent dans les centres anticancereux. *Bull Inst Nat Hyg* 1946;1:70.
6. American Joint Committee for Cancer Staging and End Results Reporting. *Clinical staging system for carcinoma of the lung.* Philadelphia: JB Lippincott, 1973.
7. Staging of Lung Cancer 1979. American Joint Committee for Cancer Staging and End-results Reporting: Task Force on Lung Cancer. Chicago, 1979.
8. Mountain CF. A new international staging system for lung cancer. *Chest* 1986;89:225S–233S.
9. Little AG, Stitik FP. Clinical staging of patients with non-small cell lung cancer. *Chest* 1990;97:1431–1438.
10. Bains MS. Surgical Treament of Lung Cancer. ACCP Section Report (part 2). *Chest* 1991;100:826–837.
11. McCaughan BC, Martini N, Bains MS, McCormick PM. Chest wall invasion in carcinoma of the lung: therapeutic and prognostic implications. *J Thorac Cardiovasc Surg* 1985;89:836–841.
12. Mountain CF. The biologic operability of stage III non-small cell lung cancer. *Ann Thorac Surg* 1985;40:60–64.
13. Paone JF, Spees EK, Newton CG, et al. An appraisal of en bloc resection of peripheral bronchogenic carcinoma involving the thoracic wall. *Chest* 1982;81:203–207.
14. Paulson DL. Carcinomas in the superior pulmonary sulcus. *J Thorac Cardiocasc Surg* 1975;70:1095–1104.
15. Piehler JM, Pairolero PC, Weiland LH. Bronchogenic carcinoma with chest wall invasion: factors affecting survival following en bloc resection. *Ann Thorac Surg* 1982;34:684–691.
16. Trastek VF, Pairolero PC, Piehler JM. En bloc (non-chest wall) resection for bronchogenic carcinoma with parietal fixation: factors affecting survival. *J Thorac Cardiovasc Surg* 1984;87:352–358.
17. Pearlberg JL, Sandler MA, Beute GH, Lewis Jr. JW, Madrazo BL. Limitations of CT in evaluation of neoplasms involving the chest wall. *J Comput Assist Tomogr* 1987;11:290–293.
18. Libshitz HI. Computed tomography in bronchogenic carcinoma. *Semin Roentgenol* 1990;25:64–72.
19. Scott IR, Müller NL, Miller RR, Evans KG, Nelems B. Resectable stage III lung cancer: CT, surgical, and pathologic correlation. *Radiology* 1988;166:75–79.
20. Pennes DR, Glazer GM, Wimbish KJ, et al. Chest wall invasion by lung cancer: limitations of CT evaluation. *AJR Am J Roentgenol* 1985;144:507–511.
21. Glazer HS, Duncan MJ, Aronberg DJ, Moran JF, Levitt RG, Sagel SS. Pleural and chest wall invasion in bronchogenic carcinoma: CT evaluation. *Radiology* 1985;157:191–194.
22. Shirakawa T, Fukuda K, Miyamoto Y, Tanabe H, Tada S. Parietal pleural invasion of lung massess: evaluation with CT performed during deep inspiration and expiration. *Radiology* 1994;192:809–811.
23. Murata K, Takahashi M, Mori M, et al. Chest wall and mediastinal invasion by lung cancer: evaluation with multisection expiratory dynamic CT. *Radiology* 1994;191:251–255.
24. Watanabe A, Shimokata K, Saka H, Nomura F, Sakai S. Chest CT combined with artificial pneumothorax: value in determining origin and extent of tumor. *AJR Am J Roentgenol* 1991;156:707–710.
25. Yokoi K, Mori K, Miyazawa N, et al. Tumor invasion of the chest wall and mediastinum in lung cancer: evaluation with pneumothorax CT. *Radiology* 1991;181:147–152.
26. Gilbert A, Deslauriers JJ, McLish A, Piraaux M. Tracheal sleeve pneumonectomy for carcinoma of the proximal left main bronchus. *Can J Surg* 1984;27:583–585.
27. Jensik RJ, Faber LP, Kittle CF, et al. Survival in patients undergoing tracheal sleeve pneumonectomy for bronchogenic carcinoma. *J Thorac Cardiovasc Surg* 1982;84:489–496.
28. Glazer HS, Kaiser LR, Anderson DJ, et al. Indeterminate mediastinal invasion in bronchogenic carcinoma: CT evaluation. *Radiology* 1989;173:37–42.
29. Baron RL, Levitt RG, Sagel SS, et al. Computed tomography in the preoperative evaluation of bronchogenic carcinoma. *Radiology* 1982;145:727–732.
30. Webb WR, Gatsonis C, Zerhouni EA, et al. CT and MR imaging in

staging non-small cell bronchogenic carcinoma: report of the Radiologic Diagnostic Oncology Group. *Radiology* 1991;178:705–713.

31. Epstein DM, Stephenson LW, Gefter WB, et al. Value of CT in the preoperative assessment of lung cancer: a survey of thoracic surgeons. *Radiology* 1986;161:423–427.

32. Primack SL, Lee KS, Logan PM, Miller RR, Müller NL. Bronchogenic carcinoma: utility of CT in the evaluation of patients with suspected lesions. *Radiology* 1994;193:795–800.

33. Herman SJ, Winton TL, Weisbrod GL, Towers MJ, Mentzer SJ. Mediastinal invasion by bronchogenic carcinoma: CT signs. *Radiology* 1994;190:841–846.

34. White PG, Adams H, Butchart EG. Preoperative staging of carcinoma of the bronchus: can computed tomography scanning reliably identify stage III tumors? *Thorax* 1994;49:951–957.

35. Naruke T, Suemasu K, Ishikawa S. Lymph node mapping and curability at various levels of metastasis in resected lung cancer. *J Thorac Cardiovasc Surg* 1978;76:832–839.

36. Naruke T, Goya T, Tsuchiya R, Suemasu K. The importance of surgery to non-small cell carciinoma of lung with mediastinal lymph node metastasis. *Ann Thorac Surg* 1988;46:603–610.

37. Kirschner PA. Lung cancer: preopertive radiation therapy and surgery. *NY State J Med* 1981;81:339.

38. Martini N, Flehinger BJ, Zaman MB, Beattie EJ. Results of resection in non-oat cell carcinoma of the lung with mediastinal lymph node metastases. *Ann Surg* 1983;198:386–397.

39. Martini N, Flehinger BJ. The role of surgery in N2 lung cancer. *Surg Clin North Am* 1987;67:1037–1049.

40. Pearson FG, DeLaure NC, Ilves Rea. Significance of positive superior mediastinal nodes identified at mediastinoscopy in patients with resectable cancer of the lung. *J Thorac Cardiovasc Surg* 1982;83:1–11.

41. Coughlin M, Deslauriers J, Beaulieu Mea. Role of mediastinoscopy in pre-treatment staging of patients with primary lung cancer. *Ann Thorac Surg* 1985;40:556–560.

42. Bergh NP, Schersten T. Bronchogenic carcinoma: a follow-up study of a surgically treated series with special reference to the prognostic significance of lymph node metastasis. *Acta Chir Scan (Suppl)* 1965;341:1–42.

43. Little AG, DeMeester TR, MacMahon H. The staging of lung cancer. *Semin Oncol* 1983;10:56–70.

44. Kirsh MM, Sloan H. Mediastinal metastases in bronchogenic carcinoma: influence of postoperative irradiation, cell type, and location. *Ann Thorac Surg* 1982;33:459–463.

45. Smith RA. The importance of mediastinal lymph node invasion by pulmonary carcinoma in selection of patients for resection. *Ann Thorac Surg* 1978;25:5–11.

46. Tisi GM, Friedman PJ, Peters RM, et al. Clinical staging of primary lung cancer. *Am Rev Respir Dis* 1983;127:659–664.

47. Wang K-P. Staging of bronchogenic carcinoma by bronchoscopy. *Chest* 1994;106:588–593.

48. Glazer HS, Aronberg DJ, Sagel SS, Friedman PJ. CT demonstration of calcified mediastinal lymph nodes: a guide to the new ATS classification. *AJR Am J Roentgenol* 1986;147:17–20.

49. Quint LE, Glazer GM, Orringer MB. Mediastinal lymph node detection and sizing at CT and autospy. *AJR Am J Roentgenol* 1986;147:469–472.

50. Genereux GP, Howie JL. Normal mediastinal lymph node size and number: CT and anatomic study. *AJR Am J Roentgenol* 1984;142:1095–1100.

51. Ashida C, Zerhouni EA, Fishman EK. CT demonstration of prominent right hilar soft tissue collections. *J Comput Assist Tomogr* 1987;11:57–59.

52. Aronberg DJ, Peterson RR, Glazer HS. The superior sinus of the pericardium: CT appearance. *Radiology* 1985;153:489–492.

53. Haramati LB, Cartagena AM, Austin JHM. CT evaluation of mediastinal lymphadenopathy: non-contrast 5 mm vs. post-contrast 10 mm. sections. *J Comput Assist Tomogr* 1995;19:375–378.

54. Rouviere H. *Anatomy of the human lymphatic system.* Ann Arbor, MI: Edwards, 1938.

55. Borrie J. Primary carcinoma of the bronchus: prognosis following surgical resection. *Ann R Coll Surg Engl* 1952;10:165–168.

56. Nohl-Oser HC. Lymphatics of the lung. In: Shields TW, ed. *General thoracic surgery.* Philadelphia: Lea and Febiger, 1989.

57. Libshitz HI, McKenna RJ, Mountain CF. Patterns of mediastinal metastases in bronchogenic carcinoma. *Chest* 1986;90:229–232.

58. Nohl-Oser HC. An investigation of the anatomy of the lymphatic drainage of the lungs. *Ann R Coll Surg Engl* 1972;51:157–176.

59. Faling LJ, Pugatch RD, Jung-Legg Y, et al. Computed tomographic scanning of the mediastinum in the staging of bronchogenic carcinoma. *Am Rev Resp Dis* 1981;124:690–695.

60. Moak GD, Cockerill EM, Farber MD, Yaw PB, Manfredi F. Computed tomography vs. standard radiology in the evaluation of mediastinal adenopathy. *Chest* 1982;82:69–75.

61. Osborne DR, Korobkin M, Ravin CE. Comparison of plain radiography, conventional tomography, and computed tomography in detecting intrathoracic lymph node metastases from lung carcinoma. *Radiology* 1982;142:157–161.

62. Lewis Jr JW, Mdrazo BL, Gross SC, et al. The value of radiography and computed tomography in the staging of lung carcinoma. *Ann Thorac Surg* 1982;34:553–558.

63. Libshitz HI, McKenna RJ. Mediastinal lymph node size in lung cancer. *AJR Am J Roentgenol* 1984;143:715–718.

64. Libshitz HI, McKenna RJ, Haynie TP, McMurtrey MJ, Mountain CT. Mediastinal evaluation in lung cancer. *Radiology* 1984;151:295–299.

65. Daly BDT, Faling LJ, Pugatch RD, et al. Computed tomography: an effective technique for mediastinal staging in lung cancer. *J Thorac Cardiovasc Surg* 1984;88:486–494.

66. Glazer GM, Orringer MB, Gross BH, Quint LE. The mediastinum in non-small cell lung cancer: CT-surgical correlation. *AJR Am J Roentgenol* 1984;142:1101–1105.

67. Breyer RH, Karstaedt N, Mills SA. Computed tomography for evaluation of mediastinal lymph nodes in lung cancer: correlation with surgical staging. *Ann Thorac Surg* 1984;38:215–220.

68. Brion JP, Depau L, Kuhn Gea. Role of computed tomography and meiastinoscopy in preoperative staging of lung carcinoma. *J Comput Assist Tomogr* 1985;9:480–484.

69. Musset D, Grenier P, Carette MF, et al. Primary lung cancer staging: prospective comparative study of MR imaging with CT. *Radiology* 1986;160:607–611.

70. Rhoads AC, Thomas JH, Hemreck AS. Comparative studies of computerized tompgraphy and mediastinoscopy for the staging of bronchogenic carcinoma. *Am J Surg* 1986;152:587–591.

71. Staples CA, Müller NL, Miller RR, Evans KG, Nelems B. Mediastinal nodes in bronchogenic carcinoma: comparison between CT and mediastinoscopy. *Radiology* 1988;167:367–372.

72. McLoud TC, Bourgouin PM, Greenberg RW, et al. Bronchogenic carcinoma: analysis of staging in the mediastinum with CT by correlative lymph node mapping and sampling. *Radiology* 1992;182:319–323.

73. Schnyder PA, Gamsu G. CT of the pretracheal retrocaval space. *AJR Am J Roentgenol* 1981;136:303–308.

74. Glazer GM, Gross BH, Quint LE, et al. Normal mediastinal lymph nodes: number and size according to American Thoracic Society mapping. *AJR Am J Roentgenol* 1985;144:261–265.

75. Kiyono K, Sone S, Sakai Fea. The number and size of normal mediastinal lymph nodes: a postmortem study. *AJR Am J Roentgenol* 1988;150:771–776.

76. Buy JN, Ghossain MA, Poirson F, et al. Computed tomography of mediastinal lymph nodes in nonsmall cell lung cancer: a new approach based on the lymphatic pathway of tumor spread. *J Comput Assist Tomogr* 1988;12:545–552.

77. Glazer GM, Gross BH, Quint LE, et al. Normal mediastinal lymph nodes: number and size according to American Thoracic Society mapping. *AJR* 1985;144:261–265.

78. Hirleman MR, Yin-Chin VS, Chin LC, Schapiro RL. The resectability of primary lung carcinoma: a diagnostic staging review. *CT* 1980;4:146–163.

79. McKenna RJ, Libshitz HI, Mountain CF. Roentgenographic evaluation of mediastinal nodes for preoperative assessment in lung cancer. *Chest* 1985;88:206–210.

80. Seely JM, Mayo JR, Miller RR, Müller NL. T1 Lung cancer: prevalence of mediastinal nodal metastases and diagnostic accuracy of CT. *Radiology* 1993;186:129–132.

81. Dales RE, Stark RM, Raman S. Computed tomography to stage lung cancer: approaching a controversy using meta-analysis. *Am Rev Respir Dis* 1990;141:1096–1101.

82. Guyatt DH, Cook DJ, Walter S. The Canadian Lung Oncology Group. Investigation for mediastinal disease in patients with apparently operable lung cancer. *Ann Thorac Surg* 1995;60:1382–1389.

83. Pearson FG. Use of mediastinoscopy in selection of patients for lung cancer operations. *Ann Thorac Surg* 1980;30:205–207.

84. Ashraf MH, Milsom PL, Walesby RK. Selection by mediastinoscopy

and lung-term survival in bronchial carcinoma. *Ann Thorac Surg* 1980;30:208–214.

85. Daly BDT, Mueller JD, Faling LJ, et al. N2 lung cancer: outcome in patients with false-negative computed tomographic scans of the chest. *J Thorac Cardidovasc Surg* 1993;105:904–911.

86. Schenk DA, Bower JH, Bryan CL. Transbronchial needle aspiration staging of bronchogenic carcinoma. *Am Rev Resp Dis* 1986;134:146–148.

87. Boring CC, Squires SS, Tong T. Lung cancer. *Cancer J Clin* 1992;42:19–38.

88. Mathews MJ, Kanhouwa S, Peckren J, Robinette D. Frequency of residual and metastatic tumor in patients undergoing curative surgical resection in lung cancer. *Chem Rep* 1973;4:63–66.

89. Winstanley DP. Fruitless resections. *Thorax* 1968;23:327.

90. Sider L, Horejs D. Frequency of extrathoracic metastases from bronchogenic carcinoma in patients with normal-sized hilar and mediastinal lymph nodes on CT. *AJR Am J Roentgenol* 1988;151:893–895.

91. Salvatierra A, Baamonde C, Llamas JM, Cruz F, Lopez-Pujol J. Extrathoracic staging of bronchogenic carcinoma. *Chest* 1990;97:1052–1058.

92. Ferrigno D, Buccheri G. Cranial computed tomography as a part of the initial staging procedures for patients with non-small cell lung cancer. *Chest* 1994;106:1025–1029.

93. Kormas P, Bradshaw JR, Jeyasingham K. Preopertive computed tomography of the brain in non-small cell bronchogenic carcinoma. *Thorax* 1992;47:106–108.

94. Silvestri GA, Littenberg B, Colice GL. The clinical evaluation for detecting metastatic lung cancer: a meta-analysis. *Am Respir Crit Care Med* 1995;152:225–230.

95. Silverman P, ed. *Helical/spiral computed tomography. A practical approach to clinical protocols.* Philadelphia: Lippincott-Raven, 1998.

96. Oliver TW, Bernardino ME, Miller JI, et al. Isolated adrenal masses in nonsmall-cell bronchogenic carcinoma. *Radiology* 1984;153:217–218.

97. Korobkin M, Brodeur FJ, Yutzy GG, et al. Differentiation of adrenal adenomas from nonadenomas using CT attenuation values. *AJR Am J Roentgenol* 1996;166:531 536.

98. Macari M, Rofsky NM, Naidich DP, Megibow AJ. Utility of noncontrast helical CT of the adrenal glands in evaluating patients with non-small-cell lung cancer in an unmonitored environment. *Radiology* 1998 (*in press*).

99. Korobkin M, Brodeur FJ, Francis IR, et al. Delayed enhanced CT for differentiation of benign from malignant adrenal masses. *Radiology* 1996;200:737–742.

100. Stahel RA, Ginsberg R, Havemann Kea. Staging and prognostic factors in small cell lung cancer: a consensus report. *Lung Cancer* 1989;5:119–124.

101. Zwischenberger JB, Cox Jr CS. Staging and surgery for lung cancer. *J Thorac Imaging* 1991;84:641–648.

102. Meyer JA, Comis RL, Ginsber SJ. Selective surgical resection in small cell carcinoma of the lung. *J Thorac Cardiovasc Surg* 1982;84:641–648.

103. Meyer JA, Comis RL, Ginsber SJ, et al. The prospect of disease control by surgery combined with chemotherapy in stage I and II small cell carcinoma of the lung. *Ann Thorac Surg* 1983;36:37–41.

104. Ginsberg RJ. Surgery and small cell lung cancer: an overview. *Lung Cancer* 1989;5:22–236.

105. Davis S, Wright PW, Schulman SF, et al. Long term survival in small cell carcinoma of the lung. A population experience. *J Clin Oncol* 1985;3:80–91.

106. Webb WR, Jansen BC, Sollitto R, et al. Bronchogenic carcinoma: staging with MR compared with staging with CT and surgery. *Radiology* 1985;156:117–124.

107. Martini N, Heelan R, Westcott J, et al. Comparative merits of conventional, computed tomographic, and magnetic resonance imaging in assessing mediastinal involvement in surgically confirmed lung cancer. *J Thorac Cardiovasc Surg* 1985;90:639–648.

108. Patterson GA, Ginsberg RJ, Poon PYea. A prospective evluation of magnetic resonance imaging, computed tomography and mediastinoscopy in the preoperative assessment of mediastinal node status in bronchogenic carcinoma. *J Thorac Cardiovasc Surg* 1987;94:679–684.

109. Poon PY, Bronskill MJ, Henkelman RM, et al. Mediastinal lymph node metastases form bronchogenic carcinoma: detection with MR imaging and CT. *Radiology* 1987;162:651–656.

110. Grenier P, Dubray B, Carette MF, et al. Preoperative thoracic staging of lung cancer: CT and MR evaluation. *Diagn Inter Radiol* 1989;1:23–28.

111. Haggar AM, Pearlberg JL, Froelich JW, et al. Chest-wall invasion by carcinoma of the lung: detection by MR imaging. *AJR Am J Roentgenol* 1987;148:1075–1078.

112. Padovani B, Mouroux J, Seksik L, et al. Chest wall invasion by bronchogenic carcinoma: evaluation with MR imaging. *Radiology* 1993;187:33–38.

113. Webb WR, Jensen BJ, Gamsu G, Sollitto R, Moore EH. Sagittal MR imaging of the chest: normal and abnormal. *J Comput Assist Tomogr* 1985;9:471–479.

114. Heelan RT, Demas BE, Caravelli JF, et al. Superior sulcus tumors: CT and MR imaging. *Radiology* 1989;170:637–641.

115. Takasugi J, Rapoport S, Shaw C. Superior sulcus tumors: the role of imaging. *J Thorac Imag* 1989;4:41–48.

116. Blair DN, Rapoport S, Sostman HD, Blair OC. Normal brachial plexus: MR imaging. *Radiology* 1987;165:763–767.

117. Castagno AA, Shuman WP. MR imaging in clinically suspected brachial plexus tumor. *AJR Am J Roentgenol* 1987;149:1219–1222.

118. Webb WR, Kameda K, Adachi S, Kono M. Detection of T factor in lung cancer using MRI and CT. *J Thorac Imag* 1988;3:73–80.

119. Tobler J, Levitt RG, Glazer HS, et al. Differentiation of proximal bronchogenic carcinoma from postobstructive lobar collapse by magnetic resonance imaging: comparison with computed tomography. *Invest Radiol* 1987;22:538–543.

120. Herold CJ, Kuhlman JE, Zerhouni EA. Pulmonary atelectasis. *Radiology* 1991;178:715–720.

121. DeGeer G, Webb WR, Sollitto R, Golden J. MR characteristics of benign lymph node enlargement in sarcoiosis and Castleman's disease. *Eur J Radiol* 1986;6:145–148.

122. Glazer G, Orringer MB, Chenevert TL, et al. Mediastinal lymph nodes: relaxation time/pathologic correlation and implications in staging of lung cancer with MR imaging. *Radiology* 1988;168:429–431.

123. Laissy JP, Gay-Depassier P, Soyer P, et al. Enlarged mediastinal lymph nodes in bronchogenic carcinoma: assessment with dynamic contrast-enhanced MR imaging. *Radiology* 1994;191:263–267.

124. Berland LL, Koslin DB, Kenney PJ, et al. Differentiation between small benign and malignant adrenal masses with dynamic incremented CT. *AJR Am J Roentgenol* 1988;151:95–101.

125. Reinig JW, Doppman JL, Dwyer AJ, Frank J. MRI of indeterminate adrenal masses. *AJR Am J Roentgenol* 1986;147:493–496.

126. Glazer GM, Woolsey EJ, Borrello J, et al. Adrenal tissue characterization using MR imaging. *Radiology* 1986;158:73–79.

127. Chang A, Glazer HS, Lee JK, Ling D, Heiken JP. Adrenal gland: MR imaging. *Radiology* 1987;163:123–128.

128. Chezmar JL, Robbins SM, Nelson RC, et al. Adrenal masses: characterization with T1-weighted MR imaging. *Radiology* 1988;166:357–359.

129. Reinig JW, Stutley JE, Leonhardt CM, et al. Differentiation of adrenal massess with MR imaging: comparison of techniques. *Radiology* 1994;192:41–46.

130. Glazer HS, Lee JK, Levitt RG, et al. Radiation fibrosis: differentiation from recurrent tumor by MR imaging. *Radiology* 1985;156:721–726.

131. Pearson FG. Lung cancer: the past 25 years. *Chest* 1986;89:200S–205S.

132. Pearlberg JL, Sandler MA, Beute GH, Madrazo BL. T1N0M0 bronchogenic carcinoma: assessment by CT. *Radiology* 1985;157:187–190.

133. Heavey LR, Glazer GM, Gross BH, Francis IR, Orringer MB. The role of CT in staging radiogarphic T1N0M0 lung cancer. *AJR Am J Roentgenol* 1986;146:285–290.

134. Conces DJ, Klink JF, Tarver RD, Moak GD. T1N0M0 lung cancer: evaluation with CT. *Radiology* 1989;170:643–646.

135. Lewis P, Griffin S, Marsden P, et al. Whole-body F-18-fluorodeoxyglucose positron emission tomography in preoperative evaluation of lung cancer. *Lancet* 1994;344:1265–1266.

136. Valk PE, Pounds TR, Hopkins DM, et al. Staging non-small cell lung cancer by whole-body positron emission tomographic imaging. *Ann Thorac Surg* 1995;60:1573–1582.

137. Hughes JMB. 18F-Fluorodeoxyglucose PET scaans in lung cancer. *Thorax* 1996;51(Suppl 2):S16–S22.

138. Bury T, Dowlati A, Paulus P, et al. Evaluation of the solitary pulmonary nodule by positron emission tomography imaging. *Eur Resp J* 1996;9:410–414.

139. Gordon BA, Flanagan FL, Dehdashti F. Whole-body positron emis-

sion tomograpny: normal variations, pitfalls, and technical considerations. *AJR Am J Roentgenol* 1997;169:1675–1679.

140. Chin R, Ward R, Keyes JW, et al. Mediastinal staging of non-small-cell lung cancer with positron emission tomography. *Am J Resp Crit Care Med* 1995;152:2090–2096.

141. Sazon DAD, Santiago SM, Soo Hoo GW, et al. Fluorodeoxyglucose-positron emission tomography in the detection and staging of lung cancer. *Am J Respir Crit Care Med* 1996;153:417–421.

142. Wahl RL, Quint LE, Greenough RL, et al. Staging of mediastinal non-small cell lung cancer with FDG PET, CT, and fusion images: preliminary prospective evaluation. *Radiology* 1994;191:371–377.

143. Patz Jr EF, Lowe VJ, Goodman PC, Herndon J. Thoracic nodal staging with PET imaging with 18FDG in patients with bronchogenic carcinoma. *Chest* 1995;108:1617–1621.

144. Rege SD, Hoh CK, Glaspy JA, et al. Imaging of pulmonary mass lesions with whole-body positron emission tomography and fluorodeoxyglucose. *Cancer* 1993;72:82–90.

145. Duhaylongsod FG, Lowe VJ, Patz EF, et al. Detection of primary and recurrent lung cancer by means of F-18 fluorodeoxyglucose positron emission tomography (FDG PET). *J Thorac Cardiovas Surg* 1995;110:130–140.

146. Hubner KF, Buonocore E, Singh SK, Gould HR, Cotten DW. Characterization of chest masses by FDG positron emission tomography. *Clin Nucl Med* 1995;20:293–298.

147. Patz Jr ER, Lowe VJ, Hoffman JM, et al. Persistent or recurrent bronchogenic carcinoma: detection with PT and 2-(F-18)-fluoro-2-deoxy-D-glucose. *Radiology* 1994;191:379–382.

148. Inoue T, Kim EE, Komaki R, et al. Detecting recurrent or residual lung cancer with FDG-PET. *J Nucl Med* 1995;36:788–793.

149. Heelan RT. Invited commentary. *Ann Thorac Surg* 1995;60:1573.

150. Shreve PD, Steventon RS, Deters EC, et al. Oncologic diagnosis with 2-(Fluorine-18) Fluoro-2-deoxy-D-glucose imaging: dual-head coincidence gamma camera versus positron emission tomographic scanner. *Radiology* 1998;207:431–437.

CHAPTER 6

Diffuse Lung Disease

Despite the well-established role of chest radiography to accurately and inexpensively display a wide range of pulmonary parenchymal pathology, equally well-established limitations have been documented (1). Epler et al., in examining 458 patients with histologically confirmed infiltrative lung disease, showed that 44, or nearly 10%, had normal prebiopsy chest radiographs (Fig. 6-1) (2). Similar results have been reported by Gaensler and Carrington (3).

Abnormalities detected by chest radiographs are frequently nonspecific. Simple, precise, and consistent guidelines for recognizing the various patterns of diffuse lung disease seem difficult to define, probably because of varia-

tions inherently associated with the visual interpretation of nonfocal and complex abnormalities (Fig. 6-2). Utilizing a semiquantitative approach based on a slight modification of the International Labour Office (ILO) classification, McLoud et al. found, in an evaluation of 365 cases of diffuse infiltrative lung disease proved with open-lung biopsy, that their first two radiologic diagnostic choices corresponded to the histologic diagnosis in only 50% of cases, improving to just 78% when the first three choices were included (4). Significantly, in this same study there was only 70% interobserver agreement as to the predominant type of opacity present or the degree of profusion.

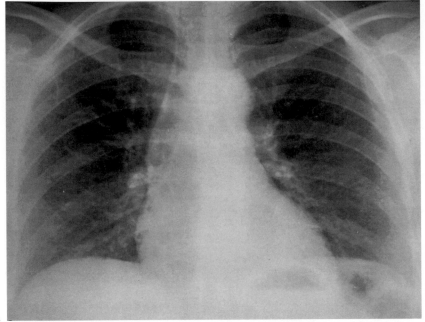

A

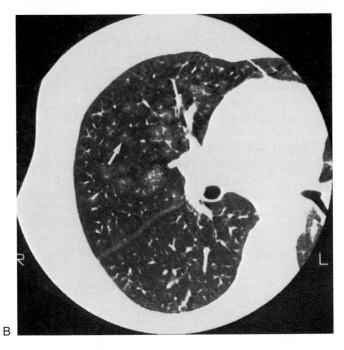

B

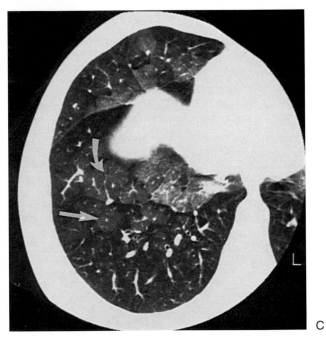

C

FIG. 6-1. Radiographically occult lung disease. **A:** Normal posteroanterior radiograph in a patient presenting with hemoptysis. **B,C:** Sequential 1.5-mm thick, target reconstructed CT sections through the mid and lower portion of the right lung, respectively. These show characteristic features of ground-glass attenuation. Note that there are numerous focal areas of increased lung density, within which normal anatomic structures can still be visualized (*curved arrow* in **C**). Note additionally that many of these densities are localized around core pulmonary arteries, identifiable as central dots within secondary pulmonary lobules (*arrows* in **B** and **C**). This distribution reflects the underlying anatomy as may be predicted in a patient clinically aspirating blood.

By eliminating superimposition of structures and enhancing attenuation discrimination, computed tomography (CT) provides a direct visual window into the lungs. Although these advantages were appreciated early after the development of CT in the diagnosis of both focal and diffuse lung disease, technical limitations, including 18-second scan times and relatively poor reconstruction algorithms, precluded widespread utilization (5–8). However, with the development of rapid scan times (1 to 2 seconds), 1- to 2-mm collimation scans and improved reconstruction algorithms, CT has become an established imaging modality in the as-

sessment of diffuse lung disease. Thin collimation (1- to 2-mm thick sections) and targeted reconstruction with a high spatial frequency (edge-enhancing) algorithm—high-resolution computed tomography (HRCT)—provides remarkably detailed images of lung architecture (9). The HRCT images provide a view of the lung parenchyma comparable to naked eye examination of lung specimens by the pathologist (10–12).

In this chapter, the role of CT in the evaluation of diffuse lung disease is reviewed; the role of CT in the evaluation of focal lung disease was considered in Chapter 4.

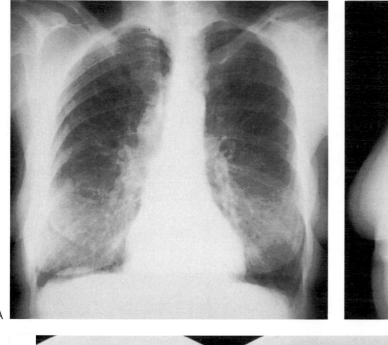

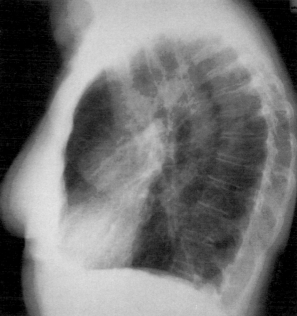

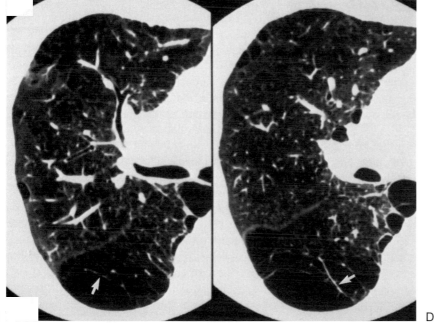

FIG. 6-2. "Dirty lung" emphysema. **A,B:** Posteroanterior and lateral radiographs show diffuse, ill-defined reticular opacities throughout both lungs. **C,D:** Retrospectively targeted high-resolution CT images of the right mid and lower lung, respectively, clearly reveal extensive emphysema without evidence of diffuse interstitial disease. The reticular pattern seen on the chest radiographs are caused by the septa separating bullae, most easily identified laterally and posteriorly (*arrows*). In addition to peripheral bullae, discrete areas of markedly low tissue attenuation without clearly definable walls can be identified within the lung parenchyma, findings compatible with diffuse emphysematous disease. Note that the intervening lung parenchyma is normal and that intrapulmonary vessels are well-defined with smooth contours.

GENERAL PRINCIPLES AND METHODOLOGY

In no other portion of the chest is the diagnostic efficacy of CT so inextricably tied to scan technique as in the evaluation of diffuse lung disease. Variations in technique so alter the appearance of the lung that in select cases, accurate diagnosis may depend on the selection of appropriate scan parameters. As a consequence, accurate evaluation of diffuse lung disease requires that a variety of protocols that specifically reflect a wide range of clinical indications be established.

The essential elements of HRCT are acquisition of thin-sections (1 to 2 mm) and use of a high spatial frequency (edge-enhancing) reconstruction algorithm. Further improvement in spatial resolution can be obtained with the use of targeted reconstructions with field-of-view (FOV) restricted to individual lungs (13). Routinely, images are acquired with the shortest possible scan time (generally 1 second) using a 512 × 512 matrix, with milliamperage (mA) typically varying between 200 and 300, depending on the patient's size. It should be noted that considerable dose reduction, to as low as 40 mAs, still allows acquisition of interpretable images of the lung parenchyma on HRCT (14) (Fig. 6-3). The low-dose HRCT technique allows better as-

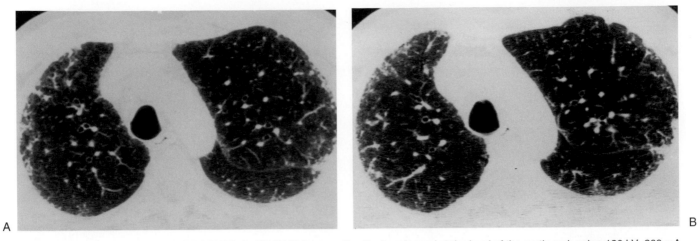

FIG. 6-3. Low-dose high-resolution CT (HRCT). **A:** HRCT (1.5-mm collimation) performed at the level of the aortic arch using 120 kV, 200 mA, and 2 seconds scan. Mild parenchymal abnormalities are present in the subpleural lung regions consisting of irregular interfaces and small irregular lines. **B:** HRCT (1.5-mm collimation) obtained at the same level using 120 kV, 40 mA, and 2 seconds scan shows the findings equally well. Increased noise is present posteriorly in the paraspinal region but this does not affect the diagnostic quality of the image. The patient was a 71-year-old man with idiopathic pulmonary fibrosis.

sessment of lung parenchyma than the chest radiograph (15). However, mild ground-glass attenuation, emphysema, and fibrosis detectable on conventional-dose HRCT can be missed on low-dose HRCT (14–16). Therefore the higher milliamperage setting (200 to 300 mAs) is recommended in the initial assessment of patients, but reduced-milliamperage HRCT can be used in the evaluation of response to treatment or disease progression in patients in whom radiation dose is a major concern.

Optimal technical parameters for individual images have been described (13,17) but there is no general agreement as to what constitutes an acceptable high-resolution study (18). Individual reports differ strikingly in overall technique, especially in determining the number and levels of necessary scans, and the indications for both prone and supine images.

Two major alternative approaches have been advocated for the assessment of patients with diffuse lung disease: HRCT as an adjunct to a complete conventional CT (CCT), and HRCT as an independent study. In the first approach a few additional HRCT images are obtained either in select areas, following evaluation of an initial sequence of 7- to 10-mm thick sections to further define regions suspected or proven to be abnormal; or, alternatively, at specific, preselected levels, such as the aortic arch, carina, or just above the diaphragm (10,11). This approach requires little additional scan time, and may be of value in select cases by further defining the nature of focal abnormalities. Unfortunately, only a very limited portion of the lung is actually sampled with HRCT using this approach. Furthermore, Leung et al. (19) demonstrated that HRCT performed at only three preselected levels (aortic arch, tracheal carina, and 2 cm above the diaphragm) was comparable to a complete CCT in the differential diagnosis of chronic infiltrative lung disease. The combination of complete CCT plus HRCT did not significantly improve the diagnostic accuracy (19).

The second approach emphasizes HRCT by using only thin sections from the outset. Images typically are obtained at preselected levels chosen to maximize evaluation of the different lung zones. There is no consensus, however, about the number of HRCT scans required for an adequate assessment of the lung parenchyma. Different investigators have used HRCT scans at 1 cm, 2 cm, and even 4 cm intervals with the patient supine, prone, or both supine and prone (20–22). The main advantage of a small number of scans is to reduce radiation exposure and cost (15,23,24). The main disadvantage with a small number of scans is that focal parenchymal abnormalities may be overlooked, the patchy distribution of many diffuse infiltrative lung diseases may not be appreciated, and small nodules may be missed between high-resolution sections (19–25). The optimal number of HRCT scans therefore depends on the clinical situation. In the initial assessment of patients with suspected infiltrative lung disease, it is recommended that HRCT scans be obtained at 1 cm intervals through the chest with the patient supine. In patients with known or suspected occupational exposure to asbestos, scans of the prone patient are often necessary to distinguish reversible gravity-dependent density and atelectasis from fixed structural abnormalities in dependent portions of the lung bases, where pulmonary fibrosis is most likely to occur (19,20,25). Although some investigators (17,25) obtain HRCT in the prone position only when dependent lung density is problematic, others (20) recommend prone scanning routinely. It should be noted that dependent density is a diagnostic dilemma only in patients with normal lungs or subtle parenchymal abnormalities. In patients with diffuse lung disease who have abnormalities visible on the chest radiograph, dependent density is seldom a diagnostic problem and therefore prone scans are usually unnecessary (26).

Although the HRCT technique should be customized to

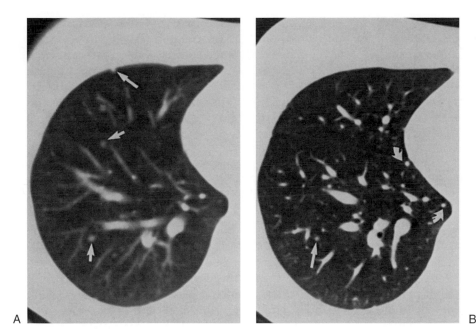

FIG. 6-4. Identifying pulmonary nodules: 10-mm versus 1.5-mm thick section. **A,B:** Target reconstructed images through the right lower lobe at the exact same levels using 10-mm and 1.5-mm thick sections, respectively. In this case, identification of individual nodules is visually easier with 10-mm thick sections (*arrows*), although close scrutiny of the 1.5-mm thick section reveals the presence of nodules within the lungs. Some may even be seen to better advantage (*curved arrows* in **B**).

each individual patient, in the routine assessment of patients with known or suspected diffuse lung disease, we recommend 1-mm thick sections obtained every 10 mm from the thoracic inlet to the diaphragm, prospectively reconstructed using a high-spatial-frequency algorithm. Select images may then be retrospectively targeted, as clinically indicated. Prone images are not routinely acquired, but are obtained in cases in which disease, in dependent portions of the lung, needs to be excluded, as when evaluating patients with suspected asbestosis or patients with suspected infiltrative lung diseases who have normal or questionable findings on the chest radiograph (26).

This approach allows more complete sampling of the lungs and permits far more precise characterization of the nature and extent of disease (27). In our experience, even with diffuse lung disease, focal alterations are the rule. These are easily missed when only a few random images are obtained. That this technique is likely to yield comparable or even higher diagnostic accuracy than routine CT studies using 10-mm thick sections has been documented (19,27,28). An important exception to this rule that "less is more" is in the evaluation of patients with suspected metastatic disease. In this setting, where the identification of even one nodule may be clinically significant, incomplete sampling is unacceptable; furthermore, nodules are easier to identify with conventional 10-mm thick sections (Fig. 6-4) or with spiral technique. These considerations are less significant when imaging diseases characterized by large numbers of nodules. As documented by Brauner et al., in patients with diffuse nodular diseases such as sarcoidosis, obtaining 1.5-mm sections every 10 mm throughout the lungs allows identification of nodules in virtually all patients (29).

It should be emphasized that there are no predetermined

"best" windows and levels for imaging the lung. Precise settings are often a matter of subjective preference. As a general guide, we recommend a window level of -600 to -700 HU and a window width of 1000 to 1500 HU for the assessment of the lung parenchyma. However, as illustrated in this chapter, a wide range of settings is employed, depending on the particular nature of the pathology to be illustrated. Narrowing the window width enhances visual resolution. This may be particularly helpful when assessing focal increases and decreases in lung attenuation, as may be seen in patients with emphysema. Conversely, wide window widths are often more informative when the disease process occupies a large area and involves a wide range of tissue-density alterations, as may occur with complex pleural-parenchymal disease. In these cases, the panoramic view afforded by a wide window width improves visual comprehension. Although rarely emphasized, it is worth noting that for the purposes of producing both slides and prints, images obtained with narrow windows are far easier to reproduce and display; this may, in part, explain the wide acceptance of narrower windows as "standard" (see Chapter 1 for a more detailed discussion).

To date, the role of volumetric CT for assessing diffuse lung disease has been limited. In fact, it is possible to selectively sample as much as 5 to 10 mm of lung using 1-mm collimation during a single breath hold. Multiplanar volume reconstructions (MPVRs), reconstructed in the axial plane, can then be used to generate both maximum (MIPS) and minimum (MIN-IPS) intensity projection images. These have the advantage of retaining high spatial resolution while preserving the anatomic cross-sectional orientation derived from thicker sections (Fig. 6-5). To date, this approach has been described as a method for evaluating patients with subtle emphysema, as well as micronodular disease. As docu-

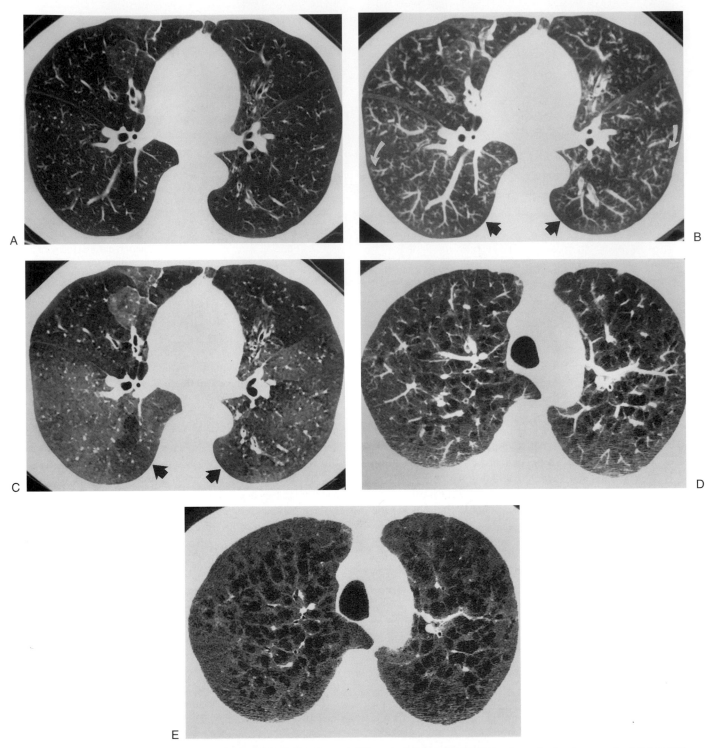

FIG. 6-5. Diffuse infiltrative lung disease: evaluation with maximum (MIP) and minimum (MinIP) intensity projection images. **A:** A 1-mm high-resolution CT (HRCT) section through the lower lobes shows pattern of subtle mosaic attenuation with suggestion of focal air-trapping within the middle lobe and lingula and the posterior segments of both lower lobes. No obvious nodules or tree-in-bud pattern identified. **B,C:** MIP and MinIP images, respectively, obtained using five contiguous 1-mm sections centered at the same level as shown in **A**. On the MIP image pattern of diffuse nodules with a tree-in-bud configuration is apparent (*curved arrows* in **B**). Focal air trapping is slightly more apparent in the posterobasilar segments of the lower lobes (*straight arrows* in **B**). Note that whereas the nodules all but disappear on the MinIP image, mosaic attenuation is much more apparent (*arrows* in **C**). These findings are all consistent with infectious bronchiolitis with accompanying air-trapping identifiable even without acquiring scans in expiration. **D,E:** HRCT and corresponding MinIP image in a different patient than in **A–C**. Note that in this case, whereas diffuse emphysema is apparent on the HRCT image, visual assessment of the extent of emphysema is easier on the corresponding MinIP image.

mented by Remy-Jardin et al., in a study of 81 patients with possible micronodular diseases (including pneumoconioses, sarcoidosis, and smoker's bronchiolitis, among others), MIPS images enabled detection of micronodules involving less than 25% of the lung surface in patients with inconclusive CCT studies, and showed to better advantage the presence and extent of nodules in patients with abnormal CCT studies (30). Similarly, Bhalla et al., in a study of all variety of diffuse infiltrative lung diseases, found MIPS images better able to demonstrate micronodular disease as well as areas of emphysema and ground-glass attenuation using MIN-IPS images (31). Although suggestive, an actual clinical role for this approach remains to be validated.

NORMAL LUNG ANATOMY

The lung is composed of anatomical units that demonstrate similar architecture at progressively smaller sizes, as described by fractal geometry; from large to small, these units are lungs, lobes, segments, subsegments, secondary lobules, and acini. At each level, these are organized around central or ''core'' supporting structures (airways and pulmonary arteries) and within peripheral or ''shell'' supporting structures (pleura and connective tissue septa).

The lobes are marginated to a variable degree by the interlobar fissures. In normal subjects, three lobes (upper, middle, and lower) are present on the right, and two (upper and lower) are present on the left. Lobes can be identified on CT by identifying the interlobular fissures or the avascular plane that mark their positions, or when fissures are incomplete or poorly localized, by identifying bronchial branches. Lobar bronchi have a consistent branching pattern in the large majority of patients; lobar bronchial anomalies are rare. Pulmonary artery branching patterns are more variable, and therefore, less valuable in indentifying individual pulmonary lobes.

Pulmonary segments are less well marginated than lobes, and do not have easily definable boundaries. Individual seg-

ments are best localized on the basis of segmental bronchi and by noting the relatively consistent location of segments within lobes and in relation to lobar fissures (32–34). Arterial anatomy is less valuable in identifying segments, as arterial branching is somewhat more variable than bronchial branching (see Chapter 3). As with pulmonary segments, subsegments are best identified on the basis of bronchial anatomy. At a subsegmental level, lung is composed of secondary pulmonary lobules and acini, which are described in detail below.

The Lung Interstitium

The lung is supported by a network of connective tissue fibers, termed the lung interstitium. The interstitium must be strong enough to maintain the patency of alveoli, airways, and vessels, but at the same time must be thin enough to allow adequate gas exchange between air in the alveolar spaces and blood in pulmonary capillaries.

The interstitium is organized into three fiber systems, the peribronchovascular interstitium, the subpleural interstitium, and the intralobular interstitium, which have been described in detail by Weibel (35). Together, these three form a continuous fiber skeleton that serves to support lung parenchyma between the hila centrally and the pleural surfaces peripherally (Fig. 6-6), and which, to a large extent, is replicated from the level of the lobes to the level of the secondary pulmonary lobules.

The peribronchovascular interstitium is a system of fibers that invests bronchi and pulmonary arteries, and serves to support the ''core'' or medullary structures of the lung (see Fig. 6-6). In the parahilar regions the peribronchovascular interstitium forms a strong connective tissue sheath that surrounds large bronchi and arteries; it continues into the lung periphery, investing centrilobular arteries and bronchioles, and continues to the level of the alveolar ducts and sacs (35). The peribronchovascular interstitium is described as the ''axial fiber system'' by Weibel.

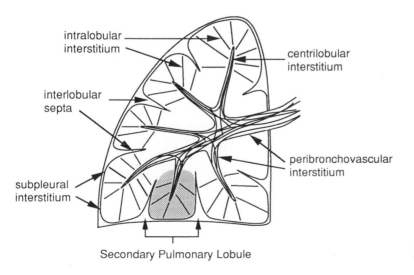

intralobular interstitium

centrilobular interstitium

interlobular septa

peribronchovascular interstitium

subpleural interstitium

Secondary Pulmonary Lobule

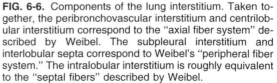

FIG. 6-6. Components of the lung interstitium. Taken together, the peribronchovascular interstitium and centrilobular interstitium correspond to the "axial fiber system" described by Weibel. The subpleural interstitium and interlobular septa correspond to Weibel's "peripheral fiber system." The intralobular interstitium is roughly equivalent to the "septal fibers" described by Weibel.

The subpleural interstitium is located beneath the visceral pleura, and envelopes the lung in a fibrous sac from which connective tissue septa penetrate the lung parenchyma (see Fig. 6-6). These septa include the interlobular septa, which are described in detail below. The subpleural interstitium and interlobular septa are both parts of the "peripheral fiber system" described by Weibel (35); they support the "shell" or cortical lung parenchyma.

The intralobular interstitium is a network of thin fibers that forms a fine connective tissue mesh in the walls of alveoli, and thus bridges the gap between the peribronchovascular interstitium surrounding vessels and bronchi in the center of lobules, and the interlobular septa and subpleural interstitium in the lobular periphery (see Fig. 6-6). These fibers keep capillaries and alveoli open for functional gas exchange. The intralobular interstitium corresponds to the "septal fibers" described by Weibel (35).

Bronchi and Pulmonary Vessels

Within the lung parenchyma, bronchi and pulmonary arteries are closely associated and branch in parallel. Each bronchus is positioned adjacent to a pulmonary artery of similar diameter, and this relationship is maintained from the hila to the level of respiratory bronchioles in the lung periphery. As indicated above, bronchi and arteries are encased by a network of fibers, the peribronchovascular interstitium or bronchovascular sheath, which also extends from the pulmonary hila into the peripheral lung. In addition to the artery and bronchus, this sheath contains amorphous collagen, lymphatics, and small lymph nodes, ranging in size from 1 mm in the lung periphery to 5 to 10 mm near the hila. It should be noted that lymphatics do not extend beyond the terminal bronchioles.

Since some lung diseases produce thickening of the peribronchovascular interstitium in the central or parahilar lung, in relation to large bronchi and pulmonary vessels, it is im-portant to be aware of the normal CT appearances of the parahilar bronchi and pulmonary vessels (Fig. 6-7). (Interested readers are referred to Chapter 3 for an in-depth discussion of normal bronchi.)

When imaged at an angle to their longitudinal axis, central pulmonary arteries normally appear as rounded or elliptical opacities on CT or HRCT, accompanied by uniformly thin-walled bronchi of similar shape (12,36,37). When imaged along their axis, bronchi and vessels should appear roughly cylindrical, or show slight tapering as they branch, depending on the length of the segment that is visible; tapering of a vessel or bronchus is most easily seen when a long segment is visible.

The diameter of an artery and its neighboring bronchus should be approximately equal, although vessels may appear slightly larger than their accompanying bronchus, particularly in dependent lung regions. Although the presence of bronchi larger than their adjacent arteries is often assumed to indicate the presence of bronchial dilatation, or bronchiectasis, bronchi may appear larger than adjacent arteries in a significant number of normal subjects. In a study of normal subjects, Lynch et al., (38) compared the internal diameters of lobar, segmental, subsegmental, and smaller bronchi to those of adjacent artery branches on HRCT. Nineteen percent of bronchi had an internal bronchial diameter greater than the artery diameter, and 59% of normal subjects showed at least one such bronchus.

The outer walls of visible pulmonary artery branches should form a smooth and sharply defined interface with the surrounding lung, whether they are seen in cross-section or along their length. The walls of large bronchi, outlined by lung on one side, and air in the bronchial lumen on the other, normally appear to be smooth and of uniform thickness. Thickening of the peribronchial and perivascular interstitium can result in irregularity of the interface between arteries and bronchi and the adjacent lung (9,39).

Assessment of bronchial wall thickness on HRCT is quite

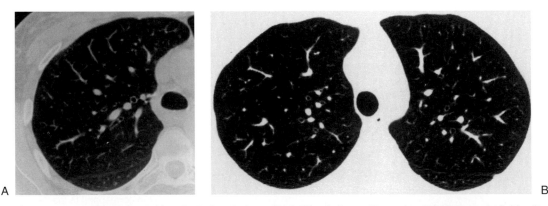

FIG. 6-7. Normal appearances of large bronchi and arteries photographed with window settings of −600/2000 Hounsfield units (HU) (**A**) and −700/1000 HU (**B**). The diameters of vessels and their neighboring bronchi are approximately equal. The outer walls of bronchi and pulmonary vessels are smooth and sharply defined. Bronchi are not visible within the peripheral 2 cm of lung despite the fact that vessels are well seen in this region.

TABLE 6-1. *Relation of airway diameter to wall thickness*

	Diameter (mm)	Wall thickness (mm)
Lobar and segmental bronchi	5–8	1.5
Subsegmental bronchi/ bronchiole	1.5–3	0.2–0.3
Lobular bronchiole	1	0.15
Terminal bronchiole	0.7	0.1
Acinar bronchiole	0.5	0.05

subjective, and is dependent on the window settings used (38,40). Also, since the apparent thickness of the bronchial wall represents not only the wall itself, but the surrounding peribronchovascular interstitium as well, peribronchovascular interstitial thickening results in apparent bronchial wall thickening (so-called peribronchial cuffing) on HRCT.

The wall thickness of conducting bronchi and bronchioles is approximately proportional to their diameter, at least for bronchi distal to the segmental level. In general, the thickness of the wall of a bronchus or bronchiole less than 5 mm in diameter should measure from 1/6 to 1/10 of its diameter (Table 6-1) (41); however, precise measurement of the wall thickness of small bronchi or bronchioles is difficult as wall thickness approximates pixel size.

Bronchi and pulmonary arteries divide by dichotomous branching. There are approximately 23 generations of airway branches, from the trachea to alveolar sacs (Fig. 6-8), and 28 generations of pulmonary artery branches. Since a bronchus is usually recognized only when its walls are visualized, it is not possible to resolve airways with a wall thickness of less than 300 microns. This corresponds to bronchi of about 1 to 2 mm in diameter and not closer than 2 cm to the pleural surface, equivalent to between the seventh and ninth generation of airways (12,42). Rarely, smaller airways approximately 1 mm in diameter can be recognized coursing perpendicularly within the plane of a very thin section by virtue of their lower density and their proximity to an adjacent pulmonary artery, even though their walls cannot be clearly seen.

Blood vessels with diameters of 300 microns can be visualized, corresponding to sixteenth generation arteries at the level of the terminal and most proximal respiratory bronchioles (see Fig. 6-8). Because vascular structures typically can be seen to within a few millimeters of the pleural surfaces and can be followed to the level of the secondary pulmonary lobule, the arterial tree is a useful landmark for defining HRCT lung anatomy (12,42).

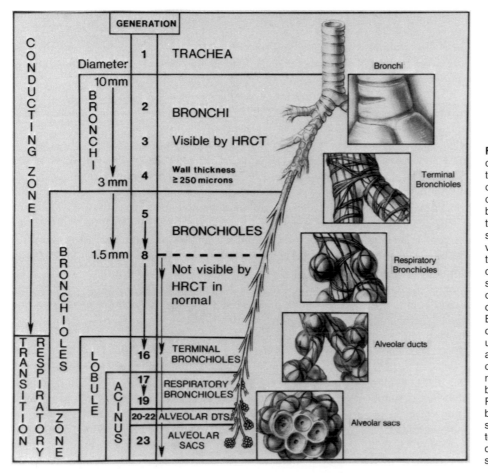

FIG. 6-8. Bronchial generations. The bronchi and airways from the first generation, the trachea, to the last generation, the alveolar sacs, are represented. Bronchi that contain cartilage within their walls measure between 10 and 3 mm in diameter and extend to the fourth generation, that is, the subsegmental branches. They are easily visible by direct high-resolution computed tomography (HRCT). Bronchioles, which contain not cartilage but rather an extensive network of fibers within their walls, are only seen to the eighth generation, which correspond to a diameter of about 1.5 mm. Beyond the eighth generation, the bronchiolar walls are not resolvable by HRCT unless abnormal. The terminal bronchioles are the sixteenth-generation airways and conduct air into the lobules. Beyond the terminal bronchiole, four to eight respiratory bronchioles lead to the formation of acini. Respiratory bronchioles are characterized by the presence of out-pouchings representing alveolar structures. Each respiratory bronchiole leads to a series of alveolar ducts and terminal groupings of alveolar sacs.

The pulmonary veins follow a course independent of the bronchial tree and lie between two pairs of bronchi and arteries (see Fig. 6-6). This position is maintained into the lung periphery, where veins are seen within the interlobular septa.

Secondary Pulmonary Lobules and Acini

The secondary pulmonary lobule, as defined by Miller, refers to the smallest unit of lung structure marginated by connective tissue septa (Figs. 6-9 and 6-10) (43). Secondary pulmonary lobules are irregularly polyhedral in shape and somewhat variable in size, measuring approximately 1 to 2.5 cm in diameter in most locations (35,41,44–47). In one study, the average diameter of pulmonary lobules measured in several adults ranged from 11 to 17 mm (45). Each secondary lobule is supplied by a small bronchiole and pulmonary artery, and is variably marginated, in different lung regions, by connective-tissue interlobular septa that contain pulmonary vein and lymphatic branches (44).

Secondary pulmonary lobules are made up of a limited number of pulmonary acini, usually a dozen or fewer, although the number of lobular acini can vary from 3 to 24 (47,48). A pulmonary acinus is defined as the portion of the lung parenchyma distal to a terminal bronchiole and supplied by a first order respiratory bronchiole or bronchioles and comprised of respiratory bronchioles, alveolar ducts, alveolar sacs, and alveoli (49). Since respiratory bronchioles are the largest airways that have alveoli in their walls, an acinus is the largest lung unit in which all airways participate in gas exchange. Acini are usually described as ranging from 6 to 10 mm in diameter (45,50).

As indicated above, Miller has defined the secondary pulmonary lobule as the smallest lung unit marginated by connective tissue septa (43). Reid has suggested an alternate definition of the secondary pulmonary lobule, based on the branching pattern of peripheral bronchioles, rather than the presence and location of connective tissue septa (44,48,49). On bronchograms, small bronchioles can be seen to arise at intervals of 5 to 10 mm from larger airways, the so-called ''centimeter pattern'' of branching; these small bronchioles then show branching at approximately 2 mm intervals, the ''millimeter pattern'' (44,48,49). Airways showing the millimeter pattern of branching are considered by Reid to be intralobular, with each branch corresponding to a terminal bronchiole (44,49). Lobules are considered to be the lung units supplied by three to five ''millimeter pattern'' bronchioles. Although Reid's criteria delineate lung units of approximately equal size, about 1 cm in diameter and containing three to five acini, it should be noted, that this definition does not necessarily describe lung units equivalent to secondary lobules as defined by Miller and marginated by interlobular septa (see Fig. 6-6) (47), although a small Miller's lobule can be the same as a Reid's lobule. Miller's

definition is most applicable to the interpretation of CT, and is widely accepted by pathologists because interlobular septa are visible on histologic sections. In this book, we use the terms ''secondary pulmonary lobule,'' ''pulmonary lobule,'' and ''lobule'' to refer to a secondary lobule as defined by Miller.

High-Resolution CT of the Secondary Lobule

An understanding of secondary lobular anatomy and the appearances of lobular structures are key to the interpretation of HRCT. HRCT can show many features of the secondary pulmonary lobule in both normal and abnormal lungs, and, in many lung diseases, particularly interstitial diseases, produce some characteristic changes in lobular structures (9–12,23,36,39). Heitzman has been instrumental in emphasizing the importance of the secondary pulmonary lobule in the radiologic diagnosis of lung disease (44), and the importance of recognizing secondary lobular abnormalities on HRCT has been clearly shown by many authors.

Interlobular Septa

Anatomically, secondary lobules are marginated by connective tissue interlobular septa, which extend inward from the pleural surface. These septa are part of the subpleural interstitium (the peripheral interstitial fiber system described by Weibel) (see Fig. 6-6) (35), which extends over the surface of the lung beneath the visceral pleura. A rich lymphatic system, referred to as the superficial lymphatic network, drains the visceral pleura and courses within the interlobular septa in parallel with septal veins; these ultimately lead to lymphatics and nodes within the hila.

It should be emphasized that not all interlobular septa are equally well defined. The interlobular septa are thickest and most numerous in the apical, anterior, and lateral aspects of the upper lobes, the anterior and lateral aspects of the middle lobe and lingula, the anterior and diaphragmatic surfaces of the lower lobes, and along the mediastinal pleural surfaces (51); thus, secondary lobules are best defined in these regions. Septa measure about 100 μm (0.1 mm) in thickness in a subpleural location (12,42). Within the central lung, interlobular septa are thinner and less well defined than peripherally, and lobules are more difficult to identify in this location.

Peripherally, interlobular septa measuring 100 μm or 0.1 mm in thickness are at the lower limit of HRCT resolution (42), but nonetheless they are sometimes visible on HRCT scans performed *in vitro* (12). On *in vitro* HRCT, interlobular septa are often visible as very thin, straight lines of uniform thickness which are usually 1–2.5 cm in length and perpendicular to the pleural surface (Figs. 6-11 and 6-12). Several septa in continuity can be seen as a linear opacity measuring up to 4 cm in length. As documented by Webb et al (12) in

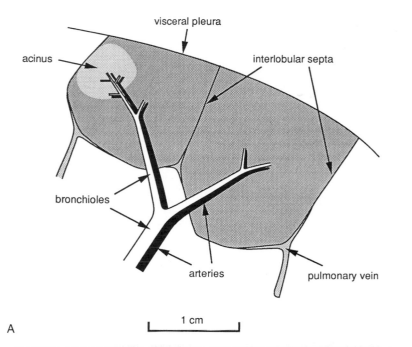

visceral pleura

acinus

interlobular septa

bronchioles

arteries

pulmonary vein

1 cm

A

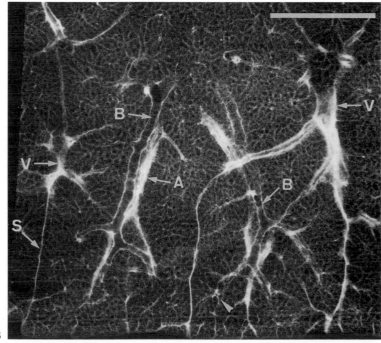

B

FIG. 6-9. A: Anatomy of the secondary pulmonary lobule, as defined by Miller. Two adjacent lobules are shown in this diagram. **B:** Radiographic anatomy of the secondary pulmonary lobule. Radiograph of a 1-mm lung slice taken from the lower lobe. Two well-defined secondary pulmonary lobules are visible. Lobules are marginated by thin interlobular septa (*S*) containing pulmonary vein (*V*) branches. Bronchioles (*B*) and pulmonary arteries (*A*) are centrilobular. Bar = 1 cm. (Courtesy of Harumi Itoh, M.D., Kyoto University, Kyoto, Japan. From ref 47, with permission.)

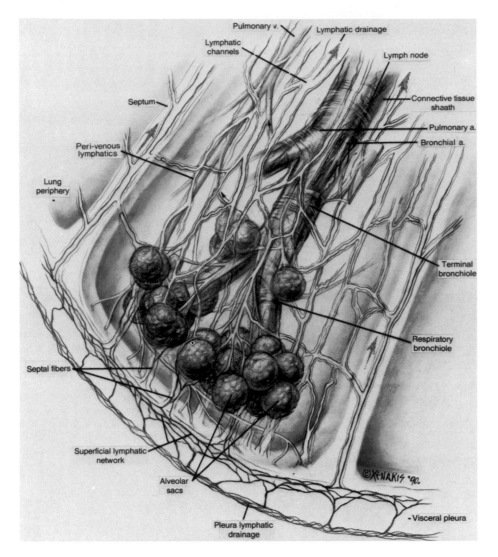

FIG. 6-10. A secondary lobule according to Miller is represented. The centrilobular structures are composed of the terminal bronchiole and pulmonary artery, enclosed in a bronchovascular sheath. The bronchial artery runs in parallel to these structures within the connective tissue sheath. A deep lymphatic system located in close apposition to the core structures drains the interstitium. Note that lymphatics are not present around alveolar sacs. In the periphery of the lobule are the visceral pleura and septa extending from the visceral pleura into the lung substance. Within these peripheral structures run the pulmonary veins and the superficial lymphatic network that drains the pleura via septal lymphatics that are perivenous in location. The functional units of the lung made up of collections of alveolar sacs are in effect suspended between the core structures and the shell structures via a network of interconnecting elastic fibers. This basic organization is self-replicated from the smallest to the largest functional lung unit.

their evaluation of inflated lung specimens, an average of only four septa at least 1 cm in length extending to the pleura were visible over the anterior and lateral surfaces of the mid and upper lung zones, while an average of only two septa could be identified over the lateral and posterior pleural surfaces.

On clinical scans in normal patients, interlobular septa are less commonly seen, and are seen less well than they are in studies of isolated lungs. A few septa are often visible in the lung periphery in normal subjects, but they tend to be inconspicuous (Fig. 6-13); normal septa are most often seen anteriorly, along the mediastinal pleural surfaces, or in the lower lobes or just above the diaphragm (20,39,52). When visible, they are usually seen extending to the pleural surface. In the central lung, septa are thinner than they are peripherally and are infrequently seen in normals; often interlobular septa, which are clearly defined in this region, are abnormally thickened.

Occasionally, when interlobular septa are not clearly visible, their locations can be inferred by locating septal pulmonary vein branches, approximately 0.5 mm in diameter. Veins can sometimes be seen as linear (see Fig. 6-13B), arcuate, or branching structures (see Fig. 6-13C), or as a row or chain of dots, surrounding centrilobular arteries, and approximately 5 to 10 mm from them.

The Centrilobular Region

The central portion of the lobule, referred to as the centrilobular region or lobular core (44), contains the pulmonary artery and bronchiolar branches that supply the lobule, as well as some supporting connective tissue (i.e., the peribronchovascular interstitium) (see Fig. 6-10 and 6-11) (12,35,42). It is difficult to precisely define lobules in relation to the bronchial or arterial trees; lobules do not arise at a specific branching generation or from a specific type of bronchiole or artery (41).

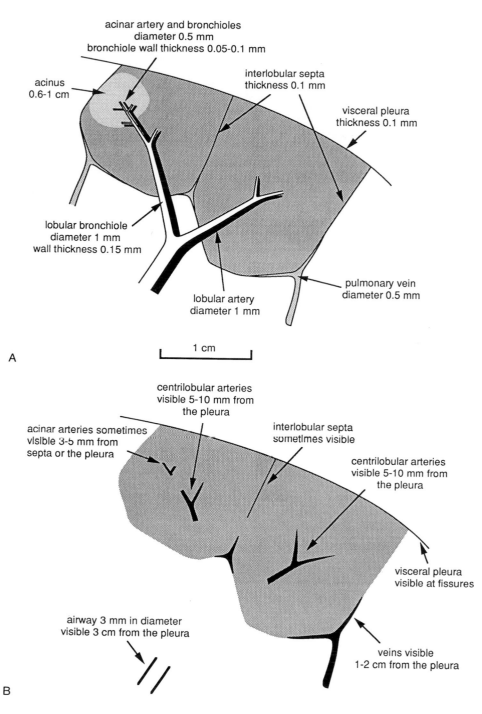

acinar artery and bronchioles
diameter 0.5 mm
bronchiole wall thickness 0.05-0.1 mm

acinus
0.6-1 cm

interlobular septa
thickness 0.1 mm

visceral pleura
thickness 0.1 mm

lobular bronchiole
diameter 1 mm
wall thickness 0.15 mm

pulmonary vein
diameter 0.5 mm

lobular artery
diameter 1 mm

1 cm

A

centrilobular arteries
visible 5-10 mm from
the pleura

acinar arteries sometimes
visible 3-5 mm from
septa or the pleura

interlobular septa
sometimes visible

centrilobular arteries
visible 5-10 mm from
the pleura

visceral pleura
visible at fissures

airway 3 mm in diameter
visible 3 cm from the pleura

veins visible
1-2 cm from the pleura

B

FIG. 6-11. Dimensions of secondary lobular structures (**A**) and their visibility on high-resolution CT (**B**).

The branching of the lobular bronchiole and artery are irregularly dichotomous (53). In other words, when they divide, they divide into two branches which are usually of different sizes; one branch is nearly the same size as the one it arose from, and the other is smaller (see Fig. 6-9B). Thus, on bronchograms or arteriograms (or HRCT), there often appears to be a single dominant bronchiole and artery in the center of the lobule, which give off smaller branches at intervals along their length.

The HRCT appearances and visibility of structures in the centrilobular region are determined primarily by their size (see Figs. 6-9 and 6-11). Secondary lobules are supplied by arteries and bronchioles measuring approximately 1 mm in diameter, whereas intralobular terminal bronchioles and arteries measure about 0.7 mm in diameter, and acinar bronchioles and arteries range from 0.3 mm to 0.5 mm in diameter. Arteries of this size can be easily resolved using HRCT technique (12,42).

On clinical scans, a linear, branching, or dot-like opacity frequently seen within the center of a lobule, or within a

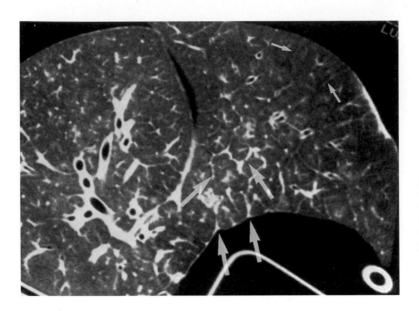

FIG. 6-12. Interlobular septa in an isolated lung. Some thin, normal interlobular septa (*small arrows*) are faintly visible in the peripheral lung. Interlobular septa along the mediastinal pleural surface (*large arrows*) are slightly thickened by edema fluid and are more easily seen. Note that a very thin line is visible at the pleural surfaces and in the lung fissure, similar in thickness and appearance to the normal interlobular septa. This line represents the subpleural interstitial compartment and visceral pleura. (From ref. 12, with permission.)

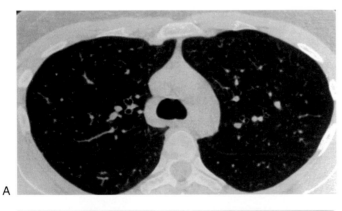

FIG. 6-13. A: High-resolution CT in a normal subject; window mean/width—600/2000 Hounsfield units (HU). Interlobular septa are inconspicuous, and the few that are visible are very thin. The major fissures appear as thin, sharply defined lines. B: Two pulmonary vein branches (*arrows*) marginate a pulmonary lobule in the anterior lung, but the interlobular septa surrounding this lobule are very thin and difficult to see. The centrilobular artery lies equidistant between the veins. C: HRCT in a normal subject (−700/1000 HU) shows few interlobular septa. A venous arcade (*arrow*) is visible in the lower lobe, with the centrilobular artery visible as a dot, centered within the arcade.

A

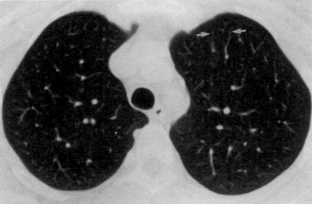

B

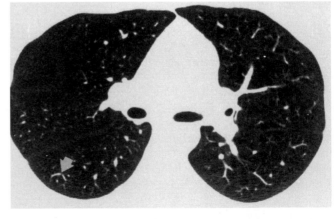

C

centimeter of the pleural surface, represents the intralobular artery branch or its divisions (see Fig. 6-13C) (23). The smallest arteries resolved extend to within 3 to 5 mm of the pleural surface or lobular margin and are as small as 0.2 mm in diameter (12,23,42). The visible centrilobular arteries are not seen to extend to the pleural surface in the absence of atelectasis. A similar branching structure, seen slightly farther from the pleural surface can represent a pulmonary vein. Although vein branches can sometimes be seen in relation to interlobular septa, whereas artery branches are centrally located relative to surrounding septa, veins and arteries cannot always be distinguished. Fortunately differentiation between these is not often necessary in clinical practice.

The thickness of the wall of an airway determines its visibility. For a 1 mm bronchiole supplying a secondary lobule, the thickness of its wall measures approximately 0.15 mm; this is at the lower limit of HRCT resolution. The wall of a terminal bronchiole measures only 0.1 mm in thickness, and that of an acinar bronchiole only 0.05 mm, both of which are below the resolution of HRCT technique for a tubular structure. In one *in vitro* study, only bronchioles having a diameter of 2 mm or more or having a wall thickness of more than 100 μm (0.1 mm) were visible using HRCT (42); and resolution is certainly less than this on clinical scans. It is important to remember that on clinical HRCT, intralobular bronchioles are not normally visible, and bronchi or bronchioles are not normally seen within 1 cm of the pleural surface.

Pulmonary acini making up the lobules (47) and the intralobular interstitium (35), a fine network of very thin fibers within the alveolar septa, are not visible on HRCT in normal subjects.

Lung Attenuation

Most of the lung, representing alveoli and their associated pulmonary capillary bed, supplied by small airways and branches of the pulmonary arteries and veins, appears featureless on HRCT, identifiable as homogeneous gray "background" density. The thickness of alveolar walls normally measures approximately 20 to 30 μm and is therefore an order of magnitude below the resolution of HRCT. On HRCT, lung parenchyma should be of greater opacity than air, but this difference may vary with window settings (see Chapter 1).

Generally speaking, lung opacity as seen on HRCT scans obtained at full inspiration appears relatively homogeneous. Measurements of lung attenuation in normal subjects can range from -700 to -900 HU, corresponding to lung densities of approximately 0.300 to 0.100 g/mL respectively (54,55). However, an attenuation gradient is normally present, if measurements are made, with the most dependent lung regions being the densest, and the most nondependent lung regions being the least dense. This gradient is largely caused by regional differences in blood volume and gas volume that, in turn, are determined by gravity, mechanical stresses

on the lung, and intrapleural pressures (54,56). Differences in attenuation between anterior and posterior lung have been measured in supine patients, and values generally range from 50 to 100 HU (54,55,57,58), although gradients of more than 200 HU have been reported (57). The anteroposterior attenuation gradient was found to be nearly linear, and was present regardless of whether the subject was supine or prone (57).

Genereaux measured anteroposterior attenuation gradients at three levels (at the aortic arch, the carina, and above the right hemidiaphragm) in normal subjects (58). An anteroposterior attenuation gradient was found at all levels, although the gradient was larger at the lung bases than in the upper lung; the anteroposterior gradient averaged 36 HU at the aortic arch, 65 HU at the carina, and 88 HU at the lung bases. The attenuation gradient was even larger if only cortical lung was considered. Within cortical lung, the attenuation differences at the 3 levels studied respectively were 45 HU, 81 HU, 113 HU.

Vock et al. analyzed CT measured pulmonary attenuation in children (54). In general, lung attenuation in children is greater than that in adults , but anteroposterior attenuation gradients were similar to those found in adults, averaging 56 HU at the subcarinal level (54,57).

Although most authors have reported that normal anteroposterior lung attenuation gradients are linear, with attenuation increasing gradually from anterior to posterior lung, the lingula and superior segments of the lower lobes can appear relatively lucent in some normal subjects (59); focal lucency in these segments should be considered a normal finding. Although the reason for this is unclear, these slender segments may be less well ventilated than adjacent lung and therefore less well perfused, or some air-trapping may be present.

PATTERNS OF ABNORMALITY ON HIGH-RESOLUTION CT

The diffuse parenchymal lung diseases include chronic and acute infiltrative lung diseases and emphysema. The definition of diffuse lung disease is somewhat arbitrary because these conditions often have a patchy or focal distribution. Findings that indicate the presence of pulmonary parenchymal abnormalities consistent with diffuse lung disease include linear and reticular opacities, nodular opacities, ground-glass attenuation, consolidation, and decreased attenuation.

Linear and Reticular Opacities

Linear and reticular opacities result from thickening of the pulmonary interstitium by fluid, fibrosis, or infiltration by cells or other material. An early finding is the interface sign that is characterized by the presence of irregular interfaces between the aerated lung and bronchi, vessels, and visceral pleura (9) (Fig. 6-14). The interface sign was visible

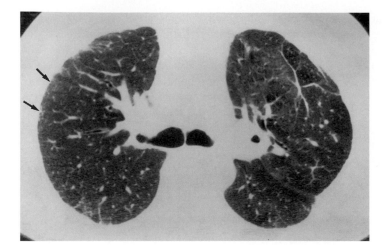

FIG. 6-14. Irregular interface sign. High-resolution CT (1.5-mm collimation) at the level of the right upper lobe bronchus demonstrates irregular interfaces between the lung parenchyma and the pleura (*arrows*). Also noted are irregular linear opacities and distortion of lung architecture particularly in the left upper lobe. The patient was a 63-year-old man with asbestosis.

in 89% of patients with interstitial lung disease reported by Zerhouni et al. (9) and 98% of patients with idiopathic pulmonary fibrosis reported by Nishimura et al. (60). Although the interface sign is a common finding, it is a nonspecific sign of interstitial lung disease. Other findings include peribronchial interstitial thickening, thickening of the interlobular septa, intralobular linear opacities, and cysts.

A common sign of infiltrative lung disease is the presence of peribronchial or perivascular interstitial thickening, that is, thickening of the connective tissue sheet surrounding the bronchi and pulmonary vessels (Fig. 6-15). Thickening of the peribronchovascular interstitium is most commonly seen in patients with interstitial pulmonary edema (12,61) or with diseases that affect predominantly the pulmonary lymphatics such as lymphangitic carcinomatosis and sarcoidosis (28,62–64). The thickening may be smooth, as typically seen in pulmonary edema, or irregular as seen in sarcoidosis, and pulmonary fibrosis. In lymphangitic carcinomatosis the thickening may be smooth or irregular. In patients with pulmonary fibrosis and peribronchovascular interstitial thicken-

ing, there is often dilatation of the bronchi caused by traction by the surrounding fibrosis. This is referred to as traction bronchiectasis (65).

A characteristic finding in patients with interstitial lung disease is the presence of thickening of the interlobular septa. This may be caused by edema, cellular infiltration, or fibrosis. Normally only a few septa are seen. Thickened septa (septal lines) are readily recognized in the lung periphery as lines 1 to 2 cm in length, 0.5 to 2 cm apart, perpendicular to the pleura and extending to the pleural surface (Fig. 6-16). In the central lung regions, thickened septa outlining one or more adjacent secondary pulmonary lobules can be seen as polygonal arcades (9,62). Septal thickening may be smooth, nodular or irregular. Smooth thickening of interlobular septa is seen most commonly in patients with pulmonary edema (61,66) and lymphangitic spread of carcinoma (28,62). Less common causes of smooth interlobular septal thickening include sarcoidosis (67), alveolar proteinosis (68,69), amyloidosis (70), and Kaposi's sarcoma (71). Nodular septal thickening characteristically occurs in patients with

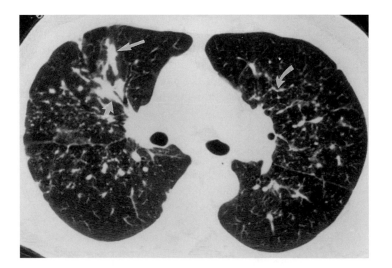

FIG. 6-15. Peribronchial and perivascular interstitial thickening. High-resolution CT (1.5-mm collimation) at the level of the bronchus intermedius demonstrates peribronchial (*short straight arrow*) and perivascular (*long straight arrow*) thickening. Also noted are small nodules and thickening of interlobular septa (*curved arrow*). The patient was a 60-year-old man with sarcoidosis.

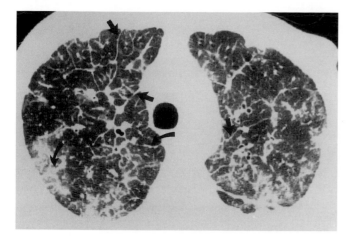

FIG. 6-16. Interlobular septal thickening. High-resolution CT (1-mm collimation) at the level of the aortic arch demonstrates smooth (*straight arrows*) and nodular (*curved arrows*) interlobular septal thickening. Also noted are subpleural nodules. The patient was a 72-year-old man with lymphangitic carcinomatosis caused by metastatic adenocarcinoma of the rectum.

lymphangitic carcinomatosis (28,72), Kaposi's sarcoma (71), sarcoidosis (73,74), silicosis and coalworkers' pneumoconiosis (73–76). In patients with interstitial fibrosis, interlobular septal thickening, when present, is usually irregular in appearance (10,12). Furthermore, in these patients the irregular thickening of the septa is usually associated with other findings of interstitial fibrosis such as intralobular linear opacities and architectural distortion (77,78).

Intralobular linear opacities are caused by thickening of the interstitium within the secondary pulmonary lobule. They result in a fine reticular pattern, a mesh of small irregular lines separated by only a few millimeters (Fig. 6-17).

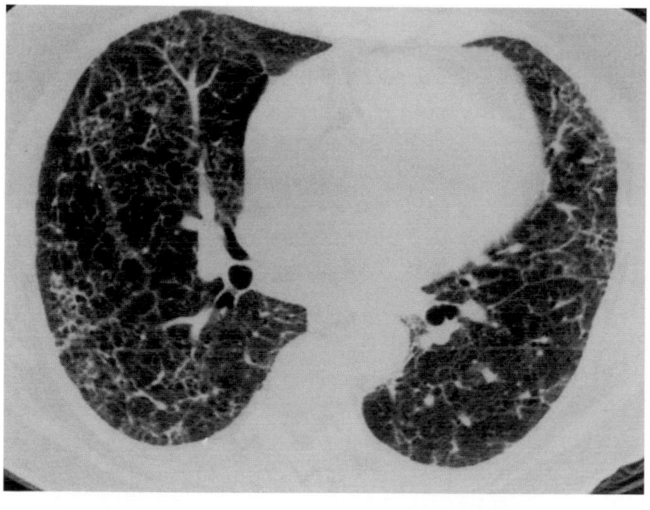

Intralobular linear opacities are most commonly caused by fibrosis. In idiopathic pulmonary fibrosis and fibrosing alveolitis associated with collagen vascular diseases, the intralobular linear opacities are characteristically most evident in the subpleural lung regions and in the lower lung zones (60,79) (Fig. 6-18). A similar pattern and distribution may be seen in asbestosis although the diagnosis can usually be suggested by the presence of associated pleural thickening (20,77). In chronic hypersensitivity pneumonitis the fibrosis is usually most severe in the mid-lung zones and is more random in distribution rather than having a subpleural predominance (80), although in some cases the findings may be similar to those of idiopathic pulmonary fibrosis (81). Although intralobular linear opacities usually indicate fibrosis, they may also occasionally be seen in the absence of fibrosis, having been described in patients with lymphangitic carcinomatosis (28) and alveolar proteinosis (68,69).

Cysts are rounded air-containing spaces surrounded by well-defined walls (Fig. 6-19). They are commonly seen in idiopathic pulmonary fibrosis (78,79), fibrosing alveolitis associated with systemic sclerosis and rheumatoid arthritis (78,82), asbestosis (20,78), and chronic hypersensitivity pneumonitis (78,81). In patients with pulmonary fibrosis cystic spaces represent honeycombing, that is, end-stage fibrosis, and are usually associated with architectural distortion and traction bronchiectasis. The honeycombing in patients with fibrosing alveolitis and asbestosis usually is most

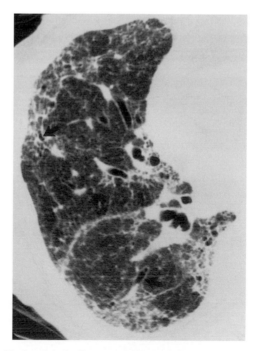

FIG. 6-18. Intralobular linear opacities in collagen vascular disease. High-resolution CT (1.5-mm collimation) targeted to the right lung, demonstrates intralobular linear opacities mainly in the subpleural lung regions. Note dilated bronchi in the areas of fibrosis, a finding known as traction bronchiectasis (*arrows*). The patient was a 73-year-old man with fibrosing alveolitis associated with rheumatoid arthritis.

FIG. 6-17. Intralobular linear opacities. High-resolution CT (1.5-mm collimation) through the lower lung zones demonstrates linear opacities separated by only a few millimeters causing a fine reticular pattern. Also noted is irregular interlobular septal thickening. The patient was a 58-year-old woman with idiopathic pulmonary fibrosis.

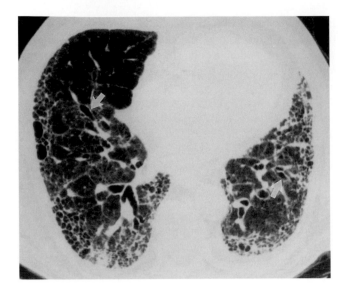

FIG. 6-19. Cystic air-spaces in idiopathic pulmonary fibrosis (IPF). High-resolution CT (1.5-mm collimation) through the lower lung zones demonstrates numerous cysts mainly involving the subpleural lung regions. The cysts range from a few millimeters to 2 cm in diameter. Also, note traction bronchiectasis (*arrows*). The patient was an 81-year-old man with honeycomb lung related to IPF.

severe in the subpleural lung regions and in the lung bases. The honeycombing in chronic hypersensitivity pneumonitis is also most marked in the subpleural lung regions but tends to be most severe in the mid-lung zones with relative sparing of the lung bases (78,80). Cystic air spaces are a characteristic finding of lymphangioleiomyomatosis (83,84). In lymphangioleiomyomatosis the cysts are seen throughout the lungs without any zonal predominance. Furthermore, the cysts in patients with lymphangioleiomyomatosis are not related to fibrosis and therefore are surrounded by relatively normal lung parenchyma (83,84). Cystic spaces similar to those seen in lymphangioleiomyomatosis have also been described in patients with Langerhans' cell histiocytosis (85–87). The

cysts in Langerhans' histiocytosis characteristically involve the upper two-thirds of the lungs with relative sparing of the lung bases and often have bizarre shapes (Fig. 6-20).

Nodular Opacities

Nodules 1 to 10 mm in diameter are seen in a number of acute and chronic infiltrative lung diseases. Nodules with sharply defined borders are usually interstitial whereas nodules with ill-defined margins or a ground-glass appearance are more likely to represent disease involving mainly the airspace (9,88). Although airspace nodules have frequently been termed "acinar" nodules, because they often measure between 5 to 10 mm in diameter, they have been shown

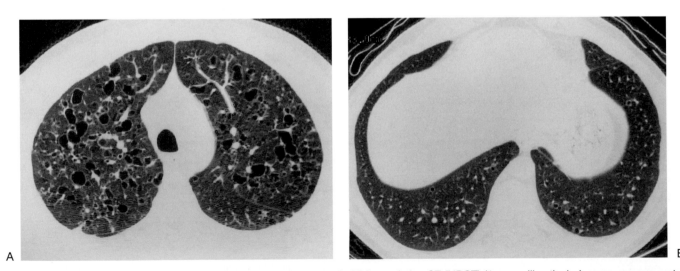

A B

FIG. 6-20. Cystic air-spaces in Langerhan's pulmonary histiocytosis. **A:** High-resolution CT (HRCT) (1 mm collimation) shows numerous cysts with well-defined walls randomly distributed in the upper lobes. Although some of the cysts are closely related to pulmonary arteries and may be difficult to distinguish from bronchiectasis several of the cysts are in the subpleural lung regions and, therefore, easily distinguished from dilated bronchi. **B:** HRCT through the lung bases shows very few cysts. The relative sparing of the lung bases is characteristic of Langerhan's pulmonary histiocytosis. The patient was a 30-year-old man.

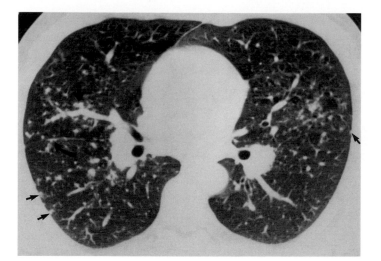

FIG. 6-21. Perilymphatic nodules. High-resolution CT (1.5-mm collimation) demonstrates nodules along vessels (*straight arrow*), interlobar fissure (*curved arrow*) and subpleural lung regions (*small arrows*). This distribution is characteristic of sarcoidosis. Also note bilateral hilar lymphadenopathy. The patient was a 37-year-old man with stage 2 sarcoidosis.

by Itoh et al. to represent centrilobular and peribronchiolar abnormalities rather than involvement of the acini (53). The distinction of interstitial from airspace nodules can often not be confidently made on CT and is of limited value in the differential diagnosis. A more useful approach to the differential diagnosis is based on the distribution of the nodules. A perilymphatic distribution along the bronchovascular interstitium, interlobular septa, and subpleural lung regions is characteristically seen in patients with sarcoidosis (63), lymphangitic carcinomatosis (28), silicosis and coalworkers' pneumoconiosis (75,76) (Fig. 6-21). In these conditions the nodules tend to be well-defined and usually measure 2 to 5 mm in diameter. Nodules in a perilymphatic distribution are frequently associated with nodular thickening of the bronchovascular bundles. Another sign helpful in assessing the perilymphatic distribution is the presence of subpleural nodules in relation to the interlobar fissures, a characteristic finding in silicosis, coalworkers' pneumoconiosis and sarcoidosis.

Small nodules in a centrilobular distribution are characteristically seen in hypersensitivity pneumonitis (22,89), endobronchial spread of tuberculosis (47,90), and various forms of bronchiolitis including Asian panbronchiolitis (91), smokers' respiratory bronchiolitis (92), and bronchiolitis obliterans with organizing pneumonia (93). Centrilobular nodules in hypersensitivity pneumonitis typically have poorly defined margins (Fig. 6-22). They may be diffuse throughout the lungs or involve mainly the middle and lower lung zones. Centrilobular nodules associated with endobronchial spread of tuberculosis have a more focal distribution and frequently present with a tree-in-bud appearance (Fig. 6-23).

Small nodules in a miliary distribution are seen most commonly in miliary tuberculosis (94,95) and miliary fungal infections (96) and less commonly in sarcoidosis (Fig. 6-24). Hematogenous miliary metastases are most numerous in the lung periphery and at the lung bases but have a random distribution regarding the lobular structures (97).

Nodules greater than 1 cm in diameter may result from

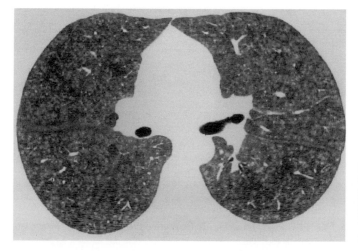

FIG. 6-22. Centrilobular nodules in hypersensitivity pneumonitis. High-resolution CT (1-mm collimation) at the level of the bronchus intermedius demonstrates numerous poorly defined centrilobular nodules. Note that the nodules are a few millimeters away from the pleura including interlobar fissures, a characteristic finding of centrilobular nodules. The patient was 35-year-old man with subacute hypersensitivity pneumonitis (bird-breeder's lung).

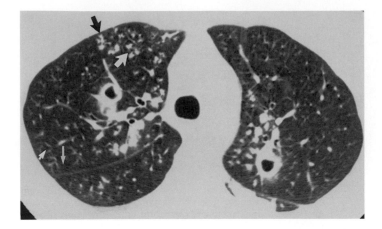

FIG. 6-23. Tree-in-bud appearance in tuberculosis. High-resolution CT (1.5-mm collimation) through the upper lobes demonstrates bilateral cavities and sharply defined centrilobular nodules. The nodules and branching lines have an appearance that resembles a tree-in-bud (*arrows*). The patient was a 29-year-old man with endobronchial spread of tuberculosis (compare with Figure 6-5B).

conglomeration of smaller nodules or from progressive fibrosis as may be seen in patients with silicosis (98), sarcoidosis (67,99), or talcosis (100). More commonly larger nodules result from pulmonary metastases, septic emboli (101), or Wegener's granulomatosis (102, 103). Pulmonary metastases tend to have smooth margins and are most numerous in the subpleural regions of the lower lung zones. Septic emboli have a similar distribution. A characteristic sign of septic emboli on HRCT is the presence of vessels in close association with the nodules ("feeding vessel" sign) (101). The nodules in Wegener's granulomatosis may range from 2 mm to 7 cm in diameter, usually have irregular margins, and frequently cavitate (102,103).

In immunocompromised patients nodules larger than 1 cm in diameter may be caused by septic embolism (101), invasive aspergillosis (104,105), posttransplant lymphoproliferative disorders (106), or lymphoma (107). Nodules caused by invasive pulmonary aspergillosis often have a characteristic

halo of ground-glass attenuation surrounding the nodule (104) (Fig. 6-25). This halo is caused by hemorrhage. Although the "halo sign" was first described in invasive aspergillosis, it may also be seen in other hemorrhagic nodules including candidiasis, Wegener's granulomatosis, metastatic angiosarcoma, and Kaposi's sarcoma (105). Posttransplant lymphoproliferative disorders and lymphomas seen in patients with AIDS often present with pulmonary nodules, which may have smooth or irregular margins (106,107). In immunocompromised patients lymphoma may often involve the lungs without associated hilar or mediastinal lymphadenopathy.

Ground-Glass Attenuation

Ground-glass attenuation is characterized by the presence of hazy increased attenuation of the lung without obscuration of the underlying bronchial and vascular outlines (108). If

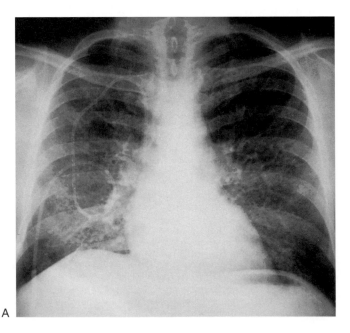

A

FIG. 6-24. Miliary disease. **A:** Posteroanterior radiograph shows pattern typical of miliary disease.

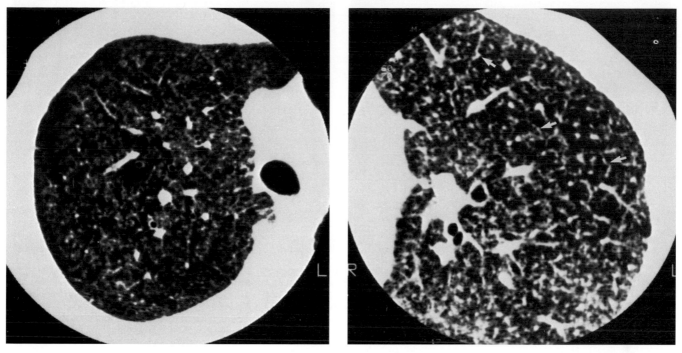

B

C

FIG. 6-24. *Continued.* **B:** Retrospectively targeted high-resolution CT (HRCT) image of the right upper lobe shows innumerable widely scattered nodules, without obvious relation to lobular anatomy. **C:** Retrospectively targeted HRCT image through the lungs of another patient with transbronchial biopsy evidence of noncaseating granulomata, presumed to be secondary to sarcoidosis. In this case, spatial resolution has been maximized by using a small field of view. There is clear accentuation of reticular structures, with miliary-sized nodules clearly identifiable causing nodular thickening of interlobular septa (*white arrows*) as a result of the presence of granulomata scattered throughout the interstitium.

the vessels are obscured, the term "consolidation" is used (109,110). Ground-glass attenuation results from volume averaging of abnormalities below the resolution of CT and may be caused by interstitial thickening, airspace filling, or both (110). Although ground-glass attenuation is a nonspecific finding, it is an important sign because it usually indicates the presence of active, potentially treatable disease (110,111). It is important to emphasize that ground-glass attenuation should only be considered to represent reversible disease if there are no other findings of fibrosis such as traction bronchiectasis, reticulation, or honeycombing (112) (Fig. 6-26). Areas of ground-glass attenuation in patients with chronic infiltrative lung disease are most commonly caused by idiopathic pulmonary fibrosis and fibrosing alveolitis associated with collagen vascular disease (19,111), desquamative interstitial pneumonia (DIP) (113), hypersensitivity pneumonitis (21), sarcoidosis (29,67), and, less commonly, alveolar proteinosis (68,69). In alveolar proteinosis the areas of ground-glass attenuation frequently have a patchy or geographic distribution with sharp demarcation between normal and abnormal lung parenchyma. In fibrosing alveolitis and in DIP, the areas of ground-glass attenuation tend to involve mainly the subpleural lung regions and the lung bases (Fig. 6-27). Ground-glass attenuation in hypersensitivity pneumonitis may be diffuse or involve mainly the mid and lower lung zones. Although ground-glass attenuation is commonly seen in sarcoidosis, it is almost always associated with other findings including

hilar and mediastinal lymphadenopathy and perilymphatic nodules.

Areas of ground-glass attenuation in patients with AIDS are highly suggestive of *Pneumocystis carinii* pneumonia (71,114) (Fig. 6-28) (see also Chapter 7). In the non-AIDS

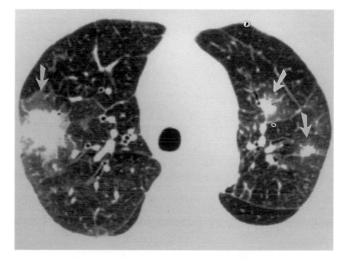

FIG. 6-25. Nodules with halo in invasive aspergillosis. High-resolution CT (1-mm collimation) through the upper lung zones demonstrates nodules ranging from 5 to 25 mm in diameter. The nodules have irregular margins and are surrounded by a halo of ground-glass attenuation (*arrows*). The patient was a 77-year-old woman with leukemia and angio-invasive aspergillosis.

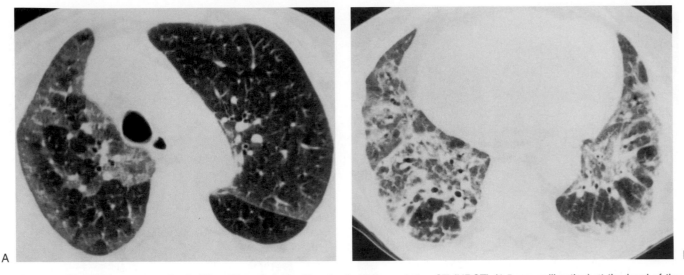

A

B

FIG. 6-26. Ground-glass attenuation in idiopathic pulmonary fibrosis. **A:** High-resolution CT (HRCT) (1.5-mm collimation) at the level of the aortic arch demonstrates areas of ground-glass attenuation involving mainly the subpleural lung regions of the right upper lobe. Mild disease is present in the left upper lobe particularly adjacent to the left interlobar fissure. On open lung biopsy, the findings in the right upper lobe were shown to be caused by alveolitis, that is, potentially reversible disease. **B:** HRCT through the lower lung zones in the same patient also show extensive areas of ground-glass attenuation. However, there is also evidence of fibrosis with irregular linear opacities and architectural distortion. Open lung biopsy of the right lower lobe demonstrated mainly fibrosis. The patient was an 82-year-old woman with idiopathic pulmonary fibrosis.

immunocompromised patient, areas of ground-glass attenuation are a relatively nonspecific finding being seen in patients with *Pneumocystis carinii* pneumonia, cytomegalovirus pneumonia, cytotoxic drug reaction, pulmonary edema, and pulmonary hemorrhage (115,116).

Consolidation

Parenchymal consolidation usually results from filling of the air spaces by fluid, protein, cells, or other material

(47,88,110). Occasionally it may result from replacement of air in the alveoli by extensive interstitial disease as may be seen in patients with sarcoidosis and usual interstitial pneumonia (UIP) (110). Essentially all conditions leading to areas of ground-glass attenuation, when severe enough, will cause consolidation and both findings are frequently present in the same patient (117,118). Diffuse diseases commonly associated with consolidation include bacterial and fungal pneumonia, adult respiratory distress syndrome (ARDS), acute interstitial pneumonia (AIP) (117), and bronchiolitis obliterans with organizing pneumonia (118). AIP is essentially the idiopathic form of ARDS, more properly classified as one of the idiopathic interstitial pneumonias (see section below on Idiopathic Interstitial Pneumonitis).

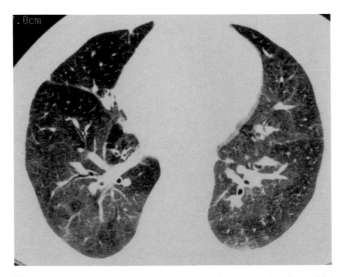

FIG. 6-27. Ground-glass attenuation in desquamative interstitial pneumonia (DIP). High-resolution CT (1.5-mm collimation) through the lower lung zones demonstrates bilateral areas of ground-glass attenuation with relative sparing of the right middle lobe. There is minimal if any evidence of fibrosis. The patient was a 63-year-old woman with DIP.

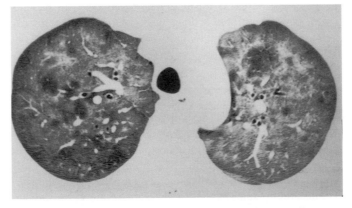

FIG. 6-28. Ground-glass attenuation in *Pneumocystis carinii* pneumonia (PCP). High-resolution CT (1.5-mm collimation) shows extensive areas of ground-glass attenuation in the upper lobes. The patient was a 41-year-old male with acquired immune deficiency syndrome (AIDS) and *Pneumocystis carinii* pneumonia (PCP).

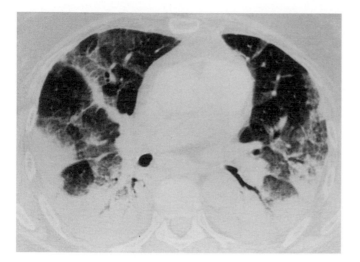

FIG. 6-29. Consolidation in acute interstitial pneumonia (AIP). High-resolution CT (1.5-mm collimation) demonstrates bilateral consolidation involving mainly the dependent regions of the lower lobes. Patchy areas of ground-glass attenuation are seen anteriorly. The patient was an 83-year-old woman with AIP.

The CT findings, therefore, are similar to those of ARDS (117,119) and consist of extensive bilateral areas of ground-glass attenuation and consolidation (Figs. 6-29 and 6-30). Bronchiolitis obliterans with organizing pneumonia (BOOP), also known as cryptogenic organizing pneumonia (COP), most frequently presents with bilateral areas of consolidation, which in approximately 60% of cases are peribronchial or subpleural in distribution (118) (Fig. 6-31).

In the majority of patients with consolidation the findings are readily apparent on the radiograph and CT adds little additional information. However, because the distribution of the consolidation is better appreciated on CT, it sometimes can be helpful in the differential diagnosis. For example, in up to 50% of patients with chronic eosinophilic pneumonia the peripheral consolidation (''reverse pulmonary edema pattern'') may not be apparent on the radiograph but can be clearly seen on CT (120). CT can also demonstrate localized collections of fat in patients with patchy or diffuse consolidation caused by lipoid pneumonia (121). It may also be helpful in patients with suspected amiodarone lung by demonstrating the characteristic increased attenuation caused by accumulation of this iodinated agent within the lung parenchyma (122) (Fig. 6-32). It is also helpful in the diagnosis of metastatic pulmonary calcification (123).

Decreased Attenuation

Decreased lung attenuation may result from lung destruction, as seen in emphysema, or from decreased blood flow caused by pulmonary vascular or airway abnormalities. Emphysema is characterized by the presence of areas of abnormally low attenuation without definable walls (124,125). It should be noted, however, that when emphysema involves

the entire secondary lobule, the interlobular septa may give the appearance of thin (1 mm or less) walls. Thin walls are also seen with bullae, which are defined as sharply demarcated areas of emphysema measuring 1 cm or more in diameter and possessing a wall of less than 1-mm in thickness (126). Bullae may therefore resemble lung cysts, although the distinction can usually be readily made because bullae are almost always associated with extensive emphysema. Three main forms of emphysema are recognized: centrilobular, typically associated with cigarette smoking; panlobular, typically associated with alpha-1 protease deficiency; and distal acinar emphysema.

Centrilobular emphysema can be diagnosed by the presence of small lucencies near the center of the secondary lobule (127) (Fig. 6-33). It is usually most severe in the upper lobes. Panlobular emphysema involves mainly the lower lobes and is characterized by the presence of diffuse areas of low attenuation with little intervening normal lung (128) (Fig. 6-34). Distal acinar emphysema is characterized by areas of low attenuation in the subpleural lung regions and adjacent to vessels and interlobular septa (125).

Decreased attenuation may also be caused by decreased perfusion resulting from vascular obstruction as seen in patients with pulmonary thromboembolism (129,130). Redistribution of blood flow away from the areas of vascular obstruction leads to increased attenuation in areas of normal lung parenchyma. This combination of areas with decreased attenuation and areas with increased attenuation is known as mosaic perfusion. More commonly, mosaic perfusion is caused by airway diseases leading to decreased ventilation, reflex vasoconstriction, and blood flow redistribution (131,132).

In some patients it may be difficult to determine whether a mosaic pattern of lung attenuation is caused by flow redistribution to areas of normal lung or whether it is caused by patchy areas of ground-glass attenuation resulting from infiltrative lung disease (133). This distinction, however, can usually be readily made by close attention to the size of the pulmonary vessels and assessment of presence of air trapping on expiratory CT. In patients with a patchy infiltrative process resulting in mosaic attenuation, the number and caliber of vessels are not appreciably different between normal and abnormal regions of lung (66) (see Fig. 6-26). A mosaic pattern of lung attenuation caused by pulmonary vascular disease, such as pulmonary arterial hypertension and chronic pulmonary thromboembolism, is associated with a decrease in the number and size of vessels in the areas of low attenuation compared to areas with increased attenuation that have an increase in the number and size of vessels caused by flow redistribution (66) (Fig. 6-35). A similar pattern is seen in patients with flow redistribution caused by primary small airway disease (66,133) (Fig. 6-36). Distinction between mosaic attenuation caused by small airway disease and vascular disease requires careful analysis of associated findings such as enlargment of central pulmonary arteries, often seen in patients with pulmonary arterial hypertension or recurrent

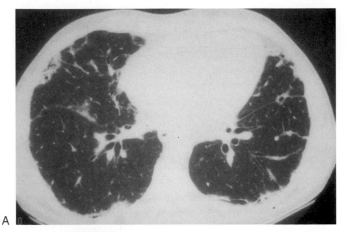

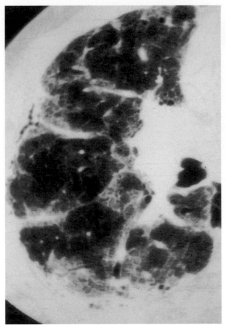

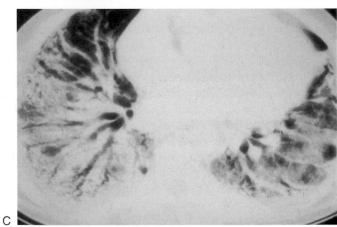

FIG. 6-30. Acute interstitial pneumonitis (AIP). **A:** CT section through the lung bases shows early changes of peripheral reticulatin and subtle honeycombing. **B:** Target reconstruction of the right mid lung approximately 1 week after **A** shows more extensive reticulation with foci of ground-glass attenuation noted. These changes accompanied progressively severe dyspnea. **C:** CT section through the lung bases approximately 1 week following **B** shows that the lower lobes now appear diffusely consolidated. Note that the bronchi appear corkscrewed, consistent with extensive traction bronchiectasis. This finding is an important indicator of the presence of extensive lung fibrosis. **D:** Open lung biopsy specimen shows extensive fibrosis replacing the lung parenchyma. This constellation of findings, in particular, the rapid appearance of diffuse lung fibrosis is characteristic of AIP.

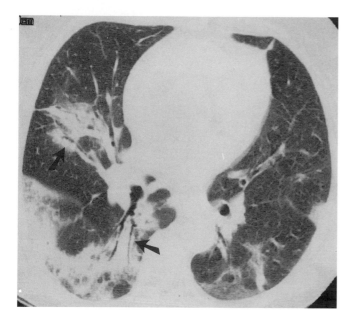

FIG. 6-31. Consolidation in bronchiolitis obliterans with organizing pneumonia. High-resolution CT (1-mm collimation) demonstrates asymmetric bilateral consolidation. The consolidation is predominantly peribronchial (*arrows*) and subpleural in distribution. The patient was an 81-year-old woman with bronchiolitis obliterans with organizing pneumonia.

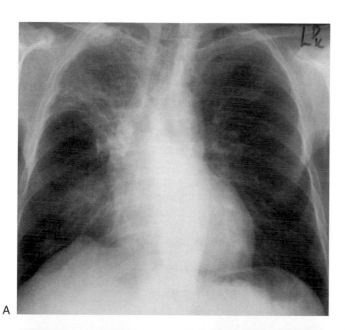

A

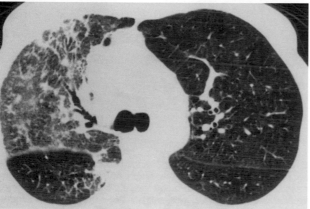

B

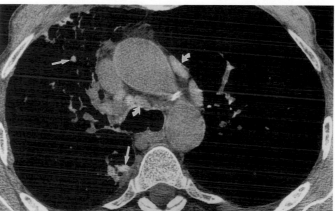

C

FIG. 6-32. Amiodarone lung. **A:** Chest radiograph demonstrates areas of parenchymal consolidation in the right upper, middle and lower lobes. Also noted are irregular linear opacities in the right and left upper lobes. **B:** High-resolution CT (1.5-mm collimation) demonstrates extensive areas of ground-glass attenuation in the right upper lobe and focal areas of consolidation in the right upper and lower lobes as well as a few irregular linear opacities. **C:** Mediastinal windows demonstrate focal areas of increased attenuation in the right upper and lower lobes (*straight arrows*) as well as increased attenuation of the mediastinal lymph nodes (*curved arrows*). Increased attenuation was also present in the thyroid, heart and liver (not shown). The patient was a 61-year-old man with amiodarone lung.

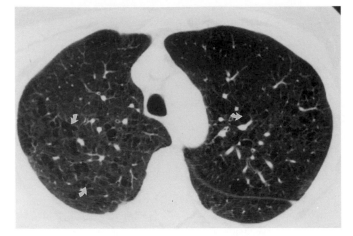

FIG. 6-33. Centrilobular emphysema. High-resolution-CT (1.5-mm collimation) demonstrates focal areas of decreased attenuation with no definable walls (compare with Fig. 6-5D,E). Note that in several areas small centrilobular vessels can be seen within the areas of decreased attenuation (*arrows*). The patient was a 59-year-old smoker with centrilobular emphysema.

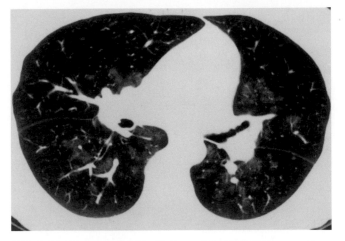

FIG. 6-35. Mosaic perfusion. High-resolution CT (1.5-mm collimation) demonstrates a pattern of mosaic perfusion with focal areas of decreased attenuation and small vessels as well as areas with increased attenuation associated with increased size and number of vessels. The patient was a 52-year-old woman with mosaic perfusion caused by chronic pulmonary arterial hypertension.

pulmonary emboli, and bronchial dilatation, often seen in patients with small airway disease (134). The distinction can also be facilitated by performing CT at suspended full expiration. In patients with airway disease the lucent areas show little change in volume and attenuation at end-expiration because of air trapping (133,135). In patients with primary vascular disease, because there is no air trapping, the attenuation in both the oligemic and hyperemic lung tends to increase to a similar degree at end-expiration. It should be noted, however, that in some cases the distinction may not be possible based only on the HRCT findings (134).

CHRONIC INFILTRATIVE LUNG DISEASE

A large number of chronic diseases may cause diffuse infiltration of the lungs. Although they are often referred to as chronic interstitial diseases, the majority involve both the interstitium and the air spaces. Therefore the term chronic infiltrative lung disease (CILD) is preferable (10,136). Although there are more than 150 different chronic lung diseases, approximately 20 conditions account for the vast majority of cases (136–138). Various classifications of chronic infiltrative lung diseases have been suggested. These have been based on etiology, pathogenesis, or pathologic findings

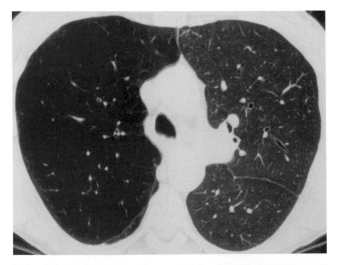

FIG. 6-34. Panlobular emphysema. High-resolution CT (1-mm collimation) demonstrates panlobular emphysema in the native right lung and a normal transplanted left lung. Note the characteristic simplification of the lung parenchyma in panlobular emphysema as compared to the normal architecture in the transplanted lung.

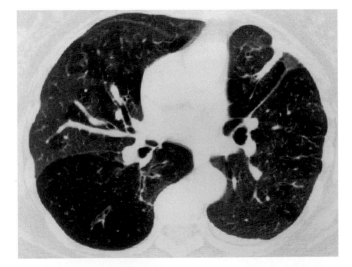

FIG. 6-36. Mosaic perfusion. High-resolution CT (1-mm collimation) demonstrates focal areas of decreased perfusion and areas with increased size and number of blood vessels characteristic of mosaic perfusion. Also noted is a localized area of scarring in the lingula. This patient was a 63-year-old woman with bronchiolitis obliterans presumably caused by childhood pneumonia.

TABLE 6-2. *Classification of most common chronic infiltrative lung diseases based on predominant pattern of abnormality on high resolution CT*

1. Linear or reticular pattern
    Interstitial pneumonitis
        Idiopathic (IPF/UIP)
        Collagen vascular disease
        Drug reaction
    Asbestosis
    Lymphangitic carcinomatosis
    CHF
2. Cystic pattern
    Langerhans cell histiocytosis
    Lymphangioleiomyomatosis
    Honeycomb lung
        IPF (UIP)
        Collagen vascular disease
        Chronic hypersensitivity pneumonitis
        Radiation
        Sarcoidosis
3. Nodular opacities
    Predominately perilymphatic
        Sarcoidosis
        Lymphangitic carcinomatosis
        Silicosis/coalworkers' pneumoconiosis
    Predominately centrilobular
        Subacute hypersensitivity pneumonitis
        Lymphocytic interstitial pneumonitis
        Bronchioloalveolar cell carcinoma
    Random
        Hematogenous metastases
        Miliary disease
4. Ground-glass attenuation
    Desquamative interstitial pneumonia
    Alveolar proteinosis
    Acute hypersensitivity pneumonitis
5. Consolidation
    BOOP
    Chronic eosinophilic pneumonia
    Lipoid pneumonia
    Bronchioloalveolar carcinoma
    Lymphoma

IPF, idiopathic pulmonary fibrosis; UIP, usual interstitial pneumonitis; CHF, congestive heart failure; BOOP, bronchiolitis obliterans with organized pneumonia.

TABLE 6-3. *Interstitial pneumonitis: pathologic classification*

Idiopathic interstitial pneumonitis
    IPF (UIP)
    DIP/RB-ILD
    AIP
    NSIP
Interstitial pneumonitis associated with infection
    Viral; mycoplasma
Interstitial pneumonitis associated with environmental
    exposure
    Asbestosis
    Hypersensitivity pneumonitis
    Drug reactions
    GIP
Interstitial pneumonitis associated with collagen vascular
    • disease
Interstitial pneumonitis associated with immunodeficiency
    LIP

IPF, idiopathic pulmonary fibrosis; UIP, usual interstitial pneumonitis; DIP, dequamative interstitial pneumonitis; RB-ILD, respiratory bronchiolitis-interstitial lung disease; AIP, acute interstitial pneumonitis; NSIP, nonspecific interstitial pneumonitis; GIP, giant cell interstitial pneumonitis; LIP, lymphocytic interstitial pneumonitis.

spiratory bronchiolitis-interstitial lung disease (RB-ILD); acute interstitial pneumonitis (AIP); and nonspecific interstitial pneumonitis (NSIP).

First characterized by Liebow, idiopathic interstitial pneumonitis was initially divided into five categories including: UIP; DIP; bronchiolitis interstitial pneumonia (BIP); lymphoid interstitial pneumonia (LIP); and giant cell interstitial pneumonia (GIP) (140). Awareness that BIP, now recognized as bronchiolitis obliterans organizing pneumonia (BOOP), represents a disorder predominantly affecting the distal airways, whereas LIP is more accurately characterized as one of the lymphoproliferative disorders often seen in association with HIV infection, and GIP represents a reaction to hard metal inhalation, has recently led to a more inclusive classification of the interstitial pneumonias (see Table 6-3).

Idiopathic Pulmonary Fibrosis (Usual Interstitial Pneumonia)

Previously considered synonymous with all patients with idiopathic interstitial pneumonitis (141,142), current understanding suggests that the term IPF should now be restricted only to patients with histologic evidence of UIP. The most common of the four histologic forms of idiopathic interstitial pneumonitis (see Table 6-4), IPF represents a distinct clinicopathologic entity defined by a combination of clinical, histological, and radiological features (139). It cannot be overemphasized that although all patients with IPF have UIP, UIP in itself is nonspecific and may be seen in patients with diffuse interstitial pneumonitis from a number of known

(103–106). From the radiologic point of view, however, it is reasonable to classify the various diseases based on the predominant pattern of abnormality on CT (Table 6-2).

Idiopathic Interstitial Pneumonitis

Few topics have caused greater confusion than idiopathic interstitial pneumonitis. Usually referred to either as idiopathic pulmonary fibrosis (IPF) or cryptogenic fibrosing alveolitis, idiopathic interstitial pneumonitis has recently been shown to encompass four distinct histologic entities, separable histologically, clinically, and radiographically (Tables 6-3 and 6-4) (139). These include: usual interstitial pneumonitis (UIP); desquamative interstitial pneumonitis (DIP)/ re-

TABLE 6-4. *Idiopathic interstitial pneumonitis: clinical-pathologic features*

	Pathologic features			
Temporal appearance	IPF (UIP) variegated	DIP/RBILD uniform	AIP uniform	NSIP uniform
Fibrosis				
fibroblast proliferation	random fibroblast foci prominent	no	diffuse fibroblast foci	rare
collagen deposition	common; patchy distribution	variable; diffuse (DIP) or focal (RBILD)	no	variable; diffuse
microscopic honey combing	common	no	no	rare
Inflammation				
Interstitial	scant	scant	scant	common
intraalveolar macrophage accumulation	occasional	diffuse (DIP) or peribronchiolar (RBILD)	no	occasional
BOOP	no	no	no	occasional

	Clinical features			
	IPF (UIP)	DIP/RBILD	AIP	NSIP
Onset	insidious	insidious	acute	subacute
Mean approx age	middle-aged	middle-aged slightly <UIP	middle-aged may occur in children	middle-aged
Response to steroids	poor	good; complete recovery possible	poor; complete recovery possible	good; complete recovery possible
Approx. mortality rate/ mean survival	60–65% (5–6 yrs)	25–30% (12 yrs)	60–65% (1–2 mo)	10–15% (17 mo)

UIP, usual interstitial pneumonitis; IPF, idiopathic pulmonary fibrosis; DIP, dequamative interstitial pneumonitis; RBILD, respiratory bronchiolitis interstitial lung disease; AIP, acute interstitial pneumonitis; NSIP, nonspecific interstitial pneumonitis; BOOP, bronchiolitis obliterans organizing pneumonia.
From ref. 139, with permission.

causes, including collagen vascular disease and asbestosis. Given its near universal usage, the term IPF, consequently, is preferred to UIP when discussing this form of idiopathic interstitial pneumonitis.

Clinically, IPF occurs most commonly in patients between 40 and 70 years of age, with a male to female ratio = 2. Notably, the disease rarely affects children. The onset of disease is typically insidious with progressive exertional dyspnea and a dry cough (143,144). Nonspecific systemic symptoms, including fever and weight loss have been reported in as many as 50% of cases (145). Laboratory findings are also nonspecific and include antinuclear antibodies, cryoglobulins and rheumatoid factor (139). Unfortunately, the prognosis of UIP is poor, with mortality rates ranging between 50% and 70%, and death occurring from progressive respiratory insufficiency typically within 6 years from the time of diagnosis, despite therapy.

Histologically, IPF results in patchy, nonuniform areas of fibrosis, inflammation, and honeycombing interspersed between areas of normal lung (139). Most of the fibrosis represents dense collagen resulting in thickened alveolar septa. Collagen is also found in association with areas of microscopic honeycombing with dilatation of respiratory bronchioles and alveolar ducts. The most characteristic finding is the presence of discrete zones of spindle cell prolifera-

tion within areas of fibrosis arranged along the long axis of alveolar septa, so-called fibroblast foci (139). These foci, representing zones of active fibrosis, are the earliest manifestation of disease and occur in response to recurrent episodes of acute lung injury. The result is focal fibroblast proliferation leading to collagen deposition and eventual honeycombing with each of these components temporally evolving at different rates. In distinction to these varying patterns of fibrosis, inflammation is usually mild and composed mainly of small lymphocytes admixed with plasma cells, and less commonly neutrophils and eosinophils. Typically these are seen in association either with areas of dense acellular collagen or microscopic honeycombing.

Traditionally, patients with IPF have been subclassified histologically based on the degree of cellularity versus fibrosis, with the notion being that the degree of inflammation or alveolitis would be predictive of response to treatment with steroids. These studies, however, included all histologic types of idiopathic interstitial pneumonitis (146–148). Not surprisingly, the definition and significance of cellularity as a prognostic factor has proved controversial (139). As emphasized by Katzenstein and Meyers, there is no convincing evidence that inflammation or alveolitis ever represents a predominant histologic finding in patients with IPF or even precedes the development of fibrosis (139). Similarly, the finding of intraalveolar macrophages, in itself a nonspecific finding, also bears no relationship to the stage of disease. In distinction, the degree of fibrosis, especially the extent of honeycombing, is predictive of a lack of response. As will be discussed, these observations are pertinent to HRCT in patients with IPF, especially for assessing the importance of ground-glass attenuation as a method for defining disease activity.

Despite numerous previous reports documenting the HRCT appearance of IPF, these studies must be interpreted cautiously as it is likely that most if not all of these include forms of idiopathic interstitial pneumonitis other than UIP. On HRCT, the main pattern of abnormality in IPF consists of intralobular linear opacities that correspond histologically to thin irregular areas of fibrosis (10,79) (Fig. 6-37). This

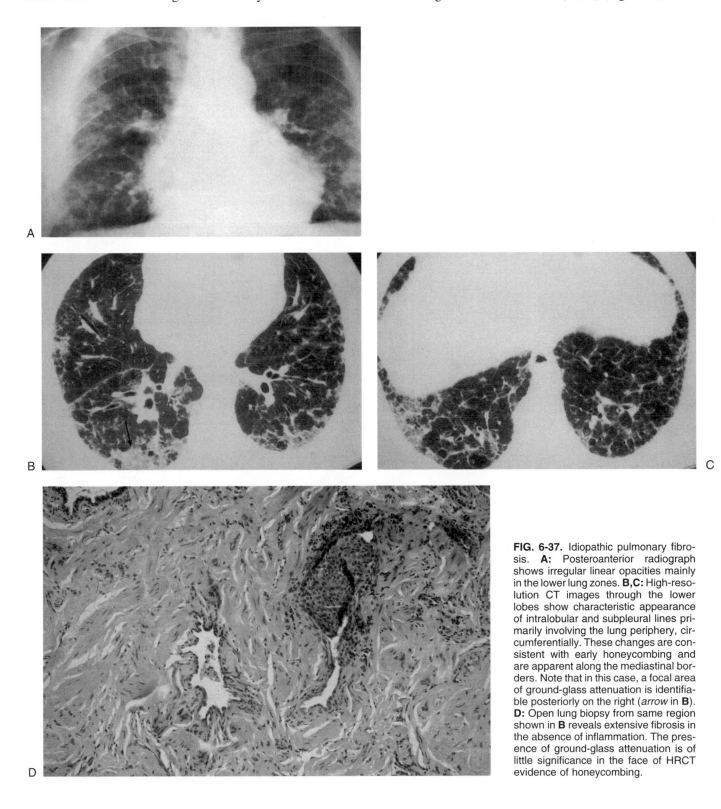

FIG. 6-37. Idiopathic pulmonary fibrosis. A: Posteroanterior radiograph shows irregular linear opacities mainly in the lower lung zones. B,C: High-resolution CT images through the lower lobes show characteristic appearance of intralobular and subpleural lines primarily involving the lung periphery, circumferentially. These changes are consistent with early honeycombing and are apparent along the mediastinal borders. Note that in this case, a focal area of ground-glass attenuation is identifiable posteriorly on the right (arrow in B). D: Open lung biopsy from same region shown in B reveals extensive fibrosis in the absence of inflammation. The presence of ground-glass attenuation is of little significance in the face of HRCT evidence of honeycombing.

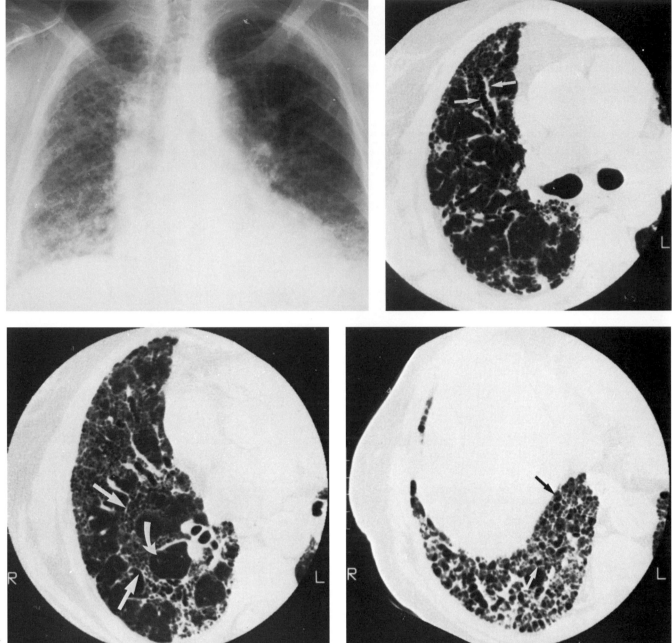

FIG. 6-38. Honeycomb lung in idiopathic pulmonary fibrosis. **A:** Posteroanterior radiograph shows evidence of diffuse reticulation throughout both lungs in a pattern suggestive of honeycombing. **B–D:** Sequential, retrospectively targeted high-resolution CT images through the right lung. These show cystic spaces which are easily identifiable (*arrows* in **C** and **D**). In portions of lung less severely involved, these areas of honeycombing can be seen to cut broad paths through the lung (*straight arrows* in **C**), in the process isolating relatively preserved, individual, secondary pulmonary lobules (*curved arrow* in **C**). The configuration of airways and vessels is now markedly irregular (*arrows* in **B**), and the pleural surfaces are more clearly irregular (compare with Fig. 6-37).

results in a fine reticular pattern that is characteristically most severe in the subpleural lung regions and in the lung bases (10,60,79). Also noted are irregular interfaces between the lung and pulmonary vessels, bronchi and pleural surfaces (9,60). Fibrosis results in dilatation and tortuosity of bronchi and bronchioles, findings referred to as traction bronchiectasis and bronchiolectasis (65,112). Late stage IPF is characterized by honeycombing (79,149) (see Figs. 6-19; Fig. 6-

38). Honeycombing, like the irregular linear pattern, is most severe in the subpleural lung regions and in the lung bases (10,79). The hallmark of IPF on HRCT, histologically, is its patchy distribution. Areas of normal lung parenchyma, ground-glass attenuation, intralobular lines, and honeycombing are frequently seen in the same patient, often in the same pulmonary segment (10,79).

Enlarged mediastinal lymph nodes may also be present

in 70% to 90% of patients with IPF (150,151). They usually measure between 10 and 15 mm in short axis diameter and involve only one or two nodal stations (151).

Areas of ground-glass attenuation are frequently present in patients with IPF and are the source of some controversy. Although Müller et al., in an early study of 12 patients demonstrated that in approximately 80% of cases areas of ground-glass attenuation reflect the presence of active, potentially treatable alveolitis, as previously noted, the prognostic significance of this finding is controversial (152). In this regard, it should be emphasized that ground-glass attenuation in itself is nonspecific and may result from areas of fibrosis or honeycombing below the resolution of HRCT (110, 152). Ground-glass attenuation resulting from fibrosis can usually be recognized on CT by the presence of other signs of fibrosis such as intralobular lines, honeycombing, and traction bronchiectasis or bronchiolectasis (see Figs. 6-26 and 6-30) (112).

It has been suggested that patients with areas of ground-glass attenuation are more likely to respond to treatment with corticosteroids than patients without areas of ground-glass attenuation (152). As a corollary finding, in patients with IPF who do not receive treatment or do not respond to therapy, it has been shown that areas of ground-glass attenuation precede and predict the development of a reticular pattern or honeycombing in the same location (153,154).

Nonetheless, the role of HRCT in predicting response to therapy remains controversial. In an early report assessing 12 patients with HRCT, Müller et al. correlated HRCT findings with disease activity assessed with open lung biopsy and found significant correlation between the extent of parenchymal opacification and tissue cellularity (152). Unfortunately, this included assessment of both intraalveolar as well as interstitial cellularity, with the former as previously noted of doubtful prognostic significance (139).

Lee et al. (149) correlated the extent of ground-glass attenuation at presentation with the improvement in pulmonary function following treatment with corticosteroids in 19 patients with IPF. The extent of ground-glass attenuation correlated significantly with the improvement in the forced vital capacity ($r = 0.71$, $p < 0.001$), and in gas transfer as assessed by the carbon monoxide diffusing capacity ($r = 0.67$, $p < 0.002$) after treatment. Taking a different tack, Wells et al. (111) correlated the predominant pattern of abnormality on CT with response to treatment and prognosis in 76 patients with IPF. The CT findings were categorized as consisting predominantly of ground-glass attenuation (n = 8), a mixed pattern (n = 18), or a predominantly reticular pattern (n = 50). Although approximately 80% of patients with predominantly ground-glass attenuation on HRCT responded to treatment compared to only 20% of patients with a mixed pattern and 4% of patients with a predominantly reticular pattern, only about 10% of patients had predominantly ground-glass attenuation, whereas 25% had equivalent extent of ground-glass attenuation and reticulation and 65% had predominant reticulation. This distribution of findings raises the question of whether or not this study actually represented a heterogeneous population of patients with varying forms of idiopathic interstitial pneumonitis (111). In particular, the finding of predominant diffuse ground-glass attenuation in the absence of other HRCT findings of fibrosis suggests that these patients represented a select subgroup most likely with DIP (see below) to account for their significantly improved response to therapy.

Hartman et al. assessed the significance of areas of ground-glass attenuation on HRCT in patients with biopsy proven IPF compared to those with DIP in a retrospective study of 23 patients (12 with UIP and 11 with DIP) who had both initial and follow-up HRCT scans (154a). Eleven patients with UIP and 11 with DIP received treatment between the initial and follow-up scans (median follow-up 10 months). Nine of the 12 patients (75%) with IPF showed an increase in the extent of ground-glass attenuation or progression to reticulation or honeycombing on follow-up, as compared with only 2 (18%) with DIP. Thus, although areas of ground-glass attenuation reflect the presence of active inflammation, in most patients with IPF they progress to fibrosis despite treatment.

Desquamative Interstitial Pneumonitis/Respiratory Bronchiolitis Interstitial Lung Disease

Previously thought to represent a subset of patients with idiopathic pulmonary fibrosis (141,155), DIP is now regarded as a separate histologic type of idiopathic interstitial pneumonitis (see Table 6-4). In distinction to IPF, DIP/RBILD is characterized histologically by the presence of a large number of macrophages within the air spaces, associated with only mild inflammation of the alveolar walls, and mild fibrosis (141,156). Importantly, regardless of location, lesions all appear temporally uniform with each portion of the lung showing monotonous uniformity. When these findings are confined primarily to the peribronchiolar air spaces, the process is termed respiratory bronchiolitis interstitial lung disease (RBILD), with DIP reserved for more diffuse parenchymal involvement. In effect the two terms describe a spectrum of findings of a likely single disease entity, hence the combined terminology DIP/RBILD. In this regard it is worth noting that although the majority of cases of DIP are idiopathic, a DIP-like reaction may also be seen in collagen vascular diseases, asbestosis, Langerhan's pulmonary histiocytosis, and drug reactions (155). As a consequence, the diagnosis of DIP/RBILD usually requires open lung biopsy for confirmation.

Because the primary abnormality in these cases is the presence of intraalveolar macrophages and not desquamated epithelial cells, as initially thought, the term desquamative interstitial pneumonitis (DIP) in fact is a misnomer (139). Nonetheless, although some have advocated dropping this term in favor of respiratory bronchiolitis interstitial lung disease alone, like other commonly used terms such as BOOP and IPF, DIP is likely to remain a standard part of the vocabulary.

Clinically, DIP/RBILD occurs almost exclusively in smokers. Similar to IPF, the onset is insidious and typically occurs in middle aged adults with a male:female ratio = 2. Patients with DIP have a much better prognosis and a better response to corticosteroid treatment than patients with UIP (141,155,157). Spontaneous remission has even been noted to occur in a minority of patients (157). The five-year mortality for patients with DIP is only 5% compared to 60% to 70% in patients with UIP.

The findings of DIP on the chest radiograph have been reported as consisting of areas of ground-glass attenuation (156) or as being similar to that of UIP, that is, a reticular pattern mainly involving the lower lung zones but having milder fibrosis than UIP (157). However, in up to 22% of patients with biopsy proven DIP the chest radiograph is normal (157).

The predominant HRCT finding in patients with respiratory bronchiolitis is the finding of ill-defined, centrilobular ground-glass nodules, usually with an upper lobe predominance (see Chapter 3). In distinction, the predominant CT findings in patients with DIP is the presence of areas of ground-glass attenuation (113,152). In the vast majority of patients the areas of ground-glass attenuation involve mainly the middle and lower lung zones (113). The ground-glass attenuation is predominantly peripheral in distribution in 60% of cases, patchy in 20%, and diffuse in 20% of patients (113) (see Figs. 6-27; Figs. 6-39–6-41). Irregular linear opacities and architectural distortion indicating the presence of fibrosis were seen in 60% of cases reported by Hartman et al. (113,152). The fibrosis was usually mild and involved mainly the subpleural lung regions of the lower lung zones. Honeycombing, when present, was limited to the subpleural regions of the lower lung zones (113). The distribution of abnormalities in DIP is therefore similar to that of UIP. However, the predominant abnormality in DIP consists of ground-glass attenuation whereas the predominant finding in UIP consists of irregular linear opacities and honeycombing (113,152,158).

Acute Interstitial Pneumonitis

More generally known as Hamman-Rich syndrome, acute interstitial pneumonitis is characterized by diffuse active interstitial fibrosis with proliferation of fibroblasts and myofibroblasts in the absence of extensive collagen deposition (159). These changes represent a response to an acute lung injury presumably sustained only weeks prior to the onset of disease and as such resemble the organizing phase of diffuse alveolar damage (DAD) (160). Unlike UIP, AIP is characterized by a diffusely uniform appearance. Unlike DIP/RBILD, intraalveolar macrophages do not constitute a major histologic component, although hyaline membranes may be prominent. With progression, microscopic foci of honeycombing may develop within a matter of weeks.

Clinically, the onset of disease is rapid and unlike UIP and DIP, may affect any group including children, without

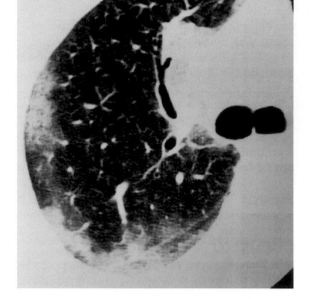

FIG. 6-39. Desquamative interstitial pneumonia (DIP). High-resolution CT in a 54-year-old woman with DIP shows areas of ground-glass attenuation in a predominantly subpleural distribution.

apparent sex predilection. The disease is usually rapidly progressive clinically resulting in the ARDS. Mortality rates are high, averaging approximately 60%, with death occurring within a few months of the onset of disease. Survival, however, is generally accompanied by near complete resolution of disease without recurrence (159).

To date, only limited data is available regarding both the radiographic and CT appearance of this entity. As noted by Primack et al. (117), chest radiographs typically show a pattern consistent with ARDS with diffuse airspace consolidation. On CT, findings include diffuse ground-glass attenuation, usually in association with abnormalities suggestive

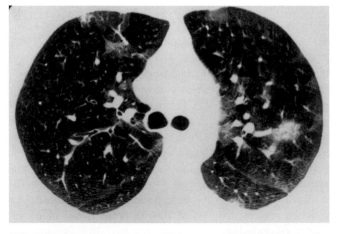

FIG. 6-40. Desquamative interstitial pneumonia (DIP). High-resolution CT in a 40-year-old man with DIP shows bilateral areas of ground-glass attenuation in a patchy distribution.

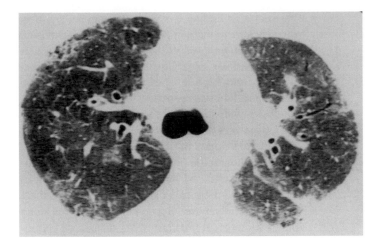

FIG. 6-41. Desquamative interstitial pneumonia (DIP). High-resolution CT in a 53-year-old man with DIP shows diffuse areas of ground-glass attenuation. Also noted is evidence of mild fibrosis in the subpleural lung regions of the upper lobes.

of underlying fibrosis, in particular, traction bronchiectasis (see Figs. 6-29 and 6-30) (117).

Nonspecific Interstitial Pneumonia and Fibrosis

Nonspecific interstitial pneumonia and fibrosis (NSIP) is characterized histologically by a relatively uniform pattern of dense cellular interstitial inflammation composed of a mixture of lymphocytes and plasma cells usually involving alveolar septa in association with variable degrees of fibrosis (142,161,162). Changes are temporally uniform and rarely associated with evidence of honeycombing. As such it represents a distinct form of idiopathic interstitial pneumonitis, clearly separable from IPF (UIP), DIP/RBILD, and AIP (139). Unlike DIP/RBILD and AIP, which are rare diseases, NSIP is a relatively common, second in frequency only to UIP (142).

Clinically, NSIP usually affects middle-aged patients, slightly more often in females. Onset is typically subacute or insidious and characterized by nonspecific respiratory symptoms. Prognosis is usually good with the majority of patients responding to treatment with corticosteroids (142,163).

Park et al. (163) described the high resolution CT findings in seven patients with NSIP. The predominant abnormalities consisted of patchy or diffuse bilateral areas of ground-glass attenuation. Associated areas of consolidation involving mainly the dependent regions of the lower lobes were present in 71% of cases. Irregular linear opacities suggestive of fibrosis were present in 29% of cases. Honeycombing was not seen in any of the patients.

Collagen Vascular Diseases

Histologic and CT findings identical to those of IPF (UIP) may be seen in patients with progressive systemic sclerosis (PSS, scleroderma), rheumatoid arthritis, and, less commonly, mixed collagen vascular disease, polymyositis, and systemic lupus erythematous (82,141,158,164) (Fig. 6-42). In a prospective study of 23 patients with PSS, evidence of interstitial disease was seen on the chest radiograph in 15 (65%) and on HRCT in 21 (91%) patients (164). The most common HRCT pattern consisted of irregular linear subpleural opacities causing fine reticulation. This pattern was seen in 17 (74%) of patients and honeycombing in seven (30%). Similarly to IPF, the fibrosis involved mainly the subpleural lung regions and the lower lung zones. There was no significant correlation between the duration of PSS and the severity of fibrosis on HRCT.

A study of 53 patients with PSS (82) revealed abnormality on HRCT in 32 (60%) cases. The most common findings included areas of ground-glass attenuation, honeycombing, and micronodules. The abnormalities had a subpleural and basal predominance. The micronodules are presumably

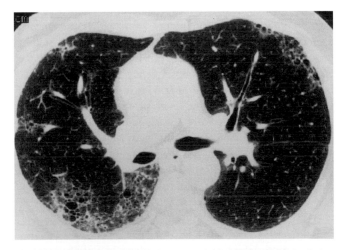

FIG. 6-42. Fibrosing alveolitis in rheumatoid arthritis. High-resolution CT (1-mm collimation) demonstrates irregular linear opacities, mild honeycombing and areas of ground-glass attenuation. The abnormalities are patchy in distribution but involve predominantly the subpleural lung regions. The appearance is identical to that of idiopathic pulmonary fibrosis. The patient was a 63-year-old man with fibrosing alveolitis associated with rheumatoid arthritis.

caused by lymphoid hyperplasia, a common finding in PSS (82,141). Other findings on HRCT include diffuse pleural thickening seen in approximately 25% of cases (82), enlarged mediastinal lymph nodes present in approximately 60% of cases (165), and asymptomatic esophageal dilatation seen in 80% of cases of PSS with interstitial fibrosis (165).

The fibrosis in PSS has a less aggressive course and a better prognosis than the prognosis in IPF (111). Similar to patients with IPF, the distinction between potentially reversible inflammation and fibrosis can be correctly made on HRCT in 80% of cases (166). Wells et al. (111) demonstrated that patients with areas of ground-glass attenuation were more likely to respond to treatment than patients with predominantly reticular opacities.

Approximately 5% of patients with rheumatoid arthritis have clinically significant fibrosis (166,167). The pattern and distribution of fibrosis in rheumatoid arthritis is similar to that of IPF (158,168). Much more common is clinical evidence of pleural involvement, usually pleural thickening, which is seen in 30% to 40% of patients (141,169). Other common findings in patients with rheumatoid arthritis include bronchiectasis, bronchiolectasis, and subpleural micronodules. Bronchiectasis is seen in approximately 10% of patients with rheumatoid arthritis (168).

Asbestosis

Asbestosis is defined as diffuse lung fibrosis caused by inhalation of asbestos fibers (170,171). The fate of inhaled asbestos fibers is determined mainly by fiber diameter (171). Fiber length plays a limited role, asbestos fibers several hundred microns in length being able to reach the alveoli (171). Fibers of 5 μm or more in diameter tend to be deposited in large airways from which clearance is relatively rapid through mucociliary action. Thinner fibers are more likely to be deposited in either the peripheral airways or, if extremely fine, the distal air spaces from which clearance is usually slower. These fibers are not likely to be ingested by the alveolar macrophages or, even less likely, the alveolar epithelial cells, and as a consequence may be transported into the interstitium of the lung with resultant formation of aggregates, usually at the level of the respiratory bronchioles. *In vitro* cell studies and research on animal models indicate that exposure to asbestos activates alveolar macrophages, which in turn causes the release of chemotactic factors derived from neutrophils, as well as a protein factor similar to a collagenase inhibitor that disturbs the balance of collagen turnover in the lung. These result in fibrogenic changes within the interstitium (172,173).

Asbestosis characteristically occurs 15 to 20 years following exposure, with disease progressing even after exposure has ceased. Initially, asbestosis affects respiratory bronchioles with development of peribronchiolar fibrosis. Fibrosis subsequently involves the alveolar walls and, when severe, leads to solid areas of scarring and honeycombing that involve large portions of the lung, predominantly in the subpleural regions of the lower lobes. Although it has been suggested that peribronchiolar fibrosis is characteristic of early asbestosis, this finding is nonspecific per se, and may result from exposure to many types of mineral dust exposure (174). The development of diffuse interstitial fibrosis is dose-related: asbestosis generally occurs only in those patients with long-term, high-level exposure, for example, asbestos miners and asbestos insulators (171).

As pathologic evaluation is not usually obtained in individual cases, assessing pulmonary parenchymal fibrosis has necessitated the development of a constellation of clinical, functional, and radiographic findings to establish the diagnosis of asbestosis *in vivo*. As determined by the American Thoracic Society, the diagnosis can be inferred when there is a reliable history of nontrivial exposure to asbestos along with a combination of: (a) restrictive lung disease on pulmonary function testing as well as a diffusion abnormality; (b) the presence of rales at auscultation; and (c) abnormal chest radiographs. It has been suggested that among these, "the findings on the chest roentgenogram are the most important" (175).

Unfortunately, there are limitations to the value of radiographic interpretation in defining a population with asbestos-induced abnormalities (Fig. 6-43). In a review of 200 admission chest radiographs interpreted according to the ILO classification of diffuse lung disease, Epstein et al. found that 22 patients (11%) without occupational exposure had abnormalities that otherwise might have been interpreted as indicative of significant dust exposure (176). Additionally, radiographic-pathologic correlative studies have shown that interstitial fibrosis may be present despite normal appearing chest radiographs in up to 20% of patients (177,178). Rockoff and Schwartz, analyzing the limitations of the ILO classification in predicting histologically verified asbestosis, also found that chest radiographs can result in a 10% to 20% probability of a normal interpretation (179). Added to these difficulties are significant problems with interobserver variability, specifically in the interpretation of opacities of mild profusion (180). Although the American Thoracic Society has specified as part of their definition of asbestosis a profusion (severity) of 1/1 or greater (175), as pointed out by Weill, it is unlikely that any one category will constitute a lower limit of abnormality that will prove diagnostic of asbestosis for all qualified readers (181).

The potential of CT to evaluate patients with documented exposure to asbestos has been noted by numerous investigators (20,52,182–194). In many cases the fibrosis is mild and limited to the dependent regions of the lower lung zones. It may be difficult, if not impossible, to distinguish mild fibrosis in these areas from normal increase in attenuation and atelectasis in the dependent lung. Therefore it is recommended that in patients being assessed for asbestosis, HRCT scans be obtained in both supine and prone position (20,190). Although in most cases the scans should be obtained at 10 or 20 mm intervals, a limited technique consisting of four or five equally spaced scans obtained from the level of the tracheal carina to the diaphragm has been shown to have good sensitivity in the detection of asbestosis and may be appropriate for screening (193).

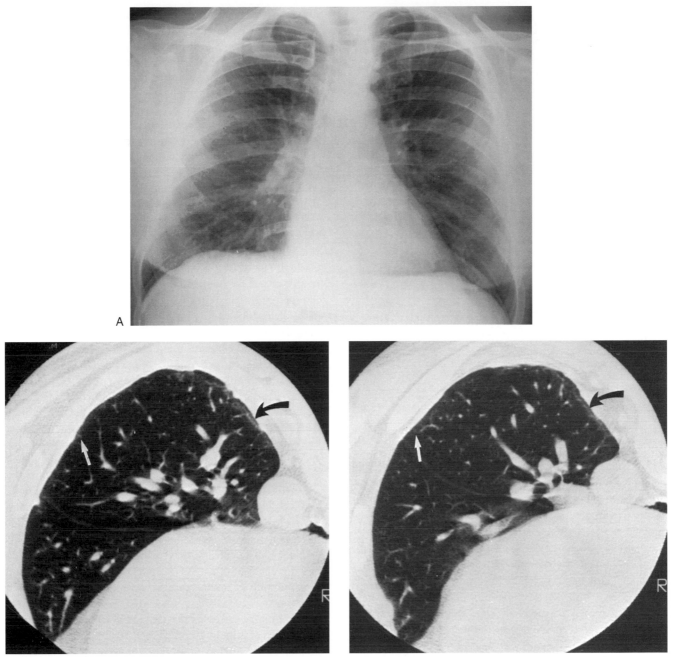

FIG. 6-43. Asbestosis. **A:** Posteroanterior radiograph shows minimal nodularity of the right hemidiaphragm. The lungs appear normal. **B,C:** Sequential 1.5-mm target reconstructed sections through the right lower lobe obtained with the patient in a prone position show subtle parenchymal changes consistent with asbestosis. In addition to pleural plaques, intralobular lines and dots (*straight arrows* in **B** and **C**) are identifiable. These result in a prominent subpleural curvilinear line posteromedial (*curved arrows* in **B** and **C**).

Asbestosis can usually be readily recognized on HRCT by the presence of fibrosis associated with pleural plaques or diffuse pleural thickening. Akira et al. assessed the earliest stage in which asbestosis could be detected on HRCT in 23 asbestos-exposed patients with radiographic profusion scores of 0 or 1 (192). The earliest abnormalities on HRCT consisted of subpleural nodules 1 mm or less in diameter (Fig. 6-44). The nodules were a few millimeters away from the pleura and occasionally appeared as fine branching struc-

tures (192). The subpleural nodules reflect the presence of centrilobular, peribronchiolar fibrosis (77,192). Confluence of nodules led to pleural based nodular irregularities and subpleural curvilinear lines (192) (Fig. 6-45). As the fibrosis progresses, extending from the peribronchiolar region to involve the alveolar walls, intralobular lines and irregular thickening of the interlobular septa are seen on HRCT (192) (Figs. 6-46 and 6-47). With further progression of fibrosis, architectural distortion, traction bronchiectasis, and eventu-

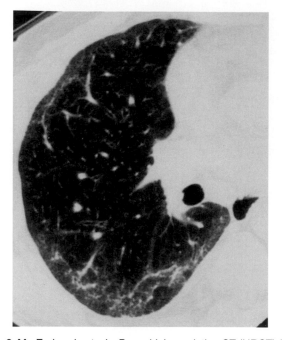

FIG. 6-44. Early asbestosis. Prone high-resolution CT (HRCT) (1.5-mm collimation) in patient with early asbestosis demonstrates ill-defined subpleural nodules and irregular linear opacities. The patient was a 54-year-old shipyard worker. HRCT done 3 years previously had been normal.

ally honeycombing are seen (78, 194) (Fig. 6-48). Pathologically and on HRCT the findings are most severe in the subpleural lung regions of the lower lung zones (171). Other common findings in asbestosis include curvilinear subpleural lines and parenchymal bands. In patients with asbestosis, curvilinear subpleural lines may be caused by early peribronchiolar fibrosis combined with collapse of alveoli caused by fibrosis (192), fine honeycombing (195), or atelectasis (196). They are, however, a nonspecific finding being seen in the dependent lung regions in up to 20% of subjects without history of exposure to asbestos (52,197). Parenchymal bands are linear densities 2 to 5 cm in length coursing through the lungs and usually attaching to the pleura (52,77) (Fig. 6-49). Parenchymal bands may be caused by thickened septa marginating several secondary lobules, fibrosis along the bronchovascular sheaths, coarse scars, or areas of atelectasis (77,197). Although parenchymal bands are common in asbestosis, being seen in 60% to 80% of patients (20,198), they are not specific, being present in 10% to 20% of patients with various lung diseases not related to asbestos (197,198).

Ground-glass attenuation is relatively uncommon in patients with asbestosis and when present usually is not extensive (198). It correlates with the presence of mild alveolar wall fibrosis or edema (77).

The diagnosis of asbestosis on HRCT is based on clinical history of exposure, findings indicative of bilateral pulmonary fibrosis and bilateral pleural plaques or diffuse pleural thickening. The specificity of the diagnosis increases with the number of parenchymal abnormalities present on HRCT

(194). In a study correlating HRCT and histopathologic findings, in 25 patients with asbestosis and 5 without, the HRCT findings in patients with confirmed asbestosis consisted of interstitial lines (84%), parenchymal bands (76%), architectural distortion of secondary pulmonary lobules (56%), subpleural lines (44%), and honeycombing (32%). The likelihood of asbestosis being present histopathologically increased from 60% in patients with one of these abnormalities on HRCT, 80% in patients with two, and 100% in patients with three or more abnormalities. However, the sensitivity decreased from 88% for a diagnosis based on the presence of only one of the five abnormalities, to 78% for two abnormalities, and 56% for three abnormalities (194).

The relationship between chest radiographic findings and HRCT has also been assessed. Aberle et al. evaluated HRCT findings in 100 occupationally exposed individuals defined clinically as having asbestosis (52). The authors found that in 85% of patients with clinical asbestosis, HRCT scans were interpreted as consistent with a high probability of asbestosis, with low probability reported in only 4% of cases. Importantly, of 55 individuals without clinical evidence of asbestosis, HRCT studies were interpreted as highly suggestive of asbestosis in nearly one-third. Similar findings have been reported by Staples et al. (191). In this study of more than 400 asbestos-exposed workers with documented latency periods of at least 10 years, evaluated clinically, physiologically, and with HRCT, these authors found that in nearly one-third of patients, HRCT findings suggestive of asbestosis could be identified despite normal radiographic appearances. Furthermore, significant differences could be documented in both vital capacity and diffusing capacity between patients with normal scans and those with HRCT evidence of parenchymal abnormalities. These findings are especially interesting as it has been suggested that changes in both vital and diffusing capacity may actually precede chest radiographic abnormalities.

In addition to finding disease within the lungs of patients with normal chest radiographs, HRCT may be of value by excluding disease in otherwise equivocal cases. As documented by Friedman et al., in their analysis of chest radiographs and HRCT scans in 60 patients with clinically suspected asbestosis, the positive predictive values of well-performed chest radiographs compared with HRCT scans for documenting the presence of significant lung disease was 79% versus 100%, respectively (185). Most important, these authors concluded that HRCT is of greatest value in eliminating false-positive diagnoses of lung disease caused by obscuration of the underlying parenchyma by pleural plaques.

Despite these reports, the role of HRCT in evaluating patients suspected of having asbestosis remains controversial (197,199). Although HRCT has been shown to be more sensitive than routine chest radiography in detecting abnormalities within the lung, the specificity of HRCT findings, in particular, has been challenged. Most of the findings reported in patients with documented asbestosis have also been described in other diseases that result in diffuse pulmonary

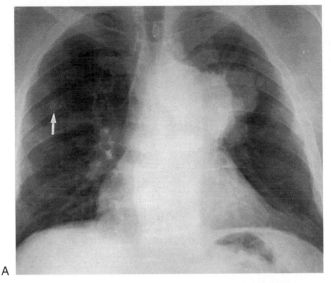

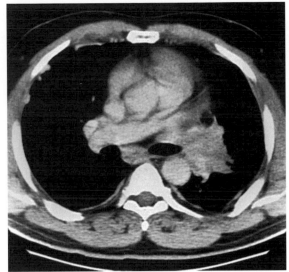

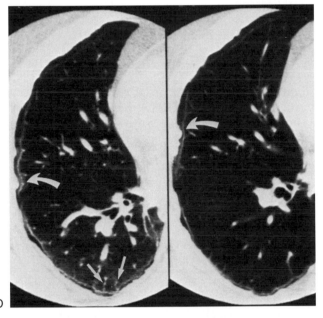

FIG. 6-45. Asbestosis. A: Posteroanterior radiograph shows a large mass in the left upper lobe and left hilum. Ill-defined contralateral densities can be seen as suggestive of pleural plaques (*arrow*). The lower lobes appear normal. **B:** Section through the left hilum imaged with mediastinal windows shows a large tumor mass associated with subcarinal adenopathy. Bilateral pleural plaques are easily identifiable, characteristic of asbestos-related pleural disease. **C,D:** Sequential, retrospectively targeted high-resolution CT sections through the right lower lobe show extensive, nearly circumferential subpleural curvilinear densities, associated with subtly thickened subpleural septal and core lines (*straight arrows* in **C**). Note that curvilinear lines can be seen both removed from as well as adjacent to pleural plaques (*curved arrows* in **C** and **D**).

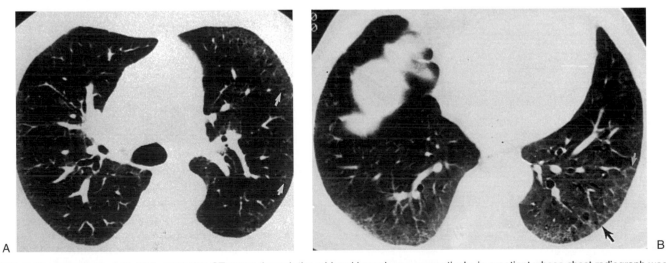

FIG. 6-46. Asbestosis. A,B: High-resolution CT scans through the mid and lower lungs, respectively, in a patient whose chest radiograph was interpreted as showing a profusion of 1/0. Abnormalities clearly predominate in the subpleural lung, including thickened subpleural intralobular lines (*straight white arrows* in **A** and **B**). Additionally, peripheral branches of the pulmonary arteries appear to extend to the pleural surfaces, suggesting that there is thickening of the interstitium surrounding the core pulmonary arteries (*black arrows* in **B**). Note that the overall effect is a fine subpleural reticulation associated with very subtle cystic changes, indicative of early honeycombing.

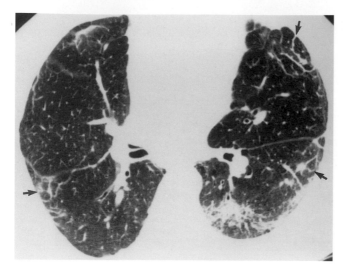

FIG. 6-47. Asbestosis. High-resolution CT (1.5-mm collimation) in 70-year-old patient with asbestosis demonstrates intralobular linear opacities and irregular thickening of interlobular septa with associated architectural distortion indicating the presence of fibrosis (*arrows*).

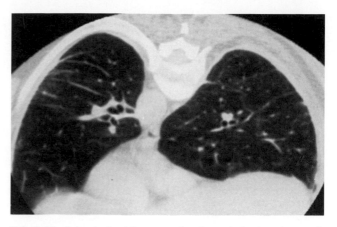

FIG. 6-49. Asbestosis. 1.5-mm section through the lung bases obtained with the patient in a prone position shows typical appearance of broad bands within both lower lobes. Note that on the left (corresponding to the right lower lobe), many of these bands have a curvilinear configuration. This finding probably represents the earliest manifestation of incipient round atelectasis.

fibrosis. Indeed, no CT finding, alone or in combination, should be interpreted as pathognomonic of asbestosis (199). Of course, given the wealth of data that has now been accumulated documenting the appearance of parenchymal fibrosis in particular, it can be argued that in patients with a history of documented nontrivial asbestos exposure, HRCT findings may be construed as significant indicators of asbestosis (200).

In summary, it is apparent that there is considerable potential for the use of HRCT in the evaluation of patients with a history of significant exposure to asbestos. At present, in our judgment, the main indications for the use of HRCT include: (a) evaluation of patients with equivocal chest radiographs, especially those in whom the presence of pleural plaques makes definitive interpretation of underlying paren-

chymal disease difficult; and (b) evaluation of patients with clinical evidence of disease in whom chest radiographs are interpreted as normal. The role of HRCT to evaluate patients with classic radiograph evidence of diffuse lung disease is less clear. Given the greater contrast resolution of CT coupled with the ability of CT to provide unobstructed views of the pulmonary parenchyma, it can be anticipated that the role of CT to evaluate patients with suspected asbestos-related parenchymal disease will continue to grow.

Lymphangitic Carcinomatosis

Pulmonary lymphangitic carcinomatosis refers to the spread of tumor within pulmonary lymphatics. In the majority of cases, lymphangitic carcinomatosis results from hematogenous tumor spread to the lungs with resultant thickening and infiltration of interlobular septa, subpleural interstitium, and bronchovascular bundles (201). In approximately 25% of cases, lymphangitic carcinomatosis is secondary to retrograde spread of tumor from infiltrated and enlarged hilar lymph nodes (201,202). Lymphangitic carcinomatosis usually results from adenocarcinoma arising from the breast, lung, gastrointestinal tract, or prostate, or less commonly from an unknown primary.

Radiographic changes are described as interstitial, with diffuse, although occasionally unilateral, reticulation, prominent Kerley's A and B lines, and effusions (201–205). As noted, hilar adenopathy occurs in a significant minority of patients. Although these findings are highly suggestive, especially in the setting of a known primary, the radiographic diagnosis of lymphangitic carcinomatosis may be problematic. In addition to a large differential of causes of interstitial disease in patients with known malignancies, in up to 50% of cases the radiograph may prove normal (203,204).

Several studies have assessed the HRCT findings in pa-

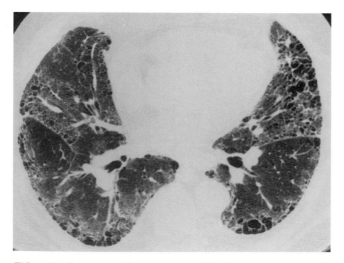

FIG. 6-48. Asbestosis. High-resolution CT in 59-year-old patient with advanced asbestosis demonstrates extensive bilateral honeycombing involving mainly the subpleural lung regions.

tients with lymphangitic carcinomatosis (9,28,62,72,206). The characteristic abnormalities consist of thickening of the interlobular septa and thickening of the peribronchovascular and subpleural interstitium with preservation of normal lung architecture (see Fig. 6-16; Fig. 6-50). The thickened interlobular septa are most commonly identified as lines 1 to 2 cm in length contacting the pleural surface or as polygonal arcades in the more central lung regions (9,28,62). The thickened septa may be smooth or have a beaded or nodular appearance caused by tumor growth along the lymphatics (9,10,28,62,206) (Fig. 6-51). Similarly, the thickening of the peribronchovascular interstitium may be smooth or nodular (28) (Fig. 6-52). Thickening of the interstitium along the centrilobular artery is frequently seen in the areas with interlobular septal thickening resulting in a prominent centrilobular dot. Smooth or nodular thickening of the subpleural inter-

stitium is also frequently present, being particularly well seen in the region of the interlobar fissures. Discrete small nodules may also be present (9,72). A distinctive feature of lymphangitic carcinomatosis is the preservation of normal lobular architecture allowing easy distinction from pulmonary fibrosis. Although lymphangitic carcinomatosis is most commonly bilateral and diffuse, it may occasionally be focal or unilateral in distribution (28,62).

Abnormalities characteristic of lymphangitic carcinomatosis have been described on HRCT in patients with normal or nonspecific findings on chest radiographs or CCT scans (28,62). In our experience the presence of thickened and beaded interlobular septal lines on HRCT in the clinical setting of known malignancy is essentially diagnostic of lymphangitic carcinomatosis. Although similar findings have been described in cases of viral pneumonia and, more importantly,

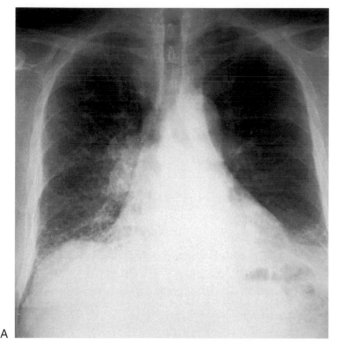

A

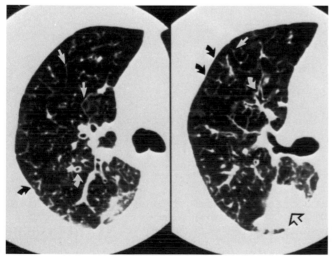

B,C

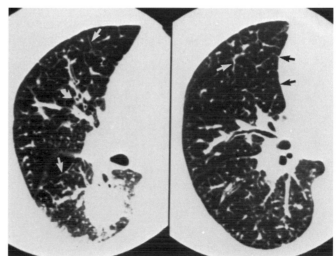

D,E

FIG. 6-50. Lymphangitic carcinomatosis. **A:** Posteroanterior radiograph shows asymmetric pulmonary infiltrates in the right lung associated with a mass in the superior segment of the right lower lobe. **B–E:** Sequential high-resolution CT sections through the right lung confirm the presence of a mass in the superior segment of the right lower lobe (*open arrow* in **C**), associated with soft-tissue fullness within the right hilum. Note thickening of peripheral interlobular septa (*curved black arrows* in **B** and **C**), thickened of central bronchial walls (*curved white arrows* in **B–D**), and most characteristic, prominent polygonal arcades, frequently traceable along central bronchovascular pathways to hilar and mediastinal surfaces (*black arrows* in **E**), characteristic of thickened secondary pulmonary lobular septa (*arrows* in **B–E**). The appearance of these has been likened to "beaded septa."

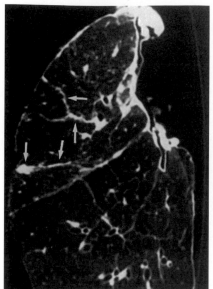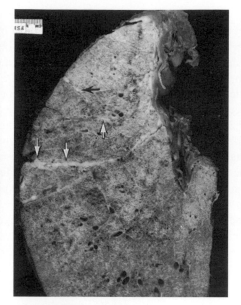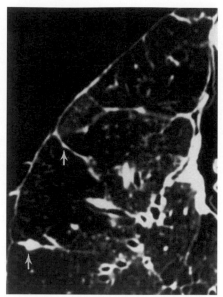

A,B

C

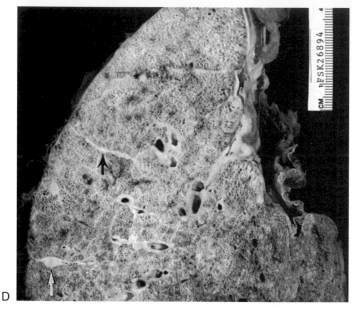

D

FIG. 6-51. Lymphangitic carcinomatosis. CT-pathologic correlation. **A,B:** CT section and corresponding inflated fixed lung specimen, respectively, in a patient with metastatic mediastinal germinoma. Coarse reticulation is apparent throughout the upper lobe, in particular, note the characteristic beaded appearance of thickened interlobular septa (*arrows*). **C,D:** Enlargements of both CT and fixed inflated lung sections in the same patient show to better extent the beaded appearance of lymphangitic carcinomatosis. *Arrows* point to thickened interlobular septa infiltrated by tumor.

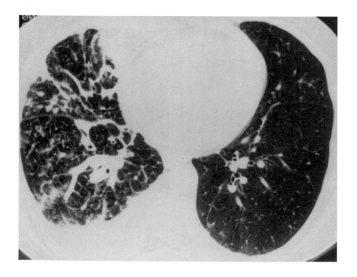

FIG. 6-52. Lymphangitic carcinomatosis. High-resolution CT (1.5-mm collimation) demonstrates marked thickening of the peribronchial and perivascular interstitium of the right lung compared with the left lung. The patient was a 67-year-old woman with lymphangitic carcinomatosis involving almost exclusively the right lung.

have been reported to occur in patients with sarcoidosis, when identified in the appropriate clinical setting, these changes are in our judgement sufficiently characteristic in select cases to obviate either transbronchial or open-lung biopsies (39).

Langerhans Cell Histiocytosis (Pulmonary Histiocytosis X)

Langerhans cell histiocytosis, also known as pulmonary histiocytosis X or eosinophilic granuloma of the lung, is a granulomatous disorder of unknown etiology that typically affects young or middle-aged adults (141). In 60% of cases, disease is isolated to the lungs; however, 20% also have bone involvement, and another 20% have multi-visceral disease. Clinically, patients usually present with nonspecific respiratory complaints; no consistent patterns of abnormality are shown on pulmonary function tests. Although up to 20% of patients present following a pneumothorax, as many as one-fifth are asymptomatic and are identified only because of abnormal chest radiographs (207,208). In most patients the course of the disease is surprisingly benign, with spontaneous resolution frequently occurring without therapy. Unfortunately, in a small percentage of patients, disease is progressive and leads to scarring and honeycombed lung.

Pathologically, Langerhans cell histiocytosis is characterized by nodules and cysts (141). Histologically, the diagnosis is made by the presence of characteristic large histiocytes (Langerhans cells) that contain rod- or racket-shaped organelles (Birbeck granules) (141,209). Although necrosis is rarely identified, nodules frequently appear cavitated; small and large cysts may also be identified (Fig. 6-53). Sequential high resolution CT studies in patients with pulmonary Langerhans cell histiocytosis have shown that at least some of the cysts represent transformation of nodular lesions.

Radiologically, pulmonary Langerhans cell histiocytosis most commonly causes a reticulonodular pattern primarily involving the mid and upper lung zones (207,208). Cysts and honeycombing have been reported on the radiograph in between 1% and 15% of cases. These findings are considerably different from the CT appearance of Langerhans cell histiocytosis (see Fig. 6-53; Fig. 6-54). The predominant finding on CT is the presence of cysts, which are seen in 70% to 90% of patients (85,86). Differentiation from emphysema is usually possible caused by the presence of identifiable walls; greater difficulty may be experienced differentiating cysts from cavitating nodules and bronchiectasis, however, as both can occasionally be present as well. Nodules, usually less than 5 mm in size, are also commonly present; as documented with HRCT, these frequently are distributed in the centers of secondary pulmonary lobules around small airways and often cavitate (Fig. 6-55). Significantly, CT showed that many lesions that appeared reticular on plain radiographs were actually cysts (85) (see Fig. 6-54). CT also showed clearly that the abundance of small nodules up to 5 mm in size was consistently underestimated on plain radiographs (85).

By comparing abnormalities identified both early and late in the course of disease, Brauner et al. documented that a predictable pattern of progression from nodules, to cavitated nodules and thick-walled cysts, to thin-walled cysts with eventual confluence could be discerned (86,87). The cysts in Langerhans cell histiocytosis may be round or have bilobed or branching shapes. Bizarre shapes result from confluence of cysts or ectatic and thick walled bronchi (85,86). Although the exact mechanism of cyst formation remains unclear, in most cases the appearance of these in cross-section is strikingly characteristic (see Figs. 6-20, 6-53 and 6-54). The cysts may range from a few millimeters to greater than 20 mm in diameter. Despite the appearance of extensive distortion and destruction, as shown in Figure 6-54, many of these changes, in fact, may be reversible. In the majority of cases, Langerhans cell histiocytosis can be readily distinguished from other causes of cystic lung disease because of the characteristic distribution throughout the upper and middle lung zones with relative sparing of the lung bases (Figs. 6-20, 6-53).

Pulmonary Lymphangioleiomyomatosis

Lymphangioleiomyomatosis (LAM) is a rare disease characterized by the disorderly proliferation within the pulmonary interstitium of benign-appearing smooth muscle resulting in thickening of the walls of the lymphatics, blood vessels, and bronchioles, the lumens of which may become partially or completely occluded (141). The disease affects only women of child-bearing age. Typically patients present with progressive dyspnea and/or hemoptysis, with either recurrent pneumothoraces caused by rupture of peripheral, dilated air spaces secondary to air-trapping from obstructed airways, or with chylous effusions secondary to dilated and obstructed lymphatics. Although clinical progression is usually characterized by progressive pulmonary insufficiency, promising results have been obtained using hormonal therapy and/or oophorectomy (210).

Radiographically, the diagnosis is suggested when there is evidence of diffuse interstitial disease in the setting of normal or increased lung volume (Fig. 6-56). Interestingly, few reports emphasize cyst identification per se. As noted, pneumothoraces and effusions are common, especially as presenting abnormalities.

CT findings in patients with this disorder have been reported and are strikingly uniform in their descriptions (83,84,211–216) (see Fig. 6-56; Fig. 6-57). Innumerable thin-walled cysts can be identified, presumably the result of airspace ectasia secondary to progressive airway obstruction. When evaluated with HRCT, cysts typically vary in size from a few millimeters to up to 5 cm. Initially, only a few scattered cysts may be identifiable (see Fig. 6-57). With progression, these become more uniformly distributed throughout the lungs (see Fig. 6-56). Characteristically, intervening lung appears strikingly normal despite almost total replacement of lung tissue in cases with advanced disease. Nodu-

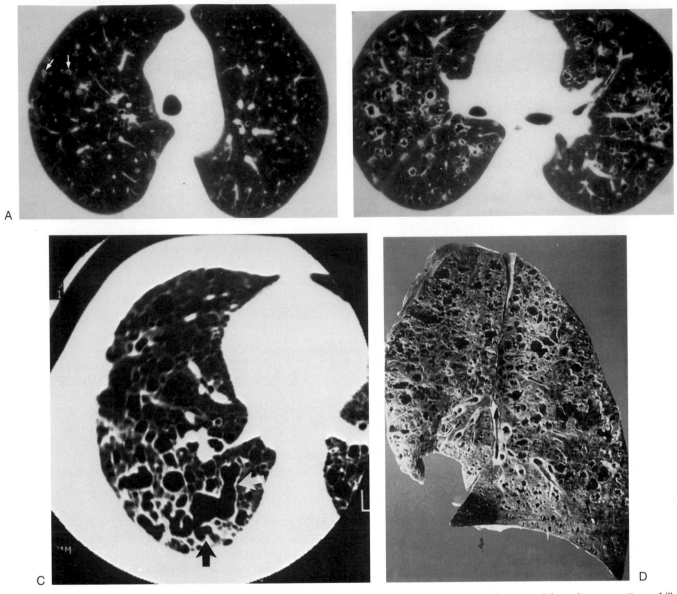

FIG. 6-53. Langerhans cell histiocytosis (LCH): disease spectrum. **A:** One-millimeter section through the upper lobes shows a pattern of ill-defined ground-glass centrilobular nodules resembling changes usually seen in patients with hypersensitivity pneumonitis (HP). Note, however, the presence of a few scattered thick-walled cysts (*arrows*)—a finding distinctly unusual in patients with HP. Findings consistent with early LCH, subsequently documented by transbronchial biopsy. **B:** One-millimeter section through a different patient than shown in **A**, demonstrates more typical appearance of scattered thick-walled irregular cysts in the absence of significant reticulation or nodularity. **C:** High-resolution CT section through the right lung in another patient with documented Langerhans cell histiocytosis. Innumerable well-defined, uniformly thick-walled cysts are scattered throughout the lung, some in bizarre, branching patterns mimicking the appearance of bronchiectasis. Presumably this appearance is caused by cyst fusion. Despite extensive disease, no obvious reticulation or fibrosis is apparent. **D:** Pathologic section from another patient with Langerhans cell histiocytosis showing multiple cysts throughout the lungs, frequently exhibiting unusual branching configurations. Note relative sparing of the lung bases. (Courtesy of Carlos R.R. de Carvalho, M.D., Universidade de Sao Paulo, Brazil.)

larity, thickened interlobular septal lines, and vascular destruction are generally notable by their absence. Not surprisingly, similar CT findings have been reported to occur in patients with tuberous sclerosis (Fig. 6-58) (84). As compared with routine radiography, these changes have consistently been reported as easier to identify with CT (83,214).

In an evaluation of eight patients with documented lymphangioleiomyomatosis, Sherrier et al. (215) reported associated mediastinal and/or retrocrural lymphadenopathy in half

of their cases. In our experience, the finding of nodular retrocrural densities in these patients should suggest also the possibility of dilatation of the thoracic duct. In these cases, differentiation may require that lymphangiography be performed.

In select cases, differentiation between LAM and pulmonary emphysema may present difficulties because of the seeming lack of an identifiable cyst wall in both disorders. However, uniform distribution throughout both lungs

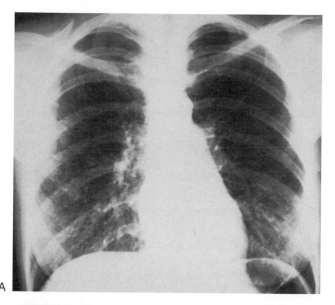

A

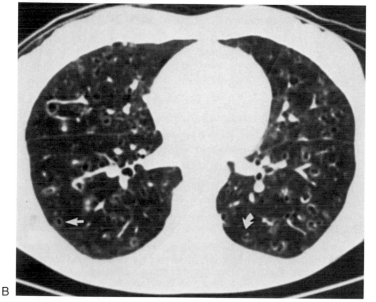

B

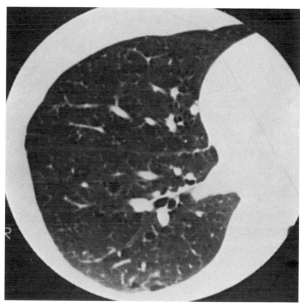

C

FIG. 6-54. Langerhans cell histiocytosis: response to therapy. **A:** Posteroanterior radiograph shows diffuse increased markings interpreted by most observers as consistent with reticular, "interstitial" lung disease. **B:** Nontargeted high-resolution CT (HRCT) section through the lower lobes shows a characteristic appearance of multiple well-defined cysts with uniformly thick walls, seemingly randomly distributed throughout the lungs (*straight arrow*). Many of the cysts are suggestive of dilated bronchi (*curved arrow*). Note the absence of diffuse reticulation within the lung. Transbronchial biopsy documented Langerhans cell histiocytosis. **C:** HRCT section through the right inferior pulmonary vein at precisely the same level as shown in **B**, following 6 months of medical therapy. Note that although some cysts are still present, they are smaller than seen previously and some mimic the appearance of centrilobular emphysema. Significantly, a large number of cysts have disappeared altogether.

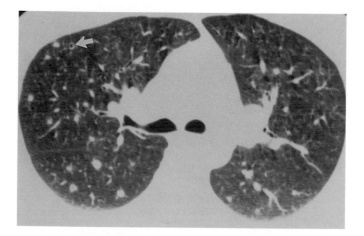

FIG. 6-55. Langerhan's pulmonary histiocytosis. High-resolution CT demonstrates several small nodules in the upper lobes. Cavitation is present in one of the nodules in the right upper lobe (*arrow*). The patient was a 30-year-old man with Langerhan's pulmonary histiocytosis (compare with Fig. 6-53A,B).

strongly favors the diagnosis of LAM. Identification of residual core lobular structures in the cyst centers, characteristic of emphysema, is also helpful in differentiating these conditions (see Fig. 6-33). The cystic changes in LAM may be identical to those of Langerhans cell histiocytosis. However, the cysts in Langerhans histiocytosis tend to show relative sparing of the lung bases whereas the cysts in LAM involve all lung zones to a similar extent (see Figs. 6-20, 6-53–6-55). Other helpful findings are the frequent presence of bizarre shaped cysts and nodules in Langerhans cell histiocytosis.

Honeycomb Lung

Honeycomb lung (end-stage lung) represents the end result of several chronic infiltrative lung diseases with replacement of normal lung by cystic spaces separated by areas of fibrosis (141). The cystic spaces represent dilated respiratory bronchioles (217,218). Honeycombing is more commonly seen on HRCT than on the chest radiograph. In a review of the findings in 23 patients with idiopathic pulmonary fibrosis, Staples et al. detected honeycombing on the chest radiograph in seven (30%) patients and on HRCT in 21 (91%) patients (158). Based on the chest radiographic findings and histopathologic assessment of small specimens obtained at open lung biopsy, it was commonly accepted that the morphologic appearance of honeycomb lung was similar regardless of etiology (219,220). However, a specific diagnosis can be made on HRCT in a majority of cases based on the distribution of abnormalities and the presence of associated

findings (78). In a review of HRCT scans of 61 consecutive patients with end-stage lung, two independent observers made a correct first choice diagnosis in 87% of cases (78). A correct first choice diagnosis in patients with honeycomb lung was made most commonly in Langerhans cell histiocytosis (100% of cases), asbestosis (90%), fibrosing alveolitis (88%), hypersensitivity pneumonitis (HP) (87%), and sarcoidosis (83%). The observers had a high degree of confidence in their first choice diagnosis in 62% of HRCT interpretations and when they were confident, they were correct in 100% of cases.

The most common disease leading to honeycomb lung is idiopathic pulmonary fibrosis, which accounted for almost 50% of cases reported by Primack et al. (78). Honeycomb lung in idiopathic pulmonary fibrosis and in fibrosing alveolitis associated with collagen vascular diseases is characterized by the presence of architectural distortion and cysts predominantly in the lung bases and subpleural lung regions (see Fig. 6-19). Although honeycombing in asbestosis may have a similar distribution, the diagnosis can usually be confidently made on HRCT based on the presence of associated pleural plaques or diffuse pleural thickening (78) (Fig. 6-59). End-stage fibrosis in sarcoidosis may result in conglomerate masses, perihilar cystic changes caused by markedly ectatic bronchi, or subpleural honeycombing. The diagnosis can usually be readily made by the characteristic predominance in the perihilar regions of the mid and upper lung zones (Fig. 6-60). The cysts in Langerhans cell histiocytosis do not have a central or peripheral predominance and involve the upper and middle lung zones with relative sparing of the lung bases (78) (see Figs. 6-20, 6-53).

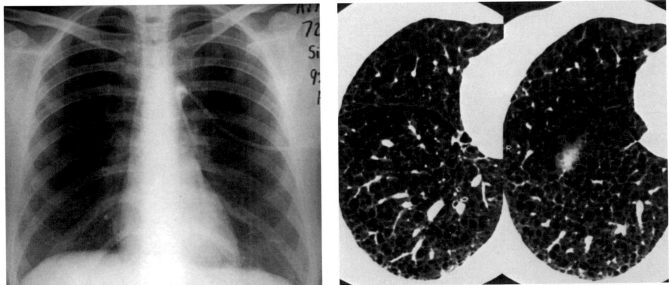

A   B,C

FIG. 6-56. Lymphangioleiomyomatosis (LAM). **A:** Posteroanterior radiograph shows only subtle suggestion of hyperaeration and a few scattered nonspecific reticular densities in this patient with open-lung biopsy-documented LAM. **B,C:** Sequential high-resolution CT sections through the right lower lobe show diffuse cystic changes throughout the lungs. Although the appearance superficially mimics emphysema, note that the cysts are uniformly distributed throughout the lungs (compare with Fig. 6-33), and have thin but definable walls in the absence of obvious reticular or nodular disease.

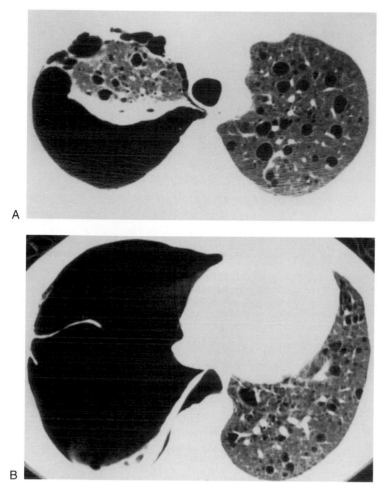

FIG. 6-57. Lymphangioleiomyomatosis (LAM). **A,B:** High-resolution CT through the upper and lower lobes demonstrates cysts with well-defined wall. Also note large right pneumothorax and several pleural adhesions. Although there are considerably fewer cysts as compared with the appearance of Figure 6-43, the morphologic appearance is otherwise indistinguishable. The diffuse distribution of cysts throughout the lungs allows distinction of LAM from Langerhan's pulmonary histiocytosis (compare with Figure 6-20).

Chronic HP is a relatively uncommon cause of honeycomb lung. The honeycombing may be subpleural or random in distribution. In the study by Primack et al., honeycomb lung caused by chronic HP was readily distinguished from idiopathic pulmonary fibrosis by the lack of lower lung zone predominance and the presence of extensive areas of ground-glass attenuation or small nodules (78). However, in approximately 10% of cases, chronic HP may cause findings indistinguishable from those of idiopathic pulmonary fibrosis (81). It cannot be overemphasized that in all cases the HRCT scans must be correlated with the clinical findings.

The ability to make a confident diagnosis on HRCT in

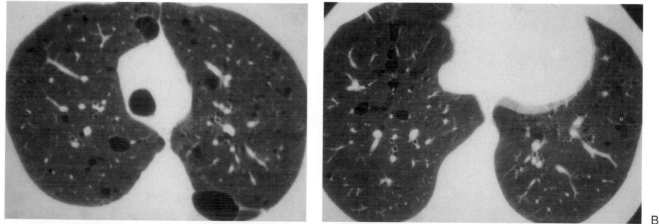

FIG. 6-58. Tuberous sclerosis. **A,B:** One-millimeter sections through the upper and lower lobes, respectively shows a pattern of seemingly randomly scattered thin-walled cysts. Although this appearance superficially resembles centrilobular emphysema, note that the cyst walls are better defined. Early in the course of this disease, cysts may not be as extensive as shown in Figure 6-56.

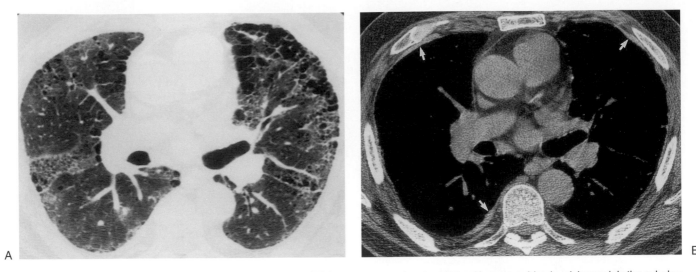

FIG. 6-59. End-stage fibrosis in asbestosis. **A:** High-resolution CT demonstrates extensive bilateral honeycombing involving mainly the subpleural lung regions. The appearance is identical to that of end-stage idiopathic pulmonary fibrosis. **B:** Mediastinal windows demonstrate bilateral pleural plaques (*arrows*) characteristic of asbestos exposure. The patient was a 59-year-old with end-stage fibrosis caused by asbestosis.

the majority of patients with honeycomb lung may be of significant clinical utility. Areas with honeycomb lung do not yield a specific histologic diagnosis and therefore should be avoided on open lung biopsy (3). In a review of the results of open lung biopsy in 502 patients with chronic infiltrative lung disease, Gaensler and Carrington reported that 3.4% of patients had a nonspecific diagnosis of honeycombing. Based on their experience, they do not recommend biopsy in patients with extensive honeycombing because biopsy is unlikely to be helpful in the diagnosis or treatment (3).

Sarcoidosis

Sarcoidosis is a multisystem disorder of unknown etiology characterized by the presence of widespread, noncaseating granulomas (141). It most commonly affects patients be-

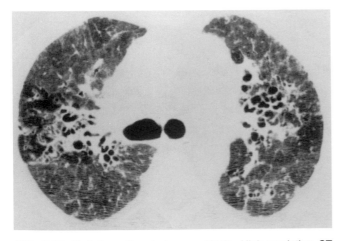

FIG. 6-60. End-stage fibrosis in sarcoidosis. High-resolution CT demonstrates perihilar cystic appearance caused by markedly ectatic bronchi. Central conglomeration of ectatic bronchi caused by perihilar fibrosis is characteristic of end-stage sarcoidosis.

tween 20 and 40 years of age, with onset before the age of 10 or after the age of 60 years being unusual (141). The granulomas may resolve spontaneously or progress to fibrosis. Although sarcoidosis may involve almost any organ, most of the morbidity and mortality is caused by pulmonary disease (221). Pulmonary manifestations are present in 90% of patients, 20% to 25% of whom have permanent functional impairment.

Approximately 60% to 70% of patients with sarcoidosis have a characteristic radiologic appearance consisting of bilateral hilar and paratracheal lymphadenopathy with or without concomitant parenchymal abnormalities (222–224). In 25% to 30% of cases, however, the radiologic findings are nonspecific or atypical, and in 5% to 10% of patients, the chest radiograph is normal in spite of the presence of pulmonary granulomas (141,221–225).

The variable and often nonspecific radiographic findings are surprising given the characteristic pathologic appearance and distribution of sarcoidosis. Sarcoid granulomas, the hallmark of the disease, are distributed mainly along the lymphatics in the bronchovascular sheath and, to a lesser extent, in the interlobular septa and subpleural lung regions (10,141). This distribution is one of the most helpful features in recognizing sarcoidosis pathologically and is responsible for the high rate of success in diagnosis by bronchial and transbronchial biopsies (141). This distribution is difficult to appreciate on the radiograph because of the superimposition of parenchymal structures, but can be clearly identified on CT (10,29,63).

The characteristic CT findings of sarcoidosis consist of small nodules and nodular thickening along the bronchovascular bundles, interlobular septa, interlobular fissures, and subpleural lung regions (29,63,74) (see Fig. 6-21; Figs. 6-61 and 6-62). The thickening of the interstitium surrounding

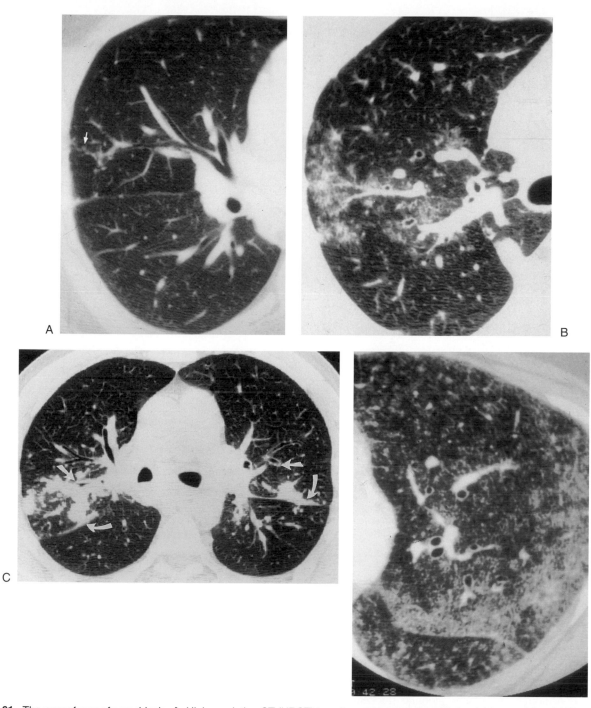

FIG. 6-61. The many faces of sarcoidosis. **A:** High-resolution CT (HRCT) target reconstruction through the right upper lobe shows small cluster of peribronchovascular nodules (*arrow*) associated with nodularity of the major fissure. This pattern, although superficially resembling tree-in-bud, is characteristic of early sarcoidosis (compare with Fig. 6-23). **B:** HRCT target reconstruction in a different patient than in **A** shows greater profusion of nodules, which nonetheless are still clearly clustered in a distinctive peribronchovascular distribution. Note the absence of obvious secondary lobular septal thickening despite the fact that sarcoidosis is a perilymphatic disease (compare with Fig. 6-16). **C:** HRCT through the upper lung zones demonstrates irregular nodules in the peribronchial (*straight arrows*) and subpleural lung regions, particularly along the interlobar fissures (*curved arrows*). The patient was a 32-year-old man with stage 2 sarcoidosis. **D:** HRCT target reconstruction through the left upper lobe shows a miliary pattern. Note that despite marked profusion, there is still a tendency of these nodules to cluster, especially peripherally (compare with Fig. 6-24).

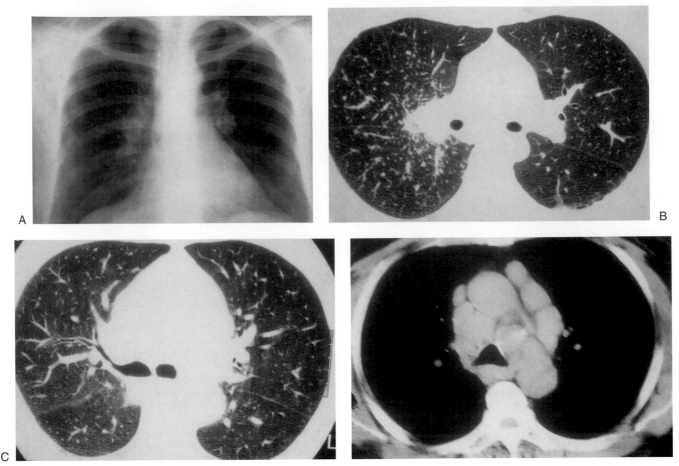

FIG. 6-62. Sarcoidosis: clinical role of CT. **A:** Posteroanterior chest radiograph shows typical pattern of bilateral hilar and right paratracheal adenopathy in this asymptomatic 20-year-old female. There is slight nonspecific asymmetric accentuation of markings in the right lung. **B:** One-millimeter section shows characteristic appearance of clusters of small peribronchovascular and subpleural nodules. Despite asymmetry, these findings in conjunction with the radiograph and clinical history were sufficient to obviate biopsy. Clinical follow-up following steroids confirmed resolution of findings consistent with clinical diagnosis of sarcoidosis. **C,D:** One-millimeter sections imaged with lung and mediastinal windows, respectively in a different patient than shown in **A** and **B**. In this case, despite mild thickening of the right upper lobe bronchial wall, routine forceps transbronchial biopsy was nondiagnostic. Follow-up transbronchial (Wang) core needle biopsy, however, yielded noncaseating granulomata. In addition to helping to select the most likely foci for transbronchial biopsy, CT is also helpful in assessing the presence and extent of mediastinal adenopathy (see text).

vessels and bronchi is most marked in the perihilar regions of the middle and upper lung zones. Thickening of the peribronchovascular interstitium is also present in the centrilobular regions leading to centrilobular nodules and branching structures. The nodules seen on HRCT represent coalescence of microscopic granulomas and usually have irregular margins (10,63). Although irregular or nodular thickening of the interlobular septa is frequently present, it is usually not extensive. Confluence of numerous granulomas may lead to nodules or large opacities measuring 1 to 4 cm in diameter. These are seen in 15% to 25% of patients and frequently contain air bronchograms (29,73,226,227). Areas of ground-glass attenuation may be present in patients with sarcoidosis. Correlation with pathologic specimens has shown that these represent extensive interstitial sarcoid granulomas below the resolution of HRCT rather than alveolitis (110,226,228). Similarly, areas of consolidation (''alveolar sarcoid'') also

represent conglomeration of interstitial granulomas (228) (Fig. 6-63).

As fibrosis develops, irregular reticular opacities including intralobular lines and irregular septal thickening become a prominent feature (29,63). Fibrosis is associated with distortion of lung architecture and characteristic posterior displacement of the upper lobe bronchi indicating loss of volume in the posterior segments of the upper lobes (29). Fibrosis also leads to abnormal conglomeration of dilated distorted parahilar bronchi, a finding known as traction bronchiectasis (65) (see Fig. 6-60; Fig. 6-64). Honeycombing may also be seen in patients with sarcoidosis. It is subpleural in distribution and involves mainly the middle and upper lung zones with relative sparing of the lung bases (78). Honeycombing is usually mild and only seen in patients with severe fibrosis and central conglomeration of bronchi (74).

Enlarged hilar and mediastinal nodes are seen on CT in

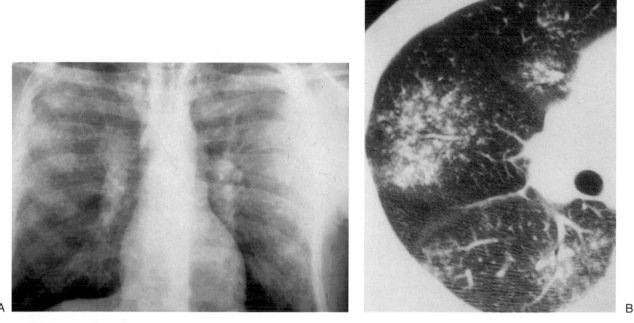

FIG. 6-63. Alveolar sarcoid. **A:** Posteroanterior radiograph shows ill-defined nodular masses scattered throughout the lungs, without evidence of mediastinal or hilar adenopathy. **B:** High-resolution CT target reconstruction through the right upper lobe shows distinctly rounded configuration of a cluster of peribronchovascular nodules otherwise indistinguishable from routine sarcoid. Bronchoscopic biopsy proved.

80% to 90% of patients with sarcoidosis, a higher prevalence than is apparent on the chest radiograph (63,151,229). Calcification of hilar and mediastinal lymph nodes is relatively commonly seen having been reported in eight of 18 (44%) of patients with longstanding sarcoidosis (67).

CT may demonstrate parenchymal abnormalities in patients with a normal chest radiograph and in patients with only hilar adenopathy apparent on the radiograph (29,63)

(Fig. 6-65). CT may also be helpful in assessing the presence and extent of complications of sarcoidosis (230). Superimposed bacterial infection and mycetomas within cavities and areas of bronchiectasis are more readily detected on CT than on the radiograph (230).

The distribution of sarcoid granulomas along the lymphatics is similar to that seen in pulmonary lymphangitic carcinomatosis. Both conditions may cause a beaded thickening of

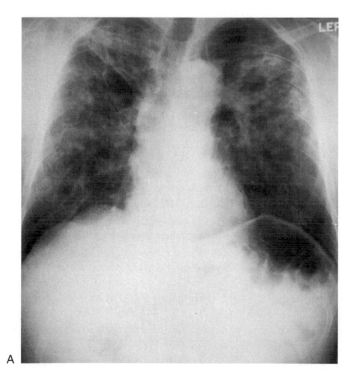

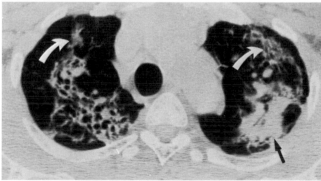

FIG. 6-64. Sarcoidosis. **A:** Posteroanterior radiograph in patient with extensive upper lobe disease, with retraction of the hila bilaterally. **B:** Nontargeted high-resolution CT section through the upper lobes shows a pattern of extensive fibrosis, with cystic spaces especially prominent in the right upper lobe. The left upper lobe is also distorted: a conglomerate density is present (*straight arrow*), in this case stable over several years. In the periphery, despite extensive scanning, the pattern of disease remains distinctly peribronchial (*curved arrows*).

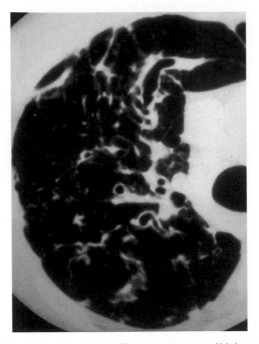

FIG. 6-65. Stage 3 sarcoidosis. Target reconstructed high-resolution CT image through the right upper lobe shows characteristic appearance of architectural distortion with associated traction bronchiectasis and focal emphysema predominantly central in location with relative sparing of the lung periphery. Note the absence of typical honeycombing.

the bronchovascular bundles and interlobular septa (62,74). However, in sarcoidosis the septal thickening is usually less extensive than seen in pulmonary lymphangitic carcinomatosis, characteristically involves mainly the middle and upper lung zones, and is often associated with distortion of the lobular architecture (63,231). The nodules in sarcoidosis often have irregular margins whereas in lymphangitic carcinomatosis they are smooth. In some patients, however, the pattern of parenchymal involvement may be similar (25).

Silicosis and Coal Worker's Pneumoconiosis

Silicosis occurs as a reaction to the inhalation of dust containing silicon dioxide and is seen most commonly in heavy metal or hard rock miners. Chronic exposure results in the formation of small, discrete, hyalinized nodules predominantly in the upper lobes. The nodules are sharply defined, tend to localize around respiratory bronchioles, and are clearly separable from surrounding alveoli, which may be either normal or show evidence of emphysema (141). The diagnosis of silicosis is usually made by correlating clinical history with characteristic plain radiographic findings, demonstrating either simple silicosis (characterized by multiple small opacities) or complicated silicosis (characterized by large coalescent pulmonary opacities resulting in so-called progressive massive fibrosis). Hilar lymphadenopathy is present in many patients and the nodes are often calcified.

A characteristic peripheral "egg-shell" calcification is seen in approximately 5% of cases of silicosis and is virtually pathognomonic of this entity (232).

Coal worker's pneumoconiosis results from inhalation of coal dust. Since a small amount of silica is present in coalmine dust, it was long assumed that coal worker's pneumoconiosis represented a form of silicosis, but this is not usually the case (233). Coal worker's pneumoconiosis can be seen in workers exposure to washed coal, which is nearly free of silica. Histologically, the characteristic lesion in coal worker's pneumoconiosis is the coal macule, which consists of a focal accumulation of coal dust surrounded by a small amount of fibrous tissue (233); however, the amount of fibrosis is much less than that seen with silicosis (234). As the disease progresses, coal macules are surrounded by small areas of emphysema. As in patients with silicosis, these abnormalities tend to surround respiratory bronchioles and are therefore primarily centrilobular in location (233,234). The characteristic radiologic findings in patients with coal worker's pneumoconiosis are similar to those of silicosis and consist of small, well-circumscribed nodules usually measuring 2 to 5 mm in diameter and involving mainly the upper and posterior lung zones (233,234). Large opacities, also known as conglomerate masses or progressive massive fibrosis, may be seen.

On HRCT, as on the radiograph, the most characteristic findings in simple silicosis and coal worker's pneumoconiosis consist of small nodules that are seen predominantly in the posterior aspects of the upper lung zones (75,98,233–237). These nodules are characteristically in a centrilobular distribution although they may also frequently be seen in the subpleural lung regions (75,76,236,237). The nodules vary in size but usually measure between 2 to 5 mm in diameter and may be calcified (Fig. 6-66).

Progressive massive fibrosis in silicosis and coal worker's pneumoconiosis is always associated with a background of small nodules visible on CT (75,235). The conglomerate masses are usually oval in shape, have irregular margins, and are associated with distortion of lung architecture and frequently surrounding emphysema (Fig. 6-67).

HRCT has been shown to be superior to both CCT and chest radiography in the detection of small nodules in patients with silicosis (98). Bégin et al. (98) compared HRCT to CCT in chest radiographs in 49 patients exposed to silica dust and chest radiograph scores of 0 or 1 as determined by the ILO criteria. Thirteen (41%) of 32 patients with chest radiographs interpreted as normal had evidence of silicosis on CT or HRCT. In 10% of the patients with silicosis, abnormalities were visible only on HRCT. In the remaining cases, the abnormalities were more clearly defined on HRCT than on CCT. Remy-Jardin et al. (75) reviewed the chest radiographs and CT scans in miners exposed to coal dust. Nodules were detected on HRCT in 11 out of 48 patients (23%) with no evidence of pneumoconiosis on chest radiographs (ILO profusion score less than 1/0).

CT can also provide useful information regarding the

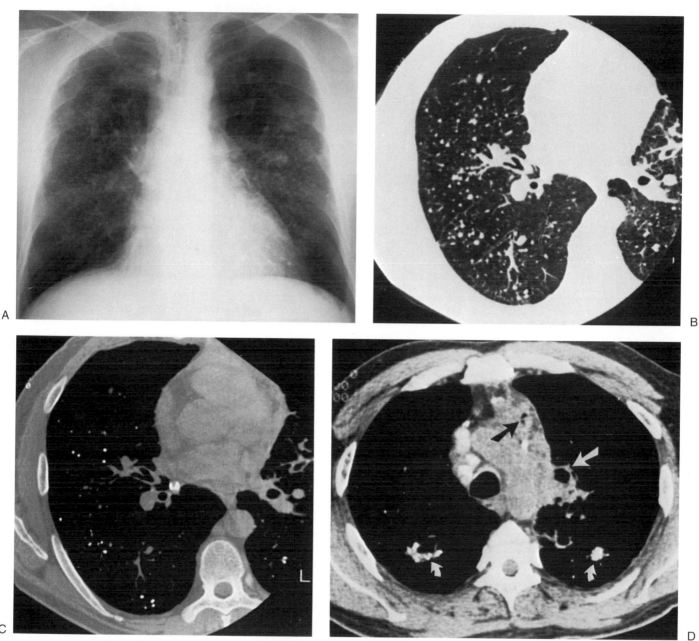

FIG. 6-66. Silicosis. **A:** Posteroanterior radiograph shows typical appearance of sharply defined opacities throughout the lungs, with a suggestion of early coalescence in the upper lobes. **B,C:** High-resolution CT section through the right lung imaged with lung and mediastinal windows, respectively. Numerous well-defined small nodules are identifiable scattered randomly throughout the lung, many of which are calcified. Note that there is no evidence of fibrosis: the pleural margins and vessels are smooth. Emphysematous changes are apparent. **D:** Section at the level of the aortic arch shows calcified mediastinal nodes, as well as clearly definable cavities in both the left hilum and anterior mediastinum (*straight white* and *black arrows*). These cavities, which were not seen on the plain radiographs, even retrospectively, proved to be tuberculous in a patient with documented silicotuberculosis. Note early progressive fibrosis in both upper lobes (*curved arrows*).

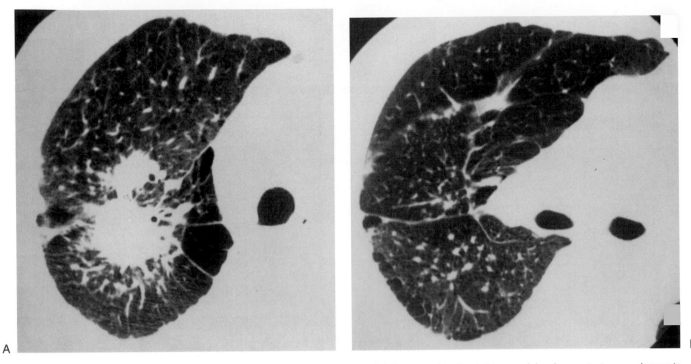

FIG. 6-67. Progressive massive fibrosis in silicosis. **A:** High-resolution CT (HRCT) targeted to the right upper lobe demonstrates conglomerate mass of fibrosis with surrounding architectural distortion and emphysema. Also noted are a few subpleural nodules. **B:** HRCT targeted to the right mid-lung zone demonstrates a few nodules mainly in the right lower lobe. Also noted is evidence of emphysema.

stage of the disease in patients with silicosis and coal worker's pneumoconiosis by allowing detection of coalescence of nodules and the development of conglomerate masses that may not be apparent on plain radiographs (235,236).

Hematogenous Metastases

In most patients, hematogenous tumor metastases to the lungs result in the presence of localized tumor nodules rather than the extensive lymphatic invasion seen in lymphangitic carcinomatosis. Hematogenous metastases usually result in multiple, large, well-defined nodules. Less commonly they may present as multiple small nodules, mimicking the appearance of diffuse interstitial disease on chest radiographs. On HRCT, as on the radiograph, hematogenous metastases tend to involve mainly the lower lung zones and frequently have a peripheral distribution (205,238). Hematogenous metastases are usually randomly distributed with respect to lobular anatomy. Murata et al. (97) assessed the relationship of metastatic nodules to lobular structures using HRCT, specimen radiographs, and stereomicroscopy in five lungs obtained at autopsy from patients with metastatic neoplasms. Nodules were widely distributed throughout pulmonary lobules; as seen on HRCT, 11% of small nodules were centrilobular, 21% were close to interlobular septa, and 68% were located in other regions within the secondary lobule.

As previously noted, although HRCT allows assessment of nodule relation to secondary pulmonary lobules, it is not the recommended technique for the evaluation of patients with suspected pulmonary metastases because metastases may be missed between HRCT sections. The recommended technique for assessment of metastases consists of 7 to 10 mm collimation spiral CT scans. Buckley et al. (239) have shown that the detection of metastases improves significantly with the use of spiral CT and narrow interscan spacing. They compared spiral CT scans obtained using 8 mm thick sections reconstructed every 8 mm with images formatted by using 4 or 5 mm interscan spacing. The narrower interscan spacing yielded more lesions and improved the confident recognition of nodules. Increased reconstruction frequency of volumetric spiral data sets also resulted in a reduction of false positive diagnosis (239).

Hypersensitivity Pneumonitis

Hypersensitivity pneumonitis (HP) (extrinsic allergic alveolitis) is an immunologically mediated lung disease caused by inhalation of antigens contained in a variety of organic dusts (141,240). It is most commonly caused by thermophilic actinomycetes present in moldy hay (farmer's lung), compost (mushroom worker's lung), and contaminated humidifiers or airconditioners (humidifier lung). Another common cause are proteins contained in birds' serum, droppings, and feathers (bird breeder's lung) (241,242).

Heavy exposure to the inciting antigen may lead to the acute form of HP characterized by dyspnea and fever developing within 4 to 6 hours after exposure (241,242). The chest radiograph may be normal or show bilateral consolidation.

The consolidation resolves within a few days to reveal a fine nodular or reticular nodular pattern characteristic of the subacute phase of HP (242,243). In patients with heavy exposure, the diagnosis is readily made by clinical history and identification of serum precipitins (141). In many patients, however, the presentation is more insidious, repeated exposures to relatively low doses of antigen leading to slowly progressive dyspnea over several weeks or months (141,242). The diagnosis of HP in these cases is often not suspected clinically prior to lung biopsy (141). Pathologically, subacute HP is characterized by the presence of ill-defined, nonnecrotizing granulomas, interstitial alveolitis, and cellular inflammation of the bronchioles (bronchiolitis) (141). Definitive histologic diagnosis requires all three components, but these are only present in 50% to 75% of cases (141). The diagnosis therefore is usually based on a combination of clinical, radiologic and pathologic findings. The radiologic and pathologic findings of the subacute stage of HP are reversible with avoidance of the offending antigen and corticosteroid therapy (141,243). The chronic phase of HP is characterized by the presence of fibrosis, which may occur after months or years of intermittent exposure (244). Repeated exposure to the antigen leads to acute and subacute changes superimposed on chronic fibrosis.

HRCT has been shown to be particularly helpful in the assessment of patients with subacute HP (21,245,246). Characteristic HRCT findings include bilateral areas of ground-glass attenuation and poorly defined centrilobular nodules (21,245–247). These correlate with the presence of interstitial alveolitis and cellular bronchiolitis (245). The areas of ground-glass attenuation may be diffuse but frequently have a mid and lower lung zone predominance (246) (Fig. 6-68). Localized areas of decreased attenuation and perfusion are often present in conjunction with areas of ground-glass attenuation, giving a pattern of mosaic attenuation. The areas of low attenuation in HP often have a lobular distribution and show air trapping on CT scans performed at end-expiration (248). Ground-glass attenuation may also be seen in conjunction with centrilobular nodules (21,246) (Fig. 6-69). The centrilobular nodules measure less than 5 mm in diameter and are also most numerous in the middle and lower lung zones. In some patients centrilobular nodules may be the only finding or the predominant abnormality seen in HP (21,247) (see Fig. 6-22).

Chronic HP is characterized pathologically by the presence of fibrosis. On HRCT the findings of fibrosis consist of intralobular linear opacities giving a reticular pattern, architectural distortion, and, eventually, honeycombing (80,245). The distribution of fibrosis in the transverse plane is variable, being patchy in distribution in some cases and predominantly subpleural in others (80). Honeycombing, when present, is usually subpleural (21,80). The fibrosis most commonly shows a mid lung zone predominance or is evenly distributed throughout the upper, middle, and lower lung zones (80) (Fig. 6-70). In the majority of patients with chronic HP evidence of acute or subacute disease is also seen on HRCT, consisting of areas of ground-glass attenuation and centrilobular nodules involving mainly the middle and lower lung zones (80,247).

Several studies have shown that HRCT may demonstrate parenchymal abnormalities in patients with HP and normal chest radiographs (21,247,249). In a study by Remy-Jardin et al. (21), 7 of 21 patients with subacute HP (30%) had normal chest radiographs and all patients had abnormal HRCT scans. However, HP may also be present in patients with normal HRCT. Out of 11 subjects with relatively mild HP reported by Lynch et al., only one (9%) had abnormal chest radiograph and five (45%) had abnormal HRCT (22). It should be noted that in this study HRCT scans were performed at 4 cm intervals (22). It cannot be overemphasized that optimal assessment of infiltrative lung disease requires HRCT scans at 1 cm intervals in the supine position, or at 2 cm intervals in both supine and prone positions.

The characteristic findings frequently allow confident diagnosis of HP on HRCT (78,81). The main differential diagnosis of patients presenting with a several month history of dry cough, progressive shortness of breath, and HRCT showing bilateral areas of ground-glass attenuation, includes HP, DIP, and alveolar proteinosis (68,113,246). Careful clinical history and serologic testing can often confirm the diagnosis of HP, thus obviating lung biopsy. DIP is rare, frequently has a subpleural predominance of the areas of ground-glass attenuation, and is not associated with centrilobular nodules (113). However, in some cases the findings of HP may be identical to those of DIP and biopsy may be required for definitive diagnosis (81). Alveolar proteinosis, also rare, is characterized by the presence of smoothly thickened interlobular septa within areas of ground-glass attenuation giving a "crazy-paving" appearance (68).

The chronic form of HP can usually be readily distinguished from other causes of pulmonary fibrosis (78,81). The main differential diagnosis is with IPF. The distinction can usually be made by the presence of centrilobular nodules and the relative sparing of the lung bases seen in HP as compared to the basal predominance seen in IPF. However, in approximately 10% of cases the findings of chronic HP may be identical to those of IPF (78,81). A definitive diagnosis requires correlation with clinical history, serologic tests and, in some cases, lung biopsy.

Alveolar Proteinosis

Pulmonary alveolar proteinosis is an infiltrative lung disease characterized by filling of the air spaces with a periodic acid Schiff (PAS)-positive lipoproteinaceous material (250). The majority of cases are idiopathic. Less commonly alveolar proteinosis may result from heavy exposure to dusts (silicoproteinosis), drug reactions, or immunologic disturbances (155). Idiopathic pulmonary alveolar proteinosis is seen most commonly in men 30 to 50 years of age. The radiographic findings usually consist of bilateral, perihilar, patchy

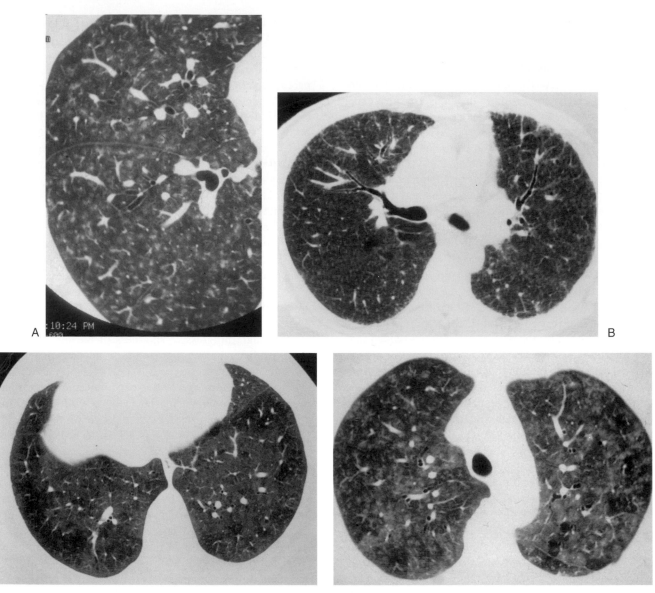

FIG. 6-68. Hypersensitivity pneumonitis (HP): CT spectrum. **A:** Target reconstructed high-resolution CT (HRCT) image through the right upper lobe shows characteristic appearance of uniformly distributed centrilobular ground-glass nodules in the absence of reticulation or cavitation. This finding is characteristic of subacute HP. **B:** HRCT demonstrates bilateral areas of ground-glass attenuation as well as poorly defined small nodular opacities in a patient with subacute HP. Incidental note is made of right mastectomy. **C:** HRCT through the lower lung zones in a 42-year-old woman with subacute HP demonstrates extensive bilateral areas of ground-glass attenuation. **D:** HRCT through the upper lobes in a different patient than **A** or **B** also shows pattern of diffuse ground-glass attenuation. In this case close inspection reveals that areas of ground-glass attenuation actually represent myriad small centrilobular nodules (compare with **B**). Note that in addition there are focal areas of apparent air-trapping, a feature commonly identified in patients with diffuse HP.

or diffuse consolidation, usually most severe in the lung bases (251).

The characteristic HRCT findings of alveolar proteinosis consist of bilateral areas of ground-glass attenuation associated with smoothly thickened interlobular septa (68) (Fig. 6-71). The ground-glass attenuation often has geographic distribution with sharp demarcation between normal and abnormal parenchyma (68,69). Thickening of the interlobular septa is only seen in areas with ground-glass attenuation or

consolidation and is presumably caused by mild edema or fibrosis (68,69). The combination of geographic distribution and interlobular septal thickening in areas of ground-glass attenuation results in a ''crazy-paving'' appearance, which is highly suggestive of alveolar proteinosis (68). Other HRCT findings include ill-defined nodular opacities and areas of airspace consolidation (69).

CT may be helpful in the diagnosis of alveolar proteinosis and in the detection of focal pneumonia (69). In patients

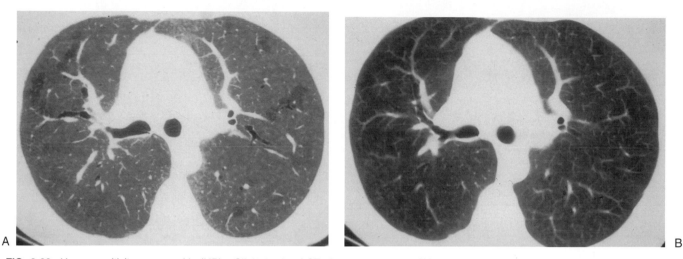

FIG. 6-69. Hypersensitivity pneumonitis (HP)—Clinical role of CT. **A:** High-resolution CT section shows pattern of apparent diffuse ground-glass attenuation. Small centrilobular nodules are apparent, however, throughout both lungs in association with focal areas of air-trapping (compare with Fig. 6-68D). In this case, detailed clinical history revealed that the patient raised pigeons. **B:** Follow-up CT scan several weeks following initiation of steroid therapy shows near complete resolution of the abnormalities. In the appropriate clinical setting, CT findings may be sufficiently specific of HP to warrant empiric therapy.

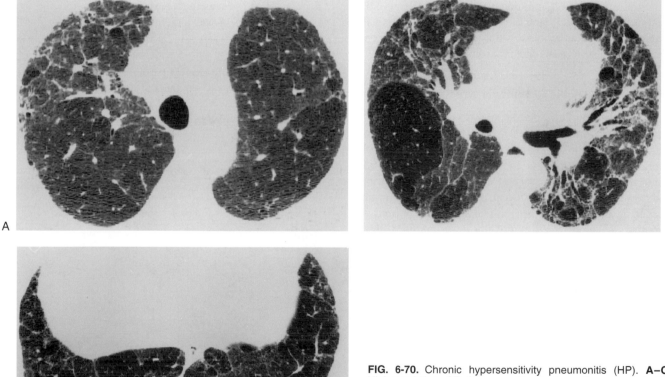

FIG. 6-70. Chronic hypersensitivity pneumonitis (HP). **A–C:** High-resolution CT (1-mm collimation) sections through the upper, middle, and lower lung zones, respectively, demonstrate irregular linear opacities mainly involving the middle lung zones. Also noted are areas of ground-glass attenuation presumably caused by superimposed subacute HP. The predominant distribution in the midlung zones with relative sparing of the lung bases in fibrosis caused by HP allows distinction from IPF in the majority of cases.

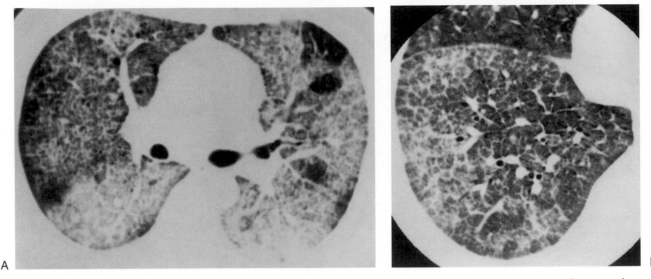

FIG. 6-71. Alveolar proteinosis. **A:** High-resolution CT (HRCT) at the level of the bronchus intermedius demonstrates extensive areas of ground-glass attenuation and consolidation. Note sharp demarcation between normal and abnormal parenchyma, particularly in the left upper lobe. Also noted is fine reticulation. **B:** HRCT targeted to the right lower lobe and performed one year later demonstrates interval improvement. Again noted are areas of ground-glass attenuation and fine reticulation. The reticulation is caused by smoothly thickened interlobular septa.

with alveolar proteinosis it may be difficult to distinguish infection from consolidation caused by the underlying disease on the chest radiograph. CT may confirm a clinically suspected infection by demonstrating focal areas of dense consolidation or abscess formation (69).

Chronic Eosinophilic Pneumonia

Chronic eosinophilic pneumonia is an idiopathic condition characterized histologically by filling of the air spaces with eosinophils and macrophages and an associated mild interstitial pneumonia (141,155). The patients present with a one month or more history of cough, fever, weight loss, and dyspnea (252,253). Chronic eosinophilic pneumonia is seen most commonly in middle aged women and the majority of patients have peripheral eosinophilia. Chronic eosinophilic pneumonia resolves rapidly with corticosteroid therapy.

The characteristic radiologic findings of chronic eosinophilic pneumonia consist of peripheral, nonsegmental areas of consolidation, the "photographic negative of pulmonary edema" involving mainly the upper lobes (254). This pattern is seen in approximately 50% of cases (253). In the remaining cases the radiographic findings are nonspecific and consist of unilateral or patchy bilateral consolidation.

On HRCT a peripheral distribution of consolidation is seen even when it is not apparent on the radiograph (120,255). Mayo et al. (120) reviewed the chest radiographs and CT scans in six patients with chronic eosinophilic pneumonia. In only one patient was the classic pattern of consolidation confined to the outer third of the lungs readily apparent on the radiograph. However, on CT a predominantly peripheral distribution of the consolidation could be clearly

identified in all cases (Fig. 6-72). In five of the six patients the consolidation was most severe in the middle and upper lung zones, and in one patient it involved mainly the mid and lower lung zones. Mediastinal lymphadenopathy was seen on CT in three of six patients.

In a review of 17 patients by Ebara et al. (255) a peripheral distribution was seen on the radiograph in 11 (65%) and on CT in all cases. The findings on CT included areas of consolidation or ground-glass attenuation or both. Less commonly, streaking or band-like opacities, nodular opacities, and lobar atelectasis may also be seen (120,255).

The combination of peripheral consolidation and eosino-

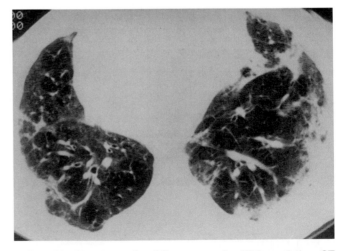

FIG. 6-72. Chronic eosinophilic pneumonia. High-resolution CT through the lower lung zones in a 43-year-old woman demonstrates bilateral subpleural areas of consolidation.

philia is virtually diagnostic of chronic eosinophilic pneumonia (see Fig. 6-72). As mentioned above, an identical peripheral distribution of consolidation may also be seen in some patients with bronchiolitis obliterans organizing pneumonia (see Chapter 3) (93). However, the consolidation in BOOP often involves mainly the lower lung zones whereas the consolidation in chronic eosinophilic pneumonia usually has an upper lobe distribution. Less commonly, peripheral distribution similar to chronic eosinophilic pneumonia may be seen in DIP (113) and sarcoidosis (256).

Lipoid Pneumonia

Exogenous lipoid pneumonia results from aspiration of mineral, vegetable, or animal oil. Histologically the early stage is characterized by a hemorrhagic bronchopneumonia (257). This is followed by an infiltrate consisting of lipid-laden macrophages filling the air spaces. Subsequently there is fibroblastic proliferation with bands of collagen surrounding the oil (257). The amount of fibrosis is variable, occasionally being dense and extensive. Radiographic findings include a solitary nodule simulating bronchogenic carcinoma, localized areas of consolidation, and extensive bilateral bronchopneumonia (258,259).

The CT findings in lipoid pneumonia have been described in a small number of cases (121,260,261). Lee et al. (121) reviewed the findings in six patients with lipoid pneumonia, three being caused by aspiration of mineral oil taken for constipation, and three being caused by shark liver oil taken as a restorative. The chest radiograph showed bilateral airspace consolidation in three patients, irregular mass-like lesions in two, and a reticulonodular pattern in one case. CT scans in the three patients with diffuse consolidation demon-strated that the consolidation had attenuation lower than that of chest wall musculature, but slightly higher than that of subcutaneous fat. These three cases were caused by intake of large amounts of shark liver oil. The two patients with mass-like lesions on the radiograph were shown on HRCT to have localized consolidation containing fat (Fig. 6-73) (see also Fig. 4-33). The consolidation in these two patients was surrounded by irregular linear opacities and architectural distortion indicating fibrosis. In the patient with reticulonodular subpleural infiltrate no areas of low attenuation were seen on CT. As the authors pointed out, in this patient the diagnosis of lipoid pneumonia was based on clinical history and transbronchial biopsy. Therefore the subpleural fibrosis may not have been caused by the lipoid pneumonia.

Drug-Induced Lung Disease

Pulmonary complications may develop in up to 20% of patients receiving cytotoxic chemotherapy (262). The diagnosis of drug-induced lung disease is primarily clinical being based on a temporal relationship between chemotherapy and a characteristic reaction after an appropriate latent period and exclusion of other causes of lung disease. The three main kinds of lung response to drug-induced injury are noncardiogenic pulmonary edema, hypersensitivity lung disease, and chronic pneumonitis/fibrosis (263).

Noncardiogenic pulmonary edema (adult respiratory distress syndrome, ARDS) has been described most commonly after administration of cytosine arabinoside, methotrexate, and cyclophosphamide (264). The clinical and radiologic findings are similar to those of ARDS caused by other causes. HRCT demonstrates widespread airspace consolidation, which may have a predominant distribution in the dependent lung regions (265).

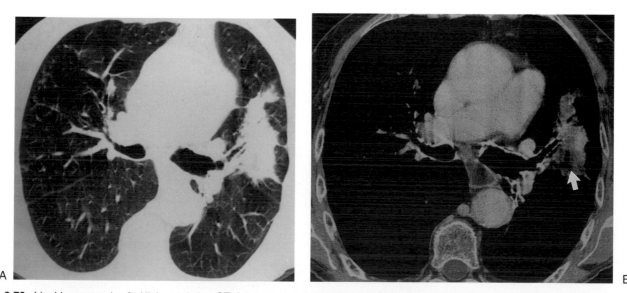

FIG. 6-73. Lipoid pneumonia. **A:** High-resolution CT demonstrates focal area of consolidation in the left upper lobe. **B:** Identical image as **A**, imaged with mediastinal windows demonstrates fat within the areas of consolidation (*arrow*). Also noted is a fluid filled esophagus. The patient was an 81-year-old woman who developed lipoid pneumonia caused by aspiration of mineral oil taken as a laxative.

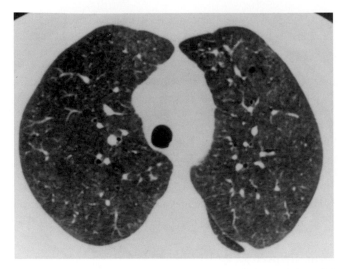

FIG. 6-74. Hypersensitivity drug reaction. High-resolution CT (HRCT) scan demonstrates diffuse bilateral areas of ground-glass attenuation and poorly defined centrilobular nodular opacities. The HRCT and the pathologic findings were those of hypersensitivity pneumonitis. The hypersensitivity reaction was caused by cyclophosphamide therapy. The CT findings resolved following discontinuation of cyclophosphamide treatment.

Hypersensitivity lung disease is seen most commonly with methotrexate but may also occur following administration of bleomycin or cyclophosphamide and carmustine (263,265). The presentation is usually acute with dry cough and progressive shortness of breath developing days or weeks after drug administration. The chest radiograph may demonstrate bilateral areas of consolidation or ground-glass opacities. The characteristic HRCT findings consist of bilateral areas of ground-glass attenuation, which may be patchy in distribution or diffuse (Fig. 6-74) (265). Localized areas of airspace consolidation may be present in some cases (265).

Chronic pneumonitis/fibrosis is the most common drug induced lung injury and has been described with virtually all categories of cytotoxic drugs (264). Pneumonitis/fibrosis is seen most commonly following treatment with bleomycin. The radiographic findings consist of patchy areas of consolidation involving the lower lobes or a progressive reticular or reticulonodular pattern involving mainly the lower lung zones (266). The HRCT findings consist of patchy areas of consolidation in the lower lobes or a reticular pattern involving mainly the lower lung zones and subpleural lung regions in a pattern and distribution similar to that seen in idiopathic pulmonary fibrosis (Fig. 6-75)(265,267).

Although the HRCT findings of drug induced pulmonary disease are nonspecific, CT is superior to chest radiography in demonstrating parenchymal abnormalities in these patients. Padley et al. (265) reviewed the chest radiographs and HRCT scans of 23 patients with drug-induced lung disease and five normal controls. Two independent observers detected abnormalities consistent with drug-induced lung disease in 17 (74%) of the 23 patients on the chest radiograph and in all cases on HRCT. Bellamy et al. (268) reviewed the chest radiographs and CT scans in 100 patients receiving bleomycin. Pulmonary abnormalities consistent with bleomycin-induced lung disease were detected on 15% of the chest radiographs and 38% of CT scans.

EMPHYSEMA

As defined by the American Thoracic Society, emphysema represents an anatomic alteration of the lung characterized by an abnormal enlargement of the air spaces distal to the terminal bronchioles accompanied by destructive changes of the alveolar walls (269). Although pulmonary functional abnormalities may be present, including an increase in total lung capacity (TLC), functional residual capacity (FRC), and residual volume (RV), and there may be a

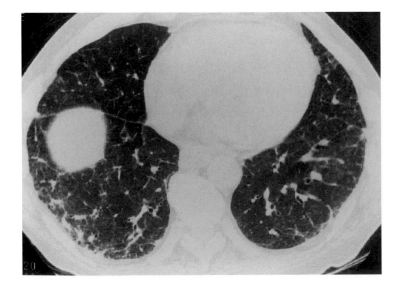

FIG. 6-75. Drug induced pulmonary fibrosis. High-resolution CT scan in a 75-year-old man demonstrates predominantly subpleural distribution of irregular linear opacities with associated architectural distortion. Also noted are patchy areas of ground-glass attenuation. The findings were caused by chronic pneumonitis/fibrosis secondary to methotrexate-induced lung disease.

decrease in elastic recoil and maximal expiratory flow rates, these changes do not constitute part of emphysema's definition. Disease confirmation has required anatomic verification at either surgery or autopsy.

Emphysema is usually classified anatomically based on the distribution of abnormalities within the acinus or secondary lobule and includes: centrilobular (proximal acinar) emphysema, if the primary focus of destruction centers on air spaces surrounding respiratory bronchioles, as typically occurs in smokers; panlobular (panacinar) emphysema if air spaces are evenly destroyed throughout the acinus, as occurs in patients with alpha-1 antiprotease deficiency; paraseptal (distal acinar) emphysema, if there is selective involvement of the distal acini, which, when confluent, leads to the formation of bullae, with resultant spontaneous pneumothorax, as occurs especially in younger patients (270). Irregular airspace enlargement, also known as irregular or paracicatricial emphysema, is seen in association with focal scars or with diffuse cicatrizing lung diseases including tuberculosis, chronic sarcoidosis, and certain pneumoconiosis, especially silicosis. It cannot be overstated that differentiation among these various forms of emphysema may be exceedingly difficult, even for the pathologist, especially when the emphysema is severe and when more than one type is present at the same time, as occurs not infrequently.

Radiographic abnormalities in patients with emphysema have been well documented. In most series the diagnosis is based on finding avascular spaces within the lung, evidence of hyperinflation, or a decrease in the caliber and number of vessels in the lung periphery, the so-called "arterial deficiency" pattern of emphysema (271–275).

Despite discrepancies in the reported significance of these signs, most radiographic-pathologic correlative studies have concluded that routine radiographs are of only limited utility and are an imprecise method of diagnosing emphysema (125). In the largest such study, Thurlbeck and Simon found that chest radiographs were positive in only 41% of cases of moderate emphysema and 67% of cases of severe emphysema, when graded pathologically (271). It should be noted that significant different results have been reported by Sutinen et al. (272) and more recently by Miniati et al. (275). Based on somewhat different radiographic criteria than those utilized by Thurlbeck and Simon, these authors concluded that when utilizing a combination of various signs, radiographs were reliable indicators of both the presence and absence of emphysema. In spite of these claims, it is difficult to believe that the radiograph has such a high accuracy when confronted with day-to-day reading of radiographs and the low accuracy demonstrated by others (125).

A number of studies have assessed the CT and HRCT findings in patients with emphysema (124,125,127,276–280). These studies have shown that CT is superior to the chest radiograph and pulmonary function tests, and HRCT is superior to CCT in the detection of emphysema. Emphysema is characterized on HRCT by the presence of localized areas of low attenuation without definable walls and easily

separable from surrounding lung parenchyma (Figs. 6-76–6-78). The pattern and distribution of emphysema on HRCT are influenced by the type of emphysema (125,127). Centrilobular emphysema is characterized by localized small areas of lucency near the center of the secondary pulmonary lobules (see Fig. 6-33). It involves mainly the upper lung zones. Panlobular emphysema is characterized by uniform destruction of the secondary lobule leading to widespread areas of abnormally low attenuation (125,279). There is also a decrease in the number and size of pulmonary vessels in the affected lung. Panlobular emphysema is almost always most severe in the lower lung zones (see Fig. 6-34). Paraseptal emphysema involves the periphery of the secondary lobule, near the interlobular septa and subpleural lung regions.

Using HRCT, it is possible to identify even mild emphysema on postmortem lung specimen (278) (Fig. 6-79). Correlation between the *in vitro* CT emphysema score and the pathologic score is excellent (r = 0.91). Although it may be possible to obtain a near one-to-one correlation between CT and pathologic specimens *in vitro*, it is not possible at the present time to obtain such a good correlation *in vivo* (125). Using a GE 9800 scanner, Miller et al. (279) obtained a CT-pathologic correlation of 0.81 when using 10-mm collimation scans and a correlation of 0.85 when using 1.5-mm collimation scans. In this series, 33 of 38 patients had emphysema; out of these 33, four patients with mild centrilobu-

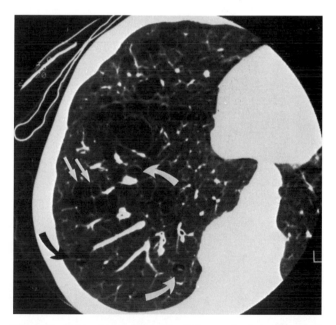

FIG. 6-76. Pulmonary emphysema. Retrospectively targeted high-resolution CT section through the right lower lobe shows characteristic pattern of emphysema, consisting of well-defined zones of decreased attenuation, without definable walls. Instead, these spaces typically are delimited peripherally by interlobular veins, which are particularly well seen along the course of large central veins (*straight arrows*). Occasionally when sectioned tangentially, central or core lobular vessels can be identified as well (*curved arrows*).

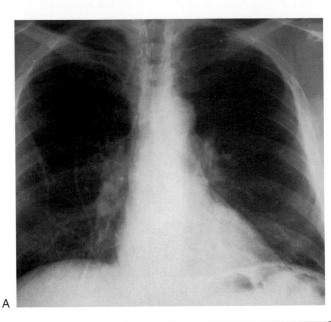

A

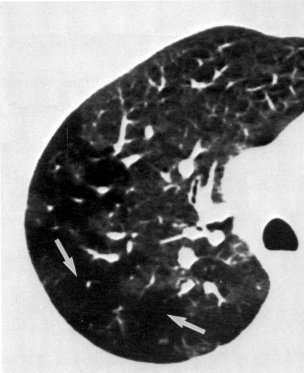

B

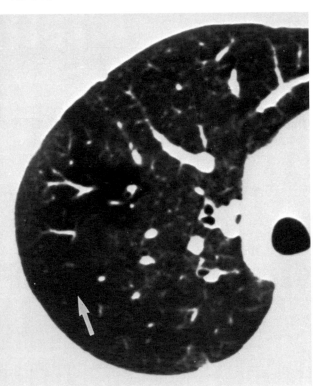

C

FIG. 6-77. Diffuse emphysema: CT-radiographic correlation. **A:** Posteroanterior radiograph shows classic appearance of arterial deficiency pattern of emphysema in both upper lobes. **B,C:** Sequential high-resolution CT sections through the right upper lobe show characteristic pattern of geographic or zonal regions of decreased attenuation within which few if any pulmonary vessels can be found (*arrows* in **B** and **C**). These findings are characteristic of more advanced emphysema as compared with Figure 6-76.

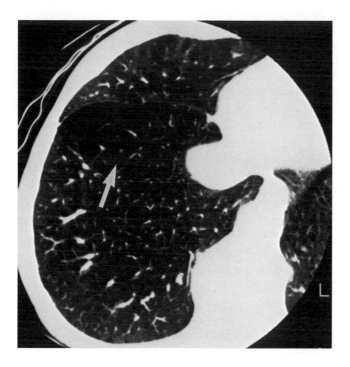

FIG. 6-78. Diffuse emphysema: differentiation from reticular lung disease. Target reconstructed 1.5-mm thick section through the right lower lobe shows diffuse emphysematous destruction of the lung, recognizable as regions of markedly low attenuation without definable walls. When extensive, emphysematous disease may take the configuration of secondary pulmonary lobules (*arrow*). Although this appearance superficially mimics diffuse reticular lung disease, differentiation is rarely problematic: unlike most reticular lung diseases, emphysema tends to be more central than peripheral. Additionally, despite their seeming prominence, interlobular septa are not actually thickened and there is no evidence of prominent or irregular bronchovascular markings. Diagnostic certainty is also enhanced by the finding of prominent central core lobular structures in otherwise destroyed secondary lobules (compare with Fig. 6-76).

lar emphysema were interpreted as showing no emphysema on CT. Kuwano et al. (280) found a lower correlation between the CT scores and the pathologic scores of emphysema (approximately 0.7) but no statistical difference between the HRCT and the pathologic scores in 42 patients with mild to moderate emphysema. Paraseptal emphysema can usually be easily detected on HRCT but mild centrilobular

emphysema or panlobular emphysema may be missed (125,127,279). Therefore, although CT is undoubtedly the most sensitive method to diagnose emphysema *in vivo*, it does not detect the early stages of emphysema and it cannot be used to definitely rule out the diagnosis (125).

The overall extent of emphysema may be difficult to estimate visually because of the wide range of volumes repre-

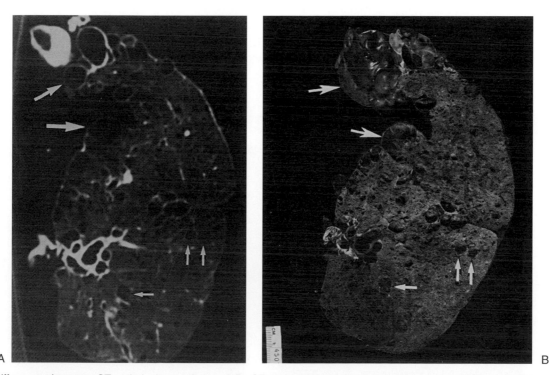

FIG. 6-79. Diffuse emphysema: CT-pathologic correlation. **A,B:** CT and corresponding fixed inflated lung specimen sections, respectively. Emphysematous disease is characterized by low-attenuation areas easily separable from surrounding normal parenchyma despite the absence of a clearly definable wall (*arrows* in **A** and **B**). These are easily differentiated from bronchiectasis because of the absence of associated pulmonary artery branches and definable wall thickness.

sented in the different images. This difficulty can be circumvented by highlighting areas of abnormally low attenuation using a computer program. The GE scanner has a standard software program called "Density Mask" that highlights voxels within any desired range. Müller et al. (281) compared the density mask with the visual assessment of emphysema on CCT in 28 patients undergoing lung resection for tumor. In each patient, a single representative CT scan was compared to the corresponding pathologic specimen of tissue. The authors assessed the accuracy of various density masks. The best correlations were observed by highlighting all voxels with attenuation equal to or less than −910 HU. The correlation between the density mask and the pathologic score of emphysema was 0.9, which was similar to the mean visual scores by the two independent observers.

Although CT is the most accurate method for diagnosing emphysema *in vivo* in most patients the diagnosis can be readily made by a combination of clinical history, pulmonary function tests, and chest radiographs. The main indication for the use of CT is in the preoperative assessment of patients being considered for bullectomy (282,283) or for lung volume reduction surgery (284). Bullectomy is most effective in patients with large bullae and absence of generalized emphysema and who have rapid progression of dyspnea and demonstrate restrictive lung function caused by compression of normal areas of lung. Large bullae can compress the remaining lung parenchyma and cause further functional and clinical impairment. CT allows assessment not only of the extent of bullae but also of the degree of compression and the severity of emphysema in the remaining lung (Fig. 6-80).

Bullectomy is applicable only to a small, highly select group of patients. Recently lung volume reduction surgery (LVRS) has become an accepted method to treat selected patients with severe emphysema and without large bullae. The procedure consists of bilateral wedge resection of the most severely involved lung (285,286). Inclusion criteria include severe emphysema with hyperinflation, forced expiratory volume in 1 second between 10% and 40% of predicted, residual volume equal or greater than 180% predicted, and total lung capacity equal or greater than 110% of predicted (284). The best surgical candidates are patients with hyperinflation caused by severe emphysema rather than airway disease, heterogeneous distribution of the emphysema with specific target areas for surgical resection in the upper lobes, and evidence of compression of relatively normal lung (286,287).

CT allows excellent assessment of the presence, extent, and localization of areas of emphysema prior to LVRS (284). The analysis may be based on subjective assessment of the images or the use of objective quantification of areas with decreased attenuation using a threshold value for emphysema, usually −900 HU (284,288,289). Optimal assessment of emphysema is obtained by the use of HRCT scans at 10 mm intervals through the chest. However, more rapid objective quantification of emphysema can be obtained by using a threshold value (−900 HU) on single breath-hold volume acquisition spiral CT (284,289).

CT may also be indicated for assessing patients who have dyspnea and decreased carbon monoxide diffusing capacity without evidence of obstruction of air flow. Klein et al. (290) reported ten such patients, all smokers with impaired gas exchange and normal findings on chest radiographs, but with evidence of emphysema on HRCT scans. In such patients, HRCT can help differentiate emphysema from pulmonary, vascular, or interstitial lung disease.

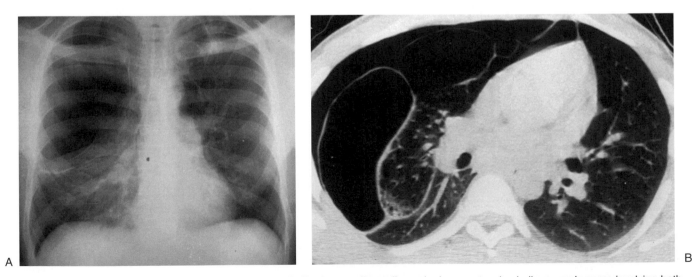

A   B

FIG. 6-80. Bullous emphysema: presurgical assessment. **A:** Posteroanterior radiograph shows extensive bullous emphysema involving both upper lung zones, more extensively on the right. **B:** High-resolution CT section through the mid lung shows large bullae on the right side, causing considerable compression of the adjacent right upper lobe. Despite this, visualized lung is normal in appearance and without evidence of diffuse emphysematous change, supporting in this case operative intervention.

It has also been suggested that CT may be useful in the early detection of apical subpleural bullae in patients with idiopathic spontaneous pneumothorax (291,292). This form of pneumothorax occurs most often in tall, young adults and is thought to be caused by rupture of a subpleural bulla. Out of 20 patients reported by Lesur et al. (291), CT demonstrated emphysema in 17 with a predominance in the lung apices and in a subpleural location in 16. Bense et al. (292) also demonstrated that emphysema is seen on CT in the majority of nonsmoking patients with spontaneous pneumothorax. They compared the CT findings in 27 nonsmoking patients with spontaneous pneumothorax to the findings in 10 healthy subjects who had never smoked. Emphysema was present on CT in 22 of the 27 nonsmoking patients with spontaneous pneumothorax and in none of the 10 control subjects. The emphysema was present mainly in the periphery of the upper lung zones, a distribution consistent with paraseptal emphysema. In none of the cases was emphysema detected on the chest radiograph.

ACUTE LUNG DISEASE IN THE NON-AIDS IMMUNOCOMPROMISED PATIENT

Acute diffuse infiltrative lung disease may result from a variety of causes including infection, cardiogenic and noncardiogenic edema, hemorrhage, drug reactions, aspiration, and inhalation injuries (293). Although CT plays a limited role in the differential diagnosis of acute lung disease in the immunocompetent host, CT and, in particular, HRCT is being used with increasing frequency in the assessment of acute lung disease in the immunocompromised patient. The role of CT to assess lung disease in AIDS patients will be addressed in Chapter 7.

Pulmonary lung disease is a major cause of morbidity and mortality in non-AIDS immunocompromised patients. Early diagnosis is important in directing treatment (294) and reducing the mortality rate from pulmonary complications in immunocompromised patients (295).

The clinical and chest radiographic findings associated with acute infectious and/or infiltrative lung disease in the non-AIDS immunocompromised host have been extensively described but in many cases a timely diagnosis proves elusive. Although the chest radiograph remains the first and foremost imaging modality in these patients, it may be normal in up to 10% of patients with proven pulmonary disease and it seldom allows a confident specific diagnosis (296,297). A number of studies have shown that HRCT may demonstrate parenchymal abnormalities in patients with normal or questionable radiographic findings and may allow confident diagnosis in patients with nonspecific radiographic findings (71,298–302) (Fig. 6-81). The HRCT findings in immunocompromised patients have been shown to closely reflect the pathologic findings (115,303–306). Because CT and HRCT are superior to the radiograph in demonstrating the presence, distribution, and extent of parenchymal abnormalities, CT may be helpful as a guide to the optimal type and site of lung biopsy (298,307,308).

Although a number of different diseases may cause diffuse pulmonary infiltrates in the immunocompromised host, the majority of cases are caused by infection (297,309). The type of complication is influenced by the specific immunologic abnormality. The most common causes of immunosuppression are the acquired immunodeficiency syndrome (AIDS), hematologic malignancy such as leukemia or lymphoma, chemotherapy of tumors , and organ transplantation. Patients with AIDS are more susceptible than nonimmunocompro-

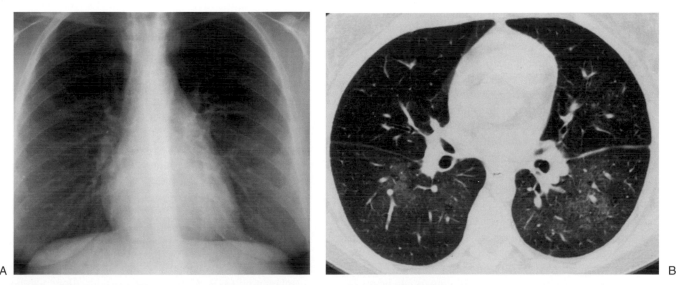

FIG. 6-81. Drug reaction. A 28-year-old woman presented with progressive shortness of breath following bone marrow transplant. **A:** Chest radiograph was interpreted prospectively as being normal. **B:** High-resolution CT demonstrates areas of ground-glass attenuation mainly in the lower lobes. Based on the CT findings the patient underwent lung biopsy. Final diagnosis: drug reaction to carmustine.

mised individuals to develop community-acquired pneumonias, but the most common organism to lead to life-threatening complications in these patients is *Pneumocystis carinii* pneumonia. Although patients with AIDS may develop invasive aspergillosis, this complication is seen much more commonly in patients with leukemia who are undergoing immunosuppressive therapy. Cytomegalovirus pneumonia, on the other hand, is seen most commonly in patients undergoing organ transplantation. The type of complication is also influenced by the severity of immunosuppression and the time elapsed since transplantation. For example, in patients undergoing solid organ or bone marrow transplantation opportunistic infection is seen most commonly during the first month after transplantation whereas posttransplant lymphoproliferative disorders and bronchiolitis obliterans occur several months to years after transplantation. It is essential, therefore, to interpret the HRCT findings in the appropriate clinical context. In this section we will review the CT manifestations of the most common intrathoracic complications seen in immunocompromised non-AIDS patients; the findings in patients with AIDS are discussed in Chapter 7.

HRCT has been shown to be particularly useful in the assessment of patients with *Pneumocystis carinii* pneumonia, cytomegalovirus pneumonia, invasive aspergillosis, septic emboli, mycobacterial infection, and bronchiolitis obliterans.

Pneumocystis carinii Pneumonia (PCP)

The vast majority of patients with PCP have a predisposing condition such as AIDS, lymphoma, leukemia, organ transplantation, or are undergoing treatment with cytotoxic drugs or corticosteroids (310). Rarely it may occur in elderly patients without identifiable risk factors (311). In contrast to the usual insidious onset seen in patients with AIDS, PCP in the non-AIDS immunocompromised host is usually acute and manifested by fever, dyspnea, and hypoxemia (312). Non-AIDS immunocompromised patients with PCP have fewer organisms than patients with AIDS (310), and therefore induced sputum and bronchoalveolar lavage are less likely to be positive. It has been shown, however, that the degree of hypoxemia in patients with PCP correlates with the degree of inflammatory reaction and not with the number of organisms. Immunocompromised non-AIDS patients with PCP tend to have more severe inflammatory reaction and therefore be more hypoxemic than patients with AIDS (310).

The typical chest radiographic findings include bilateral perihilar ground-glass, interstitial or airspace infiltrates, which are seen in up to 85% of cases (296,313–315). Atypical distributions may occur in non-AIDS patients, including upper lobe distribution simulating tuberculosis (316) and, in patients undergoing mediastinal irradiation, sparing of the regions of lung included within the radiation port (316).

In the majority of cases of PCP the diagnosis can be readily be made by a combination of clinical and radiographic findings. However, in 10% of patients, the initial chest radio-

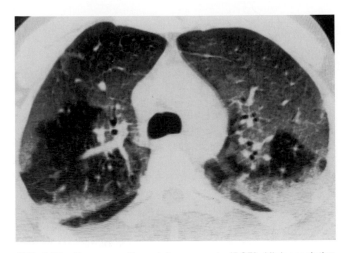

FIG. 6-82. *Pneumocystis carinii* pneumonia (PCP). High-resolution CT demonstrates bilateral areas of ground-glass attenuation. Note areas of spared lung giving a mosaic appearance.

graph may be normal despite documentation of infection (296,313). HRCT can be helpful in the assessment of symptomatic patients with normal or questionable radiographic findings and in the assessment of patients with atypical presentation.

The HRCT findings of PCP have been described in several studies (71,114,313,317). The predominant finding on CT consists of bilateral areas of ground-glass attenuation (Fig. 6-82). With more severe disease patients develop extensive bilateral consolidation. A distinct "mosaic" pattern can often be identified with areas of normal lung intervening between scattered, focal areas of ground-glass attenuation (114).

Although in patients with AIDS the presence of areas of ground-glass attenuation is virtually pathognomonic of PCP (71,301), in immunocompromised patients without AIDS, ground-glass attenuation is a less specific finding. Brown et al. (115) compared the findings on HRCT with pathologic specimens in 33 immunocompromised patients with acute pulmonary complications. Fourteen patients without AIDS had ground-glass attenuation as their main abnormality. In these 14 patients PCP accounted for the areas of ground-glass attenuation in three cases, cytotoxic drug reaction in four, cryptogenic organizing pneumonia in four, lymphoma in two cases, and cytomegalovirus pneumonia in one. Therefore a definitive diagnosis requires bronchoalveolar lavage, transbronchial or surgical biopsy.

Cytomegalovirus (CMV) Pneumonia

Cytomegalovirus (CMV) pneumonia frequently occurs in immunosuppressed patients, especially following organ transplantation (318–320). In patients with allogeneic bone marrow transplantation, CMV pneumonitis typically occurs more than two months following transplantation (321). Patients with severe graft-versus-host disease are at highest risk. CMV infection has also been frequently identified in renal transplantation patients.

Kang et al. (301) reviewed the CT findings in 10 transplant patients who had pathologically proven isolated pulmonary CMV infection. Five patients had bone marrow transplant and five had solid organ transplant. Nine of 10 patients had parenchymal abnormalities apparent at CT and one had normal CT scans. The most common finding was the presence of small nodules (1 to 5 mm in diameter) that were present in 6 of the 10 patients. The nodules were distributed symmetrically and diffusely in both lungs in all six cases. Four patients had bilateral areas of nonsegmental parenchymal consolidation involving mainly the lower lung zones. Bilateral areas of ground-glass attenuation were identified in four patients and irregular lines in one. Ill-defined small nodular opacities and areas of consolidation were also the most common finding seen on CT by Aafedt et al. in eight immunosuppressed patients with CMV pneumonia (322).

Invasive Aspergillosis

Invasive aspergillosis is a relatively common pulmonary complication in immunocompromised patients. Although it may occur in severe immunosuppression from any cause, including AIDS, it is most commonly seen in patients with prolonged granulocytopenia following treatment for acute leukemia (323–325). Most patients present with fever, cough, and progressive dyspnea. The mortality rate for invasive aspergillosis is approximately 60%. Survival depends on early diagnosis and institution of appropriate therapy (326).

Pathologically, two distinct forms of invasive aspergillosis are observed: airway invasive and angioinvasive aspergillosis (304,323,327). The angioinvasive form leads to occlusion of medium to large caliber arteries by plugs of hyphae and the development of infected infarcts (327). Less commonly, the organisms invade the airways rather than the vessels. Invasive aspergillosis centered on the airways accounts for approximately 30% of cases (304,323). The diagnosis of airways invasive aspergillosis is based on the presence of organisms deep to the basement membrane.

The radiographic findings of invasive pulmonary aspergillosis are nonspecific consisting of ill-defined nodules, mass-like infiltrates, subsegmental and segmental consolidation (325,327). The only specific radiographic finding consists of the air crescent sign. This finding, however, is a late manifestation of invasive aspergillosis being seen during the healing phase of the lesion (328).

On HRCT, invasive aspergillosis can be frequently recognized early on by the presence of a characteristic halo of ground-glass attenuation surrounding focal dense parenchymal nodules (329,330) (see Fig. 6-25; Fig. 6-83). Radiologic-pathologic correlation in patients with documented invasive pulmonary aspergillosis has shown that the halo is caused by a rim of coagulation necrosis or hemorrhage surrounding a central fungal nodule or pulmonary infarct (105,331).

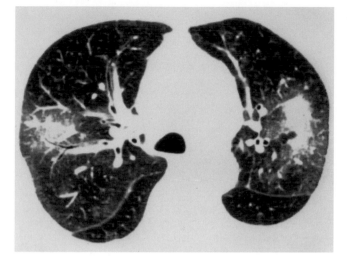

FIG. 6-83. Angioinvasive aspergillosis. High-resolution CT demonstrates irregularly marginated soft tissue nodules in the upper lobes surrounded by a halo of ground-glass attenuation. The patient was a 77-year-old woman with leukemia.

The frequency of the halo sign in angioinvasive aspergillosis is variable depending on the patient population. In the study by Blum et al. (332), out of 22 immunocompromised patients with invasive pulmonary aspergillosis in the setting of granulocytopenia, 16 (73%) demonstrated the halo sign. However, out of 10 AIDS patients with proven invasive pulmonary aspergillosis reported by Staples et al., none had the halo sign (306).

Some authors (330,331) have concluded that, in an appropriate population, the CT appearance of early invasive aspergillosis with a halo sign is sufficiently characteristic to justify a presumptive diagnosis and treatment. In the study by Blum et al. (332), the halo sign had 100% specificity for the diagnosis of angioinvasive aspergillosis. However, the halo sign may be seen with any nodule surrounded by hemorrhage (105,333). Primack et al. demonstrated the halo sign in association with cytomegalovirus and Herpes simplex pneumonia, Wegener's granulomatosis, metastatic angiosarcoma, and Kaposi's sarcoma (105).

Nodules with a surrounding halo are the most characteristic finding in angioinvasive aspergillosis. Other abnormalities on HRCT include areas of subsegmental or segmental consolidation reflecting the presence of subsegmental or segmental pulmonary infarcts (115,116). Another relatively common, although albeit late, finding in angioinvasive pulmonary aspergillosis is the presence of an air crescent representing air between retracted, infarcted lung and the adjacent lung parenchyma (328,329).

The characteristic HRCT findings of airway invasive aspergillosis consist of peribronchial consolidation reflecting the presence of aspergillus bronchopneumonia and/or centrilobular nodules measuring 2 to 5 mm in diameter caused by aspergillus bronchiolitis (Fig. 6-84) (304).

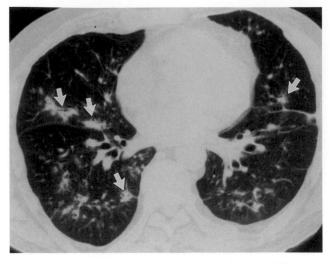

FIG. 6-84. Airway invasive aspergillosis. High-resolution CT demonstrates focal areas of peribronchial consolidation (*arrows*). The patient was a 55-year-old man with acute myelogenous leukemia who had undergone bone marrow transplantation.

The utility of CT in assessing immunosuppressed patients with suspected aspergillosis has been stressed by several investigators (116,306,329). CT is more sensitive than the radiograph in detecting findings suggestive of invasive aspergillosis and in characterizing their appearance.

Septic Emboli

Septic emboli are seen most commonly in intravenous drug abusers and in immunocompromised patients with central venous lines. The diagnosis is usually suspected based on clinical history and radiographic findings of peripheral nodules with various degrees of cavitation. However, in some patients the findings may not be readily apparent on the radiograph and be well demonstrated on CT (334). The CT and HRCT findings consist of peripheral nodules most numerous in the lower lung zones (101,334) (see Fig. 4-16). The nodules frequently show varying stages of cavitation presumably caused by intermittent seeding of the lungs by infected material. A characteristic finding on HRCT is the presence of feeding vessels seen in association with peripheral nodules (334). These have been reported in 60% to 70% of patients with septic pulmonary emboli (101,334).

Compared with plain radiographs, CT scans provided useful additional information in eight of 15 (53%) patients with septic emboli reported by Huang et al. (334). Furthermore, the diagnosis of septic embolism was first suggested on CT in 7 of 15 cases in this study, and in 6 of 18 cases in the study by Kuhlman et al. (101).

Noninfectious Complications

A large number of noninfectious complications may be seen in immunocompromised patients, including pulmonary edema, drug induced lung disease, diffuse alveolar hemor-

rhage, posttransplantation lymphoproliferative disorder, bronchiolitis obliterans, and recurrence or extension of underlying neoplasm. CT has been shown to be particularly helpful in the assessment of patients with clinically suspected drug induced lung disease and bronchiolitis obliterans.

CLINICAL UTILITY OF CT

The clinical value of CT and its role in the evaluation of patients with suspected or known diffuse lung diseases can be reviewed by addressing the following questions:

1. To what extent does CT augment the diagnostic sensitivity and specificity of chest radiography?
2. What are the advantages and disadvantages of HRCT over CCT?
3. What is the diagnostic accuracy based on the CT findings as compared to the chest radiograph in diffuse lung disease?
4. What is the role for CT in the assessment of disease activity and prognosis as compared with alternate techniques such as bronchoalveolar lavage (BAL), or gallium-67 citrate scanning?
5. How does CT compare with other modalities in predicting the accuracy of transbronchial versus open lung biopsy in the diagnosis of diffuse lung disease? Can CT ever obviate lung biopsy?

Diagnostic Sensitivity and Specificity of CT Compared to Routine Chest Radiography

Chest radiographs are important in the assessment of patients suspected of having diffuse lung disease: they are inexpensive, readily available, and often can provide information that is sufficient for diagnosis or management. Chest radiographs, however, have well known limitations in both sensitivity and specificity for evaluating patients with diffuse infiltrative lung diseases (2,3,335). Ten to 16% of patients with pathologically proven infiltrative lung disease have normal chest radiographs (2,3,335) (see Figs. 6-1, 6-81). Furthermore, between 10% and 20% of patients with radiographic findings suggestive of infiltrative lung disease have normal lungs (2,3,335).

The sensitivity of CT for detecting diffuse lung disease has been compared to that of plain chest radiography in a number of studies. Without exception these have shown that CT, and particularly HRCT, are more sensitive than chest radiography for detecting both acute and chronic diffuse lung diseases (20,29,63,83,301,335). Diseases in which HRCT has been shown to be more sensitive than plain radiographs include interstitial pulmonary fibrosis of various causes (164), sarcoidosis (29,63), asbestosis (20,191), coal worker's pneumoconiosis (75), Langerhan's pulmonary histiocytosis (85,86), lymphangioleiomyomatosis (83,216), lymphangitic carcinomatosis (62), emphysema (280,290,292), and pulmonary complications in immunocompromised patients (62, 280,290,292,298,299,301).

It should be noted, however, that a negative HRCT study does not rule out parenchymal lung disease (335,336). Averaging the results of several studies, Padley et al. concluded that the sensitivity of HRCT for detecting biopsy proven chronic infiltrative lung diseases was 94%, as compared to 80% for chest radiographs (336). Kang et al. (301) compared the sensitivity of CT scans and chest radiographs in 106 patients with pulmonary complications in AIDS and 33 patients with no active intrathoracic disease. Of the 106 patients with intrathoracic complications, 96% were correctly identified at CT as compared to 90% on the chest radiograph.

CT has also been shown to have a greater specificity allowing more confident distinction of patients with normal lungs from those with infiltrative lung disease. In the study by Padley et al., which included 86 patients with chronic infiltrative lung disease and 14 normals, the specificity in identifying normals based on CT findings was 96% compared to 82% on chest radiographs (335). In the study by Kang et al. (301), patients without intrathoracic complications were correctly identified on CT in 86% of cases compared to 73% on chest radiographs.

Based on the greater sensitivity and specificity of CT as compared to the chest radiograph, CT is indicated in the assessment of patients with normal or questionable radiographic findings who have symptoms or pulmonary function findings suggestive of diffuse lung disease.

High-Resolution versus Conventional CT Imaging

Several studies have demonstrated that HRCT is superior to CCT in the assessment of diffuse lung disease (19,20,75,337). Aberle et al. (20) demonstrated that HRCT performed in both the supine and prone positions was able to identify subtle parenchymal reticulation in 96% of patients with asbestosis compared to only 83% of cases on CCT. Leung et al. (19) randomly compared three select HRCT sections with CCT scans obtained at the same three levels and with complete CCT studies of the lungs, in 75 patients with documented diffuse lung disease. In each case, the observers provided their most likely diagnosis as well as their degrees of confidence. The highest confidence level in diagnosis was reached in 49% of interpretations based only on the three available HRCT sections, as compared with 31% of interpretations based on the corresponding three 10-mm sections and 43% of interpretations based on a complete set of contiguous 10-mm thick sections through the thorax. The correct diagnoses were made in 92%, 96%, and 94% of these readings, respectively. Surprisingly, the confidence in diagnosis and the diagnostic accuracy did not improve significantly when the findings on CCT were added to those of HRCT.

Similarly, Remy-Jardin et al. (337) in an assessment of 150 patients evaluated by both conventional 10-mm CT sections and HRCT obtained at identical levels found that HRCT was clearly superior to CCT in the identification of nodular and linear interfaces, septal and paraseptal lines, small cystic air spaces, bronchiectasis, and pleural thickening (Fig. 6-85). These authors also confirmed that reliable identification of ground-glass attenuation required the use of HRCT. They also demonstrated that acquiring HRCT sections at 15-mm intervals was significantly more accurate in evaluating the full range of abnormalities when compared to a few select HRCT sections.

Several recent studies have focused on the potential role of low-dose CT scans in the evaluation of patients with diffuse parenchymal lung disease (14,15,338) (see Fig. 6-3). HRCT scans performed at 10- and 20-mm intervals result in a skin entrance dose equivalent to 12% and 6%, respectively, of

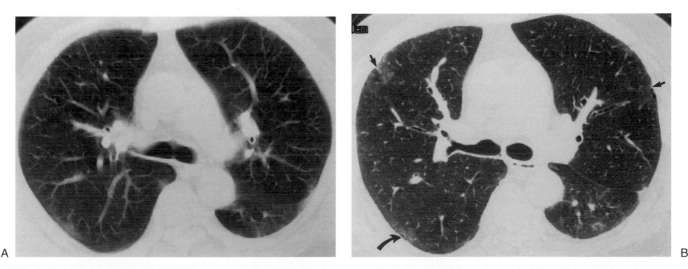

A B

FIG. 6-85. High-resolution CT (HRCT) versus conventional CT. **A:** 7-mm collimation spiral CT at the level of the right upper lobe bronchus demonstrates no definite abnormality. **B:** HRCT (1-mm collimation) at the same level demonstrates irregular interfaces (*straight arrows*) and localized areas of ground-glass attenuation mainly in the subpleural lung regions (*curved arrow*). Open lung biopsy demonstrated idiopathic pulmonary fibrosis with mild fibrosis and active alveolitis.

the radiation dose of CCT (338). HRCT scans performed at 20-mm intervals using low-dose technique (40 mAs) result in an average skin dose comparable to that of routine chest radiography. Lee et al. (15) compared the diagnostic accuracy of low-dose HRCT (80 mAs, 120 kVp), conventional dose HRCT (300 mAs, 120 kVp) and conventional chest radiographs in 10 normal controls and 50 patients with chronic infiltrative lung disease. For each HRCT technique, only three images were used, obtained at the levels of the aortic arch, tracheal carina, and 1 cm above the right hemidiaphragm. A correct first choice diagnosis was made significantly more often with either HRCT technique than with radiography. A high confidence level in making a diagnosis was reached in 42% of radiographic examinations, 61% of low-dose and 63% of conventional-dose HRCT exams ($p <$ 0.05) and these were correct in 92%, 90%, and 96% of studies, respectively. Although conventional-dose HRCT was slightly more accurate than low-dose HRCT, this difference was not statistically significant. The limited low-dose, thin-section CT used in this study was significantly superior to chest radiography and resulted in an equivalent effective radiation dose (0.03 mSv). It should be noted, however, that mild ground-glass attenuation and emphysema detectable on conventional-dose HRCT may be missed on low-dose HRCT (14). The optimal dose for HRCT has yet to be established.

HRCT (1- to 2-mm collimation) is recommended in the assessment of chronic and acute infiltrative lung diseases because it is superior to CCT and because it gives considerably lower radiation dose.

Diagnostic Accuracy of CT Compared with Routine Chest Radiography

Several studies have documented that CT is superior to the plain radiograph in allowing correct diagnosis of specific lung diseases, with considerably better interobserver agreement, both in chronic infiltrative lung diseases (14,15,25,99,335,337) and acute lung diseases in immunocompromised AIDS (301) and non-AIDS patients (302) (see Fig. 6-2). The majority of these studies has utilized an approach emphasizing blinded interpretations of a series of radiographic and CT findings in which individual observers listed their first three diagnostic choices in decreasing order of probability with degrees of confidence in those diagnoses usually expressed on a three-point scale. In the study by Mathieson et al. (25), the accuracies of chest radiographs and CT in making specific diagnoses were compared in 118 patients with various diffuse infiltrative lung diseases. A confident diagnosis was made more than twice as often on CT than on chest radiographs (49% versus 23%, respectively) and this diagnosis was more often correct on CT (93%) than on the radiograph (77%) ($p <$ 0.001). An approximately two-fold improvement in diagnostic accuracy of HRCT (53% of cases) compared to chest radiographs (27%) was also reported by Grenier et al., in a study of 140 patients

with 18 different infiltrative lung diseases (99). Slightly smaller improvement in diagnostic accuracy of CT compared to chest radiography was reported by others (335,340).

In an attempt to further refine the diagnostic accuracy, Grenier et al. (341) used Bayesian analysis to determine the relative value of clinical data, chest radiographs, and HRCT in patients with chronic diffuse infiltrative lung disease. For this study, two samples from the same population of patients with 27 different diffuse lung diseases were consecutively assessed, an initial training set of 208 cases for the development of the decision aid and a subsequent prospectively evaluated set of 100 "test" cases. Of the 208 initial cases, a correct diagnosis based on clinical data alone was obtained in 29% of cases, radiography alone in 9%, and HRCT in 36% of cases. This increased to 54% when clinical and radiographic findings were combined and 80% when all three were analyzed together ($p <$ 0.01). With prior and conditional probabilities determined from the initial set, the frequency of a high confidence level correct diagnosis based on Bayesian analysis in the 100 test cases from clinical, radiographic, and HRCT data alone was 27%, 4%, and 49%, respectively. The combination of the three tests allowed a high degree confident diagnosis in 61% of cases. HRCT made the greatest contribution to the diagnosis of sarcoidosis, Langerhans cell histiocytosis, HP, lymphangitic carcinomatosis, and silicosis. Although only minor improvement was seen in the diagnosis of idiopathic pulmonary fibrosis, as the authors noted, this probably reflected a population with advanced disease, as virtually all of these patients presented with diffuse radiographic abnormalities. Not surprisingly, the value of HRCT diminished with less common diseases: in this regard it is significant that 23 (68%) of 34 misclassified patients in this study had diseases classified as "miscellaneous."

Kang et al. (301) compared the diagnostic accuracy of CT with that of chest radiography in the detection and diagnosis of thoracic complications in patients with AIDS. CT was superior to chest radiography in the exclusion of disease in normal controls, in the detection of parenchymal abnormalities, and in the differential diagnosis. Of 89 patients with one proven pulmonary complication in AIDS, the observers were confident in their first choice diagnosis in 34% of cases at chest radiography and in 47% at CT. This diagnosis was correct in 67% of confident radiographic interpretations as compared to 87% of interpretations at CT ($p <$ 0.1). The confident first choice diagnosis at CT was most often correct in Kaposi's sarcoma, *Pneumocystis carinii* pneumonia and in the AIDS-related lymphoma.

Although all studies comparing CT with chest radiography have demonstrated that CT is superior, there has been some variation in the reported accuracy of CT. This may be related to different patient population or to different CT technique. The studies reporting the highest diagnostic accuracy of CT as compared to chest radiography have used either HRCT combined with CCT or, exclusively, 1- to 2-mm collimation HRCT sections (15,25,99,341). The studies reporting lower diagnostic accuracy of CT used 3-mm (335) or 5-mm thick sections (340). It cannot be overemphasized that accurate assessment of diffuse lung diseases requires the use of HRCT (1- to 2-mm collimation scans).

The various studies have shown that HRCT allows for a greater diagnostic accuracy than chest radiography and CCT in chronic infiltrative lung diseases and in acute infiltrative lung diseases seen in immunocompromised patients. Therefore, HRCT is indicated to make a specific diagnosis, or to limit the differential diagnosis, in patients with abnormal chest radiographs, in whom the clinical and radiographic findings are nonspecific, and further evaluation is considered appropriate.

Assessment of Disease Activity: The Significance of Ground-Glass Attenuation

Although HRCT can play an important role in the evaluation of disease activity in patients with diffuse lung disease, assessment of the true clinical value of HRCT must be individualized by disease entity. Needless to say, a potential role for HRCT to manage therapy is important as determining when and if to treat patients, particularly with corticosteroids, often proves to be a frustrating clinical dilemma.

To date, most attention has focused on the potential of HRCT to assess disease activity in patients with idiopathic interstitial pneumonitis (111,149,152,153). As noted in greater detail previously in the section on idiopathic interstitial pneumonitis, this topic is controversial as most prior reports have included a homogeneous population of patients under the general heading of IPF (139). Furthermore, there has been general lack of agreement as to the significance of cellularity in these patients, as prior studies have often included assessment of both intraalveolar macrophages as well as interstitial inflammation to histologicaly assay disease activity (139).

This is not to suggest that the finding of ground-glass attenuation is without value as means for assessing disease activity in patients with diffuse infiltrative lung disease. Leung et al., for example, in a study of 22 patients with a variety of chronic infiltrative lung diseases in which ground-glass attenuation was the predominant or exclusive CT finding, showed that 18 (82%) had active potentially reversible lung disease on lung biopsy (110) (Fig. 6-86). Similarly, Remy-Jardin et al. in a study of 26 patients with diffuse infiltrative lung diseases, demonstrated that areas of ground-glass attenuation corresponded to inflammation in 24 of 37 (65%) biopsy sites. As emphasized by these authors, ground-glass attenuation in itself is a nonspecific finding and is most valuable when seen in the absence of other findings indicative of fibrosis. In this same study, in 11 of the 13 (85%) cases in which ground-glass attenuation represented fibrosis rather than active disease, it was associated with traction bronchiectasis or bronchiolectasis, markers of interstitial fibrosis (112). It cannot be overemphasized that ground-glass attenuation can only be considered a reliable indicator of active inflammation when there are not associated findings of fibrosis in the same areas (112) (see Figs. 6-26, 6-27).

The value of CT in distinguishing potentially reversible active disease from irreversible fibrosis has also been assessed in a number of specific clinical settings other than IPF. Sequential CT findings have been assessed in 27 patients with HP (bird breeders' lung) (21). Patients in whom the main CT abnormalities consisted of diffuse micronodules, ground-glass attenuation and focal air trapping in the absence of diffuse reticulation or honeycombing uniformly improved following cessation of exposure to the inciting antigen, whereas those with a predominantly fibrotic pattern showed little if any change. Similar to patients with IPF, the prognostic significance of ground-glass attenuation in itself was less significant than the extent of underlying fibrosis.

Although alveolitis has been postulated to represent the initial stage in the development of sarcoid granulomata, it is seldom present at the time when the patients are evaluated clinically (228). The predominant histologic finding at the time of diagnosis consists of noncaseating granulomata. These account for the predominant finding on HRCT that consists of nodules in a characteristic perilymphatic distribution. Even when areas of ground-glass attenuation are present on HRCT, these have been shown to represent volume averaging of interstitial granulomata below the resolution of HRCT (63,110,228). In patients with sarcoidosis, nodules, areas of ground-glass attenuation, and parenchymal consolidation have been shown to be reversible in most patients following treatment with corticosteroids (29,67) (Fig. 6-87). Reticulation, architectural distortion, cystic spaces, and traction bronchiectasis are irreversible (29,67). It should be noted, however, that although certain findings on HRCT may indicate potentially reversible disease, it is controversial whether HRCT is helpful in predicting which patients with sarcoidosis are most likely to respond to corticosteroid therapy (342). Further studies are required to determine the role of the HRCT in the assessment of disease activity and prognosis in patients with sarcoidosis.

In patients with AIDS, bilateral areas of ground-glass attenuation are virtually diagnostic of *Pneumocystis carinii* pneumonia (71,313). Less commonly, they may be caused by cytomegalovirus pneumonia, pyogenic pneumonia, or be seen around hemorrhagic nodules in Kaposi's sarcoma (71,305).

HRCT may also be helpful in assessing disease activity in mycobacterial infections, both in immunocompromised and nonimmunocompromised patients. Im et al. (94) assessed sequential CT scans before and after antituberculous therapy in 26 patients with active tuberculosis. The most common findings at presentation consisted of centrilobular nodules and linear branching structures corresponding pathologically to the presence of mucus filled small airways. In virtually all cases, sequential studies showed these opacities to be reversible within five months after the start of treatment. Furthermore, in 11 of 12 patients with recent reactivation, CT accurately differentiated old fibrotic lesions

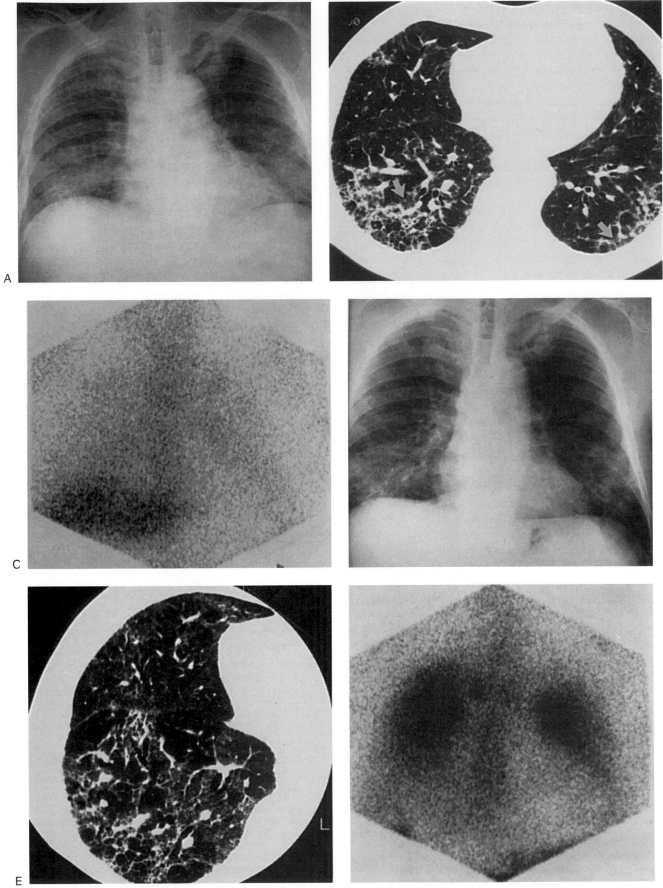

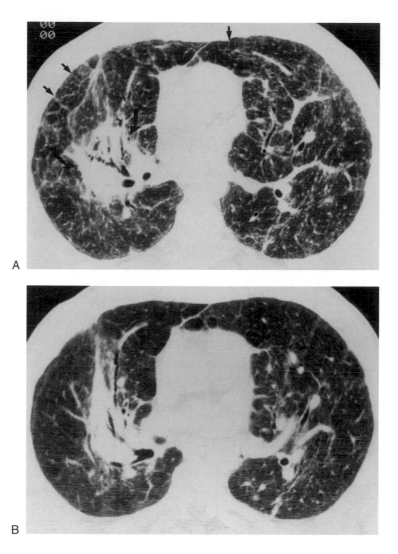

FIG. 6-87. Ground-glass reversibility in sarcoidosis. **A:** High-resolution CT (HRCT) in a 32-year-old man with sarcoidosis demonstrates extensive bilateral areas of ground-glass attenuation, interlobular septal thickening (*straight arrows*). Small nodules are present, particularly in the left lower lobe. Also noted is right peribronchial fibrosis with traction bronchiectasis and architectural distortion (*curved arrows*). **B:** HRCT two years later demonstrates marked improvement. Note almost complete resolution of ground-glass attenuation and interlobular septal thickening as well as decreased number of small nodules. However, the peribronchial fibrosis persists.

from new active ones. The authors concluded that HRCT was a reliable method for determining disease activity in patients with tuberculosis.

High Resolution CT-Guided Lung Biopsy

One of the most important indications for the use of HRCT is as a potential guide for the site and type of lung biopsy. Many diffuse lung diseases are patchy in distribution with areas of abnormal lung being interspersed among relatively normal areas of lung parenchyma. Furthermore, both active and fibrotic disease can be present in the same lung and indeed in the same pulmonary segment (141,152). Because of its ability to visualize, characterize, and determine the distribution of parenchymal disease, HRCT also provides a unique insight into the likely efficacy of transbronchial (TBBx) or open lung biopsy (via thoracotomy or video-assisted thoracoscopy) in patients with either acute or chronic diffuse lung disease and the optimal biopsy site (Figs. 6-88 and 6-89).

FIG. 6-86. Idiopathic pulmonary fibrosis (IPF): correlation between disease activity and ground-glass attenuation. **A:** Posteroanterior radiograph shows diffuse lung infiltrates, most prominent at the lung bases. **B:** A 1.5-mm section through the lung bases shows typical appearance of pulmonary fibrosis with associated honeycombing. A few focal areas of ground-glass attenuation can be identified (*arrows*). **C:** Corresponding Ga-67 scan shows faint diffuse uptake throughout the lungs, considerably less intense than the adjacent liver. At this time, an open-lung biopsy from the right lower lobe confirmed the diagnosis of IPF, and the patient was started on a course of steroids. **D:** Posteroanterior radiograph obtained 5 months after that shown in **A**. Although there clearly has been progression of disease, it is difficult to determine to what extent this reflects active, ongoing disease or progressive fibrosis. In the interval between radiographs the patient had stopped taking his medication. **E:** High-resolution CT section through the right lower lobe at approximately the same level as in **B**. Ground-glass opacification is now more prominent suggesting considerable alveolitis (compare with **B**). **F:** Corresponding Ga-67 scan shows intense bilateral uptake, consistent with extensive alveolitis.

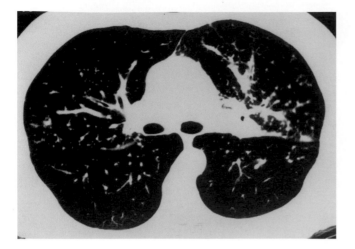

Fig. 6-88. High-resolution CT (HRCT) as a guide to transbronchial biopsy. HRCT in a 52-year-old woman demonstrates nodular thickening of the bronchovascular bundles and of the interlobar fissures. The findings are most severe in the upper lobes, particularly left upper lobe, with minimal abnormalities seen in the lower lobes. The peribronchovascular distribution of the abnormalities suggested that transbronchial biopsy would be likely to yield a definitive diagnosis. Also, given the distribution of abnormalities, a biopsy of the left upper lobe was considered to be more likely to be diagnostic than a biopsy in either lower lobe. Transbronchial biopsy of the left upper lobe was diagnostic of sarcoidosis.

Although TBBx is frequently used in an attempt to diagnose diffuse lung disease, the limitations of TBBx for establishing the etiology of diffuse pulmonary disease have been well documented. In a classic study, Wall et al. showed that TBBx was diagnostic in only 20 (38%) of 53 patients presenting with radiographic evidence of diffuse lung disease (343). In the remaining 33 cases, TTBx were reported either as normal or nonspecific, whereas open lung biopsies resulted in specific diagnoses in 92% of cases. Similar results have been reported by Wilson et al. (344) in a study of 127 patients with a variety of parenchymal abnormalities. They found that TBBx allowed a "specific" diagnosis in only 52% of patients with diffuse infiltrative processes. Also, diagnoses suggested by TTBx may bear little relationship to diagnoses subsequently made on open biopsy (343), and a nonspecific transbronchial biopsy diagnosis, such as "interstitial pneumonia" or "interstitial fibrosis" should be considered as potentially misleading (3,345).

In patients with chronic diffuse lung disease, TTBx is most accurate in patients with sarcoidosis or lymphangitic carcinomatosis (343); these entities preferentially involve peribronchial tissues and therefore are most accessible to transbronchial biopsy (343,346). In this regard, however, it should be noted that despite the efficacy of TTBx especially in patients with sarcoidosis, a significantly greater diagnostic yield may result when TBBx is coupled with transbronchial needle aspiration (TBNA) (see Fig. 6-62). As documented by Morales et al., in their study of 51 consecutive patients with combined TBBx and TBNA, overall in 33% of cases, a histologic diagnosis of sarcoidosis was established only with TBNA (346a). Interestingly, in patients with stage 1 disease, TBBx was diagnostic in 60%, and TBNA was diagnostic in 53%, the combined yield equaled 83%. Surprisingly, even in patients with stage 2 sarcoidosis, TBBx was diagnostic in only 76% of cases. These data strongly suggest a role for CT prior to bronchoscopy to optimize selection of sites for biopsy, both in the lung as well as in the mediastinum (see Fig. 6-62).

Although the accuracy of transbronchial biopsy has improved over the past decade, especially in establishing such diagnoses as Langerhans cell histiocytosis, pulmonary alveolar proteinosis, eosinophilic lung disease, Goodpasture's syndrome, and Wegener's granulomatosis, these entities represent a distinct minority of cases (138). More importantly, there has been little improvement in the ability of TBBx or BAL to assess patients with pulmonary fibrosis (345).

Open lung biopsy (OLBx) is often diagnostic, with accuracies greater than 90% generally reported (3,343,347), but this procedure is also subject to sampling error, as biopsies

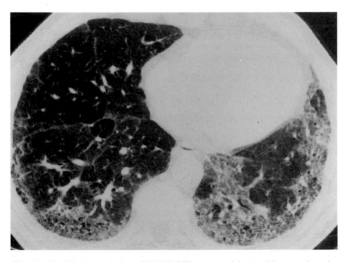

Fig. 6-89. High-resolution CT (HRCT) as a guide to video-assisted thoracoscopic biopsy. HRCT scan in a 58-year-old man with progressive shortness of breath demonstrates a reticular pattern and areas of ground-glass attenuation involving mainly the subpleural regions of the right lower lobe, left lower lobe and lingula. Also noted is honeycombing in these areas. Small focal areas of ground-glass attenuation are present in the right middle lobe. Biopsy of the right middle lobe in this patient confirmed the diagnosis of idiopathic pulmonary fibrosis but gave no indication of the extensive honeycombing present in this patient. Biopsy of the lower lobes, on the other hand, may have revealed only honeycombing but may not have yielded a specific diagnosis. In patients with chronic infiltrative lung disease, open or video-assisted thoracoscopic biopsy should be performed in areas with relatively mild involvement. Areas with honeycombing should be avoided as they may only yield nonspecific end-stage fibrosis.

taken from a small region of lung may not reflect the state of the diseased lung as a whole. This is most important when attempts are made to assess disease activity in patients with diffuse fibrotic lung diseases such as idiopathic pulmonary fibrosis or collagen vascular disease (345). It has been emphasized that the role of the surgeon at the time of open lung biopsy is to obtain representative tissue, while avoiding areas of extensive honeycombing (3). However, this may be difficult, especially in patients with idiopathic pulmonary fibrosis, owing to the predominantly subpleural distribution of the fibrosis.

Given the limitations of both transbronchial and open biopsy techniques, it is not surprising that HRCT has emerged as an important tool for assessing patients with suspected DILD prior to lung biopsy. HRCT is of considerable value in determining the most appropriate sites for biopsy by showing the regions most likely to be active and, therefore, most likely to be diagnostic (116,152,307). Also, using HRCT, areas of end-stage honeycombing can be avoided. Second, HRCT can play a decisive role in selecting among transbronchial biopsy, lavage and/or open lung biopsy as the most efficacious method for obtaining a histologic diagnosis. Of particular value is the identification of peribronchial abnormalities, as characteristically occur in patients with sarcoidosis (see Figs. 6-21, 6-61, 6-62) (29,63) and lymphangitic carcinomatosis (28,62) (see Figs. 6-50–6-52). As shown by Lenique et al., the demonstration of abnormal airways in patients with sarcoidosis correlates with the likelihood of obtaining a histologic diagnosis (346).

Not surprisingly, HRCT has proved more efficacious than chest radiographs in predicting the likely efficacy of TBBx for diagnosing DILD. Mathieson et al. (25) compared the accuracy of plain radiographs and CT in determining whether TTBx or OLBx would be most appropriate in patients with chronic infiltrative lung disease. Using CT, three observers correctly predicted that a TTBx would be likely to be diagnostic in 87% of patients in which this was appropriate. They correctly predicted the need for OLBx in 99% of cases. By comparison, plain radiographs proved significantly less valuable ($p < 0.001$).

Recently, video-assisted thoracoscopic lung biopsy (VAT) has gained acceptance as an alternate to thoracotomy for performing an OLBx. As most studies confirm equivalent diagnostic accuracy, VAT may be the preferred method given lower cost and morbidity compared with thoracotomy (347). Because the operator's field of view is rather limited when performing this procedure, HRCT has proven extremely helpful in directing the surgeon to the most appropriate biopsy site (see Fig. 6-89). Additionally, using CT guidance, needle localization of the biopsy site may be performed prior to the procedure. Although this technique has been described primarily as a localization technique for resection of lung nodules (348,349), it has proved equally applicable to the biopsy of diffuse lung disease.

HRCT has also been shown to play an important potential role in the pre-bronchoscopic assessment of immunocom-

promised patients. As documented by Janzen et al., in a retrospective study evaluating 33 consecutive immunocompromised non-AIDS patients (including 20 bone marrow transplant patients) presenting with acute pulmonary disease with both HRCT and bronchoscopy (307). Bronchoscopy provided a specific diagnosis in 17 (52%) of 33 patients. Significantly, bronchoscopy proved diagnostic more often in patients with HRCT disease involving the central versus the peripheral third of the lungs (70% versus 23%, $p = 0.02$). Results also proved more diagnostic in patients with infectious versus noninfectious disease (71% versus 17%, $p < 0.005$). Based on these findings the authors concluded that HRCT should precede bronchoscopy in immunocompromised patients in order to determine optimal sites for biopsy as well as predict likely results of bronchoscopy.

Similar studies have also concluded a role for HRCT in evaluating bone marrow transplant patients (299,300). Mori et al., in a study of 33 febrile bone marrow recipients, found that CT showed nodules in 20 of 21 episodes of documented fungal infection but none in nine bacteremic episodes (300). From these data, the authors concluded that CT studies showing the presence of nodules in this population could be taken as presumptive evidence of fungal infection warranting empiric therapy without the need for bronchoscopy. In a similar prospective study of 36 symptomatic episodes in 33 bone marrow transplant patients, Barloon et al. reported that in comparison with plain radiographs, HRCT resulted in a change of management in a total of 11 (50%) of 22 patients, including establishing the need for bronchoscopy and/or OLBx in six patients (299).

Of even greater potential clinical utility is the potential role of HRCT in evaluating patients presenting with hemoptysis (350–353) (see Chapter 3). The role of bronchoscopy in the evaluation of patients presenting with hemoptysis has proved controversial (354,355). In fact, the etiology of hemoptysis most often proves elusive; nearly 50% of cases remain undiagnosed despite radiographic and bronchoscopic evaluation (353,354). In most reported series to date, HRCT has proved of greatest value in identifying bronchiectasis as a cause of hemoptysis (350–353). As shown by McGuinness et al. (353), in a prospective study of 57 consecutive patients presenting with hemoptysis evaluated both with CT and fiber optic bronchoscopy, CT identified all cancers; furthermore, the overall diagnostic yield of bronchoscopy was documented to be less than CT (47% compared with 61%, respectively). CT proved especially valuable in diagnosing bronchiectasis, present in 25% of cases.

From the data in the literature it can be concluded that CT is indicated as a guide for the need of lung biopsy and as a guide for the optimal type and site of biopsy.

Can HRCT ever obviate biopsy? Although controversial, in our judgment there are a number of diseases whose appearances are sufficiently characteristic in cross-section to warrant empiric therapy in the absence of tissue confirmation in the appropriate clinical setting (Table 6-5) (356).

These include: patients with known causes of interstitial

TABLE 6-5. *Specific etiologies potentially established by high resolution CT*

Diagnosis	CT Findings
Silicosis	Well-defined (often calcified) nodules predominately in the posterior protions of both upper lobes usually in association with pericicitricial emphysema
Sarcoidosis	Perilymphatic nodules associated with diffuse adenopathy
Lymphangitic carcinomatosis	Beaded secondary lobular septa in association with peri-lymphatic nodules
Subacute hypersensitivity pneumonitis	Diffuse ground-glass centrilobular nodules in the absence of reticulation or a tree-in-bud appearance
Infectious bronchiolitis	Peripheral nodules with a tree-in-bud configuration
Interstitial pneumonitis secondary to a known etiology including collagen vascular disease or asbestosis	Diffuse reticular changes and/or honeycombing involving the lung bases and periphery
Idiopathic interstitial pneumonitis	Diffuse reticular changes and/or honeycombing (identical to findings in patients with interstitial pneumonitis of known etiology)
Lymphangioleiomyomatosis (specifically in women of child bearing age)	Thin-walled cystic spaces uniformly distributed throughout both lungs with or without an associated pneumothorax in the absence of reticular changes or nodules
Pneumocystis carinii pneumonia (in HIV + patients)	Diffuse and/or symmetric ground-glass attenuation with or without associated cystic changes
Langerhan's cell histiocytosis	Bilateral bizarre shaped cysts with or without associated nodules with relative sparing of the lower 1/3 of the lungs
Kaposi's sarcoma (in HIV + patients)	Ill-defined peribronchovascular nodular infiltrates extending from the perihilar regions peripherally with or without associated subpleural nodules, adenopathy or pleural effusions

HIV, human immunodeficiency virus.

pneumonitis, such as collagen vascular disease (see Figs. 6-18, 6-42) or asbestosis with predominant peripheral and basilar changes on HRCT (see Figs. 6-14, 6-43–6-48, 6-59); patients with classic features of sarcoidosis, that is, peri-lymphatic nodules in association with diffuse hilar and mediastinal adenopathy (see Figs. 6-15, 6-21, 6-61, 6-62); patients with a known history of exposure to silica or coal dust with well defined random nodules predominantly occupying the posterior portions of the upper lobes (see Fig. 6-66); patients with known malignancy with typical features of lymphangitic carcinomatosis (including a diagnosis of Kaposi's sarcoma in HIV-positive patients) (see Figs. 6-16, 6-50–6-52); patients with subacute HP, with known antigen exposure and diffuse centrilobular nodules (see Figs. 6-22, 6-68–6-69); and patients with evidence of honeycomb lung, from whatever etiology (see Figs. 6-19, 6-38, 6-60). HRCT may also be of value in select patients with classic features of Langerhans cell histiocytosis (see Figs. 6-20, 6-53–6-55), or either lymphanioleiomyomatosis or tuberous sclerosis (see Figs. 6-56–6-58). Although more controversial, in our experience the finding of marked reticular changes in the lung bases and periphery in the absence of ground-glass attenuation is sufficiently specific for the presence of lung fibrosis as to warrant empiric therapy for IPF. CT is also of value in select patients, especially those with known immunodeficiency disorders with a variety of infections, including: HIV-positive patients presenting with diffuse ground-glass attenuation, compatible with the diagnosis of *Pneumo-*

cystis carinii pneumonia (see Fig. 6-28; see Chapter 7), or with a diffuse tree-in-bud pattern indicative of infectious bronchiolitis (see Fig. 6-23; see Chapter 3). In the latter case, in our experience, the yield of transbronchial biopsy with or without lavage is sufficiently low to warrant a course of empiric antibiotic therapy (see Chapter 3). CT is also of value to direct empiric therapy in neutropenic patients presenting with findings indicative of invasive fungal infections (see Figs. 6-25 and 6-83). Clearly, use of CT to obviate lung biopsy requires thorough familiarity with the various patterns of DILD identifiable with HRCT as well as detailed clinical correlation as well as careful clinical and radiologic follow-up.

More problematic is the question of whether or not biopsies should be obtained in patients with otherwise unexplained respiratory symptoms with normal HRCT studies. Padley et al., in a study of 100 patients with documented DILD noted that in 18% of patients HRCT studies were interpreted as normal (335). Similarly, in a prospective study of 25 patients with open lung biopsy proved IPF, Orens et al. reported finding 3 (12%) patients with normal HRCT examinations (357). Lynch et al. in an assessment of patients with biopsy proved HP found that only 5 of 11 patients had HRCT evidence of centrilobular nodules, with the remainder proving to have normal CT (22). These data, although limited, confirm that a normal HRCT study does not exclude DILD in patients for whom there is a high index of suspicion of pulmonary disease.

MRI

To date, the role of MRI in the clinical evaluation of both diffuse and focal lung disease has been limited because of a number of factors. Compared with other tissues, lung has relatively low water density, with tissue per unit volume measuring only approximately one-fifth that of solid organs, resulting in a low signal-to-noise ratio (358–360). Additionally, spatial resolution is diminished by a combination of respiratory and cardiac motion. Finally, susceptibility artifacts caused by innumerable air-water interfaces within the lung result in loss of signal, especially when gradient-refocused techniques are utilized. Despite these limitations, MRI does have the potential to evolve into a powerful tool for the investigation of pulmonary disease because of markedly increased contrast resolution.

Experimental studies have documented that MRI can be used to quantitate lung water content (361–371). Using animal models, close agreement has been documented between MRI signal intensities and gravimetrically determined lung wet-to-dry weight ratios. Although determination of absolute lung water content has proven difficult *in vivo*, measurements of relative lung water changes have been shown to be proportional to true lung water content, and may prove to be a sensitive method for following the course of lung injury (359). Furthermore, using animal models, Schmidt et al. have shown documented differences in the MRI characteristics of permeability versus hydrostatic pulmonary edema; to date, however, the pattern of distribution of edema has not proven sufficiently specific to provide reliable discrimination (366).

More recently Mayo et al. demonstrated that lung water and pleural pressure gradients could be assessed in normal human volunteers using a multi-echo sequence (371). Five normal volunteers were imaged in the supine and prone positions during quiet breathing, and in the supine position at TLC using a cardiac gated multi-echo pulse sequence with echo spacing of 20 msec from TE20 to 240 msec on a Picker 0.15 T MR imager. After validating the technique, they demonstrated that there was no significant difference in average lung density in the prone (0.21 ± 0.03 g/mL) and in the supine (0.20 ± 0.03 g/mL) positions. Lung density decreased at TLC (0.12 ± 0.01 g/mL) ($p < 0.01$). Gradients in lung density were visible in all prone and supine scans at functional residual capacity and on average the gradients were decreased by 90% at TLC. The authors concluded that MRI allows measurement of lung water content and pleural pressure gradient.

Although MR has greater contrast resolution than CT, attempts to differentiate among various etiologies of parenchymal consolidation have been generally disappointing. Moore et al. in a study of 16 patients with known airspace diseases evaluated the potential of MRI to differentiate among various etiologies and found considerable overlap in both T1 and T2 values, although one case of alveolar proteinosis was distinctive because of its especially low T1

value (372). It is likely that with greater experience a wide range of appearances will be documented for this entity as well. Similar attempts to differentiate pulmonary hemorrhage from edema were also equivocal (373). A single case report of pulmonary hemosiderosis diagnosed by MR imaging demonstrated increased signal intensity on T1-weighted images with marked decrease on T2-weighted images (374). The authors suggested that the MRI finding of decreased parenchymal signal intensity on T2-weighted images with high associated signal on T1, in the appropriate clinical context, may be sufficiently specific to allow safe initiation of treatment and deferral of lung biopsy in unstable patients (374).

MRI has been shown to be helpful in distinguishing patients with atelectasis caused by central obstructing masses from nonobstructive atelectasis (interested readers are referred to Chapter 3 for a more detailed discussion) (375,376). Herold et al. compared cardiac gated standard spin-echo MRI sequences in 17 patients with obstructive atelectasis and 25 patients with nonobstructive atelectasis. No signal differences were observed between the two types of atelectasis on T1-weighted images. However, all 17 cases with obstructive atelectasis showed increased signal intensity on T2-weighted images whereas 22 of 25 cases of nonobstructive atelectasis demonstrated very low signal intensity on T2-weighted images (377). The difference in signal intensity is probably related to absorption of air and accumulation of secretions in the obstructed lung (377). The resulting increase in free fluid prolongs the T2 relaxation times and leads to high signal intensity on T2-weighted images. In nonobstructive atelectasis, on the other hand, the short T2 relaxation time is caused by the low proton density and the magnetic susceptibility effects caused by residual air.

Of considerable promise is the potential of MRI to identify active interstitial lung disease. Investigating bleomycin-induced alveolitis and pulmonary fibrosis in 18 Lewis rats, Vitinski et al. found MRI signal intensities to be markedly elevated in both disease states (376). Additionally, both T1 and T2 values of lungs with documented alveolitis and controls proved equivalent, although these values were significantly decreased in fibrotic lungs. Consistent differentiation between foci of active inflammation and fibrosis in the lung, however, has proven controversial (378–380).

McFadden et al., in a study of 34 patients with a variety of interstitial lung diseases, found a strong correlation between qualitative assessment of signal intensity within the lungs and clinical assessment of disease activity (381). In this study the most severely affected patients proved to have the greatest signal intensities, and follow-up examinations in 10 patients showed a decrease in image intensity in patients responding to treatment. Unfortunately, MRI signal characteristics were of no use in differentiating patients who responded to therapy from those whose disease remained stable or worsened with therapy.

Müller et al., compared the value of MR imaging to that of HRCT in the assessment of chronic infiltrative lung dis-

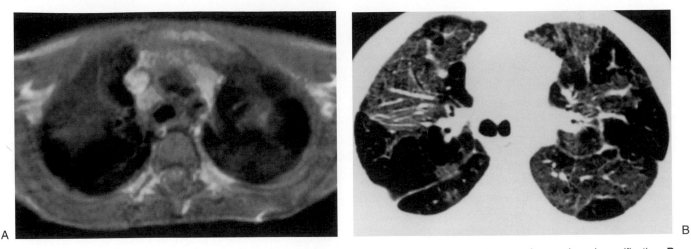

A

B

FIG. 6-90. Ground-glass opacification in hypersensitivity pneumonitis. **A:** MR demonstrates bilateral areas of parenchymal opacification. **B:** High-resolution CT (HRCT) demonstrates patchy bilateral areas of ground-glass attenuation. The appearance of the parenchymal opacification on MR is comparable to that of HRCT but the anatomic detail is much better visualized on HRCT. (From Müller NL, Mayo JR, Zwirewich CV. Value of MR imaging in the evaluation of chronic infiltrative lung diseases: comparison with CT. *AJR Am J Roentgenol* 1992;158:1205–1209, with permission.)

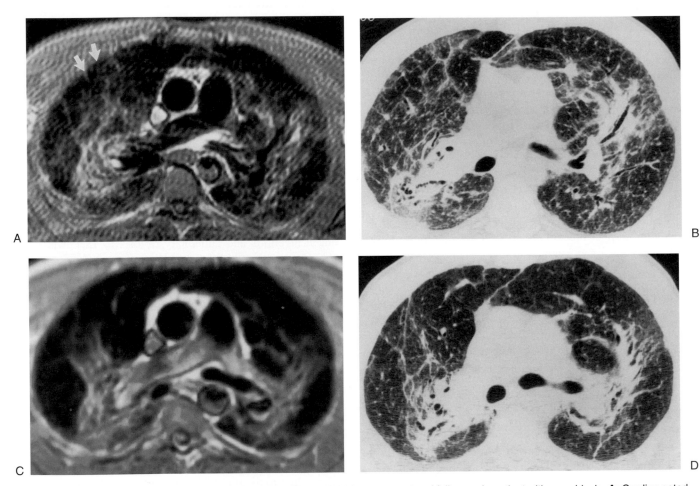

A

B

C

D

FIG. 6-91. Comparison of MRI with high-resolution CT (HRCT) in initial assessment and follow-up in patient with sarcoidosis. **A:** Cardiac gated, spin-echo T1-weighted MR (TR 857, TE 15) demonstrates extensive bilateral parenchymal opacification. Also note interlobular septal thickening (*arrows*) and extensive central peribronchial fibrosis with traction bronchiectasis. **B:** HRCT at the same level more clearly demonstrates the interlobular septal thickening and the presence of small nodules. Visualization of ground-glass attenuation on HRCT is comparable to that seen on MR. **C:** MR (TR 1000, TE 7) two years later demonstrates considerable improvement in the interlobular septal thickening and parenchymal opacification. Central peribronchial fibrosis persists. **D:** High-resolution CT performed at the same level and on the same day as follow-up MR demonstrates similar improvement but better visualization of parenchymal detail.

ease in 25 patients (382). All patients had cardiac gated spin-echo MRI and 1.5 mm collimation HRCT. HRCT was considerably better than MRI in the anatomic assessment of the lung parenchyma and in demonstrating fibrosis. However, areas of airspace opacification (ground-glass attenuation and parenchymal consolidation) were equally well seen on MR as on HRCT (Figs. 6-90 and 6-91). OLBx demonstrated that the areas of airspace opacification seen on MRI and on HRCT corresponded to areas of active alveolitis or airspace infiltrates. Follow-up demonstrated similar degrees of change in the airspace opacification over time on MRI and CT (see Fig. 6-91). The authors concluded that whereas MRI was considerably inferior to HRCT in the initial assessment of patients with chronic infiltrative lung disease, it may play a potential role in the assessment and follow-up of patients with predominantly airspace opacification. It should be noted, however, that in order to provide similar anatomic detail, MR images would have to be obtained using 1- to 2-mm thick sections in order to avoid volume averaging which may result in over estimation of areas of ground-glass attenuation similar to what occurs with CT (152,228).

Primack et al. compared the MRI with pathologic findings in 22 consecutive patients with chronic infiltrative lung disease (383). Fifteen patients had OLBx and seven had TBBx. They demonstrated that the MRI findings correlated closely with the macroscopic findings on OLBx. Evidence of parenchymal opacification was seen on MRI in 14 patients, nine interpreted as being equivalent to ground-glass intensity and five to consolidation. In 12 of the 14 patients the parenchymal opacification represented an active inflammatory process including alveolitis, pneumonia, and granulomatous infection, whereas in two patients it represented fibrosis. As the authors pointed out, a major limitation of MR in the assessment of infiltrative lung disease is the low spatial resolution compared to HRCT. Therefore MR is not recommended in the routine assessment of patients with infiltrative lung disease. It may be used as an alternate imaging modality in patients who express concern about radiation exposure or in young patients who are repeatedly scanned for assessment of response to treatment or disease progression (383).

REFERENCES

1. Felson B. A new look at pattern recognition of diffuse pulmonary disease. *AJR Am J Roentgenol* 1979;133:183–189.
2. Epler GR, McLoud TC, Gaensler EA, Mikus JP, Carrington CB. Normal chest roentgenograms in chronic diffuse infiltrative lung disease. *N Engl J Med* 1978;298:801–809.
3. Gaensler EA, Carrington CB. Open biopsy for chronic diffuse infiltrative lung disease: clinical, roentgenographic, and physiologic correlations in 502 patients. *Ann Thorac Surg* 1980;30:411–426.
4. McLoud TC, Carrington CB, Gaensler EA. Diffuse infiltrative lung disease: a new scheme for description. *Radiology* 1983;149:353–363.
5. Wegener OH, Koeppe P, Oeser H. Measurement of lung density by computed tomography. *J Comput Assist Tomogr* 1978;2:263–273.
6. Solomon A, Kreel L, McNicol M, Johnson N. Computed tomography in pulmonary sarcoidosis. *J Comput Assist Tomogr* 1979;3:754–758.
7. Robinson PJ, Kreel L. Pulmonary tissue attenuation with computed tomography: comparison of inspiration and expiration scans. *J Comput Assist Tomogr* 1979;3:740–748.
8. Kreel L. Computed tomography of interstitial pulmonary disease. *J Comput Assist Tomogr* 1982;6:181–199.
9. Zerhouni EA, Naidich DP, Stitik FP, Khouri NF, Siegelman SS. Computed tomography of the pulmonary parenchyma: Part 2. Interstitial disease. *J Thorac Imaging* 1985;1:54–64.
10. Müller NL, Miller RR. Computed tomography of chronic diffuse infiltrative lung disease: Part 1. *Am Rev Respir Dis* 1990;142:1206–1215.
11. Müller NL, Miller RR. Computed tomography of chronic diffuse infiltrative lung disease: Part 2. *Am Rev Respir Dis* 1990;142:1440–1448.
12. Webb WR, Stein MG, Finkbeiner WE, et al. Normal and diseased isolated lungs: high-resolution CT. *Radiology* 1988;166:81–87.
13. Mayo JR, Webb WR, Gould R, et al. High-resolution CT of the lungs: an optimal approach. *Radiology* 1987;163:507–510.
14. Zwirewich CV, Mayo JR, Müller NL. Low-dose high-resolution CT of lung parenchyma. *Radiology* 1991;180:413–417.
15. Lee KS, Primack SL, Staples CA, et al. Chronic infiltrative lung disease: comparison of diagnostic accuracies of radiography and low- and conventional-dose thin-section CT. *Radiology* 1994;191:669–673.
16. Majorin ML, Varpula M, Kurki T, Pakkala L. High-resolution CT of the lung in asbestos-exposed subjects. Comparison of low-dose and high-dose HRCT. *Acta Radiologica* 1994;35:473–477.
17. Murata K, Khan A, Rojas KA, Herman PG. Optimization of computed tomography technique to demonstrate the fine structure of the lung. *Invest Radiol* 1988;23:170–175.
18. Naidich DP. Pulmonary parenchymal high-resolution CT: to be or not to be. *Radiology* 1989;171:22–24.
19. Leung AN, Staples CA, Müller NL. Chronic diffuse infiltrative lung disease: comparison of diagnostic accuracy of high-resolution and conventional CT. *AJR Am J Roentgenol* 1991;157:693–696.
20. Aberle DR, Gamsu G, Ray CS, Feuerstein IM. Asbestos-related pleural and parenchymal fibrosis: detection with high-resolution CT. *Radiology* 1988;166:729–734.
21. Remy-Jardin M, Remy J, Wallaert B, Müller NL. Subacute and chronic bird breeder hypersensitivity pneumonitis: sequential evaluation with CT and correlation with lung function tests and bronchoalveolar lavage. *Radiology* 1993;198:111–118.
22. Lynch DA, Rose CS, Way D, King TE. Hypersensitivity pneumonitis: sensitivity of high-resolution CT in a population-based study. *AJR* 1992;159:469–472.
23. Webb WR. High-resolution CT of the lung parenchyma. *Radiol Clin North Am* 1989;27:1085–1097.
24. Gamsu G, Klein JS. High resolution computed tomography of diffuse lung disease. *Clin Radiol* 1989;40:554–556.
25. Mathieson JR, Mayo JR, Staples CA, Müller NL. Chronic diffuse infiltrative lung disease: comparison of diagnostic accuracy of CT and chest radiography. *Radiology* 1989;171:111–116.
26. Volpe J, Storto ML, Lee K, Webb WR. High-resolution CT of the lung: determination of the usefulness of CT scans obtained with the patient prone based on plain radiographic findings. *AJR Am J Roentgenol* 1997;169:369–374.
27. Grenier P, Maurice F, Musset D, Menu Y, Nahum H. Bronchiectasis: assessment by thin-section CT. *Radiology* 1986;161:95–99.
28. Munk PL, Müller NL, Miller RR, Ostrow DN. Pulmonary lymphangitic carcinomatosis: CT and pathologic findings. *Radiology* 1988;166:705–709.
29. Brauner MW, Grenier P, Mompoint D, Lenoir S, de Cremoux H. Pulmonary sarcoidosis: evaluation with high-resolution CT. *Radiology* 1989;172:467–471.
30. Remy-Jardin M, Remy J, Gosselin B, et al. Sliding thin slab, minimum intensity projection technique in the diagnosis of emphysema: histopathologic-CT correlation. *Radiology* 1996;200:665–671.
31. Bhalla M, Naidich DP, McGuinness G, et al. Diffuse lung disease: assessment with helical CT: preliminary observations of the role of maximum and minimum projection images. *Radiology* 1996;200:341–347.
32. Boyden EA. The nomenclature of the bronchopulmonary segments and their blood supply. *Dis Chest* 1961;39:1–6.
33. Naidich DP, Zinn WL, Ettenger NA, McCauley DI, Garay SM. Basilar segmental bronchi: thin-section CT evaluation. *Radiology* 1988;169:11–16.
34. Osborne D, Vock P, Godwin JD, Silverman PM. CT identification of

bronchopulmonary segments: 50 normal subjects. *AJR Am J Roentgenol* 1984;142:47–52.

35. Weibel ER. Looking into the lung: what can it tell us? *AJR Am J Roentgenol* 1979;133:1021–1031.

36. Webb WR. High-resolution computed tomography of the lung: normal and abnormal anatomy. *Semin Roentgenol* 1991;26:110–117.

37. Webb WR. High resolution lung computed tomography: normal anatomic and pathologic findings. *Radiol Clin North Am* 1991;29:1051–1063.

38. Lynch DA, Newell JD, Tschomper BA, et al. Uncomplicated asthma in adults: comparison of CT appearance of the lungs in asthmatic and healthy subjects. *Radiology* 1993;188:829–833.

39. Zerhouni E. Computed tomography of the pulmonary parenchyma: an overview. *Chest* 1989;95:901–907.

40. Webb WR, Gamsu G, Wall SD, Cann CE, Proctor E. CT of a bronchial phantom: factors affecting appearance and size measurements. *Invest Radiol* 1984;19:394–398.

41. Weibel ER, Taylor CR. Design and structure of the human lung. In: Fishman AP, ed. *Pulmonary diseases and disorders,* 2nd ed. New York: McGraw-Hill, 1988;1:11–60.

42. Murata K, Itoh H, Todo G, et al. Centrilobular lesions of the lung: demonstration by high-resolution CT and pathologic correlation. *Radiology* 1986;161:641–645.

43. Miller WS. *The lung.* Springfield: Charles C. Thomas, 1947.

44. Heitzman ER, Markarian B, Berger I, Dailey E. The secondary pulmonary lobule: a practical concept for interpretation of radiographs. II. application of the anatomic concept to an underastanding of roentgen pattern of in disease states. *Radiology* 1969;93:514–520.

45. Osborne DR, Effmann EL, Hedlund LW. Postnatal growth and size of the pulmonary acinus and secondary lobule in man. *AJR Am J Roentgenol* 1983;140:449–454.

46. Raskin SP. The pulmonary acinus: historical notes. *Radiology* 1982;144:31–34.

47. Itoh H, Murata K, Konishi J, et al. Diffuse lung disease: pathologic basis for the high-resolution computed tomography findings. *J Thorac Imag* 1993;8:176–188.

48. Reid L. The secondary pulmonary lobule in the adult human lung, with special reference to its appearance in bronchograms. *Thorax* 1958;13:110–115.

49. Reid L, Simon G. The peripheral pattern in the normal bronchogram and its relation to peripheral pulmonary anatomy. *Thorax* 1958;13:103–109.

50. Gamsu G, Thurlbeck WM, T. MP, Fraser RG. Peripheral bronchographic morphology in the normal human lung. *Invest Radiol* 1971;6:161–170.

51. Reid L, Rubino M. The connective tissue septa in the foetal human lung. *Thorax* 1959;14:3–13.

52. Aberle DR, Gamsu G, Ray CS. High-resolution CT of benign asbestos-related diseases: clinical and radiographic correlation. *AJR Am J Roentgenol* 1988;151:883–891.

53. Itoh H, Tokunaga S, Asamoto H, et al. Radiologic-pathologic correlations of small lung nodules with special reference to peribronchiolar nodules. *AJR Am J Roentgenol* 1978;130:223–231.

54. Vock P, Malanowski D, Tschaeppeler H, et al. Computed tomographic lung density in children. *Invest Radiol* 1987;22:627–631.

55. Millar AB, Denison DM. Vertical gradients of lung density in healthy supine men. *Thorax* 1989;44:485–490.

56. Murata K, Itoh H, Senda M, et al. Stratified impairment of pulmonary ventilation in "diffuse panbronchiolitis": PET and CT studies. *J Comput Assist Tomogr* 1989;13:48–53.

57. Rosenblum LJ, Mauceri RA, Wellenstein DE, et al. Density patterns in the normal lung as determined by computed tomography. *Radiology* 1980;137:409–416.

58. Genereux GP. Computed tomography and the lung: review of anatomic and densitometric features with their clinical application. *J Can Assoc Radiol* 1985;36:88–102.

59. Webb WR, Stern EJ, Kanth N, Gamsu G. Dynamic pulmonary CT: findings in normal adult men. *Radiology* 1993;186:117–124.

60. Nishimura K, Kitaichi M, Izumi T, Nagai S, Itoh H. Usual interstitial pneumonia: histologic correlation with high-resolution CT. *Radiology* 1992;182:337–342.

61. Storto ML, Kee ST, Golden JA, Webb WR. Pictorial essay. Hydrostatic pulmonary edema: high-resolution CT findings. *Am J Roentgenol* 1995;165:817–820.

62. Stein MG, Mayo J, Müller N, et al. Pulmonary lymphangitic spread of carcinoma: appearance on CT scans. *Radiology* 1987;162:371–375.

63. Müller NL, Kullnig P, Miller RR. The CT findings of pulmonary sarcoidosis: analysis of 25 patients. *AJR Am J Roentgenol* 1989;152:1179–1182.

64. Bessis L, Callard P, Gotheil C, Biaggi A, Grenier P. High-resolution CT of parenchymal lung disease: precise correlation with histologic findings. *RadioGraphics* 1992;12:45–58.

65. Westcott JL, Cole SR. Traction bronchiectasis in end-stage pulmonary fibrosis. *Radiology* 1986;161:665–669.

66. Primack SL, Müller NL, Mayo JR, Remy-Jardin M, Remy J. Pulmonary parenchymal abnormalities of vascular origin: high-resolution CT findings. *RadioGraphics* 1994;14:739–746.

67. Murdoch J, Müller NL. Pulmonary sarcoidosis: changes on follow-up CT examinations. *AJR Am J Roentgenol* 1992;159:473–477.

68. Murch CR, Carr DH. Computed tomography appearances of pulmonary alveolar proteinosis. *Clin Radiol* 1989;40:240–243.

69. Godwin JD, Müller NL, Takasugi JE. Pulmonary alveolar proteinosis: CT findings. *Radiology* 1988;169:609–613.

70. Graham CM, Stern EJ, Finkbeiner WE, Webb WR. High-resolution CT appearance of diffuse alveolar septal amyloidosis. *AJR Am J Roentgenol* 1992;158:265–267.

71. Hartman TE, Primack SL, Müller NL, Staples CA. Diagnosis of thoracic complications of AIDS: accuracy of CT. *AJR Am J Roentgenol* 1994;162:547–553.

72. Ren H, Hruban RH, Kuhlman JE, et al. Computed tomography of inflation-fixed lungs: the beaded septum sign of pulmonary metastases. *J Comput Assist Tomogr* 1989;13:411–416.

73. Müller NL, Mawson JB, Mathieson JR, et al. Sarcoidosis: correlation of extent of disease at CT with clinical, functional, and radiographic findings. *Radiology* 1989;171:613–618.

74. Lynch DA, Webb WR, Gamsu G, Stulbarg M, Golden J. Computed tomography in pulmonary sarcoidosis. *J Comput Assist Tomogr* 1989;13:405–410.

75. Remy-Jardin M, Degreef JM, Beuscart R, Voisin C, Remy J. Coal worker's pneumoconiosis: CT assessment in exposed workers and correlation with radiographic findings. *Radiology* 1990;177:363–371.

76. Remy-Jardin M, Beuscart R, Sault MC, Marquette CH, Remy J. Subpleural micronodules in diffuse infiltrative lung diseases: evaluation with thin-section CT scans. *Radiology* 1990;177:133–139.

77. Akira M, Yamamoto S, Yokoyama K, et al. Asbestosis: high-resolution CT-pathologic correlation. *Radiology* 1990;176:389–394.

78. Primack SL, Hartman TE, Hansell DM, Müller NL. End-stage lung disease: CT findings in 61 patients. *Radiology* 1993;189:681–686.

79. Müller NL, Miller RR, Webb WR, Evans KG, Ostrow DN. Fibrosing alveolitis: CT-pathologic correlation. *Radiology* 1986;160:585–588.

80. Adler BD, Padley SP, Müller NL, Remy-Jardin M, Remy J. Chronic hypersensitivity pneumonitis: high-resolution CT and radiographic features in 16 patients. *Radiology* 1992;185:91–95.

81. Lynch DA, Newell JD, Logan PM, King TE, Jr., Müller NL. Can CT distinguish hypersensitivity pneumonitis from idiopathic pulmonary fibrosis? *AJR Am J Roentgenol* 1995;165:807–811.

82. Remy-Jardin M, Remy J, Wallaert B, Bataille D, Hatron PY. Pulmonary involvement in progressive systemic sclerosis: sequential evaluation with CT, pulmonary function tests, and bronchoalveolar lavage. *Radiology* 1993;188:499–506.

83. Müller NL, Chiles C, Kullnig P. Pulmonary lymphangiomyomatosis: correlation of CT with radiographic and functional findings. *Radiology* 1990;175:335–339.

84. Lenoir S, Grenier P, Brauner MW, et al. Pulmonary lymphangiomyomatosis and tuberous sclerosis: comparison of radiographic and thin-section CT findings. *Radiology* 1990;175:329–334.

85. Moore AD, Godwin JD, Müller NL, et al. Pulmonary histiocytosis X: comparison of radiographic and CT findings. *Radiology* 1989;172:249–254.

86. Brauner MW, Grenier P, Mouelhi MM, Mompoint D, Lenoir S. Pulmonary histiocytosis X: evaluation with high resolution CT. *Radiology* 1989;172:255–258.

87. Brauner MW, Grenier P, Tijani K, Battesti JP, Valeyre D. Pulmonary Langerhans cell histiocytosis: evolution of lesions on CT scans. *Radiology* 1997;204:497–502.

88. Naidich DP, Zerhouni EA, Hutchins GM, et al. Computed tomography of the pulmonary parenchyma: part 1. distal air-space disease. *J Thorac Imaging* 1985;1:39–53.

89. Akira M, Kita N, Higashihara T, Sakatani M, Kozuka T. Summer-

type hypersensitivity pneumonitis: comparison of high-resolution CT and plain radiographic findings. *AJR Am J Roentgenol* 1992;158: 1223–1228.

90. Lee KS, Kim YH, Kim WS, et al. Endobronchial tuberculosis: CT features. *J Comput Assist Tomogr* 1991;15:424–428.

91. Nishimura K, Kitaichi M, Izumi T, Itoh H. Diffuse panbronchiolitis: correlation of high-resolution CT and pathologic findings. *Radiology* 1992;184:779–785.

92. Remy-Jardin M, Remy J, Gosselin B, Becette V, Edme JL. Lung parenchymal changes secondary to cigarette smoking: pathologic-CT correlations. *Radiology* 1993;186:643–651.

93. Müller NL, Staples CA, Miller RR. Bronchiolitis obliterans organizing pneumonia: CT features in 14 patients. *AJR* 1990;154:983–987.

94. Im JG, Itoh H, Shim YS, et al. Pulmonary tuberculosis: CT findings early active disease and sequential change with antituberculous therapy. *Radiology* 1993;186:653–660.

95. Oh Y-W, Kim YH, Lee NJ, et al. High-resolution CT appearance of miliary tuberculosis. *J Comput Assist Tomogr* 1994;18:862–866.

96. McGuinness G, Naidich DP, Jagirdar J, Leitman B, McCauley DI. High resolution CT findings in miliary lung disease. *J Comput Assist Tomogr* 1992;16:384–390.

97. Murata K, Takahashi M, Mori M, et al. Pulmonary metastatic nodules: CT-pathologic correlation. *Radiology* 1992;182:331–335.

98. Bégin R, Ostiguy G, Fillion R, Colman N. Computed tomography scan in the early detection of silicosis. *Am Rev Respir Dis* 1991;3:1.

99. Grenier P, Valeyre D, Cluzel P, et al. Chronic diffuse interstitial lung disease: diagnostic value of chest radiography and high-resolution CT. *Radiology* 1991;179:123–132.

100. Padley SPG, Adler BD, Staples CA, Miller RR, Müller NL. Pulmonary talcosis: CT findings in three cases. *Radiology* 1993;186: 125–127.

101. Kuhlman JE, Fishman EK, Teiger C. Pulmonary septic emboli: diagnosis with CT. *Radiology* 1990;174:211–213.

102. Weir IH, Müller NL, Chiles C, et al. Wegener's granulomatosis: findings from computed tomography of the chest in 10 patients. *Can Assoc Radiol J* 1992;43:31–34.

103. Papiris SP, Manoussakis MN, Drosos AA, et al. Imaging of thoracic Wegener's granulomatosis: the computed tomographic appearance. *Am J Med* 1992;93:529–536.

104. Kuhlman JE, Fishman EK, Burch PA, et al. CT of invasive pulmonary aspergillosis. *AJR Am J Roentgenol* 1988;150:1015–1020.

105. Primack SL, Hartman TE, Lee KS, Müller NL. Pulmonary nodules and the CT halo sign. *Radiology* 1994;190:513–515.

106. Dodd GD, Ledesma-Medina J, Baron RL, Fuhrman CR. Post-transplant lymphoproliferataive disorder: intrathoracic manifestations. *Radiology* 1992;184:65–69.

107. Carignan S, Staples CA, Müller NL. Intrathoracic lymphoproliferative disorders in the immunocompromised patient: CT findings. *Radiology* 1995;197:53–58.

108. Austin JHM, Müller NL, Friedman PJ, et al. Glossary of terms for CT of the lungs: recommendations of the Nomenclature Committee of the Fleischner Society. *Radiology* 1996;200:327–331.

109. Remy-Jardin M, Remy J, Giraud F, Wattinne L, Gosselin B. Computed tomography assessment of ground-glass opacity: semiology and significance. *J Thorac Imag* 1993;8:249–264.

110. Leung AN, Miller RR, Müller NL. Parenchymal opacification in chronic infiltrative lung diseases: CT-pathologic correlation. *Radiology* 1993;188:209–214.

111. Wells AU, Hansell DM, Rubens MB, et al. The predictive value of appearances of thin-section computed tomography in fibrosing alveolitis. *Am Rev Respir Dis* 1993;148:1076–1082.

112. Remy-Jardin M, Giraud F, Remy J, et al. Importance of ground-glass attenuation in chronic diffuse infiltrative lung disease: pathologic-CT correlation. *Radiology* 1993;189:693–698.

113. Hartman TE, Primack SL, Swensen SJ, et al. Desquamative interstitial pneumonia: thin-section CT findings in 22 patients. *Radiology* 1993; 187:787–790.

114. Bergin CJ, Wirth RL, Berry GJ, Castellino RA. *Pneumocystis carinii* pneumonia: CT and HRCT observations. *J Comput Assist Tomogr* 1990;14:756–759.

115. Brown MJ, Miller RR, Müller NL. Acute lung disease in the immunocompromised host: CT and pathologic examination findings. *Radiology* 1994;190:247–254.

116. Primack SL, Müller NL. High-resolution computed tomography in acute diffuse lung disease in the immunocompromised patient. *Rad Clin N Am* 1994;32:731–744.

117. Primack SL, Hartman TE, Ikezoe J, et al. Acute interstitial pneumonia: radiographic and CT findings in nine patients. *Radiology* 1993;188: 817–820.

118. Lee KS, Kullnig P, Hartman TE, Müller NL. Cryptogenic organizing pneumonia: CT findings in 43 patients. *AJR Am J Roentgenol* 1994; 162:543–546.

119. Greene R. Adult respiratory distress syndrome: acute alveolar damage. *Radiology* 1987;163:57–66.

120. Mayo JR, Müller NL, Road J, Sisler J, Lillington G. Chronic eosinophilic pneumonia: CT findings in six cases. *AJR Am J Roentgenol* 1989;153:727–730.

121. Lee KS, Müller NL, Hale V, Newell JDJ, Lynch DA, Im JG. Lipoid pneumonia: CT findings. *J Comput Assist Tomogr* 1995;19:48–51.

122. Kuhlman JE. The role of chest computed tomography in the diagnosis of drug-related reactions. *J Thorac Imaging* 1991;6(1):52–61.

123. Hartman TE, Müller NL, Primack SL, et al. Metastatic pulmonary calcification in patients with hypercalcemia: findings on chest radiographs and CT scans. *AJR Am J Roentgenol* 1994;162:799–802.

124. Foster WL, Pratt PC, Roggli VL, et al. Centrilobular emphysema: CT-pathologic correlation. *Radiology* 1986;159:27–32.

125. Thurlbeck WM, Müller NL. Emphysema: definition, imaging, and quantification. *AJR Am J Roentgenol* 1994;163:1017–1025.

126. Tuddenham WJ. Glossary of terms for thoracic radiology: recommendations of the Nomenclature Committee of the Fleischner Society. *AJR Am J Roentgenol* 1984;143:509–517.

127. Bergin CJ, Müller NL, Miller RR. CT in the qualitative assessment of emphysema. *J Thorac Imaging* 1986;1:94–103.

128. Spouge D, Mayo JR, Cardoso W, Müller NL. Panacinar emphysema: CT and pathologic correlation. *J Comput Assist Tomogr* 1993;17: 710–713.

129. King MA, Bergin CJ, Yeung DWC, et al. Chronic pulmonary thromboembolism: detection of regional hypoperfusion with CT. *Radiology* 1994;191:359–363.

130. Schwickert HC, Schweden F, Schild HH, et al. Pulmonary arteries and lung parenchyma in chronic pulmonary embolism: preoperative and postoperative CT findings. *Radiology* 1994;351–357.

131. Grenier P, Cordeau MP, Beigelman C. High-resolution computed tomography of the airways. *J Thorac Imag* 1993;8:213–229.

132. Marti-Bonmati L, Ruiz PF, Catala F, Mata JM, Calonge E. CT findings in Swyer-James syndrome. *Radiology* 1989;172:477–480.

133. Stern EJ, Swensen SJ, Hartman TE, Frank MS. Pictorial essay. CT mosaic pattern of lung attenuation: Distinguishing different causes. *Am J Roentgenol* 1995;165:813–816.

134. Worthy SA, Müller NL, Hartman TE, et al. Mosaic attenuation pattern on thin-section CT: differentiation between infiltrative lung, airway and vascular diseases as a cause. *Radiology* 1997;205:465–470.

135. Müller NL, Miller RR. Diseases of the bronchioles: CT and histopathologic findings. *Radiology* 1995;196:3–12.

136. Carrington CB, Gaensler EA. Clinical-pathologic approach to diffuse infiltrative lung disease. *Monogr Pathol* 1978;19:58–87.

137. Corrin B. *Pathology of interstitial lung disease.* Harasawa M, Fukuchi Y, Morinari H, eds. Tokyo: University of Tokyo Press, 1989.

138. Coultas DB, Zumwalt RE, Black WC, Sobonya RE. The epidemiology of interstitial lung diseases. *Am J Respir Crit Care Med* 1994;150: 967–972.

139. Katzenstein A-L, Myers J. Idiopathic pulmonary fibrosis. Clinical relevance of pathologic classification. *Am J Resp Crit Care Med* 1998; 157:1301–1315.

140. Liebow AA. Definition and classification of interstitial pneumonias in human pathology. *Prog Respir Res* 1975;8:1–31.

141. Colby TV, Carrington CB. *Interstitial lung disease.* Thurlbeck WM, Churg AM, eds. New York: Thieme, 1995.

142. Katzenstein ALA, Fiorelli RF. Nonspecific interstitial pneumonia/fibrosis. *Am J Surg Pathol* 1994;18:136–147.

143. Panos RJ, Mortenson RL, Niccoli SA, King TE. Clinical deterioration in patients with idiopathic pulmonary fibrosis: causes and assessment. *Am J Med* 1990;88:396–404.

144. Cherniak RM, Crystal RG, Kalica AR. Current concepts in idiopathic pulmonary fibrosis: a road map for the future. *Am Rev Resp Dis* 1991; 143:680–683.

145. Crystal RG, Fulmer JD, Roberts WC, et al. Idiopathic pulmonary fibrosis: clinical, histologic, radiographic, physiologic, scintigraphic, cytologic, and biochemical aspects. *Ann Intern Med* 1976;85: 769–788.

146. Gelb AF, Dreisen RB, Epstein JD, et al. Immune complexes, gallium lung scans, and bronchoalveolar lavage in idiopathic interstital pneumonitis-fibrosis: a structure-function clinical study. *Chest* 1983;84: 148–153.

147. Tukiainen P, Taskinen E, Holsti P, Korhola O, Valle M. Prognosis of cryptogenic fibrosing alveolitis. *Thorax* 1983;38:349–355.

148. Turner-Warwick M, Burrows B, Johnson A. Cryptogenic fibrosing alveolitis: clinical features and their influence on survival. *Thorax* 1980;35:171–180.

149. Lee JS, Im JG, Ahn JM, Kim YM, Han MC. Fibrosing alveolitis: prognostic implication of ground-glass attenuation at high-resolution CT. *Radiology* 1992;184:415–454.

150. Bergin C, Castellino RA. Mediastinal lymph node enlargement on CT scans in patients with usual interstitial pneumonitis. *Am J Roentgenol* 1990;154:251–254.

151. Niimi H, Kang EY, Kwong JS, Carignan S, Müller NL. Chronic infiltrative lung disease: prevalence of mediastinal lymphadenopathy. *J Comput Assist Tomog* 1996;20:305–308.

152. Müller NL, Staples CA, Miller RR, et al. Disease activity in idiopathic pulmonary fibrosis: CT and pathologic correlation. *Radiology* 1987; 165:731–734.

153. Terriff BA, Kwan SY, Chan-Yeung MM, Müller NL. Fibrosing alveolitis: chest radiography and CT as predictors of clinical and functional impairment at follow-up in 26 patients. *Radiology* 1992;184:445–449.

154. Akira M, Sakatani M, Ueda E. Idiopathic pulmonary fibrosis: progression of honeycombing at thin-section CT. *Radiology* 1993;189: 687–691.

154a.Hartman TE, Primack SL, Kang EY, et al. Disease progression in usual interstitial pneumonia compared with desquamative interstitial pneumonia. *Chest* 1996;110:378–382.

155. Thurlbeck WM, Miller RR, Müller NL, Rosenow ECI. *Diffuse diseases of the lung: a team approach.* Philadelphia: Decker, 1991.

156. Liebow AA, Steer A, Billingsley JG. Desquamative interstitial pneumonia. *Am J Med* 1965;38:369–404.

157. Carrington CB, Gaensler EA, Coute RE, Fitzgerald MS, Gupta RG. Natural history and treated course of usual and desquamative interstitial pneumonia. *N Engl J Med* 1978;298:801–809.

158. Staples CA, Müller NL, Vedal S, et al. Usual interstitial pneumonia: correlation of CT with clinical, functional, and radiologic findings. *Radiology* 1987;162:377–381.

159. Katzenstein ALA, Myers JL, Mazur MT. Acute interstitial pneumonia: a clinicopathologic, ultrastructural, and cell kinetic study. *Am J Surg Pathol* 1986;10:256–267.

160. Katzenstein A-L. Katzenstein and Askin's surgical pathology of nonneoplastic lung disease. In: Livolsi VA, ed. *Major problems in pathology,* vol 3. Philadelphia: WB Saunders, 1997.

161. Müller NL, Colby TV. Idiopathic interstitial pneumonias: high-resolution CT and histologic findings. *RadioGraphics* 1997;17:1016–1022.

162. Mcadams HP, Rosadodechristenson ML, Wehunt WD, Fishback NF. The alphabet soup revisited: the chronic interstitial pneumonias in the 1990s. *RadioGraphics* 1996;16:1009–1033.

163. Park JS, Lee KS, Kim JS, et al. Nonspecific interstitial pneumonia with fibrosis: radiographic and CT findings in seven patients. *Radiology* 1995;195:645–648.

164. Schurawitzki H, Stiglbauer R, Graninger W, et al. Interstitial lung disease in progressive systemic sclerosis: high-resolution CT versus radiography. *Radiology* 1990;176:755–759.

165. Bhalla M, Silver RM, Shepard JO, McLoud TC. Chest CT in patients with scleroderma: prevalence of asymptomatic esophageal dilatation and mediastinal lymphadenopathy. *AJR Am J Roentgenol* 1993;161: 269–272.

166. Wells AU, Hansell DM, Corrin B, et al. High resolution computed tomography as a predictor of lung histology in systemic sclerosis. *Thorax* 1992;47:508–512.

167. Jurik AG, Davidsen D, Graudal H. Prevalence of pulmonary involvement in rheumatoid arthritis and its relationship to some characteristics of the patients—a radiological and clinical study. *Scand J Rheumatol* 1982;11:217–224.

168. Remy-Jardin M, Remy J, Cortet B, Mauri F, Delcambre B. Lung changes in rheumatoid arthritis: CT findings. *Radiology* 1994;193: 375–382.

169. Fujii M, Adachi S, Shimizu T, et al. Interstitial lung disease in rheumatoid arthritis: assessment with high-resolution computed tomography. *J Thorac Imag* 1993;8:54–62.

170. Craighead JE. The pathology of asbestos-associated disease of the lungs and pleural cavities: diagnostic criteria and proposed grading schema. Report of the Pneumoconiosis Committee of the College of Amerian Pathologists and the National Institute for Occupational Safety and Health. *Arch Pathol Lab Med* 1982;106:544–596.

171. Churg A, Green FH. *Occupational lung disease.* Thurlbeck WM, Churg AM, eds. New York: Thieme, 1995.

172. Becklake MR, Case BW. Fiber burden and asbestos-related lung disease: determinants of dose-response relationships. *Am J Respir Crit Care Med* 1994;150:1488–1492.

173. Crystal RG, Gadek JE, Ferrans VJ, et al. Interstitial lung disease: current concepts of pathogenesis, staging and therapy. *Am J Med* 1981; 70:542–568.

174. Smith DD. What is asbestosis? *Chest* 1990;98:963,964.

175. American Thoracic Society. The diagnosis of non-malignant diseases related to asbestos. *Am Rev Respir Dis* 1986;134:363–368.

176. Epstein DM, Miller WT, Bresnitz EA, Levine MS, Gefter WB. Application of ILO classification to a population without industrial exposure: findings to be differentiated from pneumoconiosis. *AJR Am J Roentgenol* 1984;142:53–58.

177. Gaensler EA, Carrington CB, Coutu RE. Pathologic, phsyiologic, and radiologic correlations in the pneumoconioses. *Ann NY Acad Sci* 1972; 200:574–607.

178. Kipen HM, Lilis R, Suzuki Y, Valciukas JA, Selikoff IJ. Pulmonary fibrosis in asbestos insulation workers with lung cancer: a radiological and histopathological evaluation. *Br J Indust Med* 1987;44:96–100.

179. Rockoff SD, Schwartz A. Roentgenographic underestimation of early asbestosis by International Labor Organization classification: analysis of data and probabilities. *Chest* 1988;93:1088–1091.

180. Ducatman AM, Yang WN, Forman AS. 'B-readers' and asbestos medical surveillance. *J Occup Med* 1988;30:644–647.

181. Weill H. Diagnosis of asbestos-related disease. *Chest* 1987;91: 802–803.

182. Kreel L. Computed tomography in the evaluation of pulmonary asbestosis: preliminary experience with the EMI general purpose scanner. *Act Radiol Diagn (Stock)* 1976;17:405–412.

183. Katz D, Kreel L. Computed tomography in pulmonary asbestosis. *Clin Radiol* 1979;30:207–213.

184. Bégin R, Boctor M, Bergeron D. Radiographic assessment of pleuropulmonary disease in asbestos workers: posteroanterior, four view films, and computed tomograms of the thorax. *Br J Ind Med* 1984; 41:373–383.

185. Friedman AC, Fiel SB, Fisher MS, et al. Asbestos-related pleural disease and asbestosis: a comparison of CT and chest radiography. *AJR Am J Roentgenol* 1988;150:268–275.

186. Slozewizc S, Reznek RH, Herdman M. Role of computed tomography in evaluating asbestos related lung disease. *Br J Ind Med* 1989;46: 777–781.

187. Sluis-Cremer GK, Hnizdo E. Progression of irregular opacities in asbestos miners. *Br J Ind Med* 1989;46:846–852.

188. Lynch DA, Gamsu G, Aberle DR. Conventional and high resolution computed tomography in the diagnosis of asbestos related diseases. *RadioGraphics* 1989;9:523–551.

189. Murata K, Khan A, Herman PG. Pulmonary parenchymal disease: evaluation with high-resolution CT. *Radiology* 1989;170:629–635.

190. Gamsu G, Aberle DR, Lynch D. Computed tomography in the diagnosis of asbestos-related thoracic disease. *J Thorac Imaging* 1989;4: 61–67.

191. Staples CA, Gamsu G, Ray CS, Webb WR. High resolution computed tomography and lung function in asbestos-exposed workers with normal chest radiographs. *Am Rev Respir Dis* 1989;139:1502–1508.

192. Akira M, Yokoyama K, Yamamoto S, et al. Early asbestosis: evaluation with high-resolution CT. *Radiology* 1991;178:409–416.

193. Murray KA, Gamsu G, Webb WR, Salmon CJ, Egger MJ. Highresolution computed tomography sampling for detection of asbestosrelated lung disease. *Acad Radiol* 1995;2:111–115.

194. Gamsu G, Salmon CJ, Warnock ML, Blanc PD. CT quantification of interstitial fibrosis in patients with asbestosis: a comparison of two methods. *AJR Am J Roentgenol* 1995;164:63–68.

195. Yoshimura H, Hatakeyama M, Otsuji H, et al. Pulmonary asbestosis: CT study of subpleural curvilinear shadow. Work in progress. *Radiology* 1986;158:653–658.

196. Friedman AC, Fiel SB, Radecki PD, Lev-Toaff AS. Computed tomography of benign pleural and pulmonary parenchymal abnormalities related to asbestos exposure. *Semin Ultrasound, CT and MR* 1990; 11:393–408.

197. Bergin CJ, Castellino RA, Blank N, Moses L. Specificity of high-resolution CT findings in pulmonary asbestosis: do patients scanned for other indications have similar findings? *AJR Am J Roentgenol* 1994;163:551–555.

198. Al Jarad N, Strickland B, Pearson MC, Rubens MB, Rudd RM. High-resolution computed tomographic assessment of asbestosis and cryptogenic fibrosing alveolitis: a comparative study. *Thorax* 1992;47:645–650.

199. McLoud TC. The use of CT in the examination of asbestos-exposed persons (editorial). *Radiology* 1988;169:862,863.

200. Gamsu G. High resolution CT in the diagnosis of asbestos-related pleuroparenchymal disease. *Am J Ind Med* 1989;16:115–117.

201. Heitzman ER. *The lung: radiologic-pathologic correlations*. 2nd ed. St. Louis: Mosby, 1984.

202. Janower ML, Blennerhasset JB. Lymphangitic spread of metastatic tumor to lung. *Radiology* 1971;101:267–273.

203. Trapnell DH. The radiological appearance of lymphangitic carcinomatosis of the lung. *Thorax* 1964;19:251–260.

204. Goldsmith HS, Bailey HD, Callahan EL, Beattie ESJ. Pulmonary metastases from breast carcinoma. *Arch Surg* 1967;94:483–488.

205. Crow J, Slavin G, Kreel L. Pulmonary metastasis: a pathologic and radiologic study. *Cancer* 1981;47:2595–2602.

206. Johkoh T, Ikezoe J, Tomiyama N, et al. CT findings in lymphangitic carcinomatosis of the lung: correlation with histologic findings and pulmonary function tests. *AJR Am J Roentgenol* 1992;158:1217–1222.

207. Lacronique J, Roth C, Battesti JP, Basset F, Chretien J. Chest radiological features of pulmonary histiocytosis X: a report based on 50 adult cases. *Thorax* 1982;37:104–109.

208. Friedman PJ, Liebow AA, Sokoloff J. Eosinophilic granuloma of lung: clinical aspects of primary pulmonary histiocytosis in the adult. *Medicine* 1981;60:385–396.

209. Siegelman SS. Taking the X out of Histiocytosis X. *Radiology* 1997;204:322–324.

210. Eliasson AH, Phillips YY, Tenholder MF. Treatment of lymphangioleiomyomatosis. A meta-analysis. *Chest* 1989;196:1342–1355.

211. Berger JL, Shaff MI. Case Report. Pulmonary lymphangioleiomyomatosis. *J Comput Assist Tomogr* 1981;5:565–567.

212. Merchant RN, Pearson MG, Rankin RN, Morgan WKC. Computerized tomography in the diagnosis of lymphangioleiomyomatosis. *Am Rev Respir Dis* 1985;131:295–297.

213. Templeton PA, McLoud TC, Müller NL, Shepard JA, Moore EH. Pulmonary lymphangioleiomyomatosis: CT and pathologic findings. *J Comput Assist Tomogr* 1989;13:54–57.

214. Rappaport DC, Weisbrod GL, Herman SJ, Chamberlain DW. Pulmonary lymphangioleiomyomatosis: high-resolution CT findings in four cases. *AJR Am J Roentgenol* 1989;152:961–964.

215. Sherrier RH, Chiles C, Roggli V. Pulmonary lymphangioleiomyomatosis: CT findings. *AJR Am J Roentgenol* 1989;153:937–940.

216. Aberle DR, Hansell DM, Brown K, Tashkin DP. Lymphangiomyomatosis: CT, chest radiographic, and functional correlations. *Radiology* 1990;176:381–387.

217. Fraser RS, Pare JAP, Fraser RG, Pare PDE, eds. *Synopsis of diseases of the chest*. Philadelphia: W. Saunders, 1994.

218. Pimentel JC. Three-dimensional photographic reconstruction in a study of the pathogenesis of honeycomb lung. *Thorax* 1967;22:444–452.

219. Genereux GP. The end-stage lung: pathogenesis, pathology, and radiology. *Radiology* 1975;116:279–289.

220. Fraser RG, Pare JAP, Pare PD, Fraser RS, Genereux GP. *Diagnosis of diseases of the chest*. 3rd ed. Philadelphia, PA.: Saunders, 1988.

221. Crystal RG, Bitterman PB, Rennard SI, Hance AJ, Keogh BA. Interstitial lung diseases of unknown cause: disorders characterized by chronic inflammation of the lower respiratory tract. *N Engl J Med* 1984;310:154–166.

222. McLoud TC, Epler GR, Gaensler EA, Burke GW, Carrington CB. A radiographic classification for sarcoidosis: physiologic correlation. *Invest Radiol* 1982;17:129–138.

223. Scadding JG, Mitchell DN, eds. *Sarcoidosis*. London: Chapman and Hall, 1985.

224. Hillerdal G, Neu E, Osterman K, Schmekel B. Sarcoidosis: epidemiology and prognosis, a 15-year European study. *Am Rev Respir Dis* 1984;130:29–32.

225. Rockoff SD, Rohatgi PK. Unusual manifestations of thoracic sarcooidosis. *AJR Am J Roentgenol* 1985;144:513–528.

226. Nishimura K, Itoh H, Kitaichi M, Nagai S, Izumi T. Pulmonary sar-coidosis: correlation of CT and histopathologic findings. *Radiology* 1993;189:105–109.

227. Bergin CJ, Bell DY, Coblentz CL, et al. Sarcoidosis: correlation of pulmonary parenchymal pattern at CT with results of pulmonary function tests. *Radiology* 1989;171:619–624.

228. Müller NL, Miller RR. Ground-glass attenuation, nodules, alveolitis, and sarcoid granulomas (editorial). *Radiology* 1993;189:31–32.

229. Sider L, Horton ESJ. Hilar and mediastinal adenopathy in sarcoidosis as detected by computed tomography. *J Thorac Imag* 1990;5:77–80.

230. Hamper UM, Fishman EK, Khouri NF, et al. Typical and atypical CT manifestations of pulmonary sarcoidosis. *J Comput Assist Tomogr* 1986;10:928–936.

231. Bergin C, Roggli V, Coblentz C, Chiles C. The secondary pulmonary lobule: normal and abnormal CT appearances. *AJR Am J Roentgenol* 1988;151:21–25.

232. Fraser RG, Pare JAP, Pare PD, Fraser RS, Genereux GP. Pleuropulmonary disease caused by inhalation of inorganic dust (pneumoconiosis). In: *Diagnosis of diseases of the chest*. Philadelphia: W. B. Saunders, 1990:2276–2381.

233. Sargent EN, et al. Coal workers' pneumoconiosis. In: Preger L, ed. *Induced disease. Drug, irradiation, occupation*. New York: Grune & Stratton, 1980:275–295.

234. Sargent EN, et al. Silicosis. In: Preger L, ed. *Induced disease. Drug, irradiation, occupation*. New York: Grune & Stratton, 1980:297–315.

235. Bergin CJ, Müller NL, Vedal S, Chan Yeung M. CT in silicosis: correlation with plain films and pulmonary function tests. *AJR Am J Roentgenol* 1986;146:477–483.

236. Bégin R, Bergeron D, Samson L, Boctor M, Cantin A. CT assessment of silicosis in exposed workers. *AJR Am J Roentgenol* 1987;148:509–514.

237. Bégin R, Ostiguy G, Groleau S, Filion R. Computed tomographic scanning of the thorax in workers at risk of or with silicosis. *Semin Ultrasound CT MR* 1990;11:380–392.

238. Davis SD. CT evaluation for pulmonary metastases in patients with extrathoracic malignancy. *Radiology* 1991;180:1–12.

239. Buckley JA, Scott WW, Siegelman SS, et al. Pulmonary nodules: effect of increased data sampling on detection with spiral CT and confidence in diagnosis. *Radiology* 1995;196:395–400.

240. Chryssanthopoulos C, Fink JN. Hypersensitivity pneumonitis. *J Asthma* 1983;20:285–296.

241. Colby TV, Swensen SJ. Anatomic distribution and histopathologic patterns in diffuse lung disease: correlation with HRCT. *J Thorac Imag* 1996;11:1–26.

242. Fraser RG, Paré JAP, Paré PD, Fraser RS, Genereux GP. *Diseases of altered immunologic activity. Diagnosis of diseases of the chest*. Philadelphia:WB Saunders, 1989:1177–1326.

243. Cook PG, Wells IP, McGavin CR. The distribution of pulmonary shadowing in farmer's lung. *Clin Radiol* 1988;39:21–27.

244. Hapke EJ, Seal RME, Thomas GO, Hayes M, Meek JC. Farmer's lung: a clinical, radiographic, functional and serologic correlation of acute and chronic stages. *Thorax* 1968;23:451–468.

245. Silver SF, Müller NL, Miller RR, Lefcoe MS. Hypersensitivity pneumonitis: evaluation with CT. *Radiology* 1989;173:441–445.

246. Hansell DM, Moskovic E. High-resolution computed tomography in extrinsic allergic alveolitis. *Clin Radiol* 1991;43:8–12.

247. Buschman DL, Gamsu G, Waldron JA, Klein JS, King TE. Chronic hypersensitivity pneumonitis: use of CT in diagnosis. *AJR* 1992;159:957–960.

248. Hansell DM, Wells AU, Padley SPG, Müller NL. Hypersensitivity pneumonitis: correlation of individual CT patterns with functional abnormalities. *Radiology* 1996;199:123–128.

249. Genereux GP. The Fleischner lecture: computed tomography of diffuse pulmonary disease. *J Thorac Imaging* 1989;4:50–87.

250. Rosen SH, Castleman B, Liebow AA. Pulmonary alveolar proteinosis. *N Engl J Med* 1958;258:1123–1144.

251. Prakash UBS, Barham SS, Carpenter HA, Dines DE, Marsh HM. Pulmonary alveolar phospholipoproteinosis: experience with 34 cases and a review. *Mayo Clin Proc* 1987;62:499–518.

252. Carrington CB, Addington WW, Goff AM. Chronic eosinohilic pneumonia. *N Engl J Med* 1969;289:787–798.

253. Jederlinic PJ, Sicilian L, Gaensler EA. Chronic eosinophilic pneumonia: a report of 19 cases and a review of the literature. *Medicine* 1988;67:154–162.

254. Gaensler EA, Carrington CB. Peripheral opacities in chronic eosinophilic pneumonia: the photographic negative of pulmonary edema. *AJR Am J Roentgenol* 1977;128:1–13.

255. Ebara H, Ikezoe J, Johkoh T, et al. Chronic eosinophilic pneumonia: evolution of chest radiograms and CT features. *J Comput Assist Tomogr* 1994;18:737–744.

256. Glazer HS, Levitt RG, Shackelford GD. Peripheral pulmonary infiltrates in sarcoidosis. *Chest* 1984;86:741–744.

257. Wright JL, ed. *Consequences of aspiration and bronchial obstruction.* Thurlbeck WM, Churg AM, ed. New York: Thieme Medical Publishers, 1995.

258. Schwindt WD, Barbee RA, Jones RJ. Lipoid pneumonia. Its protean nature and clinical resemblance to carcinomas of the lung. *Arch Surg* 1967;95:652–657.

259. Kennedy JD, Costello P, Balikian JP, Herman PG. Exogeneous lipoid pneumonia. *AJR Am J Roentgenol* 1981;136:1145–1149.

260. Wheeler PS, Stitik FP, Hutchins GM, Klinefelter HF, Siegelman SS. Diagnosis of lipoid pneumonia by computed tomography. *JAMA* 1981;235:65–66.

261. Joshi RR, Cholankeril JV. Computed tomography in lipoid pneumonia. *J Comput Assist Tomogr* 1985;9:211–213.

262. Snyder LS, Hertz MI. Cytotoxic drug-induced lung injury. *Semin Respir Infect* 1988;3:217–228.

263. Cooper JAD, Matthay RA. Drug induced pulmonary disease. *Disease-a-Month* 1987;33:61–120.

264. Cooper JA, White DA, Matthay RA. Drug induced pulmonary disease: Part 1. Cytoxic drugs. *Am Rev Respir Dis* 1986;133:321–340.

265. Padley SPG, Adler B, Hansell DM, Müller NL. High-resolution computed tomography of drug-induced lung disease. *Clin Radiol* 1992;46:232–236.

266. Aronchick JM, Gefter WB. Drug-induced pulmonary disorders. *Semin Roentgenol* 1995;30:18–34.

267. Rimmer MJ, Dixon AK, Flower CD, Sikora K. Bleomycin lung: computed tomographic observations. *Br J Radiol* 1985;58:1041–1045.

268. Bellamy EA, Husband JE, Blaquiere RM, Law MR. Bleomycin-related lung damage: CT evidence. *Radiology* 1985;156:155–158.

269. American Thoracic Society. Chronic bronchitis, asthma, and pulmonary emphysema: statement by the Committee on Diagnostic Standards for Nontuberculous Respiratory Diseases. *Am Rev Resp Dis* 1962;85:762–768.

270. Snider GL, Kleinerman J, Thurlbeck WM, Bengali ZH. The definition of emphysema. Report of a National Heart, Lung, and Blood Institute, Division of Lung Diseases Workshop. *Am Rev Resp Dis* 1985;132:182–185.

271. Thurlbeck WM, Simon G. Radiographic appearance of the chest in emphysema. *AJR Am J Roentgenol* 1978;130:429–440.

272. Sutinen S, Christoforidis AJ, Klugh GA, Pratt PC. Roentgenologic criteria for the recognition of nonsymptomatic pulmonary emphysema: correlation between roentgenologic findings and pulmonary pathology. *Am Rev Resp Dis* 1965;91:69–76.

273. Nicklaus TM, Stowell DW, Christiansen WR, Renzetti ADJ. The accuracy of the roentgenologic diagnosis of chronic pulmonary emphysema. *Am Rev Resp Dis* 1966;93:889–900.

274. Pratt PC. Role of conventional chest radiography in diagnosis and exclusion of emphysema. *Am J Med* 1987;82:998–1006.

275. Miniati M, Filippi E, Falaschi F, et al. Radiologic evaluation of emphysema in patients with chronic obstructing pulmonary disease: chest radiography versus high resolution computed tomography. *Am J Respir Crit Care Med* 1995;151:1359–1367.

276. Hayhurst MD, MacNee W, Flenley DC, al et. Diagnosis of pulmonary emphysema by computerised tomography. *Lancet* 1984;2:320–322.

277. Bergin CJ, Müller NL, Nichols DM, al et. The diagnosis of emphysema: a computed tomographic-pathologic correlation. *Am Rev Respir Dis* 1986;133:541–546.

278. Hruban RH, Ren H, Kuhlman JE, et al. Inflation-fixed lungs: pathologic-radiologic (CT) correlation of lung transplantation. *J Comput Assist Tomogr* 1990;14:329–335.

279. Miller RR, Müller NL, Vedal S, Morrison NJ, Staples CA. Limitations of computed tomography in the assessment of emphysema. *Am Rev Respir Dis* 1989;139:980–983.

280. Kuwano K, Matsuba K, Ikeda T, et al. The diagnosis of mild emphysema: correlation of computed tomography and pathology scores. *Am Rev Respir Dis* 1990;141:169–178.

281. Müller NL, Staples CA, Miller RR, Abboud RT. Density mask: an objective method to quantitate emphysema using computed tomography. *Chest* 1988;94:782–787.

282. Morgan MDL, Strickland B. Computed tomography in the assessment of bullous lung disease. *Br J Dis Chest* 1984;78:10–25.

283. Gaensler EA, Jederlinic PJ, FitzGerald MX. Patient work-up for bullectomy. *J Thorac Imag* 1986;13:75–93.

284. Kazerooni EA, Whyte RI, Flint A, Martinez FJ. Imaging of emphysema and lung volume reduction surgery. *RadioGraphics* 1997;17:1023–1036.

285. Cooper JD, Trulock EP, Triantafillou AN, et al. Bilateral pneumectomy (volume reduction) for chronic obstructive pulmonary disease. *J Thorac Cardiovasc Surg* 1995;109:106–119.

286. Brenner M, Yusen R, McKenna RJ, et al. Lung volume reduction surgery for emphysema. *Chest* 1996;110:205–218.

287. Slone R, Gierada D. Radiology of pulmonary emphysema and lung reduction surgery. *Semin Thor Cardiovasc Surg* 1996;8:61–82.

288. Holbert JM, Brown ML, Sciurba FC, et al. Changes in lung volume and volume of emphysema after unilateral lung reduction surgery: analysis with CT lung densitometry. *Radiology* 1996;201:793–797.

289. Bae KT, Slone RM, Gierada DS, Yusem RD, Cooper JD. Patients with emphysema: quantitative CT analysis with CT lung densitometry. *Radiology* 1997;1997:705–714.

290. Klein JS, Gamsu G, Webb WR, Golden JA, Müller NL. High-resolution CT diagnosis of emphysema in symptomatic patients with normal chest radiographs and isolated low diffusing capacity. *Radiology* 1992;182:817–821.

291. Lesur O, Delorme N, Fromaget JM, Bernadac P, Polu JM. Computed tomography in the etiologic assessment of idiopathic spontaneous pneumothorax. *Chest* 1990;98:341–347.

292. Bense L, Lewander R, Eklund G, Hedenstierna G, Wiman LG. Non-smoking, non-alpha-1-antitrypsin deficiency induced emphysema in nonsmokers with healing spontaneous pneumothorax, identified by computed tomography of the lungs. *Chest* 1993;103:433–438.

293. Müller NL, Miller RR. Acute diffuse lung disease. In: Putman CE, ed. *Diagnostic imaging of the lung.* New York: Marcel Dekker, 1990:337–441.

294. Catterall JR, McCabe RE, Brokks RG, Remington JS. Open lung biopsy in patients with Hodgkin's disease and pulmonary infiltrates. *Am Rev Resp Dis* 1989;139:1274–1279.

295. Ramsey PG, Rubin RH, Tolkoff-Rubin NE. The renal transplant patient with fever and pulmonaary infiltrates: etiology, clinical manifestations and management. *Medicine* 1980;59:206–222.

296. Murray JF, Mills J. Pulmonary infectious complications of human immunodeficiency virus infection. *Am Rev Resp Dis* 1990;141:1356–1372.

297. Rosenow EC, Wilson WR, Cockerill FR. Pulmonary disease in the immunocompromised host. *Mayo Clin Proc* 1985;60:473–487.

298. Graham NJ, Müller NL, Miller RR. Intrathoracic complications following allogenic bone marrow transplant: CT findings. *Radiology* 1991;181:153–156.

299. Barloon TJ, Galvin JR, Mori M, Stanford W, Gingrich RD. High-resolution ultrafast chest CT in the clinical management of febrile bone marrow transplant patients with normal or nonspecific chest roentgenograms (see comments). *Chest* 1991;99:928–933.

300. Mori M, Galvin JR, Barloon TJ, Gingrich RD, Stanford W. Fungal pulmonary infections after bone marrow transplantation: evaluation with radiography and CT. *Radiology* 1991;178:721–726.

301. Kang EY, Staples CA, McGuinness G, Primack SL, Müller NL. Thoracic complications in AIDS: comparison of diagnostic accuracy of radiography and thin-section CT. *AJR* 1996.

302. Janzen DL, Padley SPG, Adler BD, Müller NL. Acute pulmonary complications in immunocompromised non-AIDS patients: comparison of diagnostic accuracy of CT and chest radiography. *Clin Radiol* 1993;47:159–165.

303. Worthy SA, Flint JD, Müller NL. Pulmonary complications after bone marrow transplantation: high resolution CT and pathologic findings. *Radiographics* 1997;17:1359–1371.

304. Logan PM, Primack PL, Miller RR, Müller NL. Invasive aspergilosis of the airways: radiographic, CT and pathologic findings. *Radiology* 1994;193:383–388.

305. McGuinness G, Scholes JV, Garay SM, et al. Cytomegalovirus pneumonitis: spectrum of parenchymal CT findings with pathologic correlation in 21 AIDS patients. *Radiology* 1994;192:451–459.

306. Staples CA, Kang EY, Wright JL, Phillips P, Müller NL. Invasive pulmonary aspergillosis in AIDS: Radiographic, CT, and pathologic findings. *Radiology* 1995;196:409–414.

307. Janzen DL, Adler BD, Padley SPG, Müller NL. Diagnostic success of bronchoscopic biopsy in immunocompromised patients with acute pulmonary disease: predictive value of disease distribution as shown on CT. *AJR Am J Roentgenol* 1993;160:21–24.

308. Gruden JF, Klein JS, Webb WR. Percutaneous transthoracic needle biopsy in AIDS: analysis in 32 patients. *Radiology* 1993;189:567–571.

309. Williams DM, Krick JA, Remington JS. Pulmonary infection in the compromised host. *Am Rev Resp Dis* 1976;114:359–394.

310. Limper AH, Offord KP, Smith TF, Martin WJ. *Pneumocystis carinii* pneumonia: differences in lung parasite number and inflammation in patients with and without AIDS. *Am Rev Resp Dis* 1989;140:1204–1209.

311. Jacobs JL, Libby DM, Winters RA, et al. A cluster of *Pneumocystis carinii* pneumonia in adults without predisposing illnesses. *N Engl J Med* 1991;324:246–250.

312. Godeau B, Coutant-Perronne V, Huong DLT. *Pneumocystis carinii* pneumonia in the course of connective tissue disease: report of 34 cases. *J Rheumatol* 1994;21:246–251.

313. Naidich DP, McGuinness G. Pulmonary manifestations of AIDS: CT and radiographic correlations. *Rad Clin N Am* 1991;29:999–1017.

314. Suster B, Ackerman M, Orenstein M, Wax MR. Pulmonary manifestations of AIDS: review of 106 episodes. *Radiology* 1987;161:87–93.

315. DeLorenzo LJ, Huang CT, Maguire GP, Stone DJ. Roentgenographic patterns of *Pneumocystis carinii* pneumonia in 104 patients with AIDS. *Chest* 1987;91:323–327.

316. Milligan SA, Stulbarg MS, Gamsu G, Golden JA. *Pneumocystis carinii* pneumonia radiographically simulating tuberculosis. *Am Rev Respir Dis* 1985;132:1124–1126.

317. Kuhlman JE, Kavuru M, Fishman EK, Siegelman SS. *Pneumocystis carinii* pneumonia: spectrum of parenchymal CT findings. *Radiology* 1990;175:711–714.

318. Crawford SE, Hackman RC, Clark JG. Open lung biopsy diagnosis of diffuse pulmonary infiltrates after marrow transplantation. *Chest* 1988;94:949–953.

319. Herman S, Rappaport D, Weisbrod G, et al. Single-lung transplantation: imaging features. *Radiology* 1989;170:89–93.

320. Maurer JR, Tullis E, Grossman RF, et al. Infectious complications following isolated lung transplantation. *Chest* 1992;101:1056–1059.

321. Armitage JO. Bone marrow transplantation. *N Engl J Med* 1994;330:827–838.

322. Aafedt BC, Halvorsen R, Tylen U, Hertz M. Cytomegalovirus pneumonia: computed tomography findings. *Can Assoc Radiol J* 1990;41:276–280.

323. Young RC, Bennett JE, Vogel CL, Carbone PP, DeVita VT. Aspergillosis: the spectrum of disease in 98 patients. *Medicine* 1970;49:147–173.

324. Gerson SL, Talbot GH, Hurwitz S, et al. Prolonged granulocytopenia: the major risk factor for invasive pulmonary aspergillosis in patients with acute leukemia. *Ann Intern Med* 1984;100:345–351.

325. Gefter WB. The spectrum of pulmonary aspergillus. *J Thorac Imag* 1992;7:56–74.

326. Aisner J, Schimpff SC, Wiernek PH. Treatment of invasive aspergillosis: relation of early diagnosis and treatment to response. *Ann Int Med* 1977;86:539–543.

327. Orr DP, Myerwitz RL, Dubois PJ. Pathoradiologic correlation of invasive pulmonary aspergillosis in the compromised host. *Cancer* 1978;41:2028–2039.

328. Curtis AMB, Smith GJW, Ravin CE. Air crescent sign of invasive pulmonary aspergillosis. *Radiology* 1979;133:17–21.

329. Kuhlman JE, Fishman EK, Siegelman SS. Invasive pulmonary aspergillosis in acute leukemia: characteristic findings of CT, the CT halo sign, and the role of CT in early diagnosis. *Radiology* 1985;157:611–614.

330. Kuhlman JE, Fishman EK, Burch PA, et al. Invasive pulmonary aspergillosis in acute leukemia: the contribution of CT to early diagnosis and aggressive management. *Chest* 1987;92:95–99.

331. Hruban RH, Meziane MA, Zerhouni EA, et al. Radiologic-pathologic correlation of the CT halo sign in invasive aspergillosis. *J Comput Assist Tomogr* 1987;11:534–536.

332. Blum U, Windfuhr X, Buitrago-Tellez C, et al. Invasive pulmonary aspergillosis: MRI, CT and plain radiographic findings and their contribution for early diagnosis. *Chest* 1994;106:1156–1161.

333. Gaeta M, Volta S, Stroscio S, Romeo P, Pandolfo I. CT "halo sign" in pulmonary tuberculoma. *J Comput Assist Tomogr* 1992;16:827–828.

334. Huang RM, Naidich DP, Lubat E, et al. Septic pulmonary emboli: CT-radiographic correlation. *AJR Am J Roentgenol* 1989;153:41–45.

335. Padley SPG, Hansell DM, Flower CDR, Jennings P. Comparative accuracy of high resolution computed tomography and chest radiography in the diagnosis of chronic diffuse infiltrative lung disease. *Clin Radiol* 1991;44:222–226.

336. Padley SPG, Adler B, Müller NL. High-resolution computed tomography of the chest: current indications. *J Thorac Imag* 1993;8:189–199.

337. Remy-Jardin M, Remy J, Deffontaines C, Duhamel A. Assessment of diffuse infiltrative lung disease: comparison of conventional CT and high-resolution CT. *Radiology* 1991;181:157–162.

338. Mayo JR, Jackson SA, Müller NL. High-resolution CT of the chest: radiation dose. *AJR* 1993;160:479–481.

339. Kang EY, Grenier P, Laurent F, Müller NL. Interlobular septal thickening: patterns at high-resolution computed tomography. *J Thorac Imag* 1996;11:260–264.

340. Nishimura K, Izumi T, Kitaichi M, Nagai S, Itoh H. The diagnostic accuracy of high-resolution computed tomography in diffuse infiltrative lung diseases. *Chest* 1993;104:1149–1155.

341. Grenier P, Chevret S, Beigelman C, et al. Chronic diffuse infiltrative lung disease: determination of the diagnostic value of clincial data, chest radiography, and CT with Bayesian analysis. *Radiology* 1994;383–390.

342. Remy-Jardin M, Giraud F, Remy J, et al. Pulmonary sarcoidosis: role of CT in the evaluation of disease activity and functional impairment and in prognosis assessment. *Radiology* 1994;191:675–680.

343. Wall CP, Gaensler EA, Carrington CB, Hayes JA. Comparison of transbronchial and open biopsies in chronic infiltrative lung diseases. *Am Rev Respir Dis* 1981;123:280–285.

344. Wilson RK, Fechner RE, Greenberg SD, Estrada R, Stevens PM. Clinical implications of a "nonspecific" transbronchial biopsy. *Am J Med* 1978;65:252–256.

345. Raghu G. Idiopathic pulmonary fibrosis. A rational clinical approach. *Chest* 1987;92:148–154.

346. Lenique F, Braunner MW, Grenier P, et al. CT assessment of bronchi in sarcoidosis: endoscopic and pathologic correlations. *Radiology* 1995;194:419–423.

346a. Morales CF, Patefield AJ, Strollo PJ, Schenk DA. Flexible TTNA in the diagnosis of sarcoidosis. *Chest* 1994;106:708–711.

347. Bensard DD, McIntyre RC, Waring BJ, Simon JS. Comparison of video thoracoscopic lung biopsy to open lung biopsy in the diagnosis of interstitial lung disease. *Chest* 1993;103:765–770.

348. Templeton PA, Krasna M. Localization of pulmonary nodules for thoracoscopic resection: use of needle/wire breast biopsy system. *AJR Am J Roentgenol* 1993;160:761–762.

349. Shah RM, Spirn PW, Salazar AM, et al. Role of thoracoscopy and preoperative localization procedures in the diagnosis and management of pulmonary pathology. *Semin Ultrasound Ct MRI* 1995;16:371–378.

350. Naidich DP, Funt S, Ettenger NA, Arranda C. Hemoptysis: CT-bronchoscopic correlations in 58 cases. *Radiology* 1990;177:357–362.

351. Millar A, Boothroyd A, Edwards D, Hetzel M. The role of computed tomography (CT) in the investigation of unexplained hemoptysis. *Resp Med* 1992;86:39–44.

352. Set PAK, Flower CDR, Smith IE, et al. Hemoptysis: comparative study of the role of CT and fiberoptic bronchoscopy. *Radiology* 1993;189:677–680.

353. McGuinness G, Beacher JR, Harkin TJ, et al. Hemoptysis: prospective high-resolution CT/bronchoscopic correlation. *Chest* 1994;105:1155–1162.

354. Poe RH, Levy PC, Israel RH, Ortiz CR, Kallay MC. Use of fiberoptic bronchoscopy in the diagnosis of bronchogenic carcinoma. A study in patients with idiopathic pleural effusions. *Chest* 1994;105:1663–1667.

355. Rohwedder JJ. Enticements for fruitless bronchoscopy (editorial). *Chest* 1989;96:708–710.

356. Gruden JF, Naidich DP. High-resolution CT: can it obviate lung biopsy? *Clin Pulm Med* 1998;5:23–35.

357. Orens JB, Kazerooni EA, Martinez FJ, et al. The sensitivity of high-resolution CT in detecting idiopathic pulmonary fibrosis proved by open lung biopsy: a prospective study. *Chest* 1995;108:109–115.

358. Ailion DC, Case TA, Blatter DD, et al. Applications of NMR spin imaging to the study of the lungs. *Bull Magn Reson* 1983;6:130–139.

359. Cutillo AG, Morris AH, Ailion DC, Dureny CH. Clinical implications of nuclear magnetic resonance lung research. *Chest* 1989;96:643–652.

360. Gamsu G, Sostman D. Magnetic resonance imaging of the thorax. *Am Rev Resp Dis* 1989;139:254–274.

361. Hayes CE, Cae TA, Ailion DC, Morris AH, Cutillo A, Blackburn CW. Lung water quantitation by nuclear magnetic resonance imaging. *Science* 1982;216:1313–1315.

362. Huber DJ, Adams DF. Proton NMR of acute pulmonary edema and hemorrhage (abstract). *Invest Radiol* 1984;19:S21.

363. Skalina S, Kundal HL, Wolf G, Marshall B. The effect of pulmonary edema on proton nuclear magnetic resonance relaxation times. *Invest Radiol* 1984;19:7–9.

364. Cutillo AG, Morris AH, Blatter DD, et al. Determination of lung water content and distribution by nuclear magnetic resonance. *J Appl Physiol* 1984;57:583–588.

365. Wexler HR, Nicholson RL, Prato FS, et al. Quantitation of lung water by nuclear magnetic resonance imaging. A preliminary study. *Invest Radiol* 1985;20:583–590.

366. Schmidt HC, McNamara MT, Brasch RC, Higgins CB. Assessment of severity of experimental pulmonary edema with MRI: effect of relaxation enhancement by Gd-DTPA. *Radiology* 1985;20:687–692.

367. MacLennan FM, Foster MA, Smith FW, Crosher GA. Measurement of total lung water from nuclear magnetic resonance images. *Br J Radiol* 1986;59:552–560.

368. Schmidt HC, Daw-Guey T, Higgins CB. Pulmonary edema: an MR study of permeability and hydrostatic types in animals. *Radiology* 1986;158:297–302.

369. Mayo JR, Müller NL, Forster BB, Okazawa M, Pare PD. Magnetic resonance imaging of hydrostatic pulmonary edema in isolated dog lungs: comparison with computed tomography. *Can Assoc Radiol J* 1990;41:281–286.

370. Phillips DM, Allen PS, Man SFP. Assessment of temporal changes in pulmonary edema with NRM imaging. *J Appl Physiol* 1989;66:1197–1208.

371. Mayo JR, MacKay AL, Whittall KP, Baile EM, Pare PD. Measurement of lung water content and pleural pressure gradient with magnetic resonance imaging. *J Thorac Imaging* 1995;10:73–81.

372. Moore EH, Webb WR, Müller NL, Sollitto R. MRI of pulmonary airspace disease: experimental model and preliminary clinical results. *AJR Am J Roentgenol* 1986;146:1123–1128.

373. Huber DJ, Kobzik L, Solorzano C, Melanson G, Adams DF. Nuclear magntic resonance spectroscopy of acute and evolving pulmonary hemorrhage: an *in vitro* study. *Invest Radiol* 1987;22:632–637.

374. Rubin GD, Edwards DK, Reicher MA, Doemeny JM, Carson SH. Diagnosis of pulmonary hemosiderosis by MR imaging. *AJR Am J Roentgenol* 1989;152:573–574.

375. Tobler J, Levitt RG, Glazer HS, et al. Differentiation of proximal bronchogenic carcinoma from post-obstructive lobar collapse by magentic resonance imaging. Comparison with computed tomography. *Invest Radiol* 1987;22:538–543.

376. Vitinski S, Pearson MG, Karlik SJ, et al. Differentiation of parenchymal lung disorders with in vitro proton nuclear magnetic resonance. *Magn Reson Med* 1986;3:120–125.

377. Herold CJ, Kuhlman JE, Zerhouni EA. Pulmonary atelectasis: signal patterns with MR imaging. *Radiology* 1991;178:715–720.

378. Glazer HS, Lee JKT, Levitt RG, et al. Differentitation of radiation fibrosis from recurrent pulmonary neoplasm by magnetic resonance imaging. *AJR Am J Roentgenol* 1984;143:729–730.

379. Inch WR, Prato FS, Butland TS, Frei JV. Use of nuclear magnetic resonance to monitor lung injury by x-irradiation: a preliminary study. *Resp Care* 1986;31:388–394.

380. Taylor DB, Joske D, Anderson J, Barry-Walsh C. Cavitating pulmonary nodules in histiocytosis-X high resolution CT demonstration. *Australia Radiol* 1990;34:253–255.

381. McFadden RG, Carr TJ, Wood TE. Proton magnetic resonance imaging to stage activity of interstitial lung disease. *Chest* 1987;92:31–39.

382. Müller NL, Mayo JR, Zwirewich CV. Value of MR imaging in the evaluation of chronic infiltrative lung diseases: comparison with CT. *AJR Am J Roentgenol* 1992;158:1205–1209.

383. Primack SL, Mayo JR, Hartman TE, Miller RR, Müller NL. MRI of infiltrative lung disease: comparison with pathologic findings. *J Comput Assist Tomogr* 1994;18:233–238.

CHAPTER 7

Pulmonary Complications of Acquired Immunodeficiency Syndrome

Georgeann McGuinness

Thirty million people to date are infected with human immunodeficiency virus (HIV) worldwide. This number includes estimates as high as 1 in 4 patients in some sub-Saharan nations. In the United States, an estimated 550,000 persons are infected with HIV, of whom 223,000 have clinical acquired immunodeficiency syndrome (AIDS) (1). Altogether, 68,473 new cases of AIDS were reported to the Centers for Disease Control and Prevention (CDC) in 1996 (1), thus making AIDS the leading cause of death in the United States in people between the ages of 25 and 44 years. Unfortunately, toward the close of its second decade, the AIDS epidemic continues without expectations of a vaccine in the near future.

Despite encouraging preliminary results using protease inhibitor therapy, HIV-associated and AIDS-related pulmonary complications continue to present a considerable diagnostic dilemma. Health care workers and AIDS researchers guardedly speculate that HIV positivity and AIDS may be managed as a chronic condition rather than as a premorbid condition. Whether these potentially chronically affected patients will be maintained in good health or will continue to be afflicted by a spectrum of AIDS-related diseases is unclear, however. Therefore, it seems reasonable to assume that AIDS will continue to be an important and challenging issue, whether in the management of deteriorating patients or in the long-term care of relatively well patients.

This chapter reviews diseases that affect the lungs of AIDS patients, both infectious and noninfectious, with emphasis placed on integrating computed tomography (CT) findings with pertinent clinical and laboratory data, in particular the degree of immunosuppression as reflected in the CD4 level (2).

CHANGING TRENDS: EPIDEMIOLOGY AND DISEASE PATTERNS

Pulmonary manifestations of HIV infection remained relatively unchanged during the first decade of the AIDS epidemic (3). However, a growing clinical awareness of changing or expanding disease patterns over the past decade led to the 1993 revision by the CDC of the list of surveillance diseases in the diagnosis of AIDS (4). Of particular note was the inclusion of recurrent pyogenic pneumonia and pulmonary *Mycobacterium tuberculosis* infection [tuberculosis (TB)] in the HIV-positive patient as index diseases for AIDS.

The lungs remain one of the chief target organs for HIV-associated disease, and pulmonary manifestations continue to be a significant source of morbidity and mortality. Almost 70% of AIDS patients suffer a respiratory episode during the course of their illness (5). As important, the nature of respiratory diseases, in terms of agent, severity, and duration, as well as the relative likelihood of specific diseases, continues to evolve.

To date, three factors have been proposed to account for these changing trends in the epidemiology of HIV infection. Arguably the most important of these factors is the widespread use of prophylactic therapy for *Pneumocystis carinii* pneumonia (PCP). Routine PCP prophylaxis has been administered since 1989, and changes in disease patterns attributable to its use have been traced to this time. In one study, the incidence of specific diseases in a large group of HIV-positive homosexual men who did not have AIDS and of whom only some were receiving prophylactic therapy was prospectively compared (6). Not surprisingly, PCP occurred less frequently in the group receiving therapy. In distinction, four AIDS-defining diseases did occur with increased frequency in this group, including wasting syndrome, cytomegalovirus (CMV) disease, *Mycobacterium avium* complex (MAC) disease, and esophageal candidiasis. Effective PCP prophylaxis not only led to a decrease in the incidence of PCP as an initial diagnosis and lengthened the disease-free interval between episodes, but it also decreased the lifetime occurrence of PCP in AIDS. Similar findings have been reported by Katz and coworkers (7). Examining temporal trends of opportunistic infections (OIs) and malignancies in homosexual men with AIDS, these authors noted that whereas the rate of PCP decreased from 1981 to 1990, especially between 1985 and 1990, the rates of MAC and CMV significantly increased, again a likely result of the widespread use of PCP prophylaxis.

Also contributing to changing disease trends in AIDS are shifts in population groups affected. Specifically, the incidence of AIDS is increasing in women (8), children, and ethnic minorities, whereas homosexual and bisexual men represent a decreasing percentage of cases (9). The relative proportional growth in intravenous drug abusers (IVDAs) likely reflects the finding that this group is particularly recalcitrant to modification of high-risk behavior. Variations in the incidence of specific diseases within these groups are important. Disease patterns among inner-city AIDS patients (10), a population reflecting an increasing representation of women with AIDS as well as a higher percentage of IVDAs and a lower percentage of homosexual men, have been examined in a large autopsy series. Whereas bacterial pneumonia was the most common infection of the lung in these groups, PCP, the second most common pulmonary infection, was a more frequent cause of death. CMV, the third most common lung infection and the third most common cause of death, occurred more frequently in patients infected with HIV through sexual contact. Recognition that bacterial pneumonia is of increasing importance in IVDAs has been growing (10–14).

The impact of government spending on care for AIDS patients as a proposed third factor in encouraging disease trends has been more difficult to measure. For example, the 30% decline in deaths from AIDS in New York City in 1996 despite an unchanged rate of new AIDS cases has been attributed in part by the Assistant Commissioner of Disease Intervention Research to the fact that federal funding for care of New York City's AIDS patients more than doubled

in 1994 and has remained at this higher level (15). The economic impact of this finding is obvious; access to care will undoubtedly widen the disparity in disease patterns and life expectancy noted between advantaged and disadvantaged patients. Unfortunately, basic prophylactic therapy, much less protease inhibitor therapy, remains unavailable to many patients in the United States, as well as most patients in developing countries.

The lengthening life expectancy of many AIDS patients is allowing survival at advanced levels of immunocompromise, a trend that also affects evolving disease patterns. Effective prophylaxis against more virulent organisms, as well as profound immunosuppression, allows less virulent organisms such as CMV and MAC to produce significant morbidity and mortality.

IMAGE INTERPRETATION: INTEGRATION OF CLINICAL DATA

Integration of clinical data with radiographic findings in assessing HIV/AIDS-related pulmonary diseases is critical. Knowing that a patient is HIV-positive or has AIDS should be considered insufficient clinical history. It is now possible to measure plasma HIV viral load directly and to make more specific measurements such as human herpesvirus-8 viremia in peripheral blood mononuclear cells in patients with Kaposi's sarcoma (KS). The CD4 lymphocyte level, in particular, is a well-accepted measure of the degree of immunocompromise that can be used as a marker for the onset of specific OIs and neoplasms in AIDS (5,12,16,17). In this regard, a CD4 level of 200 cells/mm^3 marks the onset of clinical AIDS in the HIV-positive patient (4), even in the absence of OIs. Specific diseases occur with increasing frequency in AIDS as particular CD4 thresholds are reached, and as a corollary, these illnesses are less likely to occur in patients who are not as severely immunocompromised. CD4 levels therefore are routinely employed as the best predictor of disease progression, and they are applied to clinical decisions regarding initiation of prophylactic therapy.

When the immune system is less severely impaired, at CD4 levels higher than 500 cells/mm^3, patients are at risk for infections from relatively virulent organisms, such as bacterial pneumonia or TB. Although an association with HIV infection remains poorly defined, as will be discussed later, lung cancer may also occur during this period. As the immune system continues to falter, additional diseases must be considered. Although patients continue to acquire recurrent bacterial pneumonias or TB when their CD4 levels are between 200 and 499 cells/mm^3, noninfectious processes increase in frequency. At CD4 levels lower than 200 cells/mm^3, PCP and disseminated TB are common. Most cases of PCP occur in patients with CD4 levels lower than 100 cells/mm^3. KS also occurs with increasing frequency in this range. When CD4 levels are lower than 100 cells/mm^3, reflecting a profoundly depressed immune system, CMV disease, MAC disease, and disseminated fungal infections are more likely to occur (17). Consideration of a patient's level of immunocompromise as measured by the CD4 level, therefore, not only is valuable in generating appropriate differential diagnoses in an AIDS patient with a given radiographic pattern, but also may be useful in understanding temporal variations in patterns of a specific disease (16,18).

In addition to assessing CD4 levels, an appropriately tailored differential diagnosis in AIDS should include consideration of the risk factors for HIV infection: KS, for example, is seen in homosexual or bisexual men and their sex partners, but it is rarely identified outside this group. CMV disease is more common when HIV has been contracted through sexual contact, either heterosexual or homosexual (10). Bacterial pneumonias are more common in IVDAs (5,10–14).

Neutropenic patients and patients receiving steroid therapy are particularly susceptible to fungal infections.

The type, severity, and chronicity of symptoms may also be of value for image interpretation. This category includes the severity and duration of dyspnea, fever, and cough, especially if the cough is productive. Also of concern are laboratory values including the degree of hypoxemia reflected by an increased alveolar–arterial oxygen gradient, serum lactate dehydrogenase levels, and the presence of leukocytosis. Coupled with the CD4 count, these findings can enhance the accuracy of radiologic diagnosis. Diffuse reticular markings, for instance, are consistent with a diagnosis of PCP (Fig. 7-1A). However, this diagnosis is unlikely in patients

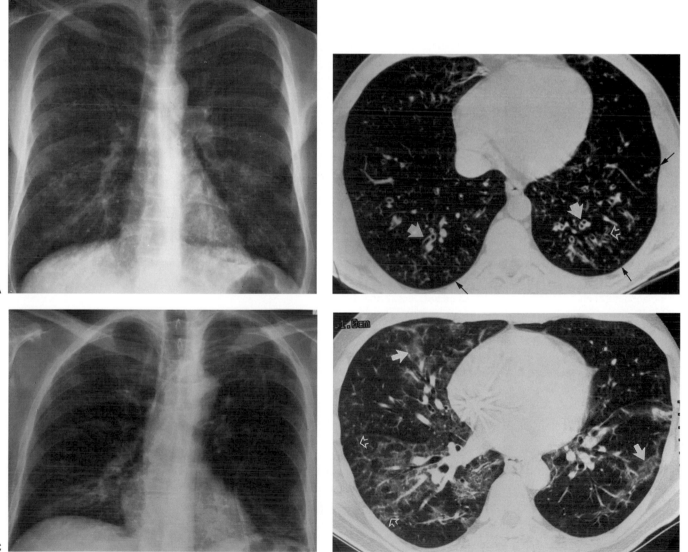

FIG. 7-1. Accuracy of CT versus radiography in diffuse AIDS-related lung disease. Infectious bronchiolitis mimicking *Pneumocystis carinii* pneumonia (PCP) on chest radiography. **A:** Chest radiograph in a 32-year-old man with a productive cough demonstrates diffusely increased coarse reticular lung markings, mimicking interstitial infiltrate seen in PCP (compare with **C**). **B:** A 1-mm section through the lung bases clearly demonstrates bronchial wall thickening (*large white arrows*), bronchiectasis (*open arrow*), and centrilobular impacted bronchioles (*black arrows*). Note the absence of interstitial disease or ground glass attenuation. Sputum culture grew mixed pyogenic organisms; no other infections were diagnosed at bronchoscopy. **C:** Chest radiograph in a 44-year-old man with PCP and a dry cough demonstrates a similar pattern of coarse interstitial markings. **D:** A 1.5-mm section through the lung bases, however, depicts a distinctly different pattern of focal areas of ground glass attenuation (*arrows*) consistent with alveolitis and reticular markings (*open arrows*) reflecting thickened interlobular septa.

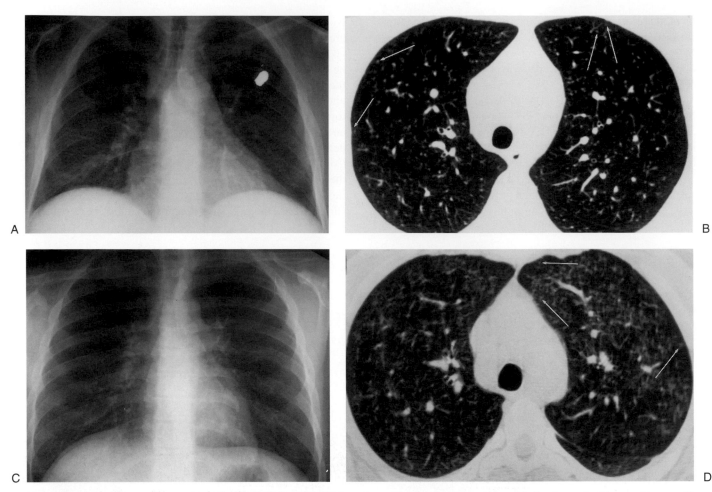

FIG. 7-2. Miliary infiltrates in symptomatic and asymptomatic AIDS patients. **A:** Chest radiograph in a febrile, dyspneic 37-year-old man with AIDS and subtle, diffuse 3-mm lung nodules. Note the incidental bullet fragments. **B:** A 1.5-mm section through the upper lungs in the same patient demonstrates innumerable tiny nodules (*arrows*), best appreciated in the lung periphery, in this patient with disseminated tuberculosis. **C:** Small nodules of 2 to 3 mm are noted diffusely on chest radiography in this 25-year-old HIV-positive man without pulmonary complaints. **D:** A 1-mm section through the upper lungs depicts 2- to 3-mm nodules (*arrows*) throughout the interstitium. Lymphocytic interstitial pneumonitis was diagnosed at transbronchial biopsy (compare with Figs. 7-10A and 7-30).

with a cough productive of purulent sputum, a clinical presentation more consistent with pyogenic small airway disease. As will be discussed later, although occasionally this disorder is difficult to distinguish from PCP radiographically, a diagnosis of small airway inflammation is easily confirmed at high-resolution computed tomography (CT) (Fig. 7-1B). As a second example, small, randomly distributed nodules of 3 to 5 mm may reflect disseminated fungal or mycobacterial infection in symptomatic patients (Fig. 7-2A,B), but these lesions are more likely to represent a more indolent process such as lymphoproliferative disorder in asymptomatic patients (Fig. 7-2C, D).

The occurrence of prior OIs also may affect the likelihood of a new OI. As documented by Finkelstein and associates (19) in a statistical analysis of a cohort of more than 1,500 HIV-positive patients, the occurrence of each OI increased the risk of developing subsequent specific OIs, even when adjusted for all other factors, including CD4 level. Whereas these data are proposed in support of revised criteria for determining the timing and relative benefit of various forms of prophylactic therapy, this information may also be useful in predicting the relative likelihood of a given diagnosis in an AIDS patient with specific imaging findings at a known CD4 level and a prior history of pulmonary OIs.

PULMONARY DISEASES

Given the protean nature of pulmonary manifestations of HIV infection and AIDS, it should come as no surprise that the various causes of pulmonary disease overlap, both clinically and radiographically. Nonetheless, distinct patterns of abnormalities can be identified, particularly for the most common diseases. This is especially true regarding CT interpretation. For this reason, individual diseases are reviewed separately, with the express purpose of emphasizing those characteristics, clinical and radiographic, that are most valuable in the differential diagnosis.

Infections

Bacterial Infections

Lower respiratory tract infections, including bacterial pneumonia (10,13,20) and bronchitis (13,20), have superseded PCP as the most common infection in the lungs of AIDS patients. In a prospective 18-month study of patients with or at risk for HIV infection, Wallace and associates (11) reported that pyogenic infections, including bronchitis (16%), acute sinusitis (5%), and bacterial pneumonia (5%), were more common than PCP (4%) in patients with both early and severe immunocompromise. Hirschtick and colleagues (13), in a study of 1,130 HIV-positive patients followed for 5 years, found acute bronchitis to be the most frequent disorder of the lower respiratory tract, with bacterial pneumonias occurring at a rate more than 5 times that of the HIV-negative control group.

The widespread use of anti-PCP prophylaxis is the primary reason for the decrease in PCP relative to bacterial infections; these regimes may also alter or obliterate the composition of normal airway-colonizing organisms, causing a selection of resistant or pathogenic organisms. Paradoxically, prophylaxis with oral trimethoprim–sulfamethoxazole for PCP may provide some protection from bacterial infections. In the study of Hirschtick and associates (13), the incidence of bacterial pneumonia in the HIV-positive cohort receiving oral prophylaxis for PCP decreased by 32% compared with HIV-positive patients who were not receiving prophylactic therapy. Other likely factors, less easy to assess, include the increasing relevance of impaired humoral immunity in AIDS compared with cell-mediated immunity, especially in IVDAs (10,12–14).

Bacterial pneumonias are most commonly due to organisms such as *Streptococcus pneumoniae, streptococcus viridans, Haemophilus influenzae,* or *Pseudomonas aeruginosa* (14,20–24). These organisms typically result in lobar or segmental consolidation (Fig. 7-3A) (18,23). Occasional series have reported atypical radiographic presentations of these infections. In a review of 60 episodes of bacterial pneumonia in HIV-positive patients by Magnenat and associates (14), 45% had classic segmental or lobar areas of consolidation radiographically, whereas 55% of cases presented with predominately interstitial infiltrates, which the authors believed mimicked OIs such as PCP. However, this likely represents a group with infectious bronchiolitis, bronchitis, or early bronchopneumonia; in our experience, diffuse airway disease can be difficult to distinguish from PCP radiographically. Areas of cavitation, particularly with gram-negative organisms such as *Pseudomonas,* may occasionally be seen (Fig. 7-3C,D). A higher propensity for multilobar and bilateral disease has been reported (23). These patients typically have episodes of bacteremia (12), and relapse is common.

Classically, *Pseudomonas aeruginosa* infection presents with acute pneumonia and septicemia. High mortality rates have been noted in AIDS patients who are at heightened risk of becoming infected because of neutropenia or long-standing use of indwelling catheters. A more indolent form of this infection has been described resembling bronchopulmonary *Pseudomonas* infection in patients with cystic fibrosis (25). This syndrome occurs in patients with advanced immunocompromise (average CD4 level, 25 cells/mm^3) but without traditional risk factors for *Pseudomonas* infection, is acquired in the community, and, despite the tendency for relapse after effective therapy, has a low mortality rate (Fig. 7-4). All patients in one report of this syndrome had advanced AIDS, a finding that led these authors to conclude that the most important factor in the development of *Pseudomonas* infection may have been prolonged survival in the face of severe immunosuppression (25).

In a special subset of patients, bacterial infections result primarily in pyogenic airway disease. In particular, an increase in the incidence of infectious bronchitis, bronchiolitis, and bronchiectasis in AIDS has been recognized (13,20–22,24,26–28). As documented by the Pulmonary Complications of HIV Infection Study Group (11), the predominant lower respiratory infection in cohort members entered into the study with CD4 levels higher than 200 cells/mm^3 was acute bacterial bronchitis. Radiographic changes, when present, typically include subtle bronchial wall thickening, appreciated as "tram tracks," and occasionally small, approximately 3-mm nodular densities, representing impacted bronchioles (Fig. 7-5). In HIV-positive patients, these changes are typically symmetric and primarily affect the lower lobes (27). However, even when classic, small airway disease can be difficult to diagnose at chest radiography. Findings may be subtle or confusing (Fig. 7-6); as a consequence, CT should be obtained when this diagnosis is considered, because CT findings are generally characteristic. Radiographic changes and clinical findings, if not recognized as small airway disease, may be attributed to other causes such as PCP (see Fig. 7-1) (24). CT findings diagnostic of this entity include bronchial wall thickening resulting from bronchial or peribronchial inflammation and bronchiolitis identifiable as small (approximately 3 mm), ill-defined centrilobular densities representing bronchioles impacted with inflammatory material (Fig. 7-7A) (29,30). Focal areas of air trapping secondary to small airway disease also may be present (Fig. 7-7B), most easily identified on images obtained at end-expiration (Fig. 7-7C). Expiratory scans also serve to differentiate heterogeneous parenchymal attenuation resulting from mosaic perfusion in small airway disease from ground glass attenuation alveolitis, which, as discussed later, is most commonly seen in patients with PCP.

The diagnosis of bacterial infection in HIV-positive patients or in those with AIDS is established on the basis of clinical presentation supported by corroborative radiographic findings and sputum culture and smear. Although bronchoscopy is rarely indicated, bronchoalveolar lavage (BAL) has proved effective in establishing the diagnosis, with sensitivities of BAL culture reported to be greater than 80% when obtained before antibiotic therapy is instituted (14). Blood cultures should be routinely performed because

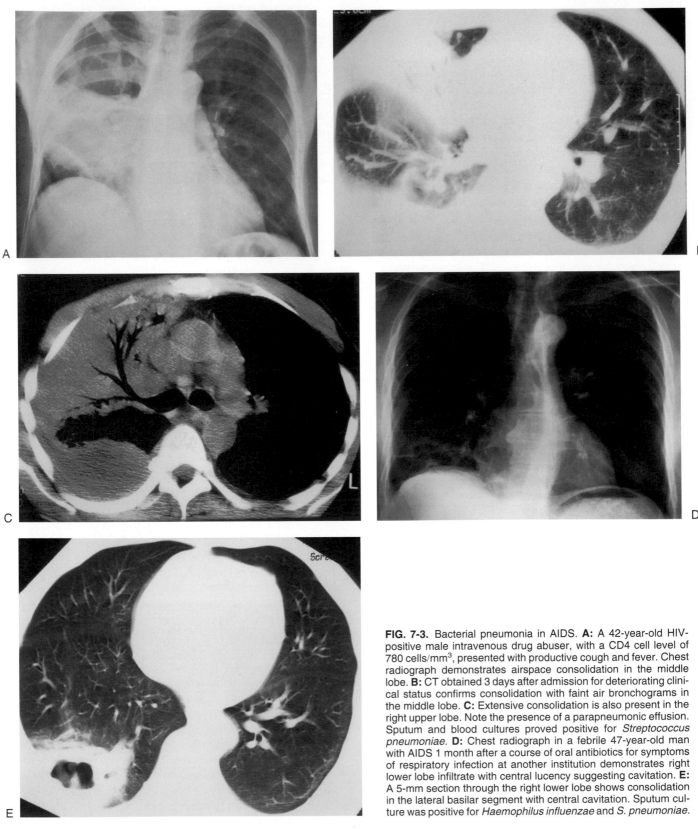

FIG. 7-3. Bacterial pneumonia in AIDS. **A:** A 42-year-old HIV-positive male intravenous drug abuser, with a CD4 cell level of 780 cells/mm^3, presented with productive cough and fever. Chest radiograph demonstrates airspace consolidation in the middle lobe. **B:** CT obtained 3 days after admission for deteriorating clinical status confirms consolidation with faint air bronchograms in the middle lobe. **C:** Extensive consolidation is also present in the right upper lobe. Note the presence of a parapneumonic effusion. Sputum and blood cultures proved positive for *Streptococcus pneumoniae.* **D:** Chest radiograph in a febrile 47-year-old man with AIDS 1 month after a course of oral antibiotics for symptoms of respiratory infection at another institution demonstrates right lower lobe infiltrate with central lucency suggesting cavitation. **E:** A 5-mm section through the right lower lobe shows consolidation in the lateral basilar segment with central cavitation. Sputum culture was positive for *Haemophilus influenzae* and *S. pneumoniae.*

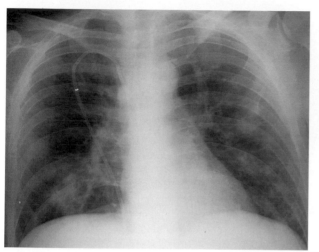

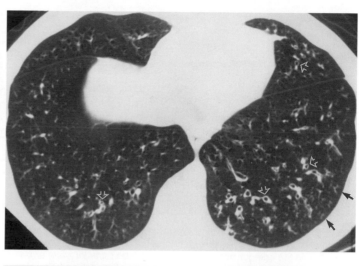

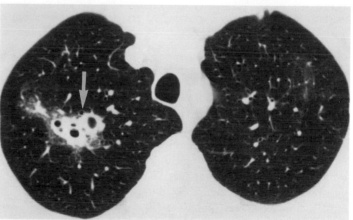

FIG. 7-4. Chronic, recurrent *Pseudomonas* infection in a 33-year-old man with AIDS. **A:** Chest radiograph depicts thick-walled bronchi, scattered nodules, some with central lucencies, and small peripheral densities attributed to impacted bronchi. **B:** A 1-mm section through the lung bases demonstrates dilated, thick-walled bronchi (*open arrows*), and peripheral impacted bronchioles (*black arrows*). **C:** A 1-mm section through the upper lobes depicts clustered, air-containing structures attributed to cystic bronchiectasis with adjacent inflammation (*arrow*). This pattern of panlobar airway involvement resembles chronic *Pseudomonas* infection seen in patients with cystic fibrosis.

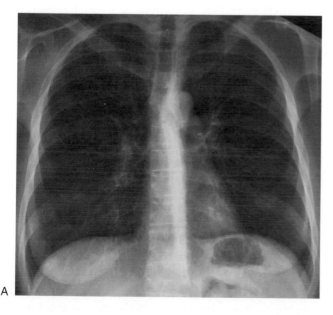

FIG. 7-5. Infectious small airway disease in a 32-year-old woman with recurrent bacterial pulmonary infections. **A:** Chest radiograph shows subtle foci of increased markings, best appreciated in the infrahilar regions, particularly on the left. Bronchial ectasia and wall thickening is noted. (*continues*)

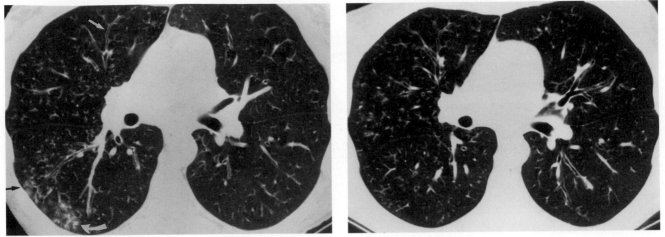

B

C

FIG. 7-5. *Continued.* **B:** A 1-mm section at the level of the bronchus intermedius reveals foci of impacted bronchioles, with peribronchiolar inflammation in the lateral basilar segment of the right lower lobe, producing a tree-in-bud pattern (*black arrow* and *curved arrow*). Mild bronchiectasis is seen in the anterior portion of the middle lobe (*straight white arrow*). Note subtle bronchiolar impaction elsewhere in the right middle lobe. Sputum cultures were positive for *Haemophilus influenzae* and *Streptococcus pneumoniae*. **C:** Follow-up CT with 1-mm collimation 2 months later after antibiotic therapy shows marked improvement in bronchiolar inflammation. Impacted bronchioles, however, have not completely cleared despite therapy, and residual bronchiectasis is extensive.

of the high incidence of bacteremia in these patients. Surprisingly, the radiographic findings may be the most problematic component in the algorithm. In a study comparing the accuracy of diagnosis based on chest radiographs for TB, PCP, and bacterial pneumonia (18), the diagnosis of bacterial pneumonia proved the least accurate and the most likely to mimic the other infections (Fig. 7-8). Atypical bacterial pneumonias have also been reported to be difficult to distinguish radiographically from PCP (14), particularly if the manifestation is primarily that of diffuse airway disease (see Fig. 7-1), or one mimicking TB presenting as a focal infiltrate with ipsilateral adenopathy (see Fig. 7-8).

Pneumocystis carinii *Pneumonia*

Effective anti-PCP prophylaxis has led to a profound decline in the incidence of this OI. Accurate measures of immunosuppression and appropriate application of PCP prophylaxis have decreased the incidence of PCP as an index disease in AIDS. This change likely represents both an absolute and a relative decrease in PCP as an index diagnosis because of the expansion of AIDS diagnostic criteria. Early in the AIDS epidemic, PCP was the index diagnosis for AIDS in nearly two-thirds of cases; currently, it accounts for approximately 40% of index diagnoses (31). A longitudinal prospective study of the natural history of HIV infection among 4,954 homosexual men showed a decrease from 47% in 1988 to 25% in 1991 in the frequency of PCP as the index AIDS diagnosis, a finding correlating with increasing use of prophylactic therapy (6). Within the 6-month period after CD4 levels had dropped below 200 cells/mm^3, a prospective study of 1,182 patients by the Pulmonary Complications of HIV Infection Study Group found PCP to be 9 times less frequent in persons using preventive therapy. Among white

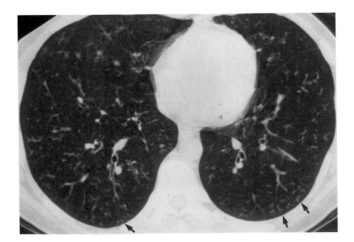

FIG. 7-6. Bacterial bronchiolitis in a 34-year-old man with AIDS, dyspnea, fever, productive cough, and a normal chest radiograph. A 1-mm section through the lower lobes in a patient with a normal chest radiograph (not shown) demonstrates clusters of nodular densities with characteristic branching V- and Y-shaped configuration (*arrows*) approximately 2 to 3 mm from pleural surfaces, which are characteristic of infectious bronchiolitis. Symptoms improved after broad-spectrum antibiotic therapy.

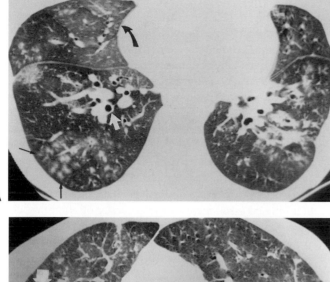

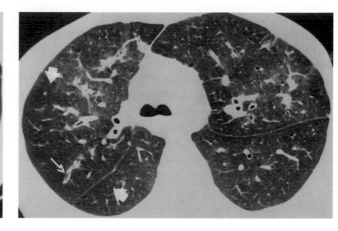

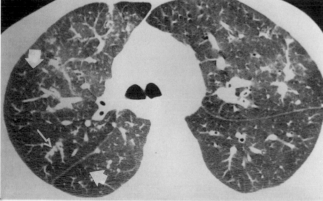

FIG. 7-7. Mosaic perfusion secondary to air trapping from small airway infection in a 32-year-old woman with AIDS. **A:** A 1-mm section through the lung bases demonstrates areas of bronchiolar impaction (*straight arrows*) and thick-walled central airways (*white arrow*). Attenuation of lung parenchyma in areas of airway disease is decreased relative to the normal parenchymal attenuation (*curved arrow*). If the lower density lung is not recognized as abnormal, secondary to air trapping, the areas of normal lung attenuation may be mistaken as representing increased lung density by comparison and misinterpreted as alveolitis. **B,C:** A 1-mm sections through the upper lung in this same patient both in deep inspiration (**B**) and expiration (**C**) demonstrate that the higher-attenuation lung increase in density and decrease in volume at expiration, whereas the areas of lower-attenuation lung do not change (*arrows*), consistent with air trapping. Note the dilated, thick-walled, impacted bronchi in this area (*open arrows*). (From ref. 2, with permission.)

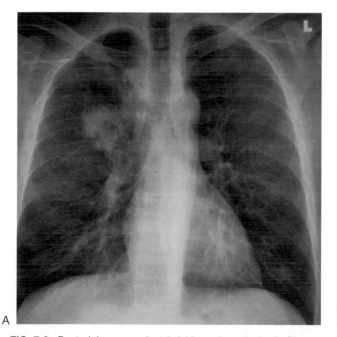

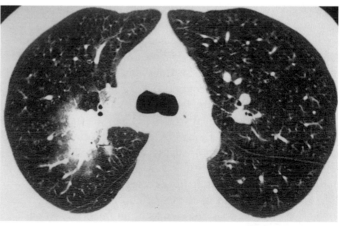

FIG. 7-8. Bacterial pneumonia mimicking tuberculosis. **A:** Chest radiograph in this 27-year-old purified protein derivative–positive woman with AIDS complaining of cough and fever depicts right paratracheal adenopathy with associated suprahilar mass or consolidation. A second smaller focus of infiltrate is also present in the left lung base. These findings are suggestive of primary tuberculosis. **B:** A 1-mm section demonstrates suprahilar area of consolidation in the right upper lobe with associated adenopathy on mediastinal windows (not shown). Blood and sputum cultures were positive for *Streptococcus pneumoniae*. There was no evidence of mycobacterial infection. (From ref. 2, with permission.)

patients, in whom the overall incidence of PCP was higher, the disparity increased to a 26.6% incidence in patients not receiving prophylactic therapy, as compared with 1.9% in those receiving therapy (32). Effective chemoprophylaxis is also contributing to the lengthened life expectancy of AIDS patients. In a large cohort study comparing survival periods from a CD4 lymphocyte count of 200 cells/mm^3 to death, those patients receiving antiretroviral therapy and PCP prophylaxis had significantly longer survival times, compared with those patients receiving antiretroviral therapy alone (33). In many more recent studies, PCP is no longer the most common lung infection in AIDS, because it has been supplanted by bacterial infections (10,13,20). It remains the most common OI of the lungs in AIDS, and 60% of patients continue to have an episode of PCP during the course of their illness (34).

Variations in the relative risk of developing PCP associated with baseline demographic characteristics have been reported (32). In a prospective study of 1,182 HIV-infected patients compared with a matched HIV-negative cohort, Stansell and associates (32) found that case rates in homosexual and bisexual men were more than twice those in IVDAs, and male subjects developed PCP more than twice as frequently as female subjects. White subjects developed PCP at a rate more than 3 times that of black subjects across all transmission group categories despite a higher prophylactic therapy utilization rate. Specifically, 85% of white patients with CD4 levels lower than 200 cells/mm^3 acquired PCP, compared with 64% of black subjects (32).

Although PCP may occur at a CD4 level higher than 200 cells/mm^3, and it remains a common AIDS-defining illness, the diagnosis should be more strongly considered in a patient with CD4 cells below this level, and it is most common in patients with CD4 levels lower than 100 cells/mm^3. Patients typically present with insidious symptoms of fever, nonproductive cough, and dyspnea. An elevated serum lactate dehydrogenase level is sensitive for PCP, but it may result from a variety of other pulmonary processes as well.

Chest radiographs classically demonstrate diffuse, often perihilar, reticular or granular opacities, which often obscure underlying vascular markings. Hazy areas of ground glass opacities are particularly common in the upper lobes (Fig. 7-9A,B). Thin-walled cystic lesions are recognized in about 10% of cases radiographically (35), but they are more commonly identified with CT (see Fig. 7-9). Cysts are responsible for the well-known propensity of these patients to develop spontaneous pneumothoraces. Equivocal or normal chest radiographs, reported in the range of 10% to 39% (34,36), are uncommon in our experience.

Unusual presentations are increasing in frequency in patients with PCP because of the effects of treatment, and they occur in 5% to 10% of cases. Atypical findings include focal or asymmetric consolidation, nodules, and even miliary opacities (Fig. 7-10) and pleural effusions (37). Adenopathy, typically associated with aerosolized pentamidine prophylaxis therapy, is now only rarely identified (Fig. 7-11) (38).

Masses (Fig. 7-12A,B), including occasional cavitary masses (Fig. 7-12C), are infrequent, and therefore, the presence of a thick-walled cavity, rarely representing a necrotic "PCP-oma," should raise the suspicion of TB, fungal infection, and even lung carcinoma. Necrotizing vasculitis resulting from PCP (39) and endobronchial lesions (40) also have been described. PCP may incite a granulomatous host response (36,41) that, when chronic, may calcify. These calcified granulomas occur in the lung parenchyma, but also in lymph nodes (see Fig. 7-11C) and, when disseminated, at extrathoracic sites (see Fig. 7-11D) (42). Despite the presence of overlapping radiographic features and atypical findings in PCP, the chest radiograph is often of diagnostic value. In a blinded assessment of the accuracy of admitting chest radiographs in establishing the diagnosis of PCP, TB, and bacterial pneumonia, Boiselle and associates (18) found that the overall accuracy for establishing the diagnosis of PCP was 75%. Patients without active lung disease were identified 100% of the time, whereas an accurate diagnosis of TB was suggested in 84% of cases, exceeding that of PCP.

On high-resolution CT, the hallmark of acute PCP is the finding of diffuse ground-glass attenuation. This finding corresponds pathologically to an exudative alveolitis associated with an accumulation of fluid, organisms, fibrin, and debris within the alveolar spaces. Usually indistinct, ground-glass attenuation may be strikingly geographic in distribution because of selective involvement of discrete secondary pulmonary lobules; this results in an unusually sharp demarcation between normal and abnormal lung (see Fig. 7-9) (36,37). At an early stage, subtle interlobular reticulation may be identified within areas of ground glass attenuation; when present, these features correlate with histologic evidence of interstitial and interlobular septal infiltration by mononuclear cells and edema (see Fig. 7-9). In distinction, during the subacute phase of infection, reticulation is more extensive and correlates with histologic evidence of dilated interlobular septal lymphatics associated with plasma cell and macrophage infiltration, presumably the result of pneumonic organization (Fig. 7-13). Permanent sequelae of PCP in the form of diffuse interstitial fibrosis with or without residual bizarre-shaped cysts or emphysema may occur even after appropriate therapy.

When the clinical suspicion of PCP is high, a negative chest radiograph, particularly in the setting of hypoxemia, should not preclude further testing to distinguish patients who may be safely observed from those who should undergo empiric therapy or further diagnostic procedures (12). In this regard, CT has consistently been found to be more accurate than chest radiographs for both diagnosing and excluding PCP (43). In our institutions, CT is commonly used for this purpose. Hartman and associates (44) reviewed CT findings in 102 AIDS patients with proved pulmonary disease compared with 20 HIV-positive patients without pulmonary disease. The presence of ground-glass opacities in particular proved highly sensitive for diagnosing PCP; when a confi-

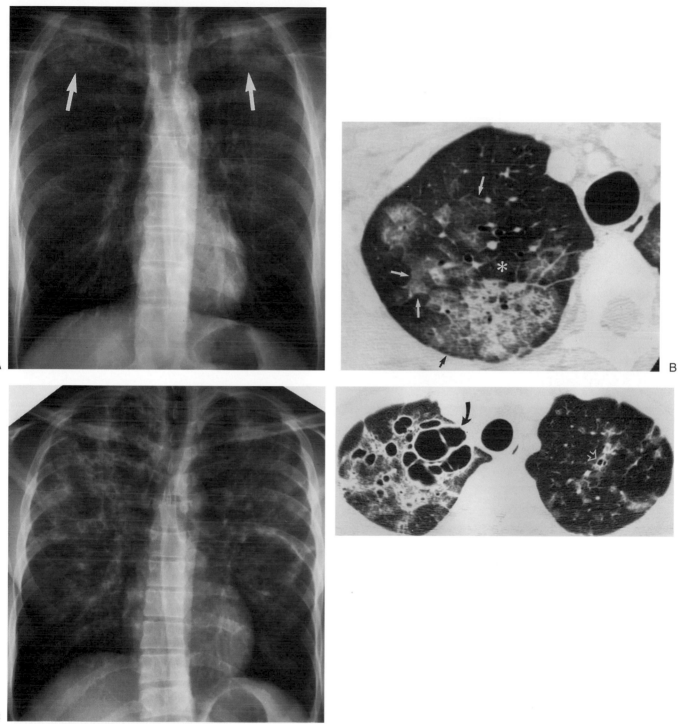

FIG. 7-9. Typical manifestations of *Pneumocystis carinii* pneumonia (PCP). **A:** Chest radiograph in a 44-year-old HIV-positive man without a history of opportunistic infection who is taking oral trimethoprim–sulfamethoxazole prophylactic therapy for PCP. Bilateral hazy areas of increased lung density are seen, primarily in the upper lobes (*arrows*). Upper lobe disease, in the past associated with aerosolized administration of pentamidine for PCP prophylaxis, is not unusual, even outside this clinical setting. This form of therapy is rarely used today. **B:** Enlargement of a a 1-mm section through the right upper lobe depicts patchy, geographic areas of ground glass attenuation conforming to secondary pulmonary lobules (*white arrows*), with scattered areas of lower attenuation, representing noninvolved lung, also outlined by secondary lobular septa (*asterisk*). Note the reticular changes secondary to interlobular septal thickening (*black arrow*) best appreciated in the lung periphery. Bronchoalveolar lavage was positive for PCP. **C:** Chest radiograph in a 48-year-old man with AIDS and a history of prior PCP demonstrates coarse increased markings throughout the lungs, with superimposed hazy areas of increased lung density. Multiple thin-walled air-containing structures are identified bilaterally consistent with cystic PCP. **D:** A 1-mm section shows areas of ground glass attenuation, within which both thin-walled and thick-walled cystic lesions are identified (*open arrow*), typically in areas of coexistent ground glass attenuation. As cysts enlarge, they coalesce to form multiseptated cystic masses (*curved arrow*).

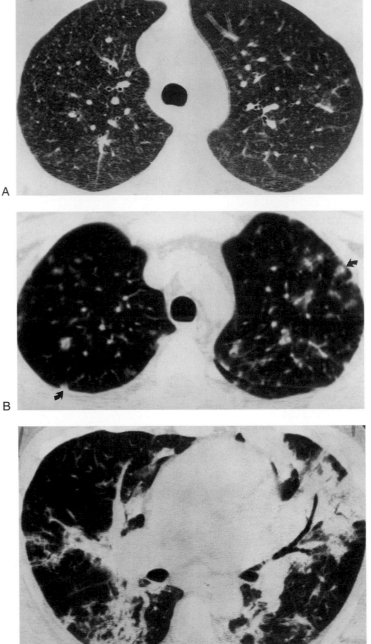

FIG. 7-10. Unusual manifestations of *Pneumocystis carinii* pneumonia (PCP). **A:** High-resolution CT with 1.0-mm collimation in a 34-year-old man with AIDS-related lymphoma demonstrates profusion of 2- to 3-mm nodules, consistent with miliary PCP. At transbronchial biopsy, poorly formed granulomas were identified in the lung interstitium, associated with *P. carinii* organisms in the airspaces. PCP occasionally incites a granulomatous response, even during acute infection. (Note the similarity in appearance with Fig. 7-2A,D.) **B:** A 34-year-old man with PCP appreciated as poorly marginated subcentimeter lung nodules (*arrows*). **C:** Dense, segmental consolidation in the lingula, middle lobe, and right lower lobe are appreciated at high-resolution CT in this 37-year-old man with PCP.

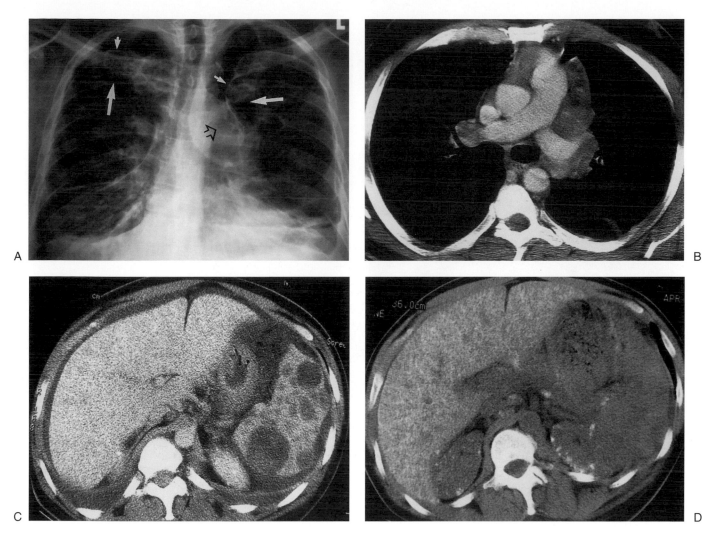

FIG. 7-11. Adenopathy, bilateral pneumothorax, effusions, and extrathoracic dissemination secondary to incompletely treated *Pneumocystis carinii* pneumonia (PCP) in a 45-year-old man with AIDS. **A:** Patient presented 3 weeks after a full course of intravenous trimethoprim–sulfamethoxazole for PCP. Chest radiograph depicts increased reticular markings and lung cysts (*large arrows*), pleural effusions, bilateral pneumothoraces (*small arrows*), and adenopathy in the aorticopulmonic window (*open arrow*). Hazy areas of increased lung density are best appreciated in the lower portions of the lungs. **B:** Contrast-enhanced CT at the level of the carina with 1-mm collimation imaged with narrow windows confirms extensive heterogeneous adenopathy in the aorticopulmonary window as well as in both hila. Bronchoalveolar lavage was positive for PCP. **C:** CT through the upper abdomen at the same time demonstrates multiple low-attenuation foci in the spleen as well as diffuse heterogeneity of the contrast-enhanced liver parenchyma (compare with Fig. 7-27D). **D:** Follow-up noncontrast CT with 10 mm-collimation 3 months later demonstrates heterogeneously high-attenuation liver parenchyma, suggesting calcifications, with low-attenuation foci and calcifications in the spleen. Calcifications secondary to granulomatous PCP are also evident in the kidneys and retroperitoneal lymph nodes.

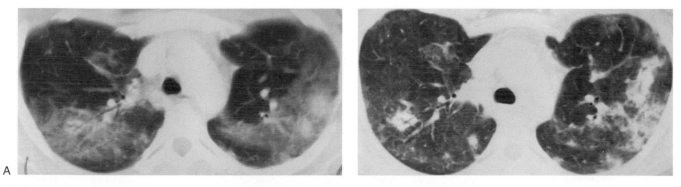

FIG. 7-12. Masslike and cavitary *Pneumocystis carinii* pneumonia (PCP). **A:** A 10-mm section in a 27-year-old woman complaining of dyspnea, but not known to be HIV-positive, demonstrates patchy areas of ground glass attenuation. PCP and HIV infection were diagnosed, and she was treated with intravenous trimethoprim–sulfamethoxazole. **B:** Follow-up CT 28 days later with 5-mm collimation shows organization of the pneumonia, with retracting areas of dense consolidation. Sequential radiographs (not shown) continued, however, to demonstrate masslike densities in the upper lungs. At transbronchial biopsy, abundant *Pneumocystis* organisms were identified in the absence of other infection. She was then treated with intravenous pentamidine. (*continues*)

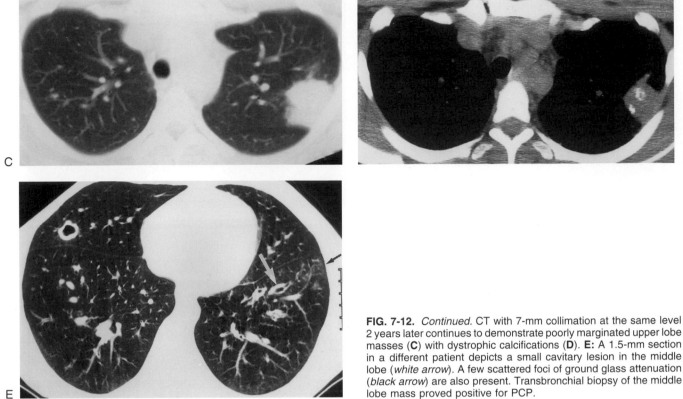

FIG. 7-12. *Continued.* CT with 7-mm collimation at the same level 2 years later continues to demonstrate poorly marginated upper lobe masses (**C**) with dystrophic calcifications (**D**). **E:** A 1.5-mm section in a different patient depicts a small cavitary lesion in the middle lobe (*white arrow*). A few scattered foci of ground glass attenuation (*black arrow*) are also present. Transbronchial biopsy of the middle lobe mass proved positive for PCP.

dent diagnosis of PCP was made on the basis of CT findings, it was correct in 94% of cases.

Similarly, in a study of patients with a high clinical suspicion of PCP but normal or equivocal radiographs, Gruden and associates (45) found a sensitivity of 100% and specificity of 86% for the diagnosis of PCP based on identification of ground glass attenuation on high-resolution CT. Further-

more, if empiric treatment had been initiated in this series based on the presence of ground glass attenuation on CT alone, the number of BALs performed in this series would have been decreased by 78% without missing any case of PCP. Based on these data, in our judgment and that of others, a positive high-resolution CT in this setting is sufficiently suggestive of the diagnosis either to base initiation of em-

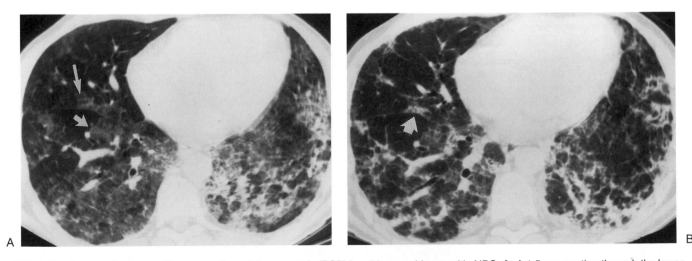

FIG. 7-13. Acute and subacute *Pneumocystis carinii* pneumonia (PCP) in a 36-year-old man with AIDS. **A:** A 1.5-mm section through the lower lobes shows patchy areas of ground glass attenuation (*arrows*). Fine reticular changes are superimposed on these areas of involved lung, attributable to interstitial and interlobular infiltration by inflammatory cells. **B:** Follow-up CT at the same level 3 weeks after initiation of antibiotic therapy demonstrates regression of ground glass attenuation as the alveolitis resolves, and replacement by coarse reticulation in the same areas (*arrow*) as the predominant finding.

piric therapy (46) or to pursue definitive diagnosis with bronchoscopy (47). The cost of a CT scan is approximately one-third that of BAL, and accordingly, whereas appropriate use of CT may prompt aggressive diagnostic procedures, it may also prevent unnecessary procedures if the CT is negative.

Fungal Infections

Fungal pulmonary infections are relatively unusual in patients with AIDS, even in those with advanced levels of immunocompromise (48,49). This is because the primary immune impairment in AIDS is due to dysfunctional T lymphocytes and cell-mediated immunity, whereas the major cells involved in host defense from fungal infection are neutrophils and, in the lungs, alveolar macrophages. Qualitative defects of neutrophil or macrophage function do occur, however, with advanced levels of immunosuppression that allow fungal infection. The most common fungal infection in AIDS overall is caused by *Cryptococcus* and occurs in 10% to 15% of AIDS patients (50–52), whereas aspergillosis is the most common pulmonary fungal infection.

Aspergillosis

The incidence of aspergillosis is increasing in AIDS, and the disease has a high associated mortality (49,53). Infection, typically with *Aspergillus fumigatus,* can take one of two forms: tissue-invasive aspergillosis, which is more common (48,54,55), or tracheobronchial aspergillosis. Patients are usually severely immunocompromised, with a CD4 cell count of less than 50 cells/mm^3 in almost all cases (49,53). Granulocytopenia and steroid use, considered classic risk factors for *Aspergillus* infection in non-AIDS patients, are absent in about 50% of AIDS patients (53).

The most common findings in tissue-invasive aspergillosis are thick-walled, cavitary lesions, seen in conjunction with areas of consolidation, nodules, and pleural effusions (49,50,53,55). Cavitary lesions, seen in 80% of cases by Staples and associates (49), were found pathologically to represent pulmonary infarcts, reflecting the well-described propensity for angioinvasion by this organism (Fig. 7-14). Pathologic examination has also demonstrated nodules resulting from infarcts or nonvascular tissue invasion, as well

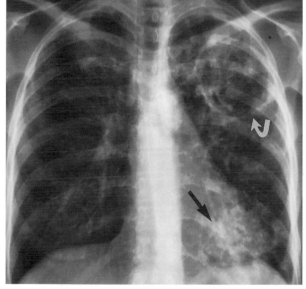

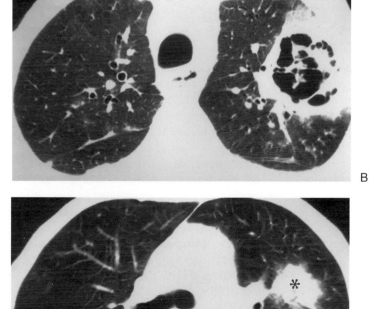

FIG. 7-14. Invasive aspergillosis in a female intravenous drug abuser with AIDS and a CD4 level of less than 100 cells/mm^3. **A:** Chest radiograph demonstrates diffuse, coarse lung markings as well as scattered ill-defined nodular densities, especially at the left lung base (*arrow*). A large, irregularly thick-walled cavity is also present in the left upper lobe (*curved white arrow*). **B:** A 1-mm section demonstrates a large cavity with an irregular, nodular wall in the left upper lobe. Internal septations are clearly present within the cavity. **C:** A 5-mm section at the level of the carina shows a poorly marginated solid nodule more inferiorly in the left upper lobe (*asterisk*). Note the presence of circumferential ground glass attenuation (so-called halo sign) consistent with hemorrhagic ischemia resulting from angioinvasion. Bronchoalveolar lavage was positive for *Aspergillus;* transbronchial biopsy within the left upper lobe confirmed tissue invasion.

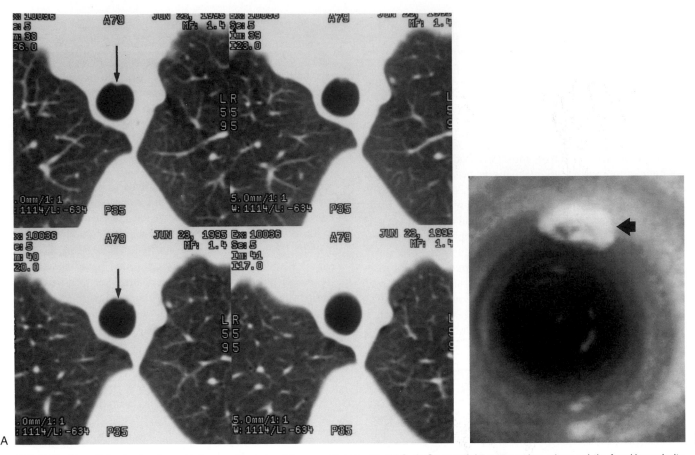

FIG. 7-15. Necrotizing tracheobronchial aspergillosis in a 39-year-old man with AIDS. **A:** Sequential 5-mm sections show subtle, focal irregularity of the anterior wall of the trachea (*arrows*) (see also Fig. 3-9). **B:** Photograph obtained at fiber optic bronchoscopy depicts a raised, white lesion with central blackened umbilication in the anterior trachea (*arrow*), corresponding to the lesion depicted in **A**. Biopsy specimen showed inflammation, necrosis, and tissue invasion, with *Aspergillus* hyphae associated with destruction of the tracheal epithelium. (From ref. 2, with permission.)

as nodules caused by impacted small airways. Areas of consolidation were due to a combination of pneumonia, infarction, and airway involvement (49).

Approximately 10% of reported cases of aspergillosis in patients with AIDS affect the airways (55). Necrotizing tracheobronchial aspergillosis is associated with nodular tracheal or bronchial wall thickening, mucosal ulcerations, and occasionally pseudomembrane formation within the airways. At CT, these changes may be appreciated as areas of nodular tracheobronchial wall thickening (Fig. 7-15; see Fig. 3-9). A more unusual pattern of airway involvement is obstructing bronchial aspergillosis, which does not involve tissue invasion, but instead occludes the distal airways by endoluminal fungus (48). Surprisingly, these patients may be more acutely ill than those with tissue-invasive aspergillosis and may suffer both hypoxemia and chest pain (48). The radiographic presentation is usually bilateral, diffuse lower lobe consolidation, presumably caused by focal postobstructive atelectasis. At CT, impacted small airways may be recognized (Fig. 7-16).

Less commonly, infection with *Aspergillus* results in the formation of intracavitary mycetomas. Addrizzo-Harris and associates (56), in a comparison of aspergillomas developing in HIV-positive patients versus HIV-negative patients, found

important differences between these populations. Whereas cavitary TB was the most common preexisting condition in both groups, in 3 of 10 HIV-positive patients studied, cavities were due to prior PCP. Hemoptysis, present in 73% of HIV-negative patients, occurred in only 40% of HIV-infected patients. Furthermore, evidence of clinical progression with the development of invasive or semiinvasive aspergillosis occurred in half the HIV-positive patients, despite concurrent antifungal therapy, whereas none of the HIV-negative patients demonstrated disease progression (56).

Confirmation of *Aspergillus* infection is complicated by the finding that patients with AIDS often have the organism in sputum or BAL fluid cultures in the absence of clinical or radiographic disease. Lortholary and associates (53) cited the value of BAL culture in establishing the diagnosis; in their series of 33 patients with tissue-invasive aspergillosis, the 28 patients who had BAL all had positive cultures from the fluid (53). Given that the incidence of *Aspergillus* colonization without tissue invasion is as high as 4% in AIDS, however (57), and the disadvantage that this study did not use a control group of patients with BAL but without tissue-invasive aspergillosis, the positive predictive value and specificity of this test require further examination (55). In 45 of

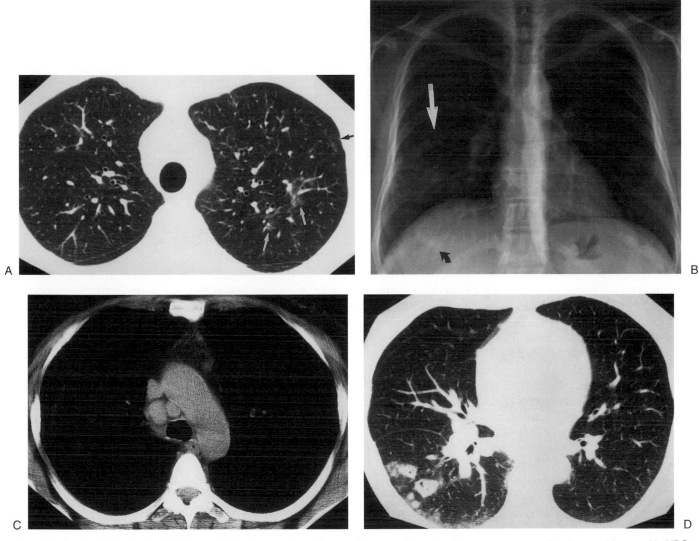

FIG. 7-16. Cryptococcal infection in AIDS. **A:** A 1-mm section through the upper lobes obtained in a symptomatic 50-year-old man with AIDS and a normal radiograph (not shown), with serum cryptantigen titers of 1:8,000. Scattered ill-defined nodular areas of ground glass attenuation are noted (*arrows*), associated with slightly increased reticular markings without evidence of parenchymal consolidation. **B:** Chest radiograph in a 37-year-old woman with AIDS demonstrates enlarged azygos nodes associated with a cluster of thin-walled cavitary lesions in the peripheral right lower lung (*white arrow*) and some ill-defined nodular densities in the right lung base (*black arrow*). **C:** A 7-mm section confirms pretracheal and paratracheal adenopathy. **D:** High-resolution image through the lung bases depicts small nodular densities with areas of early cavitation. Cryptococcal organisms were identified at transbronchial biopsy.

the 972 patients observed by Pursell and associates (57), *Aspergillus* was recovered from respiratory sites ante mortem; however, only 4 had documented tissue-invasive aspergillosis at autopsy (0.4%). Documentation of actual tissue invasion requires biopsy. Airway involvement may be detected through bronchoscopic inspection and biopsy, if involvement is proximal, or through expectoration or extraction of fungal casts in cases of obstructing bronchial aspergillosis.

Cryptococcosis

Cryptococcal pneumonia is usually associated with meningitis and disseminated disease. Although the lung is the most common site of *Cryptococcal neoformans* infection, meningitis is the most common clinical presentation (51,58).

Cryptococcal pneumonia occurs in 30% to 40% of AIDS patients with cryptococcal infection. Most patients are severely immunocompromised, with CD4 counts lower than 100 cells/mm^3.

Imaging findings in patients with cryptococcal infection are varied. Interstitial infiltrates, primarily reticular or reticulonodular, are the most common radiographic pattern, occurring in 50% to 62% of patients (51,52,58). Other parenchymal abnormalities include nodules and consolidation (see Fig. 7-16A) (51). Discrete nodules are identified in approximately 30% of cases (51). Nodules may be more common in patients with early AIDS, and, in fact, only those patients with less advanced AIDS may manifest necrotic nodules (58). Adenopathy and pleural effusions also may be present (see Fig. 7-16B,C) (58,59). Atypical findings include miliary nodules (52) as well as foci of ground glass attenuation.

Although this finding has raised the question whether crytpococcal infection should be considered in the differential diagnosis of causes of ground glass attenuation, in my experience, cryptococcal pneumonia rarely presents with diffuse ground glass attenuation and rarely, if ever, should be mistaken for PCP.

Diagnosis can be established on the basis of biopsy, including transbronchial or transthoracic biopsy (see Fig. 7-16A). If necrotic, the liquid center of the nodule center is often easily aspirated, and the diagnosis can be established in the radiology suite based on identification with India ink stain of the characteristic capsule or with positive culture, which may be obtained from sputum induction, BAL, or biopsy (58).

Histoplasmosis

In contrast to cryptococcosis, histoplasmosis, the most common fungal infection in the United States, is an AIDS index disease when it is extrathoracic. The infection is seen in approximately 5% of AIDS patients in endemic areas, but the incidence drops to approximately 2% overall. Disseminated disease occurs in approximately 75% of patients, usually with advanced immunosuppression and CD4 levels lower than 100 cells/mm^3 (50). In some series, as many as 50% of infected AIDS patients have developed respiratory disease (60,61). Even in nonendemic areas, infection may represent recrudescence of remote disease (62).

Chest radiographic findings are varied and nonspecific. Chest radiographs in 27 AIDS patients with documented disseminated histoplasmosis and evidence of lung involvement demonstrated nodular opacities to be the most frequent finding. In all but 1 case, nodules were smaller than 3 mm (Fig. 7-17). Other findings included linear or irregular opacities, airspace opacities, small pleural effusions, and adenopathy

(61). Similar findings have been reported by others, especially the finding of random small nodules (62). These characteristics are in contrast to those of acute pulmonary histoplasmosis in the immunocompetent host, in which focal airspace consolidation is seen approximately 75% of the time, and adenopathy is seen approximately 80% of the time (61).

Culture of bronchial aspirates positively identifies the organism 50% to 75% of the time; sputum cultures, however, are only positive in 10% to 15% of cases (50). Histopathologic evaluation of tissue obtained by transbronchial biopsy, or bone marrow biopsy in disseminated disease, provides the fastest means of establishing the diagnosis (62). A normal chest radiograph does not exclude the diagnosis of disseminated histoplasmosis (61).

Mycobacterial Infections

The AIDS epidemic has been linked to a coincident resurgence in TB. This is reflected in the inclusion of pulmonary TB in the revised list of index infections for HIV-positive patients for the surveillance definition of AIDS (4). The subset of AIDS patients who are IVDAs may be at particular risk (63). Some investigators believe that increased risk in this group partially reflects the finding that IVDAs tend to be concentrated in areas with a high prevalence of TB (64). A large, prospective cohort of HIV-positive patients followed over disparate geographic areas in the United States for a median of 4.5 years by the Pulmonary Complications of HIV Infection Study Group found residence in eastern states to be the strongest demographic predictor for TB, after adjustment for transmission and ethnic groups (64). Increased susceptibility to TB was not thought likely on immunologic grounds because CD4 levels were comparable among these groups, but rather, it was thought to be due to the combination of increased prevalence of latent infection

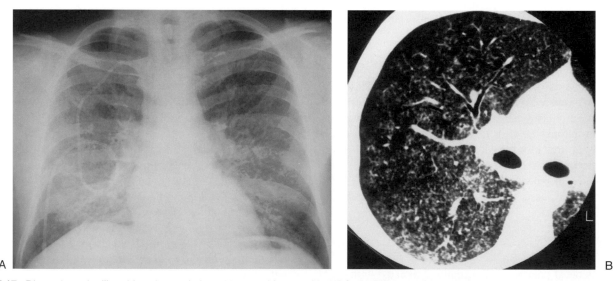

FIG. 7-17. Disseminated miliary histoplasmosis in a 44-year-old man with AIDS. **A:** Diffuse miliary nodules bilaterally are seen on the chest radiograph in this patient. **B:** High-resolution reconstruction of a 1.5-mm collimated image at the level of the carina confirms 2- to 3-mm nodules throughout the lung interstitium in this patient. Miliary nodules are the most common appearance of disseminated histoplasmosis, although tuberculosis remains the more common infectious cause of miliary infiltrates. (From ref. 2, with permission.)

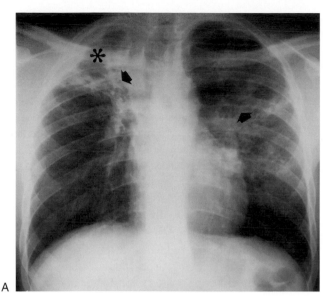

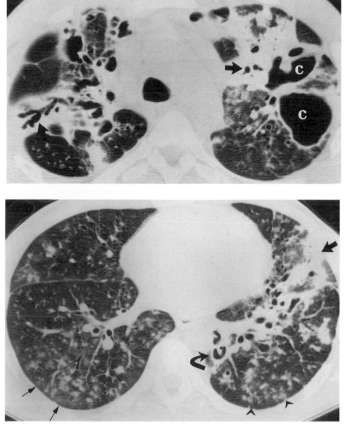

FIG. 7-18. Postprimary tuberculosis in a 30-year-old HIV-positive man with a CD4 level of 330 cells/mm³. **A:** Chest radiograph demonstrates a large, thick-walled cavity in the right upper lobe (*asterisk*), with bronchiectasis in both upper lungs (*arrows*). Scattered nodular infiltrates are present. Upper lung involvement is typical of reactivation tuberculosis. **B:** A 1-mm section at the level of the aortic arch reveals consolidation and bronchiectasis in both upper lobes (*arrows*), as well as cavities in the left upper lobe (*c*), not predicted based on the chest radiograph. **C:** A 1-mm section through the lower portions of the lungs in this patient demonstrates surprisingly extensive lower lung disease, including consolidation (*large arrow*), bronchiectasis (*curved arrow*), and bronchiolar impaction (*arrowheads*) resulting in a tree-in-bud pattern (*small arrows*) consistent with endobronchial dissemination. Lower lung involvement is more common in reactivation tuberculosis in AIDS than in the general population. (From ref. 2, with permission.)

and greater degree of exposure to TB in the eastern states.

The incidence of TB in the AIDS population is 200 to 500 times that of the general population (64); although it is one of the most curable diseases in these patients, it is also one of the most contagious. Because of the virulence of *M. tuberculosis* infection compared with other OIs, TB may affect patients who are minimally immunocompromised.

Establishing the diagnosis of TB may be particularly difficult in this patient population. Many patients with advanced AIDS are anergic, and therefore tuberculin skin test negative, even when they are infected. Adding to the difficulty is a higher incidence of negative sputum smears and cultures in AIDS patients with TB relative to the general population. Recognition of the broad spectrum of radiographic findings in this infection should increase the likelihood of making a timely diagnosis (65). Delay in establishing the correct diagnosis in this patient population is hazardous. Kramer and coworkers (66), in a series of 52 AIDS patients, found that the diagnosis of TB was delayed in 48%. Furthermore, 45% of those in whom the diagnosis was delayed died of TB, as compared with 19% with timely diagnoses. Other studies suggest that TB infection may accelerate the course

of HIV infection, in terms of both increased concurrent OIs and decreased survival (67).

The pattern of TB differs between HIV-seronegative and HIV-seropositive patients (68–70). Specifically, diffuse disease and atypical patterns including lower lung disease, miliary infiltrates, and adenopathy are seen more frequently seen in the HIV-positive population. Only occasional studies fail to support these observations (71). In AIDS, radiographic patterns reflect both primary and secondary infection with a higher incidence of progressive disease noted because of impaired immunity (63). Investigators have further observed that within the HIV-infected population the radiographic manifestations of TB reflect the level of immunocompromise, with different patterns of disease early and late in the course of AIDS (72,73). When the immune system is less severely impaired, at a level of CD4 cells greater than 200 cells/mm³, a pattern consistent with reactivation TB is most commonly seen consequent to hypersensitivity and acquired immunity. Findings include upper lobe cavities, infiltrates, and nodules. Pleural effusions are seen more commonly in patients with CD4 levels higher than 200 cells/mm³ (Fig. 7-18) (72). Some series report a relatively lower incidence of cavitary disease, and more frequent middle and lower lung infiltrates in AIDS patients as compared with reactivation TB in the immunocompetent population (see Fig. 7-18) (68,74). However, the incidence of cavitary disease has been increasing, possibly reflecting the revision of CDC criteria for the diagnosis of AIDS, which now includes TB as an index disease in HIV-positive persons. Because patients are now being reported with TB and HIV earlier, when CD4 levels are not drastically reduced, the manifestations of TB, including cavitary disease, are more consistent with those seen in the general population (73). Nonetheless, some of these patients with relatively well preserved immune function may not have had prior exposure to *Mycobacterium,* and the clinical appearance will then be typical of primary TB.

In contrast, in more severely immunocompromised patients (CD4 counts less than 200 cells/mm^3), the most common presentation is that of primary TB, with ipsilateral adenopathy and consolidation or miliary disease (Fig. 7-19). In a series by Long and associates (74), a primary pattern of disease was identified on chest radiographs in 80% of HIV-positive patients with clinical AIDS and TB, as compared with 30% of HIV-positive non-AIDS patients and 11% of HIV-negative patients. Most striking is the finding of markedly enlarged mediastinal and hilar lymph nodes. Extensive adenopathy may correlate with immunocompromise (72); it is more common with more advanced immunosuppression. Adenopathy is not only seen in primary disease, but it may be a feature of reactivation TB in the AIDS patient, a finding unusual in the non-AIDS patient (74). An increased incidence of normal chest radiographs has also been observed in these patients (68,70). Greenberg and coworkers (70) found 14% of AIDS patients with active TB to have normal chest radiographs; 91% of these patients had CD4 levels lower than 200 cells/mm^3. Because 32% of the chest radiographs in their series proved either normal or were considered atypical, these authors concluded that chest radiography is not a useful screening test in patients with AIDS (70).

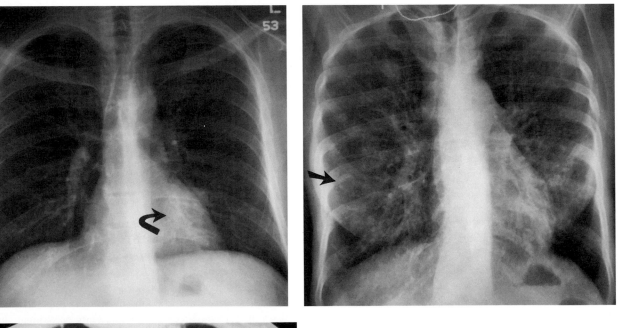

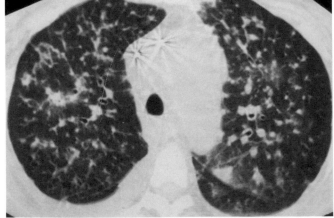

FIG. 7-19. Primary pattern tuberculosis in a 32-year-old HIV-positive man with a CD4 level of 46 cells/mm^3. **A:** Chest radiograph demonstrates the classic pattern of lower lung infiltrate (*arrow*) on the left and ipsilateral infrahilar adenopathy. This patient proved anergic. **B:** Chest radiograph in a hospital worker who became HIV seropositive after a needlestick. Diffusely increased markings consist of small nodules, at least one of which has cavitated (*arrow*), and coarse reticular markings. There is an area of consolidation in the retrocardiac left lower lobe. **C:** A 1.5-mm section shows scattered small nodules and reticular markings. Larger nodules and focal cavitation were confirmed in the lower portions of the lungs. This patient had no history of prior mycobacterial infection, and this disseminated disorder was considered a progressive primary disease.

Some studies have failed to identify a significant difference in appearance of TB depending on the level of immunocompromise. In a study by Leung and associates (68), CT findings in HIV-positive and HIV-negative patients were compared; in addition, these authors further subdivided HIV-positive patients into those with CD4 counts higher than and lower than 200 cells/mm³. Surprisingly, no significant difference could be identified in radiographic appearances between these groups (68).

Tuberculous bronchitis and bronchiolitis, resulting from endobronchial spread of infection, can be seen in either primary or postprimary TB, even in the absence of cavitary disease (27). Endobronchial disease caused by either *M. tuberculosis* or MAC may have identical CT appearances, resulting in a characteristic tree-in-bud pattern (see Fig. 7-18C). Bronchiectasis is common in both primary and reactivation disease. In distinction to bacterial airway infection, airway findings are usually asymmetric, involving both upper and lower portions of the lungs, reflecting both patterns of disease (compare with Figs. 7-1, 7-4, and 7-5). In the absence of cavities, adenopathy, or infiltrates, these changes may be subtle or absent on chest radiographs.

Adenitis from TB has been further characterized by CT. In HIV-positive patients, nodes typically have low-density centers, a feature that may be of diagnostic value. In a retrospective review of 25 HIV-positive patients with documented TB adenitis evaluated by contrast-enhanced CT, the most characteristic finding was the presence of low-density mediastinal and hilar lymph nodes in 80%, usually associated with marked rim enhancement (Fig. 7-20) (75). In this setting, the use of transbronchial needle aspiration (TBNA) has proved especially useful, often allowing the only means of rapid diagnosis (76). Other infections, especially fungal diseases, may produce a similar appearance; as a consequence, definitive diagnosis is still requisite to exclude other organisms as well as drug resistance.

A remarkable feature of TB in patients with HIV infection is the high incidence of extrapulmonary involvement. Since 1987, extrapulmonary TB has been an AIDS-defining condition in HIV-positive patients (77). Extrapulmonary TB is more frequent in advanced AIDS, and it correlates with diminishing CD4 cell counts. In a series reported by Jones and associates (72), extrathoracic TB was present in 70% of HIV-positive patients with TB and CD4 counts lower than or equal to 100 cells/mm³, as compared with 50% and 44%, respectively, in patients with levels less than 200 and less than 300 cells/mm³. Chest roentgenographic features in these patients may be consistent with either a primary or secondary pattern of disease, with miliary disease occurring in about half the cases (78). Extrathoracic disease most frequently manifests as lymphadenitis or disseminated multiorgan disease (see Fig. 7-20). Bone marrow, genitourinary, central nervous system, and spinal diseases are common.

In patients with documented disease, serial chest radiographs should be routinely used to monitor response to therapy. In the setting of AIDS, however, the possibility of unrelated pulmonary processes arising during treatment must be considered. As reported by Small and associates (79), 27% of patients with AIDS and TB developed new HIV-related lung disease during the follow-up period of 3 to 6 months while they were undergoing treatment for TB.

Mycobacterium avium *Complex*

AIDS patients are also at heightened risk for atypical mycobacterial infection. In two cohort studies (6,7), 25% to 35% of patients developed disseminated MAC infection. Those patients with advanced AIDS, usually with CD4 levels lower than 50 cells/mm³, are at particular risk. Unlike infection with *M. tuberculosis,* pulmonary disease due to MAC is rarely an AIDS-defining illness.

Imaging findings in these patients include diffuse, patchy areas of parenchymal consolidation, ill-defined nodules, and cavities (Fig. 7-21). Although adenopathy is variably present, it is not a dominant feature of MAC infection. In up to 21% of HIV-positive patients with documented pulmonary MAC, chest radiographs appear normal (80). This lack of specificity of radiographic findings thwarts the establishment of a specific diagnosis of MAC infection. When comparing the roentgenographic findings in HIV-positive patients with MAC with those of patients with *M. tuberculosis* infection, Modilevsky and colleagues (80) were able prospectively to predict the correct diagnosis in 83% of patients with TB, as opposed to only 25% of those with MAC infections.

Viral Infections

Several viruses infect the lungs of AIDS patients, including CMV and herpes simplex virus, as well as HIV itself (81,82).

Cytomegalovirus Infection

CMV is the most common viral pathogen to cause significant morbidity and mortality in AIDS patients. At autopsy, up to 80% of AIDS patients have evidence of CMV infection (83–85). Despite ubiquitous recovery from the lungs of AIDS patients, CMV has not been considered an important lung pathogen; this reflects a combination of factors, including the difficulty in establishing this diagnosis antemortum. In these same autopsy series (83–85), pulmonary CMV infection was successfully diagnosed ante mortem in only 13% to 24% of those cases with documented CMV pneumonia. Studies suggest an increase in CMV pneumonitis (83,86,87). The reasons for this increase in prevalence are multifactorial and include the routine use of PCP prophylaxis, as well as use of steroid therapy in a variety of AIDS-related clinical settings, and enhanced life expectancy at advanced levels of immunosuppression (5,6,83,86–88). Increasing prevalence may also reflect changing trends in demographics, with CMV reported more commonly as a cause of infection in

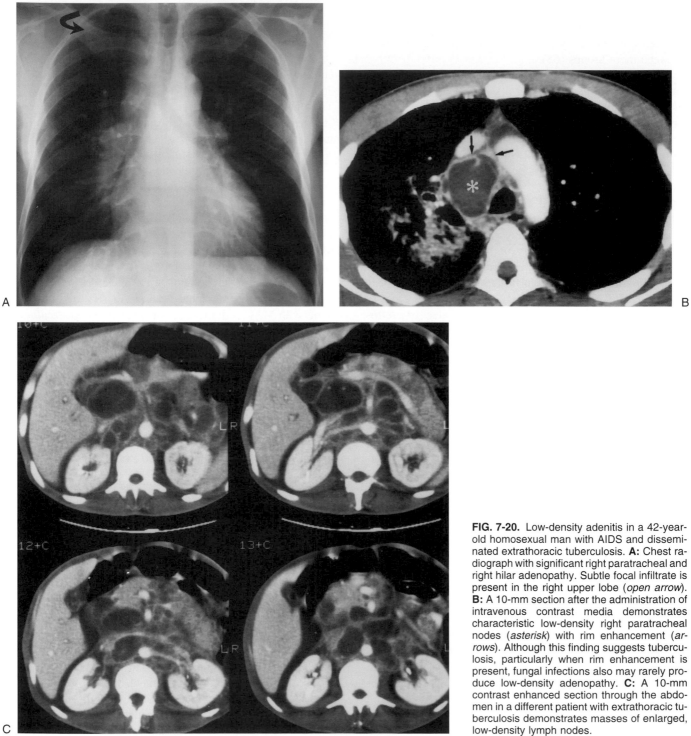

FIG. 7-20. Low-density adenitis in a 42-year-old homosexual man with AIDS and disseminated extrathoracic tuberculosis. **A:** Chest radiograph with significant right paratracheal and right hilar adenopathy. Subtle focal infiltrate is present in the right upper lobe (*open arrow*). **B:** A 10-mm section after the administration of intravenous contrast media demonstrates characteristic low-density right paratracheal nodes (*asterisk*) with rim enhancement (*arrows*). Although this finding suggests tuberculosis, particularly when rim enhancement is present, fungal infections also may rarely produce low-density adenopathy. **C:** A 10-mm contrast enhanced section through the abdomen in a different patient with extrathoracic tuberculosis demonstrates masses of enlarged, low-density lymph nodes.

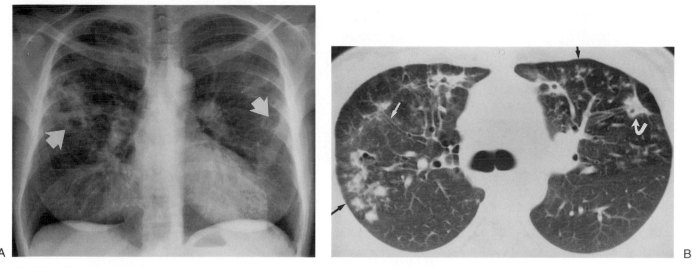

FIG. 7-21. *Mycobacterium avium* complex (MAC) infection in AIDS. **A:** Chest radiograph in a 35-year-old female prostitute with sexually contracted AIDS and MAC pulmonary infection demonstrates diffuse panlobar patchy infiltrates, poorly marginated nodules, and cavitary lesions (*arrows*). **B:** A 5-mm section at the level of the carina demonstrates bronchiectasis in the right upper lobe (*straight white arrow*), clusters of centrilobular nodules of varying sizes representing impacted bronchioles with and without surrounding consolidation (*black arrows*), and cavitary nodules (*curved white arrow*). The appearance is primarily that of infectious airway disease and would also be consistent with *M. tuberculosis* infection in AIDS, but the presence of cavitary nodules would be atypical of pyogenic airway infection.

patients who have acquired HIV through sexual relations (10). CMV occurs in patients with severe immunosuppression, usually with CD4 levels lower than 100 cells/mm^3 (87,89,90). In an evaluation by McGuinness and coworkers of 21 AIDS patients with isolated CMV pneumonia (87), two-thirds of the patients had documented extrathoracic CMV infection, almost half of the patients had KS, and nearly two-thirds of the patients were being treated prophylactically for PCP. All the patients in this series had CD4 levels lower than 50 cells/mm^3. These data suggest that, in advanced AIDS, the presence of the foregoing risk factors should prompt consideration of the rare diagnosis of CMV pneumonia.

Nine patients with AIDS and CMV pneumonia have been described. In all cases, either diffuse ground-glass attenuation or airspace consolidation could be identified. In a few cases, consolidation had a distinctly nodular configuration. Given similar clinical presentations, it is not surprising that these cases were initially thought to represent PCP (90). In a larger series evaluating the CT appearance of CMV pneumonia in 21 AIDS patients, the spectrum of parenchymal findings in the lungs was much broader, with clear overlap with other AIDS-related processes, especially PCP. In this series, the most common CT and radiographic finding was airspace disease (87), most often appearing as ground glass attenuation (Fig. 7-22A), less commonly as dense consolidation. Heterogeneous opacities, primarily reticular, were seen in a few cases. Surprisingly, nodules or masses were identified in 67% of cases (Fig. 7-22B). Small airway disease, including bronchiectasis, bronchial wall thickening, and bronchiolitis (see Fig. 7-22C), was identified in 29% of pa-

tients, in some cases occurring as the sole manifestation of disease. CT patterns of disease corresponded closely to the pathologic changes identified in each patient, especially diffuse alveolar damage, focal interstitial pneumonitis, and airway inflammation.

At present, no general clinical consensus exists regarding an acceptably sensitive and timely means for early diagnosis of CMV pneumonia. Positive viral cultures of BAL fluid have limited value because identification of cytomegalic cells in BAL fluid has a sensitivity ranging only between 3% and 44% (84,87,89). Furthermore, the presence of the virus does not necessarily correlate with organ infection (84). Identification of pathognomonic cells with intranuclear inclusion bodies is generally considered necessary for the diagnosis of CMV pneumonia (84,90). Unfortunately, the sensitivity of transbronchial biopsy is low because the infection may be focal. Transthoracic biopsy has been successfully used to assess areas of nodular consolidation (see Fig. 7-22B) (87). Establishing the diagnosis of CMV pneumonia is critical because this infection responds to antiviral therapy (90). In a series of nine AIDS patients with documented CMV pneumonitis, five underwent treatment, all with dramatic improvement in objective signs and clinical symptoms, and most important, all were discharged from the hospital. At 6-month follow-up, none had evidence of recurrence (90).

Herpes Simplex Virus Infection

Herpes simplex virus is a rare pathogen in the lungs of AIDS patients. Disease may be focal or diffuse; when focal, it often takes the form of necrotizing tracheobronchitis, and

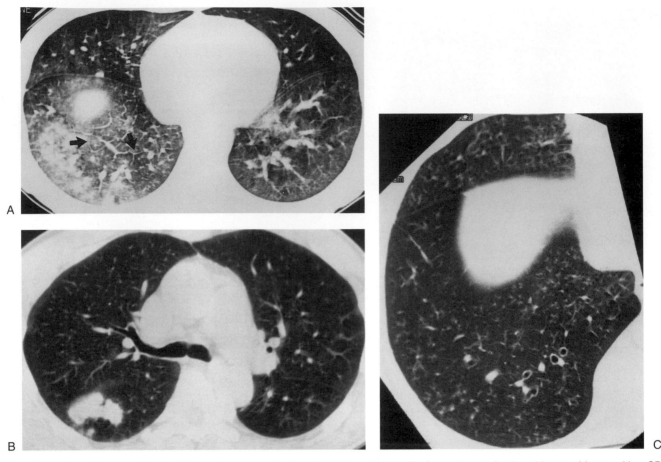

FIG. 7-22. Spectrum of findings in AIDS-related cytomegalovirus (CMV) pneumonitis. **A:** A 1.5-mm section in a 32-year-old man with a CD4 level of 35 cells/mm³ demonstrates areas of ground glass attenuation in the lower portions of the lungs, consistent with alveolitis. Within these areas, interlobular septal thickening is present (*black arrows*), best appreciated in the right lower lobe. Although the commonest manifestation of CMV pneumonia in AIDS, this appearance overlaps with other causes of alveolitis, especially due to *Pneumocystis carinii* pneumonia. **B:** A 5-mm section in a 34-year-old man with AIDS. An irregularly marginated mass is present in the right lower lobe. A transthoracic biopsy specimen (not shown) showed a solid mass of necrotic atypical lymphocytes with numerous cytomegalic inclusion bodies. **C:** Enlargement of a 1-mm section through the right lung base in another patient with CMV infection manifesting as airway disease. Thick-walled, ectatic bronchi are noted, with peripheral ill-defined centrilobular small nodules, consistent with impacted bronchi (compare with Figs. 7-1B, 7-4B, 7-5B, 7-6B, 7-18C, and 7-21B).

when diffuse, it manifests as interstitial pneumonitis (Fig. 7-23) (91). The diagnosis of herpes simplex virus infection is based on identifying typical giant cells and inclusion bodies on tissue and cytology specimens, as well as confirmatory cultures.

Rare Infections

Toxoplasmosis

Infection of the central nervous system by the parasite *Toxoplasma gondii* is a well-recognized complication in AIDS, whereas infection in the lung is rarely reported (92). In a retrospective review of 18,062 HIV-infected patients by Hanson and associates (17) and of 1,297 patients followed prospectively by the Pulmonary Complications of HIV Infection Study Group (11), no cases of pulmonary toxoplasmosis were reported in either cohort. Isolated cases, however, have been reported. In a series summarizing the chest

radiographic findings in 9 patients with this infection, a bilateral, medium to coarse nodular pattern was observed in 6 patients, whereas 3 patients had a fine reticulonodular pattern that was believed to be indistinguishable from PCP. These changes were not associated with adenopathy or effusions (92). The diagnosis can usually be established through identification of organisms in BAL fluid.

Bacillary Angiomatosis

Infection with the bacillus *Bartonella henselae* can produce multiorgan foci of vascular proliferation, seen almost exclusively in AIDS patients. Lesions are generally first recognized as cutaneous or subcutaneous angiomatous or violaceous polypoid nodules that are easily confused with the lesions of KS. The infection may produce lytic bone lesions, soft tissue masses, and low-attenuation liver and spleen lesions. Because of the vascular nature of these lesions, a char-

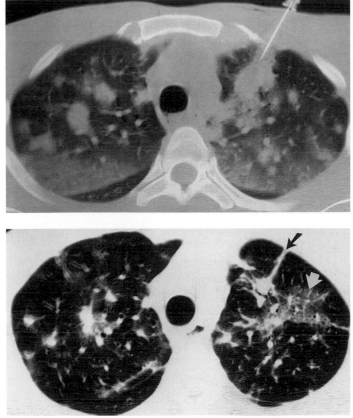

A

B

FIG. 7-23. Herpes simplex virus pneumonitis in a severely dyspneic 34-year-old man with AIDS. **A:** Initial CT with 10-mm collimation obtained during transthoracic needle biopsy demonstrates diffuse, patchy, and nodular infiltrates, with hazy areas of ground glass attenuation. The needle is entering a nodular lesion in the left upper lobe. Transbronchial and transthoracic biopsy samples were positive for characteristic inclusion cells, and culture grew herpes simplex virus, in the absence of other organisms. **B:** The patient experienced significant symptomatic improvement with antiretroviral therapy. CT 1 month later at the same level depicts regression in size of nodular lesions, with signs of organization evidenced by architectural distortion and reticulation (*white arrow*). Note the residual tract from prior transthoracic needle biopsy (*arrow*).

acteristic and strikingly dense enhancement pattern is seen after administration of an intravenous contrast agent (93,94). Thoracic involvement is frequent in this rare infection, manifested as lung nodules, mediastinal adenopathy, and pleural effusions. Intraparenchymal lung nodules may also demonstrate typical dense enhancement after intravenous contrast administration (93). The infection may also present as endobronchial polypoid nodules (95,96). Because of their violaceous appearance, these lesions may be mistaken for KS, and they require biopsy. Of the nine cases reported by Moore and associates (94), eight had lung nodules and six had pleural effusions. Mediastinal adenopathy was identified in six patients, and hilar adenopathy was noted in two patients. All these patients had advanced AIDS, with CD4 levels lower than 200 cells/mm^3 in all cases and lower than 100 cells/mm^3 in eight cases (94). Because these lesions exhibit dramatic and rapid response to antibiotic therapy, establishing pathologic proof of diagnosis is critical (94).

Rhodococcus Infection

Pneumonia in AIDS caused by *Rhodococcus equi* frequently cavitates and may cause empyema, extrapulmonary abscesses, and mediastinal invasion. Associated bacteremia is common, and although the infection is often indolent, it is characterized by frequent antibiotic failure and relapse. Although reports are few, response to prolonged treatment with at least two antibiotics proven effective against the organism has been reported (97). Radiographic findings include single or multiple segmental or lobar infiltrates, often cavitary, and frequently associated with pleural effusion or empyema. Endobronchial dissemination may be evidenced by acinar peribronchial nodules (98).

Strongylodiasis

Strongyloides stercoralis causes an intestinal infection in both immunocompromised and immune intact mammals, including humans. In the immunocompromised AIDS population, the hyperinfection syndrome, with disease dissemination including pulmonary involvement, has been described. Although reports are few (99), 2- to 5-mm lung nodules superimposed on diffuse interstitial infiltrates have been described, associated with recovery of the organism from both sputum and BAL fluid. Lung parenchymal findings regress in response to antibiotic therapy.

Noninfectious AIDS-Related Disease

Neoplastic Disease

Kaposi's Sarcoma

KS is the most common AIDS-related malignant disease. Occurring in approximately 25% of AIDS patients overall,

KS occurs almost exclusively in homosexual or bisexual men or their partners (12), with a male-to-female ratio of 50:1 (7,100). A decline in the incidence of KS has been noted (7,100,101). Presumably, this decrease represents a change in demographics, with relatively fewer patients now falling into previously well-defined risk groups for KS as a result of a reduction in transmission rates because of safe sex practices. Underreporting probably also plays a role, because in many centers mucocutaneous lesions are considered sufficiently characteristic to obviate biopsy.

These unique demographics have long led to speculation that KS in patients with AIDS may be due to an infectious agent (101) or a cofactor, rather than just HIV infection. As early as 1994, a virus in the herpes family was identified as the probable cause of KS (102), and it is referred to as KS-associated herpesvirus or human herpesvirus-8. This virus has subsequently been confirmed as the causative agent, likely in conjunction with other presumably infectious cofactors (103–105).

Pulmonary involvement occurs in up to 50% of patients with epidemic KS (106–108), and it is almost always preceded by documented cutaneous or visceral involvement. However, mucocutaneous involvement is not always recognized before lung involvement, and its absence therefore does not exclude the diagnosis. In a study of 168 AIDS patients with pulmonary KS, Huang and associates (109) found that 15% of patients had pulmonary KS in the absence of mucocutaneous involvement. KS may develop in patients with CD4 counts higher than 200 cells/mm^3, and it is considered a common initial complication of AIDS in homosexual men by some investigators (110). More commonly, however, it afflicts patients with CD4 counts lower than 100 cells/mm^3. In a study of 76 patients by Gruden and associates (106), the median CD4 level was 34 cells/mm^3. Similar results have been reported by Huang and associates (109). This finding is important because it is well established that the tumor becomes more aggressive with increasing immune impairment (104).

Attempts at diagnosis have generally been deemed warranted because palliation has been reported (111–113). Some authors believe that a combination of chemotherapy and local radiation is the most effective modality for alleviation of pain and for optimal cosmetic outcome (114). Investigators have reported that antiretroviral therapy itself may be effective. In an evaluation reported by Leebe and associates of a small cohort of 10 patients who were treated with triple therapy with protease inhibitors (115), 6 complete responses, 2 partial responses, and 2 patients with progressive disease were noted. In 7 of 8 patients, human herpesvirus-8 viremia became undetectable within 2 months of the onset of therapy.

When typical radiologic changes in the thorax are identified in a symptomatic patient with extrathoracic KS, an aggressive bronchoscopic assessment should be performed to identify potential candidates for treatment (111) and to rule out concurrent infection (109). The characteristic presenting symptoms of pulmonary KS are cough, dyspnea, and fever (109), which cannot be distinguished from superimposed infection.

Radiographic findings in pulmonary parenchymal KS have been well described and include characteristic thickening along bronchovascular bundles, often spreading peripherally from a perihilar origin as the tumor progresses (Figs. 7-24–7-26) (106). In patients with known mucocutaneous KS, even subtle radiographic or CT irregularities of the airway walls should be viewed as suspicious for early KS (see Fig. 7-24A,B) (27). With tumor progression, this thickening becomes progressively nodular. The middle and lower portions of the lungs are affected more frequently as compared with the upper portions of the lungs (106,109). Ultimately, coalescence of nodules, especially common in the lower lobes, leads to dense airspace consolidation, possibly on the basis of airway obstruction (see Fig. 7-24C,D). Poorly marinated nodules and interstitial infiltrates (109,116), often representing interlobular septal thickening, are also appreciated at later stages. Interlobular septal thickening (see Figs. 7-24D and 7-26) likely reflects either tumor infiltration or edema secondary to central lymphatic obstruction and may be strikingly asymmetric.

Airway involvement is common in KS, identified in up to 77% of cases with proven thoracic KS at bronchoscopy (see Fig. 7-25). Although endobronchial lesions have been found to predict the presence of parenchymal disease (106,107), the incidence of airway lesions in patients with parenchymal disease is uncertain (106,107). CT is an insensitive method for detecting endobronchial KS, but bulky tumors large enough to cause strider in the upper airways or atelectasis in smaller lobar or segmental bronchi are usually visible as soft tissue filling defects impinging into the lumina of the airways on CT scans (117).

Pleural effusions occur in 30% to 89% of cases (106,109,116,118,119). Lymphadenopathy, both hilar and mediastinal, occurs in 10% to 16% of patients at chest radiography, although markedly enlarged lymph nodes are an unusual manifestation except in advanced disease.

CT findings in parenchymal KS include bronchial wall thickening (117–119), often in conjunction with subtle thickening of the interface between the lung and associated vessels (106) (see Figs. 7-24B and 7-25), representing tumor infiltration along the axial interstitium. In an examination of thin-section CT findings in 53 patients with pulmonary KS, Khalil and associates (118) found spiculated nodules to be the most common abnormality seen in 79% of cases, compared with bronchovascular thickening identified in 66% of cases. In distinction, other investigators have found peribronchovascular nodular infiltrates to be more common (119). Investigators also disagree regarding the prevalence

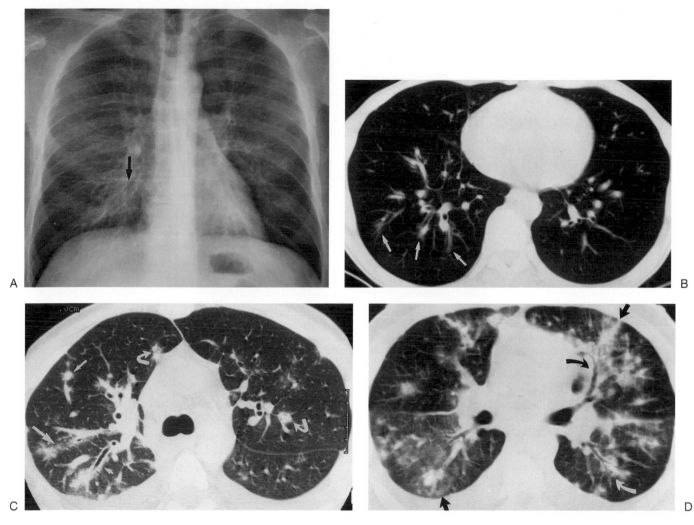

FIG. 7-24. Early and advanced pulmonary Kaposi's sarcoma (KS) in AIDS. **A:** Chest radiograph in a 30-year-old man with cutaneous KS reveals subtle bronchial wall thickening in the infrahilar regions (*arrow*). **B:** A 5-mm section demonstrates mild thickening of the bronchial walls in the right lower lobe and indistinct thickening of the interface between the vessel and the lung (*arrows*), resulting in irregularly marginated, enlarged vessels, findings suggestive of early pulmonary KS (compare with the appearance of normal contralateral airways and vessels). **C:** A 1-mm section in a different patient with more extensive tumor than shown in **A** and **B**. Peribronchovascular soft tissue infiltration is most easily recognized when the bronchi or vessels lie in the plane of section (*arrows*), but it may only be identified as a poorly defined nodular density when viewed in cross section (*curved arrows*). **D:** A 5-mm section in a 32-year-old man with extensive pulmonary KS demonstrates distinctly peribronchial flame or plume-shaped soft tissue densities extending into the lung from the hilar regions (*curved arrow*) resulting in thickened bronchial walls. Some of the poorly marginated peripheral nodules have become confluent (*straight arrows*).

of enlarged lymph nodes on CT, with reported prevalences between 15% and 53% (117–119).

Given the consistency of reported CT findings in patients with parnchymal KS, it is not surprising that KS has proved one of the AIDS-related pulmonary diseases that can be most reliably diagnosed based on imaging findings alone. Assessing the accuracy of CT interpretations in the diagnosis of thoracic complications of AIDS, Hartman and associates (44) evaluated CT scans in 102 patients with proved thoracic disease and in 20 patients without disease by using readers blinded to all clinical data. An accurate diagnosis of KS was confidently established in 90% of cases with KS, exceeded in accuracy only by the diagnosis of PCP, which was accu-

rate in 94% of cases (44). Similar findings have been reported by Kang and associates (43), who also found CT to be superior to chest radiography not only in diagnosing KS, but also in ruling out disease.

KS lesions have characteristic histologic features, comprising spindle-shaped stromal cells, abnormal endothelium lining vascular channels, and slitlike spaces of extravasated red cells (see Fig. 7-25) (104). The gross appearance of both mucocutaneous and tracheobronchial KS is also characteristic, identifiable as raised or macular, erythematous, or violaceous plaques. This appearance is considered virtually pathognomonic, mimicked only rarely by lesions associated with bacillary angiomatosis. As a consequence, although one

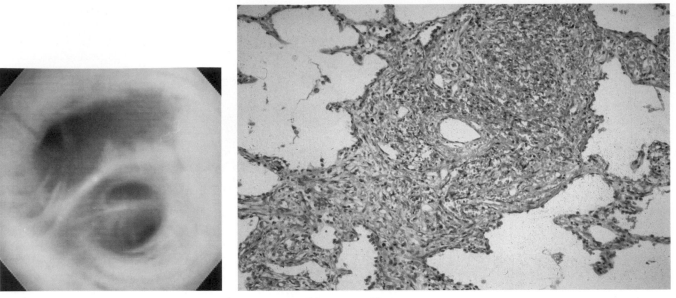

FIG. 7-25. Kaposi's sarcoma: histologic and bronchoscopic correlations. **A:** Bronchoscopic image at the level of the secondary carina shows characteristic appearance of focal erythematous lesions extending from the carina into the proximal portion of the left upper lobe bronchus. **B:** Histologic section obtained at autopsy shows aggregated spindle cells and vascular slits distinctly perivascular in distribution, characteristic of Kaposi's sarcoma. The tumor forms a poorly defined nodular mass that extends peripherally along interstitial pathways.

may safely perform biopsy of these lesions despite their vascular nature, most bronchoscopists experienced with the appearance of endobronchial KS consider the finding of characteristic endobronchial lesions sufficient for diagnosis.

Lymphoma

AIDS-related lymphoma is the second most common malignant disease identified in AIDS patients. It is especially common in the central nervous system, gastrointestinal tract, and bone marrow, but intrathoracic disease is relatively uncommon (120,121), occurring in as few as 10% of cases in some series (122). In fact, reports have suggested that the prevalence of intrathoracic lymphoma may be higher than previously thought. Eisner and associates (123), for example, found evidence of intrathoracic disease at autopsy in 71% of 38 cases, only 5.8% of whom had disease diagnosed clinically. In this series, the lungs and pleura were the most common extranodal sites of involvement. The incidence of lymphomas in AIDS patients is increasing, a trend that is likely to continue given longer life expectancies in HIV-positive patients and relatively longer latency periods required for the development of neoplasms (124).

Three histologic types have been reported: non-Hodgkin's lymphoma, Hodgkin's lymphoma, and Burkitt-type lymphoma. These tumors tend to occur at younger ages in AIDS

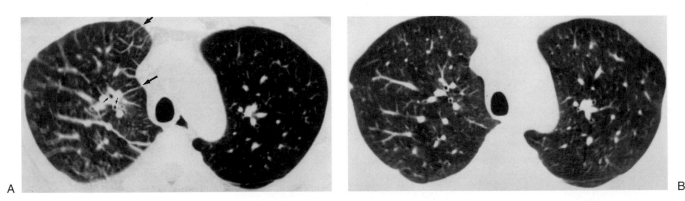

FIG. 7-26. Interlobular septal thickening in Kaposi's sarcoma (KS): before and after treatment. **A:** High-resolution CT in a 36-year-old man with pulmonary KS depicts increased markings in the right lung primarily resulting from thickened interlobular septa (*large black arrows*), but also demonstrating thickening of the right suprahilar bronchovascular bundle (*small black arrows*). Thickened interlobular septa in KS likely reflects tumor infiltration or edema secondary to central lymphatic obstruction. **B:** Follow-up CT at the same level 2 months after chemotherapy shows marked regression in the peribronchovascular tumor and resolution of interlobular septal thickening. The patient's dyspnea had also improved.

patients as compared with the general population, and 75% are at an advanced stage (stage III or IV) at presentation. Most patients have systemic symptoms of fever, night sweats, or weight loss (125). Epstien-Barr virus genome has been identified in 50% to 85% of AIDS-related non-Hodgkin's lymphomas (125,126).

Non-Hodgkin's lymphoma, which is usually of immunoblastic, large cell, small noncleaved cell, or Burkitt type, is the most common AIDS-related lymphoma, accounting for approximately 90% of cases (124). It occurs at more advanced stages of immunosuppression, usually with CD4 levels less than 100 cells/mm^3 (125). Despite advanced immunosuppression in most cases, lymphoma is an AIDS-defining diagnosis, occurring as the index disease in up to 39% of cases (123). Most of these tumors are high-grade lymphomas of B-cell origin, are highly aggressive with poorly differentiated histologic subtypes, and are associated with a poor prognosis. Fewer than than 10% of patients survive beyond 2 years after diagnosis (125). Investigators have speculated that HIV-induced immune dysregulation and chronic perturbation of the immune system lead to increased B-cell stimulation, with uncontrolled proliferation from T-cell impairment (125).

Hodgkin's lymphoma tends to occur early in AIDS, usually when the CD4 cell counts are greater than 200 cells/mm^3, and the association with Epstien-Barr virus is less clear. In some studies, Hodgkin's disease is not clearly linked to Epstien-Barr virus infection (125), whereas other studies found a higher association between Epstien-Barr virus and Hodgkin's than non-Hodgkin's lymphoma (124). Whether the incidence of Hodgkin's lymphoma is increased in the AIDS population is unclear, and consequently this disorder is not included as an index disease by the CDC. When diagnosed, Hodgkin's disease is characterized by advanced clinical stage, high histologic grade, and frequent bone marrow involvement at presentation (124).

Intrathoracic involvement of AIDS-related lymphoma is typically extranodal, with parenchymal disease and pleural effusions more commonly identified. Diffuse nodules are the most common pulmonary parenchymal presentation (120,123,127). Characteristically, nodules are discrete, single, or multiple, and they are well defined without significant adenopathy (Fig. 7-27). A solitary, well-defined pulmonary nodule is common, and it should be considered suggestive of AIDS-related lymphoma (120,128). Up to 10% of lymphomatous lung masses may cavitate (see Fig. 7-27) (128). Masses and nodules are often peripheral. In distinction, interstitial infiltrates in the absence of masses are only rarely described. Dense airspace consolidation may also be identified (121,125,127).

Whereas adenopathy is generally considered rare, especially as a presenting finding (122), studies have suggested that the incidence of thoracic adenopathy may be much higher than previously thought, especially when assessed by CT or at autopsy (123). Endoluminal airway disease is generally considered a rare manifestation of AIDS-related lymphoma (129,130). In the series of Eisner and associates (123), however, of 16 patients undergoing bronchoscopy, 19% had visible endobronchial lesions. CT findings in this group were nonspecific and included areas of tracheal irregularity and rare polypoid endobronchial lesions (Fig. 7-28) (27).

Pleural effusions are commonly associated with AIDS-related thoracic lymphoma, seen in approximately 25% to 73% of cases (120,123,128). In a series reported by Blunt and associates of 20 proved or suspected cases of AIDS-related lymphoma (128), 3 patients had extrathoracic masses that showed direct spread into the mediastinum (see Fig. 7-26).

A rare form of AIDS-related B-cell lymphoma presenting as pleural, pericardial, or peritoneal effusions in the absence of a soft tissue tumor has been described (104) and is known as body cavity–based lymphoma. A comparison of 42 patients with AIDS-related lymphomas with 151 HIV-negative patients with lymphomas found a total of 8 body cavity–based lymphomas among the AIDS patients; all 8 cases were positive for KS-associated herpesvirus, the herpesvirus implicated in KS. In distinction, all remaining 185 specimens, including all from the 151 HIV-negative patients, were negative for the virus (131).

As noted, the high incidence of thoracic AIDS-related lymphoma in autopsy series, in contrast to clinical series, suggests that this entity is underdiagnosed antemortum (123). In the autopsy series of Eisner and associates (123), only 5% of cases had thoracic involvement documented during life. This finding is not surprising, given the wide range of radiologic findings outlined earlier. As a consequence, diagnosis generally requires histopathologic confirmation. The role of transbronchial biopsy for histologic confirmation is controversial. Whereas transbronchial biopsy has been reported only rarely to provide a tissue diagnosis (122), some investigators report a diagnostic yield of 58% (123). Diagnostic material also may be obtained through transthoracic needle biopsy (128) or open lung biopsy (122,132). Flow cytometry analysis of pleural fluid or needle aspiration specimens may increase the diagnostic yield for lymphoma as well. In a series reported by Gruden and associates of 32 AIDS patients with focal lung abnormalities on which percutaneous transthoracic needle biopsy was performed (133), a specific diagnosis was obtained in 27 cases, 3 of which proved to be AIDS-related lymphoma. In distinction, none of the nondiagnostic cases proved to have lymphoma. Although numbers reported to date are small, Eisner and associates (123) noted a 75% diagnostic yield by pleural fluid cytology in 8 patients, equaling their yield from open lung biopsy. Larger prospective studies are needed to support these findings.

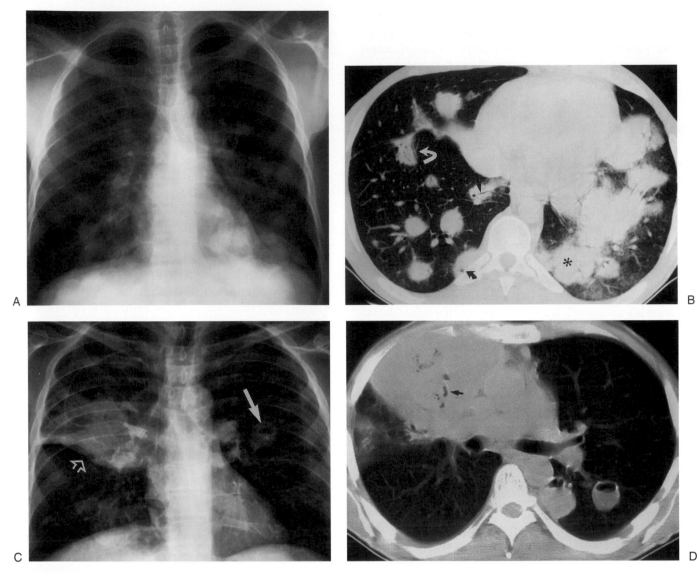

FIG. 7-27. AIDS-related lymphoma in the thorax. **A:** Chest radiograph demonstrates multiple bilateral nodules in the absence of significant adenopathy in this 34-year-old male intravenous drug abuser with non-Hodgkin's lymphoma in the lungs. This tumor was determined by immunohistochemical stains to be Epstein-Barr virus driven. **B:** A 5-mm section demonstrates well-defined multilobar lung nodules, some of which surround small peripheral airways (*small black arrow* and *curved white arrow*). Others are becoming confluent, especially in the left lower lung (*asterisk*). Note the suggestion of minimal cavitation in a right lower lung nodule (*curved black arrow*). **C:** Chest radiograph in a different AIDS patient with lymphoma demonstrates cavitary nodules in the left midlung (*arrow*) and masslike consolidation in the right upper lobe producing caudal displacement of the minor fissure (*open arrow*). **D:** A 7-mm section through the middle portions of the lungs depicts cavitary nodules in the superior segment of the left lower lobe, as well as dense consolidation in the right upper lobe, within which air bronchograms and minimal cavitation (*arrow*) are noted.

Lung Carcinoma

Because clinical differences in HIV-infected patients with lung cancer have been noted in some studies, an association with HIV infection is often raised (134). These patients often present at a younger age (135–137), and at a later stage (135,137), compared with the general population. Nonetheless, to date, despite conflicting data, no convincing evidence is available to indicate that the incidence of bronchogenic carcinoma is significantly increased in AIDS patients. Chan and associates (138) compared the incidence of bronchogenic carcinoma in young patients in risk groups for AIDS in the pre-AIDS years of 1976 to 1979 to a matched group of high-risk patients in the AIDS period of 1987 to 1990 and found no increased incidence of lung cancer. Furthermore, these same authors found no difference in clinical presentation, including age, between the two groups in their study (138). In fact, cell types of lung cancers in AIDS patients proved similar to those in young HIV-seronegative patients, with a predominance of adenocarcinoma (135–137). However, these tumors are often poorly differentiated and grow rapidly, with doubling times sometimes suggestive of an infectious process.

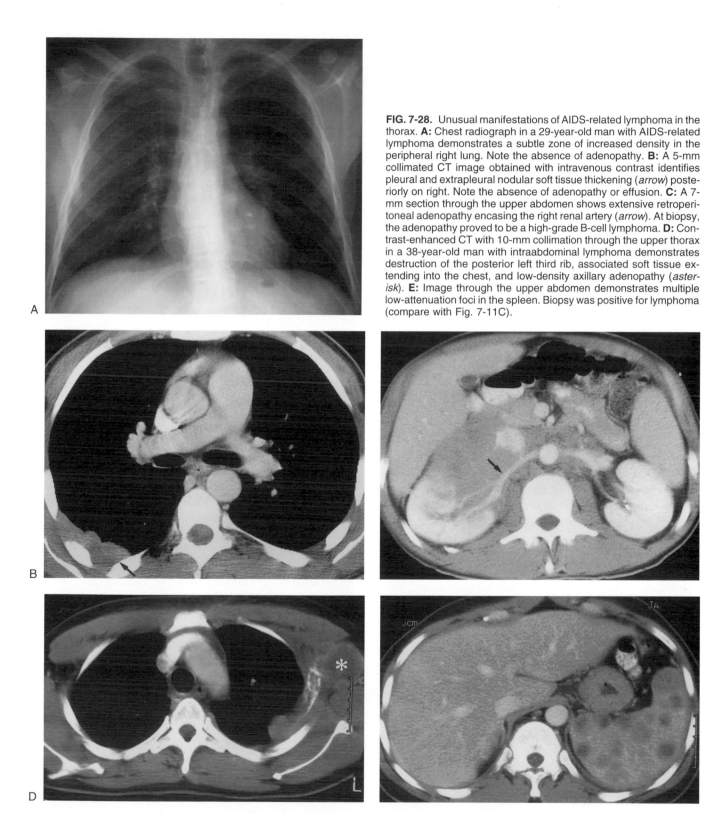

FIG. 7-28. Unusual manifestations of AIDS-related lymphoma in the thorax. **A:** Chest radiograph in a 29-year-old man with AIDS-related lymphoma demonstrates a subtle zone of increased density in the peripheral right lung. Note the absence of adenopathy. **B:** A 5-mm collimated CT image obtained with intravenous contrast identifies pleural and extrapleural nodular soft tissue thickening (*arrow*) posteriorly on right. Note the absence of adenopathy or effusion. **C:** A 7-mm section through the upper abdomen shows extensive retroperitoneal adenopathy encasing the right renal artery (*arrow*). At biopsy, the adenopathy proved to be a high-grade B-cell lymphoma. **D:** Contrast-enhanced CT with 10-mm collimation through the upper thorax in a 38-year-old man with intraabdominal lymphoma demonstrates destruction of the posterior left third rib, associated soft tissue extending into the chest, and low-density axillary adenopathy (*asterisk*). **E:** Image through the upper abdomen demonstrates multiple low-attenuation foci in the spleen. Biopsy was positive for lymphoma (compare with Fig. 7-11C).

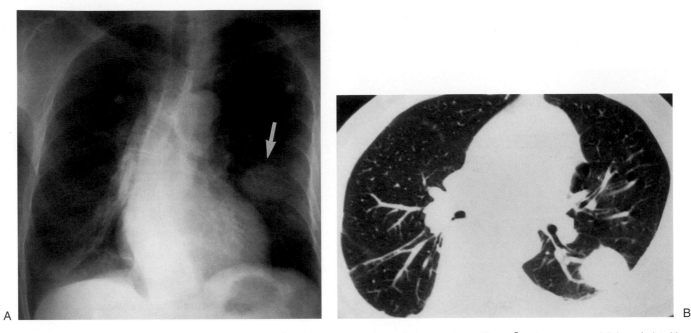

FIG. 7-29. Bronchogenic adenocarcinoma in a 46-year-old man with AIDS (CD4 cell count 270 cells/mm^3), who was complaining of pleuritic chest pain. He had a 38-pack per year smoking history. **A:** Chest radiograph demonstrates a discrete left lower lobe nodule (*arrow*). Because of immune suppression and relatively young age, infectious and neoplastic AIDS-related processes were considered, despite an appearance that would otherwise suggest lung cancer. **B:** CT confirms a solitary mass in the left lower lung. Transthoracic biopsy showed adenocarcinoma. Diagnosis of lung cancer is often delayed in AIDS patients because of the high frequency of other processes that may have similar findings.

Because these tumors may present earlier than most AIDS-related infections and neoplasms, the underlying diagnosis of HIV infection may be unknown. In a series of 13 patients identified by Gruden and associates (139), 10 patients had no history of an AIDS index disease, and in 3 patients, the HIV status was unknown before the diagnosis of lung cancer. Fewer than half of the HIV-positive patients reported by Fishman and colleagues (140) had AIDS at the time of cancer diagnosis.

Radiographic appearances usually do not differ significantly from bronchogenic carcinoma in the HIV-negative population. A lung mass or infiltrate with associated ipsilateral hilar and variable mediastinal adenopathy is the most common presentation (Fig. 7-29) (134,135,137). In the largest series to date by Fishman and colleagues (140), of 30 patients with lung cancer and HIV infection, 60% of patients had peripheral tumors, 94% of which were in the upper lobes. This pattern was more common in patients with prior TB or PCP, whereas those patients without prior OIs more characteristically had central masses, raising a potential role of postinflammatory scarring as a possible etiologic factor (140). Although other investigators have also reported an upper lung predominance, involvement of the upper lobes is also more common in non-AIDS patients with lung cancer (137).

A report by White and associates (137) described extensive pleural disease as the primary manifestation of lung cancer in 35% of 23 HIV-positive patients studied, with pleural disease the sole radiographic abnormality in 5 pa-

tients. CT evaluation proved valuable in these patients; in 7 of 8 patients with pleural disease, underlying evidence of a malignant process, obscured at chest radiography, was identified. Based on these data, investigators have suggested that lung cancer should be a diagnostic consideration in the HIV-positive patient with extensive pleural disease.

Whereas the incidence of lung cancer is not increased in the HIV-infected population, tobacco use remains the primary risk factor for developing lung carcinoma in all groups (134,135,139,140). Many patients within risk groups for HIV infection, particularly drug abusers (135,139), have a high incidence of cigarette smoking. The diagnosis of lung cancer may not be considered for two reasons: (a) these patients may be younger than usual for those with bronchogenic carcinoma; and (b) the frequency of malignant diseases and infections associated with AIDS that have radiographic findings similar to those of bronchogenic carcinoma is high (134). Even in young patients, lung carcinoma should be ruled out in those with peripheral lesions that do not respond to antibiotics (140).

Noninfectious Nonmalignant Disease

Lymphoproliferative Disorders

Various polyclonal lymphoproliferative disorders affect the lungs of HIV-positive patients (141–145). Many of these cases have been diagnosed as lymphocytic interstitial pneumonitis (LIP), the most common of these unusual disorders, despite failure to fulfill strict pathologic diagnostic criteria.

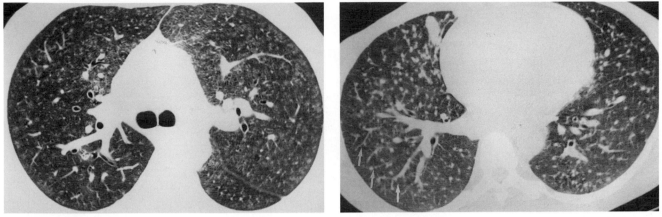

FIG. 7-30. Lymphoproliferative disorders in AIDS. **A:** A 44-year-old mildly dyspneic woman with AIDS contracted from a blood transfusion. Her CD4 cell count was 123 cells/mm³. A 1.5-mm section shows innumerable centrilobular nodules of 2 to 4 mm. These nodules are poorly marginated and of a hazy, ground glass attenuation. At biopsy, poorly formed granulomas secondary to lymphocytic interstitial pneumonitis were identified. **B:** Denser nodules in the same size range are seen on the 1.5-mm sections in this 36-year-old man with atypical lymphoproliferative disorder. Nodules are identified throughout the interstitium; the peribronchovascular distribution results in nodular vascular margins (*arrows*) (compare with Fig. 7-2C,D).

McGuinness and associates (142) examined the CT findings and pathologic findings in nine patients with AIDS or HIV infection and pulmonary lymphoproliferative disorders and found that, whereas radiographic findings were similar, pathologically three unique entities could be identified. These are classic LIP as well as two other categories, atypical lymphoproliferative disorder and mucosa-associated lymphoid tissue lymphoma.

Infrequently associated with adult AIDS patients, LIP is an AIDS-defining index disease in children less than 13 years old (146). Because LIP also occurs in adult patients who are not infected with HIV, the association in adults with AIDS has proved controversial. In fact, LIP may represent different disease entities in patients with and without AIDS. In the non-AIDS population, LIP is a prelymphomatous condition, whereas in AIDS, it follows a more indolent course, rarely, if ever, evolving into lymphoma. The process is characterized by interstitial infiltration with mature, bland, polyclonal lymphocytes, which may form poorly defined nodules or granulomas. Whereas the infiltrate has some predilection for the peribronchovascular tissue, the lesion is notable for the absence of airspace disease.

Atypical lymphoproliferative disorder is defined by diffuse interstitial infiltration with a polymorphous population of atypical lymphoid cells, including immunoblasts and occasional mitotic figures. Mucosa-associated lymphoid tissue lymphoma, previously referred to as pseudolymphoma, is defined as multiple small, nodular masses of atypical lymphoid cells, which demonstrate infiltration of the bronchial epithelium resulting in so-called lymphoepithelial lesions. Although the disease is considered a low-grade lymphoma, its lesions may also be polyclonal.

Lymphoproliferative disorders may be an early manifestation of HIV infection and may predate OIs. McGuinness and coworkers (142) found that only one of the patients in their series had a history of pulmonary OI, although eight of their nine patients had clinical AIDS. Symptoms range from mild complaints, such as cough and mild dyspnea, to marked respiratory compromise. Because the typical clinical course is indolent, patients may remain stable for months to years without treatment.

In the series reported by McGuinness and associates (142), the predominant finding at CT was ill-defined 2- to 4-mm nodules, frequently peribronchovascular in distribution, seen in 89% of cases regardless of histologic subtype (Fig. 7-30). Two patients in this series also had areas of ground glass attenuation. Similar findings have been reported by Carignan and associates (127). Of the 3 AIDS patients included in this assessment of lymphoproliferative disorders in immunocompromised patients, 2 had LIP, whereas the other had documented lymphoid hyperplasia. In another series of 16 patients with LIP and AIDS or HIV infection reported by Oldham and associates (147), both fine and coarse reticular or reticulonodular opacities were seen in 7 patients, whereas 9 patients had reticular or reticulonodular opacities with superimposed alveolar infiltrates on chest radiographs.

Bronchiolitis Obliterans

Bronchiolitis obliterans with and without organizing pneumonia in the absence of infection is a rare cause of pulmonary disease in AIDS patients (148–151). Because a definitive diagnosis usually requires an open lung biopsy, the true incidence of this disease is unknown. Bronchiolitis obliterans has been described at autopsy in 36% of patients with AIDS and PCP, presumably as a response to the pulmonary infection (41). Other authors have speculated that unsuspected bronchiolitis may cause the small airway disease commonly detected at pulmonary function testing in these

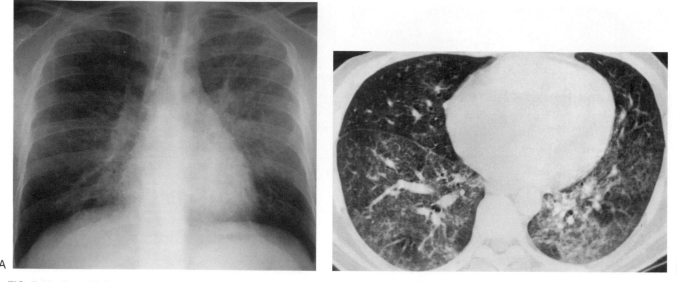

FIG. 7-31. Bronchiolitis obliterans in a dyspneic 35-year-old man with AIDS. **A:** Chest radiograph demonstrates hazy and reticular increased lung markings. The pattern resembles that seen in *Pneumocystis carinii* pneumonia (PCP). **B:** CT scan with 1.5-mm collimation through the lung bases confirms areas of hazy ground glass attenuation, within which reticulonodular markings are noted. The CT appearance also mimics that of PCP (compare with Fig. 7-1C,D). Pathognomonic endoluminal inflammatory polyps were identified at biopsy. No infectious organisms were isolated.

patients, in the absence of infection (152,153). Pathologic differentiation between bronchiolitis obliterans with organizing pneumonia and more frequent causes of pulmonary infiltrates is important clinically because patients typically respond well to steroid therapy, as do patients with bronchiolitis obliterans with organizing pneumonia associated with other underlying causes (148–151).

Bronchiolitis obliterans with organizing pneumonia is similar in appearance in both AIDS and non-AIDS populations. Most commonly, it appears as bilateral foci of parenchymal consolidation, occasionally migratory (Fig. 7-31) (148–151); less commonly, this condition may manifest either as ill-defined nodular infiltrates (151) or on CT as subtle diffuse reticular infiltrates and scattered centrilobular nodules.

DIAGNOSTIC STRATEGIES

Diagnostic pathways, designed to be practical and cost-effective, vary among institutions (154). This practice variation reflects potential differences in the relative cost and availability of various tests, the sensitivity of a given test within a specific institution, patient and physician preferences and experience, and the local prevalence and pretest probability of a given disease. Modifications of imaging strategies also reflect relative weighting of diagnostic possibilities based on clinical considerations and risk factors, as discussed in preceding sections.

Screening of asymptomatic HIV-positive persons and AIDS patients with chest radiography has a low diagnostic yield. Periodic radiographs obtained in more than 1,000 asymptomatic HIV-positive people over 1 year resulted in

a yield of only 2% with abnormal radiographs. Only 5.2% developed a new pulmonary diagnosis within 2 months of a screening radiograph, and in only 20% of these patients was the screening radiograph abnormal (155). Although it is apparent that such a low diagnostic yield does not warrant the use of routine screening, the CDC does recommend that screening radiographs be obtained in anergic HIV-positive patients or in those who are positive for purified protein derivative, even when they are asymptomatic (156).

In distinction, symptomatic patients are always evaluated with chest radiographs and, most often, sputum culture. If no pathogen is identified, or if treatment of a known pathogen fails, further evaluation is requisite. In this setting, CT may play a central role (a) to identify occult disease (see Fig. 7-6; Fig. 7-32), (b) to provide specific diagnostic information, or (c) to rule out significant intrathoracic disease.

Occult diseases for which CT may play a role include early PCP as well as miliary TB and fungal infections. CT is also of value by disclosing unsuspected adenopathy. In patients with nonspecific radiographic findings, CT may allow specific diagnoses in cases of pyogenic airway disease, including patients with endobronchial spread of TB, as well as cystic PCP. Also included in this category are patients with characteristic CT findings of peribronchvascular disease indicative of pulmonary KS. When CT findings are nonspecific, CT may still play an invaluable role by further directing the diagnostic workup by identifying optimal sites and methods for obtaining biopsies and or performing BAL. In our experience, CT is especially valuable in patients for whom TBNA is planned. Equally important, a negative high-resolution CT confidently allows exclusion of active disease (44,45).

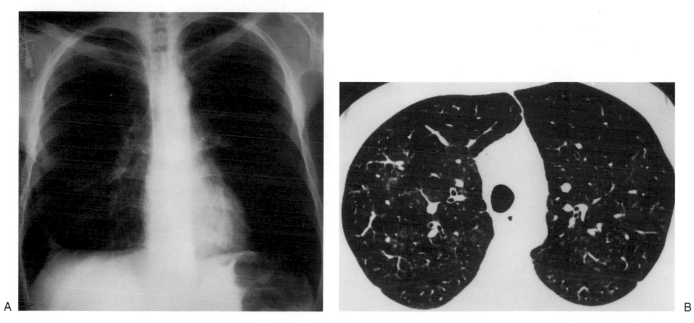

FIG. 7-32. Radiographically occult *Pneumocystis carinii* pneumonia (PCP). **A:** Chest radiograph in a 44-year-old HIV-positive man with no history of opportunistic infection. The right hemidiaphragm is tenting after remote pyogenic infection. The lungs are otherwise clear. **B:** High-resolution CT through the upper portions of the lungs demonstrates small foci of ground glass attenuation, not visible on chest radiograph, but suspicious in this setting for PCP. Bronchoalveolar lavage confirmed *Pneumocystis carinii* infection.

As documented by Gruden and associates (45), even when one has a high clinical suspicion of PCP, this diagnosis is frequently inaccurate. In this series, only 12% of patients with clinically suspected disease proved to have PCP. In distinction, CT revealed findings characteristic of infectious small airway disease in 45% of cases for which empiric treatment with antibiotics alone was indicated.

Assessing the accuracy of CT in the diagnosis of thoracic complications of AIDS, Hartman and associates (44) noted that an accurate diagnosis of PCP could be confidently established in 94% of cases, and a correct diagnosis of KS was established in 90% of cases. Similar findings have been reported by Kang and associates (43). Given the greater accuracy of CT for evaluating disease in HIV-positive persons and in AIDS patients, in our experience, it is of value to subdivide findings further into select radiographic and CT categories. Acknowledging that multiple combinations of these findings are frequently present, these include patients with predominant findings of reticular or ground-glass infiltrates, diffuse nodules, solitary or multiple masses, lobar or segmental consolidation, and intrathoracic adenopathy (Table 7-1).

Diagnostic considerations for small nodules include infections such as disseminated TB and fungal diseases such as histoplasmosis or cryptococcosis. Noninfectious lymphoproliferative disorders such as LIP may also present as small lung nodules. Occasionally, infectious airway disease is appreciated as small nodules at chest radiography, representing impacted small airways, although other signs of airway dis-

ease, including bronchial wall thickening, are usually present. Rarely, PCP may present with a nodular pattern.

In patients presenting with miliary disease, diagnostic considerations include both mycobacterial and fungal infections, especially histoplasmosis. Adenopathy, when present, typically appears necrotic, with central low density and rim enhancement after intravenous contrast enhancement. As mentioned previously, the yield of sputum examination in AIDS with miliary TB and histoplasmosis is low, often necessitating biopsy. Rarely, miliary disease is the predominant finding in patients with PCP.

Diagnostic considerations in AIDS patients with solitary or multiple masses again include fungal infections, including aspergillosis and cryptococcosis. Mycobacterial infection also may present as poorly marginated lung nodules, occasionally with surrounding zones of ground glass attenuation (so-called halo sign). Another infectious cause to be considered in the appropriate clinical setting is pyogenic infection from septic emboli. Rarely, PCP can present as large nodules. Non-Hodgkin's lymphoma and occasionally KS also may present as lung masses. Although direct association with HIV infection remains controversial, lung cancer should always be included as a possible diagnosis (137).

Given the large number of potential causes of single or multiple masses, in most cases biopsy is indicated for definitive diagnosis, assuming bacteriologic studies are negative. If lesions are accessible, in our experience and that of others, transthoracic biopsy is generally preferable to fiber optic bronchoscopy (133,157). When bronchoscopy is planned, CT may play an additional role by providing a guide before

TABLE 7-1. *Radiographic patterns in AIDS: differential diagnosis*

Pattern	Diseases	CT correlations
Normal	PCP	Patchy ground glass attenuation
	Mycobacterial or fungal infections	Miliary disease; occult cavities; low-density nodes; isolated nodules
Diffuse reticular or ground glass infiltrates	PCP	Diffuse ground glass attenuation +/− cysts; emphysema; occult pneumothorax
	Pyogenic airway disease	Diffuse, symmetric tree-in-bud appearance
	CMV	Diffuse ground glass attenuation
	PCP plus other infections (CMV, MAI, MTb, fungi)	Diffuse ground glass +/− cavities; nodules; bronchiectasis; adenopathy
	KS	Peribronchovascular infiltrates or nodules +/− coalescence; subpleural nodules +/− effusions; diffuse consolidation; thickened secondary lobules; diffuse adenopathy
Focal infiltrates	Pyogenic bacteria PCP	Occult cavitation; parapneumonic effusions
	Mycobacterial or fungal infections Non-Hodgkin's lymphoma	Low-density nodes; occult cavitation; endobronchial spread
Diffuse nodules	Mycobacterial infection	Focal endobronchial spread (tree-in-bud appearance); miliary disease
	LIP	Random centrilobular ground glass nodules
	Lymphoma	Typically well-defined nodules +/− cavitation
	Fungal infection	Miliary disease
	Septic emboli	Subpleural nodules in varying stages of cavitation
	KS	Peribronchovascular infiltrates or nodules +/− adenopathy, effusions
Solitary nodule	Fungal infection	Usually well defined; low-density (nonenhancing) after intravenous contrast, +/− cavitation, halo sign
	Lymphoma	Usually well defined +/− cavitation
	Lung cancer	+/− Spiculation, cavitation
Adenopathy	Mycobacterial or fungal infection	Low-density nodes +/− rim enhancement
	Lymphoma	Nonspecific appearance
	KS	Nonspecific appearance

CMV, cytomegaloviral pneumonia; KS, Kaposi's sarcoma; LIP, lymphocytic interstitial pneumonitis; MAI, *Mycobacterium avium-intracellulare;* MTb, *Mycobacterium tuberculosis;* PCP, *Pneumocystis carinii* pneumonia.

TBNA in patients with coexistent adenopathy (76). If flexible bronchoscopy and biopsy fail to establish a diagnosis, then open lung biopsy or video assisted thoracoscopic surgery should be performed.

Dense lobar or segmental consolidation in the AIDS patient is primarily due to infectious causes, including bacterial, mycobacterial, and fungal disease. Rarely, neoplasms such as KS and lymphoma may result in dense areas of consolidation (see Fig. 7-27). CT is indicated when the diagnosis is not established based on clinical examination and sputum or blood cultures of sputum or when empiric antibiotic therapy fails. CT may suggest specific diagnoses such as TB when low-density lymph nodes are identified; however, in this setting, the main value of CT is in assessing airway patency.

Although adenopathy in the absence of parenchymal disease can be seen in association with fungal infections, in particular with cryptococcosis or histoplasmosis, mycobacterial infection remains most common (76,158). Rarely, lymphoma and KS may present as isolated adenopathy; the clinician should also include lung cancer in the differential

diagnosis (76,137). As previously mentioned, CT is indicated in patients with adenopathy primarily to provide a guide for bronchoscopy. Investigators have shown that TBNA biopsy may be an efficacious and cost-effective method for establishing both histologic and bacteriologic diagnoses. In a series of 44 procedures in 41 HIV-positive patients, Harkin and associates (76) reported that a diagnosis was established 52% of the time at TBNA. In 48% of patients, this was the only diagnostic specimen. All these patients had at least 3 negative sputum samples.

Isolated pleural effusions typically occur in patients with TB. The differential diagnosis includes KS and lymphoma, including body cavity–based lymphoma. Underlying bacterial pneumonia should also be considered. In most cases, the finding of a lymphocytic exudative effusion is sufficiently suggestive of mycobacterial infection to warrant empiric anti-TB therapy pending the results of pleural fluid cultures and biopsy. Immediate diagnosis of TB based on smear of pleural fluid is achieved in only 15% of cases, whereas pleural biopsy demonstrates acid-fast bacillus (AFB) in 69% of cases, and granulomas are identified in 88% of cases

(159). Although pleural fluid culture is positive in 91% of cases, reliance on this results in unacceptable delay in diagnosis (159). Whereas pleural biopsy or cytology is rarely diagnostic in patients with KS, the presence of hemorrhagic fluid is strongly suggestive of the diagnosis. In this setting, CT may be of considerable value by demonstrating characteristic parenchymal lesions, supporting initiation of therapy. In distinction, pleural lymphoma may be diagnosed at thoracentesis. Although the numbers are small, Eisner and associates (123) reported a 75% diagnostic yield by pleural fluid cytology in eight patients, a finding equaling their yield from open lung biopsy.

REFERENCES

1. Centers for Disease Control and Prevention. Update: trends in AIDS incidence, deaths, and prevalence—United States, 1996. *MMWR Morb Mortal Wkly Rep* 1997;46:165–173.
2. McGuinness G. Changing trends in the pulmonary manifestations of AIDS. *Radiol Clin North Am* 1997;35:1029–1082.
3. Naidich DP, McGuinness G. Pulmonary manifestations of AIDS: CT and radiographic correlations. *Radiol Clin North Am* 1991;29: 999–1017.
4. Centers for Disease Control and Prevention. 1993 revised classification system for HIV infection and expanded surveillance definition for AIDS among adolescents and adults *MMWR Morb Mortal Wkly Rep* 1993;41:1–19.
5. Miller R. HIV-associated respiratory diseases. *Lancet* 1996;348: 307–312.
6. Hoover DR, Saah AJ, Bacellar H, et al. Clinical manifestations of AIDS in the era of *Pneumocystis* prophylaxis. *N Engl J Med* 1993; 329:1922–1926.
7. Katz MH, Hessol NA, Buchbinder SP, Hirozawa A, O'Malley P, Holmberg SD. Temporal trends of opportunistic infections and malignancies in homosexual men with AIDS. *J Infect Dis* 1994;170: 198–202.
8. Centers for Disease Control and Prevention. Update: AIDS among women. *JAMA* 1995;273:767–768.
9. Centers for Disease Control and Prevention. Update: acquired immunodeficiency syndrome—United States, 1994. *JAMA* 1995;273:692.
10. Markowitz GS, Concepcion L, Factor SM, Borczuk AC. Autopsy patterns of disease among subgroups of an inner-city Bronx AIDS population. *J Acquir Immune Defic Syndr Hum Retrovirol* 1996;13: 48–54.
11. Wallace JM, Hansen NI, Lavange L, et al. Respiratory disease trends in the pulmonary complications of HIV infection study cohort. *Am J Respir Crit Care Med* 1997;155:72–80.
12. Huang L, Stansell JD. AIDS and the lung. *Med Clin North Am* 1996; 80:755–800.
13. Hirschtick RE, Glassroth J, Jordan MC, et al. Bacterial pneumonia in persons infected with the human immunodeficiency virus. *N Engl J Med* 1995;333:845–851.
14. Magnenat J-L, Nicod LP, Auckenthaler R, Junod AF. Mode of presentation and diagnosis of bacteria pneumonia in human immunodeficiency virus–infected patients. *Am Rev Respir Dis* 1991;144: 917–922.
15. Chaisson M, Berenson L, Li W, Schwartz J, Mojica B, Hamburg M. *Declining AIDS mortality in New York City*. Alexandria, VA: Infectious Diseases Society of America for Retrovirology and Human Health, 1997.
16. Shah RM, Kaji AV, Ostrum BJ, Friedman AC. Interpretation of chest radiographs in AIDS patients: usefulness of CD4 lymphocyte counts. *Radiographics* 1997;17:47–58.
17. Hanson DL, Chu SY, Farizo KM, Ward JW. Distribution of CD4 lymphocytes at diagnosis of acquired immunodeficiency syndrome–defining and other human immunodeficiency virus–related illnesses. *Arch Intern Med* 1995;155:1537–1542.
18. Boiselle PM, Tocino I, Hooley RJ, et al. Chest radiograph interpreta-

19. Finkelstein DM, Williams PL, Molenberghs G, et al. Patterns of opportunistic infections in patients with HIV infection. *J Acquir Immune Defic Syndr Hum Retrovirol* 1996;12:38–45.
20. Wallace JM, Rao AV, Glassroth J, et al. Respiratory illness in persons with human immunodeficiency virus infection. *Am Rev Respir Dis* 1993;148:1523–1529.
21. Verghese A, Al-Samman M, Nabhan D, Naylor AD, Rivera M. Bacterial bronchitis and bronchiectasis in human immunodeficiency virus infection. *Arch Intern Med* 1994;154:2086–2091.
22. Obregon RG, Lynch DA, Kaske T, Newell JD, Kirkpatrick CH. Radiologic findings of adult primary immunodeficiency disorders: contribution of CT. *Chest* 1994;106:490–495.
23. Miller RF, Foley NM, Kessel D, Jeffrey AA. Community acquired lobar pneumonia in patients with HIV infection and AIDS. *Thorax* 1994;49:367–368.
24. Chechani V, Allam AA, Smith PR, Webber CA, Kamholz SL. Bronchitis mimicking opportunistic lung infection in patients with human immunodeficiency virus infection/AIDS. *N Y State J Med* 1992;92: 297–300.
25. Baron AD, Hollander H. *Pseudomonas aeruginosa* bronchopulmonary infection in late human immunodeficiency virus disease. *Am Rev Respir Dis* 1993;148:992–996.
26. Holmes AH, Trotman-Dickenson B, Edwards A, Peto T, Luzzi GA. Bronchiectasis in HIV disease. *Q J Med* 1992;85:875–882.
27. McGuinness G, Gruden JF, Bhalla M, Harkin TJ, Jagirdar JS, Naidich DP. AIDS-related airway disease. *AJR Am J Roentgenol* 1997;168: 67–77.
28. McGuinness G, Naidich DP, Garay SM, Leitman BS, McCauley DI. AIDS associated bronchiectasis: CT features. *J Comput Assist Tomogr* 1993;17:260–266.
29. Gruden JF, Webb WR, Warnock M. Centrilobular opacities in the lung on high-resolution CT: diagnostic considerations and pathologic correlation. *AJR Am J Roentgenol* 1994;162:569–574.
30. Murata K, Itoh H, Todo G, et al. Centrilobular lesions of the lung: demonstration by high-resolution CT and pathologic correlation. *Radiology* 1986;161:641–645.
31. Centers for Disease Control and Prevention. HIV/AIDS surveillance report. *MMWR Morb Mortal Wkly Rep* 1994;6:1–27.
32. Stansell JD, Osmond DH, Charlebois E, et al. Predictors of *Pneumocystis carinii* pneumonia in HIV-infected persons. *Am J Respir Crit Care Med* 1997;155:60–66.
33. Osmond D, Charlebois E, Lang W, Shiboski S, Moss A. Changes in AIDS survival time in two San Francisco cohorts of homosexual men, 1983–1993. *JAMA* 1994;271:1083–1087.
34. Kuhlman JE. Pneumocystic infections: the radiologist's perspective. *Radiology* 1996;198:623–635.
35. Sandhu JS, Goodman PC. Pulmonary cysts associated with *Pneumocystis carinii* pneumonia in patients with AIDS. *Radiology* 1989;173: 33–35.
36. Bergin CJ, Wirth RL, Berry GJ, Castellino RA. *Pneumocystis carinii* pneumonia: CT and HRCT observations. *J Comput Assist Tomogr* 1990;14:756–759.
37. Kuhlman JE, Kavuru M, Fishman EK, Siegelman SS. *Pneumocystis carinii* pneumonia: spectrum of parenchymal CT findings. *Radiology* 1990;175:711–714.
38. Mayor B, Schnyder P, Giron J, Landry M, Duvoisin B, Fournier D. Mediastinal and hilar lymphadenopathy due to *Pneumocystis carinii* infection in AIDS patients: CT features. *J Comput Assist Tomogr* 1994;18:408–411.
39. Liu YC, Tomashefski JF Jr, Tomford JW, Green H. Necrotizing *Pneumocystis carinii* vasculitis associated with lung necrosis and cavitation in a patient with acquired immunodeficiency syndrome. *Arch Pathol Lab Med* 1989;113:494–497.
40. Gagliardi AJ, Stover DE, Zaman MK. Endobronchial *Pneumocystis carinii* infection in a patient with acquired immune deficiency syndrome. *Chest* 1987;91:463–464.
41. Travis WD, Pittaluga S, Lipschik GY, et al. Atypical pathologic manifestations of *Pneumocystis carinii* pneumonia in the acquired immune deficiency syndrome. *Am J Surg Pathol* 1990;14:615–625.
42. Radin DR, Baker EL, Klatt EC, et al. Visceral and nodal calcification

in patients with AIDS-related *Pneumocystis carinii* infection. *AJR Am J Roentgenol* 1990;154:27–31.

43. Kang EY, Staples CA, McGuinness G, Primack SL, Müller NL. Detection and differential diagnosis of pulmonary infections and tumors in patients with AIDS: value of chest radiography versus CT. *AJR Am J Roentgenol* 1996;166:15–19.

44. Hartman TE, Primack SL, Müller NL, Staples CA. Diagnosis of thoracic complications in AIDS: accuracy of CT. *AJR Am J Roentgenol* 1994;162:547–553.

45. Gruden JF, Huang L, Turner J, et al. High-resolution CT in the evaluation of clinically suspected *Pneumocystis carinii* pneumonia in AIDS patients with normal, equivocal, or nonspecific radiographic findings. *AJR Am J Roentgenol* 1997;169:967–975.

46. Miller RF, Mitchell DM. *Pneumocystis carinii* pneumonia. *Thorax* 1995;50:191–200.

47. Huang L, Hecht FM, Stansell JD, Montanti R, Hadley WK, Hopewell P. Suspected *Pneumocystis carinii* pneumonia with a negative induced sputum examination. *Am J Respir Crit Care Med* 1995;151: 1866–1871.

48. Denning DW, Follansbee SE, Scolaro M, Norris S, Edelstein H, Stevens DA. Pulmonary aspergillosis in the acquired immunodeficiency syndrome. *N Engl J Med* 1991;324:654–662.

49. Staples CA, Kang EY, Wright J, Phillips P, Müller NL. Invasive pulmonary aspergillosis in AIDS: radiographic, CT and pathologic findings. *Radiology* 1995;196:409–414.

50. Kirchner JT. Opportunistic fungal infections in patients with HIV disease. *Postgrad Med* 1996;99:209–216.

51. Sider L, Westcott MA. Pulmonary manifestations of cryptococcosis in patients with AIDS: CT features. *J Thorac Imaging* 1994;9:78–84.

52. Miller WT, Edelman JM, Miller WT. Cryptococcal pulmonary infection in patients with AIDS: radiographic appearance. *Radiology* 1990; 175:725–728.

53. Lortholary O, Meyohas M-C, Dupont B, et al. Invasive aspergillosis in patients with acquired immunodeficiency syndrome: report of 33 cases. *Am J Med* 1993;95:177–187.

54. Kemper CA, Hostetler JS, Follansbee SE, et al. Ulcerative and plaque-like tracheobronchitis due to infection with aspergillus in patients with AIDS. *Clin Infect Dis* 1993;17:344–352.

55. Klapholz A, Salomon N, Perlman DC, Talavera W. Aspergillosis in the acquired immunodeficiency syndrome. *Chest* 1991;100: 1614–1618.

56. Addrizzo-Harris D, Harkin TJ, McGuinness G, Naidich DP, Rom WN. Pulmonary aspergilloma and AIDS: a comparison of HIV-infected and HIV-negative individuals. *Chest* 1997;111:612–618.

57. Pursell KJ, Telzak EE, Armstrong D. *Aspergillus* species colonization and invasive disease in patients with AIDS. *Clin Infect Dis* 1992;41: 141–148.

58. Friedman EP, Miller RF, Severn A, Williams JG, Shaw PJ. Cryptococcal pneumonia in patients with the acquired immunodeficiency syndrome. *Clin Radiol* 1995;50:756–760.

59. Wasser L, Talavera W. Pulmonary cryptococcosis in AIDS. *Chest* 1987;92:692–695.

60. Johnson PC, Khardori N, Najjar AF, Butt F, Mansell PWA, Sarosi GA. Progressive disseminated histoplasmosis in patients with acquired immunodeficiency syndrome. *Am J Med* 1988;85:152–158.

61. Conces DJ, Stockberger SM, Tarver RD, Wheat LJ. Disseminated histoplasmosis in AIDS: findings on chest radiographs. *AJR Am J Roentgenol* 1993;160:15–19.

62. Salzman SH, Smith RL, Aranda CP. Histoplasmosis in patients at risk for the acquired immunodeficiency syndrome in a nonendemic setting. *Chest* 1988;93:916–921.

63. Chin DP, Hopewell PC. Mycobacterial complications of HIV infection. *Clin Chest Med* 1996;17:697–711.

64. Markowitz N, Hansen NI, Hopewell PC, et al. Incidence of tuberculosis in the United States among HIV-infected persons. *Ann Intern Med* 1997;126:123–132.

65. Barnes PF, Bloch AB, Davidson PT, Snider DE. Tuberculosis in patients with human immunodeficiency virus infection. *N Engl J Med* 1991;324:1644–1650.

66. Kramer F, Modilevsky T, Waliany AR, Leedom JM, Barnes PF. Delayed diagnosis of tuberculosis in patients with human immunodeficiency virus infection. *Am J Med* 1990;89:451–456.

67. Whalen C, Horsburgh CR, Hom D, Lahart C, Simberkoff M, Ellner J. Accelerated course of human immunodeficiency virus infection after tuberculosis. *Am J Respir Crit Care Med* 1995;151:129–135.

68. Leung AN, Brauner MW, Gamsu G, et al. Pulmonary tuberculosis: comparison of CT findings in HIV-seropositive and HIV-seronegative patients. *Radiology* 1996;198:687–691.

69. Haramati LB, Jennyavital ER, Alterman DD. Effect of HIV status on chest radiographic and CT findings in patients with tuberculosis. *Clin Radiol* 1997;52:31–35.

70. Greenberg SD, Frager D, Suster B, Walker S, Stavropoulos C, Rothpearl A. Active pulmonary tuberculosis in patients with AIDS: spectrum of radiographic findings (including a normal appearance). *Radiology* 1994;193:115–119.

71. Theur CP, Hopewell PC, Elias D. Human immunodeficiency virus infection in tuberculosis patients. *J Infect Dis* 1990;162:8–12.

72. Jones BE, Young SMM, Antoniskis D, Davidson PT, Kramer F, Barnes PF. Relationship of the manifestations of tuberculosis to CD4 cell counts in patients with human immunodeficiency virus infection. *Am Rev Respir Dis* 1993;148:1292–1297.

73. Goodman PC. Tuberculosis and AIDS. *Radiol Clin North Am* 1995; 33:707–717.

74. Long R, Maycher B, Scalcini M, Manfreda J. The chest roentgenogram in pulmonary tuberculosis patients seropositive for human immunodeficiency virus type 1. *Chest* 1991;99:123–127.

75. Pastores SM, Naidich DP, Aranda CP, McGuinness G, Rom WN. Intrathoracic adenopathy associated with pulmonary tuberculosis in patients with human immunodeficiency virus infection. *Chest* 1993; 103:1433–1437.

76. Harkin TJ, Ciotoli C, Addrizzo-Harris DJ, et al. Transbronchial needle aspiration (TBNA) in patients infected with HIV. *Am J Respir Crit Care Med* 1998;157:1913–1918.

77. Centers for Disease Control and Prevention. Revision of the case definition for acquired immunodeficiency syndrome for national reporting: United States. *MMWR Morb Mortal Wkly Rep* 1987;34: 373–375.

78. Hill AR, Somasundaram P, Brustein S, et al. Disseminated tuberculosis in the acquired immunodeficiency syndrome. *Am Rev Respir Dis* 1991;144:1164–1170.

79. Small PM, Hopewell PC, Schecter GF, Chaisson RE, Goodman PC. Evolution of chest radiographs in treated patients with pulmonary tuberculosis and HIV infection. *J Thorac Imaging* 1994;9:74–77.

80. Modilevsky T, Sattler FR, Barnes PF. Mycobacterial disease in patients with human immunodeficiency virus infection. *Arch Intern Med* 1989;149:2201–2205.

81. Salahuddin SZ, Ropse RM, Groopman JE, Markham PD, Gallo RC. Human T lymphotropic virus type II infection of human alveolar macrophage. *Blood* 1986;68:281–284.

82. Beck JM. Effects of human immunodeficiency virus on pulmonary host defenses. *Semin Respir Infect* 1989;4:75–84.

83. McKenzie R, Travis WD, Dolan SA, et al. The causes of death in patients with human immunodeficiency virus infection: a clinical and pathologic study with emphasis on the role of pulmonary diseases. *Medicine* 1991;70:326–343.

84. Wallace MJ, Hannah J. Cytomegalovirus pneumonitis in patients with AIDS: findings in an autopsy series. *Chest* 1987;92:198–203.

85. Klatt EC, Shibata D. Cytomegalovirus infection in the acquired immunodeficiency syndrome: clinical and autopsy findings. *Arch Pathol Lab Med* 1988;112:540–544.

86. Nelson MR, Erskine D, Hawkins DA, Gazzard BG. Treatment with corticosteroids: a risk factor for the development of clinical cytomegalovirus disease in AIDS. *AIDS* 1993;7:375–378.

87. McGuinness G, Scholes JV, Garay SM, Leitman BS, McCauley DI, Naidich DP. Cytomegalovirus pneumonitis: spectrum of parenchymal CT findings with pathologic correlation in 21 AIDS patients. *Radiology* 1994;192:451–459.

88. Amundson DE, Murray KM, Brodine S, Oldfield EC. High-dose corticosteroid therapy for *Pneumocystis carinii* pneumonia in patients with acquired immunodeficiency syndrome. *South J Med* 1989;83: 711–714.

89. Squire SB, Lipman MCI, Bagdades EK, et al. Severe cytomegalovirus pneumonitis in HIV infected patients with higher than average CD4 counts. *Thorax* 1992;47:301–304.

90. Waxman AB, Goldie SJ, Brett-Smith H, Matthay RA. Cytomegalovirus as a primary pulmonary pathogen in AIDS. *Chest* 1997;111: 128–134.

91. Wallace JM. Viruses and other miscellaneous organisms. *Clin Chest Med* 1996;17:745–754.

92. Goodman P, Schnapp LM. Pulmonary toxoplasmosis in AIDS. *Radiology* 1992;184:791–793.

93. Coche E, Beigelman C, Lucidarme O, Finet J-F, Bakdach H, Grenier P. Thoracic bacillary angiomatosis in a patient with AIDS. *AJR Am J Roentgenol* 1995;165:56–58.

94. Moore EH, Russell LA, Klein JS, et al. Bacillary angiomatosis in patients with AIDS: multiorgan imaging findings. *Radiology* 1995;197:67–72.

95. Foltzer MA, Guiney WB, Wager GC, Alpern HD. Bronchopulmonary bacillary angiomatosis. *Chest* 1993;104:973–975.

96. Slater LN, Kyung-Whan M. Polyploid endobronchial lesions: a manifestation of bacillary angiomatosis. *Chest* 1992;102:972–974.

97. Cury JD, Harrington PT, Hosein JK. Successful medical therapy of *Rhodococcus equi* pneumonia in a patient with HIV infection. *Chest* 1992;102:1619–1621.

98. Mayor BJ, R-M., Wicky S, Giron J, Schnyder P. Radiologic findings in two AIDS patients with *Rhodococcus equi* pneumonia. *J Thorac Imaging* 1995;10:121–125.

99. Makris AN, Sher S, Bertoli C, Latour MG. Pulmonary strongyloidiasis: an unusual opportunistic pneumonia in a patient with AIDS. *AJR Am J Roentgenol* 1993;161:545–547.

100. Beral V, Peterman TA, Berkelman RL, Jaffe HW. Kaposi's sarcoma among persons with AIDS: a sexually transmitted infection? *Lancet* 1990;335:123–128.

101. Drew WL, Mills J, Hauer LB, Miner RC, Rutheri GW. Declining prevalence of Kaposi's sarcoma in homosexual AIDS patients paralled by fall in cytomegalovirus transmission. *Lancet* 1988;1:66.

102. Chang Y, Cesarman EP, Lee F, Culpepper J, Knowles DM, Moore PS. Identification of herpesvirus-like DNA sequences in AIDS-associated Kaposi's sarcoma. *Science* 1994;266:1865–1869.

103. Huang YQ, Kaplan MH, Poiesz B, et al. Human herpesvirus-like nucleic acid in various forms of Kaposi's sarcoma. *Lancet* 1995;345:759–761.

104. Fife K, Bower M. Recent insights into the pathogenesis of Kaposi's sarcoma. *Br J Cancer* 1996;73:1317–1322.

105. Cathomas G, Tamm M, McGandy CE, Perruchoud AP, Mihatsch MJ, Dalquen P. Detection of herpesvirus-like DNA in the bronchoalveolar lavage fluid of patients with pulmonary Kaposi's sarcoma. *Eur Respir J* 1996;9:1743–1746.

106. Gruden JF, Huang L, Webb WR, Gamsu G, Hopewell PC, Sides DM. AIDS-related Kaposi sarcoma of the lung: radiographic findings and staging system with bronchoscopic correlation. *Radiology* 1995;195:545–552.

107. Meduri GU, Stover DE, Lee M, Myskowski PL, Caravelli JF, Zaman MB. Pulmonary Kaposi's sarcoma in the acquired immunodeficiency syndrome: clinical, radiographic, and pathologic manifestations. *Am J Med* 1986;81:11–18.

108. Ognibene FP, Steis RG, Mahcer AMN, et al. Kaposi's sarcoma causing pulmonary infiltrates and respiratory failure in the acquired immunodeficiency syndrome. *Ann Intern Med* 1985;102:471–475.

109. Huang L, Schnapp LN, Gruden JF, Hopewell PC, Stansell JD. Presentation of AIDS-related pulmonary Kaposi's sarcoma diagnosed by bronchoscopy. *Am J Respir Crit Care Med* 1996;153:1385–1390.

110. Wang CYE, Schroeter AL, Su WPD. Acquired immunodeficiency syndrome–related Kaposi's sarcoma. *Mayo Clin Proc* 1995;70:869–879.

111. Cadranel JL, Kammoun S, Chevret S, et al. Results of chemotherapy in 30 AIDS patients with symptomatic pulmonary Kaposi's sarcoma. *Thorax* 1994;49:958–960.

112. James ND, Coker RJ, Tomlinson D, et al. Liposomal doxorubicin (Doxocil): an effective new treatment for Kaposi's sarcoma in AIDS. *Clin Oncol* 1994;6:294–296.

113. Simpson JK, Miller RF, Spittle MF. Liposomal doxorubicin for treatment of AIDS-related Kaposi's sarcoma. *Clin Oncol* 1993;5:372–374.

114. Swanton RG, Kuske RR, Hawkins RB, et al. Disseminated epidemic Kaposi's sarcoma treated with radiation and chemotherapy. *South Med J* 1996;89:718–722.

115. Leebe C, Blum LC, Pellet C, et al. Clinical and biologic impact of antiretroviral therapy with protease inhibitors on HIV-related Kaposi's sarcoma. *AIDS* 1998;12:F45–F49.

116. Davis SD, Henschke CI, Chamides BK, Westcott JL. Intrathoracic Kaposi's sarcoma in AIDS patients: radiographic-pathologic correlation. *Radiology* 1987;163:495–500.

117. Naidich DP, Tarras M, Garay SM, Birnbaum B, Rybak BJ, Schinella R. Kaposi sarcoma: CT-radiographic correlation. *Chest* 1989;96:723–728.

118. Khalil AM, Carette MF, Cadranel JL, Mayaud CM, Bigot JM. Intrathoracic Kaposi's sarcoma: CT findings. *Chest* 1995;108:1622–1626.

119. Wolff SD, Kuhlman JE, Fishman EK. Thoracic Kaposi sarcoma in AIDS: CT findings. *J Comput Assist Tomogr* 1993;17:60–62.

120. Sider L, Weiss AJ, Smith MD, Von Roenn JH, Glassroth J. Varied appearance of AIDS-related lymphoma in the chest. *Radiology* 1989;171:629–632.

121. Heitzman ER. Pulmonary neoplastic and lymphoproliferative disease in AIDS: a review. *Radiology* 1990;177:347–351.

122. Polish LB, Coh DL, Ryder JW, Myers AM, O'Brien RF. Pulmonary non-Hodgkin's lymphoma in AIDS. *Chest* 1989;96:1321–1326.

123. Eisner MD, Kaplan LD, Herndier B, Stuhlberg MS. The pulmonary manifestations of AIDS-related non-Hodgkin's lymphoma. *Chest* 1996;110:729–736.

124. Ioachim HL, Dorsett B, Cronin W, Maya M, Wahl S. Acquired immunodeficiency syndrome–associated lymphomas: clinical, pathologic, immunology, and viral characteristics in 111 cases. *Hum Pathol* 1991;22:659–673.

125. Wang CY, Snow JL, Su WPD. Lymphoma associated with human immunodeficiency virus infection. *Mayo Clin Proc* 1995;70:665–672.

126. Collins J, Müller NL, Leung AN, et al. Epstein Barr virus driven lymphoproliferative disorders of the lung: CT and histologic findings. *Radiology* 1998 (*in press*).

127. Carignan S, Staples CA, Müller NL. Intrathoracic lymphoproliferative disorders in the immunocompromised patient: CT findings. *Radiology* 1995;197:53–58.

128. Blunt DM, Padley SPG. Radiographic manifestations of AIDS related lymphoma in the thorax. *Clin Radiol* 1995;50:607–612.

129. Chaouat A, Fraisse P, Kessler R, Lang JM, Weitzenbaum E. A life-threatening tracheal localization of lymphoma in a patient with AIDS. *Chest* 1993;103:297–299.

130. Keys TC, Judson MA, Reed CE, Sahn SA. Endobronchial HIV-associated lymphoma. *Thorax* 1994;49:525–526.

131. Cesarman E, Chang Y, Moore P, Said J, Knowles D. Kaposi's sarcoma-associated herpesvirus-like DNA sequences in AIDS-related body-cavity–based lymphomas. *N Engl J Med* 1995;332:1186–1191.

132. Trachiotis GD, Hafner GH, Hix WR, Aaron BL. Role of open lung biopsy in diagnosing pulmonary complications of AIDS. *Ann Thorac Surg* 1992;54:898–902.

133. Gruden JF, Klein JS, Webb WR. Percutaneous transthoracic needle biopsy in AIDS: analysis in 32 patients. *Radiology* 1993;189:567–571.

134. Braun MA, Killam DA, Remick SC, Ruchkdescher JC. Lung cancer in patients seropositive for human immunodeficiency virus. *Radiology* 1990;175:341–343.

135. Karp J, Profeta G, Marantz PR, Karpel JP. Lung cancer in patients with immunodeficiency syndrome. *Chest* 1993;103:410–413.

136. Sridhar KS, Flores MR, Raub WA, Saldana M. Lung cancer in patients with human immunodeficiency virus infection compared with historic control subjects. *Chest* 1992;102:1704–1708.

137. White CS, Haramati LB, Elder NH, Karp J, Belani CP. Carcinoma of the lung in HIV-positive patients: findings on chest radiographs and CT scans. *AJR Am J Roentgenol* 1995;164:593–597.

138. Chan TK, Aranda CP, Rom WN. Bronchogenic carcinoma in young patients at risk for acquired immunodeficiency syndrome. *Chest* 1993;103:862–864.

139. Gruden JF, Webb WR, Dorcas CY, Klein JS, Sandhu JS. Bronchogenic carcimona in 13 patients infected with the human immunodeficiency virus (HIV): clinical and radiographic findings. *J Thorac Imaging* 1995;10:99–105.

140. Fishman JE, Schwartz DS, Sais GJ, Flores MR, Sridhar KS. Bronchogenic carcinoma in HIV-positive patients: findings on chest radiographs and CT scans. *AJR Am J Roentgenol* 1995;164:57–61.

141. Ettensohn DB, Mayer KH, Kessimian N, Smith PS. Lymphocytic bronchiolitis associated with HIV infection. *Chest* 1988;93:201–202.

142. McGuinness G, Scholes JV, Jagirdar JS, et al. Unusual lymphoproliferative disorders in nine adults with HIV or AIDS: CT and pathologic findings. *Radiology* 1995;197:59–65.

143. Travis WD, Fox CH, Devaney KO, et al. Lymphoid pneumonitis in 50 adult patients infected with the human immunodeficiency virus:

lymphocytic interstitial pneumonitis versus nonspecific interstitial pneumonitis. *Hum Pathol* 1992;23:529–541.

144. Saldana MJ, Mones JM. Lymphoid interstitial pneumonia in HIV infected individuals. *Prog Surg Pathol* 1992;12:181–215.

145. Guillon J-M, Autran B, Denis M, et al. Human immunodeficiency virus-related lymphocytic alveolitis. *Chest* 1988;94:1264–1270.

146. Centers for Disease Control and Prevention. Revision of case definitions of acquired immunodeficiency syndrome for national reporting: United States. *MMWR Morb Mortal Wkly Rep* 1985;34:373–375.

147. Oldham SAA, Castillo M, Jacobson FL, Mones JM, Saldana MJ. HIV-associated lymphocytic interstitial pneumonia: radiologic manifestations and pathologic correlation. *Radiology* 1989;170:83–87.

148. Allen JN, Wewers MD. HIV-associated bronchiolitis obliterans organizing pneumonia. *Chest* 1989;96:197–198.

149. Joseph J, Harley RA, Frye MD. Bronchiolitis obliterans with organizing pneumonia in AIDS [Letter]. *N Engl J Med* 1995;332:273.

150. Leo YS, Pitchon HE, Messler G, Meyer RD. Bronchiolitis obliterans organizing pneumonia in a patient with AIDS. *Clin Infect Dis* 1994; 18:921–924.

151. Sanito NJ, Morley TF, Condoluci DV. Bronchiolitis obliterans organizing pneumonia in an AIDS patient. *Eur Respir J* 1995;8: 1021–1024.

152. Gagliardi AJ, White DA, Meduri DE, Stover DE. Pulmonary function

153. Shaw RJ, Croussak C, Forster SM, et al. Lung function abnormalities in patients infected with the human immunodeficiency virus with and without overt pneumonitis. *Thorax* 1988;43:436–440.

154. McGuinness G, Gruden JF, Garay SM, Naidich DP. Thoracic complications of AIDS: imaging findings and diagnostic strategies. *Semin Respir Crit Care Med* 1998;19:543–560.

155. Schneider RF, Hansen NI, Rosen MJ, et al. Lack of usefulness of radiographic screening for pulmonary disease in asymptomatic HIV-infected adults. Pulmonary Complications of HIV Study Group. *Arch Intern Med* 1996;156:191–195.

156. El-Sadir W, Oleske JM, Agins BD. *Evaluation and management of early HIV infection: Clinical practice guideline No. 7.* Washington, DC: US Department of Health and Human Services Publication, 1994; 94:40–41.

157. Scott WW, Kuhlman JE. Focal pulmonary lesions in patients with AIDS: precutaneous transthoracic needle biopsy. *Radiology* 1991; 180:419.

158. Haramati LB, Choi Y, Widrow CA, Austin JH. Isolated lymphadenopathy on chest radiographs of HIV-infected patients. *Clin Radiol* 1996; 51:345–349.

159. Relkin F, Aranda CP, Garay SM. Pleural tuberculosis and HIV infection. *Chest* 1994;105:1338–1341.

abnormalities in AIDS patients with respiratory illness. *Am Rev Respir Dis* 1985;131:A75.

CHAPTER 8

Aorta, Arch Vessels, and Great Veins

Over the past decade, rapid changes in imaging technology have revolutionized our ability to study the cardiovascular system. Parallel developments in computed tomograpy (CT), magnetic resonance (MR) and transesophageal echocardiography (TEE) now present referring clinicians with a wide range of options for evaluating diseases of the aorta and great vessels.

All of these techniques provide excellent diagnostic accuracy for a wide range of thoracic aortic diseases (1,2). Because it is widely available, can be performed in the intensive care unit or the operating room, and is extremely versatile in the appropriate hands, TEE has emerged as a valuable tool for evaluating the thoracic aorta in the acute setting (1,3,4). In addition to being indispensable for evaluating the aortic valve, the introduction of multiplane probes has extended the utility of TEE in the diagnosis of protruding aortic atheromas of the thoracic aorta, a newly recognized etiology for stroke and peripheral embolization. It should also be recognized that because many elderly patients with acquired thoracic aortic disease have concomitant coronary artery dis-

ease, catheterization with angioplasty with or without stenting is now routinely performed by cardiologists who may also perform diagnostic aortography in the same examination.

Simultaneously, contrast-enhanced volumetric (helical/spiral) CT has become widely available. It is easy to perform, relatively noninvasive, and less operator-dependent than TEE. Helical CT offers a range of reconstruction and display options. Most important, unlike TEE, CT allows simultaneous evaluation of the entire thorax, markedly extending the range of potential diagnoses, especially in patients with nonspecific symptoms only indirectly suggestive of cardiovascular disease.

Although less commonly employed, MR angiography (MRA) has also emerged as a versatile tool for the evaluation of both congenital and acquired diseases of the thoracic aorta. This is a result of the rapid technologic advances in both hardware and pulse sequences as well as the use of contrast agents that shorten the T1 relaxation rate of blood (5). This evolution is now reflected in many institutions where MRA has replaced diagnostic thoracic aortography in stable patients with nontraumatic thoracic aortic disease.

Given this wide range of potential choices, the purpose of this chapter is to focus on a review of disease entities affecting the aorta and great vessels, with special emphasis placed on the advantages and limitations of CT and MR in clinical practice. In this regard, recent advances in therapeutic techniques that have equally revolutionized our approaches to these disorders will also be discussed.

IMAGING TECHNIQUES

CT Angiography

Despite considerable recent enthusiasm, CT angiography (CTA) is actually a poorly defined concept that includes a variety of rendering techniques derived from volumetric data acquisition.

Optimization of image quality for CTA requires careful attention to methods of data acquisition. The ability to acquire data volumetrically has resulted in a wide variety of potential scan protocols for axial imaging. Variables that need to be selected include collimation, pitch, breath-hold period, field of view (FOV), reconstruction interval (or index), rate and volume of intravenous contrast administration, reconstruction algorithm, and radiation dose.

To date, numerous articles have addressed the issue of optimal data acquisition protocols (6–8). Unfortunately, no single set of optimal scan parameters currently suffice for all intrathoracic CTA applications. CTA techniques often reflect a combination of personal or institutional preferences coupled with individual manufacturer capabilities. Nonetheless, general guidelines can be derived from review of the literature (Table 8-1).

Scan Parameters

In practice, it is necessary to compromise between use of the thinnest possible collimation, smallest reconstruction interval, and largest available pitch. In our experience this is most usefully accomplished by obtaining 3- to 5-mm sections with scans obtained in a cephalocaudad direction during a single breath-hold period using a pitch of 2. In patients for whom the primary indication of the study is to evaluate the aorta, scans may be obtained beginning approximately 2 cm above the aortic arch. Although 3-mm sections are especially helpful when assessing the origins of the great vessels, 5-mm sections are often more practical in order to scan the entire thorax in a single breath-hold period. As recently noted by Fishman (10), the introduction of subsecond (0.75 second) scanners makes acquisition of thinner sections throughout the entire thorax more practicable, increasing the scan volume by as much as 33% while maintaining the same collimation and pitch. Unfortunately, routine use of thin sections is often limited owing to marked increases in image processing time, storage requirements, and most

TABLE 8-1. *CT of the thoracic aorta: Technique*

Scanner settings:	kVp: 120
	mAs: 250
Rotation time:	0.75–1 second
Phase of respiration:	Suspended inspiration (quiet breathing acceptable if necessary)
Slice thickness:	3–5 mm
Pitch:	2
Reconstruct interval:	2–3 mm
Reconstruct algorithm:	Standard body FOV may be reduced to 20–25 cm for optimal 3D rendering.
Helical exposure time:	Single breath-hold period (24–30 secs usually obtainable with coaching or supplemental oxygen)
Scan direction:	Craniocaudad starting 2 cm above arch and extending to the diaphragm (or lower if thoracoabdominal aneurysm or dissection is present)
IV contrast:	
Concentration:	LOCM 300–320 mg iodine/mL or HOCM 282 mg iodine/mL (60% solution)
Rate:	3–4 mL/sec
Scan delay:	Test bolus recommended (see text)
Volume:	120 mL–150 mL

Comments:
1. Initial 10 mm noncontrast scans through the thorax at 2 cm intervals should be obtained, especially in studies performed to rule out dissection, to look for displaced intimal calcifications or intramural hematoma.
2. Multiple breath-hold acquisitions may be obtained without sacrificing the ability to obtain multiplanar reconstructions or 3D renderings provided that the same collimation, field of view and center are maintained.
3. Retrospective or prospective "segmentation" may be useful to avoid pitfall of motion at the aortic root. This pulsatile artifact has been reported when scans are performed in less than 1.5 sec. Alternatively, axial clusters can be performed with a 2 sec scan time to avoid this pitfall immediately following helical scans.

LOCM, low osmolar contrast media; HOCM, high-osmolar contrast media; FOV, field-of-view.
Modified from ref. 8.

importantly, image review time. These disadvantages are the direct result of the marked increase in the number of scans generated using thinner sections. It may be anticipated that with further technologic improvements, routine studies may result in literally hundreds of images. Clearly, selection of optimal scan parameters will continue to necessitate compromise with the exigencies of image storage, display, and interpretation. For those patients for whom scanning the entire thoracic aorta in a single breath-hold period is not feasible, even following hyperventilation or the use of supplemental oxygen, multiple acquisitions may be obtained without sacrificing the ability to perform retrospective multiplanar reconstructions or three-dimensional (3D) renderings, provided that all scan parameters remain constant. This includes the FOV, slice thickness and, often overlooked, patient centering.

Contrast Administration

Iodine Concentration, Flow Rate and Volume

Optimal contrast administration is critical to the successful performance of CTA (11–15). Considerations include: volume, route and rate of injection, iodine concentration and osmolality, and timing of scan acquisition as well as methods to diminish scan artifacts related to contrast administration.

Although Costello and colleagues have shown that adequate vascular opacification can be obtained with as little as 60 cc of 300 mg I/mL contrast media, most investigators use a considerably higher volume of contrast for CT angiographic applications. A typical protocol for contrast administration, derived from a review of recent CTA literature, is shown in Table 8-1. As a rule, 125 to 150 cc of nonionic contrast material (averaging 300 mg I/mL) is injected through an antecubital vein in the left arm using an 18- to 20-gauge catheter, at rates varying between 3 and 5 cc/second with images obtained following an approximately 20 second delay in a craniocaudad direction (7,8,16–19). Nonionic contrast agents are typically recommended to minimize the effects of nausea and vomiting as well as complications arising from extravasation caused by the rapid infusion of ionic contrast agents. Recent studies have also demonstrated both subjective and objective evidence of less patient motion with nonionic contrast agents when compared with ionic agents (20,21).

In fact, there is little agreement on optimal iodine concentration or osmolality for performing CTA. Schnyder et al., comparing the use of 125, 150 and 300 mg I/mL injected at rates varying between 1.5 to 5 mL/second found that, whereas 125 mg I/mL was unsatisfactory at any rate of injection, comparable images could be obtained using either 150 or 300 mg I/mL, assuming appropriately adjusted flow rates, with fewer streak artifacts from adjacent venous structures (14). This was calculated using either of the following formulas:

$$\text{volume} = \text{flow rate (cc/second)} \qquad (1)$$
$$\times [\text{scan delay} - \text{scan time} - 7]$$

where 7 seconds corresponds to the average transit time of contrast to the pulmonary artery; or

$$\text{volume (300 mg I/mL)} = \text{body weight (kg)} \qquad (2)$$

in which the volume is doubled if 150 mg I/mL is used (14).

Similar results have been reported by Rubin et al. In a study of 138 patients receiving a total dose of either 150 mg or 225 g of iodine (iodine concentrations varying between 75 and 300 mg/mL), with flow rates and volumes adjusted to insure delivery of the entire dose within 40 seconds, the investigators found that 100 mL of 150 mg I/mL (total dose of 15 grams) injected at a rate of 2.5 mL/second was superior for diminishing venous artifacts while maintaining adequate arterial opacification (13). It should be noted that this may require diluting a 50-mg vial of 300 mg I/mL contrast medium with 50 cc of normal saline, as this concentration of iodine has not generally been commercially available in North America (14). Whether or not self-dilution increases the rate of infectious complications resulting from contamination remains controversial.

Also controversial is the use of injectable saline solution via a power injector as a means to deliver contrast material. This technique, described in detail by Hopper et al. (11), involves first loading 75 mL of 60% nonionic contrast medium into a power injector in a vertical position, followed by 50 mL of normal saline solution loaded so as to lie on top of the denser nonionic contrast material. Meant to decrease the volume and cost of nonionic contrast material utilization, while using the saline to clear the syringe and intravenous catheter of contrast material following the injection, this approach proves to have the added benefit of significantly decreasing the number of streak artifacts from adjacent venous structures. It should be noted that other methods for diminishing streak artifacts, including caudal to cranial scan acquisition and the use of a femoral venous injection, although advocated by some, have proved largely impractical.

Scan Delay

In addition to considerations of flow rates and volume, it is also essential to optimize scan delay to insure adequate opacification of targeted vessels. Although a 20 to 30 second scan delay most often is sufficient to insure adequate opacification of the thoracic aorta, large variations between patients will be encountered. As reported by Van Hoe et al., in their evaluation of scan delay times in spiral CTA using a test bolus injection, the time to peak attenuation within the aorta varied between 11 and 32 seconds (mean 20, standard deviation 6.1 seconds) (22). This problem is easily resolved by administering 20 cc of contrast media injected at the same rate as the planned injection, with images obtained at the same preselected level (usually the middle ascending aorta or arch) using 80 to 90 mAs. As will be discussed in Chapter 9, a similar approach may be used to optimize evaluation of the pulmonary arteries. Following an 8 second delay, images are obtained every 2 to 5 seconds for a total of 25 to 30 seconds in order to generate a time-density curve (7,14). Alternatively, it is now possible to obtain equivalent data using automated scan acquisitions to monitor vascular opacification without the use of a test dose [C.A.R.E bolus (Siemens) or Smartprep (GE Medical Systems, Milwaukee, WI)]

(23). Although administration of a test dose of contrast does have the deleterious effect of increasing the background attenuation of abdominal organs rendering visualization of small vessels more difficult with CTA, this consideration is of much less concern within the thorax. Given only a slight increase in the time of examination and radiation dose, use of a timed bolus or its equivalent is strongly recommended to insure optimum vascular opacification.

MR

It cannot be overemphasized that optimal use of MR requires meticulous attention to technique. Considerable emphasis will be placed on the many fine points of scan technique that must be mastered in order to insure diagnostic accuracy. Once mastered, it should be apparent that MR represents an extraordinarily powerful tool for the evaluation of cardiovascular disease.

The advantages of MR for evaluation of the aorta include: (a) nonreliance on the use of iodinated contrast agents to image blood vessels; (b) the ability to image in multiple planes; (c) a lack of ionizing radiation; (d) the ability to evaluate valvular competency and to quantify flow and determine pressure gradients across stenotic regions; and (e) the availability of MRA techniques. Limitations of MR compared with CT include: (a) insensitivity to calcification; (b) decreased spatial resolution; (c) restriction in the numbers of patients eligible to be scanned owing to the presence of various life-support systems and monitoring devices, such as pacemakers or ventilators; and (d) cost and availability.

MR Angiography Techniques

Contemporary MR imaging of the thoracic aorta usually includes axial and oblique sagittal electrocardiographic (ECG) triggered spin-echo (SE) "black blood" imaging supplemented with a "bright blood" MRA technique. Whereas SE MR imaging of the thoracic aorta is an effective diagnostic tool in evaluating a wide range of anatomic and pathologic conditions (24–27) images may be degraded by pulsatility and flow artifacts, and this technique cannot accurately evaluate aortic arch vessel disease. In addition, because acquisition times are determined by heart rate, patients with bradycardia have long acquisition times and patients with abnormal cardiac rhythms often have poor ECG-triggering resulting in suboptimal or even nondiagnostic examinations.

MR angiographic techniques used in evaluating the thoracic aorta and arch vessels include cine gradient-echo (GRE) (28–33), two-dimensional (2D) segmented k-space time-of-flight (TOF) (30,34), 2D gadolinium-enhanced rapid GRE imaging (35–38) and gadolinium-enhanced three-dimensional (3D) MRA (5,39–41). These bright blood techniques can differentiate slow flow from thrombus, demonstrate branch vessel disease and supply additional physiological information that complements SE MR imaging. Perhaps most important, these images resemble conventional angiograms and therefore are easier for referring clinicians to interpret.

Before the advent of gadolinium enhanced MRA, TOF techniques were widely used (34). However, this approach requires ECG-gating and breath holding to maximize flow-related enhancement, minimize saturation effects and eliminate respiratory misregistration. When performed in the oblique sagittal (LAO equivalent) plane this technique may be limited by low spatial resolution, in-plane saturation effects and TOF signal loss in areas of turbulent flow or stasis. Nevertheless, when combined with SE imaging, very high diagnostic accuracy rates have been achieved for a wide range of congenital and acquired thoracic aortic diseases (30).

Two-dimensional (2D) Cine GRE MRA, with or without segmented k-space acquisition schemes, provides the capability of imaging a single slice throughout multiple cardiac cycles. Although this technique is widely used to assess aortic valvular disease and to differentiate slow flow from thrombus, it too is hindered by the display limitations of 2D techniques.

Gadolinium-enhanced 3D MR angiography depends on infusion of paramagnetic contrast agents, which results in a decreased T1 relaxation of blood (42). Using this approach, anatomic images of blood vessels are generated and distinguished from background tissues based solely on T1 relaxation rates. This contrast mechanism minimizes saturation effects and allows for rapid in-plane imaging of large anatomic segments. The intravascular signal enhancement of gadolinium chelates allows the use of 3D Fourier-transform imaging with intrinsically high spatial resolution and high signal-to-noise ratio (42). This technique results in excellent aortic enhancement, irrespective of the patients cardiac output or hemodynamic status.

Early studies using a slow infusion of 0.2 to 0.3 mmol/kg gadolinium during a 2 to 4 minute acquisition demonstrated high sensitivity and specificity for a both congenital and acquired thoracic aortic disease (5,39). However, images are often degraded by respiratory artifacts that result in considerable image blurring, especially of the arch vessels (Fig. 8-1) and the aortic root (39). In a small percentage of cases image quality of nonbreath-hold gadolinium-enhanced 3D MRA is so poor that the examination is entirely nondiagnostic. Significant enhancement of the brachiocephalic veins is almost always present and may result in obscuration of the aortic arch vessels on maximum-intensity-projection (MIP) images. In addition, because of the long acquisition times this technique provides no physiologic information regarding flow dynamics; this precludes the differentiation between true and false lumen in aortic dissection based on preferential enhancement. The advantage of the long acquisition time is the uniform, excellent aortic enhancement, which is virtually always achieved.

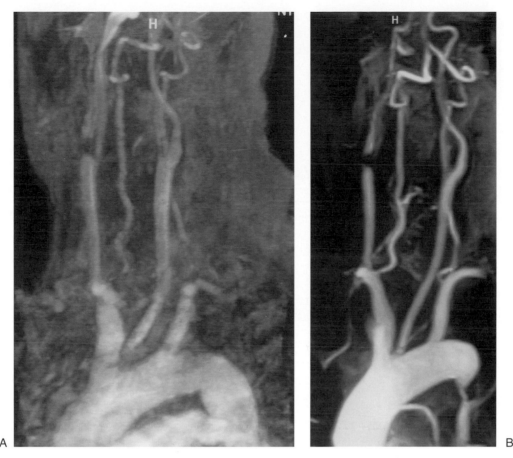

FIG. 8-1. The effects of breath holding on image quality of gadolinium-enhanced three-dimensional (3D) MR angiography. **A:** Oblique sagittal maximum-intensity-projection (MIP) image from nonbreath-hold gadolinium-enhanced 3D MR angiogram (TR/TE/FA 21/6/30°) performed in the body coil, during slow infusion of 40 mL of contrast over the first 90 seconds of a 2 minute acquisition, demonstrates blurring and ghosting artifacts resulting in poor image quality and a nondlagnostic examination. **B:** Oblique sagittal MIP image from breath-hold, gadolinium-enhanced 3D MR angiogram (TR/TE/FA 5/2/50°) performed with 20 mL of gadolinium in conjunction with a phased-array coil and a timing examination demonstrates vastly improved image quality and normal aortic arch vessels. (From ref. 289, with permission.)

Optimization and Timing of Gadolinium-Enhanced Three-Dimensional MR Angiography

With high performance gradient systems now increasingly available, the TR and TE can be shortened such that an entire 3D acquisition can be obtained in a single breath-hold (41,43). It is well established that there is only a small temporal window between peak brachiocephalic arterial enhancement and jugular venous enhancement (44,45). Rapid acquisition times may allow for a "pure" arterial study without confounding venous enhancement, and breath holding eliminates most of the artifacts seen with the longer, non-breath-hold strategies. Optimized thoracic aortic studies should demonstrate excellent arterial enhancement, minimal or no venous enhancement, and sufficient spatial resolution to resolve vessels as small as the vertebral arteries (see Fig. 8-1). In addition, optimized timing, with or without phased array multicoils, allows for a reduction in the dose of contrast used without compromising image quality or signal to noise (45) (Fig. 8-2).

However, with shorter acquisition times, new constraints regarding coordination of data acquisition with timing of the contrast injection have become apparent. Peak arterial enhancement should coincide with the acquisition of low spatial frequency lines of k-space for optimal contrast between the aortic lumen and background tissues. However, it may be difficult to predict a given patient's circulation time. Earls et al., using a 1-cc test bolus of gadolinium administered at 2 mL/second, demonstrated that the time to peak arterial enhancement (circulation time from injection site to peak aortic enhancement) can vary from 10 to 60 seconds (46). By using a timing examination in conjunction with a MR compatible power injector all patients had diagnostic quality thoracic aortograms with only 20 mL of gadolinium administered. Many centers use a timing examination because it can be performed with any MR machine (i.e., it is not a vendor specific product) and requires no additional capital purchase. However, the most widely used technique is the "best guess" technique. This is based on the premise that the majority of patients will have a circulation time from

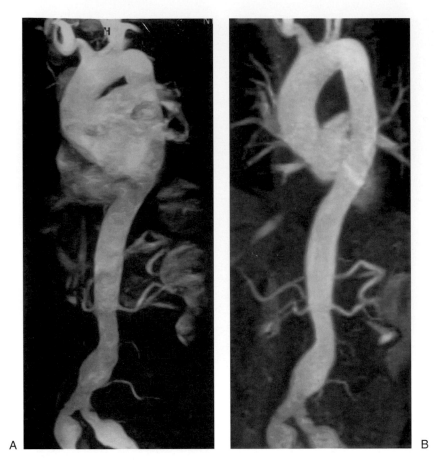

FIG. 8-2. Total body aortography: comparison of maximum-intensity-projection images from non-breath-hold, gadolinium-enhanced three-dimensional (3D) MR angiography with standard gradient strength (TR/TE/Flip angle = 21/6/30°) obtained during slow infusion of 30 mL of gadolinium (**A**) with breath-hold gadolinium-enhanced 3D MR angiography with high performance gradient strength (TR/TE/Flip angle = 5/2/30-50°) and bolus administration of 15 mL of gadolinium with a timing examination (**B**). The latter demonstrates less confounding venous enhancement and no central pulmonary arterial enhancement, both of which degrade (**A**). (From ref. 290, with permission.) All figures in this chapter using nonbreath-hold MR angiography were performed using the body coil with identical imaging parameters, gadolinium dose and infusion rate as used in Figure 8-1A. Figures describing breath-hold MR angiography were performed with either the body coil or the body phased-array coil with use of 20–30 mL of gadolinium administered at 2–3 mL/sec in conjunction with a timing examination.

peripheral vein to aorta of 12 to 20 seconds. By using a formula described in detail below, the 3D acquisition should start approximately 10 to 15 seconds after the infusion of 40 mL of gadolinium at 2 mL/second. This higher dose is necessary as a buffer to prevent mistimed examinations in patients with longer circulation times. With this technique, because of the longer bolus duration, contrast is often present within the pulmonary arteries and veins as well as the aorta.

Other more sophisticated methods of optimizing first pass contrast-enhanced MR angiography have been recently described. A novel technique developed at the Mayo Clinic uses fluoroscopic or real time triggering (47). Following the bolus injection of contrast multiple 2D GRE images are acquired with a temporal resolution of approximately 1 frame per second. When the leading edge of the contrast bolus is visually detected, breath holding instructions are given and the 3D acquisition is performed. Another approach developed by Foo et al. uses an automated sequence that detects the arrival of gadolinium with subsequent triggering of the 3D acquisition (48). The latter technique uses an SE sequence with a large voxel placed over the vessel of interest. The arrival of the gadolinium bolus is detected and triggers a 3D GRE sequence with centric phase-encoding. Therefore, the important low spatial frequency lines of k-space (which determine image contrast) are acquired at the beginning of the acquisition, coinciding with peak arterial enhancement.

Alternatively, a time-resolved approach (MR-DSA) can be used, which eliminates the need for these techniques by acquiring an entire 3D data set with sufficient temporal resolution (every 5 seconds) (49) and excellent spatial resolution. This ensures that at least 1 frame of the data set will demonstrate a selective arterial study of the vessel of interest. Even greater temporal resolution can be achieved with a time-resolved 2D technique (50), but at the expense of decreased spatial resolution.

Technical Aspects of Gadolinium-Enhanced Three-Dimensional MR Angiography

Coil Selection

Gadolinium-enhanced 3D MRA examinations are usually performed on a 1.5 T system with a high performance gradient system that allows a TR of less than 10 msec and a TE of less than 3 msec. The quadrature phased-array body coil is often used, as it provides an advantage over the body coil by virtue of increased signal-to-noise. This benefit, however, is proportional to the patient's body habitus; the increase in signal to noise is substantial in thin patients but may be negligible in obese patients. There are distinct disadvantages in using the phased-array coil, which do not apply to the body coil. The FOV is limited in the craniocaudad

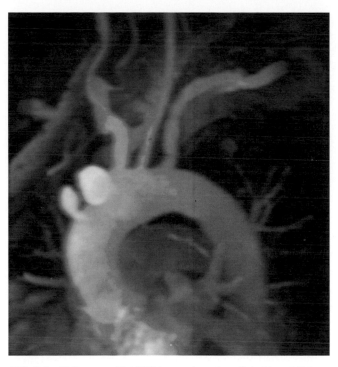

FIG. 8-3. Oblique sagittal MIP image from breath-hold gadolinium-enhanced three-dimensional MR angiogram demonstrates two pseudoaneurysms arising from the ascending aorta. These appear brighter than the descending aorta because of their proximity to the anterior elements of the phased-array coil.

When studying infants or neonates, head coils should be used and spine coils may be used for young children and adolescents with thin body habitus. Larger children and adolescents can be studied in either the body phased-array coil or the body coil.

Patient Positioning

Regardless of the coil selected, the patient's arms are positioned at the sides, and the right antecubital fossa is catheterized so that contrast draining the injection site is not present in the left brachiocephalic vein (which could obscure arch vessels on MIP images). Although some authors advocate placing the patients' arms over their heads (to minimize aliasing artifacts), this should not be performed for arch studies, as this position may cause compression of the subclavian artery and vein against the first rib. This compression can be significant in normal patients (without pathologic thoracic outlet syndrome) and can lead to a false positive diagnosis of occlusive disease in the subclavian arteries as well as susceptibility artifacts from concentrated gadolinium in the axillary vein draining the injection site (Fig. 8-4). For this reason, when specifically evaluating the subclavian, axillary, or brachial arteries, the injection should be administered in

dimension, which may result in the need for a second angiogram to evaluate the infrarenal aorta in patients with aortic dissection and diffuse aneurysmal disease. The bright signal of the subcutaneous fat may also obscure vessels of interest on MIP images, especially if a strong rectangular FOV is used. However, use of subtraction algorithms can minimize this problem if there is good coregistration between the precontrast and gadolinium-enhanced acquisitions (51). In addition, portions of the aorta closest to the coil often have more signal than segments deeper in the chest, making the MIP images difficult to window appropriately (Fig. 8-3). This can also be minimized with the use of a postprocessing filter function. The data reconstruction time, especially when performing multiple dynamic acquisitions with high resolution matrices, can be as long as ten minutes. During this reconstruction time, the machine is practically "frozen," as no further sequences can be performed. Finally, in some patients (especially children), the weight of the anterior component of the coil is uncomfortable and may potentiate claustrophobia. For these reasons, many centers use the body coil when evaluating the thoracic aorta (see Fig. 8-2). However, the body coil is clearly suboptimal when evaluating small vessels, such as the vertebral arteries, because the small field-of-view needed to resolve these vessels (25 cm) results in poor signal-to-noise. This is compounded by the fact that the very short echo time intrinsic to these 3D sequences (1–2 msec) necessitates the use of high bandwidths. This in turn also results in a signal-to-noise penalty.

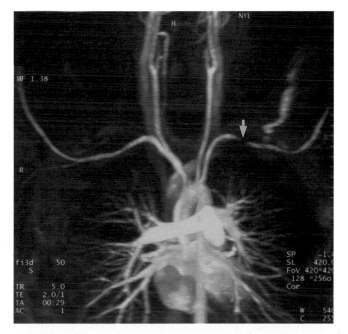

FIG. 8-4. Artifactual stenosis of the subclavian artery, caused by T2 shortening effects from concentrated gadolinium, secondary to transient venous obstruction from abducted arms (arms over the head position). Coronal maximum-intensity projection image from breath-hold gadolinium-enhanced three-dimensional MR angiogram demonstrates artifactual stenosis of the left subclavian artery (*arrow*). This results from compression of the axillary vein draining the injection site because of abduction of the arms. A second acquisition, after an additional saline flush, failed to demonstrate an abnormality. Of note is that some patients, without thoracic outlet compression, can occlude their subclavian vessels with arm abduction. (From ref. 289, with permission.)

the side contralateral to the expected pathology so that concentrated gadolinium in the draining vein will not result in artifactual signal loss from susceptibility artifacts. In addition, the use of a large volume saline flush (20 mL) will help minimize these artifacts. If bilateral disease is anticipated the lower extremity should be catheterized.

Scan Parameters

Given the wide range of variables currently available for performing MR angiography, we recommend a 3D GRE sequence using the following parameters: (3–5/1–2/30–500 [TR/TE/flip angle]), matrix of 256 × 128–192 with frequency encoding superiorly to inferiorly, a 4/8 to 7/8 rectangular field of view with a maximum dimension of 25 to 45 cm (dedicated arch vessel studies require a smaller field-of-view than thoracic aorta examinations). A coronal or oblique sagittal/left anterior oblique equivalent slab is used (thickness 9–12 cm), 50 to 80 partitions, effective section thickness of 1 to 2.2 mm, 1 acquisition (acquisition time of 10–32 seconds). Saturation pulses and gradient moment nulling are not used. ECG triggering is not routinely used as it may increase the acquisition times resulting in lengthy breath-holds. However, some find this technique to minimize motion artifacts at the aortic root and it provides for excellent anatomic images of the proximal coronary arteries (52).

It is important to position the slab from axial images at multiple levels to avoid excluding portions of extremely ectatic aortas. An unenhanced acquisition is initially performed to ensure that the vessels of interest are included in the imaging volume, to optimize the rectangular FOV that can be used without aliasing artifacts, to determine the patient's ability to suspend respiration and for use as a mask for subsequent image subtraction. This subtraction technique is helpful in eliminating the bright, subcutaneous fat, which may degrade the quality of MIP images (51).

Timing Examination

To precisely match peak arterial enhancement to the acquisition of the central lines of k-space, a timing examination is performed to measure circulation time to the region of interest (antecubital vein to aortic arch). This technique employs a 1 mL bolus of Gd-DTPA followed by 20 mL of saline, both infused at 2 to 3 mL/second while 1 cm axial magnetization-prepared GRE images (TR/TE/FA/inversion time = 11 msec/ 4.2 msec/15 degrees /300 msec/), one every 2 seconds for 60 seconds, are obtained (46). If a dark blood GRE pulse sequence is not available, one can use an ordinary GRE pulse sequence performed in the sagittal plane. Under these circumstances, because of in-plane saturation effects, a test bolus of gadolinium will result in transient aortic enhancement significantly greater than the precontrast image.

The time to peak arterial enhancement is determined by selecting the slice with the greatest qualitative enhancement.

This is less cumbersome than drawing region of interest cursors over the desired vessel.

Using the circulation time, an imaging delay between the start of the infusion of contrast and the start of the 3D acquisition is calculated with the following equation (43):

$$\text{Imaging delay} = \text{circulation time} - (\text{infusion time}/2) - (\text{imaging time}/2)$$

Once the imaging delay time is calculated, the identical 3D gradient-echo sequence is repeated with injection of 20 mL of gadolinium at 2 to 3 mL/second with an MR compatible power injector followed by a 20 mL saline flush; an inadequate flush may result in artifactual signal loss from concentrated gadolinium, as previously described (see Fig. 8-4). The examination is performed at end-inspiration as most patients find this more comfortable than breath holding at end-expiration, although the latter usually provides for better subtraction imaging with less misregistration. A second acquisition is performed after a 10 to 15 second respite during which patients can catch their breath. The purpose of this second acquisition is to better opacify the false lumen in patients with communicating dissection and as a "bail-out" if the first acquisition is suboptimal from acquiring data too early.

Following gadolinium-enhanced 3D MRA breath-hold T1-weighted gradient-echo images can be acquired through the chest to evaluate for extralumenal disease and as a general anatomic survey. These images are easy to interpret as they are very similar in appearance to contrast-enhanced CT.

Black Blood Imaging

Prior to gadolinium-enhanced MRA, axial and either oblique sagittal or coronal ECG triggered black blood T1-weighted SE images are acquired through the chest. This technique provides excellent anatomic images and is extremely useful to evaluate for mural pathology, such as intramural hematoma and the presence of pleural or pericardial effusions. Although it is not always possible to achieve high quality black blood lumenal images because of poor ECG triggering or flow artifacts, the use of longer echo times (<15 msec) and specialized dephasing gradients may be helpful. Some authors believe that aortic diameter is more reproducibly measured using black blood techniques, because of the excellent contrast between the aortic wall and the adjacent lung, unless the aorta is extremely tortuous. In this situation, true short axis aortic measurements can be achieved with reformatted images from the gadolinium-enhanced 3D data set. Although many centers still routinely perform ECG-triggered T1-weighted SE MR for black blood imaging, some institutions have replaced this time consuming technique with dark blood half-fourier single shot turbo spin-echo (HASTE) imaging (53). This technique is insensitive to patient motion, can provide excellent image quality even with poor ECG-gating, does not require breath holding, and takes less than one minute to acquire 20 images. Because of the limited signal-to-noise inherent in single shot imaging, a phased-array coil must be used. Contrast is also different with this technique and reflects the echo time of the pulse sequence used.

ECG-triggered turbo SE T2-weighted or turbo STIR images have a limited role in the evaluation of aortic disease with the exception of patients suspected of having graft infections or aortitis. In the latter clinical setting, high signal intensity within the aortic wall may correlate with disease activity.

Contrast-enhanced MRA provides excellent anatomic images but cannot quantify flow or pressure gradients. Under these circumstances, cine phase contrast MR with velocity encoding can supply additional information including measurement of pressure gradients across stenotic valves and areas of aortic narrowing (coarctation) (54). These sequences can also be used to differentiate the true from false lumen in aortic dissection and to determine if flow in the false lumen is antegrade or retrograde.

The insensitivity of MR to the presence of calcium has both advantages and disadvantages. One advantage when compared with CT is the relative ease of postprocessing MRA data as calcium does not interfere with the enhanced lumen on MIP images. Insensitivity to the detection of intimal calcifications may make characterization of pathology as intimal or medial more difficult. Another limitation is that MR is unable to detect the very heavy vascular calcifications that make certain vessels very difficult, if not impossible, to sew grafts or perform anastamoses.

Techniques of Reconstruction

CT angiography (and MRA) can be performed using either multiplanar reformations (MPR) or 3D renderings (Fig. 8-5) (55).

Multiplanar Reconstructions

As reviewed in greater depth in Chapters 1 and 3, multiplanar reconstructions (MPRs) are one voxel thick 2D ''tomographic'' sections interpolated along an arbitrary plane or curved surface (see Fig. 8-5A). These have the considerable advantage of computational efficiency, requiring only a few seconds to reconstruct, as well as the advantage of instantaneous window width and level manipulation. Offsetting any potential decrease in spatial resolution caused by partial volume averaging, it is possible to interactively obtain a series of single oblique reconstructions derived from corresponding transverse images allowing individual vessels to be displayed to best advantage along their nearest long axes. Unfortunately, MPRs are still susceptible to stair-step artifacts limiting their interpretation. Characteristically, these manifest as irregularities along the surfaces of airways that

course obliquely (6). This effect may be overcome to some degree by decreasing the reconstruction interval.

Three-Dimensional Rendering

Under this heading are included a number of different techniques all of which have in common the use of an entire volume (or preselected subvolume) of scan data to generate 2D images that convey 3D spatial information (56). Three broad categories may be identified: multiplanar volume reconstructions, including MIPs, shaded surface displays (SSDs), and volumetric rendering. Of these, the latter two may be adapted to allow both external an internal rendering of vessels.

Multiplanar Volume Reconstructions

Multiplanar volume reconstructions (MPVRs) are a variant of MPRs that allow a user to obtain 2D representations from a 3D volume (or slab) at any angle using either average, ray sum, MIP or even minimum (MINIP) intensity projections (see Fig. 8-5 B–D). Familiar as a common method for visualizing both MRA and CTA data, MPVRs may be obtained in any direction, including the axial plane, thereby simulating true cross-sectional images (57). Of these, the most commonly used for imaging vessels are MIP (58). MIPs are derived by projecting onto an imaging plane the highest density voxel encountered in a ray through the scan volume. The result is a 2D image in which blood vessels are typically highlighted. Alternatively, pixel values along individual rays may be either averaged, or summed: averaged images mimic the appearance of routine MPRs, whereas summed vessels appear translucent (see Fig. 8-5C). MIPs encode variations in pixel attenuation, allowing differentiation between calcium and thrombus: they are not threshold dependent. As a result, they also may be of value by depicting differences in flow rates as for example occurs in aortic dissection (see Fig. 8-5C), or even within single vessels as a result of antegrade flow. However, unlike other volume rendering techniques, those derived using multiplanar volume reconstructions have no depth cues. As a consequence, MIPs are best suited for displaying anatomy in which superimposition of structures is minimized. This limitation may be overcome in part by multiple projections viewed in a cine mode as well as volume editing, restricting MIPs to only a few transaxial images—so-called thin slab MIPs—to remove unwanted overlying structures. Nonetheless, MIP images, as all other multiplanar volume reconstructions, are best interpreted in conjunction with the original axial source images (58).

Shaded Surface Displays and Volumetric Rendering

Included in this category are external and internal image renderings. External rendering allows visualization of structures from an external vantage point using a simulated exter-

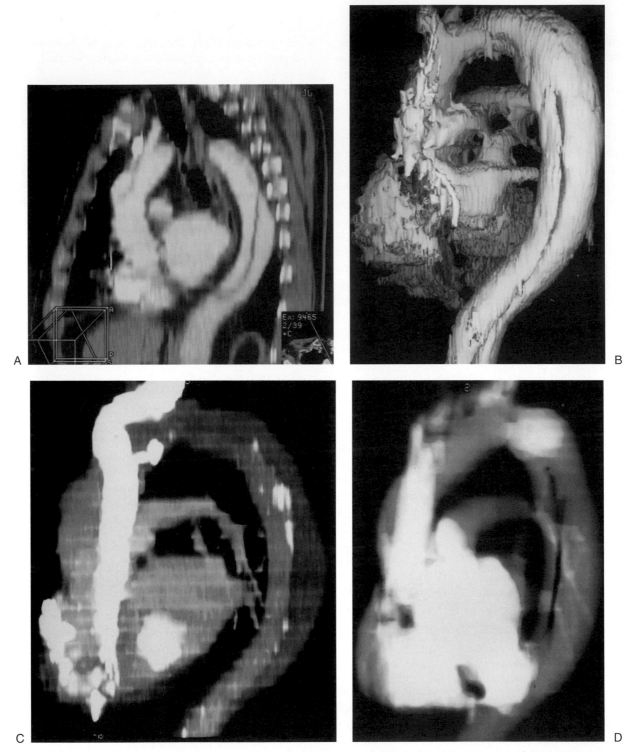

FIG. 8-5. Aortic dissection: reconstruction options. **A:** Multiplanar reconstruction (MPR) in the sagittal plane obtained using 5-mm helical CT sections with a pitch = 1.6, and reconstruction interval = 4 mm following administration of 125 cc nonionic contrast media (300 mg I/mL) at a rate of 3 cc/sec shows an intimal flap within both the ascending and descending aorta with seemingly equal opacification of both lumens. MPRs have the advantage of rapid reconstruction without extensive editing. **B:** Three-dimensional (3D) shaded surface display (SSD) again shows presence of an intimal flap extending into the ascending aorta, identifiable as a disruption in the surface contour of the vessel. Although SSDs can provide exquisite delineation of anatomy, these images require extensive editing, especially when assessing the thoracic aorta. They are also susceptible to both noise and artifacts related to partial volume averaging, and are of no use for detecting calcifications or metallic stents. **C:** Maximum intensity projection image (MIP) in the same plane as **A** and **B**. Although MIPs encode variations in pixel intensity, allowing identification of calcification and subtle differences in density between the true and the false lumen, they are limited by a lack of three-dimensionality in this image resulting in superimposition of the superior vena cava and resulting loss of delineation of the intimal flap (compare with **A** and **B**). This limitation can be overcome in part by use of multiple projections from varying angles as well as use of volume editing to create so-called thin-slab MIPs. **D:** Ray-sum projection in the same plane as **A–C**. This technique renders the aorta translucent and as such has been favored by some for assessing aortic dissection. Like MIPs, however, these too suffer from a lack of three-dimensionality and necessitate viewing in multiple projections.

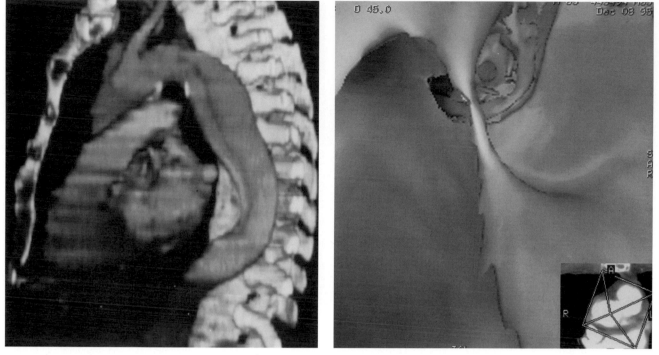

FIG. 8-5. *Continued.* **E:** Volumetric rendering in the same plane as **A–D**. These have the advantage of retaining the full range of tissue densities represented within the volume scanned, allowing a greater range of 3D images resulting in improved anatomic orientation. **F:** Internal rendering (virtual angioscopy) viewed from within the proximal ascending aorta looking toward the aortic arch using shaded-surface rendering technique clearly shows the presence of the intimal flap, as well as the origins of the great vessels, which are patent. Internal rendering may be of particular value in assessing the relationship between aneurysms and aortic branches as a roadmap prior to surgery. (From ref. 55, with permission.)

nal light source. This can be accomplished using either surface thresholding or volume rendering techniques. In the former, a single threshold is selected and used to generate surfaces at the boundaries of structures, effectively discarding all other data within the scan volume. The result is often exquisite depictions of the relationships between anatomic structures, including vascular branches. Unfortunately, despite the striking visual appearance of these images, external rendering techniques usually require time-consuming editing to create appropriate subvolumes for analysis using either manual trace or connectivity-based editing techniques. In addition, the use of a single threshold makes shaded surface techniques susceptible to both noise and to artifacts related to partial volume averaging; this can result in surface discontinuities or holes, jagged edges, and floating pixels. More important, focal areas of high density, in particular, vascular calcifications and metallic stents, may be completely obscured (7). It cannot be overemphasized that surface rendering techniques reflect voxel boundaries, not true tissue interfaces.

In distinction to shaded surface displays (SSDs), volume rendering uses linear or continuous scaling techniques in which every voxel within the original data set is assigned a proportional value based on the full range of tissue densities represented (59). By use of a transfer function, Hounsfield numbers may then be mapped to brightness, color and opac-

ity (see Fig. 8-5E) (60). This approach results in fewer artifacts and allows a greater range of possible 3D images (including the ability to create transparent tissue planes allowing anatomic structures to be viewed at various depths, as well as stereoscopic imaging). Most important, volumetric rendering allows depiction of vascular calcifications and thrombus, and provides improved visualization of small vessel anatomy (see Fig. 8-5E). Although previously limited by the need for extensive, time-consuming image processing, three-dimensional CT now can be performed using real-time interactive volume rendering (56,60,61).

Similar to external rendering, internal renderings can be performed using either volumetric rendering or 3D surface shaded reconstructions to simulate the endolumenal appearance of vessels—so-called virtual angioscopy (62). Internal rendering allows visualization of the internal structures of organs from a point source at a finite distance, simulating human perspective ostensibly as seen through an endoscope (see Fig. 8-5F). Images are viewed through the tip of a cone with either a narrow (15 degree) or wide (60 degree) field of view (63). A flight path of sequential images can also be constructed and navigated either sequentially or in a cine loop, further simulating endoscopy.

Although 3D shaded-surface reconstructions are relatively fast, they are limited by their greater susceptibility to noise and partial volume averaging; this can result in surface dis-

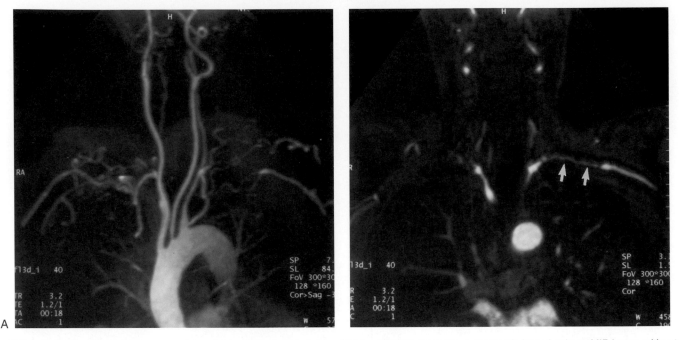

FIG. 8-6. Artifactual occlusion on maximum-intensity-projection image (MIP)—Pitfall in rendering a diagnosis based only on MIP image without evaluation of source data. **A:** Coronal MIP image from breath-hold gadolinium-enhanced three-dimensional (3D) MR angiogram in a patient with giant cell arteritis demonstrates apparent chronic, bilateral subclavian artery occlusions with extensive collateral vessels in the shoulder region. **B:** Source image from same acquisition shows a patent but severely stenotic left subclavian artery (*arrows*). (From ref. 289, with permission.)

continuities, jagged edges, and floating pixels. Volumetric rendering also has the advantage of allowing perivascular tissues to be seen through vessel walls, allowing more precise anatomic localization, although shaded surface reconstructions also allow precise localization of perivascular structures by means of simultaneous annotated displays of corresponding axial, coronal, and sagittal images oriented to conform to any given plane identified from the endoluminal display (62,63).

MR Image Analysis

Similar to CT, multiple display options and postprocessing techniques can be used to evaluate the gadolinium-enhanced acquisition and ultimately, to present the imaging information to the referring clinician in a user friendly fashion. To maximize diagnostic accuracy and minimize interpretation error the source data, MPR, and MIP images should be evaluated on an interactive console. Because the MIP algorithm only includes the voxels with the greatest signal intensity within a given ray tracing, structures of lower signal intensity, such as thrombus or intimal flap, may be excluded. Therefore, evaluation of the source data with pertinent reformations is mandatory for diagnosis of branch vessel involvement in aortic dissection and for detection and accurate measurement of aneurysmal disease. Furthermore, MIP images interpreted in isolation may be unreliable in estimating vessel caliber and can overestimate the degree of stenosis in a

given vessel. In addition, diminutive vessels may not be readily identified on MIP images but easily seen on source data (Fig. 8-6). When overlapping vessels (usually veins) obscure the artery of interest, a restricted or subvolume MIP can often eliminate the obscuring vessel. Multiplanar reformations are invaluable in demonstrating abnormalities of small vessels, such as vertebral artery ostial lesions, and in detecting aortic arch atheromata. Other postprocessing capabilities include SSD algorithms, volume rendering and virtual endoscopic renderings (63,64). However, it is unclear whether these time-consuming techniques provide any incremental diagnostic yield when compared with evaluation just the MIP and MPR images (65).

NORMAL ANATOMY

Regional anatomy of the mediastinal great vessels and their relationships to each other and other mediastinal structures are discussed in Chapter 2. In this section, the appearances of specific vascular structures will be reviewed.

The Aorta and Its Branches

The appearance of the aorta is characteristic although it can vary somewhat in size and shape in different individuals (66). The thoracic aorta is usually considered to consist of an ascending segment, a transverse segment or arch, and a descending segment (Fig. 8-7).

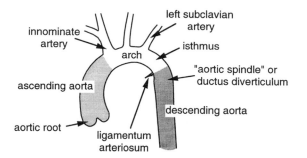

FIG. 8-7. Anatomy of the thoracic aorta and significant landmarks. The ascending aorta extends from the aortic valve to the origin of the innominate artery. Its proximal portion, in relation to the aortic valve and sinuses of Valsalva, is termed the aortic root. The aortic arch begins at the innominate artery and ends at the ligamentum arteriosum. Its most distal part, which is often slightly narrowed is termed the aortic isthmus. The descending aorta begins at the ligamentum. Its proximal portion may appear slightly dilated, and has been termed the aortic "spindle."

The proximal portion of the ascending aorta is termed the aortic root; it consists of the aortic valve, annulus, and the sinuses of Valsalva. The right and left coronary arteries arise from the right and left sinuses of Valsalva; the posterior sinus is unassociated with a coronary artery and is referred to as the noncoronary sinus. The aortic root is surrounded by cardiac structures, with the right atrium to its right, the right ventricle and pulmonary outflow tract anterior to it, and the left atrium posterior. The aortic valve and sinuses of Valsalva are occasionally seen on contrast-enhanced CT scans. Above the aortic root, the ascending aorta continues for a distance of 4 to 5 cm. This segment of the aorta is well demonstrated on CT.

The aortic arch begins at the innominate artery, and consists of two segments. The proximal part of the arch is the longest, and gives rise to the innominate, left carotid, and left subclavian arteries, although variations in the branching pattern of these vessels and their divisions are common. The distal part of the arch, between the origin of the left subclavian artery and the ligamentum arteriosum is known as the aortic isthmus; it is relatively short, measuring 1 to 2 cm in length, and its lumen may be a few millimeters narrower in adults than the aorta immediately distal to the ligamentum. Slight narrowing of the isthmus is most common in young children.

Distal to the ligamentum arteriosum is the descending thoracic aorta. The most proximal portion of the descending aorta may appear slightly dilated, a finding that is more common in children than adults. This dilated segment of the proximal descending aorta has been termed the "aortic spindle" because of its fusiform shape (see Fig. 8-7) (67); a more focal dilatation of the anterior aorta at this level may be caused by a "ductus diverticulum." The largest branches of the descending aorta are the intercostal and bronchial arteries.

Usually, narrowing of the aortic lumen in the region of the aortic isthmus is not visible on transverse images; however, this finding may be seen on oblique sagittal CT reformations or MRI. It is important to keep in mind that the aortic arch also varies in appearance depending upon its curvature and orientation relative to the scan plane. Scans traversing different parts of the arch along its length can result in a false representation of aortic arch diameter. When scans are centered through the lower portion of the arch, it may appear constricted in its mid or posterior portions. Also, although the diameter of the aortic arch decreases gradually from anterior to posterior, the arch may appear elliptical in shape on scans through the top of the arch.

Normal Aortic Diameter

The thoracic aorta tapers progressively from its origin, and consequently varies in diameter at different levels, with the ascending aorta and anterior arch being about 1 cm larger than the posterior arch and descending aorta; in unusual cases, the descending aorta appears larger than the ascending aorta.

The ascending and descending aorta appear rounded in shape, and in these locations, the diameter of the aorta can be accurately determined. As measured in more than 100 normal subjects (68) the average diameter of the proximal ascending aorta is 3.6 cm (range 2.4–4.7 cm), the ascending aorta just below the arch is 3.51 cm (range 2.2–4.6 cm), the proximal descending aorta is 2.63 cm (range 1.6–3.7 cm), the middle descending aorta is 2.48 cm (range 1.6–3.7 cm), and the distal descending aorta is 2.42 cm (range 1.4–3.3 cm) (Fig. 8-8). Aortic diameters have also been shown to increase with age, correlate with vertebral size, and be larger in men then women (Table 8-2).

It is important to recognize that the aorta can vary considerably in its diameter in different patients, as indicated by the ranges of values listed above. However, in an individual patient, the aorta should taper in a consistent fashion along its length. Any significant deviation from this should be considered suspicious of an aneurysm.

In children, the aortic diameters at these same levels have been shown to correlate closely with age, and increase in a linear fashion with growth (Fig. 8-9) (69). In every case, the diameter of the ascending aorta was greater than that of the descending aorta at the same level.

The wall of the aorta measures several millimeters in thickness in normal subjects, but increases with age. On unopacified CT scans, the aortic wall usually appears with the same attenuation as blood in the aortic lumen, and cannot be distinguished from it. However, in some anemic patients, the wall may appear slightly denser than aortic blood on unopacified scans; focal or concentric increased density of the aortic wall associated with thickening can also be seen in patients with intramural hematoma (70) and arteritis (71). In the presence of atherosclerosis and aortic plaques, focal areas of wall thickening may appear lower in attenuation than adjacent aortic wall and aortic blood because of their

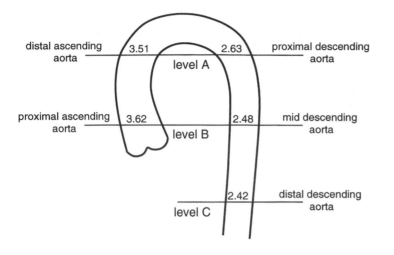

FIG 8-8. Mean values for aortic diameter measured using CT in 100 normal subjects of varying age. At each level, the range of values seen in normals was approximately 1 cm more or less than the mean. (From ref. 68, with permission.)

TABLE 8-2. *Average aorta diameter at different levels, by age and sex*

Level	Men (age)			Women (age)		
	21–40	41–60	>60	21–40	41–60	>60
Proximal ascending aorta (level A) (cm)	3.47	3.63	3.91	3.36	3.72	3.50
Distal ascending aorta (level B) (cm)	3.28	3.64	3.80	2.80	3.47	3.68
Proximal descending aorta (level A) (cm)	2.21	2.64	3.14	2.06	2.63	2.88
Middle descending aorta (level B) (cm)	2.25	2.39	2.98	1.91	2.45	2.64
Distal descending aorta (level C) (cm)	2.12	2.43	2.98	1.89	2.43	2.40

Modified from ref. 67.

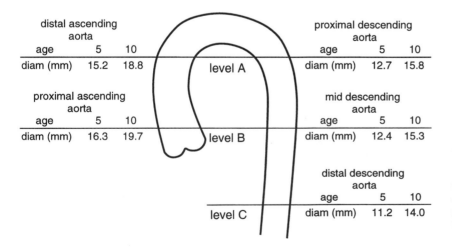

FIG. 8-9. Approximate mean values for aortic diameter in children aged 5 and 10 years. Ninety-five percent confident limits include values approximately 3 mm above and below the values shown. (From ref. 69, with permission.)

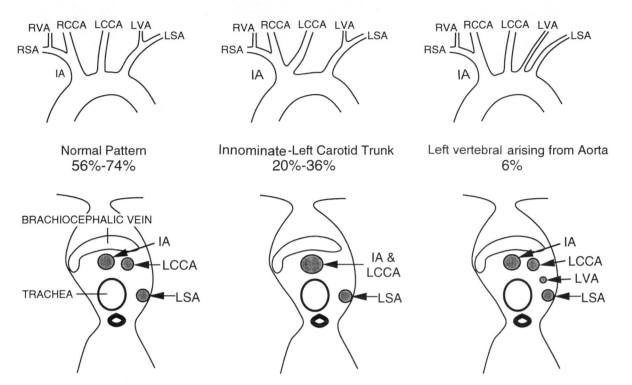

FIG. 8-10. Most common branching patterns of the arch great vessels, with their approximate frequencies, and typical CT appearances. *IA,* innominate artery; *LCCA,* left common carotid artery; *LSA,* left subclavian artery; *LVA,* left ventricle artery; *RVA,* right ventrcle artery; *RSA,* right subclavian artery.

lipid content (72); these plaques are often irregular in attenuation. On contrast opacified scans, the aortic wall may sometimes be seen as lower in attenuation than blood in the aortic lumen.

Aortic Branching

The three great arterial branches of the aorta arise sequentially, and are often seen at different levels. The innominate artery arises as the first branch of the arch, and is usually seen more caudally than the other branches. It is located near the midline of the trachea or slightly to the right of midline in most normal patients, and is in close proximity to the anterior tracheal wall (Fig. 8-10). The innominate artery is usually the largest aortic branch, as it gives rise to the right subclavian, common carotid, and vertebral arteries. The left common carotid artery arises next, and at a more cephalad level. It lies to the left and slightly posterolateral to the innominate artery; generally it has the smallest diameter of the three major arterial branches. The left subclavian artery is the last arch branch and arises from the posterosuperior portion of the aortic arch; it is usually visible at the most cephalad aspect of the arch seen on CT. The left subclavian artery is a relatively posterior structure throughout most of its course, lying to the left of, and frequently directly lateral to the trachea. The lateral border of the left subclavian artery typically indents the mediastinal surface of the left upper lobe. At the level of origin of the left subclavian artery, the posterior portion of the arch should not be confused with a mediastinal mass.

Although this pattern of branching is typical, variations are common (73,74). A "normal" branching pattern was found in only 74% of 300 arteriograms reviewed by Sutton and Rhys Davies and in from 56% to 70% of autopsy cases (see Fig. 8-10) (73,74). The most common variation is a combined origin of the innominate and left common carotid arteries (see Fig. 8-10; Fig. 8-11), which is seen in about 20% of patients at arteriography and in from 22% to 36% of cases at autopsy. In about 6% of cases, the left vertebral artery arises as a separate branch of the aorta, between the left common carotid and subclavian branches, instead of arising from the left subclavian artery itself (see Fig. 8-10; Fig. 8-12).

Above the level of the innominate artery bifurcation, the right subclavian and right common carotid arteries can be identified as separate structures and although usually located somewhat more anteriorly, may appear quite similar to the left subclavian and common carotid arteries in size and location. The exact position of the bifurcation of the brachiocephalic artery is variable, depending on the length and degree of tortuosity of this vessel. In a significant percentage of cases, the brachiocephalic artery bifurcates somewhat distally; in these cases the right subclavian artery has an oblique course, and if thin sections are not obtained near the thoracic inlet, it may not be seen at all. When the right common carotid and right subclavian arteries are visible, they nor-

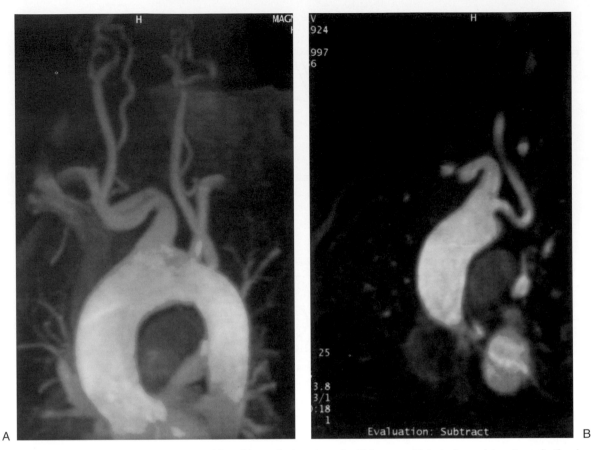

FIG. 8-11. Common origin of the left common carotid and innominate artery. **A:** Oblique sagittal maximum-intensity-projection image from breath-hold gadolinium-enhanced three-dimensional MR angiogram fails to demonstrate the origin of the left common carotid artery because of extreme tortuosity. **B:** Reformatted image from same data set demonstrates that the left common carotid does arise from a common trunk with the innominate artery and loops inferiorly just after its origin.

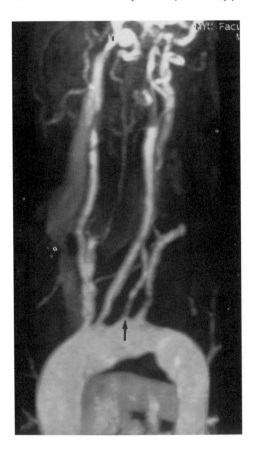

FIG. 8-12. Oblique sagittal maximum-intensity-projection image from breath-hold gadolinium-enhanced three-dimensional MR angiogram demonstrates a direct origin of the left vertebral artery from the aortic arch (*arrow*).

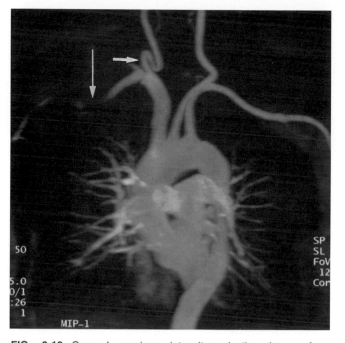

FIG. 8-13. Coronal maximum-intensity-projection image from breath-hold gadolinium-enhanced three-dimensional MR angiogram in a patient referred for a palpable neck mass demonstrates the mass as a common carotid artery loop (*short arrow*). Diffuse signal loss in the right subclavian artery (*long arrow*) is artifactual and caused by stagnant, concentrated gadolinium in the adjacent vein draining the injection site. This resulted from failure to administer a flush after the gadolinium bolus. (From ref. 289, with permission.)

CONGENITAL AORTIC DISEASE

Aortic Arch Anomalies

To recognize anomalies of the aorta and great vessels it is helpful to have a working knowledge of embryology. These anomalies are most easily understood if the hypothetical double arch system, described by Edwards (76) is used as a framework. As shown in Figure 8-14, in this system there is an aortic arch and a potential ductus arteriosus on each side; the descending aorta is in the midline posteriorly. Interruption of this arch at different locations can explain the various aortic arch anomalies. These can be divided into three main groups: left aortic arch anomalies, right aortic arch anomalies, and double aortic arch anomalies.

Normally, there is interruption of the hypothetical right arch distal to the right subclavian artery. The right common carotid and subclavian arteries fuse to become the right brachiocephalic artery as the proximal portion of the embryologic right arch becomes incorporated into the left arch. The result is the normal left-sided aortic arch. This is demonstrated in Figure 8-15.

Left Aortic Arch Anomalies

The most common congenital anomaly of the aorta is an aberrant right subclavian artery originating from an otherwise normal left-sided arch. This occurs in approximately 0.5% of the normal population (76). According to Edward's model this occurs when there is interruption of the embryologic right aortic arch between the right common carotid and the right subclavian arteries. The right subclavian artery then originates from the posterior portion of the left-sided arch and crosses the mediastinum obliquely from left to right, lying posterior to the trachea and esophagus (Figs. 8-16 and 8-17). Dilatation of the artery at its origin (kommerell diverticulum) is common (Fig. 8-18), occurring in up to 60% of cases and may present as dysphagia. True aneurysms of an aberrant right subclavian artery (Fig. 8-19) have a mortality as high as 50% and should be surgically repaired (77). Many arch vessel anatomic variants coexist with aberrant subclavian arteries; the most frequent is a common origin of both carotid arteries, which occurs in 48% of cases (Fig. 8-20) (78). Less common is a direct origin of the vertebral artery from its ipsilateral carotid artery; this occurs almost exclusively in patients with aberrant subclavian arteries (78).

Right Aortic Arch Anomalies

Using Edward's double aortic arch model, five potential anomalies can occur, although only two are relatively common. The type of anomaly encountered will depend on the exact point at which the left aortic arch is interrupted.

The most common right aortic arch anomaly is a right aortic arch with an aberrant left subclavian artery (Fig. 8-

mally are found only in sections through the uppermost portion of the superior mediastinum. Visualization of these vessels in a more inferior position, just above the aortic arch, frequently indicates the presence of some type of vascular mediastinal anomaly, usually involving the aortic arch. This has been termed the "four vessel sign" by McLoughlin et al. (75); it is common in double aortic arch.

Although the great vessels should be recognizable by their characteristic appearances and locations, tortuosity or ectasia of these vessels may present a confusing picture and be easily mistaken as pathologic. Use of intravenous contrast media, with or without multiplanar reformations, will almost always resolve this problem. Alternatively, MRA readily demonstrates tortuosity (see Fig. 8-11), ectasia, and vessel loops that may present clinically as a palpable neck mass (Fig. 8-13).

The subclavian arteries exit and enter the mediastinum by crossing over the first ribs, behind the proximal portions of the clavicles. The subclavian vein lies anterior and the subclavian artery lies posterior to the anterior scalenus muscle, which attaches to the superior border of the first rib. The transition from the mediastinal to the axillary portions of the subclavian arteries is difficult to visualize because they angle sharply as they cross over the first rib. The axillary portions of the subclavian arteries lie posterior to the corresponding veins.

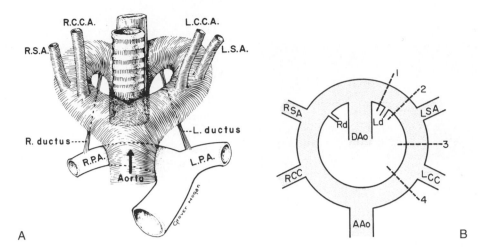

A   B

FIG. 8-14. A: Hypothetical double aortic arch of Edwards. (From Shuford WH, Sybers RG. The aortic arch and its malformations, 1974. Courtesy of Charles C. Thomas, Springfield, IL.) **B:** Schematic representation of embryonic double aortic arch. Normally, there is interruption of the right arch distal to the right subclavian artery. The result is a normal left arch. Right aortic arches result when there is interruption of some portion of the left aortic arch. Five potential sites of interruption have been identified. If there is interruption distal to the left subclavian (at either 1 or 2), the result is a right aortic arch with mirror-image branching (types 1 and 2). If there is interruption between the left subclavian and left common carotid arteries (at 3), the result is a right aortic arch with an abberant left subclavian (type 3). If the arch is interrupted proximal to the left common carotid artery (at 4), the result is a right arch with an abberant innominate artery (type 4). Finally, interruption may occur both distal to the left subclavian artery and proximal to the left subclavian artery (at 1 and 3); this results in an isolated left subclavian artery, connected to the left pulmonary artery through the left ductus arteriosus (type 5). *DAo,* descending aorta; *AAo,* ascending aorta; *LSA,* left subclavian artery; *LCC,* left common carotid artery; *Ld,* left ductus arteriosus; *Rd,* right ductus; *RCC,* right common carotid artery; *RSA,* right subclavian artery.

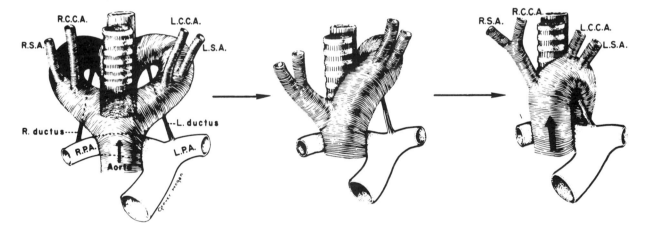

FIG. 8-15. Hypothesized embryologic development of the normal left arch. The shaded portion of the right arch, distal to the right subclavian artery, is interrupted. (From Shuford WH, Sybers RG. *The aortic arch and its malformations,* 1974. Courtesy of Charles C. Thomas, Springfield, IL.)

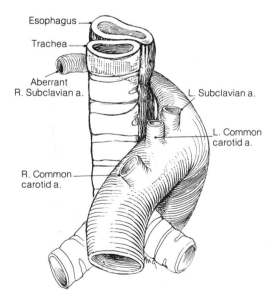

FIG. 8-16. Schematic representation of an aberrant right subclavian artery.

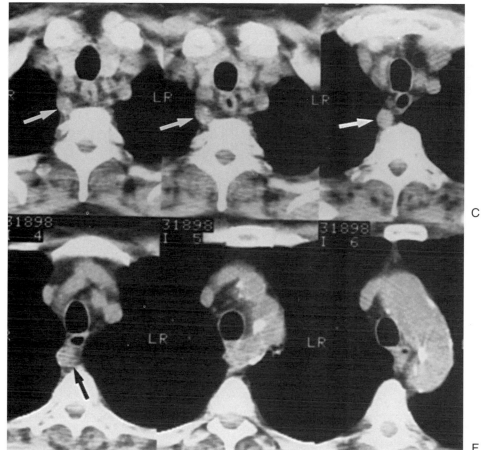

A,B

C

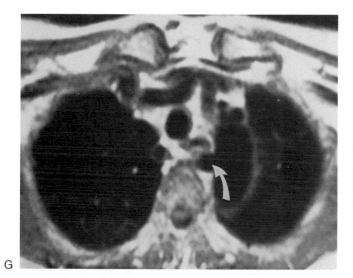

D,E

F

FIG. 8-17. Aberrant right subclavian artery. **A–F:** Enlargements of sequential CT images through the mediastinum from the great vessels to the aortic arch, inferiorly, respectively. An abberant right subclavian artery is present, arising from the medial-posterior portion of the aortic arch on the left. This artery passes posterior to the espohagus and trachea (*arrow* in **D**) and then proceeds superiorly to eventually lie in a normal position in the superior mediastinum (*arrows* in **A–C**). **G,H:** Axial and saggital MR images, respectively, in another patient with an abberant right subclavian artery. Again, the abberant artery is easily identified arising from the aorta (*arrow* in **G**), posterior to the esophagus and trachea (*arrow* in **H**).

G

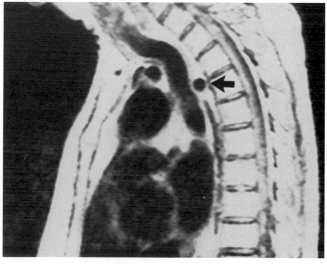

H

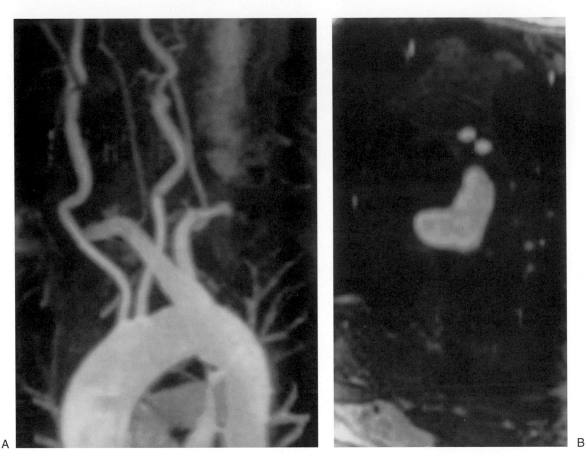

A   B

FIG. 8-18. Enlargement of an aberrant subclavian artery at its origin (diverticulum of Kommerell) **(A)**. Oblique sagittal maximum-intensity-projection image and axial reformation **(B)** from breath-hold gadolinium-enhanced three-dimensional MR angiogram show enlargement of the origin of an aberrant right subclavian artery. (From ref. 289, with permission.)

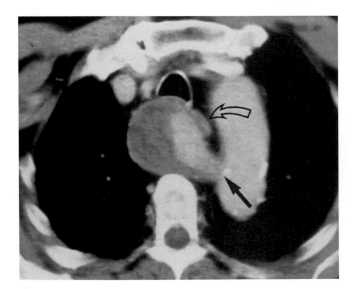

FIG. 8-19. Aneurysm, aberrant right subclavian artery. Contrast-enhanced CT image at the level of the aortic arch demonstrates an aneurysm of an aberrant right subclavian artery (*arrow*) with considerable amount of thrombus. The aneurysm causes considerable mass effect on the adjacent esophagus (*curved arrow*).

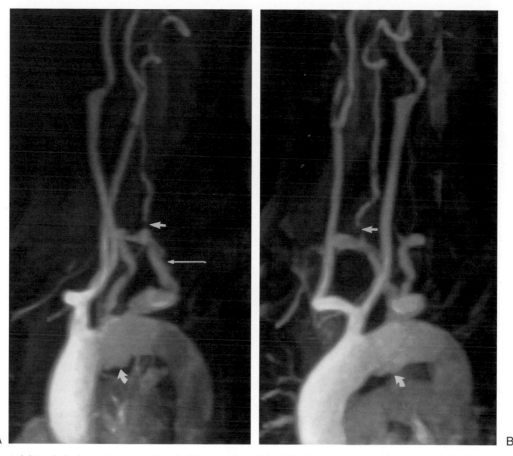

FIG. 8-20. Aberrant right subclavian artery associated with common origin of both common carotid arteries. **A,B:** Oblique sagittal maximum-intensity-projection images from breath-hold, gadolinium-enhanced three-dimensional MR angiogram demonstrate plaque within an aberrant right subclavian artery (*long arrow* in **A**), which is stenotic at its origin. There is a severe stenosis of the ipsilateral vertebral artery (*straight arrows*) and the origin of the left subclavian artery. Both carotid arteries arise from a common trunk. There is a deep ulcerated plaque on the inferior aspect of the aortic arch (*curved arrows*). (From ref. 289, with permission.)

21). This occurs in approximately one in 2,500 patients. The sequence of events leading to this malformation is illustrated in Figure 8-22. In this case, there is interruption of the left arch between the left common carotid and left subclavian arteries. This results in an anterior left common carotid artery as the first branch of the ascending aorta, and a retroesophageal left subclavian artery, which may also result in dysphagia (Fig. 8-23). This variant is usually not associated with congenital heart disease. In both aberrant right and left subclavian arteries the portion of the aberrant artery that is adjacent to the spine may be compressed resulting in vessel narrowing. A right aortic arch with mirror-image branching occurs if the hypothetical left arch is interrupted distal to the left subclavian artery (Fig. 8-24). This anomaly is significant because of the high incidence of concomitant congenital heart disease, usually tetrology of fallot. Other rare left aortic arch anomalies may result in the syndrome of the interrupted aortic arch, which is discussed in detail elsewhere in this chapter.

In the usual case of right aortic arch with mirror image branching, interruption of the left arch occurs distal to the ductus arteriosus. The result is that there is no structure posterior to the trachea or esophagus. Rarely, interruption occurs distal to the left subclavian artery but proximal to the ductus (79). If the ductus on the left side persists the result is a true vascular ring.

Symptomatic Arch Anomalies

Symptomatic arch anomalies include double aortic arch, right arch with aberrant left subclavian artery and persistent left ligamentum arteriosum, and cervical arch. All of these abnormalities can result in tracheal and esophageal compression but the former two, often present in infancy with respiratory or feeding problems. Cervical aortic arches are rare anomalies that are usually right sided and are associated with unusual great vessel origins (80). The innominate artery may fail to form and there are usually separate origins of the subclavian and carotid arteries. They are often circumflex, crossing the chest or lower neck in a near coronal orientation that may result in compression of the esophagus (81) and may present as a pulsatile neck mass.

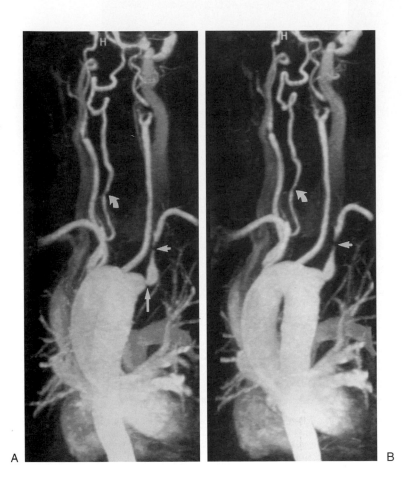

FIG. 8-21. Coronal **(A)** and oblique sagittal **(B)** maximum-intensity-projection images from breath-hold, gadolinium-enhanced three-dimensional MR angiogram show a right sided aortic arch with a stenosis at the origin (*long arrow* in **A**) and midportion (*short arrows*) of an aberrant left subclavian artery. The left vertebral artery is occluded and the right vertebral artery is prominent with a focal stenosis (*curved arrows*). The injection of contrast was administered through the right arm. (From ref. 289, with permission.)

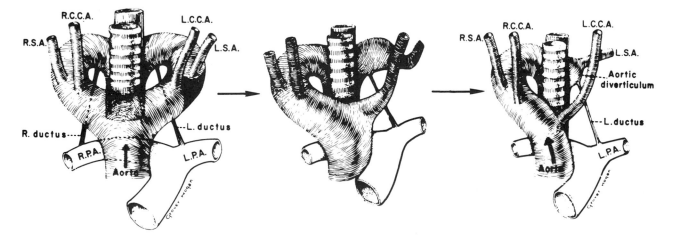

FIG. 8-22. Hypothesized embryonic development of a right aortic arch with an aberrant left subclavian artery. *RSA*, right subclavian artery; *RCCA*, right common carotid artery; *LCCA*, left common carotid artery; *LSA*, left subclavian artery; *LPA*, left pulmonary artery; *RPA*, right pulmonary artery. (From Shuford WH, Sybers RG. The aortic arch and its malformations, 1974. Courtesy of Charles C. Thomas, Springfield, IL.)

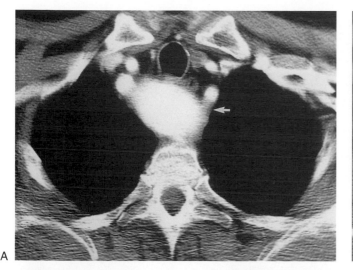

A

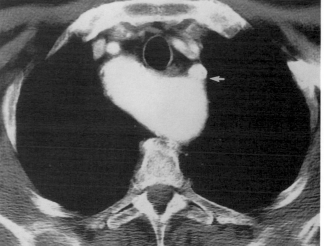

B

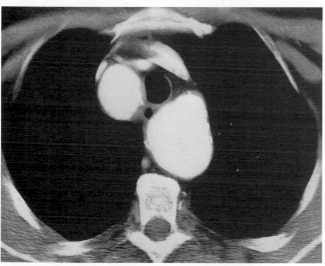

C

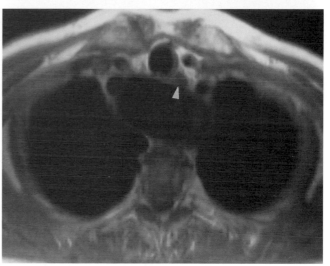

D

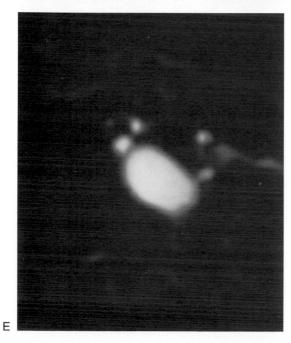

E

FIG. 8-23. Aneurysmal dilatation of a right sided aortic arch with aberrant left subclavian artery, CT and MR demonstration. **A–C:** Sequential contrast-enhanced helical CT images through the mediastinum from the great vessels to the aortic arch, inferiorly, respectively. There is aneurysmal dilatation of the ascending, arch, and descending portion of a right aortic arch. The left subclavian artery arises from the descending aorta (*arrows* in **A** and **B**). **D:** T1-weighted SE MR image at the same level as **A** demonstrates displacement of the esophagus anteriorly (*arrowhead*). **E:** Axial reformation from breath-hold gadolinium-enhanced three-dimensional MR angiogram at the same level as **A** and **D** demonstrates a four vessel arch configuration. Note that because of the arch aneurysm the superior most portion of the aorta is at the thoracic inlet and appears similar to a cervical aortic arch.

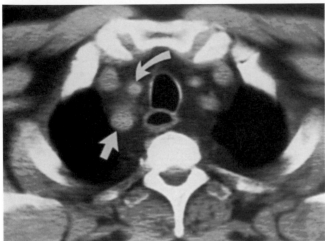

A

B

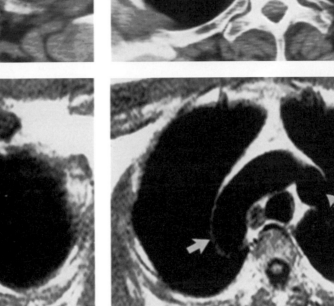

C

D

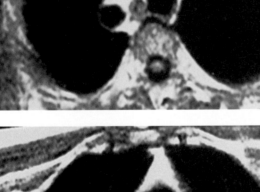

E

FIG. 8-24. Right aortic arch, mirror-image branching. **A, B:** Sequential intravenous contrast-enhanced CT images through the great vessels and aortic arch, respectively. A right-sided aortic arch is easily identified (*arrow* in **B**), lying just to the right of the trachea and esophagus. Mirror-image branching of the great vessels is present; a right bracheocephaic artery (*not shown*) has given rise to an otherwise normally positioned right subclavian artery (*arrow* in **A**) and a right common carotid artery (*curved arrow* in **A**). **C–E:** Sequential MR images through the great vessels, the aortic arch, and the aortico-pulmonary window, respectively, in a different patient than **A** and **B**. Again note the presence of a right-sided aortic arch (*arrow* in **D**) with mirror-image branching, identifiable by the presence of a left brachiocephalic artery (*arrow* in **C**). Note that in this case there is complete situs, with a left-sided superior vena cava (*curved arrows* in **D** and **E**) as well as a reversal of normal lung segmentation, identifiable by the presence of an anatomic right upper lobe bronchus on the left (*arrow* in **E**).

Double aortic arches have been classified into two types, depending on the patency of the arches (79). The most frequent form is a functional double aortic arch. In this case, both arches remain patent: the right common carotid and subclavian arteries arise from the right arch, whereas the left common carotid and subclavian arteries arise from the left arch. Both arches join posteriorly to form one descending aorta, which may be midline or, more usually, left sided. The two arches may be of equal size, although the right arch is generally larger (Figs. 8-25–8-27). Less common is the

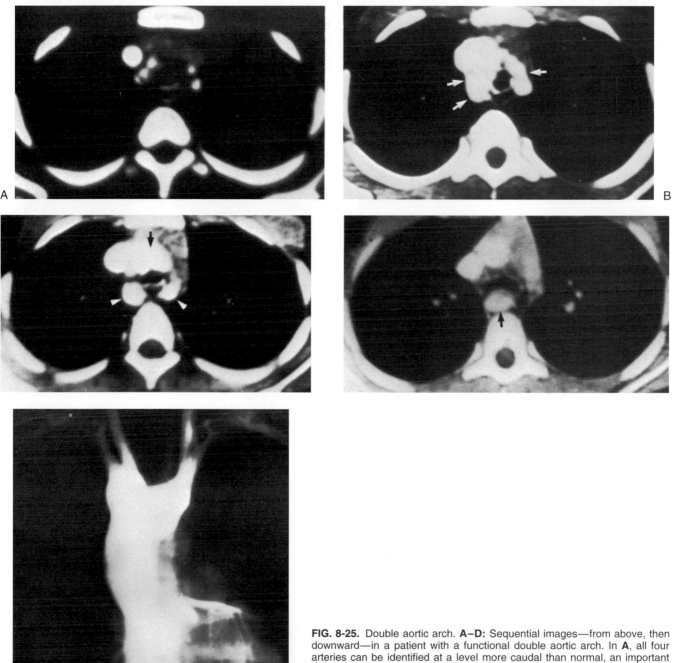

FIG. 8-25. Double aortic arch. **A–D:** Sequential images—from above, then downward—in a patient with a functional double aortic arch. In **A**, all four arteries can be identified at a level more caudal than normal, an important clue to the presence of an arch anomaly. **B:** A section through both arches; the right arch (*two arrows*) is larger than the left arch (*single arrow*). **C:** A section through the ascending aorta (*arrow*) and the posterior portions of both the right and left arches, which lie behind the trachea and esophagus in close proximity (*arrowheads*). Below this level, the descending portions of both arches fuse to form one descending aorta (*arrow* in **D**). **E:** The corresponding angiogram. (Case courtesy of Ina L.D. Tonkin, M.D., University of Tennessee Center for the Health Sciences. Images obtained by Bennett A. Alford, M.D., University of Virginia Hospital.)

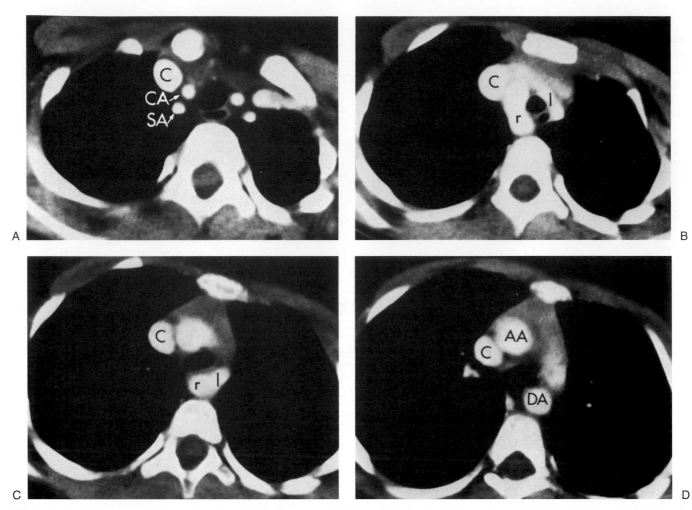

FIG. 8-26. Double aortic arch 3 mm slices. **A:** Level 1 shoes carotid (*CA*) and subclavian (*SA*) vessels on both sides of the trachea. **B:** Level 2, 6 mm inferior, shoes a larger right aortic arch (*r*) and a smaller left aortic arch (*l*) giving rise to the great vessels. **C:** Level 3 shows the right aortic arch (*r*) crossing to the left of the midline and joining with the descending left aortic arch (*l*). Note that the trachea is not severely compressed at this level. **D:** Level 4 at the level of the aortic pulmonary window.

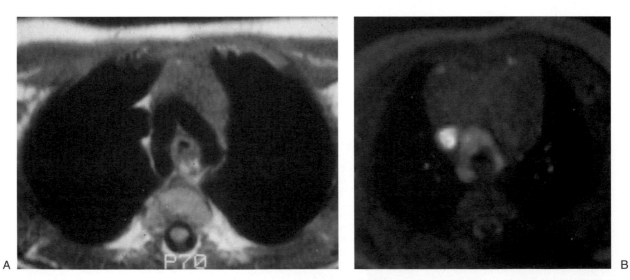

FIG. 8-27. Double aortic arch MR demonstration in 2 patients. **A:** T1-weighted SE MR image demonstrates a double aortic arch. In this case both arches are the same size. **B:** Cine gradient-echo MR image in a different child demonstrates a double aortic arch.

double arch in which atresia of some portion of the left arch has occurred. There is similarity between this condition and some of the right aortic arch anomalies. Theoretically the major difference is that with double aortic arches, some portion of the left arch persists despite atresia, and a vascular ring around the trachea and esophagus is present. With right aortic arch anomalies there is true interruption of the left aortic arch, and a true vascular ring is rarely formed.

ECG triggered SE MR (82–84), 2D TOF, cine MR or phase contrast MR (85,86) can readily demonstrate symptomatic arch anomalies, but require multiple imaging planes, which are time consuming to perform, and result in limited postprocessing potential. A single volume gadolinium-enhanced 3D MRA acquisition offers higher spatial resolution, higher signal-to-noise, faster acquisition times, and provides for high quality surgically pertinent multiplanar reformations (87). However, without breath holding, respiratory-induced blurring can result in significant degradation of image quality with this technique (88).

Conventional CT (80,89) and helical CT angiography also have been successfully used in the evaluation of pediatric great vessel anomalies (18,90,91). Advantages over MR imaging include rapid scanning times, which allows for examination of critically ill children without the constraints of a closed-bore magnet, and better evaluation of the relationships of aberrant vessels with the airways and the esophagus. Hopkins and colleagues evaluated 15 children (aged 1 month to 12 years) with helical CTA using 3-mm collimation and a bolus of 2 mL/kg of nonionic contrast injected by hand at 1 mL/second. Scanning began immediately after the infusion of contrast finished and was performed with breath holding in two children and during quiet reparation in 13. Using 2D axial images and 3D SSD they were able to diagnose anomalies correctly in 13 children (87%), including double and right-sided aortic arches, aberrant subclavian arteries, innominate artery compression syndrome, and pulmonary artery abnormalities (91). CT angiography was unable to differentiate a right aortic arch with an aberrant left subclavian artery and a ligamentum arteriosum from a double aortic arch with an atretic segment between the left common carotid and subclavian arteries. It is often very difficult to distinguish these entities, and both require surgery.

Interrupted Aortic Arch

Interrupted aortic arch (IAA) is an interruption in the continuity of the aortic arch, often with a fibrous cord between the two segments. It occurs in three places: (a) just distal to the origin of the left subclavian artery, (b) between the origins of the left common carotid and left subclavian arteries (Fig. 8-28), and (c) between the origins of the innominate and left common carotid arteries (92). These correspond to types A (25%), B (70%), and C (5%) in the Celoria and Patton classification (93). A large patent ductus arteriosus invariably supplies blood to the descending aorta. IAA is also associated in the majority of cases with intracardiac

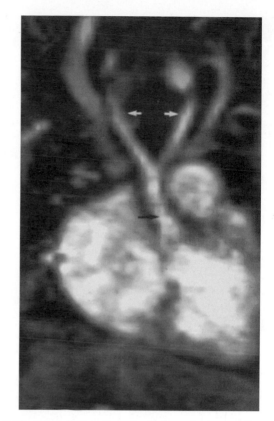

FIG. 8-28. Interrupted aortic arch with hypoplastic acending aorta in a 10-day-old infant. Coronal reformation from non–breath-hold gadolinium-enhanced three-dimensional MR angiogram, performed in the head coil, demonstrates a hypoplastic, 4-mm ascending aorta (*black arrow*), which bifurcates into both common carotid arteries (*white arrows*). The arch was interrupted distal to the common carotid arteries. (From ref. 88, with permission.)

defects and subaortic outflow obstruction. IAA usually presents within the first few days of life, as the ductus closes. Rapidly progressive congestive heart failure ensues. The mortality rate at 10 days is 50%, and by the end of the first month, 75%. Initial management includes prostaglandin therapy to maintain the patency of the PDA. Echocardiography has traditionally been used to quickly diagnose IAA, but distinguishing between IAA type A and severe coarctation is difficult. Hemodynamically stable patients, as well as those who have undergone surgical repair, can be evaluated with cine (94) or gadolinium-enhanced 3D MRA (88).

Coarctation

Clinical Features

Coarctation of the aorta represents a focal narrowing in the proximal descending thoracic aorta, usually in the region of the ductus arteriosus. When associated with tubular hypoplasia of the aortic arch or descending aorta (Fig. 8-29) it is usually referred to as preductal or infantile. Patients with aortic coarctation may present with congestive heart failure as infants when a patent ductus arteriosus closes; alterna-

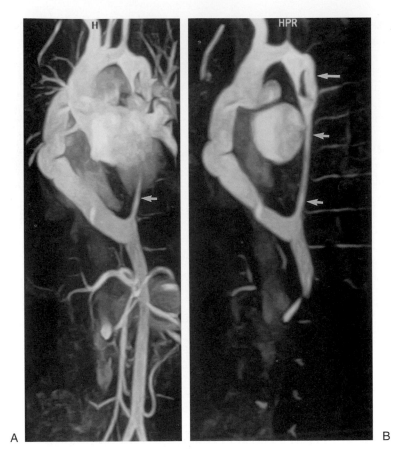

A B

FIG. 8-29. An 18-year-old man with aortic coarctation and a hypoplastic descending aorta treated with extraanatomic bypass from the ascending to descending aorta. This case represents the importance of subvolume maximum-intensity-projection (MIP) images to remove extraneous anatomy that may obscure the vessels of interest. Oblique sagittal MIP image from breath-hold gadolinium-enhanced three-dimensional (3D) MR angiogram (**A**) demonstrates an extraanatomic bypass graft from the ascending aorta to the descending aorta. *Small arrow* represents a portion of the distal hypoplastic native aorta. Subvolume oblique sagittal MIP image from breath-hold gadolinium-enhanced 3D MR angiogram (**B**) demonstrates the complete extent of the coarctation and hypoplastic aorta (*short arrows*) as well as the initial bypass graft (*long arrow*) that was unable to adequately decrease left ventricular afterload and hypertension. The extraanatomic bypass graft from the ascending aorta to the descending aorta was subsequently placed and resulted in normalization of blood pressure and a decrease in left ventricular mass. (From ref. 290, with permission.)

tively, the condition may be discovered during workup of a coexistent cardiac anomaly, the most common being a bicuspid aortic valve, which occurs in 75% to 85% of patients (95). In 2% of patients coarctation may occur as an isolated segment of narrowing of the abdominal aorta (96).

Multiple surgical techniques have been used to repair coarctation in the pediatric population. A widely used repair in infants is an extended end-to-end anastomosis after resection of the coarctation (97). Alternatively, the left subclavian artery can be mobilized proximal to the internal mammary artery and reflected down as a flap to bridge the coarctation. Dacron patch aortoplasty was a commonly used repair technique that resulted in a low rate of recurrence and stenosis, but because of an alarming incidence of late aortic rupture and sudden death resulting from aneurysm formation (98), this technique is no longer performed. More recently, transluminal balloon angioplasty has been used succesfuly in selected cases. This nonsurgical treatment works best when the stenosis is focal and located just distal to the left subclavian artery.

Adults usually present with hypertension and discrepant blood pressure measurements in the arms and legs. Almost all patients with coarctation of the aorta will have concomitant left ventricular hypertrophy. Coarctation in adults is often associated with medial degenerative disease of the aorta; thus resection with interposition graft is a widely used surgical approach. If primary resection is not feasible, extraanatomic bypass grafting from the ascending to descending aorta can be performed (see Fig. 8-29; Fig. 8-30). A less invasive alternative is transluminal angioplasty but long term results are inferior to definitive surgical repair.

Pseudocoarctation of the aorta results from a congenital elongation of the aortic arch with resultant redundancy and kinking (Figs. 8-31 and 8-32) (99). Unlike coarctation, however, there is no obstruction to blood flow and therefore little or no demonstrable pressure gradient and no evidence of collateral circulation (100,101).

Imaging Features

MR Evaluation

Although both CT and MR have been successfully used to diagnose coarctation, in our opinion, MR has proved of greater value, especially in the pediatric age group as well as for routine postsurgical evaluation.

Various traditional MRI techniques, performed in the axial and oblique sagittal plane, have been successfully used in the evaluation of coarctation, to assess both the location, the degree of anatomic narrowing and the extent of collateral circulation. These include multiplanar ECG-triggered TI-weighted SE techniques (102) supplemented by phase-con-

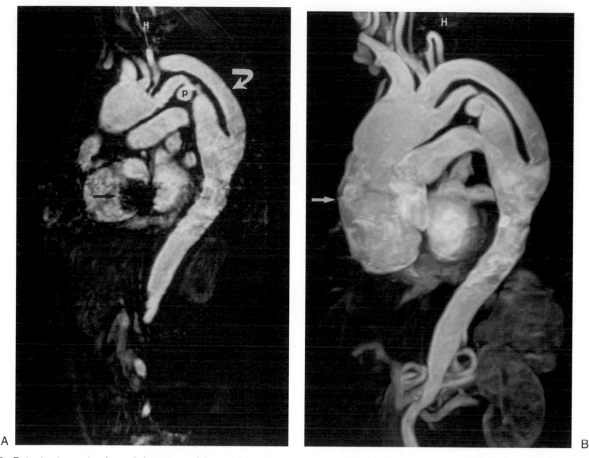

FIG. 8-30. Patent extraanatomic aortic bypass graft in an adult patient with untreated aortic coarctation associated with a native aortic pseudoaneurysm. The patient was being evaluated for an ascending aortic aneurysm and aortic valve insufficiency. **A:** Oblique sagittal source image from nonbreath-hold gadolinium-enhanced three-dimensional acquisition clearly demonstrates an extraanatomic graft (*curved arrow*) and pseudoaneurysm (*p*) of the native aorta. There is also narrowing of the proximal left subclavian artery. Susceptibility artifact is present from a prosthetic valve mitral valve (*arrow*). **B:** Oblique sagittal MIP image shows an ascending aortic aneurysm (*arrow*) and a normal abdominal aorta. Note the susceptibility artifact is obscured in the MIP image. (From ref. 39, with permission.)

trast (103) or cine MRA (104,105). The latter technique, when performed in the oblique sagittal plane, can readily demonstrate the dephasing that occurs from turbulent flow across the site of narrowing. Cine phase-contrast techniques, including velocity-encoded cine MR, are used to measure the peak velocity across the site of coarctation (106). With this information, the pressure gradient across the coarctation can be estimated. One study demonstrated that peak coarctation jet velocity measured by MR velocity mapping was comparable to results obtained with continuous wave Doppler sonography (54). This technique can also be used to determine the extent of collateral circulation by measuring flow immediately distal to the coarctation and at the level of the diaphragm. In normal aortas, flow will decrease by an average of 8% as it reaches the diaphragm, whereas in patients with hemodynamically significant coarctation, the flow will be augmented by an average of 80% (107).

Gadolinium-enhanced 3D MRA can readily demonstrate the presence of collateral circulation (Fig. 8-33) as well as the degree of associated arch hypoplasia (see Fig. 8-29) and concomitant branch vessel abnormalities. It also provides excellent anatomic images of the extent of coarctation without dephasing artifacts from turbulent flow and allows reformation of 3D data into multiple surgically pertinent imaging planes in patients with associated tubular hypoplasia (see Fig. 8-29). CT and CTA can also demonstrate the anatomic segment of coarctation and the presence of collateral vessels (108) (Fig. 8-34).

MR may be used to predict the response of patients who are candidates for balloon angioplasty (109,110). The best results with balloon angioplasty occur when the stenosis is focal and located just distal to the left subclavian artery. When the stenosis involves the proximal arch or involves a long segment, balloon angioplasty is less successful. As documented by Bank et al. in their study of 12 children with suspected coarctations evaluated both before and after surgical repair, MR proved accurate in identifying those patients who were unlikely to benefit from angioplasty (110). In addition, MR proved valuable by determining the appropriate balloon size for angioplasty.

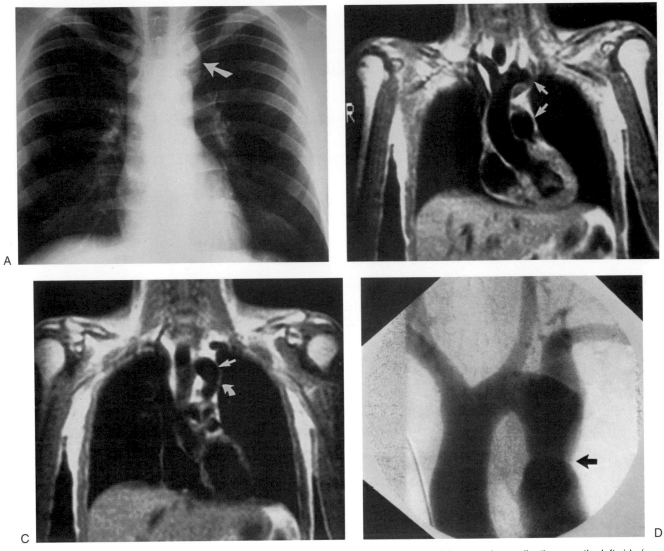

FIG. 8-31. Pseudocoarctation. **A:** Posreroanterior radiograph shows unusual configuration of the superior mediastinum on the left side (*arrow*). Differentiation between an aneurysm and a mediastinal mass is difficult. **B, C:** Sequential coronal MR images through the root of the aorta and posterior portion of the aortic arch, respectively. The ascending aorta is elongated as indicated by the considerable distance between the arch superiorly and the main pulmonary artery inferiorly (*arrow* in **B**). There is aneurysmal dilation of the aorta (*arrow* in **C**), below which there is abrupt narrowing of the lumen, suggesting possible coarctation (*curved arrow* in **C**). **D:** Coned-down view from a subtraction aortogram shows characteristic kink in the course of the aorta (*arrow*) without actual narrowing. No pressure gradients could be measured across this region. (Case coutresy of Patricia Redmond, M.D., Staten Island, NY.)

All patients with surgically repaired coarctation should undergo surveillance either with MR (105) or CT imaging to detect recurrent coarctation and pseudoaneurysm formation (Fig. 8-35). One study using ECG-triggered 2D TOF MRA with 3D surface renderings demonstrated a sensitivity of 100% for the detection of aneurysms (98). Recurrent coarctation after primary repair may result from multiple causes including inadequate removal of ductal tissue, failure to repair associated aortic arch hypoplasia and suture line tension (111). These patients can be treated with transluminal angioplasty with success rates as high as 90% (112). Alternatively, coarctation resection and extraanatomic bypass grafting from the aortic arch to the descending aorta can be performed with excellent long term results (111).

Pulmonary Sequestration

Pulmonary sequestrations are defined as nonfunctioning lung tissue that are not in continuity with the tracheobronchial tree and derive their blood supply from systemic vessels. Traditionally divided into intra- and extralobar forms, most authors consider these two entirely separate entities. Intralobar sequestrations are contiguous with normal lung parenchyma, enclosed by normal pleura. In distinction, extralobar pulmonary sequestrations lie outside the normal pleura, frequently appearing as solid masses of tissue. Intralobar sequestrations are only rarely associated with other malformations, and typically are first identified in later life, often as an asymptomatic finding on routine chest radiographs. In distinction, extralobar pulmonary sequestrations

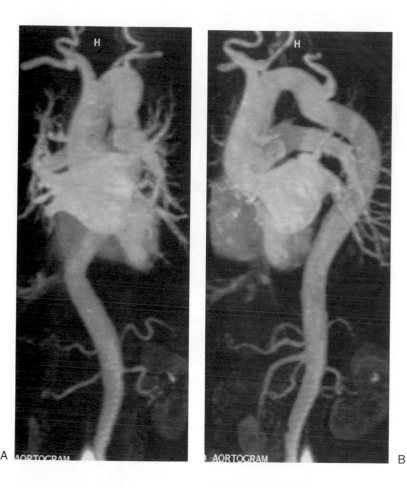

A AORTOGRAM

AORTOGRAM B

FIG. 8-32. A,B: Coronal (**A**) and oblique sagittal (**B**) maximum-intensity-projection images from breath-hold gadolinium-enhanced three-dimensional MR angiogram demonstrates pseudocoarction. Note the redundant aorta associated with buckling and inferior displacement of the left subclavian artery and the complete absence of collateral vessels. (From ref. 290, with permission.)

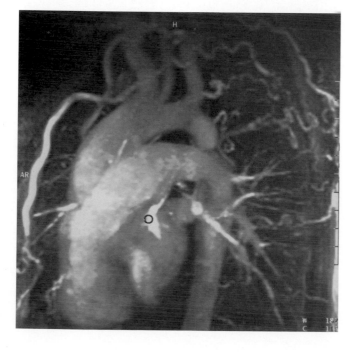

FIG. 8-33. Oblique sagittal maximum-intensity-projection image from breath-hold gadolinium-enhanced three-dimensional MR angiogram demonstrates aortic coarctation with extensive collateral circulation. (From ref. 290, with permission.)

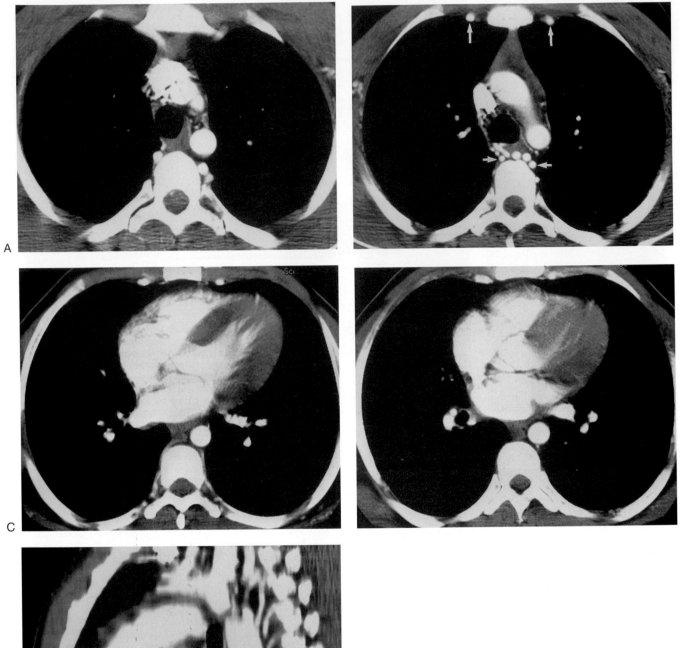

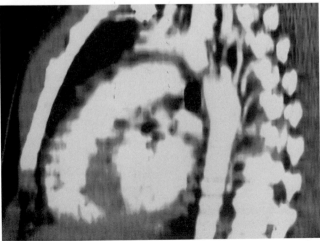

FIG. 8-34. Aortic coarctation-CTA evaluation. **A–D:** Sequential contrast-enhanced helical CTA from superior to inferior demonstrates multiple collateral vessles including intercostal (*short arrows* in **B**) and internal mammary (*long arrows* in **B**) arteries. Left ventricular hypertrophy is present as well. The site and degree of narrowing is not well visualized. **E:** Oblique sagittal multiplanar volume reconstruction better demonstrates the anatomic site and degree of narrowing, as well as the collateral blood supply.

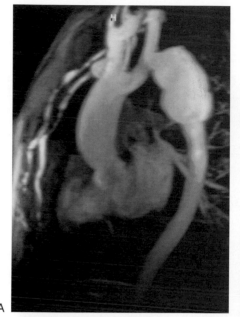

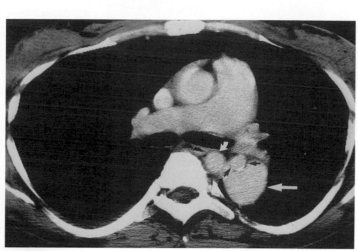

A

B

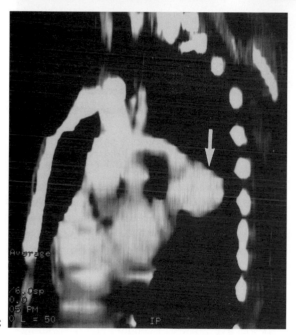

C

FIG. 8-35. Aortic coarctation-postoperative pseudoaneurysm formation detected by CT and MR. **A:** Oblique sagittal maximum-intensity-projection image from breath-hold gadolinium-enhanced three-dimensional MR angiogram demonstrates an aneurysm at the site of previous coarctation repair. Note the enlarged, tortuous internal mammary arteries with areas of focal stenosis. (From ref. 290, with permission.) **B:** Axial contrast-enhanced CT image through the level of the right pulmonary artery demonstrates a pseudoaneurysm (*long arrow*) adjacent to the aortic graft (*small arrows*). *Curved arrow* denotes the native aorta. **C:** Oblique sagittal reformation from same data set demonstrates pseudoaneurysm as well (*arrow*).

are frequently seen in association with other congenital abnormalities and are most often identified in either the neonatal period or early childhood. In patients with intralobar sequestration, the feeding artery arises from the thoracic aorta in 73% of cases, the abdominal aorta in or celiac axis in 20% and the intercostal arteries in 4% (113). Venous drainage typically is to normal pulmonary veins. Although extralobar sequestrations also typically derive blood from the arterial circulation, these frequently are considerably smaller vessels than seen in patients with intralobar sequestrations: unlike intralobar sequestrations, however, venous drainage is almost always to systemic veins, including the azygos and hemiazygos veins as well as the inferior vena cava and even the portal vein.

Regardless of the type of sequestration, both aberrant arteries and veins are easily identified using either CT or MR (114,115) (Fig. 8-36). A potential advantage of CT in these cases is the ability to simultaneously evaluate lung parenchymal abnormalities that frequently are present especially in patients with intralobar sequestrations (116).

AORTIC ANEURYSMS

Clinical Features

Aortic aneurysm is defined as an irreversible dilatation of the aorta to twice its normal diameter with all components of the aortic wall present in the dilated segment (117,118).

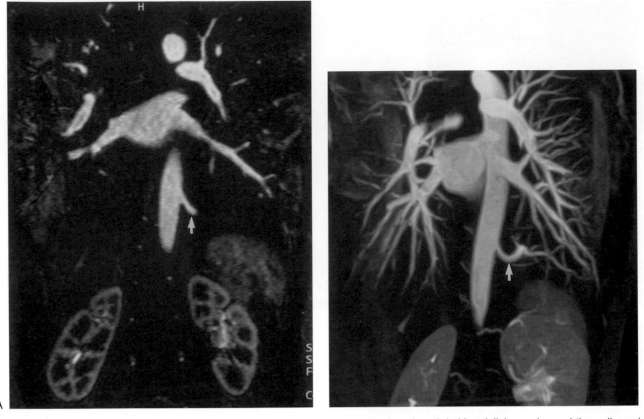

FIG. 8-36. A,B: Coronal source (**A**) and maximum-intensity-projection (**B**) images from breath-hold gadolinium-enhanced three-dimensional MR angiogram demonstrates a feeding vessel (*arrows* in **A** and **B**) to a pulmonary sequestration.

As previously discussed, aortic size is age-related and a 4-cm ascending aorta is clearly aneurysmal in a 30-year-old but normal in an octogenarian. The etiology of aneurysmal disease is broad, including degenerative disease, connective tissue disorder, trauma, aortitis (infective and inflammatory), previous surgery, hemodynamic alterations (from aortic stenosis and regurgitation), and congenital abnormalities. The histologic changes occurring in the diseased aorta include medial degeneration, medial necrosis, atherosclerosis, and inflammatory infiltration. Pseudoaneurysms, or false aneurysms, represent saccular dilatations of the aorta that do not contain an intimal layer and are usually associated with previous penetrating atheromatous ulcers, aortic surgery, trauma or infections (Fig. 8-37).

The overall incidence of thoracic aortic aneurysms from a large autopsy series over a 27 year period was 489 per 100,000 men and 437 per 100,000 women (119). This study also demonstrated an increasing prevalence of asymptomatic thoracic aneurysms with advancing age. Aneurysmal disease often is multifocal or diffuse; up to 28% of patients with thoracic aneurysms have concomitant infrarenal abdominal aortic aneurysms making evaluation of the entire aorta mandatory in patients presenting with nontraumatic thoracic aneurysms (117,120).

The most serious complication of aneurysmal disease of the thoracic aorta is death from rupture, the incidence of which varies from 42% to 70% depending upon the series (121). The overall 5 year survival rate of patients who are not surgically repaired is only 13% to 39% after diagnosis (121). A recent study reported the following observations: an average size at presentation of 5.2 cm, a mean growth rate of 0.12 cm/year, median size at time of dissection or rupture of 6.0 and 7.2 cm for ascending and descending aortic aneurysms, respectively, and an operative mortality of 9% for elective repairs (ascending and descending) and 21.7% for emergent repairs (122). In a series of 198 patients with descending aortic aneurysms, Coselli reported a 5% operative mortality rate and only a 1.5% incidence of paraplegia (123). A longitudinal CT study demonstrated growth rates of 0.42 cm a year for thoracic aneurysms and 0.56 cm per year for aneurysms involving the aortic arch (124); these expansion rates are faster than those reported for abdominal aortic aneurysms. As with abdominal aortic aneurysms, the size at presentation can be used to stratify the cohort at risk for rupture; the cumulative five-year risk of rupture increases fivefold for thoracic aneurysms greater than 6 cm in diameter. Because of the high mortality rate from rupture, combined with steadily decreasing operative morbidity and mortality rates, most centers will repair ascending aortic aneurysms at 5 to 5.5 cm, and aortic arch and or descending

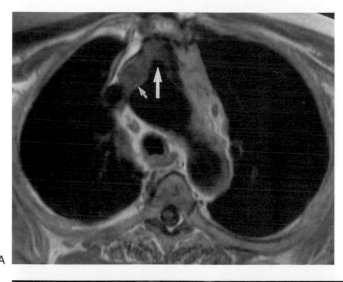

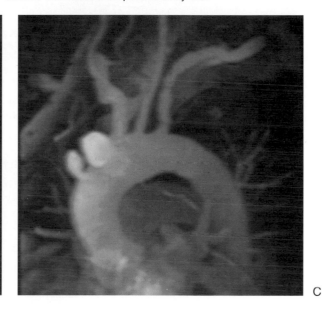

FIG. 8-37. Ascending aortic pseudoaneurysm resulting from prior mediastinitis complicating previous aortic surgery. **A:** Axial electrocardiogram triggered T1-weighted SE MR image shows pseudoaneurysm arising from the anterior portion of the ascending aorta (*long arrow*) and associated thrombus (*short arrow*). **B:** Oblique sagittal source image from breath-hold gadolinium-enhanced three-dimensional (3D) MR angiogram demonstrates the larger superior pseudoaneurysm (*long arrow*) and the neck of the inferior, smaller pseudoaneurysm (*short arrow*). **C:** Oblique sagittal maximum-intensity-projection image from breath-hold gadolinium-enhanced 3D MR angiogram demonstrates both pseudoaneurysms. These appear brighter than the descending aorta because of their proximity to the anterior elements of the phased-array coil.

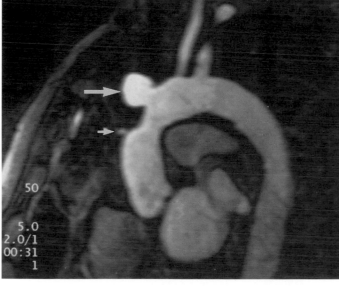

aortic aneurysms at 5.5 to 6.5 cm in uncomplicated patients without significant comorbid medical disease. Debilitated patients who are poor surgical candidates may be treated with percutaneously placed aortic stent grafts (125) (Fig. 8-38).

The operative technique for aortic aneurysms, as with dissection of the aorta, depends on the extent of involvement. Previously, conventional angiography was required for preoperative planning, but CTA or a combination of MR techniques can supply more information, with the noted limitation of inability to evaluate the coronary arteries and the intercostal arteries that supply the spinal cord (T8-L1). These techniques can readily evaluate aortic size, mural disease, thrombus and the proximal and distal extent of aneurysms. The last is extremely important as this dictates the operative approach and technique used. For aneurysms involving the ascending aorta, the type of proximal repair is determined by whether or not the sinotubular ridge and aortic valve are

compromised, and the distal extent may determine the need for hypothermic circulatory arrest. If the distal ascending aorta is not aneurysmal or diseased, and the aortic root is relatively normal, then simple aortic cross clamping with cardiopulmonary bypass without hypothermic circulatory arrest may be performed. In distinction, if the aneurysm extends to within 1 cm of the innominate artery, involves the aortic arch or is associated with extensive atheromatous plaque, then hypothermic circulatory arrest with or without retrograde brain perfusion are commonly performed. The morphology of aneurysms of the ascending aorta and aortic arch are predictable based upon the disease process. Typically, patients with cystic medial necrosis will have aneurysmal involvement of the sinuses of Valsalva with smooth tapering to a normal sized aortic arch. This results in the classic tulip or pear shaped aorta seen in patients with Marfans disease (Fig. 8-39). In contrast, atherosclerotic aneurysms or those that result from long standing aortic valve

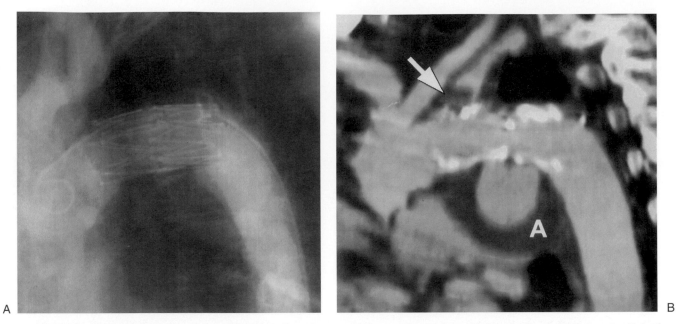

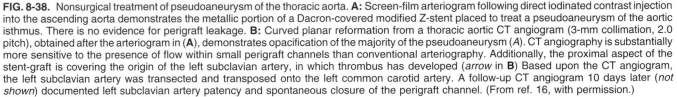

FIG. 8-38. Nonsurgical treatment of pseudoaneurysm of the thoracic aorta. **A:** Screen-film arteriogram following direct iodinated contrast injection into the ascending aorta demonstrates the metallic portion of a Dacron-covered modified Z-stent placed to treat a pseudoaneurysm of the aortic isthmus. There is no evidence for perigraft leakage. **B:** Curved planar reformation from a thoracic aortic CT angiogram (3-mm collimation, 2.0 pitch), obtained after the arteriogram in (**A**), demonstrates opacification of the majority of the pseudoaneurysm (*A*). CT angiography is substantially more sensitive to the presence of flow within small perigraft channels than conventional arteriography. Additionally, the proximal aspect of the stent-graft is covering the origin of the left subclavian artery, in which thrombus has developed (*arrow* in **B**) Based upon the CT angiogram, the left subclavian artery was transected and transposed onto the left common carotid artery. A follow-up CT angiogram 10 days later (*not shown*) documented left subclavian artery patency and spontaneous closure of the perigraft channel. (From ref. 16, with permission.)

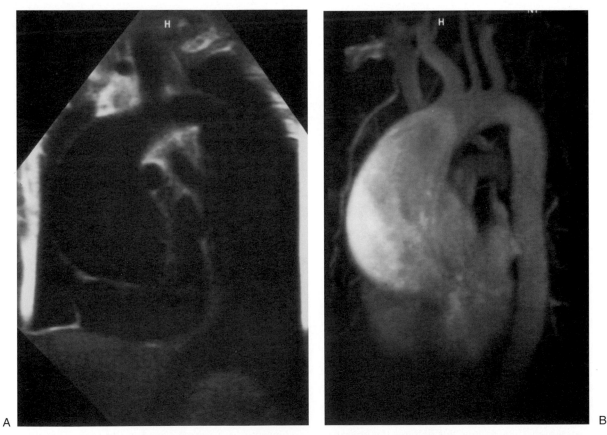

FIG. 8-39. Ascending aortic aneurysm with involvement of the sinus segment in a patient with cystic medial necrosis. **A:** Oblique sagittal black blood half-fourier single shot turbo-SE (HASTE) image performed with electrocardiogram triggering (TR/TE = 800 msec/42 msec) and oblique sagittal maximum-intensity-projection image from breath-hold gadolinium-enhanced three-dimensional MR angiogram (**B**) demonstrate the tulip shaped aortic root characteristic of cystic medial necrosis. Note the smooth tapering to a relatively normal aortic arch.

disease usually spare the sinus segment but extend into the transverse arch (Fig. 8-40).

The distinction is not always so clear cut as atherosclerotic aneurysms may also involve the sinus segment (Fig. 8-41), especially when associated with aortic regurgitation. However, they will almost never demonstrate the complete effacement of the sinotubular junction seen with cystic medial necrosis.

For thoracoabdominal aneurysms it is essential that imaging includes a complete evaluation of the renal and visceral vessels as aneurysmal involvement or occlusive disease may alter surgical management (Fig. 8-42). These aneurysms invariably contain thrombus and at times may be difficult to distinguish from chronic, thrombosed aortic dissections. The presence of a sharp, spiraling interface with compression of the patent lumen and extension over a 7 cm segment mitigates for the latter diagnosis (Fig. 8-43).

Complete replacement of the thoracic aorta may be necessary in aneurysms that involve both the ascending aorta, aortic arch, and proximal descending aorta (Fig. 8-44). This can be performed in a single operation or as a two stage procedure (126). Because patients who have undergone re-

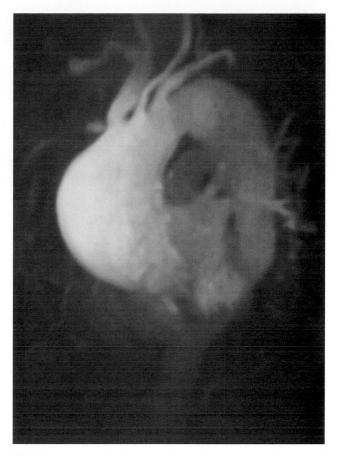

FIG. 8-41. Atherosclerotic ascending aortic aneurysm with some dilatation of the sinus segment. Oblique sagittal maximum-intensity-projection image from breath-hold gadolinium-enhanced three-dimensional MR angiogram demonstrates fusiform dilatation of the ascending aorta, with some involvement of the sinus segment, which extends into the transverse arch. This patient had significant aortic regurgitation. Note the concomitant proximal desending aortic aneurysm. Involvement of the transverse arch are characteristic of atherosclerotic aortic aneurysms and aneurysms resulting from longstanding aortic valvular disease. Because of the aortic arch involvement, surgical repair would require hypothermic circulatory arrest.

pair of thoracic aneurysms are at risk for a second noncontiguous aneurysm (117), as well as anastomotic pseudoaneurysms, they require follow-up surveillance imaging.

Imaging Features

CT Evaluation

Early CT literature using nonhelical scanning demonstrated high accuracy rates for the diagnosis of thoracic aneurysms and their complications (65,127–129). Contrast-enhanced CT can demonstrate all the gross pathologic features of aortic aneurysms, including dilatation, intraluminal thrombi, displacement or erosion of adjacent structures (Fig. 8-45), and perianeurysmal thickening and hemorrhage (65,127–129). CT has also proven valuable in detecting unu-

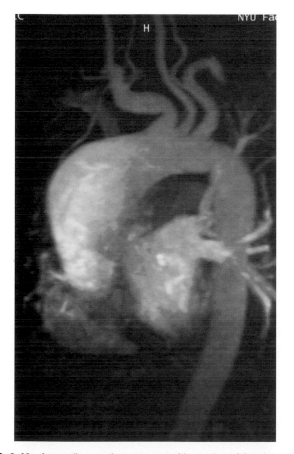

FIG. 8-40. Ascending aortic aneurysm with sparing of the sinus segment. Oblique sagittal maximum-intensity-projection image from breath-hold gadolinium-enhanced three-dimensional MR angiogram demonstrates fusiform dilatation of the ascending aorta, with relative sparing of the sinus segment, which extends into the transverse arch.

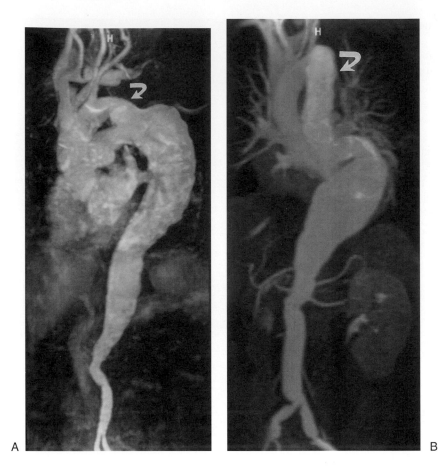

FIG. 8-42. Thoracoabdominal aneurysms. Oblique sagittal maximum-intensity-projection images from nonbreath-hold (**A**) and breath-hold (**B**) gadolinium-enhanced three-dimensional MR angiograms demonstrate thoracoabdominal aneurysms with sufficient proximal necks for cross clamping (*curved arrows*). Poor visualization of the renal and visceral vessels in (**A**) results from a combination of severe renal insufficiency and the known limitations of evaluation of branch vessels using a nonbreath-hold technique. (From ref. 290, with permission.)

sual types of aneurysms, including mycotic (Fig. 8-46) and ductus aneurysms (Fig. 8-47), as well as complications arising from aneurysms, including those secondary to rupture (130–135). CT also plays an important role in distinguishing thoracic aortic aneurysms from pulmonary masses adjacent to the mediastinum.

Thoracic aneurysms secondary to atherosclerosis are readily demonstrated as fusiform dilatation of a segment of the aorta, which usually contains mural thrombus, and may demonstrate calcification of the thrombus or the aortic wall (Fig. 8-48). The pattern of mural thrombi and calcifications within aortic aneurysms has been described (136,137). Calcification within aneurysms is common, occurring in up to 85% of cases, both mural (see Fig. 8-45) and within the thrombus itself. The latter type of calcification has been reported to

occur in approximately 25% of patients both with thoracic and abdominal aortic calcifications (137). The significance of calcification within thrombi is that this appearance can be mistaken for the displaced intimal calcification seen in aortic dissection and intramural hematoma.

Aortic thrombi may be crescentic in shape (Figs. 8-49, 8-50A) or circumferential, in which case the residual lumen appears circular. As a rule, the residual aortic lumen is smooth, although the aortic lumen may develop a very irregular contour, especially in large aneurysms, depending on the extent of thrombus (see Fig. 8-48). Unlike intramural hematomas (which will be discussed later), thrombus is often circumferential and does not displace a calcified intima. When the thrombus forms a sharp margin with the enhanced lumen, and no displaced intimal calcifications are present,

FIG. 8-43. Thoracoabdominal aneurysm with thrombus and chronic thrombosed type B dissection (**A** and **B**). Oblique sagittal maximum-intensity-projection (MIP) image from breath-hold gadolinium-enhanced three-dimensional MR angiogram (**A**) and axial, breath-hold gradient-echo image (**B**) performed immediately after (**A**) demonstrate crescentic thrombus in the descending thoracic aorta, without mass effect on the lumen. Findings are most consistent with a thoracoabdominal abdominal aneurysm. **C–E:** Chronic thrombosed dissection with aneurysmal dilatation of false lumen. **C:** Oblique sagittal source image from nonbreath-hold gadolinium-enhanced three-dimensional MR angiogram shows low signal intensity thrombus (*arrow*) with sharp luminal interface, typical for thrombosed dissection. Note secondary aneurysm formation in the abdominal aorta (*curved arrow*). **D:** MIP image is deceptively normal appearing. **E:** Axial reformation from same data set better demonstrates the sharp interface (*arrow*) between the enhanced true lumen and the thrombosed false lumen. (From ref. 88, with permission.)

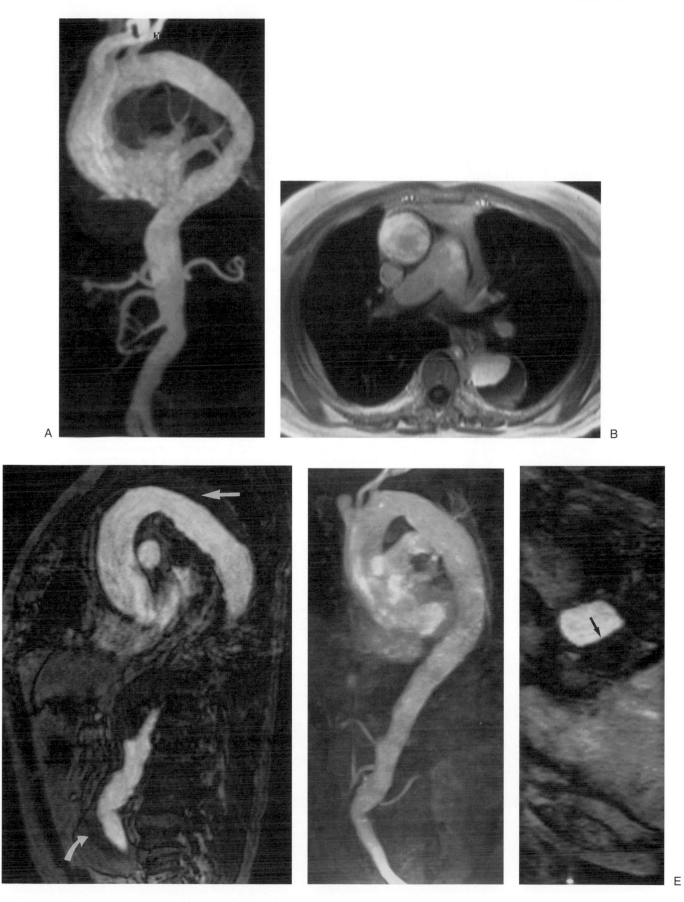

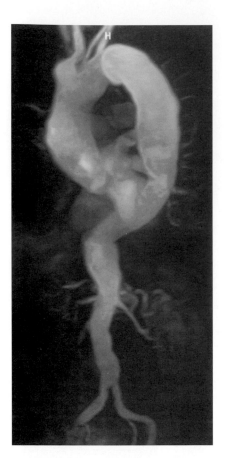

FIG. 8-44. Oblique sagittal maximum-intensity-projection image from breath-hold gadolinium-enhanced three-dimensional MR angiogram demonstrates aneurysmal dilatation of the entire thoracic aorta (megaaorta). (From ref. 290, with permission.)

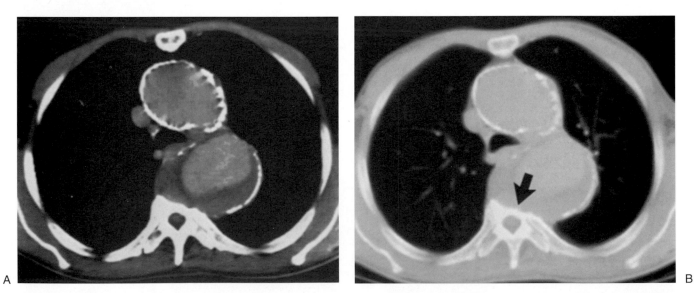

A

B

FIG. 8-45. A,B: Long standing thoracic aortic aneurysm resulting in bone erosion. Contrast-enhanced CT scans at the same level imaged with narrow and wide windows, respectively. There is dense calcification of the walls of both the ascending and descending aorta. An aneurysm is present within the proximal descending aorta, with considerable surrounding thrombus. The adjacent vertebral body has been significantly eroded (*arrow* in **B**).

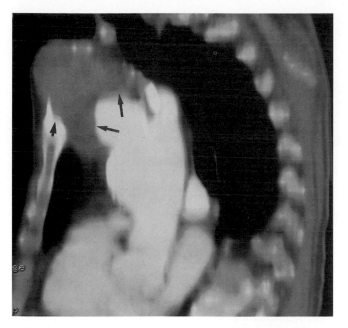

FIG. 8-46. Long standing mycotic aneurysm of the ascending aorta. Sagittal reformation from contrast-enhanced helical CT demonstrates a mycotic aneurysm of the ascending aorta with thrombus (*long arrows*) that eroded through the sternum (*short arrow*) to present as a chest wall mass.

it may be difficult to distinguish a thoracic aneurysm from a chronic aortic dissection with a thrombosed false lumen (see Fig. 8-50B).

CT can be used to follow up aneurysms, although this involves repeated use of intravenous contrast. An increasing diameter is readily detected with serial scans and helps prompt a surgical decision. CT may also have value in assessing patients with iatrogenic pseudoaneurysms, which may occur following aortic valve replacement, cardiopulmonary bypass, or coronary artery bypass grafting (138,139).

With the introduction of volumetric CT, interest has focused on the potential use of retrospective reconstruction techniques to evaluate aortic aneurysms. To date, results have been mixed (140,141). In a recent study, Quint and colleagues (140) evaluated the diagnostic contribution of helical CT with multiplanar reformations in the evaluation of 49 patients with thoracic aortic disease (36 aneurysms, 6 penetrating ulcers, 5 dissections, and 2 pseudoaneurysms). Overall diagnostic accuracy was 92%, both with and without multiplanar reconstructions. Although MPRs were of value by displaying pathology in a format more accessible to nonradiologists, their addition failed to change the diagnosis in any patient (140) (Fig. 8-51). Furthermore, whereas in two patients extension of an aneurysm into the aortic arch necessitating the use of hypothermic circulatory arrest was shown more clearly using MPRs, in a third patient multiplanar reconstructions incorrectly predicted this need.

In distinction, Kimura and coworkers have recently shown that both SSD and especially CT angioscopy were both superior to axial images for assessing the relationship between distal arch aneurysms and the origin of the great vessels (141). Comparing the accuracy of 2D axial source images with SSDs and endoscopic renderings in 12 patients with distal aortic arch aneurysms, these authors found that depiction of the relationship between the aneurysm and the orifice of the left subclavian artery was correctly diagnosed in only five (42%) of 12 patients using axial images: in distinction, using 3D display only, this relationship could be discerned in nine of the 12 (75%), whereas use of 3D endoscopic renderings allowed accurate assessment in 11 of 12 (92%) of patients (141). Reasons for failure of axial images to accurately identify the anatomic relationship between aneurysms and the left subclavian artery included the presence of atheromas obscuring continuity or gradual sloping of the proximal portion of the aneurysm obscuring its precise margin. Of the

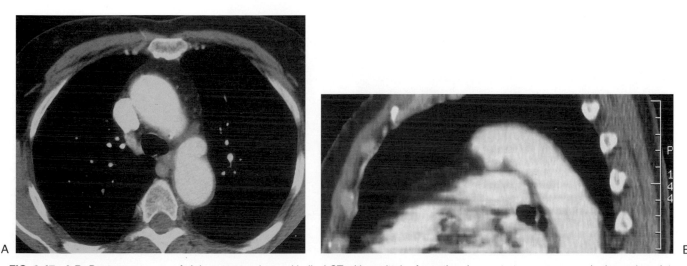

A   B

FIG. 8-47. A,B: Ductus aneurysm. Axial contrast-enhanced helical CT with sagittal reformation demonstrate an aneurysm in the region of the ductus arteriosus.

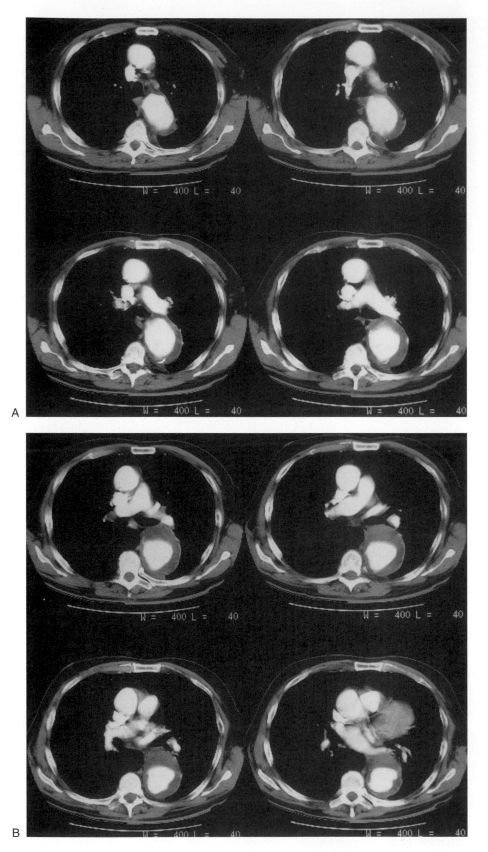

FIG. 8-48. A,B: Atherosclerotic thoracic aortic aneurysm. Sequential images (superior to inferior) from contrast-enhanced helical CT demonstrate a fusiform aneurysm of the descending thoracic aorta with irregular, mostly circumferential thrombus.

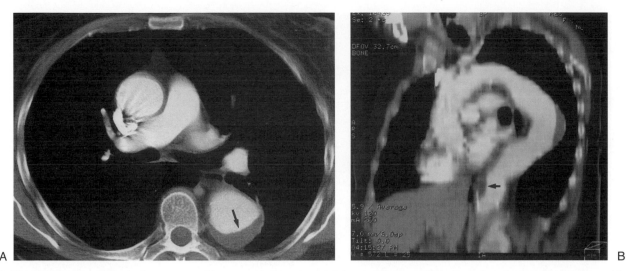

FIG. 8-49. A,B: Thoracoabdominal aneurysm with crescentic thrombus. Axial and oblique sagittal reformation from contrast-enhanced helical CT demonstrate crescentic mural thrombus in both the midthoracic aorta (*arrow* in **A**) and at the level of the diaphragm (*arrow* in **B**). Note the similar morphology as in Fig. 8-43.

three renderings, CT angioscopy most clearly delineated the distance between the arterial orifice and the border of the aneurysm.

An even more compelling use of CT for evaluating aortic aneurysms has recently been published by Rubin et al. (142). Using helical computed tomographic (CT) angiographic data, these authors demonstrated that it is possible to auto-matically derive accurate quantitation of arterial cross sections, segment lengths and absolute curvature by continuously describing variations in cross-sectional dimensions and as a function of position along the median vessel path. Previously limited, especially in patients with markedly tortuous aortas, use of quantitative vascular CT should now allow more accurate assessment of longitudinal changes in

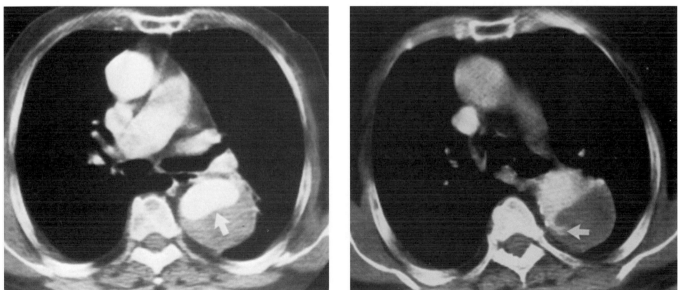

FIG. 8-50. Aortic aneurysm, CT assessment of thrombus morphology. **A:** Contrast-enhanced CT section through the carina shows characteristic appearance of a descending aortic aneurysm. Dense contrast enhancement identifies the lumen as distinct from adjacent crescentic thrombus (*arrow*). **B:** Contrast-enhanced CT section through the carina in a different patient than shown in **A**. In this case the enhanced lumen forms a sharp margin with the thrombus similar to Fig. 8-43E. This morphology can be seen in both thoracic aneurysms and thrombosed aortic dissections. The presence of displaced intimal calcifications would favor the latter diagnosis. Note that in this case, however, there is a focal area of ulceration that can be identified within the thrombus (*arrow*). This finding is worrisome and may represent the earliest sign of contained rupture; bleeding into a degenerated thrombus. These findings should always be correlated with the patient's clinical symptoms.

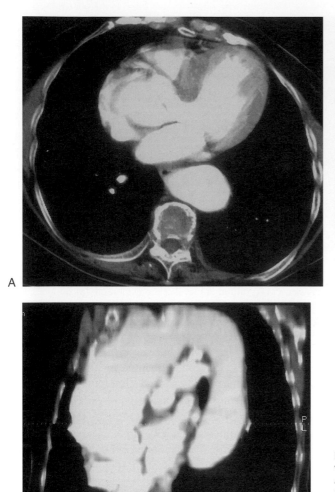

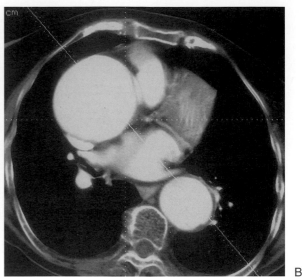

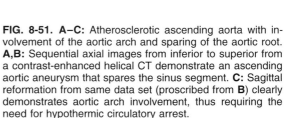

FIG. 8-51. A–C: Atherosclerotic ascending aorta with involvement of the aortic arch and sparing of the aortic root. **A,B:** Sequential axial images from inferior to superior from a contrast-enhanced helical CT demonstrate an ascending aortic aneurysm that spares the sinus segment. **C:** Sagittal reformation from same data set (proscribed from **B**) clearly demonstrates aortic arch involvement, thus requiring the need for hypothermic circulatory arrest.

aortic dimensions with time, as well as more accurate treatment planning, especially in those cases for which endoluminal stent-grafts are planned. This is in addition to the already well established role of CT for pre- and postoperative evaluation of patients with both surgical and endovascular stent-graft repair of thoracic aortic aneurysms (see Fig. 8-38) (143,144).

In our experience, the extent of aortic aneurysms, and in particular their relationship to adjacent structures, are better visualized using either MPRs or 3D renderings. In this regard, the use of MIPs to delineate the exact location of calcification may be of particular value in assessing the necks of aneurysms.

CT does have some recognized limitations in the evaluation of aneurysmal disease, aside from the risks of iodinated contrast and radiation. Evaluation of the aortic root is often difficult secondary to motion artifacts. Extreme tortuosity may preclude an accurate true short axis aortic measurement from the axial source images. Although this is readily ob-

tained by using reformatted images, not all radiologists have the requisite equipment to perform this function. Evaluation of thoracoabdominal aneurysms may be difficult as accurate assessment of the status of the renal and visceral vessels requires thin section collimation (<3 mm). With a single detector, it is currently not possible to achieve this resolution in both the thoracic and abdominal aorta from a single bolus of contrast, even using a pitch of up to 2 combined with a machine capable of subsecond scanning. However, this is not a problem with multidetector systems (145).

MR Evaluation

Aortic aneurysms and pseudoaneurysms are easily identified on ECG-triggered SE MR because of the signal void usually associated with flowing blood (27,146,147). When present, organized thrombi within the lumen of aneurysms usually appear as areas of intermediate signal intensity on T1-weighted SE images, and unorganized thrombi may appear hyperintense. As documented by Glazer et al., measurements of the maximum diameter of aneurysms with MR show near-perfect correlation with the measurements obtained with CT scans (148). In addition, MR provides accurate information concerning the relationships of aneurysms to surrounding mediastinal structures. Because of the relatively large FOV (50 cm) available in MR, in most patients the entire aorta can be studied without having to reposition the patient (see Fig. 8-2). These complete aortograms are extremely helpful when evaluating patients with thoracoabdominal aneurysms (see Figs. 8-42–8-44) or multiple, noncontiguous aneurysms (see Fig. 8-41). As already noted, an important limitation of MR is its inability to detect calcifications.

ACUTE AORTIC SYNDROMES

Aortic Dissection

Clinical Features

Dissection of the aorta most often presents as a clinical catastrophe, sometimes difficult to distinguish from myocardial infarction or pulmonary embolization. An insidious onset, however, is, not infrequent. The chest radiograph usually demonstrates a widened aortic shadow; rarely, it may remain normal. The pathology of aortic dissection represents a separation of the aortic media by a stream of blood that usually is associated with a primary intimal tear. This stream creates a false lumen that may remain contained or dissect longitudinally in an antegrade or retrograde manner and potentially reenter the true aortic lumen at a point distant from the initial intimal tear. It is unclear whether the intimal tear is the inciting factor that results in aortic dissection or whether the tear is a secondary phenomenon from hydraulic stress on an aorta weakened from a spontaneous medial hematoma (149).

Predisposing factors to the development of aortic dissection include hereditary and congenital disorders (syndromes such as Marfan's, Turner's and Ehlers–Danlos), aortic valve defects, coarctation, and aneurysmal disease. Pathologic substrates that are associated with dissection include medial degenerative disease of the aorta secondary to cystic medial necrosis, infection (syphilitic and bacterial), and arteritis. Atherosclerotic disease may cause aortic dissection, after the development of a penetrating ulcer, but is not likely a cause of typical aortic dissection. Most patients have a history of systemic hypertension. Iatrogenic causes of aortic dissection include manipulation of the aorta during surgery (aortic cross clamping or cannulation) or during percutaneous procedures including catheterization and placement of intraaortic balloon pumps (121).

Dissection of the aorta has been classified in various ways. Acute dissection refers to dissections less than 2 weeks old; chronic, older than 2 weeks. Early studies on mortality involving aortic dissection found that 75% of deaths from dis-

section occur in this 2 week period, making the distinction prognostically significant (150). In addition, dissections are classified according to the extent of involvement of the thoracic aorta according to the DeBakey or Stanford classification (151). Acute proximal dissections involve the ascending aorta (Stanford A, Debakey I and II) and account for 75% of all cases of aortic dissection (Fig. 8-52). These dissections are repaired immediately to prevent potentially fatal complications that include rupture into the pericardial or pleural space or extension into the coronary arteries or aortic root; the latter two complications can result in myocardial infarction and aortic insufficiency, respectively. Because these patients are often clinically unstable the majority will undergo operative repair based on the results of TEE alone as this modality can usually provide all of the surgically pertinent information at the patient's bedside in intensive care settings.

Chronic proximal dissections are usually associated with cystic medial necrosis and are repaired as soon as possible. Acute dissections that begin distal to the left subclavian artery (Stanford B, Debakey III) are initially treated medically primarily by controlling hypertension, unless complications such as rupture, end organ ischemia, refractory pain and or progression of dissection develop (Fig. 8-53). A small percentage of patients with medically treated distal dissections will require early surgery. Surgery is indicated in chronic distal dissections in symptomatic patients, or when an associated aneurysm exceeds 5 cm in diameter or is growing at a rate exceeding 1 cm in diameter per year (149) (Fig. 8-54).

Imaging Features

CT Evaluation

CT is a reliable means for diagnosing or excluding aortic dissection. The diagnosis rests on findings observed both on noncontrast-enhanced and contrast-enhanced scans.

Unenhanced images are helpful in detecting blood within the aortic wall from either dissection or intramural hematoma. Rarely, an intimal flap itself can be identified with a nonopacified aortic lumen in patients with severe anemia (152). More commonly, displaced intimal calcifications are seen. Unfortunately, although this finding may be helpful as a further confirmatory sign in patients with acute dissections also studied with contrast-enhanced images, in itself this finding frequently is problematic, especially when attempting to differentiate chronic thrombosed aortic dissections with displaced intimal calcifications from aortic aneurysms with calcification with thrombi (136,137). This differentiation may also be difficult when the aorta is extremely tortuous (153).

Following contrast enhancement diagnosis of aortic dissection rests on identification of two lumens separated by an intimal flap (Fig. 8-55). Ancillary findings, such as differential flow through the two lumens, compression of or irregularity in the contour of the true lumen, increase in size of

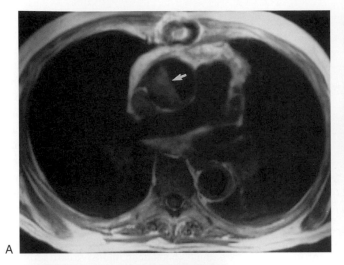

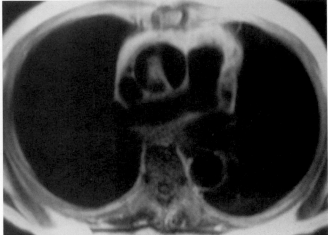

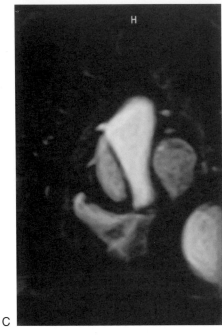

FIG. 8-52. Acute Stanford type A dissection. **A:** Electrocardiogram (ECG) triggered turbo SE T1-weighted image demonstrates an intimal flap within the ascending aorta. It is unclear if the right sided lumen (*arrow*) is patent or thrombosed. **B:** ECG triggered black blood half-fourier single shot turbo spin-echo image demonstrates flow within the right sided lumen. **C:** Coronal reformation from gadolinium-enhanced three-dimensional MR angiography data set demonstrates both lumens are patent. A single coronary bypass graft arises from the false lumen on the right and the true lumen on the left (which enhances to a greater degree). Differential signal intensity in the lumena results from the rapid acquisition time (<20 seconds) of this first pass technique.

the aorta, and the presence of a hemopericardium, are less. The most specific marker of the false lumen is the presence of aortic cobwebs; these represent residual ribbons of media incompletely sheared from the aortic wall during the dissection process (154).

Williams has recently demonstrated that the shape of the true lumen may be a marker for a dynamic form of branch vessel ischemia (155). When the true lumen is ''C-shaped'' or concave toward the false lumen (see Fig. 8-55A) there is a higher incidence of a pressure deficit in the true lumen and its tributaries, a situation that may result in end organ ischemia (155). Conversely, a flap that is oriented convex towards the false lumen is usually associated with absence of a pressure deficit in the true lumen.

There is a strong emphasis in the radiologic literature on the detection of intimal flap extension into the great vessels

(2). Although the presence of arch vessel extension may be pertinent to the management of the small number of patients with type A dissection who present with acute neurological deficits (5%) (see Fig. 8-55), in patients who are otherwise neurologically intact, this information will usually not alter surgical management. Because concomitant replacement of the aortic arch in patients with acute type A dissection is associated with higher mortality rates than simple ascending aortic graft replacement, it is usually reserved for patients whose primary intimal tear is in the transverse arch or those with arch extension resulting in weakening of the outer wall, fragmentation of the inner layer, aneurysmal dilatation, and or transmural rupture (121,156–158).

Numerous studies have documented a role for conventional and electron beam CT in assessing aortic dissection (66,127,159–167). As late as 1993, Nienaber et al. reported

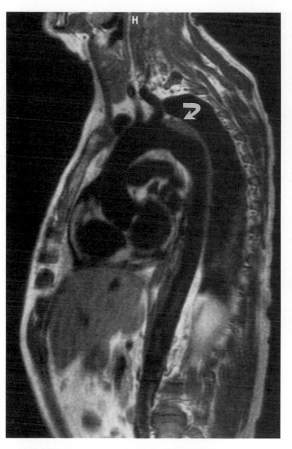

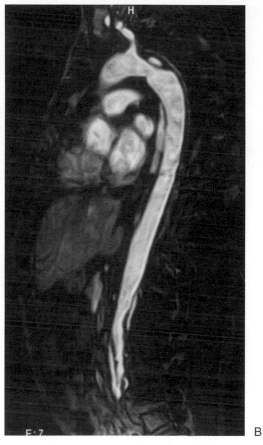

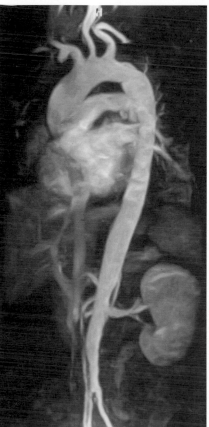

FIG. 8-53. Acute Stanford type B dissection with a normal size aorta. **A:** Oblique sagittal electrocardiogram-triggered T1-weighted SE MR image demonstrates abnormal signal (*curved arrow*) just distal to the left subclavian artery. **B:** Oblique sagittal source image from nonbreath-hold gadolinium-enhanced three-dimensional MR angiogram shows an intimal flap starting just distal to the left subclavian artery and spiraling through the abdomen. **C:** The origin of the dissection is poorly visualized on this maximum-intensity-projection and only the inferior extent of the intimal flap is definitively identified in the right iliac artery. The signal intensity within each lumen are equal as the long acquisition time (2 minutes) results in a recirculation technique whereby the gadolinium concentration in each lumen equilibrates. (From ref. 39, with permission.)

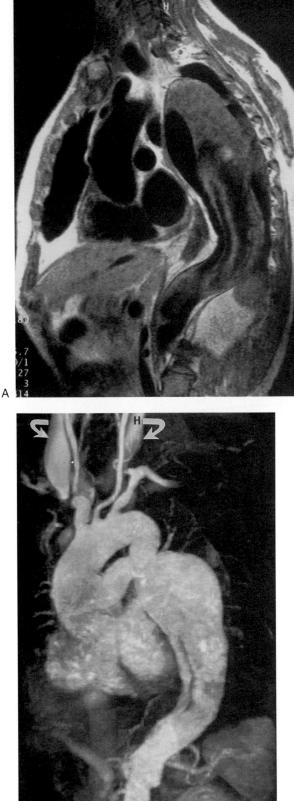

A

B

C

FIG. 8-54. Chronic Stanford type B dissection with aneurysmal dilatation of the false lumen and thrombus formation. **A:** Oblique sagittal
electrocardiogram triggered turbo SE MR image shows enlargement
of the descending thoracic aorta with differential luminal signal intensities. **B:** Oblique sagittal source image from nonbreath-hold gadolinium-
enhanced three-dimensional MR angiogram distinguishes enhancing
slow flow from unenhanced thrombus (*T*) and better delineates the
intimal flap. **C:** Oblique sagittal maximum-intensity-projection image
fails to demonstrate thrombus and the majority of the intimal flap. Overlapping high signal intensity jugular venous blood (*curved arrows*) ob-
scures portions of the left vertebral and right common carotid artery.
This overlap can be eliminated with a more restricted subvolume maximum-intensity-projection or by changing the angle of projection. Evaluation of source data is not degraded by overlapping vessels. (From
ref. 39, with permission.)

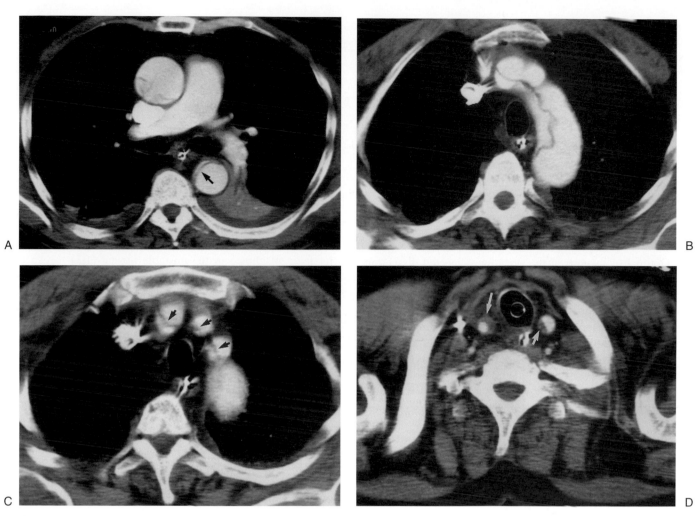

FIG. 8-55. Acute Stanford type A dissection with resultant ischemic brain injury—CT evaluation. **A–D:** Sequential contrast-enhanced helical CT scans from the mediastinum to the thoracic inlet demonstrate thin intimal flap in both the ascending aorta, arch and descending aorta. Intimal flap is present in all three proximal arch vessels (*arrows* in **C**) and thrombus is present within both common carotid arteries. Thrombus in the right common carotid artery (*long arrow* in **D**) is crescentic and in the left common carotid artery results in a sharp interface with the enhanced lumen (*short arrow* in **D**). Note also the presence of an endotracheal tube as the patient was obtunded from an acute stroke as a result of the dissection. Also note that the anterior true lumen of the descending thoracic aorta (*arrow* in **A**) is virtually collapsed with the "C-shape" appearance.

a sensitivity of 93.8% and a specificity of 87.1% using non-volumetric technique (1). More recently, the benefits of volumetric CT for assessing aortic dissection have been documented by Sommer et al. (2). Comparing the efficacy of spiral CT with TEE and MR imaging in 49 symptomatic patients with clinically suspected aortic dissection, these authors found the sensitivity of all three to be 100% with corresponding specificities of 100% and 94% for spiral CT compared with both TEE and MRI, respectively (2).

By comparison, the role of CT angiography is less well defined. Zeman et al. in a study including seven patients with proved aortic dissections found that although the extent of the intimal flap was difficult to identify in three of seven patients using axial images only, multiplanar reformations or 3D renderings clarified the relevant anatomy in all (168,169). Interestingly, of the various reformations available at that time, these authors found ray-sum projections

to be superior to both 3D surface renderings and MIPs for identifying intimal flaps. Not surprisingly, despite clear delineation of calcifications and differential flow rates, MIPs proved of least value because of decreased sensitivity for delineating intimal flaps.

More recently, Kimura et al., in a comparison of 3D surface reconstructions and endoluminal CT angioscopy with 2D axial source images found that 3D reformations were statistically of no additional benefit in patients with aortic dissection (141). Although the relationship between the intimal flap and arterial orifices was depicted by both 3D display and 3D endoscopy, these relationships were deemed better visualized on axial images. It should be noted, however, that in this study 2D images correctly identified only four of five (80%) patients with type A dissections (owing to obscuration of the orifice of the left subclavian artery by the boundary of the true and false lumens in a single case). In distinction, whereas shaded surface displays also were limited, successfully classifying only two cases (40%) caused by superimposition of the left brachiocephalic vein, 3D endoscopy allowed a correct diagnosis in all cases (141).

When evaluating the aortic root for suspected dissection with both conventional and spiral CT, motion of the aortic wall between end diastole and end systole may simulate an aortic dissection (170–174). This curvilinear motion artifact is commonly seen when using a 360 degree linear interpolation algorithm. If it remains a diagnostic dilemma, segmentation of the helical data set with use of a 180 degree linear interpolation algorithm may eliminate the artifact (173).

MR Evaluation

Optimal evaluation of the aorta for suspected dissection with MR mandates imaging from the aortic root to the iliac vessels to define the presence and location of intimal flap, to assess overall aortic diameter and branch vessel patency and to evaluate for the presence of intramural, mediastinal, pericardial and pleural hematomas. Evaluation of aortic valvular competence is readily achieved with cine GRE MR; however, virtually all patients who present to tertiary care centers with suspected acute dissection and valvular incompetence will undergo TEE for this purpose.

Differentiation of true from false lumen can be accomplished with many techniques. Morphologically, the true lumen is generally smaller, oval in configuration, hugs the inner curvature of the aorta, and rarely harbors thrombus, whereas the false lumen is usually larger, crescent shaped, extends along the outer curvature of the aorta and often contains thrombus (43). The true lumen usually demonstrates faster flow—this can be demonstrated with cine GRE, phase contrast, rapid acquisition 2D gadolinium-enhanced MRA (35) or gadolinium-enhanced 3D MRA (see Fig. 8-52) (43). However, only phase contrast (175) or rapid acquisition 2D gadolinium-enhanced MRA techniques (36) can demonstrate the presence of retrograde flow in the false lumen, if present.

Nonbreath-hold gadolinium-enhanced 3D MRA has been shown to be both sensitive and specific for the diagnosis of aortic dissection (39,176), but is insensitive to intramural hematoma and extralumenal pathology (39). Therefore, black blood techniques should always be employed in the setting of acute dissection to evaluate the aortic wall and pleural and pericardial spaces for evidence of hemorrhage. The use of breath holding vastly improves the image quality of gadolinium-enhanced 3D MRA, especially when evaluating the aortic root for dissection; it is now possible to demonstrate from which lumen the native coronary arteries, or bypass grafts, originate (see Fig. 8-52).

The interpreting radiologist should be aware of certain artifacts with gadolinium-enhanced MRA, which can result in a false positive diagnosis of aortic dissection. Differentiation of these artifacts from true dissection can be accomplished by analysis of the geometry of the suspected intimal

flap: In aortic dissections the intimal flap virtually always maintains a spiral course, whereas ghosting and ringing artifacts will not change configuration over their craniocaudad course (Fig. 8-56). On SE MR images, the superior pericardial recess should not be confused with a proximal aortic dissection (Fig. 8-57).

Aortic Dissection: Imaging Overview

Given the techniques currently available for assessing patients with suspected aortic dissection, choice of an appropriate imaging modality usually depends on a combination of factors including the hemodynamic status of the patient, the referring clinician's personal preference, and the modalities most readily available. For a variety of reasons, TEE is the modality of choice in the unstable patient (1,3). It can be performed at the bedside in an intensive care unit or in the operating room. Not only can it readily diagnose and stage aortic dissection, it is extremely accurate for evaluating complications, which include valvular incompetency and pericardial and pleural effusions. It can also render some alternative diagnoses when dissection is refuted, which cannot be evaluated with CT, MR or thoracic angiography. These would include complications from acute myocardial infarction such as pump failure, ventricular septal rupture or papillary muscle dysfunction.

In unstable patients in whom TEE cannot be performed either for technical reasons, or because of contraindications or lack of availability or expertise, CT should be performed. In distinction, in hemodynamically stable patients, in our opinion either CT or MRI can be performed.

Conventional catheter angiography is no longer routinely used in the diagnosis of acute dissection but in conjunction with interventional techniques can be used to relieve symptoms of branch vessel ischemia. This would include performing fenestrations and stent deployment as needed in patients with stable type B dissections (155, 177). Branch vessel ischemia in patients with acute type A dissections will usually be relieved by performing the proximal repair and resecting the intimal flap. Whether or not coronary angiography should be performed in the setting of acute dissection is controversial and depends on the patient's age, clinical history, and hemodynamic status.

Penetrating Ulcer

Clinical Features

Penetrating atherosclerotic ulcer is a distinct radiologic/pathologic entity in which ulceration penetrates the internal elastic lamina into the aortic media and is invariably associated with intramural hematoma and, rarely, aortic rupture (178–182). Although the clinical symptoms of chest or back pain may be identical to those seen in classic aortic dissection, most penetrating ulcers are diagnosed in asymptomatic patients who undergo aortic imaging for other reasons (178) (Fig. 8-58). Penetrating ulcers usually occur in elderly pa-

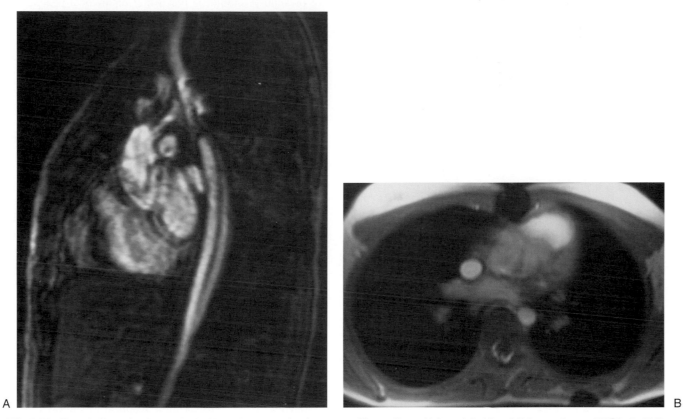

FIG. 8-56. Pseudodissection in a patient with aortic coarctation from central line artifact with breath-hold gadolinium-enhanced MRA. **A:** Oblique sagittal maximum-intensity-projection image from breath-hold gadolinium-enhanced three-dimensional MR angiogram in a patient with aortic coarctation demonstrates a linear structure in the center of the ascending and descending aorta. This does not spiral, unlike an intimal flap from an aortic dissection. This artifact likely results from acquiring the central lines of k-space during a period of rapidly rising arterial concentrations of gadolinium as described by Maki et al. (291). (From ref. 290, with permission.) **B:** Axial cine GRE image through the ascending and descending aorta, performed immediately after (**A**), is normal.

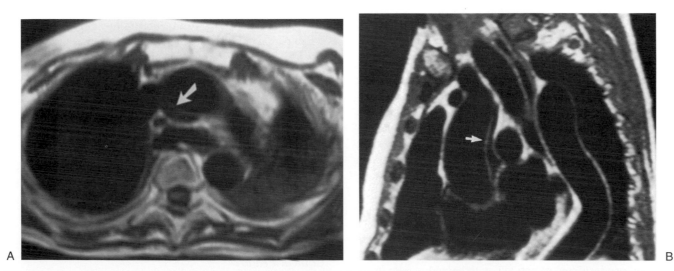

FIG. 8-57. Pseudodissection from the superior pericardial recess. **A,B:** Axial and oblique sagittal electrocardiogram triggered SE MR images demonstrate a prominent superior pericardial recess (*curved arrow* in **A**) and (*straight arrow* in **B**). This normal configuration should not be confused with an intimal flap.

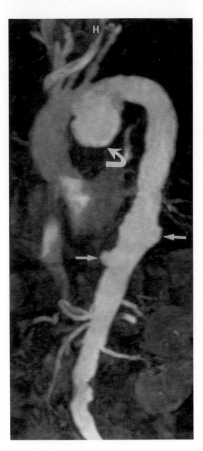

FIG. 8-58. Incidental, asymptomatic aortic ulcers. Oblique sagittal maximum-intensity-projection image from breath-hold gadolinium-enhanced three-dimensional MR angiogram demonstrates a saccular arch aneurysm (*curved arrow*) and concomitant penetrating atherosclerotic ulcers (*arrows*).

tients with severe atherosclerotic disease and typically occur in the descending thoracic aorta although they often occur in the aortic arch (Fig. 8-59), and, rarely, in the ascending aorta.

The natural history of penetrating atherosclerotic ulcers is one of progressive aortic enlargement that includes the development of saccular and fusiform aneurysms or pseudoaneurysms (Fig. 8-60) (178). For these reasons, some form of imaging surveillance is necessary to depict these abnormalities and to stratify patients who may be at risk for aortic rupture from enlarging pseudoaneurysms (178). Although an early report advocated surgical repair of all symptomatic patients (178,180), a more conservative approach has emerged (178,179) as this cohort of patients often has significant comorbid atherosclerotic disease involving the heart, brain and peripheral vasculature. The current consensus is that all patients receive aggressive antihypertensive therapy with surgery restricted to patients with hemodynamic instability, refractory pain, frank or contained aortic rupture, distal embolization or rapidly enlarging aneurysm or pseudoaneurysm. Patients with penetrating ulcers of the ascending aorta associated with intramural hematoma should probably undergo surgery as soon as possible if no contraindications are present. It should be noted that repair of a penetrating ulcer requires more extensive surgery than a Stanford B dissection and often long segments of an ulcerated, atherosclerotic thoracic aorta need to be excised (179).

Imaging Features

CT Evaluation

A penetrating ulcer is usually depicted on contrast-enhanced CT as a focal collection of contrast material that projects beyond the confines of the expected aortic lumen (see Figs. 8-59; Figs. 8-61, 8-62) (179). These lesions can be isolated or multifocal (see Fig. 8-61). An intramural hematoma (discussed in detail later in the chapter) is invariably present (179) and may be localized either to a short segment (see Fig. 8-62) or alternatively may be quite extensive (see Figs. 8-59, 8-61). Displaced intimal calcifications are often present, which confirm that the hematoma is subintimal or within the media (see Fig. 8-62). The aortic wall may be thickened and may demonstrate enhancement. An aneurysm or pseudoaneurysm may also be present.

CT findings which should be suspicious of aortic rupture include the presence of high attenuation mediastinal (see Figs. 8-59 and 8-61) or pleural/pericardial fluid collections. A retrocrural hematoma may be present as well (see Fig. 8-62). Rarely, active extravasation of contrast material into the mediastinum or pleural space may be visualized. Under these circumstances it is often difficult if not impossible to differentiate a ruptured thoracic aneurysm from a penetrating ulcer, however, both entities would require immediate surgical management.

MR Evaluation

Optimal MR evaluation of penetrating ulcers requires a combination of black blood imaging (182) and MR angiography: Although the former technique better demonstrates the concomitant intramural hematoma and allows evaluation of pleural or pericardial surfaces, the latter technique can better depict the ulcer crater. Rapid magnetization-prepared GRE images performed after gadolinium-enhanced aortography can also demonstrate enhancement within the wall of a pseudoaneurysm or contained rupture (Fig. 8-63). It should be emphasized that MR remains inferior to CT in detecting displaced intimal calcifications (179), which clearly define the aortic hematoma as subintimal or intramural in nature.

Intramural Hematoma

Clinical Features

Intramural hematoma (IMH), or aortic dissection without intimal flap, is a pathological entity with similar risk factors and clinical findings as conventional aortic dissection (70,183–185). Whereas classic dissection usually results

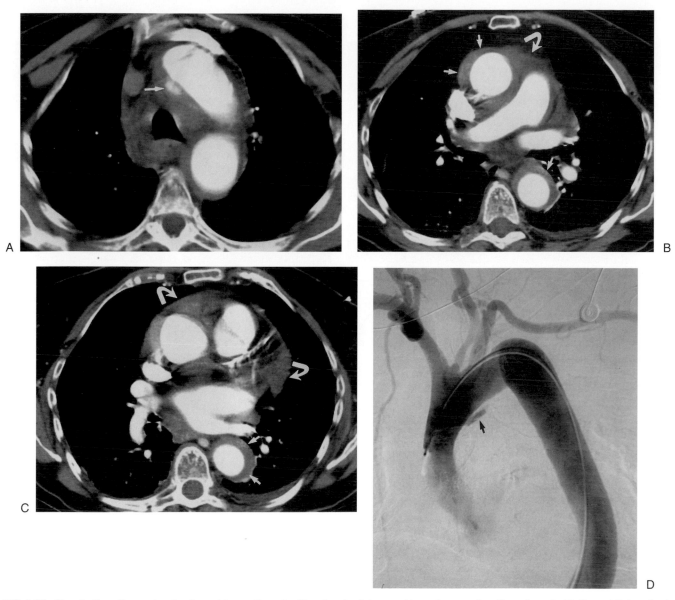

FIG. 8-59. Penetrating atherosclerotic ulcer of the aortic arch with extensive intramural hematoma and aortic rupture. **A–D:** Sequential contrast-enhanced helical CT images from superior to inferior demonstrate a penetrating atherosclerotic ulcer (*arrow* in **A**) associated with extensive aortic intramural hematoma (*small arrows* in **B** and **C**) mediastinal hematoma and a hemorrhagic pericardial effusion (*curved arrows* in **B** and **C**). **D:** Aortogram confirms the ulcer (*arrow*) arising from the undersurface of the aortic arch.

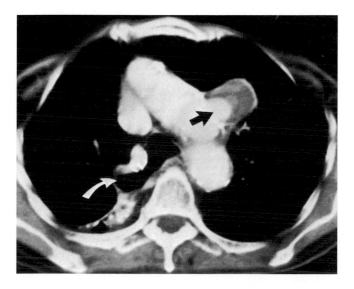

FIG. 8-60. Aortic arch pseudaneurysm resulting from penetrating atherosclerotic ulcer. Contrast-enhanced CT image at the level of the aortic arch demonstrates a pseudoaneurysm resulting from a previous penetrating ulcer (*arrow*). Note that the right upper lobe bronchus is displaced posteriorly (*curved arrow*). This is characteristic of cicatrization atelectasis within the right upper lobe secondary to previous granulomatous infection with resultant scarring.

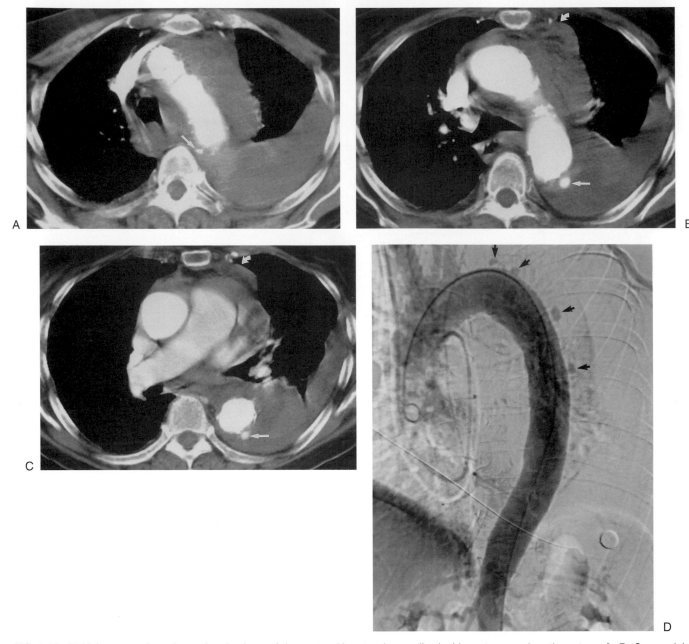

FIG. 8-61. Multiple penetrating atherosclerotic ulcers of the aorta with extensive mediastinal hematoma and aortic rupture. **A–D:** Sequential contrast-enhanced helical CT images from superior to inferior demonstrate multiple penetrating atherosclerotic ulcers (*straight arrows* in **A–C**) associated with extensive aortic intramural hematoma, mediastinal hematoma and a hemorrhagic pericardial effusion (*curved arrows* in **B** and **C**). **D:** Aortogram confirms the presence of multiple ulcers (*arrows*). It is unclear which ulcer led to the extensive hemorrhage and aortic rupture.

from a primary intimal tear, with subsequent separation of aortic wall components, IMH represent localized hemorrhage confined to the aortic media (183,186). The etiology of IMH is not well defined; theories include intimal fracture of an atherosclerotic plaque with propagation of blood into the media (penetrating ulcer), spontaneous rupture of the vasa vasorum with subsequent aortic wall weakening (70,183–185) and complete thrombosis of the false lumen in classic aortic dissection in which an intimal tear is not identified by imaging modalities. Wilson and Hutchins reviewed the autopsy results

from 204 patients with aortic dissection and 13% had no identifiable intimal tear (187); this mitigates the theory that these represent classic dissections in which the intimal flap was "missed" by imaging studies.

There remains considerable clinical and imaging overlap among the entities referred to as IMH, penetrating atherosclerotic ulcer and limited aortic dissection with thrombosed false lumen. Nevertheless, both CT, MRI and TEE have greater than 96% sensitivity in the diagnosis of intramural hematoma (188).

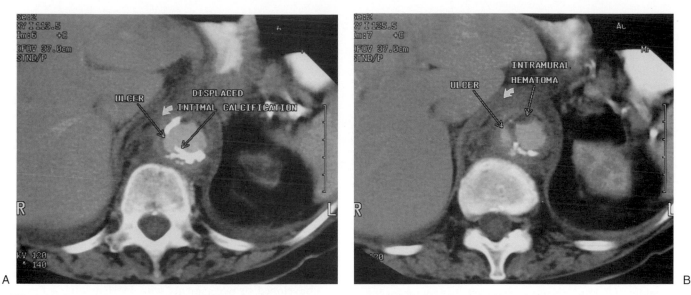

FIG. 8-62. Penetrating atherosclerotic ulcer of the distal thoracic aorta with displaced intimal calcifications. **A,B:** Two contiguous, sequential images from a contrast-enhanced helical CT examination demonstrate a penetrating atherosclerotic ulcer resulting in an intramural hematoma. Note how the ulcer has undermined the media resulting in displaced intimal calcifications. Retrocrural hematoma is present (*curved arrows* in **A** and **B**) consistent with focal aortic rupture.

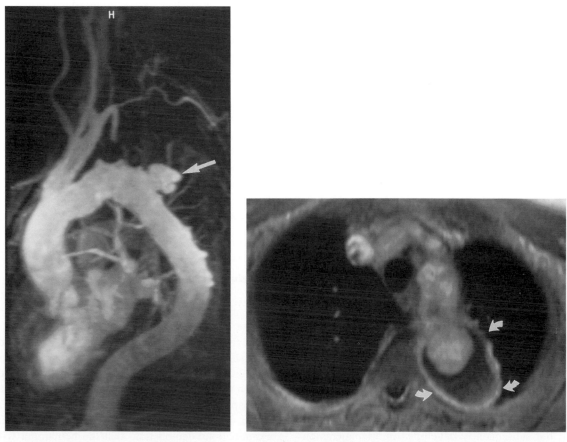

FIG. 8-63. A: Oblique sagittal maximum-intensity-projection image from breath-hold gadolinium-enhanced three-dimensional MR angiogram demonstrates multiple penetrating ulcers and a giant ulcer (*arrow*) resulting in contained aortic rupture in this patient with chest pain. **B:** The thrombus and enhancing adventitial tissue (*curved arrows*) are better demonstrated on this magnetization prepared, rapid gradient-echo sequence performed after the aortogram. (From ref. 290, with permission.)

Because the literature regarding the natural history and clinical management of IMH is sparse there is no clear consensus on treatment. In Nienaber's study (184), aortic regurgitation and pericardial or mediastinal effusions were present in 42% of patients with IMH that involved the ascending aorta and in 18% of patients with IMH limited to the descending aorta. Four of the five patients with IMH involving the ascending aorta who were treated medically died within 30 days, whereas the seven patients who underwent early surgical repair survived. Patients with IMH limited to the descending aorta did well with conservative therapy. The Cleveland Clinics group reported similar findings (183); four of five patients with involvement of the ascending aorta developed classic aortic dissections necessitating surgical repair, whereas only two of 17 patients with IMH limited to the descending aorta required surgical intervention. Robbins et al. documented IMH in 13 patients using multiple imaging modalities. Of three patients with involvement of the ascending aorta all required surgical intervention, and two died. Of 10 patients with involvement of the descending aorta only two required surgical intervention (189). In another study of 15 patients with IMH documented by TEE, two of three patients with involvement of the ascending aorta died of rupture within three days of diagnosis. Overall, five patients (33%) progressed to typical aortic dissection with recognizable intimal flap during follow-up imaging (190). In Wolff's MRI study of nine patients with IMH, both patients with involvement of the ascending aorta underwent surgery, which demonstrated classic aortic dissection with an intimal flap (185). In three patients with IMH of the descending aorta an intimal flap was detected only in the abdominal aorta (185) supporting the argument that the entire thoracoabdominal aorta should be evaluated in the setting of an acute aortic syndrome.

Sueyoshi et al. evaluated 32 patients with acute IMH with both CT and MR imaging (186). These patients had a mean age of 70 years and all presented with acute chest or back pain; 28 of these patients had hypertension and none had stigmata of Marfan's syndrome. Thirteen patients had involvement of the ascending aorta or transverse arch (type A) and 19 patients had involvement of the aorta distal to the left subclavian (type B). Fifteen of 32 patients had pleural effusions and 6 of 13 patients with type A disease had pericardial effusions.

Using serial CT and MR examinations, Sueyoshi et al. made the following important observations concerning the fate of IMH:

1. The IMH itself decreased in size in all patients and completely resolved without sequella in 13 patients.
2. Penetrating ulcer was present in six patients on the initial examination (five of which were located in the distal aortic arch) but subsequently developed in 14 patients on follow-up study between 4 and 163 days. Of these 14 patients who developed penetrating ulcers after an initial IMH 9 developed into saccular aneurysms. The majority of these developed in the distal aortic arch; this gives credence to the theory that hydraulic stress may have caused a new intimal defect in an aortic wall previously weakened by an IMH as the distal arch appears to be a region prone to hydraulic stress. The appearance of a penetrating ulcer presenting after the initial IMH was also documented by Williams et al. (168) and further supports this theory.
3. In 6 patients in whom penetrating ulcers never developed fusiform aneurysms developed 30 days to 26 months after onset. These resemble the typical atherosclerotic fusiform thoracoabdominal aneurysms, which begin in the proximal descending aorta.
4. The overall aneurysm growth rate (both saccular and fusiform) was an alarming 1.2 cm per year. This is significantly higher than previously reported.
5. Classic type A dissection (with recognizable intimal flap) developed in two patients with IMH involving the ascending aorta, a smaller number than reported by Murray (183). In contrast to Murray (183) and Nienebar findings (184) seven patients with ascending aorta involvement survived without surgery demonstrating that involvement of this segment of the aorta is not invariably fatal.

Using the data from multiple published studies (183,184,186,191,192) it appears that patients with involvement of the ascending aorta, unless they have significant comorbid disease, should undergo early surgical intervention to prevent potentially fatal complications, which include aortic rupture and pericardial tamponade. Because the natural history of patients with type B disease is unpredictable routine serial imaging at least every three months during the first year should be performed to evaluate for spontaneous progression to classic dissection (185,190), early saccular aneurysm (Fig. 8-64) or pseudoaneurysm formation. Long term follow up is required for the detection of fusiform aneurysms, which may develop in the cohort of patients without penetrating ulcers (186).

Imaging Features

CT Evaluation

The CT appearance of acute intramural hematoma are characteristic. Noncontrast examination demonstrates a crescent-shaped area along the wall of the aorta that has higher attenuation than blood, without mass effect on the patent lumen (Fig. 8-65) (70,168,186). Intimal calcifications may be displaced by the hematoma as seen in 25 of 32 patients in the largest study to date (186). Contrast-enhanced CT examinations demonstrate that the hematoma will not enhance, appears hypodense when compared with the enhanced lumen, and a recognizable intimal flap is absent (see Fig. 8-65; Fig. 8-66). Contrast is clearly necessary to define

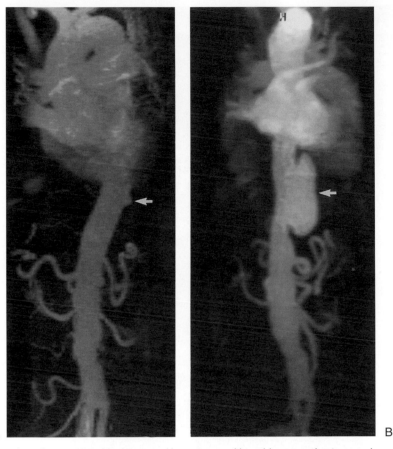

A   B

FIG. 8-64. Penetrating ulcer ocurring after spontaneous intramural hematoma, with rapid progression to pseudoaneurysm formation. **A:** Oblique sagittal maximum-intensity-projection image from breath-hold gadolinium-enhanced three-dimensional MR angiogram demonstrates a small atherosclerotic ulcer (*arrow*). This ocurred 3 months after an intramural hematoma (*not shown*). **B:** Coronal MIP image from breath-hold gadolinium-enhanced three-dimensional MR angiogram obtained 18 months after **A**, demonstrates rapid progression to large saccular pseudoaneurysm (*arrow*).

penetrating ulcers, which may be the etiology of the hematoma (180,179).

MR Evaluation

The MR appearance of IMH consists of focal crescentic wall thickening without mass effect on the aortic lumen or evidence of intimal flap (Figs. 8-67 and 8-68) (183–185). In a series of 25 patients with IMH, aortic wall thickening was 2cm + 1.2 cm and length was 8.5cm + 5cm (184). The signal characteristics reflects the age of the hemorrhage; acute intramural hematoma (symptoms <7 days) is usually isointense to muscle on T1-weighted images (see Fig. 8-67), whereas subacute intramural hematoma (symptoms >7 days) is usually bright from methemoglobin (see Fig. 8-68; 182). These "black blood" T1-weighted images are essential for the diagnosis because as previously mentioned, IMH may be occult on gadolinium-enhanced MR angiography (see Fig. 8-68) (193). Magnetization-prepared, rapid gradient-echo sequences performed after gadolinium-enhanced MRA will usually demonstrate IMH as a crescentic area of relatively low signal intensity when compared with adjacent gadolinium-enriched blood.

Ruptured Aortic Aneurysms

As previously stated, the risk of rupture of a thoracic aneurysm increases with the size of the aneurysm (122). Patients with ruptured thoracic aneurysms often have chest and/or back pain associated with hypotension.

Imaging Features

CT Evaluation

Noncontrast or contrast-enhanced CT may demonstrate a high attenuation crescent of blood within a mural thrombus. This has been called the crescent sign in abdominal aortic aneurysms (194,195) and represents acute hemorrhage into a preexisting mural thrombus or aneurysm wall; this sign usually implies acute or impending contained rupture (196). Another recently described CT finding of

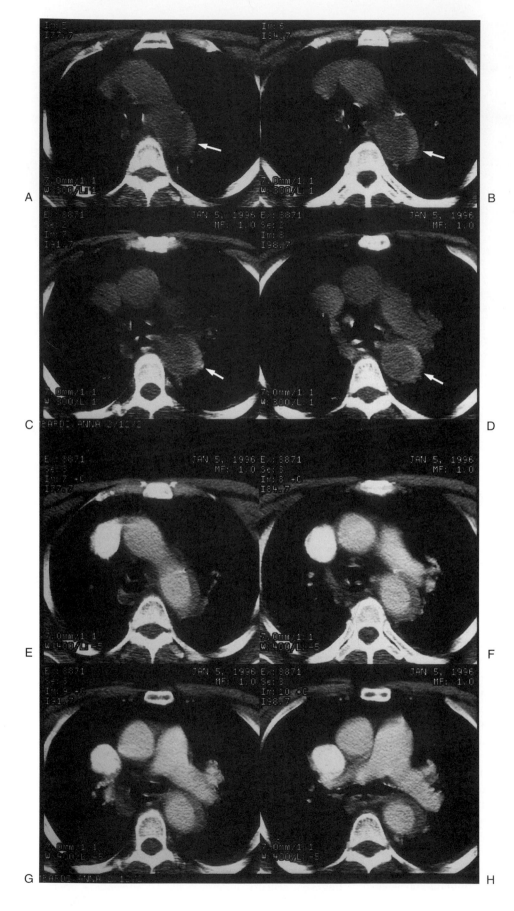

FIG. 8-65. Acute intramural hematoma limited to the descending aorta (type B) demonstrated on CT. **A–D:** Sequential images through the mediastinum, superior to inferior, from a non–contrast-enhanced helical CT examination demonstrates a crescent of high attenuation blood within the descending thoracic aorta (*arrows* in **A–D**). Note the crescent shape and the absence of mass effect on the residual aortic lumen. **E–H:** The same images after the administration of intravenous contrast demonstrate that the hematoma has not enhanced and is now hypodense when compared with the contrast-enhanced lumen.

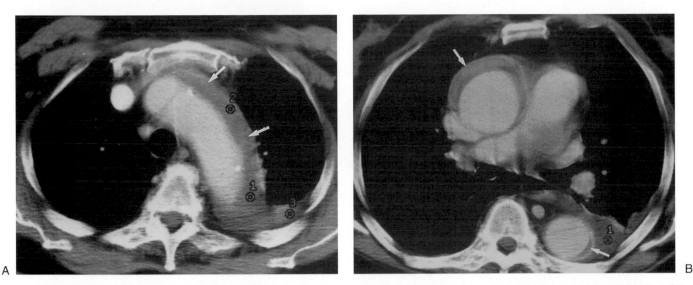

A   B

FIG. 8-66. Acute intramural hematoma involving the entire thoracic aorta (type A) demonstrated on CT. **A,B:** Contrast-enhanced helical CT images at the level of the aortic arch (**A**) and right pulmonary artery (**B**) demonstrate crescent of blood involving the ascending aorta, arch and descending aorta (*arrows*) diagnostic of aortic intramural hematoma. The blood within the wall of the aortic arch measured 60 Hounsefield units. There is a hemorrhagic left pleural effusion in (**A**).

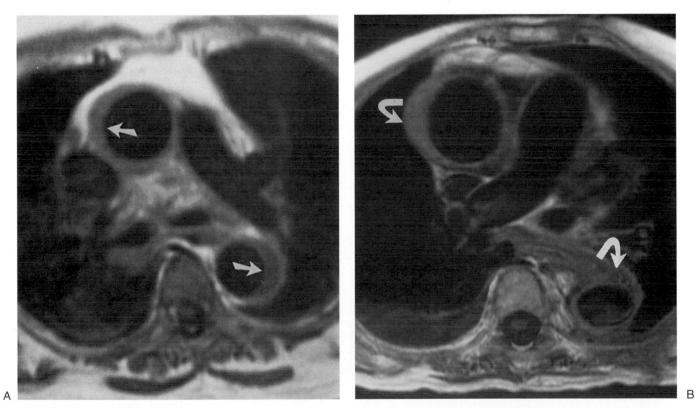

A   B

FIG. 8-67. Acute intramural hematoma involving the ascending aorta (type A) MR demonstration. **A,B:** Axial electrocardiogram triggered T1-weighted SE MR images demonstrate acute aortic intramural hematoma involving both the ascending and descending aorta (*arrows* in **A**) and (*curved arrows* in **B**). Note that the hematoma is isointense to skeletal muscle in both patients. Unlike classic aortic dissection the hematoma is crescent shaped without mass effect on the aortic lumen. Involvement of the ascending aorta portends a poor prognosis.

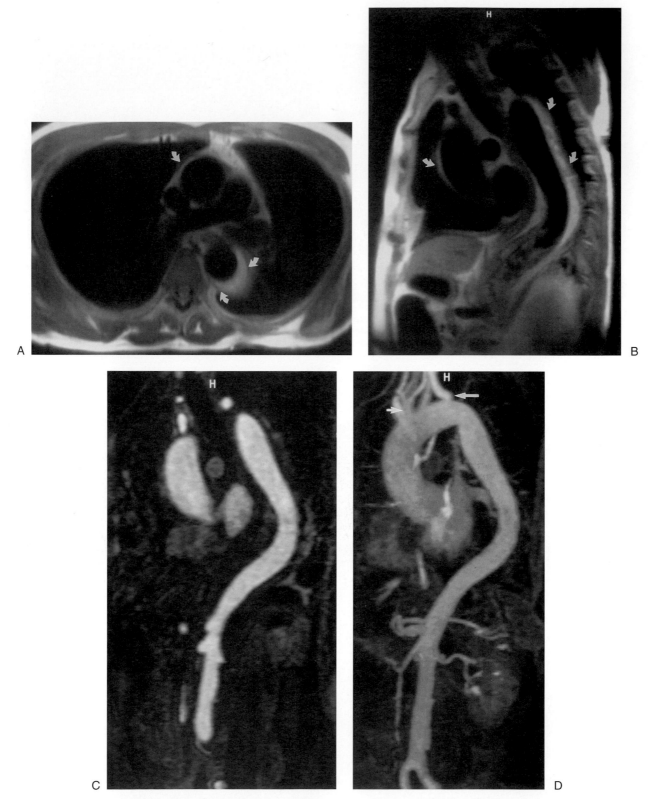

FIG. 8-68. Subacute intramural hematoma MR demonstration. **A,B:** Axial and oblique sagittal electrocardiogram black blood HASTE images demonstrate subacute aortic intramural hematoma involving both the ascending and descending aorta (*arrows* in **A** and **B**). Note the high signal intensity of the subacute hematoma, the crescentic shape, and the absence of mass effect on the aortic lumen. **C,D:** Oblique sagittal source (**C**) and maximum-intensity-projection (**D**) image from breath-hold gadolinium-enhanced three-dimensional MR angiogram fail to demonstrate the hematoma. This case demonstrates the importance of obtaining black blood images in the setting of an acute chest syndrome. Note the presence of an aberrant right subclavian artery (*long arrow* in **D**) and the common trunk of both common carotid arteries (*short arrow* in **D**).

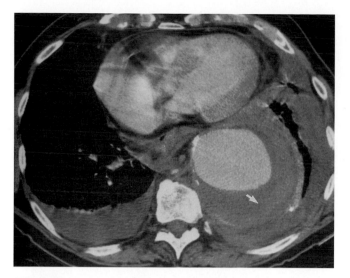

FIG. 8-69. Ruptured thoracic aortic aneurysm, CT evaluation axial contrast-enhanced helical CT image through the lower mediastinum demonstrates a ruptured thoracic aortic aneurysm. Note the enlarged deformed lumen, and the subtle hemorrhage within the wall of thrombus (*arrow*). This would be more obvious on a non–contrast-enhanced examination. Mediastinal and left pleural hematomas are present.

a contained rupture, or a deficient posterior aortic wall, is the draped aorta sign (197). This occurs when the posterior aspect of the aneurysm is in close apposition to the spine and drapes around a vertebral body. Of the 10 patients with this sign, seven had contained rupture of their aneurysm (197).

Mediastinal, pericardial and pleural hematomas may also be present and should strongly suggest the presence of rupture (Figs. 8-69 and 8-70). Contrast-enhanced CT may demonstrate deformities of the enhanced lumen, with or without active extravasation of contrast. It is likely that many cases of previously reported ruptured thoracic aneurysms actually represented penetrating ulcers that had ruptured. Often the history of a thoracic aortic aneurysm is the only clear cut way to differentiate these two surgical emergencies.

MR Evaluation

Caution should be used when evaluating the signal intensity of thrombus at MR imaging to diagnose rupture. Because methemoglobin may remain within an unorganized thrombus for much longer than has been reported in the brain, a portion of thrombus may be high signal intensity on T1-weighted SE images and should not be interpreted as evidence of contained rupture. However, this high signal intensity unorganized thrombus (198) is usually in a lamelated configuration. Clefts of high signal intensity thrombus within outer layers of low signal intensity degenerated thrombus may represent contained rupture.

AORTIC ATHEROMATA AND EMBOLIZATION

Clinical Features

Complex atherosclerotic plaques, also referred to as aortic atheromas, have recently been described as a distinct etiology for cerebral and peripheral embolization (199–204). These atheromas can result in end organ damage if diagnosis and subsequent therapy are delayed. In an autopsy study of 500 patients, Amarenco (199) found ulcerated plaques in the aortic arch in 26% of patients who died of cerebrovascular disease and in 61% of patients with cryptogenic stroke. In another study using TEE, Amarenco (200) found atheromas at least 4 mm thick in 14% of patients with stroke and in only 2% of controls. In a prospective study of 521 patients, Tunick (203) demonstrated protruding atheromas in 42 patients. Over a subsequent two year period one third of these patients experienced end artery embolic events. Among patients who undergo coronary artery bypass grafting and other cardiac procedures, embolization of atheromas from the ascending aorta is an important cause of postoperative stroke (Fig. 8-71) (202). The aortic arch is a common site of atheromas (Fig. 8-72); cross clamping of this segment in patients who undergo aortic or cardiac operations may also dislodge atherosclerotic debris. Because of these complications, many surgeons now use deep hypothermia in conjunction with circulatory arrest for aortic surgery associated with severe atherosclerotic disease. This technique allows graft placement without cross clamping a diseased aorta. Some investigators even advocate endarterectomy or graft replacement of nonaneurysmal but severely atherosclerotic aortic segments discovered at surgery that is initially performed for other aortic or cardiac pathology (121).

Imaging Features

CT Evaluation

A recent paper comparing thin section noncontrast helical CT with multiplane TEE for the diagnosis of aortic atheroma in 32 patients with clinical signs of embolization demonstrated that the two techniques were complementary (72). Although TEE was more sensitive and specific for atheromas overall, six protruding atheromas were detected only at CT (72). These all occurred in the region between the distal ascending aorta and the proximal arch, an area very difficult to image with TEE. Because unenhanced helical CT may underestimate the amount of noncalcified thrombus, the use of intravenous contrast could likely increase diagnostic yield (Fig. 8-73). Furthermore, real-time CT fluoroscopy has the potential to detect mobile components of atheromas.

MR Evaluation

To date, no study has compared TEE with MRA for the detection of aortic atheromas. Intraoperative epiaortic ultrasound may be the most accurate modality for the detection

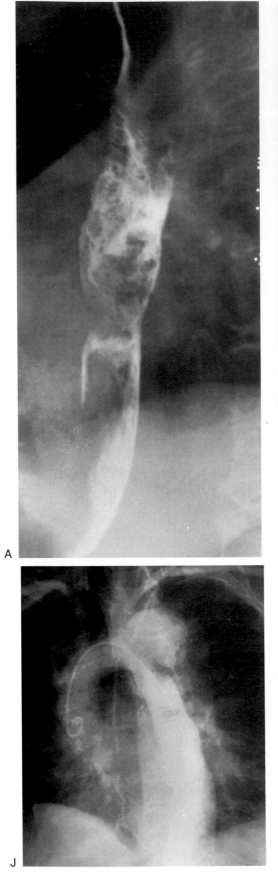

A

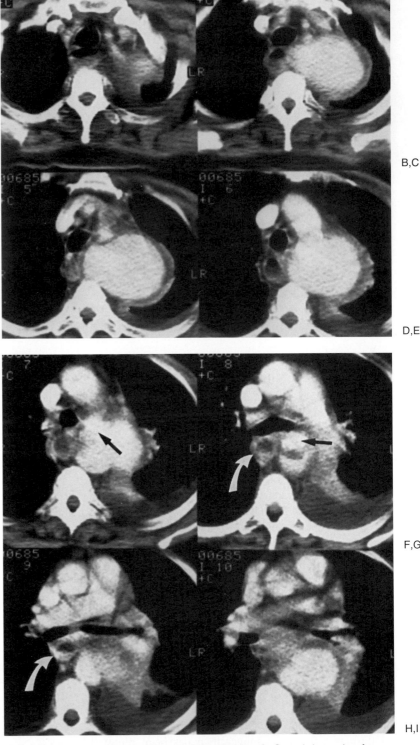

B,C

D,E

F,G

H,I

FIG. 8-70. Ruptured aortic aneurysm, CT evaluation. **A:** Coned-down view from an esophagram obtained in a patient who presented with hematemesis. A large filling defect is conspicuous within the esophageal lumen. **B–I:** Sequential contrast-enhanced CT sections from above-downward shows a large aortic aneurysm involving the proximal portion of the descending aorta. At the level of the distal trachea and carina, disruption in the wall of the aneurysm can be identified (*arrows* in **F** and **G**) with resultant mediastinal hematoma and associated left pleural effusion. A blood-fluid level can also be seen within the esophageal lumen (*curved arrow* in **H**). **J:** Corresponding aortogram showing a large aneurysm of the aorta without apparent leak. This patient died shortly thereafter despite attempts at surgical repair.

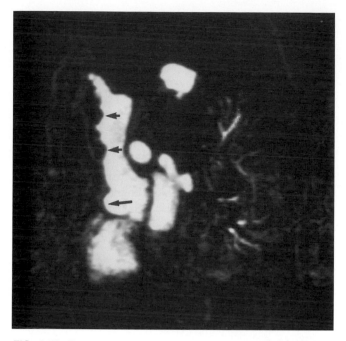

FIG. 8-71. Protruding atheromas of the ascending aorta. Oblique sagittal source image from breath-hold gadolinium-enhanced three-dimensional MR angiogram demonstrates multiple protruding atheromas of the ascending aorta (*small arrows*). *Large arrow* demonstrates the sinus of valsalva.

of aortic atheromas; it is more accurate than direct palpation or TEE (121). We have found that atheromas are readily distinguished with breath-hold gadolinium-enhanced 3D MRA as uniformly low signal intensity masses that produce an irregular surface contour and are contiguous with the aortic wall but protrude into the aortic lumen (see Figs. 8-71 and 8-72) (40,193). In contrast, thrombus, associated with aortic aneurysm, usually has a smooth lumenal contour.

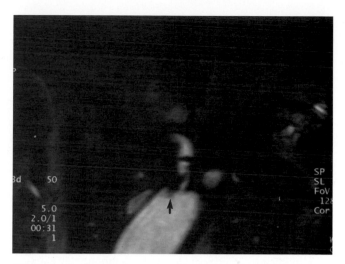

FIG. 8-72. Protruding atheromas of the aortic arch resulting in innominate artery narrowing. Oblique sagittal source image from breath-hold gadolinium-enhanced three-dimensional MR angiogram demonstrates a protruding atheroma of the aortic arch that extends into the innominate artery (*arrow*). Additional plaque is present in the distal vessel. Of note is that the region just proximal to the innominate artery is a blind area that is poorly visualized with transesophageal echocardiography. (From ref. 290, with permission.)

Because plaque mobility is an independent risk factor for embolization (201), 2D cine GRE MRA should be performed through large atheromas to detect a mobile component.

AORTIC TRAUMA

Clinical Features

The majority of aortic trauma results from blunt trauma caused by high speed motor vehicle accidents (205), plane crashes, and falls from great heights. Injury to the thoracic

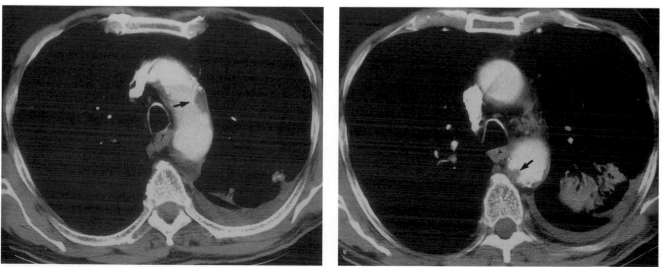

A   B

FIG. 8-73. Protruding aortic atheroma, diagnosis with contrast-enhanced CT. **A,B:** Axial images from contrast-enhanced helical CT at the level of the aortic arch and mid descending aorta demonstrate protruding atheromas measuring >4mm (*arrows*). A left pleural effusion and left upper lobe consolidation is also present.

aorta or arch vessels is present in approximately 15% of road-traffic deaths and as such represents a major cause of out-of-hospital mortality (206–208). Rupture of the thoracic aorta is immediately lethal in 75% to 90% of cases (208,206). Of the patients with thoracic aortic injury who reach the hospital alive, 60% to 70% will survive if appropriately treated. Interestingly, those who survive until hospitalization do not usually die from their aortic injury but from concomitant trauma to other vascular or organ injuries.

The mechanism of thoracic aortic injury results from deceleration or traction. Ninety percent of thoracic aortic injuries occur in the region of the aortic isthmus, the portion of the descending thoracic aorta between the origin of the left subclavian artery and the site of attachment of the ligamentum arteriosum (see Fig. 8-7) (209). Horizontal deceleration results in shearing forces at the aortic isthmus, the junction between the relatively mobile aortic arch and the fixed descending aorta (207). Bending stress may also occur as the aorta is flexed over the left pulmonary artery and left main stem bronchus (210,211). Some advocate that aortic isthmus injuries result from an osseous pinch; the aorta is squeezed between the anterior bony thorax and the spine from anterior compression.

The ascending aorta is the second most common site of injury and is involved in 5% to 20% of cases (208,209). These injuries are invariably fatal because of associated cardiac tamponade, aortic valve rupture, and coronary artery compromise. Injuries to the ascending aorta may result from sudden vertical deceleration, which displaces the heart inferiorly and into the left pleural cavity. This torsion results in traction on the ascending aorta just above the aortic valve. Another hypothesis is the water-hammer effect, caused by a rapid increase in intraaortic pressure, which may lead to rupture into the pericardium (211). Rarely, aortic injury may occur at the level of the diaphragmatic hiatus.

These injuries may result in a spectrum of pathology from benign intimal tears with medial hematomas to complete aortic transection and or arch vessel avulsion (208). Dissection, hemorrhage and vascular thrombosis may subsequently occur. Traumatic pseudoaneurysms develop when the intima and media are disrupted and the adventitia bulges outward but remains intact (208). Thrombi usually form within these false aneurysms and can serve as a nidus for embolization. These pseudoaneurysms tend to expand over time and may cause mass effect on nearby structures, fistulize to adjacent organs, and may spontaneously rupture (212).

Imaging Features

Radiographic Evaluation

In most patients, the initial radiographic examination will be a chest radiograph, usually a supine portable film. The most important findings are a loss of the normal aortic contour with widening of the mediastinum, tracheal deviation, deviation of a nasogastric tube to the right of the T-4 spinous

process and depression of the left main-stem bronchus (211). If the patient is hemodynamically unstable with an abnormal chest radiograph either aortography or surgical exploration may be performed. This will vary by the clinical scenario, the suspicion of other life threatening injuries and the treating institution's trauma protocol. If the patient is stable, an erect posterioanterior chest radiograph should be performed.

The presence of mediastinal abnormalities has a diagnostic sensitivity of 90% to 95% for a thoracic arterial injury but a low specificity (5–10%) and positive predictive value (10%–15%) (213,214). The specificity can be markedly improved when using a formula including three critical signs-loss of aortic contour, tracheal deviation, and ratio of mediastinal width to chest width (215). Although a normal chest radiograph can never exclude an aortic injury its negative predictive value is 96% for supine films and 98% for erect films (216).

CT Evaluation

Contrast-enhanced helical CT has become an important test in the algorithm of the diagnosis of traumatic aortic rupture because a completely normal examination in a stable patient virtually excludes a significant injury (217–220). This in turn has dramatically reduced the number of aortograms performed. Mirvis et al. has demonstrated that reliance on findings at admission CT rather than chest radiography resulted in a $365,000 savings owing to the elimination of unnecessary aortograms.

CT signs of aortic injury are best classified as direct or ancillary. Direct findings include active extravasation of contrast material, pseudoaneurysms, intimal flaps (Fig. 8-74), abrupt caliber change, pseudocoarctation, and focal occlusion of segments of the aorta or arch vessels. Indirect signs are those that are supportive of the diagnosis, but not specific, and include mediastinal and or retrocrural hematomas (see Fig. 8-74), which are more likely to be caused by a bony fracture or a venous injury than an aortic injury. However, if the hematoma is periaortic and obliterates the fat planes surrounding the aorta, the specificity is markedly increased to 77% (221).

Mirvis et al. evaluated 677 patients with contrast-enhanced CT with positive or equivocal findings at chest radiography. For aortic injury and mediastinal hemorrhage respectively, specificity for traumatic aortic injury was 99% and 87% and sensitivity was 90% and 100%. Therefore, the CT finding of mediastinal hemorrhage alone was sensitive for traumatic aortic injury, but the findings of direct aortic injury were more specific. Gavant et al. prospectively evaluated 1,518 patients with blunt chest trauma of which 21 patients had aortic injuries (222). Helical CT was more sensitive than aortography (100% versus 94.4%) but less specific (81.7% versus 96.3 %) in detection of aortic injuries in patients who underwent both examinations (222). Potential causes of false positive or indeterminate CT examinations were caused by motion artifacts, prominent mediastinal vessels, and protruding aortic atheromata. The same authors used CTA to evaluate traumatic aortic disease in 3,229 patients and demonstrated that MPR and MIP reconstructions offered no additional diagnostic information when compared with the axial source images (223). However, the use of overlapping reconstructed axial images was helpful in depicting subtle intimal injuries confined to the distal aortic arch above the level of the pulmonary artery (223).

ADVANCES IN SURGICAL AND INTERVENTIONAL TECHNIQUES/THE POSTOPERATIVE AORTA

Advances in the imaging of aortic disease have been paralleled by advances in surgical treatment of many of these diseases. In addition to diagnosing aortic disease, it is incumbent on the radiologist to provide pertinent information to the referring clinician that may influence operative approach and technique. To that end, the radiologist must be familiar with various operative techniques and understand the pathologic and anatomic conditions that dictate the operative approach. In addition, it is helpful to be aware of common postoperative complications and to know the follow-up imaging schedule most appropriate to each postoperative situation. This will help the referring clinician in monitoring the patient for disease evolution or progression.

The ability to induce deep hypothermia with circulatory arrest has led to profound reductions in morbidity and mortality in surgical repair of aneurysms and dissection of the thoracic aorta, especially those that involve the aortic arch (126,224,225). With this technique, core body temperature is cooled to below 18°C, the patient is placed in Trendelenberg position and cardiopulmonary bypass is halted or slowed. Aortic cross clamping, which may result in embolization of atherosclerotic debris, tearing of a fragile aorta (especially in patients with cystic medial necrosis) and aortic dissection, is avoided. It also provides for a relatively bloodless surgical field, minimizes the amount of surgical dissection needed and provides for cardiac, visceral and neurologic protection. Further cerebral protection can be achieved through cannulation of the SVC with retrograde cerebral perfusion (149). When these techniques are performed for up to 45 minutes, the incidence of subsequent neurologic deficit, primarily stroke, is below 5% (126). In a multivariate analysis, age and duration of arrest were predictive of temporary neurologic deficit, whereas age and disease involving the aortic arch and descending aorta were predictive of stroke (225).

In descending aortic repairs, including aortic dissection and thoracoabdominal aneurysms, aortic cross clamping has profound effects on perfusion of the spinal cord depending on hemodynamic alterations and on the nature of vascular supply from the descending aorta to the cord. During cross clamping, dysfunction of auto-regulatory circuits results in decreased perfusion; this has been postulated as an etiology for the significant rate of postoperative paraplegia. From a practical standpoint, the risk of paraplegia increases with the amount of aorta replaced, cross-clamp time and operation for rupture or acute dissection (225–227).

Multiple strategies have been advocated to decrease the incidence of spinal cord ischemia resulting from aortic cross clamping. Some advocate deep hypothermia with circulatory arrest, thus completely avoiding cross clamping entirely (228) although this method is not widely used because of the threat of coagulopathy and perioperative hemorrhage with systemic heparinization (229). Routine re-implantation of the largest backbleeding intercostal arteries from T8-L1, as the sole method to prevent spinal cord ischemia, has fallen out of favor at many institutions because it increases clamp times and may be technically difficult in an acutely dissected or heavily calcified aorta. Adjuncts that have dramatically

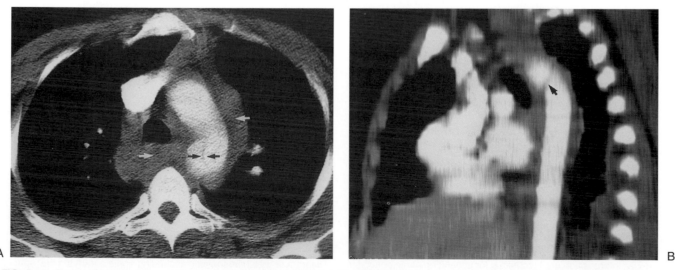

FIG. 8-74. Traumatic aortic injury at the level of the isthmus. **A,B:** Axial image from contrast-enhanced helical CT demonstrates subtle intimal flap (*black arrows*) and extensive mediastinal hematoma (*white arrows*). Image is grainy owing to the use of detail (bone) algorithm. **B:** Oblique sagittal reformat better demonstrates the aortic transection (*arrow*).

decreased the incidence of spinal cord ischemia are based on the paradigm of maximizing collateral blood flow in an attempt to improve spinal cord perfusion during aortic occlusion. These include the use of cerebrospinal fluid drainage (126,228,230–232), monitoring of spinal somatosensory evoked potentials (121), distal perfusion (232–234), administration of low dose nalaxone (228), direct epidural cooling (235) and mild hypothermia (without circulatory arrest). Most institutions favor some form of intercostal reimplantation when used with the aforementioned adjuncts as they allow for a longer clamp time without inducing critical cord ischemia (236). Using various combination of these techniques has resulted in a marked decrease in postoperative paraplegia to about 5% to 10%, a considerable improvement when compared with 16% in the largest surgical series (233).

In some institutions the interventional radiologist now plays an important role in the management of patients with aortic dissection complicated by end organ compromise. Procedures performed by these specialists include percutaneous fenestration of the dissecting membrane to equalize pressures in the true and false lumens and placement of stents to relieve critical ischemia to the kidneys, bowel, and lower extremities (155,177). In addition, the use of stent grafts for definitive treatment of thoracic aneurysms (143) and traumatic pseudoaneurysms (see Fig. 8-38) (144,237) in poor operative candidates, is now widely used in some academic centers. Successful endovascular treatment of aortic dissec-

tion involving the descending aorta (238) and ascending aorta (239) has been described in patients who are otherwise poor surgical candidates.

The Postoperative Aorta

Precise knowledge of the surgical technique performed, and its anatomic consequences, is crucial to an accurate postoperative imaging evaluation. This will enable the radiologist to differentiate normal postoperative findings from those indicative of postoperative complications, possibly requiring intervention. Two techniques are widely used for repair of aortic dissection or aneurysm: placement of a simple interposition graft (Fig. 8-75) or use of an inclusion graft technique (Fig. 8-76). With an interposition graft, the diseased segment of aorta is excised and a graft is sewn end-to-end between the two segments using full thickness bites (see Fig. 8-75). Critical vessels are usually directly reimplanted into the graft. Advocates of this technique argue that sewing the graft to all three layers of the aortic wall provides greater durability, thus minimizing the risk of anastamotic pseudoaneurysms (149,156).

The inclusion graft technique involves aortotomy, graft insertion and subsequent enclosure of the graft within the remnant of diseased aorta; this results in a potential space between the graft and the aortic wall (see Fig. 8-76). The perigraft space, defined as the potential space between the

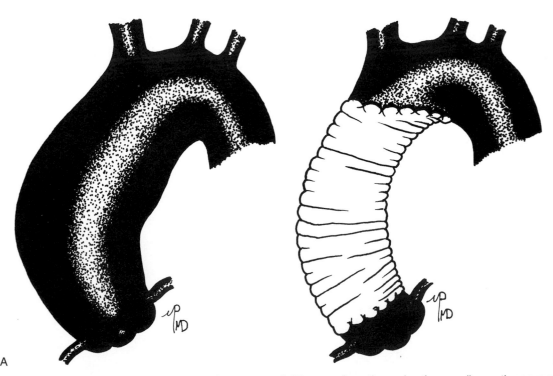

FIG. 8-75. Interposition graft technique for ascending aortic aneurysm. **A:** Diagram of an atherosclerotic ascending aortic aneurysm that spares the sinus segment but involves the transverse arch. This will require hypothermic circulatory arrest to avoid cross clamping the aortic arch and to operate in a bloodless field. **B:** Completed repair after aortic transection and supracoronary proximal anastomosis with a beveled distal anastomosis to the transverse arch.

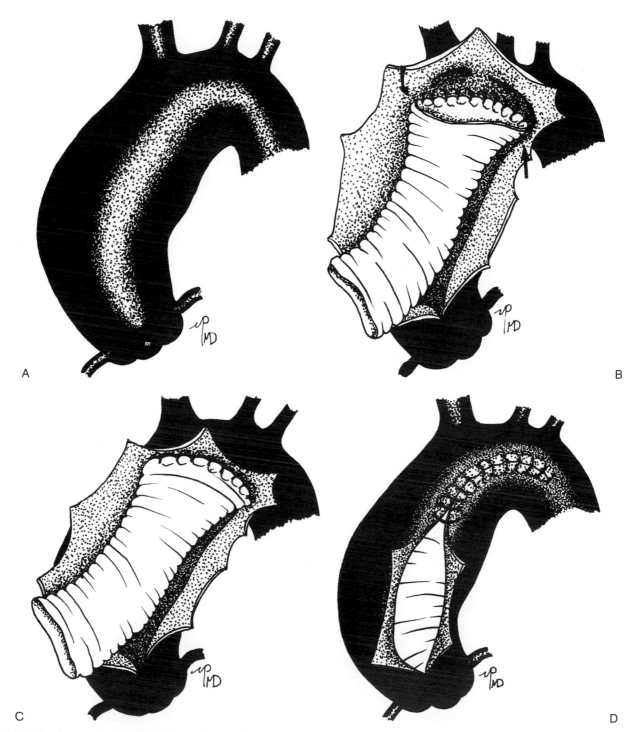

A

B

C

D

FIG. 8-76. Continous suture graft inclusion technique. **A–D:** Using hypothermic circulatory arrest the aneurysm is opened and the distal anastomosis is performed first (**B** and **C**) and followed by the proximal anastomosis, both with continous suture technique. In this illustration the hemiarch technique is shown with a tongue of graft material extending along the inferior surface of the aortic arch, beyond the origins of the great vessels (*straight arrow* in **B**). The superior edge of the graft material does not extend beyond the origin of the brachiocephalic artery (*curved arrow* in **B**). **D:** The native aortic sac is trimmed and wrapped around the prosthesis and its cut edges are sutured together. (From ref. 240, with permission.)

graft and the native aortic wrap may contain thrombus, flowing blood or both (Fig. 8-77) (240). Pseudoaneurysm formation, or persistent flow within the perigraft space, usually results from partial dehiscence of either the proximal or distal suture line (or the coronary anastomosis if reimplantation was performed) but can also result from leakage created

from needle holes with an otherwise intact suture line. Advocates of this technique believe that wrapping the graft provides for an extra measure of hemostasis if bleeding is severe, and can prevent fatal exsanguination from suture dehiscence.

In patients who undergo the inclusion graft technique, a

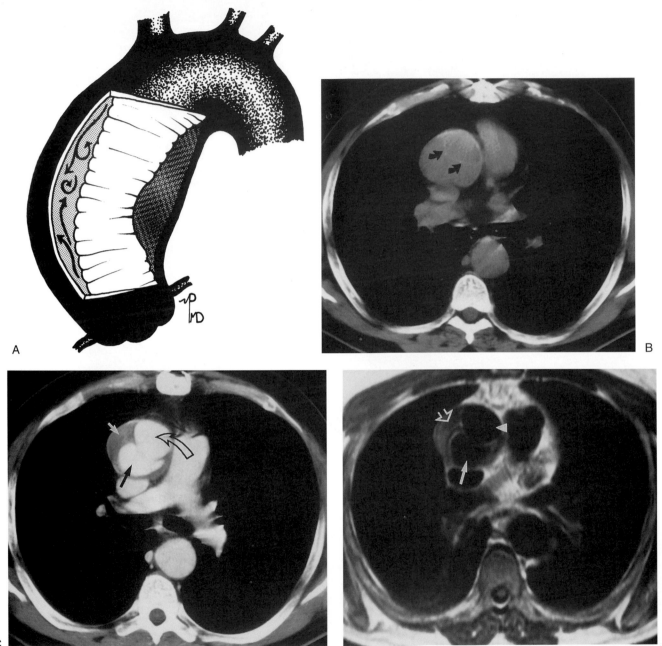

FIG. 8-77. Periprosthetic flow and thrombus, CT and MR demonstration. **A:** Diagram demonstrates the potential space between the native aorta and the aortic wrap termed the perigraft space. Perigraft flow is present anteriorly and perigraft thrombus is present posteriorly. **B:** Axial image from non–contrast-enhanced CT demonstrates enlargement of the ascending aorta with a thin, oval rim of high attenuation material (*arrows*) depicting the graft is identified in a portion of the lumen. **C:** Contrast-enhanced CT at the same level demonstrates flow within the graft (*open arrow*) and adjacent to the graft (*black arrow*). The perigraft flow as well as the adjacent thrombus (*white arrow*) is contained within the adventitial wrap. **D:** Axial electrocardiogram triggered T1-weighted SE MR image at the same level demonstrates the signal void characteristic of flow within the graft (*arrowhead*) and in the perigraft space (*arrow*). Intermediate signal intensity thrombus in the perigraft space is seen as well (*open arrow*). If this patient did not have a surgical history one could mistake these findings for a chronic aortic dissection. Note that the presence of perigraft flow and or thrombus is not an indication for reoperation unless there is symptomatic mass effect or rapid growth. (From ref. 240, with permission.)

Cabrol procedure (241) may be performed. This involves anastomosing the native aortic wrap to the right atrial appendage; the goal of this shunt is to decompress a potentially tense perigraft space, which could compromise the coronary artery ostia. Patients who undergo the Cabrol shunt may have a small amount of perigraft flow, however, this technique may prevent progression to large pseudoaneurysm formation (240).

In patients with aortic dissection or aneurysm that involve the aortic root, graft placement may be supplemented by reimplantation of the coronary arteries and resuspension of the aortic valve. Alternatively, a composite graft that includes a prosthetic valve (Bentall procedure) may be placed. A specific composite graft designed by Cabrol includes both an aortic valve and a prosthetic conduit, which is anastomosed directly to the proximal right and left main coronary arteries (241). Recognition of this type of graft is important because if imaged in an axial plane it may resemble a focal dissection at the aortic root (Fig. 8-78).

In the ascending aorta, especially after insertion of composite grafts, false aneurysm formation at the site of coronary anastomosis may lead to cardiac ischemia, infarction and sudden death. Pseudoaneurysms resulting from dehiscence of the proximal or distal suture line are commonly seen during routine postoperative surveillance (38), especially in patients with cystic medial necrosis. Of patients who undergo reoperative repair of a graft pseudoaneurysm, morbidity and mortality have been reported to be as high as 75% and 25%, respectively, and higher in the case of emergent repair (242, 243). Thus, it is essential to maintain close follow-up after ascending aortic repair, especially in patients prone to develop postoperative aneurysmal complications such as those with Marfan's syndrome, so that repair of developing pseudoaneurysms can be performed in a nonemergent setting (244). With inclusion graft techniques, the presence of a postoperative pseudoaneurysm (perigraft flow) does not always mandate surgical repair unless the patient is symptom-

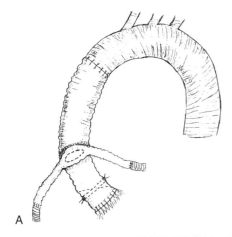

FIG. 8-78. A: Diagram of a cabrol composite graft for aortic root replacement. It consists of a graft with a prosthetic aortic valve and an end-to-side coronary tube graft. The remaining native aorta is then wrapped around the graft and a fistula between the perigraft space and right atrial appendage may be created (not shown). **B:** Axial reformation from breath-hold gadolinium-enhanced three-dimensional MR angiogram demonstrates the left coronary tube from a Cabrol graft that mimics a focal aortic dissection. **C:** Oblique axial reformation from same acquisition demonstrates the true configuration of the end-to-side coronary tube graft with patent limbs. (From ref. 290, with permission.)

A

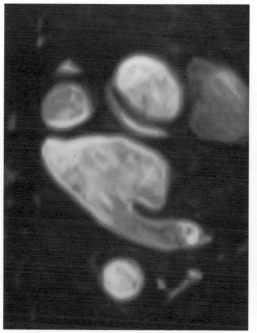

B

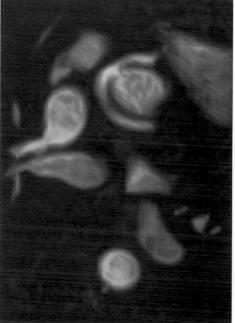

C

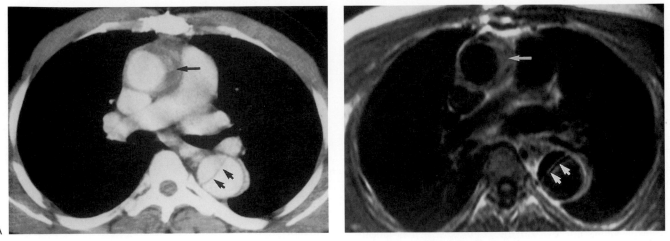

FIG. 8-79. Perigraft thrombus after inclusion graft technique repair of aortic dissection CT-MR findings. **A:** Axial contrast-enhanced CT demonstrates perigraft thrombus (*long arrow*) and persistent intimal flap distal to the graft site in the descending aorta (*small arrows*). **B:** Axial electrocardiogram triggered T1-weighted SE MR image at the same level demonstrates intermediate signal intensity thrombus in the perigraft space (*arrow*) and intimal flap in the descending aorta (*small arrows*).

atic from mass effect or hemodynamic compromise, or significant growth is documented on serial imaging (240).

In patients who have undergone repair of aortic dissection, CT or MR may demonstrate persistent intimal flap distal to the graft site in up to 75% to 100% of cases and in virtually all cases of repaired chronic dissection (Figs. 8-79–8-81) (149,245–247). Despite tacking down the intima proximally,

distal communications between the true and false lumen are common and result in persistence of the false channel. In chronic dissections, the distal anastamosis is usually made to both lumena, thus intentionally maintaining false lumen patency because it may provide critical blood supply to the kidneys or viscera. All patients with native or postoperative communicating dissections are at risk for secondary aneu-

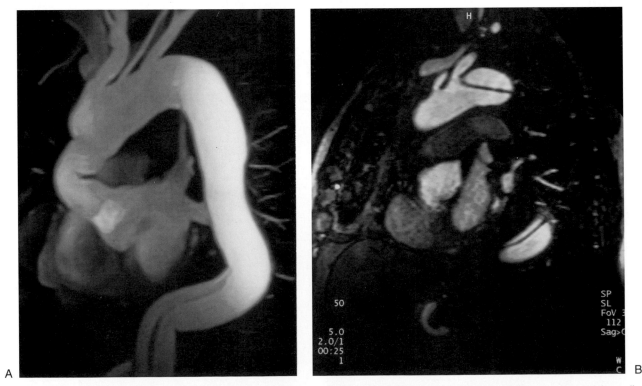

FIG. 8-80. Oblique sagittal source image (**A**) and maximum-intensity-projection image (**B**) from breath-hold gadolinium-enhanced three-dimensional MR angiogram demonstrate the typical postoperative appearance of a repaired Stanford A dissection with an interposition graft. The residual, distal intimal flap is a common postoperative finding and is best visualized on the source image. (From ref. 290, with permission.)

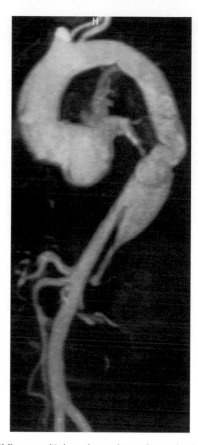

FIG. 8-81. Oblique sagittal maximum-intensity-projection image from breath-hold gadolinium-enhanced three-dimensional MR angiogram demonstrates a normal postoperative appearance of a repaired Stanford B dissection. Note that the false lumen terminates in the upper abdomen. (From ref. 290, with permission.)

rysm formation from an enlarging false lumen. In a longitudinal MR study in patients with repaired type A dissection, 25% developed aneurysms distal to the graft site (Fig. 8-82) (38).

Patients with Marfan's disease are at an even higher risk for enlarging aneurysms from progressive dilatation of the false lumen distal to the repair site (40%) (157) or the development of a separate noncontiguous aneurysm (244). These patients also have a high incidence of new dissection, distal to the graft site, in segments of the aorta that had previously appeared normal.

Imaging Features

In patients who have undergone inclusion graft techniques, enlargement of the perigraft space is readily visualized with contrast-enhanced CT, TEE and MRI and perigraft flow is reliably distinguished from thrombus with either contrast-enhanced CT or TEE.

With MR imaging, distinction between perigraft flow from thrombus may be difficult as perigraft flow is often turbulent. This may result in dephasing with artifactual signal loss on GRE imaging. A study comparing cine GRE

with 2D gadolinium-enhanced magnetization-prepared GRE MRA found the latter technique more sensitive in distinguishing perigraft flow from thrombus (292). The use of breath-hold, gadolinium-enhanced 3D MR angiography can better differentiate perigraft flow from thrombus (Fig. 8-83) for three separate but distinct reasons. First, these sequences often have a very short echo time (1–2 msec), which minimizes signal loss from turbulent flow. Second, their intrinsic high spatial resolution with small voxels minimizes artifactual signal loss from intravoxel phase dispersion. Third, the magnitude of T1 shortening of gadolinium may also partially compensate for the dephasing phenomenon.

On unenhanced CT prosthetic graft often appears as a ring of high attenuation contiguous with the aortic wall (see Fig. 8-77). Postoperative complications are readily diagnosed with similar criteria as previously discussed with MR (Fig. 8-84). A significant advantage of CT over MR is in the evaluation of patients who have had endovascular stents and stent-grafts placed as these may cause significant susceptibility artifacts with resultant artifactual signal loss. The relationship of a stent to an aortic branch vessel can be demonstrated with MIP and MPR images (see Fig. 8-38). MPRs

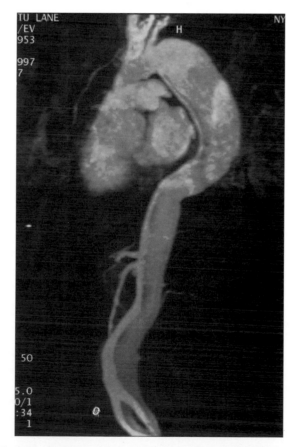

FIG. 8-82. Oblique sagittal maximum-intensity-projection image from breath-hold gadolinium-enhanced three-dimensional MR angiogram demonstrates aneurysmal dilatation of the false lumen in a patient who underwent previous repair of a Stanford type A dissection. Note the presence of higher signal intensity within the smaller, anterior true lumen.

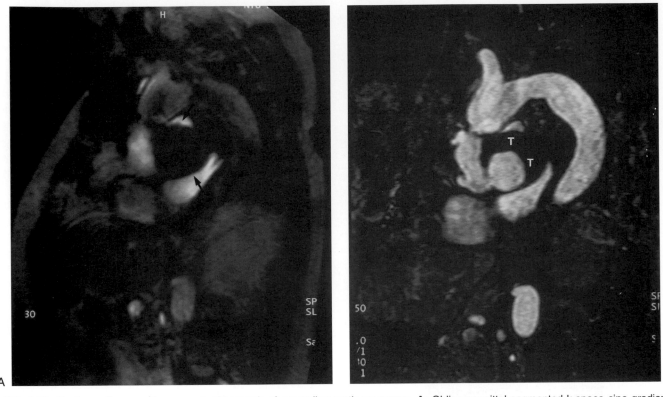

FIG. 8-83. Postoperative pseudoaneurysm after repair of ascending aortic aneurysm. **A:** Oblique sagittal segmented k-space cine gradient-echo MR image demonstrates a large area of signal void from turbulent flow posterior to the ascending aorta (*arrows*). **B:** Oblique sagittal source image from breath-hold gadolinium-enhanced three-dimensional MR angiogram demonstrates a pseudoaneurysm at the proximal suture line with concentric thrombus (*T*). This case demonstrates the importance of using gadolinium in conjunction with an ultrashort echo time (1–2 msec) to minimize signal loss from intravoxel dephasing resulting from turbulent flow. (From ref. 290, with permission.)

are invaluable for assessing the interior of the metallic prosthesis and determining the presence of intimal hyperplasia or stent deformation (18,248). Complications such as stent migration, perigraft leaks, and progressive dilatation of an aneurysm sac can be detected (144).

Coronary Artery Bypass Grafts

Although a full discussion of coronary artery imaging is outside the intended scope of the present volume, assessing coronary artery bypass grafts will be discussed as these are often present in patients who have undergone simultaneous aortic surgery.

The ability to directly visualize and assess patency of coronary artery bypass grafts (CABG) with MRA techniques is an area of great clinical interest because of the large number of patients who undergo these procedures and because postoperative graft occlusion is common. Coronary angiography is the gold standard for evaluation of these grafts but is expensive and not without inherent risks. Because of the widespread use of these grafts and the relatively common development of anginal syndromes after bypass surgery, repeated catheterizations with each new or progressive anginal syndrome are not feasible. Therefore, many clinicians rely on indirect methods of determining vessel patency, which can only suggest the presence or absence of occlusion. These are based upon changes in regional myocardial perfusion or wall contraction abnormalities (52). Clearly, a noninvasive imaging modality that could directly assess graft patency, with both high sensitivity and specificity, is needed.

Early studies using cine GRE MRA were able to demonstrate graft patency at selected levels (249,250). Recently, cine phase contrast MRA with velocity mapping has been shown to be an accurate technique in evaluating patency of saphenous vein bypass grafts. Sensitivity and specificity for graft patency with this technique were 98% and 85% (251) and 100% and 85% (252) respectively. Vrachliotis et al. (52) used a novel, ECG-triggered breath-hold gadolinium-enhanced 3D acquisition in which an experienced radiologist achieved a sensitivity and specificity of 93% for assessing graft patency (Fig. 8-85). Breath holding and ECG triggering virtually eliminated motion and pulsation artifacts respectively, and the ultrashort echo time (2 msec) minimized susceptibility artifacts from surgical clips, metal sutures and coronary stents. Perhaps of greater importance is that examination time was short, requiring only a single breath-hold, and reformatted images and subvolume MIP demonstrated long segments of tortuous graft that actually resembled conventional angiograms (52). Further ad-

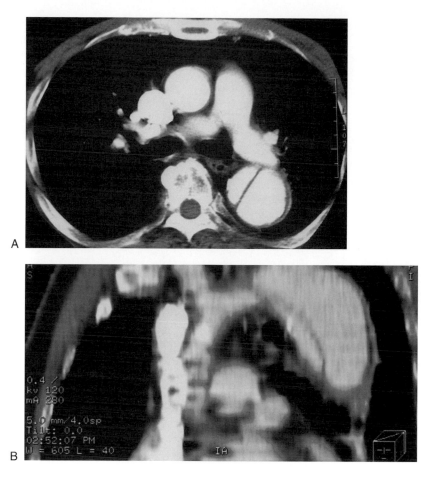

A

B

FIG. 8-84. CT examination from same patient in Fig. 8-82 demonstrating aneurysmal dilatation of the aorta distal to the repair site. **A:** Axial contrast-enhanced helical CT image at the level of the left pulmonary artery demonstrates intimal flap in an aneurysmal descending aorta. **B:** Oblique sagittal reformation better demostrates that aneurysmal dilatation begins just distal to the aortic arch.

vances in hardware, pulse sequence implementation and optimized contrast administration are likely to result in a greater role for MRA in the postoperative surveillance of coronary artery bypass grafts.

AORTITIS

Clinical Features

Takayasu's disease is the most common cause of aortitis, usually afflicting young women of Asian descent. It is an inflammatory vasculitis of unknown etiology and is categorized in one of two ways, based on clinical course or anatomic location. Sites of disease may include the aortic arch vessels, the thoracoabdominal aorta and branch vessels, and the pulmonary arteries. The disease involves the vessel walls and results in luminal abnormalities including stenoses, occlusion, dilatation, and aneurysm, all of which may coexist within the same patient (253).

The acute or systemic/prepulseless phase usually presents as an acute systemic illness with manifestations including fever, night sweats, arthralgia, myalgia, anemia, and elevation of the erythrocyte sedimentation rate (ESR) (254). Early diagnosis may be difficult because of the nonspecific symptoms but is important because the time at which treatment

is initiated can affect prognosis (254). During this phase mural thickening of the affected vessels likely results from inflammation of the tunica media and tunica adventitia.

Imaging Features

CT Evaluation

Helical CTA has been successfully used in the evaluation of arteritis (Figs. 8-86 and 8-87) (18,71). A small study of 12 patients (eight patients with active disease and four with inactive disease) examined with CTA in the evaluation of Takayasu arteritis demonstrated high attenuation of the aortic wall on precontrast images in 10 patients and mural calcifications in nine patients (71). Of these nine patients calcifications were intimal in location in three patients and mural in six (71). In six of eight patients with active disease mural enhancement was demonstrated during the arterial phase of contrast injection (71). No patients with inactive disease had arterial phase mural enhancement; thus this finding is specific but not sensitive for the detection of disease activity. Delayed CT images (performed 7 minutes after arterial phase imaging) demonstrated mural enhancement in eight patients, seven of whom had clinically active disease (71). Mural thickness can persist, even with inactive disease, as healed

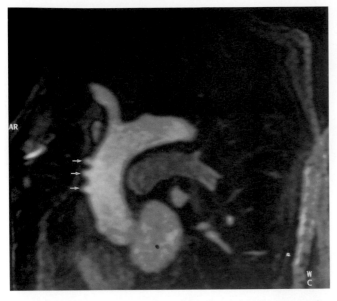

FIG. 8-85. MR evaluation of the origin of coronary bypass grafts. Oblique sagittal source image from breath-hold gadolinium-enhanced three-dimensional MR angiogram demonstrates the proximal portion of three patent coronary artery bypass grafts from the ascending aorta (*arrows*).

lesions often contain a proliferation of fibrous and connective tissue that may undergo dystrophic calcification.

MR Evaluation

MR features of the sytemic phase of aortitis are best visualized with T1-weighted SE images (255) supplemented by breath-hold STIR or T2-weighted images (Fig. 8-88). The presence of increased signal intensity within the aortic wall on the latter 2 pulse sequences may represent active disease although this has not been proven histologically.

Yamada et al. studied 77 patients with Takayasu's arteritis using T1-weighted SE and cine MR imaging. Aortic lesions included stenosis, dilatation, aneurysm, wall thickening and mural thrombi. The most frequent site of stenosis was in the descending aorta and dilatation was seen predominately in the ascending aorta. In addition aortic valve regurgitation was seen in 45% of patients and pulmonary artery involvement was seen in 70% of patients. However, no attempt was made to correlate imaging findings with disease activity in this study (255).

Treatment of acute episodes of arteritis include steroids and cytotoxic agents, but a significant percentage of patients will not respond. Both CT (256) and MR (254) case reports, involving one patient each, have demonstrated a decrease in wall thickening following steroid therapy. With CTA and MRA techniques currently available both mural disease (wall thickening or enhancement) and lumenal abnormalities, including stenoses and aneurysms, can be evaluated

with a single examination (see Figs. 8-86 and 8-87; Fig. 8-89). Angiography should be reserved for patients with symptomatic branch vessel disease, which would require surgical or radiological intervention. Angioplasty and/or stenting may be useful in treating focal disease with surgery reserved for long segment lesions and aneurysms. Because patients with arteritis have a significantly higher incidence of developing aneurysms and aortic dissections (257) than the gen-

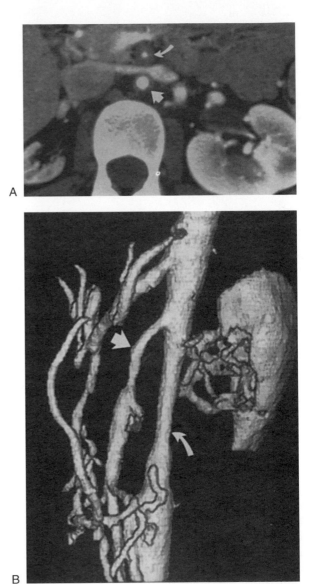

FIG. 8-86. Takayasu's arteritis. A 17-year-old woman with Takayasu's disease developed an increasing sedimentation rate. Computed tomographic angiography was performed using dual-slice technique (Elscint) with a nominal slice width of 2.5 mm and an effective pitch of 2. **A:** Transverse image shows marked thickening of the walls and narrowing of the lumina of the aorta (*straight arrow*) and the superior mesenteric artery (*curved arrow*) and atrophy of the right kidney because of renal artery occlusion. **B:** Shaded surface display image confirms the arterial narrowing. Because of disease progression (compared with prior angiography), steroid pulse therapy was administered. (Courtesy of Kenyon Kopecky Indianapolis, Indiana; from ref. 145, with permission.)

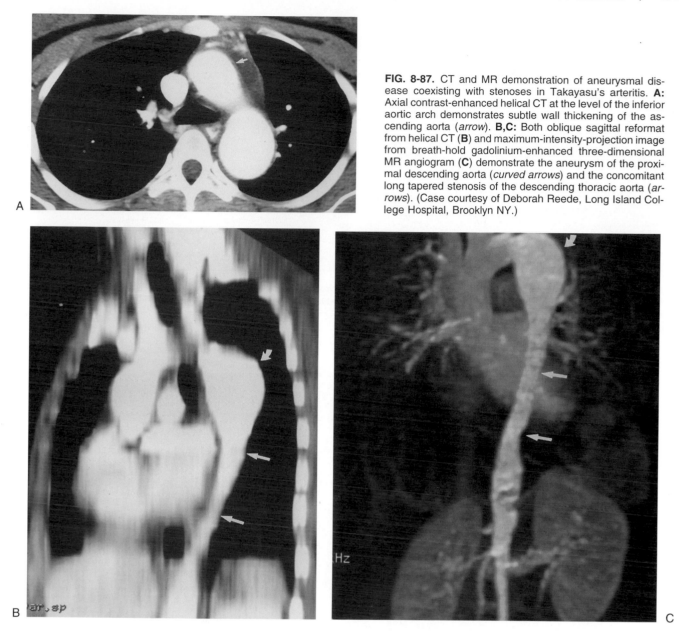

FIG. 8-87. CT and MR demonstration of aneurysmal disease coexisting with stenoses in Takayasu's arteritis. **A:** Axial contrast-enhanced helical CT at the level of the inferior aortic arch demonstrates subtle wall thickening of the ascending aorta (*arrow*). **B,C:** Both oblique sagittal reformat from helical CT (**B**) and maximum-intensity-projection image from breath-hold gadolinium-enhanced three-dimensional MR angiogram (**C**) demonstrate the aneurysm of the proximal descending aorta (*curved arrows*) and the concomitant long tapered stenosis of the descending thoracic aorta (*arrows*). (Case courtesy of Deborah Reede, Long Island College Hospital, Brooklyn NY.)

eral population they should undergo some form of follow-up imaging.

GREAT VEINS INCLUDING THE AZYGOS AND HEMIAZYGOS SYSTEMS

The superior vena cava is most important among thoracic veins, serving as the final tributary for drainage of systemic venous flow from many intrathoracic veins (Fig. 8-90). It is formed by the junction of the brachiocephalic veins in the upper mediastinum and terminates inferiorly in the right atrium. Although its position and appearance are characteristic, it is variable in size, and because of its relatively thin wall, can show transient variations in diameter with changes in fluid status or patient position. Following contrast infusion into a single arm vein, streaming or layering of contrast in the superior vena cava is commonly seen, and should not be misinterpreted as thrombus (258). Inflow of unopacified blood can also be seen at the level of the azygos vein. Because of its thin wall and intimate relationship to mediastinal and right hilar lymph nodes, obstruction is common in the presence of lymph node enlargement.

Cross-sectional anatomy of thoracic veins is complex, but has been described in detail (259–263) (see Fig. 8-90; Fig. 8-91). A knowledge of thoracic venous anatomy is important in order to understand alterations in venous flow occurring in the presence of superior vena cava obstruction (263). Important veins include the subclavian veins, brachiocephalic veins, the azygos and hemiazygos veins, accessory hemiazygos vein, the superior intercostal veins.

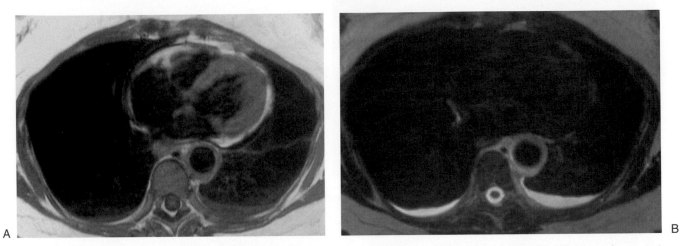

A B

FIG. 8-88. MR evaluation of arteritis-active/systemic phase. **A:** Axial electrocardiogram triggered T1-weighted SE MR image demonstrates circumferential thickening, without narrowing, of the descending thoracic aorta. **B:** Axial electrocardiogram triggered T2-weighted Turbo SE MR imaging demonstrates high signal intensity of periaortic rind. After a three month course of prednisone the patients symptoms resolved and the MR appearance of the descending aorta returned to normal.

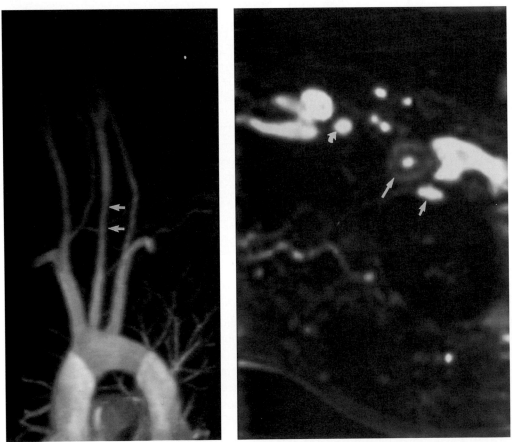

A B

FIG. 8-89. MR angiography of branch vessel disease in Takayasu's arteritis. **A:** Oblique sagittal maximum-intensity-projection image from breath-hold gadolinium-enhanced three-dimensional MR angiogram demonstrates subtle, smooth narrowing of the left common carotid artery (*arrows*). **B:** Axial reformation from delayed gadolinium-enhanced three-dimensional MR data set demonstrates marked thickening of the wall of the left common carotid artery (*long arrow*) resulting in narrowing of the lumen compared with the right common carotid artery (*curved arrow*). *Short arrow* denotes normal left subclavian artery.

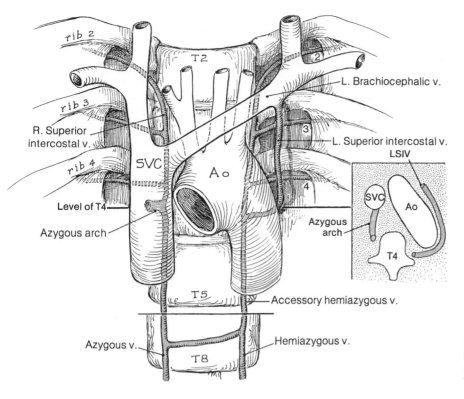

FIG. 8-90. Schematic drawing of the azygos, hemiazygos, and superior intercostal venous systems. Inset is a schematic cross-section at the level of the aortic arch.

The brachiocephalic veins are formed by the junction of the subclavian and internal jugular veins in the superior mediastinum (11) (see Figs. 8-90 and 8-91, Figs. 8-92–8-94). The subclavian veins enter the mediastinum by crossing over the first ribs, anterior to the anterior scalenus muscles, which attach to the superior borders of the first ribs, and posterior to the proximal portions of the clavicles. The internal jugular veins can be traced into the neck from the point they join the brachiocephalic veins.

The azygos and hemiazygos veins represent the thoracic continuations of the right and left ascending lumbar veins, respectively, and serve to drain many of the intercostal and lumbar veins and systemic veins of the mediastinum. The azygos and hemiazygos venous systems and their branches serve as important collateral pathways when there is obstruction or interruption of blood flow through either of the brachiocephalic vessels or the superior or inferior vena cava (263) (see Fig. 8-94).

The azygos vein lies on the right, anterior and slightly lateral to the vertebral column; it is almost always visible on CT. The azygos vein drains the lower intercostal veins (see Fig. 8-91; Fig. 8-95). On the left side, the hemiazygos vein lies posterior to the descending aorta and adjacent to the spine, draining the left lower intercostal veins. It is smaller than the azygos vein, and less commonly seen. The hemiazygos vein terminates in the azygos vein through communicating branches that cross the midline, posterior to the descending aorta, in the vicinity of the T8 vertebral body. These are sometimes seen on CT (264).

Superiorly, the azygos vein arches over the medial aspect of the right upper lobe bronchus and then courses anteriorly to terminate in the posterior portion of the superior vena cava (see Figs. 8-91G–I and 8-93). Just below its arch, the azygos vein is joined by the right superior intercostal vein (see Fig. 8-91D–F, Fig. 8-96). This vein drains the right second to fourth intercostal veins, and then courses inferiorly in a paraspinal location to its junction with the azygos. It is occasionally seen on CT in normals.

The arch of the azygos is variable in size, but can measure up to 15 mm in diameter in normal subjects in the supine position. Dilatation of the arch may be caused by central venous hypertension, as may occur with right ventricular heart failure, obstruction of the superior or inferior vena cava, or azygos continuation of an anomalous inferior vena cava (Fig. 8-97). In some normal subjects, the azygos arch appears dilated or contacts the posterior wall of the right upper lobe or right main bronchus; in either instance the azygos arch may be mistaken for a mass lesion (265,266). In most subjects the azygos vein remains unopacified following intravenous contrast administration, but occasional reflux into the azygos arch and azygos vein occurs in normals (Fig. 8-98).

On the left side, the accessory hemiazygos vein continues above the point of termination of the hemiazygos vein, ascending posterior to the descending aorta (see Fig. 8-94). At the level of the aortic arch, the accessory hemiazygos is joined by the left superior intercostal vein (which drains the second to fourth intercostal veins) in approximately 75%

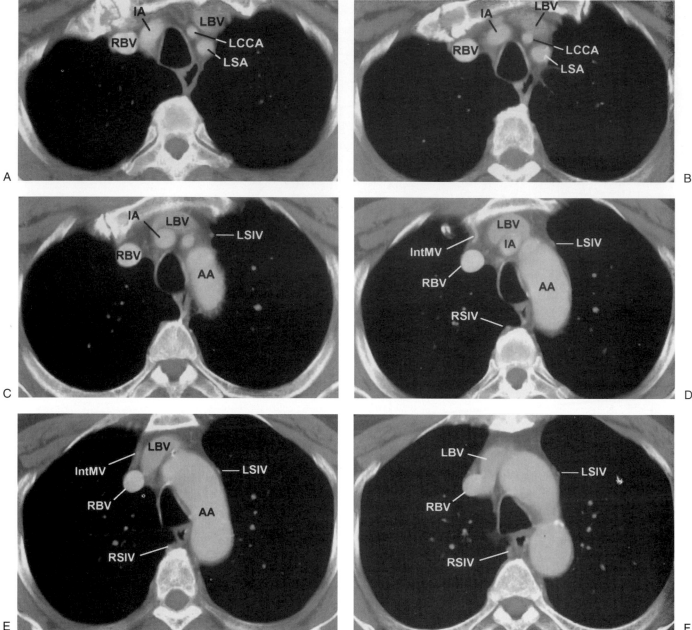

FIG. 8-91. Normal venous anatomy on CT. **A–C:** Above the level of the aortic arch, the innominate artery (*IA*), the left common carotid artery (*LCCA*), the left subclavian artery (*LSA*), the right brachiocephalic vein (*RBV*), and the left brachiocephalic vein (*LBV*) are the most conspicuous normal structures. At or near the thoracic inlet, the brachiocephalic veins are the most anterior and lateral vascular branches visible, lying immediately behind the clavicular heads and articulations of the first ribs. Although they vary in size, their positions are relatively constant. Below the thoracic inlet, the left brachiocephalic vein crosses the mediastinum from left to right, anterior to the arterial branches of the aorta. The two brachiocephalic veins have very different configurations. The right brachiocephalic vein has a nearly vertical course throughout its length; the left brachiocephalic vein is longer, and courses horizontally as it crosses the mediastinum. In **C**, the left superior intercostal vein (*LSIV*) is visible posterior to the left brachiocephalic and beneath the mediastinal pleura. **D–F:** At the level of the aortic arch (*AA*), the brachiocephalic veins are again visible, and can be seen to join to form the superior vena cava (*SVC*). Small veins visible at these levels include the right internal mammary vein (*IntMV*), left superior intercostal vein (*LSIV*), and right superior intercostal vein (*RSIV*). Internal mammary veins are often visible, and in some patients can be traced from their point of origin from the brachiocephalic veins, or on the right, the superior vena cava. The left superior intercostal vein forms a venous arch, sometimes referred to as the arch of the hemiazygos vein, the courses anteriorly around the aortic arch, near the level of T3-4, to join the left brachiocephalic vein superiorly. The right superior intercostal vein drains the right second to fourth intercostal veins, and then courses inferiorly in a paraspinal location to its junction with the azygos. It appears to represent the continuation of the azygos vein above the azygos arch, and lies anterior and to the right of the spine.

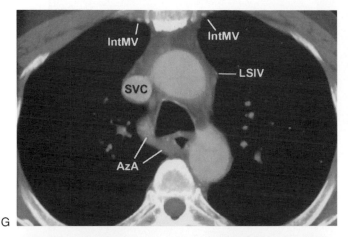

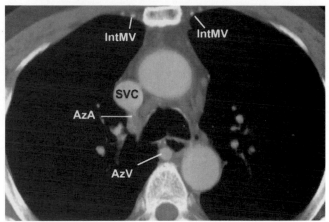

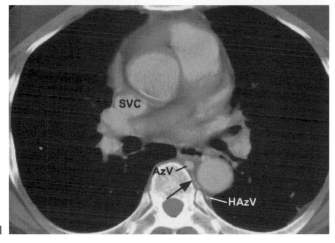

FIG. 8-91. *Continued.* **G–I:** The superior vena cava (*SVC*), the arch of the azygos vein (*AzA*), and the azygos vein (*AzV*) are visible. The azygos vein lies on the right, anterior and slightly lateral to the vertebral column; it is almost always visible on CT. The azygos vein drains the lower intercostal veins. At a lower level, the hemiazygos vein (*HAzV*) is visible to the left of the spine, posterior to the aorta. It is smaller than the azygos vein, and less commonly seen. The small vein branch connecting the hemiazygos and azygos veins is visible (*arrow* in **I**) between the aorta and the vertebral column.

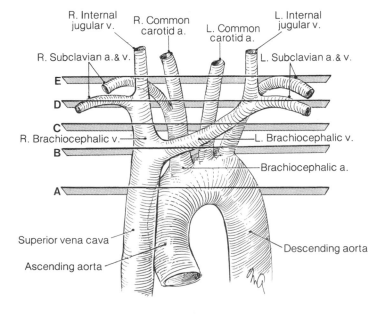

FIG. 8-92. Schematic drawing of the aortic arch and great vessels. Characteristic levels have been labeled *A* through *E*.

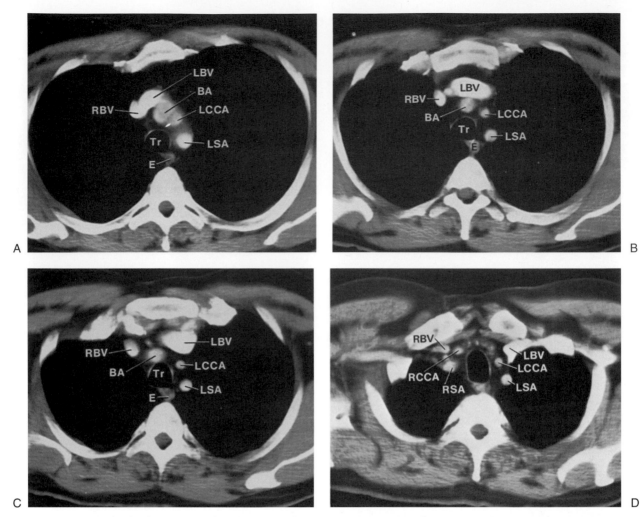

FIG. 8-93. Cross-sectional CT anatomy, great vessels. **A–D:** Sequential contrast-enhanced CT images through the great vessels, from below-upward, corresponding to levels *B*, *C*, *D*, and *E* in FIG. 8-92, respectively. Note that the left brachiocephalic vein (*LBV*) has a much more horizontal course than the right brachiocephalic vein (*RBV*) as it crosses the mediastinum. The left brachiocephalic vein is an important landmark, dividing the mediastinum into pre- and retrovascular compartments. *Tr*, trachea; *LSA*, left subclavian artery; *LCCA*, left common carotid artery; *BA*, brachiocephalic artery; *RSA*, right subclavian artery; *RCCA*, right common carotid artery; *E*, espohagus.

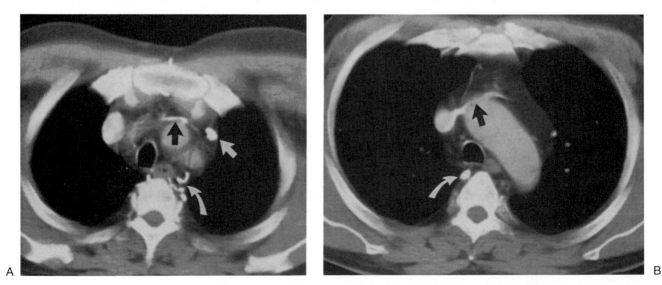

FIG. 8-94. Obstruction, braciocephalic vein. **A,B:** Sequential images through the great vessels and the aortic arch, respectively, following a bolus of intravenous contrast media administered through a left-sided antecubital vein. The left brachiocephalic vein is markedly attenuated, the result of a previous indwelling venous catheter (*black arrows* in **A** and **B**). Note that there is bright opacification of both the azygos (*curved arrows* in **A** and **B**) and hemiazygos systems (*curved arrow* in **A**), including the left superior intercostal vein beginning at the left brachiocephalic vein (*straight white arrow*). The azygos and hemiazygos venous system serves as an important collateral pathway when there is obstruction either of the brachiocephalic veins or the vena cavae.

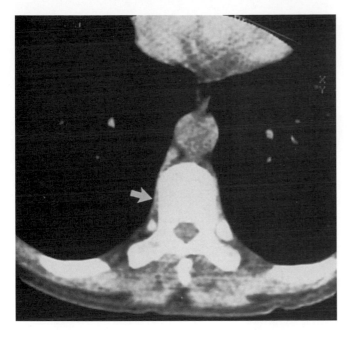

FIG. 8-95. Enlargement of a section through the lower thorax shows a normal-sized intercostal vein draining into the azygos vein (*arrow*).

of patients (261). The left superior intercostal vein forms a venous arch, sometimes referred to as the arch of the hemiazygos vein, that courses anteriorly around the aortic arch, near the level of T3-4, to join the left brachiocephalic vein superiorly (Fig. 8-99). The left superior intercostal vein is occasionally seen in normal subjects (see Fig. 8-91); it may opacify in some normals following contrast injection into the left arm. On routine radiographs, the left superior intercostal vein is most often seen end-on, adjacent to the aortic knob. Because of its appearance, it has been termed the "aortic nipple," and can be seen in up to 10% of normal patients (261). Prominence of the aortic nipple has been reported

secondary to congenital absence of the azygos vein (267) or more importantly, in presence of superior vena cava obstruction (267) (see Fig. 8-95, Fig. 8-100).

Small intrathoracic veins can sometimes be seen, even when unopacified. Intercostal veins are commonly visible in the paravertebral regions, in association with the azygos or hemiazygos veins. Internal mammary veins are also often visible, and in some patients can be traced from the point they communicate with the brachiocephalic veins, or on the right, the superior vena cava. Paraesophageal veins, veins in the paravertebral venous plexus, and chest wall veins occasionally opacify after contrast infusion, even in the ab-

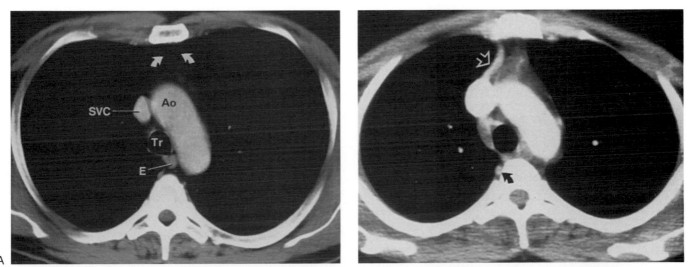

FIG. 8-96. A: CT section through the aortic arch (*Ao*), corresponding to level *A* in Fig. 8-92. At this level, the anterior mediastinum has a triangular configuration, with the apex pointing anteriorly (*arrows*). *SVC*, superior vena cava; *Tr*, trachea; *E*, esophagus. **B:** CT section at the level of the aortic arch shows a prominent right internal mammary vein draining into the superior vena cava (*open arrow*). This appearance should not be mistaken for residual thymic tissue. The *curved arrow* points to the right superior intercostal vein, which characteristically lies in a paravertebral location.

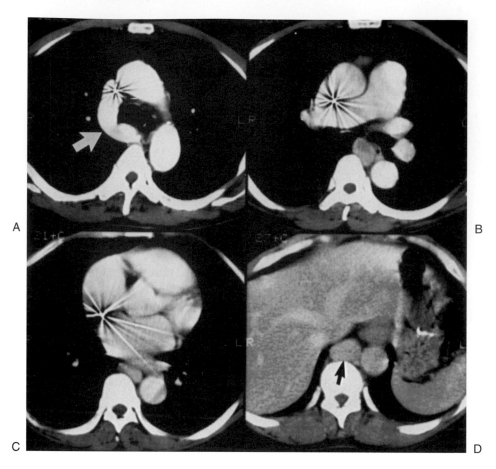

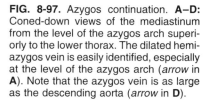

FIG. 8-97. Azygos continuation. **A–D:** Coned-down views of the mediastinum from the level of the azygos arch superiorly to the lower thorax. The dilated hemiazygos vein is easily identified, especially at the level of the azygos arch (*arrow* in **A**). Note that the azygos vein is as large as the descending aorta (*arrow* in **D**).

sence of venous obstruction, but are not easily seen on unopacified scans.

Intrathoracic veins, other that the superior vena cava and brachiocephalic veins commonly enlarge in the presence of venous obstruction, serving as important collateral pathways. Four major collateral pathways between the superior and inferior vena cava have been identified and described (263), including the (a) azygos and hemiazygos veins, (b) the vertebral venous plexus, (c) the internal mammary veins, and (d) the lateral thoracic veins in the thoracic and abdominal walls. Opacification of these veins following peripheral contrast infusion suggests venous obstruction, but can also be seen in normals. In a CT study by Kim et al. (269) of patients with intrathoracic venous obstruction, the presence of opacified venous collaterals was 96% sensitive and 92% specific for the diagnosis of symptomatic superior vena cava syndrome; the most common collateral veins to opacify were parascapular (71%), vertebral (58%), lateral thoracic (50%), internal mammary (38%), right superior intercostal (38%), azygos and hemiazygos (29%), anterior cervical (25%), and left superior intercostal (21%) (269). Periesophageal and intercostal vein opacification can also be seen, but is less common (263). In 5% to 10% of normals, some opacification of collateral veins can be expected on CT following peripheral contrast injection, but in recent studies, opacification of one or two veins has been reported in as many as 34% of normal

FIG. 8-98. Reflux of contrast agent into the azygos arch (*arrows*) following intravenous contrast infusion. This is occasionaly seen in normals.

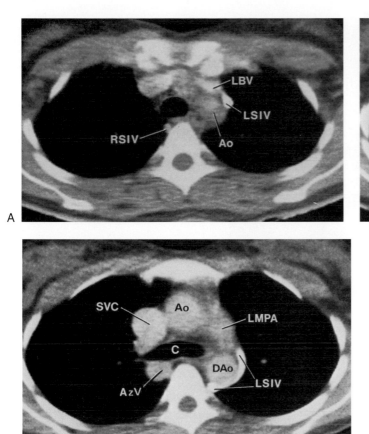

A

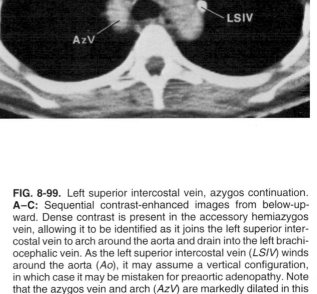

B

C

FIG. 8-99. Left superior intercostal vein, azygos continuation. A–C: Sequential contrast-enhanced images from below-upward. Dense contrast is present in the accessory hemiazygos vein, allowing it to be identified as it joins the left superior intercostal vein to arch around the aorta and drain into the left brachiocephalic vein. As the left superior intercostal vein (LSIV) winds around the aorta (Ao), it may assume a vertical configuration, in which case it may be mistaken for preaortic adenopathy. Note that the azygos vein and arch (AzV) are markedly dilated in this patient, with azygos continuation of the inferior vena cava. SVC, superior vena cava; LMPA, left main pulmonary artery; DAo, descending aorta; C, carina; LBV, left brachiocephalic vein; RSIV, right superior intercostal vein.

subjects (270). Three (6%) of 50 normal subjects studied by Kim et al. (269) showed opacification of parascapular chest wall veins or veins in the vertebral venous plexus following contrast infusion. In general, opacification of collateral veins should be considered normal unless associated with significant dilatation or other evidence of obstruction of the superior vena cava or brachiocephalic veins.

Dilatation of the azygos and hemiazygos veins is classically associated with anomalies of the inferior vena cava (Fig. 8-101), although idiopathic aneurysms have been reported (24–29). When there is developmental failure of the hepatic or infrahepatic (prenatal) segment of the inferior vena cava, blood returns to the heart via the cranial portion of the supracardinal veins (i.e., the azygos and hemiazygos veins). This anomaly has been reported in up to 2% of cases in patients with congenital heart disease undergoing cardiac catheterization. The association between azygos continuation and the asplenia and polysplenia syndromes has been well-documented. Azygos continuation may also be present in otherwise asymptomatic patients, and in this setting may be misinterpreted as some other form of pathology, specifically, a right paratracheal mass, a posterior mediastinal mass (if the dilated azygos or hemiazygos vein is identified along the paravertebral pleural reflections), or a retrocrural mass or adenopathy.

The appearance of azygos continuation is easily defined on CT by the following constellation of findings: enlargement of the arch of the azygos, enlargement of the paraspinal portions of the azygos and hemiazygos veins (especially if confluent at higher sections with the azygos arch), and enlargement of the retrocrural portions of these same veins in the absence of a definable inferior vena cava. It should be noted that once an abnormality of the inferior vena cava is diagnosed, careful examination of the abdomen should be performed to further define and clarify its specific nature.

In addition to congenital (and acquired) abnormalities of the azygos-hemiazygos venous system, the most common, clinically significant venous anomaly is persistence of the left superior vena cava. The left superior vena cava forms from a confluence of the left sublavian and left jugular veins and courses inferiorly in a position analogous to the normal superior vena cava on the right side (Figs. 8-102 and 8-103). Inferiorly, the left superior vena cava lies anterior to the left hilum and always drains into a markedly dilated coronary sinus. The anatomic course of the left superior vena cava reflects embryologic retention of the left anterior and common cardinal veins and the left horn of the sinus venosus, structures that ordinarily regress. A right superior vena cava may or may not be present. The clinical significance of this anomaly is minimal unless there is an associated atrial septal defect, with a resultant left-to-right shunt.

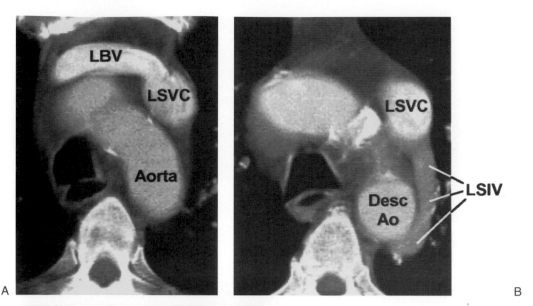

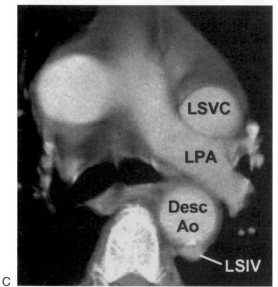

FIG. 8-100. Dilated left superior intercostal vein forming a hemiazygos arch in a patient with a left superior vena cava. **A:** The most cephalad scan shows the left brachiocephalic vein (*LBV*) and left superior vena cava (*LSVC*). These opacified after contrast infusion into the right arm. There is no evidence of a right superior vena cava. **B:** At the level of the proximal descending aorta (*Desc Ao*), the left superior intercostal vein (*LSIV*) is easily seen passing lateral to the aorta. The azygos arch is absent. **C:** At the level of the left pulmonary artery (*LPA*), the posterior portion of the left superior intercostal vein (*LSIV*) is visible posterior to the descending aorta. In this patient, the left superior intercostal vein is serving the same function as the azygos arch in a normal patient.

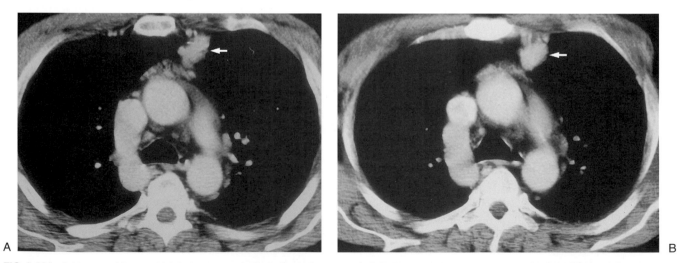

FIG. 8-101. A 32-year-old man with inferior vena cava thrombosis (not shown). **A,B:** Sequential contrast-enhanced helical CT scans demonstrate a massive azygos arch and the presence of a giant varix of the left internal mammary vein (*arrows*).

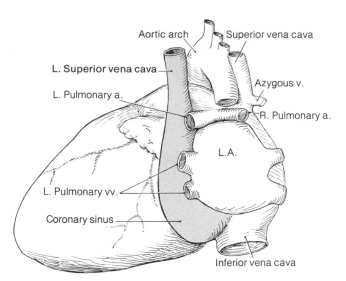

FIG. 8-102. Schematic drawing of a persistent left-sided superior vena cava, posterior view. The left-sided cava passes in front of the left hilum to drain inferiorly into an enlarged coronary sinus. *LA,* left atrium.

Acquired Venous Abnormalities

Venous obstruction, caused by extrinsic processes, is easily detected with both CT and MR (271,272). Most often there is direct visualization of the cause of obstruction. SVC obstruction most often results from bronchogenic carcinoma. Less frequently, obstruction results from either primary me-

diastinal tumors, including lymphoma, thymoma, or seminoma, or from metastatic disease, especially breast cancer. Rarely, venous obstruction results from primary vascular neoplasms, in particular angiosarcomas (Figs. 8-104 and 8-105). On occasion, the diagnosis of superior vena cava thrombosis actually may precede the diagnosis of lung cancer (Fig. 8-106). Other rare causes of venous obstruction include homocystinuria, which results in diffuse arterial and venous calcifications (Fig. 8-107).

Indirect signs of superior vena cava obstruction such as collateral circulation in the veins of the chest wall or azygos vein also are useful. However, it should be emphasized that venous enlargement alone should not be relied on as a sign of obstruction because it is dependent on the respiratory cycle or a Valsalva maneuver and sometimes represents a normal variant.

Intrinsic obstruction, caused by thrombosis, is becoming more common owing to the increasing use of central venous catheters, larger bore catheters for hyperalimentation, and the increasing number of procedures involving passage of tubes into the upper body veins. These include Swan-Ganz catheterization, pacemaker placement, dialysis catheters and more recently, peripherally inserted central lines.

The classic CT signs of venous thrombosis are: (a) enlargement of the vein, (b) a relatively lucent center, and (c) enhancing vein wall on contrast-enhanced studies. If the thrombus itself enhances it may be neoplastic in origin. Caution should be exercised so that venous thrombosis is not diagnosed on scans obtained during or immediately after a

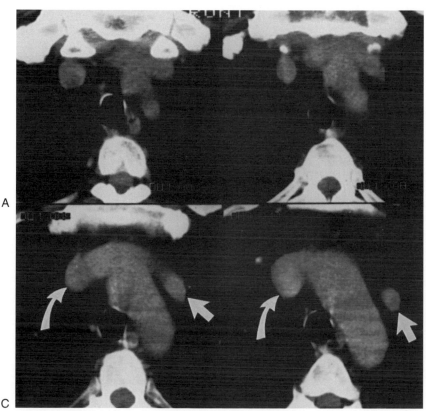

FIG. 8-103. Left-sided superior vena cava. **A–D:** Enlargements of sequential CT images from the great vessels superiorly to the aortic arch inferiorly, respectively. In addition to a left-sided vena cava (*arrows* in **C** and **D**), there is persistence of a right-sided vena cava.

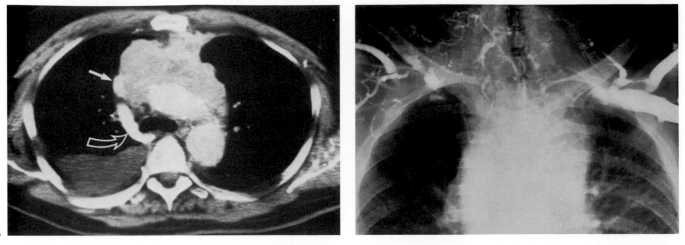

FIG. 8-104. Superior vena caval obstruction: thymic carcinoid. **A:** Contrast-enhanced CT section at the level of the carina shows a bulky, somewhat heterogeneous soft-tissue mass within the prevascular space obliterating the left brachiocephalic vein and invading the superior vena cava (*arrow*). There is dense opacification of the azygos vein (*curved arrow*) serving as a collateral. **B:** Coned-down view from simultaneous bilateral antecubital fossa venous injections shows complete obstruction of the brachiocephalic veins bilaterally. At surgery this proved to be a primary thymic carcinoid.

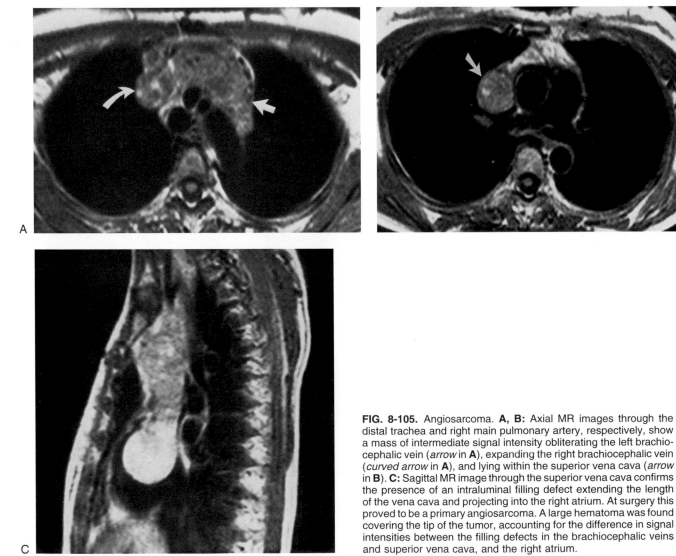

FIG. 8-105. Angiosarcoma. **A, B:** Axial MR images through the distal trachea and right main pulmonary artery, respectively, show a mass of intermediate signal intensity obliterating the left brachiocephalic vein (*arrow* in **A**), expanding the right brachiocephalic vein (*curved arrow* in **A**), and lying within the superior vena cava (*arrow* in **B**). **C:** Sagittal MR image through the superior vena cava confirms the presence of an intraluminal filling defect extending the length of the vena cava and projecting into the right atrium. At surgery this proved to be a primary angiosarcoma. A large hematoma was found covering the tip of the tumor, accounting for the difference in signal intensities between the filling defects in the brachiocephalic veins and superior vena cava, and the right atrium.

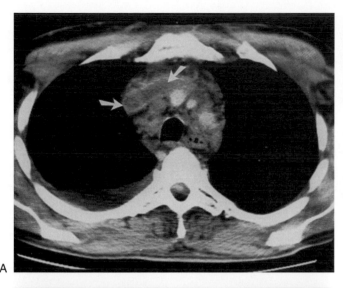

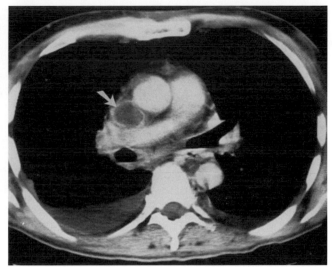

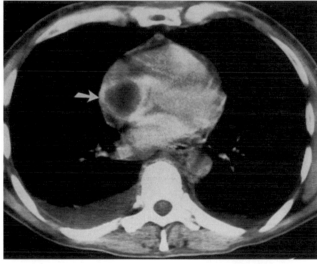

FIG. 8-106. Superior vena caval thrombosis, metastatic lung cancer. **A–C:** Sequential contrast-enhanced CT sections through the left brachiocephalic vein, the superior vena cava, and the right atrium, respectively. A well-defined filling defect is apparent (*arrows* in **A–C**) extending from the left brachiocephalic vein to the right atrium. There is considerable nodularity within the mediastinal fat, especially at the level of the great vessels. These were initially thought to represent dilated collateral mediastinal veins. Subsequent mediastinoscopy disclosed these to be metastatic lymph nodes consistent with a primary lung cancer.

bolus injection of contrast agent, since flow phenomena may mimic filling defects in mediastinal veins. This may be especially problematic in the superior vena cava adjacent to the azygos arch, as densely enhanced superior vena cava blood draining the injection mixes with unenhanced azygos blood returning from the lower body.

A peculiar abdominal manifestation of superior vena cava occlusion is the presence of a wedge-shaped region of increased density within the anterior aspect of the left lobe of the liver (273–275) (Fig. 8-108). This likely occurs because of the development of systemic-portal collaterals likely from the internal thoracic vein and the paraumbilical vein (276). Other findings on abdominal CT examinations when a central chest vein is obstructed include the presence of dense enhancement in azygos, hemiazygos, intercostal, epigastric, subcutaneous and intramuscular veins (275).

Involvement of the IVC from either thrombus or neoplasm is evaluated in a similar fashion (277). An anatomic variant, which can be mistaken for an intracaval mass, is the presence of prominent pericaval fat (278,279) (Fig. 8-109). This is

seen more frequently in patients with cirrhosis and is best evaluated using coronal reformations.

MR Venography

Technical Considerations

Recent improvements in MR technology not only have led to the need to seriously reconsider the role of MR for routine aortic imaging, but for routine imaging of intrathoracic venous structures, as well. Presently, 2D TOF venography is increasingly used for the evaluation of the thoracic and upper extremity veins (Fig. 8-110). Arterial signal is readily eliminated with a traveling presaturation pulse. In order to optimize image quality and to minimize in-plane saturation effects the slice orientation should be perpendicular to the vessel of interest. The subclavian vein runs in a horizontal direction and is best imaged with a sagittally oriented scan to maximize inflow of unsaturated blood. Similarly, the jugular veins and SVC runs in a near vertical course and are optimally imaged with axial slices. The brachioceph-

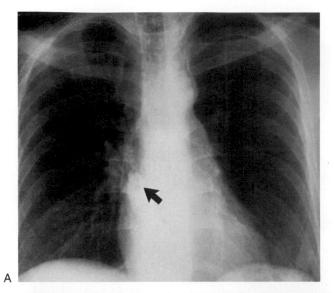

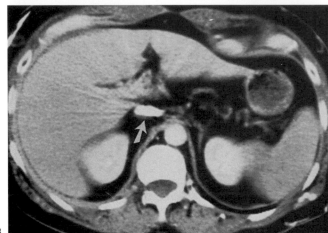

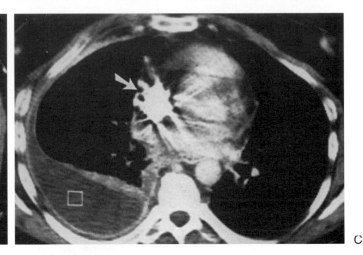

FIG. 8-107. Homocystinuria. **A:** Posteroanterior chest radiograph shows dense calcifications overlying the medial aspect of the right hilum, inferiorly (*arrow*). **B:** Contrast-enhanced CT section through the upper abdomen shows dense calcification with resultant obliteration of the inferior vena cava (*arrow*). Despite this, no obvious enlarged collateral veins are appreciated. **C:** Contrast-enhanced CT section through the aortic root shows dense calcification within the superior vena cava, causing streak artifacts (*arrow*). A moderate-sized right pleural fluid collection is present. This patient had documented homocystinuria.

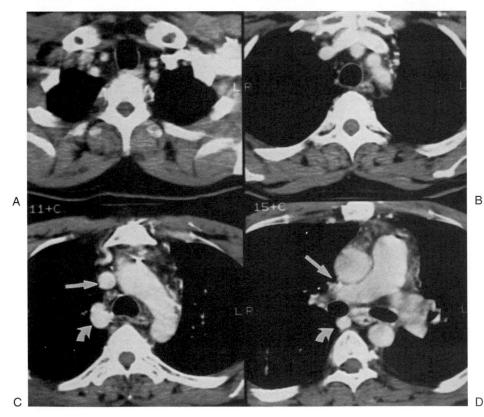

FIG. 8-108. Superior vena caval ligation. **A–D:** Sequential contrast-enhanced scans through the mediastinum from the great vessels to the subcarinal space, respectively. The superior vena cava (*arrow* in **C**) had been surgically ligated just below the aortic arch (*arrow* in **D**). There is marked enlargement of the azygos vein (*curved arrows* in **C** and **D**) as well as enlargement of numerous small mediastinal veins, especially in the prevascular space anteriorly. **E, F:** Sequential images through the liver in the same patient as shown in **A–D** are shown. There is marked contrast enhancement of the azygos and hemiazygos veins. In addition, there is dense opacification of the inferior vena cava (*open arrows*), which is presumable filling through retrograde flow through intercostal and phrenic veins (*arrows* in **E** and **F**). Finally, there is an area of density in the anterior portion of the liver (*curved arrow*), probably the result of focal systemic-portal collaterals.

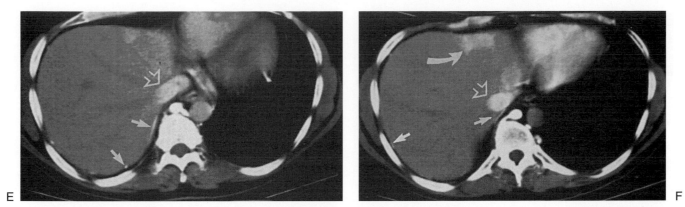

FIG. 8-108. *Continued.*

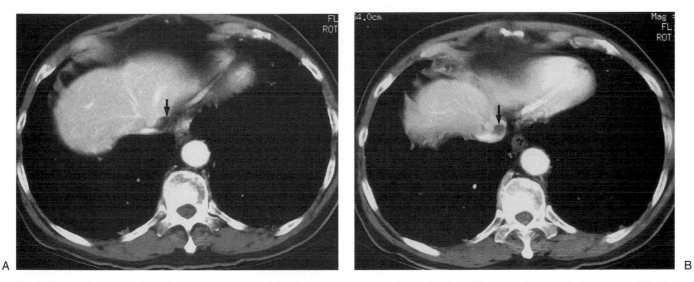

FIG. 8-109. Pericaval fat mimicking intracaval mass. **A,B:** Sequential contrast-enhanced helical CT scans at the level of the dome of the liver demonstrates pericaval fat (*arrows*) that appears to be within the inferior vena cava. This is quite common and is best demonstrated as pericaval with coronal reformations.

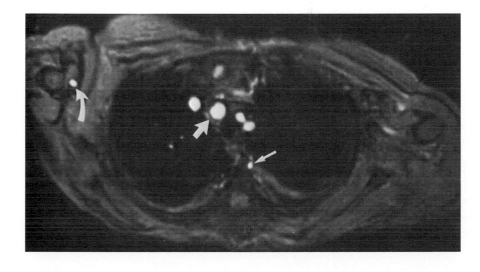

FIG. 8-110. Mediastinal MR imaging. Section through the great vessels using gradient-recalled echoes (TR = 25 msec, TE = 13 msec, flip angle = 20 degrees). In these images, flowing blood results in considerable signal within vessels, not only in the mediastinum (*straight arrows*) but in the chest wall as well (*curved arrow* at right). *TR*, repetition time; *TE*, echo time.

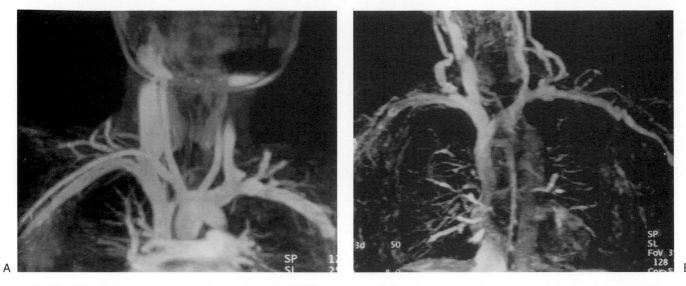

FIG. 8-111. Normal gadolinium-enhanced three-dimensional MR venogram. **A:** Breath-hold coronal source image from gadolinium-enhanced three-dimensional MR venogram obtained 40 seconds after the injection of 40 mL of gadolinium demonstrates both arteries and veins. The initial arterial phase examination is not shown. **B:** Coronal source image from later acquisition demonstrates mostly venous enhancement.

alic veins run in an oblique course and is more difficult to image for these anatomic reasons.

A slice thickness of 3 to 4 mm should be adequate and either the body or body phased-array coil can be used. Breath holding is useful for evaluation of the proximal thoracic veins as it eliminates respiratory artifacts that degrade the MIP images.

Because the venous structures that form the SVC are oriented in different planes and may have varying velocities and flow patterns, TOF imaging may be suboptimal in evaluating the entire thoracic venous system. Flow artifacts at branch points and in-plane saturation effects may result in suboptimal image quality with artifactual signal loss that can mimic thrombus. Finally, 2D TOF is unable to visualize collapsed veins with little or no flow.

As an alternative approach, excellent opacification of the venous system is attainable (without bothersome flow artifacts or saturation effects) by using intravenously administered gadolinium chelates in conjunction with 3D gradient-echo pulse sequences (280). As previously described with arterial imaging this technique obviates the need for flow-related-enhancement as image quality simply depends on the shortened T1-relaxation time of gadolinium-enhanced venous blood. In contrast to first pass arterial imaging, longer scan delay time is needed to evaluate the great veins. Because this is a recirculation technique (peripheral vein-aorta-central vein) a dose of 0.2 mmol/kg of gadolinium is required. These 3D venograms may contain both arterial and venous signal. A selective venogram can be generated using a subtraction technique, in which an arterial phase image is subtracted from a mixed venous-arterial image. These 3D data sets provide for high quality multiplanar reformations that can demonstrate long segment thrombosis with a single image. An additional benefit of gadolinium-enhanced techniques is that in the setting of acute or subacute deep venous

thrombosis periadvential venous enhancement may be present. This can further increase diagnostic confidence in difficult cases.

When performing dynamic gadolinium-enhanced 3D-GRE studies, several acquisitions may be acquired sequentially. The initial acquisition is timed with the gadolinium's first pass through the arterial system, but prior to substantial venous enhancement. A second acquisition is acquired immediately following the arterial phase; this phase usually has both arterial and venous enhancement (Fig. 8-111). The subtraction technique requires special software, which performs a pixel-by-pixel subtraction of the arterial-phase study from a mixed venous-arterial phase study. The arterial signal is nullified, whereas the subtracted data set contains only venous signal (280).

Recently, a new MR venography technique, similar to conventional venography, has been advocated. This requires the injection of dilute gadolinium (3 mL of gadolinium in 57 mL of saline) into the extremity of interest, while performing multiple, dynamic 3D gradient-echo sequences (281). Limitations of this technique include potentially difficult intravenous access in the extremity ipsilateral to the expected abnormality and only a single unilateral drainage system is typically assessed. Finally, nonvisualization of the deep venous system may occur without inherent pathology in these vessels.

Clinical Applications

As in the lower extremities, conventional contrast venography is limited in the chest and upper extremities. Patients may have limited or no venous access, veins may be obscured by adjacent masses, and high flow in the SVC may make adequate opacification difficult. Sonography is limited by poor acoustical access from the chest wall and air-filled lungs. Because of these limitations MR venography is a useful modality that eliminates the need for other imaging studies (282).

Finn et al. evaluated 30 patients with suspected thoracic venous occlusion and found MR imaging provided more comprehensive information on central venous anatomy and blood flow than catheter venography (283). MR venography also provided useful clinical information in patients without venous access.

MR venography is often useful when attempting to assess complex venous anatomy in postoperative patients or in patients with congenital anomalies. MR venography can also assist in determining suitable sites for venous access. Hartnell et al. evaluated 84 patients using breath-hold TOF MR in order to identify sites for central venous access or to diagnose and stage central venous occlusion (282). Although MRA predicted a patent site for central venous access in 28 of 28 patients, contrast venography did not show all patent veins. The authors concluded that both patent and occluded chest veins are reliably defined with MRA, including potential sites for central line placement, in a way that is not possible with other techniques and proposed that MRA may be the new "gold standard" for defining systemic venous anatomy in the chest (282).

Rose et al. also used 2D TOF MR venography to assess central vein status (284). MR angiography had 97% sensitivity and 94% specificity for detection of occlusion, and accurately predicted 100% of successful central venous catheter placements and 80% of failures and influenced therapy in 19 of 21 studies (284). However, the authors did note that interpretation of MR venograms may be difficult in patients with extensive occlusions because of complex collateral drainage patterns.

Evaluation of the subclavian and upper extremity veins with MR venography has also demonstrated good results (285–287) (Fig. 8-112). Initially, Haire et al. had a high number of false negative studies in patients with partial subclavian obstruction (285). Hansen et al. had better results, reporting 83% sensitivity and 100% specificity (286). They had two false negatives, both associated with indwelling central venous catheters.

Neoplastic involvement of the IVC from intraabdominal malignancies usually occurs from hepatocellular carcinoma, renal cell carcinoma (Fig. 8-113), adrenal cortical carcinoma (Fig. 8-114), retroperitoneal neoplasms and endometrial carcinoma. Less commonly, primary sarcomas may arise from the wall of the IVC. Using 2D TOF MR venography, demonstration of thrombus within the IVC is readily achieved but tumor thrombus may not be distinguished from bland thrombus (288). The ability to differentiate bland thrombus from tumor thrombus is predicated on the notion that tumor thrombus will enhance after the administration of gadolinium owing to tumor angiogenesis, whereas bland thrombus will not. This is best demonstrated using breath-hold gadolinium-enhanced 3D MR imaging acquired in the coronal plane. When the precontrast image is subtracted from a delayed postcontrast acquisition, enhancement of tumor thrombus is more easily visualized (see Fig. 8-114).

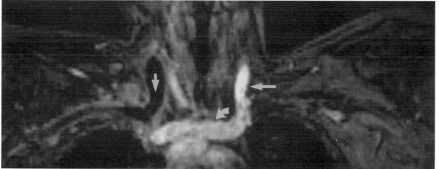

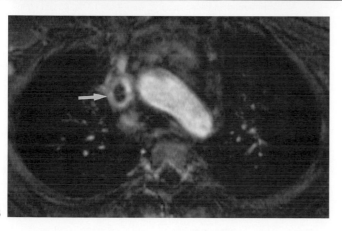

FIG. 8-112. Extensive catheter induced venous thrombosis. **A:** Coronal reformation from axial gadolinium-enhanced three-dimensional MR venogram obtained 40 seconds after the injection of 40 mL of gadolinium demonstrates low signal intensity thrombus within the right jugular vein (*short arrow*) and the right axillary and subclavian vein. Note the extensive periadventitial enhancement. The left jugular (*long arrow*) and left brachiocephalic (*curved arrow*) are normal. **B:** Axial source image at the level of the aortic arch, from same acquisition, demonstrates low signal intensity thrombus within the superior vena cava (*arrow*).

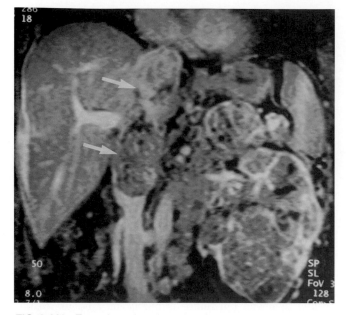

FIG. 8-113. Extensive enhancing tumor thrombus in the inferior vena cava from renal cell carcinoma-MR demonstration. Coronal source image from venous phase of gadolinium-enhanced three-dimensional MR venogram demonstrates enhancing tumor thrombus (*arrows*) expanding the inferior vena cava.

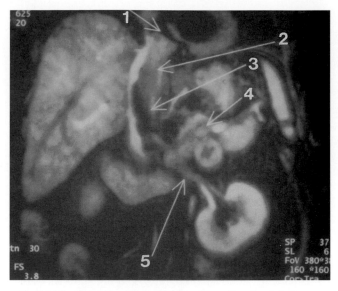

FIG. 8-114. Adrenal cortical carcinoma invading the inferior vena cava and right atrium-morphologic findings and descrimination between tumor and bland thrombus based on enhancement with gadolinium-subtracted coronal image (venous phase-precontrast acquisition), demonstrates a large thrombus in the inferior vena cava (*arrows 2 and 3*) and right atrium (*arrow 1*). Note the differentiation between the enhancing tunor thrombus superiorly (*arrow 2*) and the nonenhancing bland thrombus just inferior to it (*arrow 3*). The neoplasm is depicted in *arrow 4* and the left renal vein is *arrow 5*.

REFERENCES

1. Nienaber CA, von Kodolitsch Y, Nicholas V. The diagnosis of thoracic aortic dissection by noninvasive imaging procedures. *N Engl J Med* 1993;328:1–9.
2. Sommer T, Fehske W, Holzknecht N, et al. Aortic dissection: a comparative study of diagnosis with spiral CT, multiplanar transesophageal echocardiography, and MR imaging. *Radiology* 1996;199: 347–352.
3. Adachi H, Omoto R, Kyo S, et al. Emergency surgical intervention of the acute aortic dissection with the rapid diagnosis by transesophageal echocardiography. *Circulation* 1991;84:14–19.
4. Erbel R, Engberding R, Daniel W, et al. Echocardiography in diagnosis of aortic dissection. *Lancet* 1989;1:457–461.
5. Prince MR, Narasimham DL, Jacoby WT, et al. Three-dimensional gadolinium-enhanced MR angiography of the thoracic aorta. *Am J Roentgenol* 1996;166:1387–1397.
6. Brink JA, Mcfarland EG, Heiken JP. Helical/spiral computed body tomography. *Clin Radiol* 1997;52:489–503.
7. Rubin GD, Dake MD, Semba CP. Current status of three-dimensional spiral CT scanning for imaging the vasculature. *Radiol Clin North Am* 1995;33:51–70.
8. Costello P. Spiral CT of the thoracic aorta and its branches. In: Remy-Jardin M, Remy J, eds. *Spiral CT of the thorax*. Frankfurt: Springer-Verlag, 1996;283–305.
9. Costello P, Naidich DP. Protocols for helical CT of the chest. In: Silverman PM, ed. *Helical (spiral) computed tomography*. Philadelphia: Lippincott-Raven, 1998;65–101.
10. Fishman EK. High-resolution three-dimensional imaging from subsecond helical CT data sets: applications in vascular imaging. *Am J Roentgenol* 1997;169:441–443.
11. Costello P, Dupuy DE, Ecker CP, Tello R. Spiral CT of the thorax with reduced volume of contrast material: a comparative study. *Radiology* 1992;183:663–666.
12. Hopper KD, Mosher TJ, Kasales CJ, et al. Thoracic spiral CT: delivery of contrast material pushed with injectable saline solution in a power injector. *Radiology* 1997;205:269–271.
13. Rubin GD, Lane MJ, Bloch DA, Leung AN, Stark P. Optimization of thoracic spiral CT: effects of iodinated contrast medium concentration. *Radiology* 1996;201:785–791.
14. Schnyder P, Meuli R, Wicky S. Injection techniques. In: Remy-Jardin M, Remy J, eds. *Spiral CT of the chest*. Berlin: Springer, 1996: 41–57.
15. Storto ML, Ciccotosto C, Patea RL, Spinazzi A, Bonomo L. Spiral CT of the mediastinum: optimization of contrast medium use. *Eur J Radiol* 1994;18(Suppl.):S83–S87.
16. Rubin GD. Helical CT angiography of the thoracic aorta. *J Thorac Imag* 1997;12:128–149.
17. Dillon EH, van Leeuwen MS, Fernandez MA, Mali WPTM. Spiral CT angiography. Pictorial essay. *AJR Am J Roentgenol* 1993;160: 1273–1278.
18. Chung JW, Park JH, Im J-G, et al. Spiral CT angiography of the thoracic aorta. *RadiogGraphics* 1996;16:811–824.
19. Stehling MK, Lawrence JA, Weintraub JL, Raptopoulos V. CT angiography: expanded clinical applications. *AJR Am J Roentgenol* 1994; 163:947–955.
20. Stockberger SM, Hicklin JA, Liang Y, Wass JL, Ambrosius WT. Spiral CT with ionic and nonionic contrast material: evaluation of patient motion and scan quality. *Radiology* 1998;206:631–636.
21. Stockberger SM, Liang Y, Kicklin JA, et al. Objective measurements of motion in patients undergoing spiral CT examinations. *Radiology* 1998;206:625–629.
22. Vanhoe L, Marchal G, Baert AL, Gryspeerdt S, Mertens L. Determination of scan delay time in spiral CT-angiography: Utility of a test bolus injection. *J Comput Assist Tomogr* 1995;19:216–220.
23. Silverman P, Roberts S, Tiffl MC, Brown B, Fox SH. Helical CT of the liver: clinical application of a computer automated scanning technique—Smartprep—for obtaining images with optimal contrast enhancement. *AJR Am J Roentgenol* 1995;165:73–78.
24. Amparo EG, Higgins CB, Hricak H, et al. Aortic dissection: magnetic resonance imaging. *Radiology* 1985;155:399–406.
25. Akins EW, Carmichael MJ, Hill JA, et al. Preoperative evaluation of the thoracic aorta using MRI and angiography. *Ann Thorac Surg* 1987; 44:499–507.
26. Kersting-Sommerhoff BA, Higgins CB, White RD, Sommerhoff CP, Lipton MJ. Aortic dissection: sensitivity and specificity of MR imaging. *Radiology* 1988;166:651–655.

27. Dinsmore RE, Liberthson RR, Wismer GL. Magnetic resonance imaging of thoracic aortic aneurysm: comparison with other imaging methods. *AJR Am J Roentgenol* 1986;146:309–314.

28. Fruhwald FXJ, Neuhold A, Fezoulidis J. Cine-MR in dissection of the thoracic aorta. *Eur J Radiol* 1989;9:37–41.

29. Atkinson DJ, Edelman RR. Cine angiography of the heart in a single breath-hold with a segmented turbo-FLASH sequence. *Radiology* 1991;178:357–360.

30. Hartnell GG, Finn JP, Zenni M, et al. MR imaging of the thoracic aorta: comparison of spin-echo, angiographic and breath-hold techniques. *Radiology* 1994;191:697–704.

31. Seelos KC, Funari M, Higgins CB. Detection of aortic arch thrombus using MR imaging. *J Comput Assist Tomogr* 1991;15:244–247.

32. Sakuma H, Bourne MW, O'Sullivan M, et al. Evaluation of thoracic aortic dissection using breath-holding cine MRI. *J Comput Assist Tomogr* 1996;20:45–50.

33. Sonnabend SB, Coletti PM, Pentecost M. Demonstration of aortic lesions via cine magnetic resonance imaging. *Magn Reson Imaging* 1990;8:613–618.

34. White RD, Obuchowski NA, VanDyke CW, et al. Thoracic aortic disease: evaluation using a single MRA volume series. *J Comput Assist Tomogr* 1994;18:843–854.

35. Revel D, Loubeyre P, Delignette A, et al. Contrast-enhanced magnetic resonance tomoangiography: a new imaging technique for studying thoracic great vessels. *Magn Reson Imaging* 1993;11:1101–1105.

36. Fischer U, Vosshenrich R, Kopka L, et al. Dissection of the thoracic aorta: pre-and postoperative findings on Turbo-FLASH MR images obtained in the plane of the aortic arch. *AJR Am J Roentgenol* 1994;163:1069–1072.

37. Summer RM, Sostman HD, Spritzeer CE, et al. Fast spoiled gradient-recalled MR imaging of thoracic aortic dissection: preliminary clinical experience at 1.5 T. *Magn Reson Imaging* 1996;14:1–9.

38. Gaubert JY, Moulin G, Mesana T, et al. Type A dissection of the thoracic aorta: use of MR imaging for long-term follow-up. *Radiology* 1995;196:363–369.

39. Krinsky GA, Rofsky NM, Decorato DR, et al. Thoracic aorta: Comparison of gadolinium-enhanced three-dimensional MR angiography with conventional MR imaging. *Radiology* 1997;202:183–193.

40. Krinsky G, Rofsky N, Flyer M, et al. Gadolinium-enhanced three-dimensional MR angiography of acquired arch vessel disease. *AJR Am J Roentgenol* 1996;167:981–987.

41. Leung DA, Mckinnon GC, Davis CP, et al. Breath-hold, contrast-enhanced, three-dimensional MR angiography. *Radiology* 1996;200:569–571.

42. Prince MR. Gadolinium-enhanced MR aortography. *Radiology* 1994;191:155–164.

43. Prince MR, Narasimham DL, Stanley JC, et al. Breath-hold gadolinium-enhanced MR angiography of abdominal aorta and its major branches. *Radiology* 1995;197:785–792.

44. Levy R, Prince M. Arterial-phase three-dimensional contrast-enhanced MR angiography of the carotid arteries. *AJR Am J Roentgenol* 1996;167:211–215.

45. Krinsky G, Maya M, Rofsky N, et al. Gadolinium-enhanced 3D MRA of the aortic arch vessels in the detection of atherosclerotic cerebrovascular occlusive disease. *J Comput Assist Tomogr* 1998;22:167–178.

46. Earls J, Rofsky N, DeCorato D, Krinsky G, Weinreb J. Breath-hold single-dose gadolinium-enhanced MR aortography: usefulness of a timing examination and MR power injector. *Radiology* 1996;201:705–710.

47. Wilman A, Riederer S, King B, et al. Fluoroscopically triggered contrast-enhanced three-dimensional MR angiography with elliptical centric view order: application to the renal arteries. *Radiology* 1997;205:137–146.

48. Prince MR, Chenevert TL, Foo TK, et al. Contrast-enhanced abdominal MR angiography: Optimization of imaging delay time by automating the detection of contrast material arrival in the aorta. *Radiology* 1997;203:109–114.

49. Korosec F, Frayne R, Grist T, Mistretta C. Time-resolved contrast-enhanced 3D MR angiography. *Magn Reson Med* 1996;36:345–351.

50. Hennig J, Scheffler K, Laubenberger J, Strecker R. Time-resolved projection angiography after bolus injection of contrast agent. *Magn Reson Med* 1997;37:341–345.

51. Lee VS, Flyer MA, Weinreb JC, Krinsky GA, Rofsky NM. Image subtraction in gadolinium-enhanced MR imaging. *AJR Am J Roentgenol* 1996;167:1427–1432.

52. Vrachliotis TG, Bis KG, Aliabadi D, et al. Contrast-enhanced breath-hold MR angiography for evaluating patency of coronary artery bypass grafts. *AJR Am J Roentgenol* 1997;168:1073–1080.

53. Simonetti OP, Finn JP, White RD, Laub G, Henry DA. "Black blood" T2-weighted inversion-recovery MR imaging of the heart. *Radiology* 1996;199:49–57.

54. Mohiaddin RH, Kilner PJ, Rees S, et al. Magnetic resonance volume flow and jet velocity mapping in aortic coarctation. *J Am Coll Cardiol* 1993;22:1515–1521.

55. Naidich DP, Berman P. CT angiography of the thorax. In: RSNA categorical course in vascular imaging. RSNA Publications, 1998 (in press).

56. Johnson PT, Heath DG, Kuszyk BS, Fishman EK. CT angiography thoracic vascular imaging with interactive volume rendering technique. Pictorial essay. *J Comput Assist Tomogr* 1997;21:110–114.

57. Napel S, Marks MP, Rubin GD, et al. CT angiography with spiral CT and maximum intensity projection. *Radiology* 1992;185:607–610.

58. Prokop M, Shin HO, Schanz A, Schaeferprokop CM. Use of maximum intensity projections in CT angiography: a basic review. *RadioGraphics* 1997;17:433–451.

59. Fishman EK, Magid D, Ney DR, et al. Three-dimensional imaging. *Radiology* 1991;181:321–337.

60. Smith PA, Heath DG, Fishan EK. Virtual angioscopy using spiral CT and real-time interactive colume-rendering techniques. *J Comput Assist Tomogr* 1998;22:212–214.

61. Johnson PT, Fishman EK, Duckwall JR, Calhoun PS, Heath DG. Interactive three-dimensional volume rendering of spiral CT data: current applications in the thorax. *RadioGraphics* 1998;18:165–187.

62. Rubin GD, Beaulieu CF, Argiro V, et al. Perspective volume rendering of CT and MR images: applications for endoscopic imaging. *Radiology* 1996;199:321–330.

63. Davis CP, Ladd ME, Romanowski BJ, et al. Human aorta: preliminary results with virtual endoscopy based on three-dimensional MR imaging data sets. *Radiology* 1996;199:37–40.

64. Davis CP, Hany TF, Wildermuth S, Schmidt RT, Debatin JF. Postprocessing techniques for gadolinium-enhanced three-dimensional MR angiography. *RadioGraphics* 1997;17:1061–1067.

65. Hany TF, Schmidt M, Davis CP, Gohde SC, Debatin JF. Diagnostic impact of four postprocessing techniques in evaluating contrast-enhanced three-dimensional MR angiography. *AJR Am J Roentgenol* 1998;170:907–912.

66. White RD, Dooms GC, Higgins CB. Advances in imaging thoracic aortic disease. *Invest Radiol* 1986;21:761–778.

67. Goss CM. *Gray's anatomy*. Philadelphia: Lea & Febiger, 1996:579.

68. Aronberg DJ, Glazer HS, Madsen K, Sagel SS. Normal thoracic aortic diameters by computed tomography. *J Comput Assist Tomogr* 1984;8:247–250.

69. Fitzgerald AW, Donaldson JS, Poznanski AK. Pediatric thoracic aorta: normal measurements determined with CT. *Radiology* 1987;165:667–669.

70. Yamada T, Tada S, Harada J. Aortic dissection without intimal rupture: diagnosis with MR imaging and CT. *Radiology* 1988;168:347–352.

71. Park JH, Chung JW, Im JG, et al. Takayasu arteritis: Evaluation of mural changes in the aorta and pulmonary artery with CT angiography. *Radiology* 1995;196:89–93.

72. Tenenbaum A, Garniek A, Shemesh J, et al. Dual-helical CT for detecting aortic atheromas as a source of stroke: comparison with transesophageal echocardiography. *Radiology* 1998;208:153–158.

73. Bosniak MA. Analysis of some anatomic-Roentgenologic aspects of the brachiocephalic vessels. *AJR Am J Roentgenol* 1964;91:1222–1231.

74. Sutton D, Rhys Davies E. Arch aortography and cerebro vascular insufficiency. *Clin Radiol* 1966;17:330–345.

75. McLoughlin MJ, Weisbrod G, Wise DJ, Yeung HPH. Computed tomography in congenital anomalies of the aortic arch and great vessels. *Radiology* 1981;138:399–403.

76. Edwards J. Anomalies of derivatives of the aortic arch system. *Med Clin North Am* 1948;32:925–949.

77. Akers D, Fowl R, Plettner J, et al. Complications of anomalous origin of the right subclavian artery: case report and review of the literature. *Ann Vasc Surg* 1991;5:385–388.

78. Kieffer E, Bahnini A, Koskas F. Aberrant subclavian artery: Surgical treatment in thirty-three adult patients. *J Vasc Surg* 1994;19:100–111.

79. Shuford WH, Sybers RG, Weens HS. The angiographic features of double aortic arches. *AJR Am J Roentgenol* 1972;116:125–140.

80. Kennard DR, Spigos D, Tan WS. Cervical aortic arch: CT correlation with conventional radiologic studies. *AJR Am J Roentgenol* 1983;141:295–297.

81. Flamm SD, VanDyke CW, White RD, et al. MR imaging of the throacic aorta. *Magn Reson Imaging Clin North Am* 1996;4:217–235.

82. Bissett GSI, Strife JL, Kirks DR, Bailey WW. Vascular rings: MR imaging. *AJR Am J Roentgenol* 1987;149:251–256.

83. Gomes AS, Lois JF, George B, Alpan G, Williams RG. Congenital abnormalities of the aortic arch: MR imaging. *Radiology* 1987;165:691–695.

84. Kersting-Sommerhoff BA, Sechten UP, Fisher MR, Higgins CB. MR imaging of congenital anomalies of the aortic arch. *AJR Am J Roentgenol* 1987;149:9–13.

85. Azarow KS, Pearl RH, Hoffmann MA, et al. Vascular rings: does magnetic resonance imaging replace angiography? *Ann Thorac Surg* 1992;53:882–886.

86. Jaffe RB. Magnetic resonance imaging of vascular rings. *Semin Ultrasound CT MR* 1990;11:206.

87. Lam WW, Chan JHM, Hui Y, Chan FL. Non-breath-hold gadolinium-enhanced MR angiography of the thoracoabdominal aorta; experience in 18 children. *AJR Am J Roentgenol* 1998;170:478–480.

88. Krinsky G, Weinreb J. Gadolinium-enhanced three-dimensional MR angiography of the thoracoabdominal aorta. *Sem Ultrasound CT MR* 1996;17:280–303.

89. Webb WR, Gamsu G, Speckman JM, et al. CT demonstration of mediastinal aortic arch anomalies. *J Comput Assist Tomogr* 1982;6:445–51.

90. Katz M, Konen E, Rozenman J, Szeinberg A, Itzchak Y. Spiral CT and 3D image reconstruction of vascular rings and associated tracheobronchial anomalies. *J Comput Assist Tomogr* 1995;19:564–568.

91. Hopkins KL, Patrick LE, Simoneaux SF, et al. Pediatric great vessel anomalies: initial clinical experience with spiral CT angiography. *Radiology* 1996;200:811–815.

92. Bailey WW. Interrupted aortic arch. *Advances in Cardiac Surgery* 1994;5:97–114.

93. Celoria G, Patton R. Congenital absence of the aortic arch. *Am Heart J* 1959;58:407–412.

94. Hernandez RJ, Aisen AM, Foo TKF, Beekman RH. Thoracic cardiovascular anomalies in children: evaluation with a fast gradient-recalled-echo sequence with cardiac-triggered segmented acquisition. *Radiology* 1993;188:775–780.

95. Tawes RL, Berr CL. Congenital bicuspid aortic valves associated with coarctation of the aorta in children. *Br Heart J* 1969;31:127–128.

96. Hallett JW Jr, Brewster DC, Darling RC, O'Hara PJ. Coarctation of the abdominal aorta: current opinions in surgical management. *Ann Surg* 1980;191:430–437.

97. Merrill VM, Hoff SJ, Stewart JR, et al. Operative risk factors and durability of repair of coarctation of the aorta in the neonate. *Ann Thorac Surg* 1994;58:399–403.

98. Parks WJ, Ngo TD, Plauth WH Jr, et al. Incidence of aneurysm formation after dacron patch aortoplasty repair for coarctation of the aorta: long-term results and assessment utilizing magnetic resonance angiography with three-dimensional surface rendering. *J Am Coll Cardiol* 1995;26:266–271.

99. Soler R, Pombo F, Bargiela A, Gayol A, Rodriguez E. MRI of pseudocoarctation of the aorta: morphological and cine-MRI findings. *Comput Med Imaging Graph* 1995;19:431–434.

100. Gay WA, Young WG. Pseudocoarctation of the aorta, a reappraisal. *J Thorac Cardiovasc Surg* 1969;58:739–745.

101. Gaupp RJ, Fagan CJ, Davis M, Epstein ME. Case report. Pseudocoarctation of the aorta. *J Comput Assist Tomogr* 1981;5:571–573.

102. Von Schulthess GK, Higashino SM, Higgins CB, et al. Coarctation of the aorta: MR imaging. *Radiology* 1986;158:469–474.

103. Julsrud PR, Breen JF, Felmlee JP, et al. Coarctation of the aorta: collateral flow assessment with phase-contrast MR angiography. *AJR Am J Roentgenol* 1997;169:1735–1742.

104. Simpson IA, Chung KJ, Glass RF, et al. Cine magnetic resonance imaging for evaluation of anatomy and flow relations in infants and children with coarctation of the aorta. *Circulation* 1988;78:142–148.

105. Rees S, Somerville J, Ward C, et al. Coarctation of the aorta: MR imaging in late postoperative assessment. *Radiology* 1989;173:499–502.

106. Szolar DH, Sakuma H, Higgins CB. Cardiovascular applications of magnetic resonance flow and velocity measurements. *J Magn Reson Imaging* 1996;6:78–89.

107. Steffens JC, Courne MW, Sakuma H, et al. Quantification of collateral blood flow in coarctation of the aorta by velocity-encoded cine magnetic resonance imaging. *Circulation* 1994;90:937–943.

108. Ketyer S, Cholankeril MV. CT detection of coarctation of the aorta. *CT* 1981;5:355–358.

109. Soulen RI, Kan J, Mitchell S, White RI. Evaluation of balloon angioplasty of coarctation restenosis by MR imaging. *Am J Cardiol* 1987;60:343–345.

110. Bank ER, Aisen AM, Rocchini AP, Hernandez RJ. Coarctation of the aorta in children undergoing angioplasty: pretreatment and posttreatment MR imaging. *Radiology* 1987;162:235–240.

111. Rajasinghe HA, Reddy VM, Van Son JA, et al. Coarctation repair using end-to-side anastomosis of descending aorta to proximal aortic arch. *Ann Thorac Surg* 1996;61:840–844.

112. Shaddy RE, Boucek MM, Sturtevcant JE, et al. Comparison of angioplasty and surgery for unoperated coarctation of the aorta. *Circulation* 1993;87:793–799.

113. Stocker JT. Sequestrations of the lung. *Semin Diagn Pathol* 1986;3:106–121.

114. Cho SY, Kim HC, Bae SH, et al. Demonstration of blood supply to pulmonary sequestration by MR and CT angiography. *J Comput Assist Tomogr* 1996;20:993–995.

115. Donovan CB, Edelman RR, Vrachliotis TG, et al. Bronchopulmonary sequestration with MR angiographic evaluation: a case report. *Angiology* 1994;45:239–244.

116. Buckwalter KA, Gros BH, Hernandez RJ. Bolus dynamic computed tomography in the evaluation of pulmonary sequestration. *J Comput Assist Tomogr* 1987;11:335–340.

117. Pressler V, McNamara JJ. Aneurysm of the thoracic aorta: review of 260 cases. *J Thorac Cardiovasc Surg* 1985;89:50–54.

118. Fomon JJ, Kurzweg FT, Broadway RK. Aneurysms of the aorta: a review. *Ann Surg* 1967;165:557–563.

119. Svensjo S, Bengtsson H, Bergqvist D. Thoracic and thoracoabdominal aortic aneurysm and dissection: an investigation based on autopsy. *Br J Surg* 1996;83:68–71.

120. Bickerstaff LK, Pairolero PC, Hollier LH, et. al. Thoracic aortic aneurysms. A population-based study. *Surgery* 1982;92:1103–1108.

121. Kouchoukos NT, Dougenis D. Medical progress: surgery of the thoracic aorta. *N Engl J Med* 1997;336:1876–1888.

122. Coady MA, Rizzo JA, Hammond GL, et al. What is the appropriate size criterion for resection of thoracic aneurysms? *J Thorac Cardiovasc Surg* 1997;113:476–491.

123. Cosselli JS, Plestis KA, La Francesca S, et al. Results of congtemporary surgical treatment of descending thoracic aortic aneurysms: experience in 198 patients. *Ann Vasc Surg* 1996;10:131–137.

124. Hirose Y, Hamada S, Takamiya M, et al. Aortic aneurysms: growth rates measured with CT. *Radiology* 1992;185:249–252.

125. Mitchell RS, Dake MD, Semba CP, et al. Endovascular stent-graft repair of thoracic aortic aneurysms. *J Thorac Cardiovasc Surg* 1996;111:1054–1062.

126. Svensson LG, Crawford ES. *Cardiovascular and vascular diseases of the aorta.* Philadelphia: WB Saunders, 1997.

127. Godwin JD, Herfkens RL, Skioldebrand CG, Federle MP, Lipton MJ. Evaluation of dissections and aneurysms of the thoracic aorta by conventional and dynamic scanning. *Radiology* 1980;136:125–163.

128. Godwin JD. Examination of the thoracic aorta by computed tomography. *Chest* 1984;85:564–567.

129. White RD, Lipton MJ, Higgins CB. Noninvasive evaluation of thoracic aortic disease by contrast-enhanced computed tomography. *Am J Cardiol* 1986;57:282–290.

130. Gonda RL, Gutierrez OH, Azodo MV. Mycotic aneurysms of the aorta: radiologic features. *Radiology* 1988;168:343–346.

131. Cohen BA, Efremidis SC, Dan SJ, Robinson B, Rabinowitz JG. Aneurysm of the ductus arteriosus in an adult. *J Comput Assist Tomogr* 1981;5:421–423.

132. Kurich VA, Vogelzang RL, Hartz RS, Locicero J, Dalton D. Ruptured thoracic aneurysm: unusual manifestation and early diagnosis using CT. *Radiology* 1986;160:87–89.

133. Landtman M, Kivisari L, Bondestom S, et al. Diagnostic value of ultrasound, computed tomography, and angiography in ruptured aortic aneurysms. *Eur J Radiol* 1984;4:248–253.

134. Coblentz CL, Sallee DS, Chiles C. Aortobronchopulmonary fistula complicating aortic aneurysm: diagnosis in four cases. *AJR Am J Roentgenol* 1988;150:535–538.

135. Taneja K, Gulati M, Jain M, et al. Ductus arteriosus aneurysm in the adult: role of computed tomography in diagnosis. *Clin Radiol* 1997;52:231–234.

136. Torres WE, Maurer DE, Steinberg HV, Robbins S, Bernadino ME. CT of aortic aneurysms: the distinction between mural and thrombus calcification. *AJR Am J Roentgenol* 1988;150:1317–1319.

137. Heiberg E, Wolverson MK, Sundaram M, Shields JB. CT characteristics of atherosclerotic ancurysm versus aortic dissection. *J Comput Assist Tomogr* 1985;9:78–83.

138. Moore EH, Farmer DW, Geller SC, Golden JA, Gamsu G. Computed tomography in the diagnosis of iatrogenic false aneurysms of the ascending aorta. *AJR Am J Roentgenol* 1984;142:1117–1118.

139. Thorsen MK, Goodman LR, Sagel SS, Olinger GN, Youker JE. Ascending aorta complications after cardiac surgery. *J Comput Assist Tomogr* 1986;10:219–225.

140. Quint LE, Francis IR, Williams DM, et al. Evaluation of thoracic aortic disease with the use of helical CT and multiplanar reconstructions: comparison with surgical findings. *Radiology* 1996;201:37–41.

141. Kimura F, Shen Y, Date S, Azemoto S, Mochizuki T. Thoracic aortic aneurysm and aortic dissection: new endoscopic mode for three-dimensional CT display of aorta. *Radiology* 1996;198:573–578.

142. Rubin GD, Paik DS, Johnston PC, Napel S. Measurement of the aorta and its branches with helical CT. *Radiology* 1998;206:823–829.

143. Mitchell RS, Dake MD, Semba CP, et al. Endovascular stent-graft repair of thoracic aortic aneurysms. *J Thorac Cardiovasc Surg* 1996;111:1054–1060.

144. Kato N, Dake MD, Miller DC, et al. Traumatic thoracic aortic aneurysm: treatment with endovascular stent-grafts. *Radiology* 1997;205:657–662.

145. Kopecky KK, Gokhale HS, Hawes DR. Spiral CT angiography of the aorta. *Seminars in Ultrasound, CT and MRI* 1996;17:304–315.

146. Zeitler E, Kaiser W, Schuirer G, et al. Magnetic resonance imaging of aneurysms and thrombi. *Cardiovasc Intervent Radiol* 1986;8:321–328.

147. Lois JF, Gomes AS, Brown K, Mulder DG, Laks H. Magnetic resonance imaging of the thoracic aorta. *Am J Cardiol* 1987;60:358–362.

148. Glazer HS, Gutierrez FR, Levitt RG, Lee JKT, Murphy WA. The thoracic aorta studied by MR imaging. *Radiology* 1985;157:149–155.

149. Ergin MA, Griepp RB. Dissections of the aorta. In: Baue E, ed. *Glenn's thoracic and cardiovascular surgery*. New York: Appleton and Lange, 1996;2273–2298.

150. Hirst AE, Jr., Johns VR, Jr., Klime SW, Sr. Dissecting aneurysm of the aorta: a review of 505 cases. *Medicine* (Baltimore) 1958;37:217–279.

151. Dailey PO, Trueblood HW, Stiinson EB, et al. Management of acute aortic dissections. *Ann Thorac Surg* 1970;10:237–247.

152. Demos TC, Posniak HC, Churchill RJ. Detection of the intimal flap of aortic dissection on unenhanced CT images. *AJR Am J Roentgenol* 1986;146:601–603.

153. Godwin JD, Breimin RS, Speckman JM. Problems and pitfalls in the evaluation of thoracic aortic dissection by computed tomography. *J Comput Assist Tomogr* 1982;6:750–756.

154. Williams DM, Joshi A, Dake MD, et al. Aortic cobwebs: an anatomic marker identifying the false lumen in aortic dissection-imaging and pathologic correlation. *Radiology* 1994;190:167–174.

155. Williams DM, Lee DY, Hamilton BH, et al. The dissected aorta: 3. Anatomy and radiologic diagnosis of branch-vessel compromise. *Radiology* 1997;203:37–44.

156. Kouchoukos NT, Marshall WG, Jr. Eleven-year experience with composite graft replacement of the ascending aorta and aortic valve. *J Thorac Cardiovasc Surg* 1986;92:691–705.

157. Bachet JE, Termignon JL, Dreyfus G, et al. Aortic dissection—Prevalence, cause, and results of late reoperations. *J Thorac Cardiovasc Surg* 1994;108:199–206.

158. Crawford ES, Kirklin JW, Naftel DC, et al. Surgery for acute dissection of ascending aorta: should the arch be included? *J Thorac Cardiovasc Surg* 1992;104:46–59.

159. Egan TJ, Neimen HL, Herman RJ, Malave SR, Sanders JH. Computed tomography in the diagnosis of aortic aneurysm dissection of traumatic injury. *Radiology* 1980;136:141–146.

160. Larde D, Belloir C, Vasile N, Frija J, Ferrane J. Computed tomography of aortic dissection. *Radiology* 1980;136:147–151.

161. Moncada R, Salinas M, Churchill R, et al. Diagnosis of dissecting aortic aneurysm by computed tomography. *Lancet* 1981;1:238–241.

162. Heiberg E, Wolverson MK, Sundaram M, Connors J, Sussman N. CT findings in thoracic aortic dissection. *AJR Am J Roentgenol* 1981;136:13–17.

163. Thorsen MK, San Dretto MA, Lawson TL. Dissecting aortic aneurysms: accuracy of computed tomographic diagnosis. *Radiology* 1983;148:773–777.

164. Singh H, Fitzgerald E, Ruttley MS. Computed tomography: the investigation of choice for aortic dissection. *Br Heart J* 1987;56:171–175.

165. Vasile N, Mathieu D, Keita K, et al. Computed tomography of thoracic aortic dissection: accuracy and pitfalls. *J Comput Assist Tomogr* 1986;10:211–215.

166. Stanford W, Rooholamini SA, Galvin JR. Ultrafast computed tomography in the diagnosis of aortic aneurysms and dissections. *J Thor Imaging* 1990;5:32–39.

167. Hamada S, Takamiya M, Kimura K, et al. Type A aortic dissection: evaluation with ultrafast CT. *Radiology* 1992;183:155–158.

168. Williams MP, Farrow R. Atypical patterns in the CT diagnosis of aortic dissection. *Clin Radiol* 1994;49:686–689.

169. Zeman RK, Berman PM, Silverman PM, et al. Diagnosis of aortic dissection: value of helical CT with multiplanar reformation and three-dimensional rendering. *AJR Am J Roentgenol* 1995;164:1375–1380.

170. Burns MA, Molina PL, Gutierrez ER, et al. Motion artifact simulating aortic dissection on CT. *AJR Am J Roentgenol* 1991;157:465–467.

171. Posniak HV, Olson MC, Demos TC. Aortic motion artifact simulating dissection on CT scans: elimination with reconstructive segmented images. Technical note. *AJR Am J Roentgenol* 1993;161:557–558.

172. Duvernoy O, Coulden R, Ytterberg C. Aortic motion: a potential pitfall in CT imaging of disssection in the ascending aorta. *J Comput Assist Tomogr* 1995;19:569–572.

173. Loubeyre P, Angelie E, Grozel F, Abidi H, Van ATM. Spiral CT artifact that simulates aortic dissection: image reconstruction with use of 180 degree and 360 degree linear-interpolation algorithms. *Radiology* 1997;205:153–157.

174. Loubeyre P, Grozel F, Carrillon Y, et al. Prevalence of motion artifact simulating aortic dissection on spiral CT using a 180 degrees linear interpolation algorithm for reconstruction of the images. *European Radiol* 1997;7:320–322.

175. Inoue T, Watanabe S, Masuda Y, et al. Evaluation of blood flow patterns of true and false lumens in dissecting aneurysms using MR phase-contrast techniques. *Clin Imag* 1996;20:262–268.

176. Prince M, Grist TM, Debatin JF. *3D contrast MR angiography*. New York: Springer-Verlag, 1997.

177. Slonim SM, Nyman UR, Semba CP, et al. Aortic dissection: percutaneous management of ischemic complications with endovascular stents and balloon fenestration. *J Vasc Surg* 1996;23:241–253.

178. Harris JA, Bis KG, Glover JL, et al. Penetrating atherosclerotic ulcers of the aorta. *J Vasc Surg* 1994;19:90–99.

179. Kazerooni EA, Bree RI, Williams DM. Penetrating athersclerotic ulcers of the descending thoracic aorta: evaluation with CT and distinction from aortic dissection. *Radiology* 1992;183:759–765.

180. Stanson AW, Kazmier FJ, Hollier LH, et al. Penetrating atherosclerotic ulcers of the thoracic aorta: natural history and clinicopathologic corelations. *Ann Vasc Surg* 1986;1:15–23.

181. Welch TJ, Stanson AW, Sheedy PF, II, et al. Radidologic evaluation of penetrating aortic athersclerotic ulcer. *RadioGraphics* 1990;10:675–685.

182. Yucel EK, Steinberg FL, Efflin TK, et al. Penetrating aortic ulcers: diagnosis with MR imaging. *Radiology* 1990;177:779–781.

183. Murray JG, Manisali M, Flamm SD, et al. Intramural hematoma of the thoracic aorta: MR image findings and their prognostic implications. *Radiology* 1997;204:349–355.

184. Nienaber CA, von Kodolitsch Y, Peterson B, et al. Intramural hemorrhage of the thoracic aorta: diagnostic and therapeutic implications. *Circulation* 1995;92:1465–1472.

185. Wolff KA, Herold CJ, Tempany CM, et al. Aortic dissection: atypical patterns seen at MR imaging. *Radiology* 1991;181:489–495.

186. Sueyoshi E, Matsuoka Y, Sakamoto I, et al. Fate of intramural hematoma of the aorta: CT evaluation. *J Comput Assist Tomogr* 1997;21: 931–938.

187. Wilson SK, Hutchins GM. Aortic dissecting aneurysms: causative factors in 204 subjects. *Arch Pathol Lab Med* 1982;106:175–180.

188. Patrick TO, Roman WD. Acute aortic dissection and its variants: toward a common diagnostic and therapeutic approach. *Circulation* 1995;92:1376–1378.

189. Robbins R, McManus R, Mitchell R, et al. Management of patients with intramural hematoma of the thoracic aorta. *Circulation* 1993;88: 1–10.

190. Mohr-Kahaly S, Erbel R, Kearney P, Puth M, Meyer J. Aortic intramural hemorrhage visualized by transesophageal echocardiography: findings and prognostic implications. *J Am Coll Card* 1994;23: 658–664.

191. Mulak S, Kaufman J, Torchiana D. Diagnosis and treatment of thoracic intramural hematoma. *J Vasc Surg* 1996;24:1022–1029.

192. Keren A, Kim CB, Hu BS, et al. Accuracy of biplane and multiplane transesophageal echocardiography in diagnosis of typical aortic dissection and intramural hematoma. *J Am Coll Cardiol* 1996;28: 627–636.

193. Krinsky G, DeCoroto DR, Sadler M, et al. Breath-hold gadolinium-enhanced three-dimensional MRI of intraarterial masses: findings in two patients. *J Comput Assist Tomogr* 1997;21:631–634.

194. Mehard WB, Heiken JP, Sicard GA. High-attenuating crescent in abdominal aortic aneurysm wall at CT: a sign of acute or impending rupture. *Radiology* 1994;192:359–362.

195. Siegel CL, Cohan RH, Korobkin M, et al. Abdominal aortic aneurysm morphology: CT features in patients with ruptured and non-ruptured aneurysms. *AJR Am J Roentgenol* 1994;163:1123–1129.

196. Arita T, Matsunaga N, Takano K, et al. Abdominal aortic aneurysm: rupture associated with the high-attenuating crescent sign. *Radiology* 1997;204:765–768.

197. Halliday KE, Alkutoubi A. Draped aorta: CT sign of contained leak of aortic aneurysms. *Radiology* 1996;199:41–43.

198. Castrucci MC, Mellone R, Vanzulli A. Mural thrombi in abdominal aortic aneurysms: MR imaging characterization-useful before endovascular treatment. *Radiology* 1995;197:135–139.

199. Amarenco P, Duyckaerts C, Tzourio C, et al. Prevalence of ulcerated plaques in the aortic arch in patients with stroke. *N Engl J Med* 1992; 326:221–225.

200. Amarenco P, Cohen A, Tzourio CP. Atherosclerotic disease of the aortic arch and the risk of ischemic stroke. *N Engl J Med* 1994;331: 1474–1478.

201. Karalis DG, Chandrasekaran K, Victor MF, et al. Recognition and embolic potential of intraaortic atherosclerotic debris. *J Am Coll Cardiol* 1991;17:73–78.

202. Kronzon I, Tunick PA. Atheromatous disease of the thoracic aorta: pathologic and clinical implications. *Ann Intern Med* 1997;126: 629–637.

203. Tunick PA, Perez JL, Kronzon I. Protruding atheromas in the thoracic aorta and systemic embolization. *Ann Int Med* 1991;115:423–427.

204. Tunick PA, Rosensweig BP, Katz ES, et al. High risk for vascular events in patients with protruding aortic atheromas: a prospective study. *J Am Coll Cardiol* 1994;23:1085–1090.

205. Greendyke RM. Traumatic rupture of the aorta: special reference to automobile accidents. *JAMA* 1966;195:527–530.

206. Williams JS, Graff JA, Uku JM, Steinig JP. Aortic injury in vehicular trauma. *Ann Thorac Surg* 1994;57:726–730.

207. Pretre R, Chilcott M. Blunt trauma to the heart and great vessels. *N Engl J Med* 1997;336:626–632.

208. Parmley LF, Mattingly TW, Manion WC, Jahnke EJJ. Nonpenetrating traumatic injury of the aorta. *Circulation* 1958;17:1086–1101.

209. Groskin SA. Selected topics in chest trauma. *Semin Ultrasound CT MRI* 1996;17:119–141.

210. Sevitt S. The mechanisms of traumatic rupture of the thoracic aorta. *BR J Surg* 1977;64:166–173.

211. Creasy JD, Chiles C, Routh WD, Dyer RB. Overview of traumatic injury of the thoracic aorta. *RadioGraphics* 1997;17:27–45.

212. Pretre R, LaHarpe R, Cheretakis K, et al. Blunt injury to the ascending aorta: three patterns of presentation. *Surgery* 1996;119:603–610.

213. Woodring JH. The normal mediastinum in blunt traumatic rupture of the thoracic aorta and brachiocephalic arteries. *J Emerg Med* 1990; 8:467–476.

214. Kram HB, Wohlmuth DA, Appel PL, Shoemaker WC. Clinical and radiographic indications for aortography in blunt chest trauma. *J Vasc Surg* 1987;6:168–176.

215. Huang P, Fong C, Rademaker A. Prediction of traumatic aortic rupture from plain chest film findings using stepwise logistic regression. *Ann Emerg Med* 1987;16:1330–1333.

216. Mirvis SE, Bidwell JK, Buddemeyer EU, et al. Value of chest radiography in excluding traumatic aortic rupture. *Radiology* 1987;163: 487–493.

217. Mirvis SE, Bidwell JK, Buddemeyer EU, et al. Imaging diagnosis of traumatic aortic rupture: a review and experience at a major trauma center. *Investigative Radiol* 1987;22:187–196.

218. Raptopoulos V. Tramatic aortic tear: screening with chest CT. *Radiology* 1992;182:667–673.

219. Fisher RG, Chasen MH, Lamki N. Diagnosis of injuries of the aorta and brachiocephalic arteries caused by blunt chest trauma: CT vs aortography. *AJR Am J Roentgenol* 1994;162:1047–1052.

220. Mirvis SE, Shanmuganathan K, Miller BH, White CS, Turney SZ. Traumatic aortic injury: diagnosis with contrast-enhanced thoracic CT— Five-year experience at a major trauma center. *Radiology* 1996; 200:413–422.

221. Wong YC, Wang LJ, Lim KE. Periaortic hematoma on helical CT of the chest: A criterion for predicting blunt traumatic aortic rupture. *AJR Am J Roentgenol* 1998;170:1523–1525.

222. Gavant ML, Menke PG, Fabian T, et al. Blunt traumatic aortic rupture: detection with helical CT of the chest. *Radiology* 1995;197:125–133.

223. Gavant ML, Flick P, Menke P, Gold RE. CT aortography of thoracic aortic rupture. *AJR Am J Roentgenol* 1996;166:955–961.

224. Svensson LG, Crawford ES, Hess KR, et al. Deep hypothermia with circulatory arrest: determinations of stroke and early mortality in 656 patients. *J Thorac Cardiovasc Surg* 1992;106:19–31.

225. Ergin MA, Galla JD, Lansmann SL, et al. Hypothermic circulatory arrest in operations on the thoracic aorta: determinations of operative mortality and neurologic outcome. *J Thorac Cardiovasc Surg* 1994; 107:788–799.

226. Crawford E, Crawford J, Safi H, et al. Thoracoabdominal aortic aneurysms: preoperative and intraoperative factors determining immediate and long-term results of operations in 605 patients. *J Vasc Surg* 1986; 3:389–404.

227. Cosselli JS, Lemaire SA, de Figueiredo LP, Kirby RP. Paraplegia after thoracoabdominal aortic aneurysm repair: is dissection a risk factor? *Ann Thorac Surg* 1997;63:28–36.

228. Acher CW, Wynn MM, Hoch JR, Kranner PW. Cardiac function is a risk factor for paralysis in thoracoabdominal aortic replacement. *J Vasc Surg* 1998;27:821–830.

229. Grabenwoger M, Ehrlich M, Simon P, et al. Thoracoabdominal aneurysm repair: spinal cord protection using profound hypothermia and circulatory arrest. *J Cardiac Surg* 1994;9:679–684.

230. Miyamoto K, Ueno A, Wada T, Kimoto S. A new and simple method of preventing spinal cord damage following temporary occlusion of the thoracic aorta by draining cerebrospinal fluid. *J Cardiovasc Surg* 1960;1:188–197.

231. Blaisdell F, Cooley D. The mechanism of paraplegia after temporary thoracic aortic occlusion and its relationship to spinal fluid pressure. *Surgery* 1962;51:351–355.

232. Safi HJ, Bartoli S, Hess KR, et al. Neurologic deficit in patients at high risk with thoracoabdominal aortic aneurysms: the role of cerebrospinal fluid drainage and distal aortic perfusion. *J Vasc Surg* 1994;20: 434–443.

233. Svensson LG, Crawford ES, Hess KR, Coselli JS, Safi HJ. Experience with 1509 patients undergoing thoracoabdominal aortic operations. *J Vasc Surg* 1993;17:357–370.

234. Verdant A, Cossette R, Page A, et al. Aneurysms of the descending thoracic aorta: three hundred and sixty-six consecutive cases without paraplegia. *J Am Coll Cardiol* 1995;23:1085–1090.

235. Davison JK, Cambria RP, Vierra DJ, Columbia MA, Koustas GA. Epidural cooling for regional spinal cord hypothermia during thoracoabdominal aneurysmal repair. *J Vasc Surg* 1994;20:304–310.

236. Safi HJ, Miller III CC, Carr C. Importance of intercostal artery reattachment during thoracoabdominal aortic aneurysm repair. *J Vasc Surg* 1998;27:58–68.

237. Desgranges P, Mialhe C, Cavillon A, et al. Endovascular repair of posttraumatic thoracic pseudoaneurysm with a stent graft. *Am J Roentgenol* 1997;169:1743–1745.

238. Inoue K, Sato M, Iwase T, et al. Clinical endovascular placement of branched graft for type B aortic dissection. *J Thorac Cardiovasc Surg* 1996;112:1111–1113.

239. Shimono T, Kato N, Tokui T, et al. Endovascular stent-graft repair for acute type A aortic dissection with an intimal tear in the descending aorta. *J Thorac Cardiovasc Surg* 1998;116:171–173.

240. Rofsky NM, Weinreb JC, Grossi EA, et al. Aortic aneurysm and dissection: Normal MR imaging and CT findings after surgical repair with the continuous-suture graft-inclusion technique. *Radiology* 1993; 186:195–201.

241. Cabrol C, Pavie A, Mesnildrey P, et al. Long-term results with total replacement of the ascending aorta and reimplantation of the coronary arteries. *J Thorac Cardiovasc Surg* 1986;91:17–25.

242. Allen RC, Schneider J, Longenecker L, et al. Paraanostomotic aneurysms of the abdominal aorta. *J Vasc Surg* 1993;18:424–432.

243. Kouchoukos NT, Robicsek F, Griepp RB. Prospective study of the natural history of thoracic aortic aneurysms—Discussion. *Ann Thorac Surg* 1997;63:1544–1545.

244. Kawamoto S, Bluemke DA, Traill TA, Zerhouni EA. Thoracoabdominal aorta in Marfan syndrome: MR imaging findings of progression of vasculopathy after surgical repair. *Radiology* 1997;203:727–732.

245. Yamaguchi T, Naito H, Ohta M, et al. False lumen in type III aortic dissections: progress CT study. *Radiology* 1985;156:757–760.

246. Yamaguchi T, Guthaner DF, Wexler L. Natural history of the false channel of type A aortic dissection after surgical repair. CT study. *Radiology* 1989;170:743–747.

247. Mathieu D, Keta K, Loisance D. Post-operative CT follow-up of aortic dissection. *J Comput Assist Tomogr* 1986;10:216–218.

248. Rubin GD, Walker PJ, Dake MD et al. 3D spiral CT angiography: an alternative imaging modality for the abdominal aorta and its branches. *J Vasc Surg* 1993;18:656–666.

249. Aurigemma GP, Reichek N, Axel L, et al. Noninvasive determination of coronary artery bypass graft patency by cine magnetic resonance imaging. *Circulation* 1989;80:1595–1602.

250. White RD, Pfugfelder PW, Lipton MJ, et al. Coronary artery bypass grafts: evaluation of patency with cine MR imaging. *AJR Am J Roentgenol* 1988;150:1271–1274.

251. Galjee MA, Van Rossumk AC, Doesberg T, et al. Value of magnetic resonance imaging in assessing patency and function of coronary artery bypass grafts: an angiographically controlled study. *Circulation* 1996;93:660–666.

252. Hoodendoorn LI, Pattynama PMT, Buis B, et al. Noninvasive evaluation of aortocoronary bypass grafts with magnetic resonance flow mapping. *Am J Cardiol* 1995;78:845–848.

253. Sharma S, Sharma S, Taneja K, Gupta AK, Rajani M. Morphologic mural changes in the aorta revealed by CT in patients with nonspecific aortoarteritis (Takayasu's arteritis). *AJR Am J Roentgenol* 1996;167: 1321–1325.

254. Tanikawa K, Eguchi K, Kitamura Y, et al. Magnetic resonance imaging detection of aortic and pulmonary artery wall thickening in the acute stage of Takayasu arteritis: improvement of clinical and radiologic findings after steroid therapy. *Arthritis Rheum* 1992;35: 476–480.

255. Yamada I, Numano F, Suzuki S. Takayasu arteritis: evaluation with MR imaging. *Radiology* 1993;188:89–94.

256. Hayashi K, Fukushima T, Matsunaga N, Hombo Z. Takayasu's arteritis: decrease in aortic wall thickening following steroid therapy, documented by CT. *BR J Radiol* 1986;59:281–283.

257. Evans JM, Ofallon WM, Hunder GG. Increased incidence of aortic aneurysm and dissection in giant cell (temporal) arteritis—A population-based study. *Ann Intern Med* 1995;122:502–507.

258. Godwin JD, Webb WR. Contrast-related flow phenomena mimicking pathology on thoracic computed tomography. *J Comput Assist Tomogr* 1982;6:460–464.

259. Smathers RL, Buschi AJ, Pope TL, Brenbridge AN, Williamson BR. The azygos arch: normal and pathologic CT appearance. *AJR Am J Roentgenol* 1982;139:477–483.

260. Friedmand AC, Chambers E, Sprayregen S. The normal and abnormal left superior intercostal vein. *AJR Am J Roentgenol* 1978;131: 599–602.

261. Ball JB, Proto AV. The variable appearance of the left superior intercostal vein. *Radiology* 1982;144:445–452.

262. Lane EJ, Heitzman ER, Dinn WM. The radiology of the superior intercostal veins. *Radiology* 1976;120:263–267.

263. Engel IA, Auh YH, Rubenstien WA, et al. CT diagnosis of mediastinal and thoracic inlet venous obstruction. *AJR Am J Roentgenol* 1983; 141:521–526.

264. Takasugi JE, Godwin JD. CT appearance of the retroaortic anastomoses of the azygos system. *AJR Am J Roentgenol* 1990;154:41–44.

265. Landay MJ. Azygos vein abutting the posterior wall of the right main and upper lobe bronchi: a normal CT varient. *AJR Am J Roentgenol* 1983;140:461–462.

266. Rockoff SD, Druy EM. Tortuous azygos arch simulating a pulmonary lesion. *AJR Am J Roentgenol* 1982;138:577–579.

267. Hatfield MK, Vyborny CJ, MacMahon H, Chessare JW. Case report. Congenital absence of the azygos vein: a cause for "aortic nipple" enlargement. *AJR Am J Roentgenol* 1987;149:273–274.

268. Carter MM, Tarr RW, Mazer MJ, Carroll FE. The "aortic nipple" as a sign of impending superior vena caval syndrome. *Chest* 1985; 87:775–777.

269. Kim H-J, Kim HS, Chung SH. CT diagnosis of superior vena cava syndrome: importance of collateral vessels. *AJR Am J Roentgenol* 1993;161:539–542.

270. Trigaux J-P, Van Beers B. Thoracic collateral venous channels: normal and pathologic CT findings. *J Comput Assist Tomogr* 1990;14: 769–773.

271. Herold CJ, Bankier AA, Fleisgnman D. Spiral CT of the superior vena cava. In: Remy-Jardin M, Remy J, eds. *Spiral CT of the chest*. Berlin: Springer-Verlag, 1996;265–283.

272. Tello R, Scholz E, Finn JP, Costello P. Subclavian vein thrombosis detected with spiral CT and three-dimensional reconstruction. *AJR Am J Roentgenol* 1993;160:33–34.

273. Ishikawa T, Clark RA, Tokuda M, Ashida H. Focal contrast enhancement on hepatic CT in superior vena caval and brachiocephalic vein obstruction. *AJR Am J Roentgenol* 1983;140:337–338.

274. Maldjian PD, Obolevich AT, Cho KC. Focal enhancement of the liver on CT: A sign of SVC obstruction. *J Comput Assist Tomogr* 1995; 19:316–318.

275. Bashist B, Parisi A, Frager DH, Suster B. Abdominal CT findings when the superior vena cava, brachiocephalic vein, or subclavian vein is obstructed. *AJR Am J Roentgenol* 1996;167:1457–1463.

276. Muramatsu T, Miyamae T, Mashimo M, et al. Hot spots on liver scans associated with superior or inferior vena caval obstruction. *Clin Nucl Med* 1994;19:622–629.

277. Sonin AH, Mazer MJ, Powers TA. Obstruction of the inferior vena cava: a multiple-modality demonstration of causes, manifestations, and collateral pathways. *RadioGraphics* 1992;12:309.

278. Miyake H, Suzuki K, Ueda S, et al. Localized fat collection adjacent to the inferior vena cava: a normal variant on CT. *AJR Am J Roentgenol* 1992;158:423–425.

279. Han BK, Im JG, Jung JW, Chung MJ, Yeon KM. Pericaval fat collection that mimics thrombosis of the inferior vena cava: Demonstration with use of multi-directional reformation CT. *Radiology* 1997;203: 105–108.

280. Lebowitz JA, Rofsky NM, Krinsky GA, Weinreb JC. Gadolinium-enhanced body MR venography with subtraction technique. *AJR Am J Roentgenol* 1997;169:755–758.

281. LI WL, David V, Kaplan R, Edelman RR. Three-dimensional low dose gadolinium-enhanced peripheral MR venography. *J Magn Res Imag* 1998;8:630–633.

282. Hartnell GG, Hughes LA, Finn JP, Longmaid HE. Magnetic resonance angiography of the central chest veins—A new gold standard? *Chest* 1995;107:1053–1057.

283. Finn J, Zisk J, Edelman R, et al. Central venous occlusion: MR angiography. *Radiology* 1993;187:245–251.

284. Rose S, Gomes A, Yoon H. MR angiography for mapping potential central venous acess sites in patients with advanced venous occlusive disease. *AJR Am J Roentgenol* 1996;166:1181–1187.

285. Haire WD, Lynch TG, Lund GB, et al. Limitations of magnetic resonance imaging and ultrasound-directed (duplex) scanning in the diagnosis of subclavian vein thrombosis. *J Vasc Surg* 1991;13:391–397.

286. Hansen M, Spritzer C, Sostman H. Assessing the patency of mediastinal and thoracic inlet veins: value of MR imaging. *AJR Am J Roentgenol* 1990;155:1177–1182.

287. Erdman WA, Jayson HT, Redman HC, et al. Deep venous thrombosis of extremities: Role of MR imaging in the diagnosis. *Radiology* 1990; 174:425–431.

288. Roubidoux MA, Dunnick NR, Sostman HD, Leder RA. Renal carcinoma: detection of venous extension with gradient-echo MR imaging. *Radiology* 1992;182:269–272.

289. Krinsky G, Rofsky N. MR angiography of the aortic arch vessels and upper extremities. *Magn Reson Imaging Clin North Am* 1998;6:269–292.

290. Krinsky G, Reuss P. MR angiography of the thoracic aorta. *Magn Reson Imaging Clin North Am* 1998;6:293–320.

291. Maki JH, Prince MR, Londy FJ, et al. The effects of time-varying intravascular signal intensity and k-space acquisition order on three-dimensional MR angiography image quality. *J Magn Reson Imaging* 1996;6:642–651.

292. Loubeyre P, Delignette A, Bonefoy L, et al. Magnetic resonance imaging evaluation of the ascending aorta after graft-inclusion surgery: Comparison between an ultrafast contrast-enhanced MR sequence and conventional cine MRI. *J Magn Reson Imaging* 1996;6:478–483.

CHAPTER 9

Pulmonary Arteries and Hila

Accurate interpretation of computed tomographic (CT) and magnetic resonance (MR) scans of the pulmonary arteries and hila require detailed knowledge of normal anatomy, coupled with careful attention to scan techniques. The purpose of this chapter is to review pertinent normal CT and MR anatomy, as well as to explore how this knowledge can be applied to interpreting hilar abnormalities, with particular attention paid to assessing current concepts in the diagnosis of venous thromboembolism.

NORMAL ANATOMY

A detailed understanding of the cross-sectional anatomy of the pulmonary arteries and veins is important in the diagnosis of vascular abnormalities and is also necessary for the accurate interpretation of CT or MR images of the hila.

Central Pulmonary Arteries

The main pulmonary artery arises at the base of the right ventricle and extends superiorly for a distance of approximately 5 cm before dividing into the right and left pulmonary arteries. The main, right, and left pulmonary arteries are intrapericardial. Pulmonary arteries are elastic and, in comparison with systemic arteries, are thin-walled vessels.

Main Pulmonary Artery

On CT, the main pulmonary artery is recognizable as the most anterior vascular structure arising from the heart and is often immediately retrosternal at its point of origin (Figs. 9-1 and 9-2). In most normals, the main pulmonary artery should appear slightly smaller than the ascending aorta at the same level (see Fig. 9-1A, B). A slight tendency exists for the pulmonary artery to increase in diameter with age.

The main pulmonary artery measures up to 30 mm in diameter in normals. This measurement is best made at a right angle to the long axis of the pulmonary artery, lateral to the ascending aorta, and at the level of its bifurcation (see Fig. 9-1B). In a CT study of anatomically normal subjects by Guthaner and associates (1), the main pulmonary artery diameter was found to average 28 ± 3 mm. Kuriyama and associates (2) measured pulmonary artery diameters in both anatomically normal persons and patients with pulmonary hypertension. In normals, the main pulmonary artery averaged 24.2 ± 2.2 mm in diameter at a level near its bifurcation (2). Based on these data, the authors concluded that

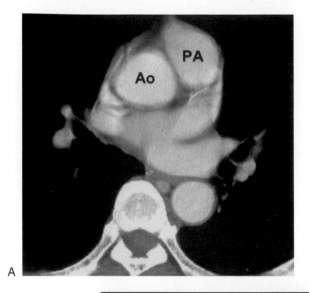

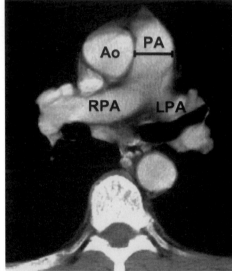

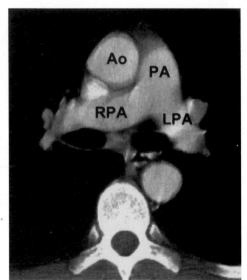

FIG. 9-1. Normal appearances of the main pulmonary artery and its branches on contrast-enhanced CT, obtained using 7-mm collimation and a pitch of 1. (**A**) is most caudal, and (**C**) is most cephalad. **A:** On the most caudal scan, the main pulmonary artery (*PA*) is the most anterior vascular structure arising from the heart. In most normals, the main pulmonary artery should appear slightly smaller than the ascending aorta (*Ao*) at the same level. **B:** Lateral to the ascending aorta, the main pulmonary artery measures up to 30 mm in diameter in normal, as indicated by the marker. The right pulmonary artery (*RPA*) arises at nearly a right angle and passes posterior to the ascending aorta and anterior to the right main bronchus as it crosses the mediastinum. The right pulmonary artery lies approximately in the scan plane; therefore, it is well seen along its length. **C:** The left pulmonary artery (*LPA*) passes slightly to the left and cephalad from its point of origin and arches over the left main bronchus as it enters the left hilum.

A

B

C

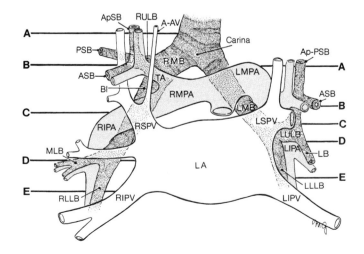

FIG. 9-2. Schematic representation of the pulmonary hila derived from anteroposterior hilar tomograms, as described by Yamashita (170). Characteristic sections are labeled *A–E*.

28.6 mm (mean plus 2 standard deviations [S.D.]) should be considered the upper limits of normal for main pulmonary artery diameter; this value was found to distinguish patients with pulmonary hypertension from healthy persons accurately. In addition, Kuriyama and coworkers (2) found that the main pulmonary artery diameter correlated well with pulmonary artery pressure.

In a more recent study of patients with chronic lung disease or pulmonary vascular disease (3) who were awaiting lung or heart–lung transplantation, considerably more overlap in pulmonary artery diameter was seen between patients with normal and with elevated pulmonary artery pressure. Main pulmonary artery diameter measured 28 ± 7 mm in patients with normal pulmonary artery pressure (≤18 mm Hg) and 33 ± 11 mm in those with pulmonary hypertension (>18 mm Hg).

Right and Left Pulmonary Arteries

The main pulmonary artery divides into right and left pulmonary arteries lateral to the ascending aorta (see Fig. 1B, C). The right pulmonary artery arises at nearly a right angle and passes posterior to the ascending aorta and anterior to the right main bronchus as it crosses the mediastinum. The right pulmonary artery lies approximately in the scan plane; therefore, it is well seen along its length on CT or MR. The left pulmonary artery appears to be a direct continuation of the main pulmonary artery, and a clear distinction between them is impossible without noting the origin of the right pulmonary artery. The left pulmonary artery passes slightly to the left and cephalad from its point of origin and arches over the left main bronchus as it enters the left hilum. The right and left pulmonary arteries should be of approximately equal size, although the left pulmonary artery appears slightly larger in most persons. In the study by Kuriyama and associates (2), the proximal right pulmonary artery measured 18.7 ± 2.8 mm in diameter in normals, and the left pulmonary artery averaged 21.0 ± 3.5 mm. In the study by Ackman Haimovici and coworkers (3), of patients undergoing organ transplantation, the left pulmonary artery averaged 21 ± 5 mm in those with normal pulmonary artery pressure.

Pulmonary Artery Branching

Pulmonary arteries divide by dichotomous branching; the 2 branches may be of approximately equal size, or one branch may be significantly larger than the other. The pulmonary artery has approximately 17 divisions from its bifurcation to the level of a diameter of 10 to 15 mm (4).

The right main pulmonary artery usually divides into an ascending trunk (truncus anterior) and a descending trunk (interlobar branch) posterior to the superior vena cava and anterior to the right main bronchus (see Fig. 9-2; Fig. 9-3). The truncus anterior supplies the right upper lobe, primarily the apical and anterior segments. Although the right interlobar branch largely supplies the right middle and lower lobes,

in about 90% of persons, a branch of the interlobar artery supplies the posterior segment of the right upper lobe (5). The interlobar branch of the right pulmonary artery largely lies within the major fissure, thus accounting for its name.

The left pulmonary artery, after passing over the left main bronchus, usually continues as the descending or interlobar left pulmonary artery, which gives rise to segmental branches of the left upper and lower lobes (see Fig. 9-2). On occasion, the left pulmonary artery gives rise to a short ascending branch that divides into segmental branches supplying the upper lobe.

The branching patterns of lobar, segmental, and subsegmental pulmonary artery branches show considerable variation. Although it is typical for the lobar, segmental, and subsegmental bronchi to be paired with a pulmonary artery branch, the origins of these branches are variable, and supernumerary or accessory artery branches supplying a lobe or segment are often present. Variation is more common in the upper lobes than in the lower lobes. To identify a specific lobar or segmental artery branch, it is usually necessary to identify its associated bronchus. Opacification of segmental pulmonary arteries can be readily seen on CT, and opacified subsegmental branches are sometimes visible.

Pulmonary arteries as small as 300 μm in diameter can be seen on high-resolution CT (6,7); these vessels roughly correspond to acinar arteries, being the 16th generation of branches, at the level of the terminal and most proximal respiratory bronchioles. However, these vessels are visible only as soft tissue attenuation structures on lung window scans, and their opacification is not visible after contrast administration. An increase or a decrease in the size of small peripheral pulmonary arteries is sometimes seen in patients with pulmonary vascular disease associated with increased or decreased blood flow.

Pulmonary Veins

The pulmonary veins arise from alveolar capillaries. Although pulmonary arteries and bronchi or bronchioles lie in the center of lung units, such as lobules, subsegments, segments, and lobes, pulmonary veins are located in their periphery. At the lobular level, veins lie within the interlobular septa (6,7).

Although the branching pattern of veins is more variable than that of the pulmonary arteries, usually two superior and two inferior pulmonary veins are found on each side (see Figs. 9-2 and 9-3; Figs. 9-4 and 9-5). On the right, the superior pulmonary vein drains the upper and middle lobes, whereas on the left, this vein drains the upper lobe. On the right, the vein draining the middle lobe (middle lobe vein) usually joins the superior vein near the left atrium. On occasion, it enters the left atrium separately and is referred to as the middle pulmonary vein. The inferior pulmonary veins drain the lower lobes.

The right superior pulmonary vein passes anterior to the right pulmonary artery and hilar bronchi to enter the left

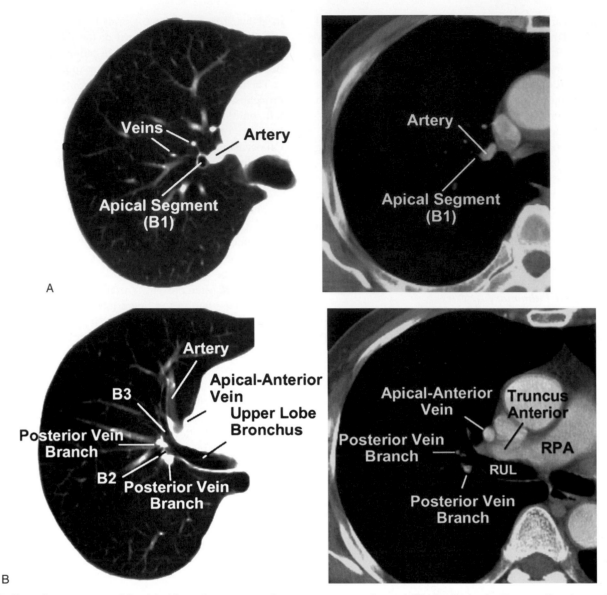

FIG. 9-3. Normal appearances of the right hilar pulmonary vasculature on contrast-enhanced CT, obtained using 7-mm collimation, a pitch of 1, and reconstruction at 7-mm intervals, and shown in a cephalocaudal direction. Both lung and tissue windows are represented. Characteristic levels shown in Fig. 9-2 are illustrated. **A:** Carina and apical segmental bronchus of the right upper lobe. Near the level of the carina, a branch or branches of the truncus anterior supplying the apical segment of the right upper lobe and a branch or branches of the right superior pulmonary vein draining the apical segment are visible in cross section; typically, arteries lie just medial to the apical segmental bronchus, and the veins lie lateral to it. **B:** Right upper lobe bronchus level. At the level of the right upper lobe bronchus, the undivided truncus anterior is visible anterior to the right upper lobe bronchus. The artery supplying the anterior upper lobe segment is visible adjacent to the corresponding segmental bronchus. Segmental upper lobe arteries are typically medial to their corresponding bronchi. Two branches of the right superior pulmonary vein, the posterior vein, lie within the angle formed by the bifurcation of the right upper lobe bronchus into anterior and posterior segmental bronchi and posterior to the posterior segment. Additionally, anterior and medial to the truncus anterior, a small convexity represents the apical-anterior vein. **C–E:** The bronchus intermedius. The bronchus intermedius is characteristically seen at two or three levels, and the contours of the pulmonary vessels can vary depending on the level of scan. **C:** At the level of the upper bronchus intermedius, the right superior pulmonary vein branches make up the anterolateral border of the right hilum, causing the right hilum at this level to have a somewhat nodular contour. Frequently, two veins can be identified in this location. Normal lymph nodes are often seen at this level, lateral to the right pulmonary artery and medial to the vein branches. **D:** Once the interlobar pulmonary artery reaches the lateral border of the bronchus intermedius, it is not unusual for the artery to have a variable appearance. This normal variation is caused by a change in the course of the pulmonary artery, as it turns inferiorly and enters the major fissure, and by the origin of the artery supplying the superior segment of the lower lobe. Two superior pulmonary vein branches remain visible in the anterior hilum. **E:** At the level of the inferior bronchus intermedius, the artery supplying the superior segment of the lower lobe arises posteriorly. The shape of the pulmonary artery at this level has been likened to the head of an elephant, with the elephant's trunk representing the superior segment artery.

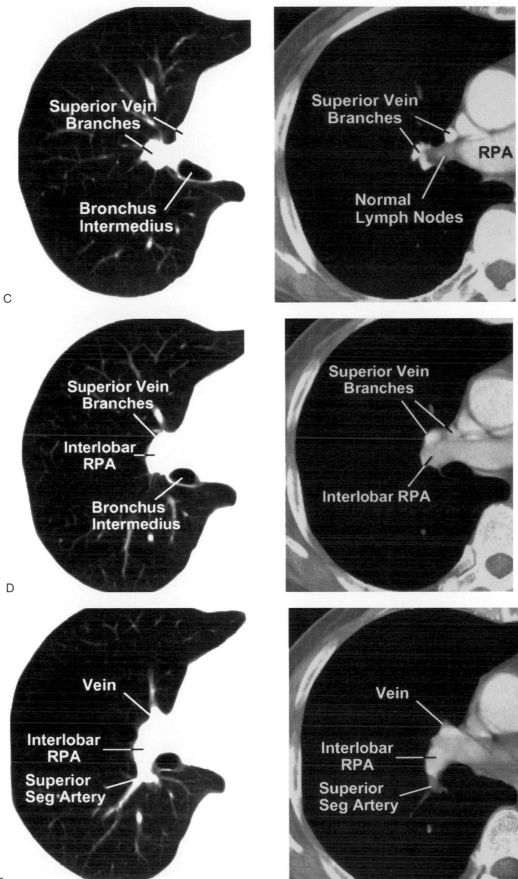

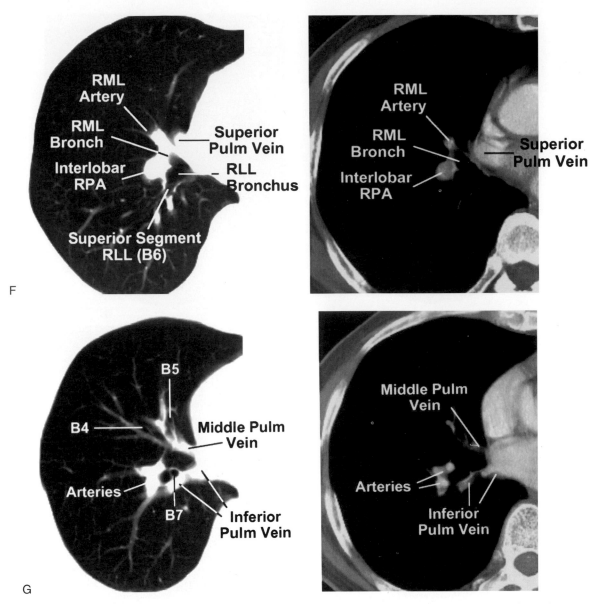

FIG. 9-3. *Continued.* **F:** The middle lobe bronchus. At the level of the origin of the middle lobe bronchus, the interlobar pulmonary artery lies immediately lateral to the middle and lower lobe bronchi. The interlobar artery at this point is oriented perpendicular to the scan plane and is thus seen in cross-section as an elliptic structure. The right superior pulmonary vein, now a single vessel, passes anterior and then medial to the middle and lower lobe bronchi and can be seen entering the upper portion of the left atrium. **G–I:** The lower lobe basilar segmental bronchi. **G:** Below the level of the origin of the middle lobe bronchus, the middle lobe vein is visible entering the left atrium anteriorly. The lower lobe pulmonary artery is beginning to divide; it lies lateral to the basal lower lobe bronchi. In this patient, the medial basal segment (*B7*) is the first branch of the basal lower lobe bronchus. The inferior pulmonary vein is oriented in the transverse plane and passes posterior to the lower lobe bronchi and arteries before entering into the lower portion of the left atrium.

atrium separate from the inferior pulmonary veins, which pass posterior to the lower lobe bronchi and arteries. Analogous to the right side, the left pulmonary veins usually enter the left atrium separately; less commonly, they join intrapericardially to form a single trunk.

Pulmonary Hilar Vessels

The pulmonary hila are complex structures composed of the lobar, segmental, and in some cases, subsegmental bron-chi, pulmonary arteries and veins, bronchial arteries and veins, soft tissue, and lymph nodes. However, the appear-ances of bronchi, vessels, and nodes, and their consistent relationships at different hilar levels allow for the reliable identification of hilar structures (8–14).

A thorough knowledge of cross-sectional bronchial anat-omy is important in the assessment of pulmonary vasculature on CT. Bronchi are easily identified because of the air they contain, and they form a framework on which the pulmonary arteries and veins are draped in a characteristic fashion. De-

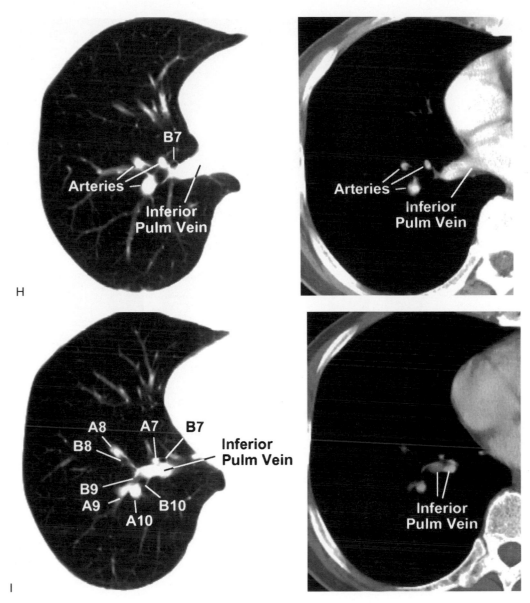

FIG. 9-3. *Continued.* **H, I:** At lower levels, the basal pulmonary artery divides into its basal segmental branches, which accompany segmental bronchi. In the lower lobe, arteries are characteristically lateral to the bronchi, and veins are medial.

spite significant variation in the appearances of segmental hilar vessels, most can be identified by noting their close association with specific segmental bronchi, by following their courses on sequential images, and by determining their sites of origin. Identification of vessels is easiest after the bolus injection of contrast material, but it is usually possible even on unopacified scans.

Evaluation of the hila is simplified by the recognition of certain characteristic sections (see Fig. 9-2) (8–14). These are most easily definable by reference to visible bronchi. On the right side, these sections include (a) the carina and apical segmental bronchus of the right upper lobe, (b) the right upper lobe bronchus, (c) the bronchus intermedius, (d) the middle lobe bronchus, and (e) the lower lobe basilar segmen-

tal bronchi. On the left side, these sections include (a) the apical-posterior segmental bronchus of the left upper lobe, (b) the upper portion of the left upper lobe bronchus, (c) the lower portion of the left upper lobe bronchus at the level of the left upper lobe spur, and (d) the lower lobe basilar segmental bronchi.

On scans obtained using 7- to 10-mm collimation and reconstructed at 7- to 10-mm intervals, most, if not all, of these characteristic sections are identifiable (see Figs. 9-3 and 9-5). Contiguous scans obtained with 3- to 5-mm collimation or reconstructions of spiral scans at intervals of 2 to 3 mm, respectively, provide a more detailed analysis of hilar anatomy, as is necessary for evaluating pulmonary emboli (PEs), for example.

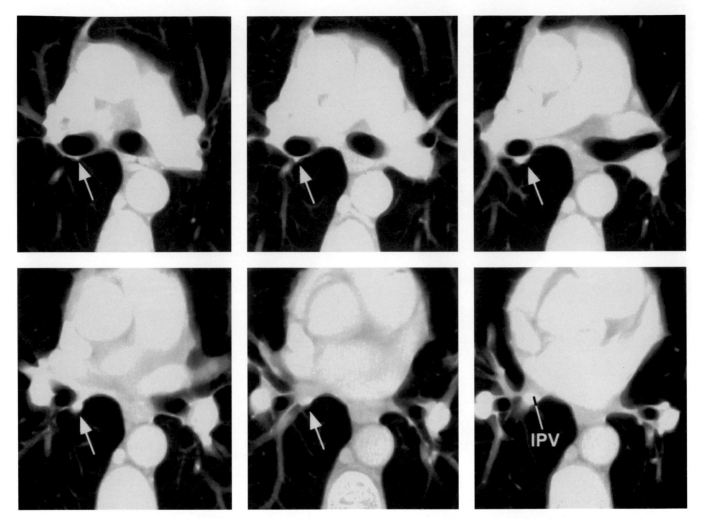

FIG. 9-4. Variation in venous drainage of the right upper lobe. In an occasional patient, a small vein branch *(arrows)* draining a portion of the posterior segment of the upper lobe passes posterior to the bronchus intermedius. At successive levels, it can be seen to pass medially behind the bronchus, to join the inferior pulmonary vein *(IPV)*.

Right Hilum

Carina and Apical Segmental Bronchus of the Right Upper Lobe

At the level of the carina, a branch or branches of the truncus anterior supplying the apical segment of the right upper lobe and a branch or branches of the right superior pulmonary vein draining the apical segment are visible coursing cephalocaudad, adjacent to the apical segmental bronchus. Typically, arteries lie just medial to the apical segmental bronchus, and the veins lie just lateral to it (see Fig. 9-3A).

Right Upper Lobe Bronchus

At the level of the right upper lobe bronchus, the undivided truncus anterior is usually identifiable. This large vessel is the first major branch of the right main pulmonary artery, arising within the pericardium (see Fig. 9-3B), and

it characteristically lies just anterior to the right upper lobe bronchus. At or slightly above this level, artery branches supplying the anterior and posterior upper lobe segments are usually visible adjacent to the corresponding segmental bronchi. They are typically medial to the bronchi.

Typically, a large branch of the right superior pulmonary vein, the posterior vein, lies within the angle formed by the bifurcation of the right upper lobe bronchus into anterior and posterior segmental bronchi. Additionally, anterior and medial to the truncus anterior, a small convexity is frequently visible, representing another right upper lobe vein, the apical-anterior vein, which is often identifiable without the injection of contrast material.

Bronchus Intermedius

At the level of the bronchus intermedius, the right superior pulmonary vein lies alongside the anterolateral border of the right interlobar pulmonary artery, causing the right hilum at

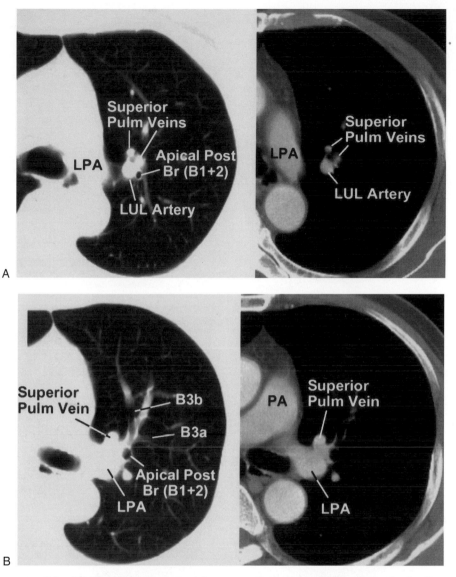

FIG. 9-5. Normal appearances of the left hilar pulmonary vasculature on contrast-enhanced CT, obtained using 7-mm collimation, a pitch of 1, and reconstruction at 7-mm intervals, and shown in a cephalocaudal direction. This is the same patient as shown in Fig. 9-3. **A–C:** Apical-posterior segment bronchus. At the level of the carina and the apical-posterior segmental bronchus (*B1 + 2*), the left upper lobe (*LUL*) pulmonary artery branch arises from the superior aspect of the left pulmonary artery (*LPA*) (the main branch to the left upper lobe). The left superior pulmonary vein draining the apical-posterior segment of the left upper lobe can be recognized as a convexity in the anterior hilum (**A, B**) and as two branches at a higher level (**A**). At a lower level (**C**), the left pulmonary artery lies posterolateral to the left main bronchus, and the superior pulmonary vein is medial to the anterior segmental bronchus (*B3*) of the left upper lobe. **D:** Upper portion of the left upper lobe bronchus. At the level of the upper portion of the left upper bronchus, the bronchial wall is slightly indented superiorly and posteriorly by the interlobar left pulmonary artery. The left superior pulmonary vein invariably lies anterior to the left upper lobe bronchus, passing medially to enter the left atrium at a lower level. **E, F:** Lower portion of the left upper lobe bronchus. At the level of the lower portion of the left upper lobe bronchus (*LUL*), through the left upper lobe spur (*arrow*) and often at the level of the superior segmental bronchus of the left lower lobe (*F*), the left interlobar pulmonary artery is oriented perpendicular to the scan plane and always lies just lateral to the bronchial spur and left lower lobe bronchus (*LLL*), posterolateral to the lingular bronchus, and anterolateral to the superior segmental bronchus (*B6*). The interface between the artery and the adjacent pulmonary parenchyma is generally smooth, and as on the right, the artery appears round or elliptic. Anteriorly, the inferior portion of the left superior pulmonary vein also can be recognized lying directly anterior to the left upper lobe bronchus and is visible entering the left atrium. **A–I:** Lower lobe basilar segmental bronchi. **G, H:** Below the level of the lingular bronchus, the basal lower lobe bronchus (truncus basalis *LLL*) is visible, with pulmonary artery branches lateral to it, and the inferior pulmonary vein is posterior and medial, at the point at which it enters the left atrium (*LA*). **I:** At the level of the basilar segmental bronchi (*B7-8, B9, B10*), the anatomy of the inferior portion of the left hilum is similar to that on the right side at the same level. Segmental pulmonary artery branches lie lateral to the segmental bronchi. The left inferior pulmonary vein is medial to the bronchial branches.

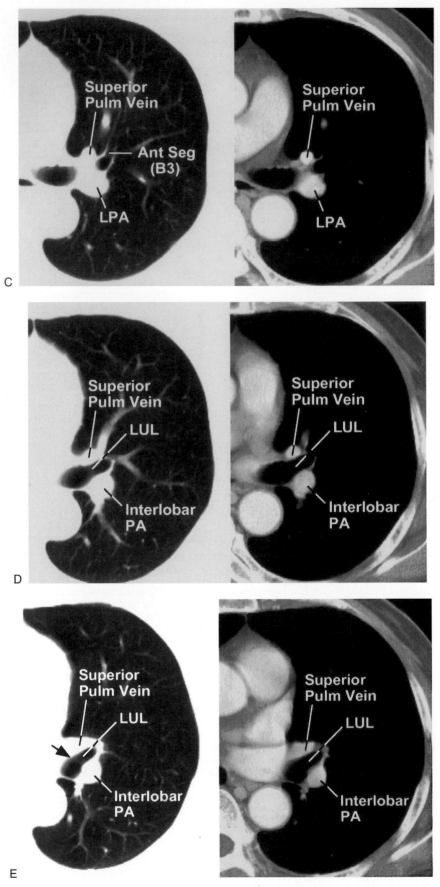

FIG. 9-5. *Continued.*

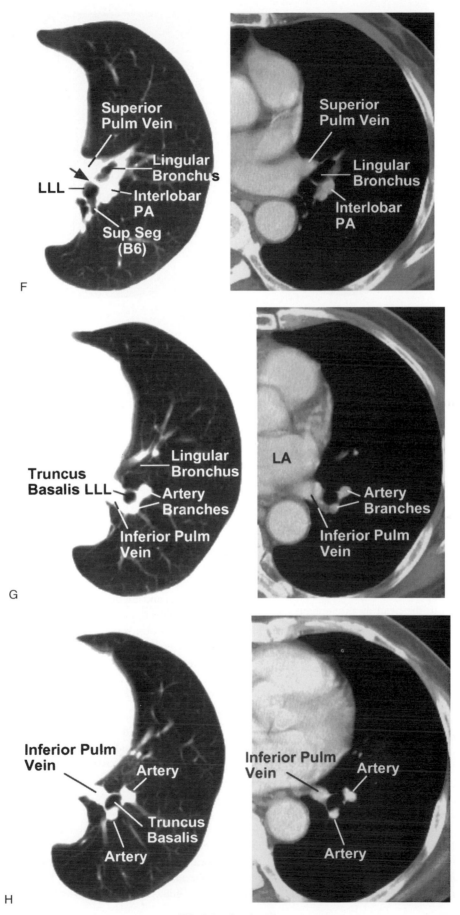

FIG. 9-5. *Continued.*

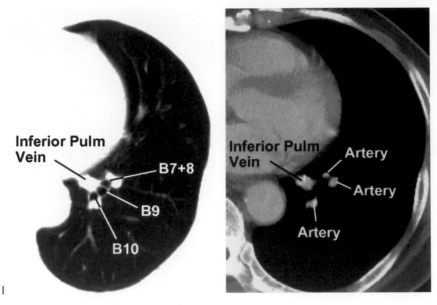

FIG. 9-5. *Continued.*

this level to have a nodular contour. Frequently, two veins can be identified in this location; these veins should not be mistaken for adenopathy (see Fig. 9-3C–E). Infrequently, a small vein branch draining a portion of the posterior segment of the upper lobe passes posterior to the bronchus intermedius; it can be seen to pass medially at successively lower levels, to join the inferior pulmonary vein (see Fig. 9-4).

Once the interlobar pulmonary artery reaches the lateral border of the bronchus intermedius, it is not unusual for the artery to have an irregular, triangular configuration (see Fig. 9-3E). This normal variation is caused by a change in its course, as it turns inferiorly and enters the major fissure, and by the origin of the artery supplying the superior segment of the lower lobe. The shape of the pulmonary artery at this level has been likened to the head of an elephant (see Fig. 9-3E), with the elephant's trunk representing the artery supplying the superior segment of the lower lobe.

Middle Lobe Bronchus

At the level of the origin of the middle lobe lobe bronchus (see Fig. 9-3F), the interlobar pulmonary artery lies immediately lateral to the lateral borders of both the middle and lower lobe bronchi. The interlobar artery at this point is oriented perpendicular to the scan plane and is thus seen in cross section as an elliptic structure. Kuriyama and associates (2) found the interlobar artery to measure 13.0 ± 1.9 mm in diameter at this level, and enlargement of the interlobar artery correlated well with the presence of pulmonary hypertension.

The right superior pulmonary vein passes anterior and then medial to the middle and lower lobe bronchi and can

be seen entering the upper portion of the left atrium. The middle lobe vein can sometimes be seen joining the superior pulmonary vein at this level.

Basal Segmental Bronchi

Below the level of the origin of the middle lobe bronchus, the lower lobe pulmonary artery often bifurcates into two short trunks, which, in turn, divide into the four basilar segmental pulmonary arteries (see Fig. 9-3G–I). These have a characteristic, rounded configuration, lying posterolateral to the proximal portions of the basilar segmental bronchi. Unlike the basilar pulmonary arteries, which are oriented cepalocaudad and are imaged in cross section, the inferior pulmonary veins are oriented in the transverse plane. They join to form the inferior pulmonary vein, which passes posterior to the lower lobe bronchi and arteries before entering into the lower portion of the left atrium.

Left Hilum

On the left side, although characteristic relationships between vessels and airways are also present, far more anatomic variation occurs than on the right.

Apical-Posterior Segment Bronchus

At the level of the carina and the apical-posterior segmental bronchus (see Fig. 9-5A–C), the left superior pulmonary vein draining the apical-posterior segment of the left upper lobe and the left upper lobe pulmonary artery branch (the main branch to the left upper lobe) can be recognized as two distinct vessels. In general, at this level, the left upper lobe pulmonary artery can be traced to its origin from the main left pulmonary artery and lies posterolateral to the left superior pulmonary vein. An arterial branch extending anteriorly and accompanying the anterior upper lobe segmental bronchus is often seen, with the superior pulmonary vein visible as a rounded opacity, lying between it and the mediastinal portion of the left pulmonary artery. At higher levels, the artery supplying the apical posterior segment is visible in cross section as a discrete branch.

Upper Portion of the Left Upper Lobe Bronchus

At the level of the upper portion of the left upper lobe bronchus, the bronchial wall is slightly indented superiorly and posteriorly by the left main pulmonary artery (see Fig. 9-5D). Posterior to the left upper lobe bronchus, the left pulmonary artery continues as the left interlobar pulmonary artery, which, as on the right, typically appears triangular and even slightly irregular at this level. The left superior pulmonary vein invariably lies anterior to the left upper lobe bronchus, passing medially to enter the left atrium, and, frequently, it lies in the transverse plane.

Lower Portion of the Left Upper Lobe Bronchus

At the level of the lower portion of the left upper lobe bronchus (see Fig. 9-5E, F), through the left upper lobe spur and often at the level of the superior segmental bronchus of the left lower lobe, the left interlobar pulmonary artery is oriented perpendicular to the scan plane and always lies just lateral to the bronchial spur posterolateral to the lingular bronchus and anterolateral to the superior segmental bronchus. Kuriyama and colleagues (2) found the interlobar artery to measure 13.0 ± 2.0 mm in diameter at this level. The interface between the artery and the adjacent pulmonary parenchyma is generally smooth, and, as on the right, the artery appears round or elliptic. Adjacent and just lateral to the origin of the lingular bronchus, the pulmonary artery to the lingula frequently can be identified. Anteriorly, the inferior portion of the left superior pulmonary vein also can be recognized lying directly anterior to the left upper lobe bronchus. As on the right, an anomalous vein draining the posterior aspect of the upper lobe may occasionally be seen passing posterior to the upper lobe bronchus to join the inferior pulmonary vein.

Lower Lobe Basilar Segmental Bronchi

At the level of the basilar segmental bronchi (see Fig. 9-5G–I), the anatomy of the inferior portion of the left hilum is essentially a mirror image of that on the right side. Branches of the pulmonary artery to the left lower lobe lie lateral and posterior to the left lower lobe basilar bronchi. The left inferior pulmonary vein passes anterolateral to the descending aorta and posterior to the bronchi and arteries as it enters the left atrium.

Normal Hilar Anatomy: MR

To date, MR has largely been used clinically as an alternate to CT to rule out hilar masses in patients who have contraindications to the use of intravenous contrast. Typically, these studies have been performed using routine, electrocardiogram (ECG)-gated, spin-echo (SE) pulse sequences. With these sequences, the appearance of the hila on MR is identical to that shown on CT. Because no signal is generated either within vessels or by air in the bronchi, and little if any signal is generated by the adjacent pulmonary parenchyma, only the walls of these structures can usually be distinguished (Fig. 9-6). As such, most hilar abnormalities are easily identifiable as foci of intermediate signal intensity.

On relatively T1-weighted, SE images through normal hila, signal generated by normal hilar fat and lymph nodes may be prominent enough to be confused with enlarged nodes or masses in a significant percentage of cases (see Fig. 9-6) (15). These entities occur most frequently in the right hilum at the point at which the right main pulmonary artery crosses in front of the bronchus intermedius to become the right interlobar pulmonary artery, at the level of the middle lobe bronchus, anterolaterally, and on the left side through the left upper lobe bronchus, especially at the level of the left upper lobe spur. Signal from within the hila also may be vascular in origin, further limiting accuracy.

Bronchial Arteries

In addition to pulmonary arteries, veins, and airways, on occasion one can also identify bronchial arteries coursing through the hila, especially when these are enlarged, as often occurs in patients with chronic thromboembolic pulmonary hypertension (CTEPH). Galen and Leonardo da Vinci described the bronchial circulation in detail and suggested its nutrient function; bronchial arteries supply bronchi, peribronchial lymph nodes, and the esophagus. Bronchial arteries, numbering from two to four, arise from the aorta or its branches. One artery is usually present on the right, arising from the third intercostal artery; in about 70% of cases, two bronchial left arteries are present, arising directly from the aorta (16). The bronchial arteries lie along the main bronchi and branch with the airways. Anatomically, they are present to the level of the terminal bronchioles.

Bronchial arteries are usually less than 2 mm in diameter. However, when enlarged, bronchial arteries may be visualized especially in the retrotracheal, retrobronchial, or retroesophageal mediastinum (16).

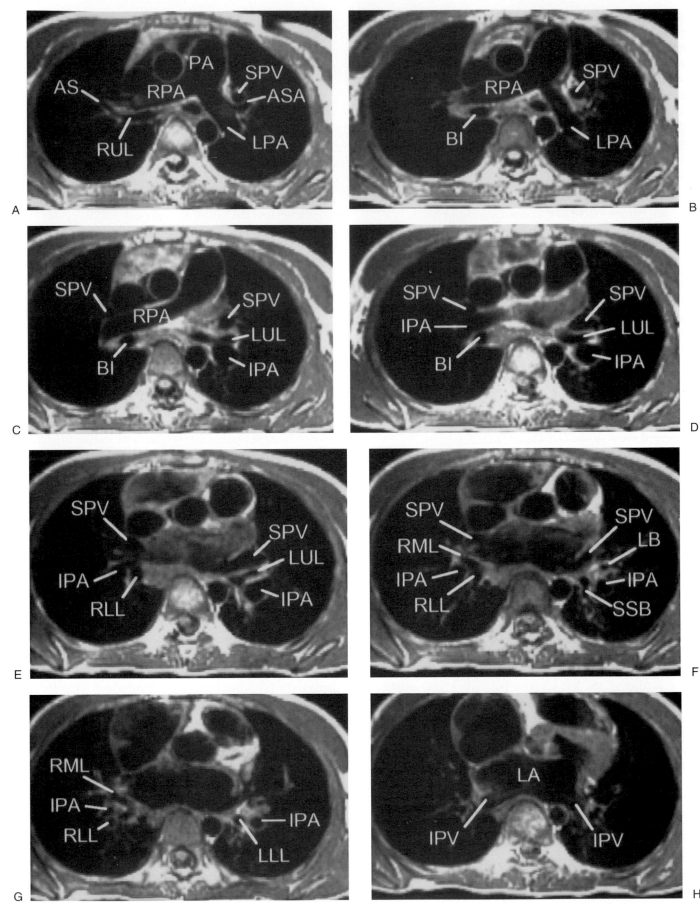

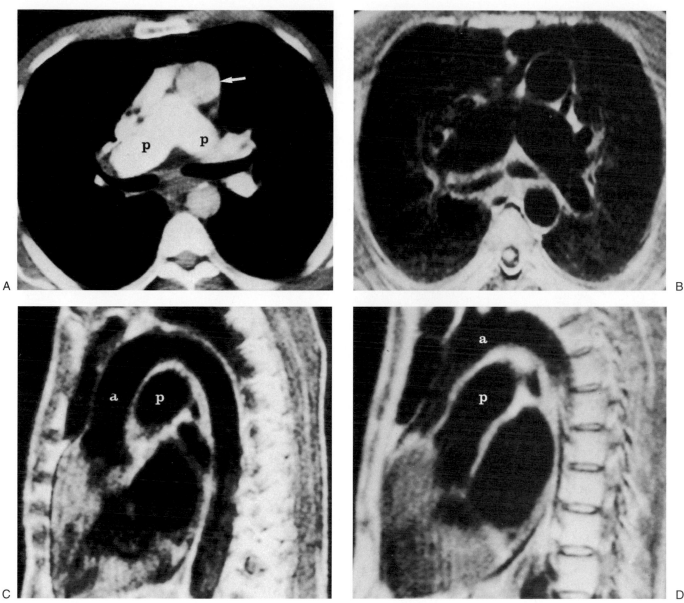

FIG. 9-7. Corrected L-transposition. **A:** CT section at the level of the right upper lobe bronchus after a bolus of intravenous contrast medium. Both the right and left main pulmonary arteries are dilated and occupy the same axial plane (*p*). They are clearly anomalous in position, lying posterior and slightly to the right of the ascending aorta (*arrow*). **B:** Every-beat gated, axial MR section at the same level as **B**, showing identical anatomic relationships (compare with **B**). **C, D:** Every-beat gated, sagittal MR sections through the root of the aorta and origin of the main pulmonary artery, respectively. In both sections, the aorta (*a*) lies anterior to the main pulmonary artery and is related to the anterior ventricle.

CONGENITAL ANOMALIES

Pulmonary Arteries

Many different congenital abnormalities may affect the main and the right and left pulmonary arteries, with and without associated cardiac abnormalities (Figs. 9-7–9-10) (17–19).

The radiologic features of "absence" or agenesis of a pulmonary artery are frequently characteristic and include a small hemithorax, ipsilateral displacement of the mediastinum, absence of the corresponding pulmonary artery, and reticular densities along the pleura and within the lung, usually attributed to systemic collateral circulation (Fig. 9-8). Resulting from embryologic disappearance of the proxi-

FIG. 9-6. A–H: Spin-echo MR of the normal hila at contiguous levels from cephalad (**A**) to caudad (**H**). The appearance of the hila on MR is identical to that shown on CT. With spin-echo imaging, only the walls of vessels and bronchi can usually be identified. As a consequence, it may be more difficult to identify specific hilar levels using MR, and a thorough knowledge of hilar anatomy is essential. Normal lymph nodes and soft tissue are recognized as areas of increased signal intensity. *AS*, anterior segment bronchus; *ASA*, anterior segment artery; *BI*, bronchus intermedius; *IPA*, interlobar pulmonary artery; *IPV*, inferior pulmonary vein; *LA*, left atrium; *LB*, lingular bronchus; *LLL*, left lower lobe bronchus; *LPA*, left pulmonary artery; *LUL*, left upper lobe bronchus; *PA*, main pulmonary artery; *RLL*, right lower lobe bronchus; *RML*, right middle lobe bronchus; *RPA*, right pulmonary artery; *RUL*, right upper lobe bronchus; *SPV*, superior pulmonary vein; *SSB*, superior segment bronchus.

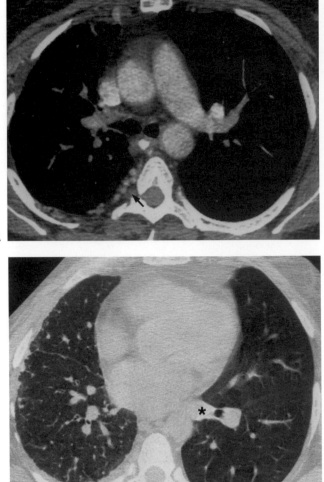

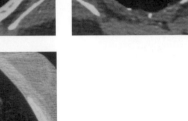

FIG. 9-8. Congenital absence of the right pulmonary artery. **A, B:** Contrast-enhanced, 1. 5-mm sections through the carina and subcarinal space, respectively, show the lack of an identifiable right pulmonary artery. Note the presence of markedly enlarged intercostal arteries serving as collateral vessels to the right lung (*arrows*). **C:** A 1. 5-mm section obtained through the lower lobes imaged with wide windows shows marked volume loss in the right lung. The pleural surface appears beaded because of the presence of prominent intercostal arteries serving as collateral vessels. Note the presence of smaller than usual branches of the right inferior pulmonary vein compared with the normal-sized left inferior pulmonary vein (*asterisk*).

mal portions of either the right or the left sixth arch, respectively, agenesis of a pulmonary artery may occur either as an isolated event or in association with congenital heart disease, typically tetralogy of Fallot.

Both absent and hypoplastic pulmonary arteries are easily identified with both CT and MR (see Fig. 9-8) (20,21). In selected cases, not only can the diagnosis be established, but also additional information concerning the presence and extent of collateral circulation may be evaluated (see Fig. 9-8). Anomalies of the right pulmonary artery may be seen in association with hypoplasia of the right lung associated with partial anomalous pulmonary venous return to the inferior vena cava, the so-called scimitar syndrome (Fig. 9-9) (21).

Another rare pulmonary arterial anomaly is the pulmonary artery sling, or anomalous left pulmonary artery (22–24). In this condition, an anomalous, retrotracheal left pulmonary artery arises from the extrapericaridal segment of the right pulmonary artery and wraps around the junction of the trachea and right main stem bronchus to pass in front of the

esophagus on its way to the left lung (Fig. 9-10). En route, the anomalous artery may cause compression of the right main stem bronchus and may result in chronic stridor. In these cases, respiratory symptoms may be dramatically relieved by surgical repair of the anomalous artery.

Berden and associates (24) coined the term ''ring-sling'' to describe the association of an aberrant left pulmonary artery with diffuse long segment tracheal stenosis. In these cases, tracheal stenosis is due to complete cartilage rings with absence of any significant pars membranacea. Unlike cases of isolated aberrant left pulmonary arteries, in cases with the ring-sling complex, repair of the anomalous pulmonary artery does not lead to symptomatic relief of stridor. Identification of anomalies of the pulmonary arteries is especially important in the evaluation of patients with cyanotic heart disease (25,26). In these cases, information concerning the presence and size of the pulmonary arteries is frequently of vital importance in determining operative strategy. This evaluation may be accomplished using either volumetric CT with or without multiplanar reformations (MPRs) (27) or MR (28).

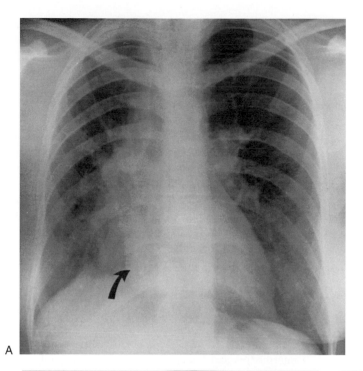

FIG. 9-9. Scimitar (hypogenetic lung) syndrome. **A:** Posteroanterior chest radiograph shows volume loss on the right side, with shift of the heart and mediastinum. An ill-defined linear density is apparent in the right lower lobe, medially, suggesting aberrant venous drainage (*arrow*). **B–D:** Every-beat gated axial images through the carina and the middle and lower thorax, respectively. Marked volume loss is apparent on the right. The right main pulmonary artery is well defined and is normal in caliber (*arrow* in **B**). The right inferior pulmonary vein cannot be identified in its normal location (compare with the normal left inferior pulmonary vein, *arrow* in **C**). Instead, one sees anomalous drainage of the right inferior pulmonary vein into the inferior vena cava (*arrow* in **D**). **E:** CT scan through the right lower lobe, imaged with lung windows, shows enlarged inferior pulmonary veins coalescing within the right lower lobe (*arrow* in **E**). These are easily defined with CT, unlike MR (compare with **A**). (From ref. 21, with permission.)

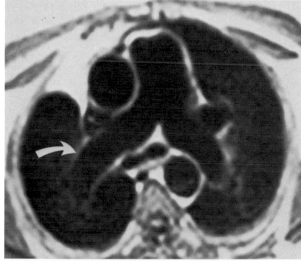

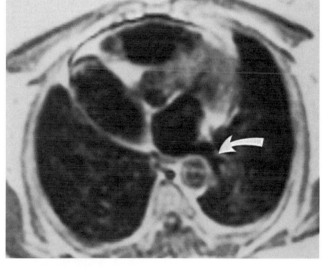

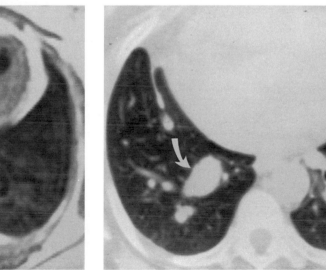

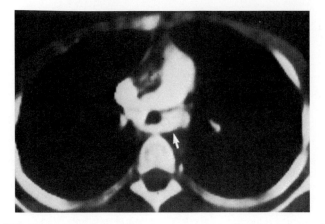

FIG. 9-10. Anomalous left pulmonary artery. Contrast-enhanced scan outlining the anomalous course of the left pulmonary artery swinging behind the trachea to reach the left hilum (*arrow*). (From ref. 23, with permission.)

Pulmonary Veins

Anomalies of the pulmonary veins are uncommon developmental abnormalities in which blood is returned either entirely or in part to the right atrium. The CT (29) and, especially, the MR appearances of anomalous pulmonary veins have been well described (30–33). Best known among these is the scimitar syndrome, in which aberrant drainage of the right inferior pulmonary vein occurs below the diaphragm, often to the inferior vena cava (see Fig. 9-9). Usually associated with a small ipsilateral hemithorax and a small or hypoplastic pulmonary artery, this diagnosis is typically made in asymptomatic patients and is of little clinical significance (21,34).

HILAR LYMPH NODES

Although direct lymphatic communications exist between lung and some mediastinal lymph node groups (i.e., paratracheal, aorticopulmonary, subcarinal, and paraesophageal), hilar lymph nodes are most important in lymph drainage from the lungs.

The use of bolus contrast enhancement usually allows the accurate identification of hilar arteries and veins on CT and the differentiation of a hilar mass or lymph nodes from normal structures. However, a knowledge of hilar lymph node anatomy can be essential in the accurate identification of vascular branches and in the differentiation of unopacified vessels from lymph nodes and normal hilar soft tissue. As pointed out by Remy-Jardin and coworkers (8), normal hilar lymph nodes can be confused with unopacified hilar arteries in CT studies obtained for the purpose of diagnosing possible PEs.

Standard nomenclature for the identification of regional lymph nodes, including hilar nodes, has been proposed by the American Thoracic Society for the purpose of staging lung cancer (35). As discussed in greater detail in Chapter 5, right hilar nodes are included in the tracheobronchial group

(10R; nodes to the right of the tracheal midline, between the cephalic border of the azygos arch and the right upper lobe bronchus), whereas left hilar nodes are included in the left peribronchial group (10L; nodes to the left of the tracheal midline, between the carina and the left upper lobe bronchus, medial to the ligamentum arteriosum); on each side, bronchopulmonary or intrapulmonary nodes (11R and 11L; distal to the main stem bronchi or secondary carina) are also considered hilar.

Although hilar lymph nodes are often portrayed as being peribronchial in location (36), this is largely a misconception. Investigators have clearly shown in surgical studies that hilar lymph nodes are related to both bronchi and vessels, and CT studies of hilar lymph node anatomy have confirmed these anatomic relationships.

Hilar lymph nodes are not located randomly, but are found in consistent locations. These nodes have been classified differently by different authors. Engel (36) described the hilar lymph nodes as belonging to anteromedial and posterolateral groups. Anteromedial nodes lie adjacent to the bifurcations of upper and lower lobe bronchi, medial to the bronchus intermedius and lower lobe bronchi on the right, and medial to the lower lobe bronchus on the left. Posterolateral nodes are located posterolateral to the interlobar and lower lobe pulmonary arteries and in relation to bifurcations of the upper and middle lobe arteries. Chang and Zinn (37) described hilar lymph nodes relative to the bronchial tree as belonging to superior, inferior, anterior, and posterior node groups. Knowledge of these classifications is of limited use in the interpretation of CT.

The distribution of hilar lymph nodes as shown on CT, making use of both bronchial and vascular landmarks, has been described by several investigators (6,8,10,12,15,38,39). Sone and associates (39), in a study of cadavers and patients, classified several hilar lymph node groups. On the right, they identified four lymph node groups. These consist of nodes grouped (a) around the upper lobe and segmental bronchi and vessels, (b) medial and lateral to the intermediate bronchus and interlobar pulmonary artery, (c) around the origin of the middle lobe bronchus and artery, and (d) around the basal trunk of the lower lobe and inferior pulmonary vein. On the left side, three characteristic node groups were identified. These consisted of nodes (a) around the upper lobe and lingular bronchi and lateral to the left pulmonary artery, (b) posterior to the left main bronchus and medial to the descending left pulmonary artery in the region of the left retrobronchial stripe, and (c) as on the right, around the basal trunk and inferior pulmonary vein.

Remy-Jardin and associates (8) suggested a modification of the classification proposed by Sone and colleagues (39), by describing four lymph node groups on the right (upper lobe, interlobar, middle lobe, and lower lobe) and four lymph node groups on the left (culminal, interlobar, lingular, and lower lobe). Based on a review of contrast-opacified spiral CT rather than anatomic specimens, in each of the regions described, unenhancing soft tissue could be seen identified

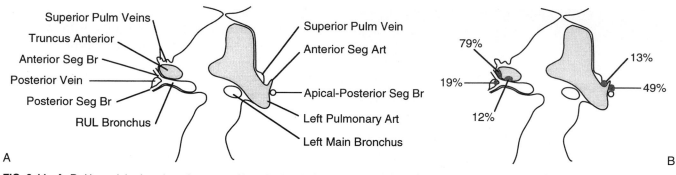

FIG. 9-11. A, B: Upper lobe lymph node groups. Near the level of the right upper lobe bronchus on the right and the apical-posterior segment bronchus on the left, soft tissue is most commonly identified adjacent to the lateral borders of the pulmonary arteries. Percentages indicate the approximate frequency with which unenhancing soft tissue is visible in the sites indicated. (Modified from ref. 8, with permission.)

corresponding to conglomerates of small lymph nodes and connective tissue. Although these regions of normal unopacified soft tissue have not been proven to represent normal lymph nodes, the assumption seems warranted, because enlarged lymph nodes are commonly seen in these same locations.

Although normal lymph nodes or soft tissue can be seen in many different locations in the hila, they are particularly common in several specific locations at easily recognizable hilar levels (10,12). Familiarity with these is of value in the interpretation of hilar CT.

Upper Lobe Node Groups

Near the levels of the upper lobe bronchi, soft tissue is most commonly identified adjacent to the lateral borders of the pulmonary arteries. On the right, a linear region of unenhancing soft tissue lateral to the truncus anterior, usually between the upper lobe bronchus and the anterior segment artery, was seen in 79% of 45 patients studied by Remy-Jardin coworkers (8), whereas on the left, nodes and soft tissue were seen lateral to the anterior segmental branch of the left main pulmonary artery in 49%, with an additional

7% showing nodes lateral to the artery itself (Fig. 9-11). At this level, nodes in other locations were much less frequent.

In addition, on the right, slightly below the right upper lobe bronchus, lateral to the bifurcation of the main pulmonary artery, anterolateral to the bronchus intermedius, and medial to superior pulmonary vein branches, it is common to see a large area of unenhanced soft tissue, composed of small nodes and fat (Figs. 9-12 and 9-13) (6,15,40). This collection can range up to 1.5 cm in diameter in some anatomically normal persons. It corresponds to part of the right upper lobe group described by Sone and associates (39), and it represents part of the "lymphatic sump" of the right lung described by Nohl (41). The term lymphatic sump has been used to indicate the important function of nodes in this group in draining the lung. This collection can be easily mistaken for a hilar mass or thrombus in the right pulmonary artery.

Interlobar Node Groups

At more caudal levels, normal lymph nodes and soft tissue are primarily found lateral to bronchi and adjacent to, or medial to, pulmonary artery branches. At the level of the right interlobar group, soft tissue is visible between the bron-

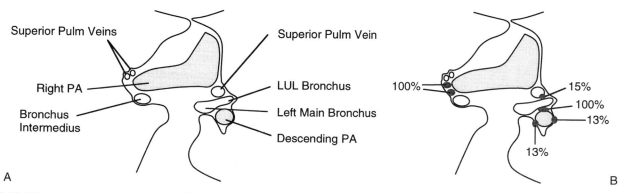

FIG. 9-12. Upper lobe lymph node groups. Slightly below the right upper lobe bronchus, lateral to the bifurcation of the main pulmonary artery, anterolateral to the bronchus intermedius, and medial to superior pulmonary vein branches, a large area of unenhanced soft tissue, composed of small nodes and fat is nearly always visible, ranging up to 1.5 cm in diameter in some normal subjects. This tissue can be easily mistaken for a hilar mass or thrombus in the right pulmonary artery. At the level of the upper portion of the left upper lobe bronchus, a rim of soft tissue is always seen between the posterior bronchial wall of the left upper lobe bronchus and the interlobar pulmonary artery, whereas nodes are less often visible medial or lateral to the artery or anterior to the bronchus. (Modified from ref. 8, with permission.)

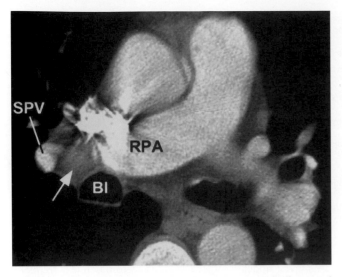

FIG. 9-13. Normal right hilar lymph nodes. In an anatomically normal patient, contrast-enhanced CT shows a large unenhanced collection of soft tissue and lymph nodes (*arrow*), lateral to the right pulmonary artery (*RPA*), anterior to the bronchus intermedius (*BI*), and medial to the superior pulmonary vein (*SPV*). (From ref. 8, with permission.)

chus intermedius and the medial aspect of the interlobar artery in 69% of cases (Fig. 9-14) (8). At the level of the upper portion of the left upper lobe bronchus, a rim of soft tissue is always seen between the posterior bronchial wall and the interlobar artery (see Fig. 9-12; Fig. 9-15).

Although not described by Remy-Jardin and associates (8), hilar lymph nodes medial to the bronchus intermedius are commonly present (36). These structures are often difficult to distinguish from adjacent subcarinal lymph nodes.

Middle Lobe and Lingular Groups

At the level of the right middle lobe bronchus and node group, it is most common to see soft tissue lateral to the

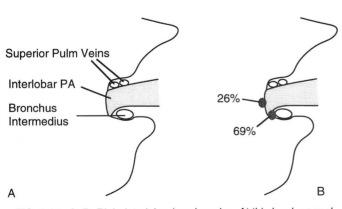

Superior Pulm Veins

Interlobar PA

Bronchus
Intermedius

26%

69%

A   B

FIG. 9-14. A, B: Right interlobar lymph nodes. At this level, normal lymph nodes and soft tissue are primarily found lateral to bronchi and adjacent to or medial to pulmonary artery branches. At the level of the right interlobar group, soft tissue is visible between the bronchus intermedius and the medial aspect of the interlobar artery. (Modified from ref. 8, with permission.)

origin of the middle lobe or lower lobe bronchi and medial to the interlobar pulmonary artery (Figs. 9-16 and 9-17). This tissue was visible in 69% of cases reported by Remy-Jardin and coworkers (8), and it can be larger than 5 mm in some patients. Slightly more posteriorly, lateral to the lower lobe bronchus and posteromedial to the interlobar artery, soft tissue was visible in 48%. At the level of the lingular bronchus (see Figs. 9-15 and 9-16), similar anatomic features are seen, with soft tissue lateral to the lingular bronchus and medial to the interlobar pulmonary artery visible in 60%. Soft tissue between the lower lobe bronchus and the artery was seen in 31% to 40% of cases. In addition, lymph nodes in the anteromedial groups described by Engel (36) are commonly present medial to the proximal lower lobe bronchi at this level.

Lower Lobe Groups

At the level of the lower lobe bronchial segments, most nodes are interposed between bronchi and medial pulmonary arteries (Fig. 9-18); small nodes were seen in about 20% of cases on the right and in 27% to 40% of cases on the left in the study by Remy-Jardin and associates (8).

Lymph nodes anterior to the truncus basalis and basal lower lobe bronchi are also commonly present, visible in about 15% to 20% of anatomically normal persons. These nodes, described as occupying the inferior hilar window, are commonly seen in patients with hilar lymph node enlargement.

Lymph Node Size

In most regions, normal nodes or collections of hilar soft tissue measure only a few millimeters in thickness as shown on CT, with a short axis diameter of less than 3 mm reliably seen (8). In three locations described previously, however, larger conglomerates of nodes and soft tissue are sometimes visible. These three regions are found at the levels of (a) the bronchus intermedius and pulmonary artery bifurcation on the right, (b) the middle lobe bronchus on the right, and (c) the upper lobe or lingular and bronchus on the left (6,15). In only the first of these, however, can unenhanced soft tissue exceeding 1 cm in least diameter be seen. Except in this one region, it would seem appropriate to use a least node diameter of 1 cm as the upper limit of normal.

PULMONARY THROMBOEMBOLISM

Few topics have inspired more controversy than the potential use of CT to assess pulmonary thromboembolism (42–45). This is the direct consequence of the introduction of volumetric (spiral/helical) CT. Since the introduction of this technique, it has been apparent that properly performed spiral CT allows uniform, high-quality opacification of all central pulmonary arteries, frequently leading to identifica-

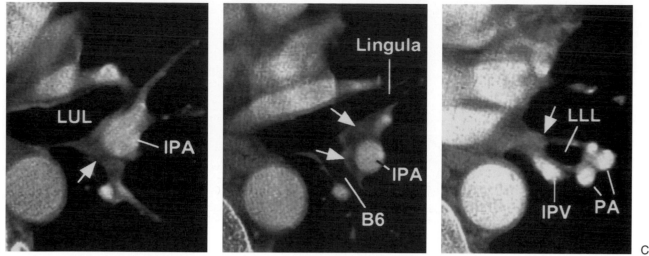

FIG. 9-15. A–C: Normal left hilar lymph nodes. Contrast-enhanced CT shows the characteristic locations of normal soft tissue and lymph nodes (*arrows*) in relation to the left upper lobe bronchus (*LUL*), interlobar pulmonary artery (*IPA*), lingular bronchus (*lingula*), superior segment bronchus (*B6*), basal left lower lobe bronchus (*LLL*), inferior pulmonary vein (*IPV*), and lower lobe arteries (*PA*). (From ref. 8, with permission.)

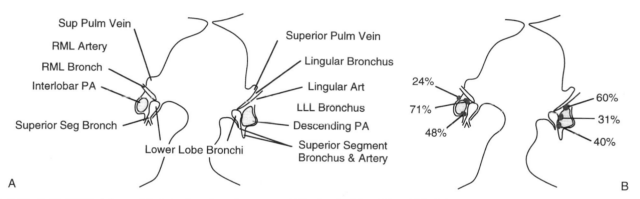

FIG. 9-16. A, B: Middle lobe and lingular lymph node groups. At the level of the right middle lobe bronchus, it is most common to see soft tissue lateral to the origin of the middle lobe or lower lobe bronchi and medial to the interlobar pulmonary artery. This node can be more than 5 mm in diameter in some patients. At the level of the lingular bronchus, similar anatomy is seen, with nodes and soft tissue lateral to the lingular bronchus and medial to the interlobar pulmonary artery. (Modified from ref. 8, with permission.)

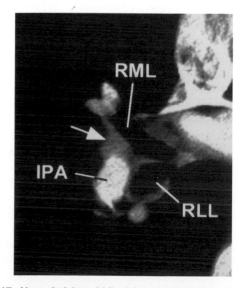

FIG. 9-17. Normal right middle lobe lymph nodes. Contrast-enhanced CT shows the location normal soft tissue and lymph nodes (*arrow*) anterior to the interlobar pulmonary artery (*IPA*), lateral to the basal lower lobe bronchus (*RLL*), and posterolateral to the right middle lobe bronchus (*RML*).

tion of otherwise unsuspected PEs (Fig. 9-19) (46–48). In a review of 1,879 consecutive contrast-enhanced helical CT scans, 18 (1%) of cases proved to have unsuspected PEs, leading to a change in management in 11 (61%) (47).

To date, some prospective studies have concluded, despite differences in technique, that properly performed and interpreted, CT can exceed 90% sensitivity and specificity for the diagnosis of central PEs (49–54).

CT Technique

Accurate assessment of patients with suspected PEs requires meticulous CT scan technique. Factors to be considered include those relating to data acquisition such as collimation, pitch, reconstruction interval, reconstruction algorithm, and scan volume, as well as those relating to contrast administration including osmolarity, dose, volume, rate of administration, and scan delay. Methods for display and interpretation also need to be selected.

To date, optimal scan parameters have yet to be defined; a review of current reports shows that variation among these

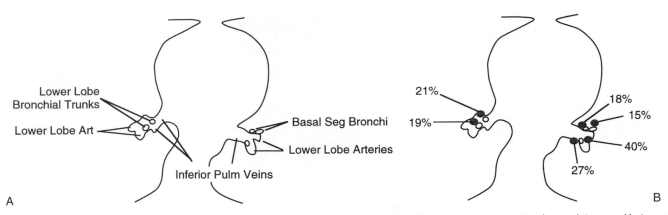

FIG. 9-18. A, B: Lower lobe lymph node groups. At the level of the lower lobe bronchi and basal segments, most nodes are interposed between bronchi and pulmonary arteries. Lymph nodes anterior to the truncus basalis and basal lower lobe bronchi are also commonly present. (Modified from ref. 8, with permission.)

factors is the rule (49–54). Nonetheless, general guidelines can be derived from both a review of the literature and personal experience (Table 9-1) (55,56).

Data Acquisition

Noncontrast Images

It has been argued that noncontrast-enhanced images, both conventional and high-resolution, be performed before contrast administration to assess pleural and parenchymal abnormalities as well as to identify calcified hilar lymph nodes (57,58). In our experience, this procedure should be consid-

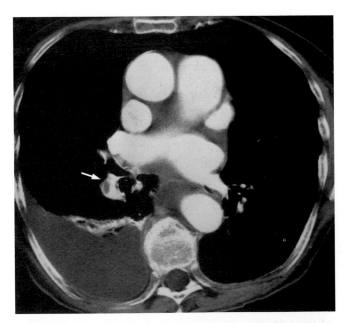

FIG. 9-19. Unsuspected acute pulmonary embolus. Contrast-enhanced 7-mm section (pitch, 1.6) obtained to evaluate a patient with a bloody right-sided pleural effusion to rule out possible occult malignancy shows unanticipated thrombus within the right interlobar pulmonary artery (*arrow*). Serendipitous identification of otherwise unexpected pulmonary emboli has dramatically increased after the introduction of helical CT.

ered optional because, in most cases, pleural and parenchymal abnormalities are equally apparent on contrast-enhanced images. When additional high-resolution images are required, these may always be added later. Although investigators have suggested that initial noncontrast-enhanced images are necessary to localize the anatomic volume of interest accurately, this is usually easily identified from the accompanying scanogram.

Collimation, Pitch, Reconstruction Interval, and Algorithm of Reconstruction

Collimation. Increasing awareness of the limitations of helical CT to assess subsegmental pulmonary arteries led to greater emphasis on the need for thinner sections. Although adequate evaluation of central pulmonary arteries has been obtained using 5- and even 7-mm sections (49,51,59,60), thinner sections are generally preferable. In this regard, the advantage of even 2-mm versus 3-mm sections has been documented. In a retrospective assessment of 800 segmental and 1,600 subsegmental pulmonary arteries, Remy-Jardin showed significant improvement in the mean number of both visualized segmental (93% versus 85%; $p < .001$) and subsegmental arteries (61% versus 37%; $p < .0001$) comparing 2-mm collimation (0.75 second per revolution; pitch, 2) with 3-mm collimation (1 second per revolution; pitch, 1.7), respectively (61). In distinction, use of 5-mm sections represents a substantially less accurate method for assessing smaller pulmonary arteries. As shown by these same authors in an earlier study, 42 of (10%) of 432 segmental arteries in 53 (71%) of 75 patients could not be adequately assessed using 5-mm sections (52). Similar findings using 5-mm collimation have been reported by other investigators (62,63).

Pitch. Pending an increase in availability of subsecond CT scanners, especially those capable of 2-mm collimation, 3-mm sections (with or without subsecond scan capability) should be routinely used (see Table 9-1). Because one must cover a total scan volume of between 10 and 12 cm (corresponding approximately to the distance between the aortic

TABLE 9-1. *Pulmonary emboli: CT technique*

Scanner settings:	kVp: 120
	mA: 250
Rotation time:	0.75–1 sec
Phase of respiration:	Suspended inspiration (quiet breathing acceptable if necessary)
Slice thickness:	3 and 5 mm
Pitch:	1.6–2
Reconstruct interval:	2 and 4 mm, respectively
Reconstruct algorithm:	Edge-enhancing or standard
Field-of-view:	Standard body FOV: may be reduced to 25 cm for optimal evaluation
Helical exposure time:	Single breath-hold period (24–30 s, usually obtainable with coaching or supplemental oxygen)
Scan direction:	Craniocaudad from the middle of the aortic arch to the inferior pulmonary veins using 3-mm sections followed by 5-mm sections to the lung bases reconstructed every 4 mm
IV contrast:	Concentration: LOCM 300–320 mg iodine/mL
	or HOCM 282 mg iodine/mL (60% solution)
	Rate: 3–4 mL/s
	Scan delay: Test bolus recommended (see text)
	Volume: 120–150 mL
Comments:	1. Initial 7–8-mm noncontrast scans through the thorax are optional to identify coexistent pleural/parenchymal disease. When initial noncontrast images are not acquired, images through the lung apices to the level of the aortic arch may be acquired on completion of the study.
	2. Multiple breath-hold acquisitions may be obtained in patients unable to hold their breath.
	3. LOCM is recommended in patients with history of prior allergy, cardiac or renal insufficiency, or pulmonary hypertension.
	4. Following completion of imaging through the chest, 10-mm sections every 50 mm from the diaphragms to the knees may be of value for detection of peripheral venous thrombi (55).

HOCM, high-osmolar contrast medium; FOV, field-of-view. LOCM, low-osmolar contrast medium.
Modified from ref. 56.

arch and the inferior pulmonary veins), using either 2- or 3-mm collimation, the examiner must use a pitch of at least 1.6 to 1.7. In fact, in our experience, routine use of a pitch of 2 is recommended because it ensures maximum coverage with acceptable image quality in most cases. Investigators have suggested that in patients who are unable to hold their breath for more than 10 seconds, multiple acquisitions using 5-mm collimation with a pitch of 2 may be preferable (57). In our experience, it is equally feasible to scan patients using 3-mm collimation with a pitch of 2 during quiet respiration, as outlined in Table 9-1.

Reconstruction Interval. Optimal spatial resolution in the Z-axis requires overlapping reconstructions. Although improved visualization of smaller arteries may be obtained when images are reconstructed every 1 mm, for most cases, 3-mm sections reconstructed every 2-mm represent a reasonable compromise between Z-axis resolution and the total number of images to be interpreted and stored. If 5-mm collimation is used, images may be reconstructed every 3 to 4 mm.

Reconstruction Algorithm. To our knowledge, no systematic evaluation of the effect of various reconstruction algorithms on detection of PEs has been reported to date. Although some studies have used high-spatial-frequency algorithms (64,65), others have used standard reconstruction algorithms (54), and still others have routinely used both (61). In lieu of a more definitive evaluation, we routinely reconstruct images prospectively using a high-spatial-resolution algorithm, pending further evaluation.

Contrast Media Administration

Iodine Concentration, Flow Rate, and Volume

Optimal contrast administration is critical to the successful performance of CT evaluation of the pulmonary arteries and invariably requires use of a power injector. To date, various protocols have been proposed. These can be divided into two groups: those that use a low concentration of iodine (24% to 30%) administered at a fast rate (between 4 and 5 mL per second) versus those that use a high concentration of iodine (60%) administered at relatively slower rate (2 to 3 mL per second) (57).

The use of low concentration protocols has theoretic advantages. These include, in particular, diminution of streak artifacts from the superior vena cava and avoidance of overshadowing small emboli resulting from "too" dense opacification of pulmonary vessels. As a practical matter, however, in our experience, these factors rarely cause clinical confusion, provided images are evaluated directly on video monitors or computer workstations in place of or in addition to hard copy (48). Viewing cases directly on a video monitor allows instantaneous electronic window manipulation that effectively minimizes artifacts. In addition, high-volume protocols also require good venous access, typically requiring use of a 20-gauge or larger peripheral intravenous catheter. Although this requirement usually presents little difficulty, in some cases venous access may be limited. Investigators have shown that adequate opacification of pulmonary arteries may be obtained using a 22-gauge antecubital venous catheter with flow rates as low as 2.0 to 2.5 mL per second using high-concentration contrast agents (48).

Some investigators have suggested that streak artifacts from the superior vena cava may also be minimized by scanning from below-upward, starting from above the diaphragms and proceeding toward the aortic arch. Although this technique has the additional advantage of minimizing artifacts from respiratory motion by first obtaining images through the lower lobes during the phase of optimal breathholding, this approach has not been universally adopted.

Costello and associates (66) have shown that adequate vascular opacification can be obtained with as little as 60 mL of 300 mg iodine per milliliter of contrast media; however, for CT evaluation of the pulmonary arteries, most investigators use between 100 and 150 mL (57,61).

Scan Delay

Optimal evaluation of the pulmonary arteries requires that an appropriate scan delay be chosen. Unfortunately, little

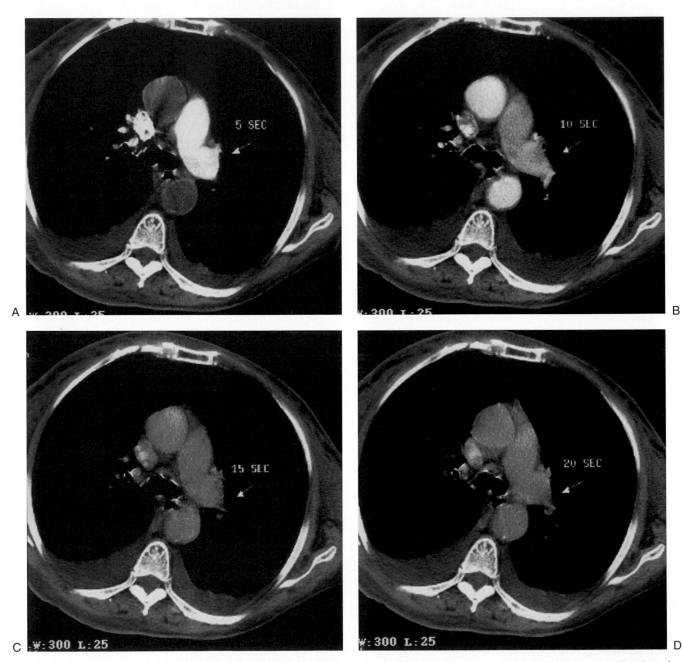

FIG. 9-20. CT technique: Use of a test bolus. **A–D:** Identical sections through the left main pulmonary artery using 3-mm collimation after administration of 20 mL 60% noniodinated contrast media at a rate of 3 mL per second obtained at 5, 10, 15, and 20 seconds, respectively. In this case, peak opacification of the pulmonary artery occurs at 5 seconds; by 15 seconds, almost complete washout of contrast occurs within the pulmonary artery. Given marked variations in circulation time among individual patients, it is strongly recommended that an initial test bolus be administered in every case.

agreement exists on appropriate scan delay. Although most investigators have used 20 seconds as an acceptable compromise, recommendations vary from as short a time as 10 to 12 seconds (57) to as long as 30 seconds when using a 22-gauge venous catheter (48). In fact, large variations among patients are encountered. Vanhoe and associates (67), for example, using a test bolus, showed that the time to peak attenuation within the aorta varied as much as between 11 and 32 seconds (mean, 20 seconds; S.D., 6.1 seconds). We have also noted considerable variation in the time of peak enhancement of pulmonary arteries (Fig. 9-20).

This problem is easily resolved by use of a test bolus of 20 mL of contrast media injected at the same rate as the planned injection, with sequential axial images obtained at the level of the right main pulmonary artery. Although some investigators have advocated obtaining as many as 10 images over a 20-second interval (58), we have found sufficient data necessary to determine that optimal scan delay may be derived from as few as 4 images obtained at 5, 10, 15, and 20 seconds after initiation of a test bolus (see Fig. 9-20). As a rule, we add 5 seconds to the time of peak pulmonary artery opacification, to ensure opacification of peripheral small pulmonary arteries as well as adequate filling of pulmonary veins. This filling is important because simultaneous opacification of pulmonary arteries and veins minimizes the chance of misinterpreting a partially opacified pulmonary vein as a PE.

Alternatively, one can now obtain equivalent data using automated scan acquisitions to monitor vascular opacification without the use of a test dose (C.A.R.E. bolus [Siemens, Iselin, NJ] or Smartprep [GE Medical Systems, Milwaukee, WI]) (68). Given only a slight increase in the time of examination and radiation dose, use of a timed bolus or its equivalent helps to ensure optimum evaluation of the pulmonary arteries.

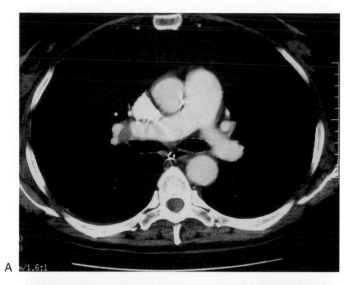

A

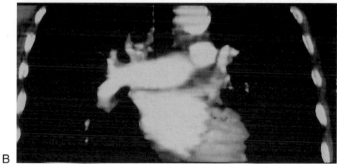

B

FIG. 9-21. Use of multiplanar reconstructions. **A:** A 3-mm section at the level of the bronchus intermedius shows an apparent filling defect in the right interlobar pulmonary artery. **B:** Multiplanar reconstruction shows that the right main, right interlobar, and right upper lobe pulmonary arteries are normal. The apparent filling defect in **A** is due to partial volume averaging (compare with Fig. 9-13). In select cases, use of multiplanar reconstructions may add to diagnostic certainty.

Data Display

As previously mentioned, viewing cases directly from the video monitor or computer workstation in place of hard copy has certain clear advantages. First, the ability to page through images in a cine mode, in particular, may be advantageous by determining whether a particular vessel is an artery or a vein. In addition, as already mentioned, instantaneous electronic windowing allows optimal selection of imaging parameters to enhance identification of partial volume artifacts that may mimic the appearance of small emboli. In one study comparing evaluation of studies on a dedicated workstation versus hard copy review, 25% more cases of PE were identified using cine paging (48).

An additional rationale for evaluating cases directly on computer workstations is the ability to generate multiplanar reconstructions. These require only minimal time and operator skill to generate and may be of particular value for assessing pulmonary arteries that course obliquely through the axial plane such as the middle lobe and lingular lobar arteries. As noted by Remy-Jardin and associates (69), in addition

to more precisely identifying the extent of thromboemboli, multiplanar reformations are of particular benefit for excluding PEs in otherwise inconclusive axial studies, especially when these studies are performed using 5-mm collimation (Fig. 9-21).

When hard-copy alone is available for interpretation, the clinician must use appropriate electronic windowing because small emboli may be obscured if windows or levels that are too narrow are used. Specifically, emboli are not identified when their attenuation exceeds the upper bound of the display window (Fig. 9-22). Brink and associates (70), using autologous emboli in 10 pigs, showed that whereas PEs typically have CT attenuation values of approximately 50 HU, their attenuation increases because of partial volume averaging with high-attenuation contrast material within the pulmonary artery. This potential pitfall can be avoided by using a display window referenced to the attenuation of a second-order pulmonary artery. Specifically, an optimal window width is obtained by selecting the mean attenuation value of the reference pulmonary artery plus 2 S.D., whereas an

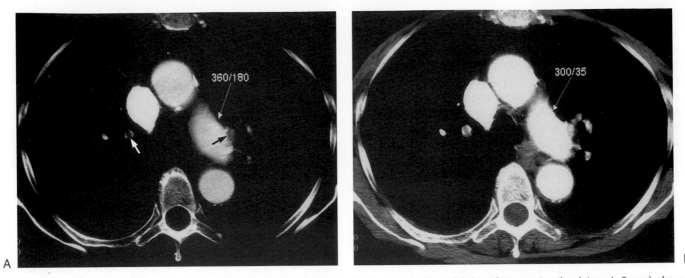

FIG. 9-22. Pulmonary emboli: role of electronic windowing. **A, B:** Identical 7-mm sections (pitch, 1.6; reconstruction interval, 6 mm) show evidence of pulmonary emboli within the right upper lobe apical segmental pulmonary artery and the left pulmonary artery (*arrows* in **A**). Theoretically, emboli are best visualized using a window width obtained by selecting the mean attenuation value of the reference pulmonary artery plus 2 S.D., with a window level obtained by dividing this number by two. In this case, the left main pulmonary artery measured 320 HU (S.D. = 20). Although images obtained by following the foregoing formula (i.e., a window of 360, and a level of 180) allow accurate identification of both right- and left-sided emboli, as shown in (**B**), identification of emboli in the left pulmonary artery is more difficult when images are evaluated with a narrower window and lower level (compare with **A**). Practically, this limitation is obviated when images are evaluated directly on screen monitors instead of on hard copy.

optimal level is obtained by dividing this number by two (70). Although window modification in this fashion should enhance identification of small PEs, as emphasized by Kuzo and Goodman (58), potential limitations include an increase in the conspicuity of artifacts resulting from image noise and especially motion. Again, these problems are obviated when studies are evaluated directly on the screen monitors instead of on film.

MR Technique

Whereas MR angiography (MRA) is a prolific topic from a research perspective, it has only recently demonstrated any relevant clinical utility for evaluating the pulmonary arteries. Although still rarely performed, MR apparently can be competitive with CT in a variety of clinical settings relating to pulmonary arterial disease. As a consequence, it is worthwhile exploring this technique in depth.

Early techniques, including cine gradient-echo (71–74), two dimensional (2D) (73,75–77) and three dimensional (3D) time-of-flight MRA (78,79), were ostensibly limited to the diagnosis of proximal disease because respiratory and cardiac motion precluded the evaluation of the distal pulmonary vasculature. Although image quality and diagnostic accuracy improved when 2D time-of-flight MRA was performed in conjunction with gadolinium chelates (80,81) and breath-holding (82–84), pulmonary MRA was still considered an orphan modality limited to research centers.

With the advent of high-performance gradient systems, an entire 3D data set, with higher spatial resolution than could be achieved with 2D techniques, can be obtained within a single breath-hold (85–92). This approach eliminates respiratory motion and thus allows visualization of distal vessels that would otherwise be obscured by blurring. In addition, signal averaging from multiple excitations of the 3D slab minimizes cardiac motion. These sequences also have short echo times (1 to 3 milliseconds), a feature that is advantageous because it results in less signal loss from flow-related spin dephasing and susceptibility artifacts resulting from air-tissue interfaces in the lungs (87). Because of saturation effects, these sequences must be performed with contrast agents that shorten the T1-relaxation rate of blood, usually gadolinium chelates (82,85). In addition, the development of specialized torso phased-array coils improves image quality by providing higher signal-to-noise ratio than available with the standard body coil (93,94). This increased signal-to-noise ratio can be traded off for higher spatial resolution, thus allowing imaging of the peripheral pulmonary vasculature as far distal as sixth-order branches (93).

Optimization of contrast-enhanced pulmonary MRA is technically challenging because multiple parameters need to be addressed (86). The patient's ability to suspend respiration is essential; at least a 20-second period of apnea is required. The use of supplemental oxygen by nasal cannula, during hyperventilation before scanning, can often augment breath-holding capabilities in debilitated patients. The longer the breath-hold, the more partitions can be performed, resulting in greater spatial resolution. However, because transit time through the pulmonary circulation is so rapid, longer acquisition times place considerable constraints on bolus timing. Because saturation pulses are generally ineffective in nulling the signal from gadolinium-enhanced blood, it is not currently possible to achieve pulmonary arterial enhancement, without concomitant pulmonary venous enhancement, unless a rapid, 2D time-resolved sequence with limited spatial resolution is performed.

Although these sequences have sufficient temporal resolution to demonstrate selective pulmonary artery enhancement and subsequent perfusion (95–98), poor spatial resolution precludes their use in depicting peripheral emboli. The use of partial fourier imaging, in conjunction with sequences that share the important central lines of k-space data, can offset the decreased spatial resolution inherent with ultrafast (<10-second) imaging (99).

At present, the optimal dose of gadolinium necessary to provide for consistent, high-quality pulmonary angiography has yet to be established. Meaney and colleagues (91) used 40 to 60 mL of gadolinium in conjunction with a coronal 3D gradient-echo sequence to diagnose PEs. The following parameters were used: TR/TE, 6.5/1.8 milliseconds; flip angle, 45 degrees; slab thickness, 8.4 to 11.2 cm with 32 partitions (3- to 4-mm slice thickness); 30- to 36-cm field-of-view resulting in a 27-second acquisition and a 2-mL per second injection rate; data acquisition commenced 7 to 10 seconds after the start of the bolus infusion. When compared with conventional pulmonary angiography, three blinded readers achieved sensitivities of 100%, 87%, and 75% and specificities of 95%, 100%, and 95%, respectively, for the diagnosis of PE. With optimized timing, lower doses of gadolinium chelates can probably be used without a reduction in image quality.

In addition to mastering the technical nuances of MRA, a firm knowledge of the benefits and disadvantages of the various postprocessing techniques currently available is also requisite. Although maximum intensity projection images most closely resemble conventional pulmonary angiograms, they may obscure emboli; this is because although this algorithm only detects those voxels with the highest signal intensity in a given ray tracing, emboli are uniformly low in signal intensity (Fig. 9-23A). As a consequence, emboli are best demonstrated as filling defects on the source images and multiplanar reformations (see Fig. 9-23B–D). Other postprocessing techniques have been used to evaluate CT angiography data, including surface rendering and virtual intraluminal endoscopy (100); although these techniques are currently available, their clinical utility has yet to be validated.

Acute Pulmonary Embolism

CT Findings

Accurate identification of acute PE requires thorough familiarity with hilar vascular anatomy. As noted in the section on normal anatomy, this identification is clearly facilitated by reference to bronchial anatomy. With the exception of the posterior subsegmental artery to the left upper lobe and the proximal portions of the lingular artery, all lobar, seg-

mental, and subsegmental arteries lie adjacent to corresponding bronchi. As a consequence, scans should always be interpreted using both narrow and wide windows. As a rule, arteries to the lower lobes, lingula, and middle lobe run lateral to their corresponding airways and medial to upper lobe bronchi and share with airways the fact that their appearance depends on their orientation (61). CT findings in patients with acute PEs have been extensively reviewed (57,58,101).

Vascular Changes

The most reliable criterion for diagnosing acute PE is the finding of an intraluminal filling defect. Characteristically, these defects are outlined at least in part by a thin rim of contrast and appear either as circular defects in vertically oriented arteries (or as free-floating masses in larger central arteries) or as serpiginous defects in horizontally oriented arteries (also described as a railroad track sign) (Fig. 9-24). This latter appearance is most commonly seen in patients with saddle PEs (Fig. 9-25). When present in obliquely oriented arteries, PEs may appear as eccentric filling defects, frequently forming acute angles with the contrast-filled lumen (see Fig. 9-25) (58). Less frequently, PEs result in complete cutoff of the lumen (Fig. 9-26). Diagnosis is facilitated in this setting by the realization that acute PEs usually result in expansion of the arterial lumen, a sign more easily recognized when assessed with lung windows (Fig. 9-27). As discussed later, nonfilling of a peripheral pulmonary artery, especially when seen only on a single axial image, should not be misinterpreted as evidence of a PE.

Parenchymal and Pleural Changes

In addition to vascular changes, certain ancillary parenchymal changes may be identified in patients with acute PEs. These changes include areas of both increased and decreased lung attenuation, as well as wedge-shaped pleural-based areas of parenchymal consolidation, linear bands, and atelectasis (Fig. 9-28). Coche and associates (102), in assessing the diagnostic value of these findings in 88 patients with suspected PE, found that peripheral wedge-shaped densities suggestive of pulmonary infarcts could be identified in 16 (62%) of 26 patients subsequently documented to have PE. In comparison, wedge-shaped areas of consolidation were identified in only 17 (27%) of 62 without PE. This finding is especially surprising given that pulmonary infarction has been estimated to occur in only approximately 10% of patients with acute PEs (101). In this regard, although most of the wedge-shaped areas of consolidation noted by Coche and associates corresponded to the distribution of segmental emboli, this association was not invariable. Not surprisingly, none of the other CT signs mentioned earlier proved to be significant indicators of acute PE. Similarly, whereas pleural effusions are commonly identified in patients with documented PE, this finding in itself is of limited diagnostic value.

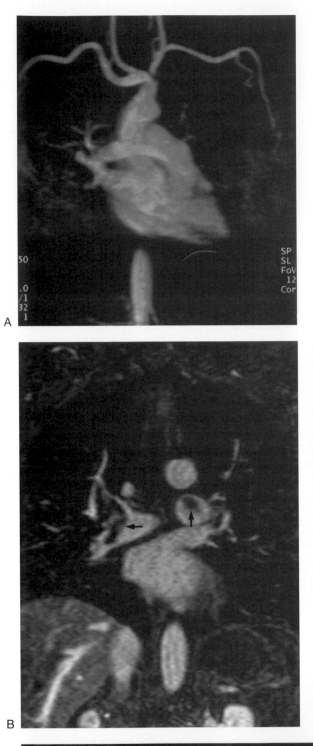

A

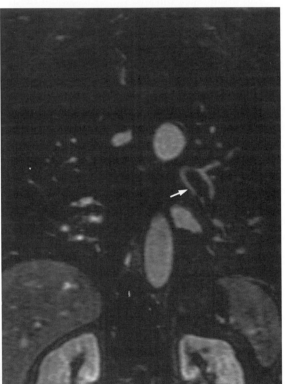

FIG. 9-23. Acute pulmonary embolus: MR evaluation. **A:** Maximum intensity projection image from a breath-hold gadolinium-enhanced three dimensional MR angiogram (TR/TE 5/2 ms) demonstrates almost no peripheral pulmonary vasculature, with the exception of some right upper lobe vessels. **B, C:** Source images from same three dimensional data set demonstrate emboli in the main, right, and left pulmonary arteries (*arrows*). **D:** Axial reformation from same three dimensional data set demonstrates emboli in the right and left main pulmonary arteries.

B

C

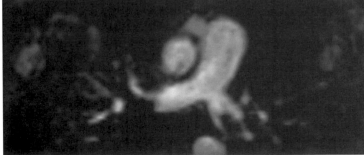

D

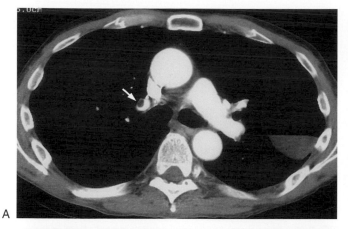

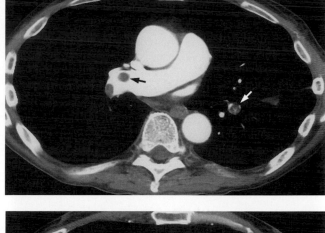

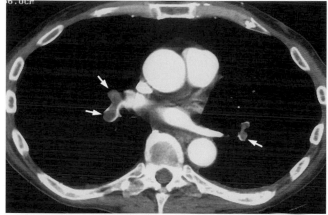

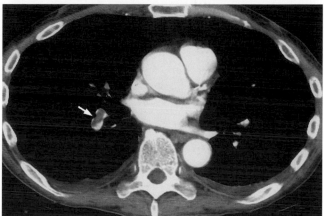

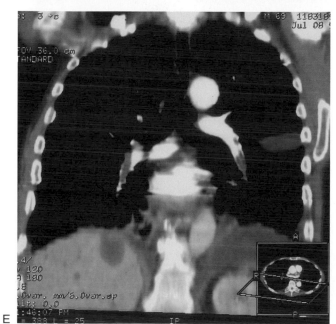

FIG. 9-24. Acute pulmonary emboli: CT findings. **A–D:** Select images from a pulmonary embolism study (3-mm collimation; pitch, 2; reconstruction interval, 2 mm), obtained after bolus administration of 120 mL 60% nonionic contrast media (15-second delay). Multiple pulmonary emboli are present (*arrows*) identifiable as discrete filling defects outlined, at least in part, by a thin rim of contrast. A small loculated effusion is present within the left major fissure. **E:** Multiplanar reconstruction shows to good advantage that the circular filling defects identified in **A–D** actually represent elongated thrombi, presumably originating from the deep femoral veins.

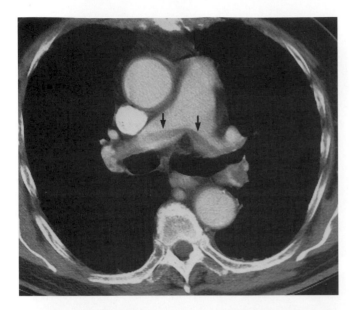

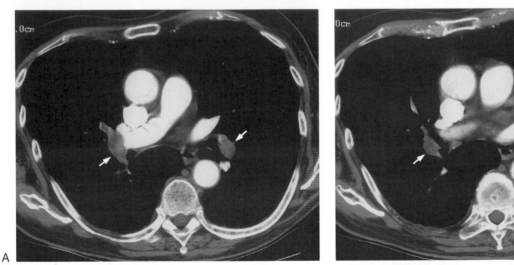

A   B

FIG. 9-26. Acute pulmonary emboli: CT appearance. A, B: Select images obtained from a pulmonary embolism study (3-mm collimation; pitch, 2; reconstruction interval, 2 mm) after a bolus of 120 mL 60% nonionic contrast media (20-second delay). In this case, clot obliterates both the left and right pulmonary arteries (*arrows* in A and B). Note the presence of a serpiginous filling defect within the middle lobe bronchus outlined by a thin rim of contrast (*curved arrow* in A).

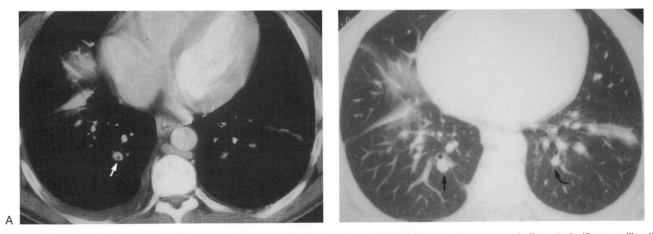

A   B

FIG. 9-27. Acute pulmonary emboli: CT appearance. A, B: Identical sections obtained from a pulmonary embolism study (5-mm collimation; pitch, 2; reconstruction interval, 4 mm), obtained after bolus administration of 120 mL 60% nonionic contrast media (20-second delay) imaged with narrow and wide windows, respectively. A discrete filling defect is present within the posterobasilar segmental artery on the right (*arrow* in A). This results in expansion of the pulmonary artery (*arrow* in B) easily identifiable on wide windows, especially by comparison with the contralateral normal basilar pulmonary arteries (*curved arrow* in B). Bilateral foci of nonspecific linear atelectasis are also apparent.

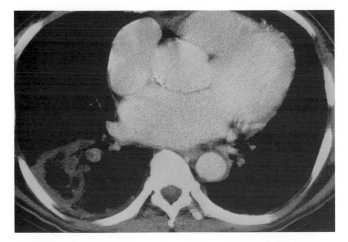

FIG. 9-28. Acute pulmonary emboli: pulmonary infarction. A 5-mm section through the right lower lobe shows a sharply defined, wedge-shaped peripheral density in the right lower lobe associated with a discrete filling defect within the right lower lobe pulmonary artery characteristic of pulmonary infarction.

Diagnostic Pitfalls

Certain potential pitfalls may lead to an erroneous diagnosis of acute PEs. These may result both from technical and patient-related factors.

Technical Factors. Despite its proved accuracy for assessing PE, it has nevertheless been estimated that in approximately 5% to 10% of cases, CT scans are nondiagnostic because of technical factors (58). Among these, most important are those related to breathing artifacts and suboptimal contrast enhancement (57). Variation in respiration may occur both in studies performed with quiet breathing as well as during ostensibly breath-held acquisitions. The result is partial volume averaging, especially of smaller arteries that course in the same plane as the CT scan causing an abrupt change in the attenuation of arteries in two contiguous sec-

tions. Avoidance of this pitfall is usually possible, provided suspect arteries are further evaluated using wide windows to confirm the presence of breathing artifacts.

Also problematic are pitfalls related to suboptimal contrast enhancement. Clearly, improperly timed acquisitions after contrast administration may lead to incomplete vascular opacification, because of the arrival of contrast material either too early (resulting in incomplete opacification of lower lobe arteries) or too late (resulting in potential pseudofilling defects in upper lobe arteries) (Fig. 9-29). As important, improper timing may lead to unnecessary confusion between arteries and veins. As previously noted, these problems may be obviated by use of a timed bolus; alternatively, additional images may be obtained after completion of initial scan acquisition using a second bolus of contrast material.

Patient Factors. Less well appreciated are problems that arise as a consequence of hemodynamic alterations within the pulmonary circulation. These have been extensively reviewed by Remy-Jardin and Remy (103). Most important are unilateral alterations in pulmonary vascular resistance resulting from atelectasis or pleural effusions (51). Local alterations in pulmonary artery pressure may result in incomplete opacification of peripheral pulmonary arteries, in particular. Similar changes have been described in patients with congestive heart failure who also may be found to have peripheral rims of low density surrounding central pulmonary arteries as a result of interstitial edema. Despite this problem, one of the clear advantages of CT compared with other imaging modalities is the ability to identify peripheral emboli in patients with underlying pleural and parenchymal abnormalities. The presence of these abnormalities should not discourage one from performing CT pulmonary angiography.

In addition to changes caused by alterations in pulmonary vascular resistance, intraluminal filling defects may also result from infection (Fig. 9-30) or, more commonly, malig-

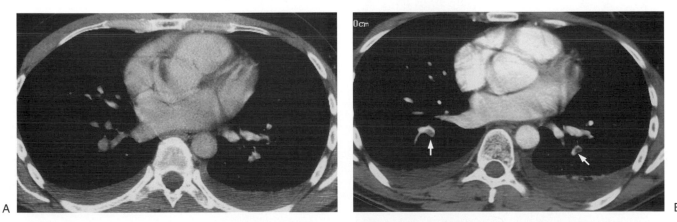

A   B

FIG. 9-29. Diagnostic pitfalls: suboptimal contrast enhancement. **A:** Section through the inferior pulmonary hila (3-mm collimation; pitch, 1.6) reconstructed using an edge-enhancing algorithm obtained after administration of 120 mL 60% nonionic contrast media using a 20-second delay. Note the suboptimal enhancement of the pulmonary arteries, thus making a definitive diagnosis of pulmonary emboli difficult. **B:** Section at nearly the identical level as in (**A**) the following day, obtained with the same technique, shows unequivocal evidence of bilateral pulmonary emboli (*arrows*). In this case, an initial test bolus showed that optimal contrast enhancement of the pulmonary arteries occurred at 10 seconds. Although these images were reconstructed with a standard instead of an edge-enhancing algorithm, improved visualization of the emboli is clearly due to improved contrast enhancement.

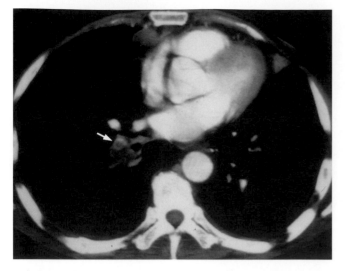

FIG. 9-30. Diagnostic pitfalls: invasive aspergillosis. A 5-mm section shows evidence of an ill-defined heterogeneous mass in the right hilum associated with a discrete filling defect within the right lower lobe pulmonary artery (*arrow*). In this case, these changes were due to invasive aspergillosis in a patient with AIDS.

nancy (Fig. 9-31). In this latter category are included patients with direct arterial encasement or invasion, as well as patients with intraluminal metastases (Fig. 9-32). Rarely, intraluminal filling defects may be the result of primary neoplasia, in particular pulmonary artery sarcomas (Fig. 9-33) (104,105). In these rare cases, a diagnosis of tumor may be suggested by noting contrast enhancement within intraluminal masses, indicative of neovascularity (106,107). Another potential pitfall in diagnosing acute PE is the presence of focal areas of mucoid impaction (Fig. 9-34) (58). These areas

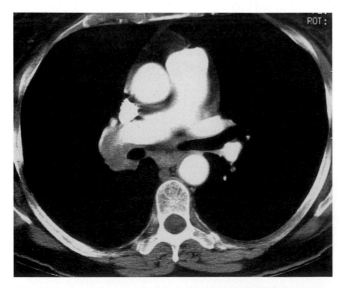

FIG. 9-31. Acute pulmonary emboli: diagnostic pitfalls. A 5-mm section through the right hilum shows increased soft tissue density associated with narrowing of the right interlobar pulmonary artery. In this case, these changes were due to bronchogenic carcinoma arising in the right hilum.

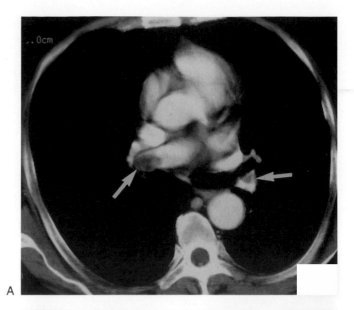

A

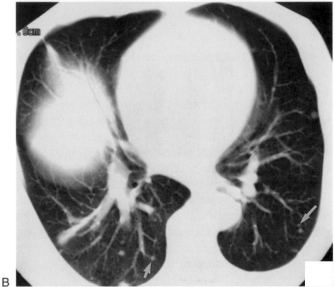

B

FIG. 9-32. Diagnostic pitfalls: tumor emboli. **A:** A 5-mm section through the lower lobes in a patient with known duodenal carcinoma shows the presence of bilateral small, well-defined nodules either adjacent to vessels or subpleural in location (*arrows*). This appearance strongly suggests metastatic disease. **B:** Section through the hilum shows discrete filling defects in both the right and left interlobar pulmonary arteries (*arrows*) consistent with the presence of tumor thrombi. In this case, 10-mm thick sections were obtained with a pitch of 1 after a bolus of 100 mL 60% nonionic contrast media after a 20-second delay. Overlapping reconstructions every 5 mm were retrospectively obtained only after recognition of intrapulmonary artery filling defects. With the increase in use of volumetric scanners, serendipitous identification of pulmonary thrombi is being increasingly reported. One of the advantages of volumetric data acquisition is the ability to reconstruct images retrospectively anywhere within the initial data set without the need for acquiring new images or reinjecting contrast. (From ref. 172, with permission.)

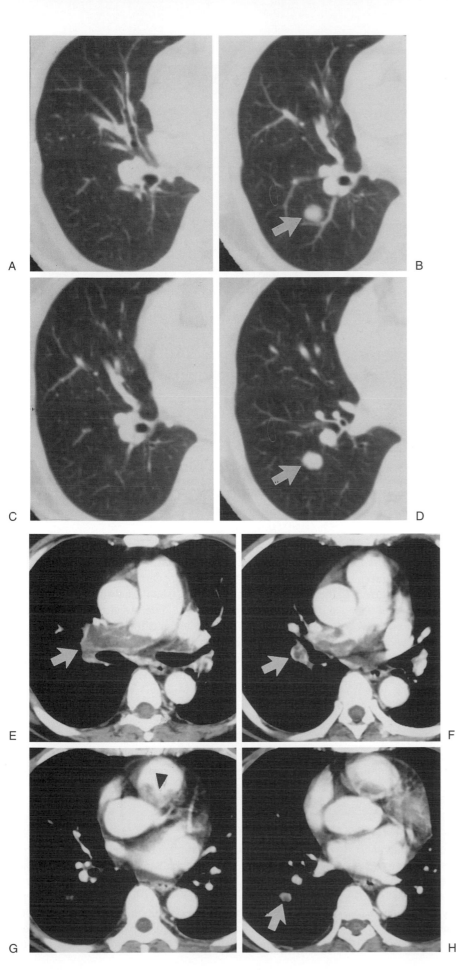

FIG. 9-33. Diagnostic pitfalls: pulmonary artery sarcoma. **A–D:** Enlargements of sequential volumetrically obtained 5-mm sections through the inferior portion of the right hilum shows two discrete, otherwise nondescript nodules in the right lower lobe (*arrows* in **B** and **D**). **E–H:** Select 5-mm images obtained 20 seconds after a bolus of 100 mL 60% nonionic contrast media at a rate of 2 mL per second show the presence of an irregular filling defect within the main (*arrowhead* in **G**) and both the right (*arrows* in **E** and **F**) and left pulmonary arteries. At biopsy, this lesion proved to be a primary pulmonary artery sarcoma. At least one of the nodules identified in the right lower lobe has the same density as the tumor noted throughout the right and left main pulmonary arteries (compare *arrow* in **H** with *arrow* in **D**), a finding suggesting that this may actually represent tumor within a focally distended pulmonary artery branch. (From ref. 172, with permission.)

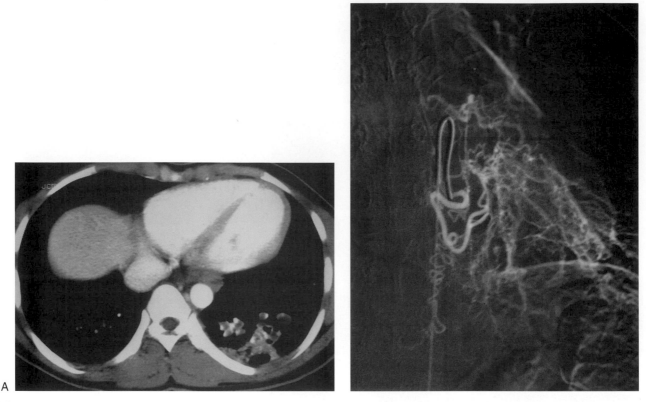

FIG. 9-34. Diagnostic pitfalls: mucoid impaction. **A:** A 5-mm section shows apparent filling defects within the left lower lobe in this patient presenting with hemoptysis. Although this appearance superficially mimics pulmonary emboli, in fact, this patient has long-standing bronchiectasis with extensive mucoid impaction of the lower lobe airways. **B:** Select view from a bronchial arteriogram shows marked hypertrophy of bronchial arteries accounting for this patient's hemoptysis.

result in tubular or branching structures that superficially mimic the appearance of thrombi. Again, evaluation is simplified when abnormalities are viewed with wide (lung) windows that allow precise delineation of bronchial anatomy.

Most important as a cause of potential interpretive errors, however, is the presence of lymphatic tissue within the hila. Differentiation between nodes and eccentric mural thrombi, in particular, may be especially difficult. Thorough familiarity with the cross-sectional appearance of hilar nodes is a prerequisite to accurate evaluation of PE (8,39). In this regard, investigators have noted that nodes in particular locations are most likely to cause confusion, especially in patients with suspected chronic PE (58). Most problematic is the level just lateral to the point at which the right main pulmonary artery bifurcates into the anterior trunk and the right interlobar pulmonary artery (40), especially in cases evaluated with 5-mm or greater collimation (see Fig. 9-21). Other difficult areas to interpret include the area between the superior segmental artery of the right lower lobe and the bronchus intermedius (see Fig. 9-14), the area between the apicoposterior segmental bronchus and the posterior subsegmental artery to the left upper lobe (see Fig. 9-16), and the area between the trunk of the pulmonary artery to the anterior segment of the right upper lobe and the anterior aspect of the right upper lobe bronchus and proximal portion of the

anterior segmental bronchus to the right upper lobe (see Fig. 9-11). Familiarity with the appearance of small nodes in these locations, in particular, should help to minimize the number of false-positive CT interpretations. In selected cases, especially those in which 5-mm sections have been obtained, use of multiplanar reconstructions may be of value; alternatively, these same areas may be rescanned using 2- to 3-mm sections with a pitch of 1, reconstructed every 1 mm.

Diagnostic Evaluation

Traditionally, the diagnosis of acute PE has rested on a combination of clinical, radiographic, scintigraphic, angiographic, and venographic criteria.

Clinical Evaluation

Clinical diagnosis is contingent on recognition of a combination of symptoms and signs related to both the chest and lower extremities. Because PEs almost always result from deep venous thrombosis (DVT), it is more appropriate to discuss venous thromboembolism than PE. Investigators have estimated that more than 500,00 patients a year develop acute PEs, corresponding to a population-based estimate of

21 patients in 100,00. Venous thromboembolism is the third most common cardiovascular disease and, as such, is a frequent cause of morbidity and mortality (108). Investigators have estimated that approximately 10% of patients with acute PE do not survive their initial event; of those who survive, nearly 70% are estimated to go undiagnosed, resulting in a mortality of 30% (109).

Although initial clinical assessment is critical to diagnosis, unfortunately signs and symptoms are neither sensitive nor specific. This includes the finding of both a widened alveolar-arterial oxygen pressure gradient as well as elevated arterial carbon dioxide. Although these findings are present in nearly 90% of cases of acute PE, investigators nevertheless have estimated that only approximately 30% of patients clinically suspected of having PE actually prove to have PE (110).

Of considerable clinical importance is recognition that certain populations are at greater risk for developing venous thromboembolism. These include patients with a history of recent surgery, trauma, congestive heart failure, immobilization, pregnancy, use of oral contraceptives, and underlying malignancy (110). Patients with previously documented venous thromboembolism are also at greater risk.

Chest Radiography

Chest radiographic findings have been described and include regional oligemia (Westermark sign), peripheral, pleural-based, wedge-shaped areas of increased lung density (Hampton hump), and prominence of central pulmonary arteries (Fleischner sign). Unfortunately, these signs are neither sensitive or specific. Although cavitation may occur in patients with infarction, the presence of a cavity should raise the possibility of coexisting infection.

Pulmonary Scintigraphy

In most institutions, the mainstay for the diagnosis of PE has been ventilation/perfusion (V/Q) lung scanning. Although perfusion lung scanning is extremely sensitive, the specificity of this test is low. As documented by the Prospective Investigation of Pulmonary Embolism Diagnosis (PIOPED) study, V/Q studies are of greatest utility when interpreted as either normal or near normal, effectively ruling out PE, or high probability, in which the likelihood of PE is greater than 95% (111). Together, however, these categories represent only approximately 40% of cases. Of the 755 patients in the PIOPED study in whom pulmonary angiographic correlation was available, only 116 (13%) with documented PE had a high-probability scan (overall specificity only 10%).

The finding of a low- or intermediate-probability scan does not constitute sufficient evidence upon which to base treatment (110). Altogether, 66% of patients with indeterminate V/Q scans and 40% of patients with low-probability scans in the PIOPED study subsequently proved to have PE

(Fig. 9-35) (111). The value of lung scans is further limited in patients with underlying emphysema, or a history of prior PE. The value of low-probability lung scan in particular has been questioned especially in patients with underlying cardiopulmonary disease. As documented by Hull et al. in a prospective study of 77 consecutive patients with low-probability lung scans and impaired cardiorespiratory reserve, 6 (7.8%) died within days of their scans with autopsy evidence of pulmonary emboli (112).

The value of an indeterminate lung scan is further diminished by the finding of considerable interobserver variability, even among experienced readers. While agreement in the PIOPED study proved excellent for high-probability (95%) and normal or near normal scans (94% and 92%, respectively), reader agreement for indeterminate scans ranged only between 70% and 75% (111). More recently, in a preliminary report from a European multicenter evaluation of PE, of the first 401 patients meeting the study protocol criteria for inclusion (including evaluation with lung scans, spiral CT and angiography), interobserver variability for V/Q scintigraphy also proved to be low [k = 40 (range: 0.3–0.49)] (113).

Attempts to improve the accuracy of V/Q scans have led to proposals for revising the original PIOPED criteria. The specific intent of these proposals has been to decrease the number of intermediate probability scans, mainly by reassigning patients with multiple matched defects and normal chest radiographs to a low-probability category (114). Applying these criteria to a select population of patients specifically referred for pulmonary angiography, Sostman and coworkers (115) have documented significant improved accuracy. For example, 20 patients who previously would have been interpreted as having intermediate-probability scans using the original PIOPED criteria, were reclassified in this study as having low-probability scans using revised criteria. None proved to have angiographic evidence of PE (115). Altogether, there was a 15% decrease in the number of intermediate-probability scans reported. Furthermore, as noted by the authors, it is likely that their results would have been still better if additional revisions had been employed, including in particular reclassifying scans as low-probability with matched ventilation, perfusion, and radiographic abnormalities restricted to the mid- and upper lung fields (115). Perhaps most important has been the realization that criteria for interpreting scans should be stratified according to patients' underlying cardiopulmonary status and clinical likelihood of having PE (116).

Despite these modifications, however, significant differences between readers of varying skill levels persist. In fact, as reported by Sostman et al., among experienced readers, so-called "gestalt" estimates of the percentage of probability of PE outperformed both the standard and revised PIOPED criteria. In part this reflects the fact that accurate interpretation of V/Q scans is dependent on recognition of indirect signs, and not direct identification of the presence of PEs. As recently confirmed by Breslaw et al., of 185

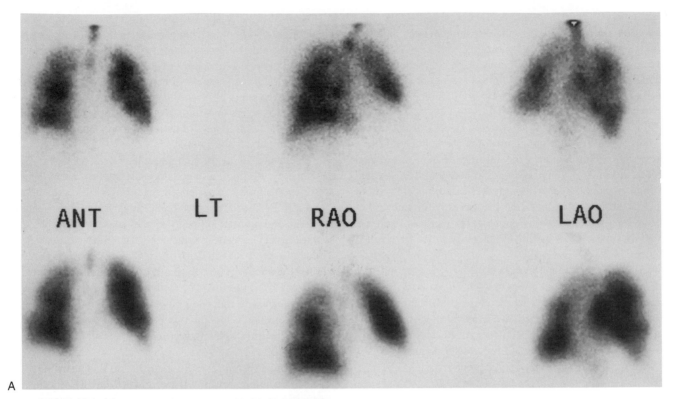

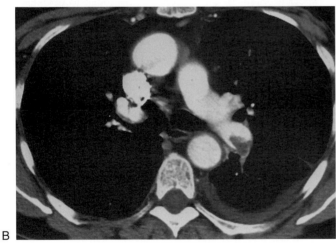

FIG. 9-35. Acute pulmonary emboli: correlation between CT and ventilation–perfusion (V/Q) study. **A:** Select anterior and oblique views from a V/Q study interpreted as intermediate probability for pulmonary embolism. **B:** A 3-mm section demonstrates a large filling defect through the left interlobar pulmonary artery.

perfusion defects identified in 68 patients, only 16% correlated anatomically with angiographic findings (117). Specifically, only 10 of 35 segmental or larger ventilation-perfusion mismatches proved to be due to angiographically documented emboli, while 43 segmental defects identified angiographically had no evidence of mismatches on corresponding V/Q studies.

Pulmonary Angiography

Pulmonary angiography traditionally has been held up as the standard for the diagnosis of PE. In fact, this examination has important limitations. First, pulmonary angiography is grossly underused. Investigators have estimated that only

between 15% and 50% of patients with indeterminate V/Q studies go on to pulmonary angiography. As documented by Khorasani and associates (118), in a retrospective review of 214 patients with clinically suspected PE and indeterminate V/Q scans, pulmonary angiograms were obtained in only 55 (26%), 19 of which proved positive. This, despite the fact that pulmonary angiography is well documented to have low morbidity (2%) and mortality (<1%) (111).

As important, interobserver agreement should be deemed unacceptably low. As documented in the PIOPED study, although the overall interobserver agreement for the diagnosis of central PE was 81%, this decreased to only 66% in patients with subsegmental emboli (111). Although various techniques have been proposed to enhance the accuracy of pulmonary angiography including cineangiography, balloon-occlusion angiography, and superselective angiography (119), these techniques are not widely used. When pulmonary angiography is indicated, reliance on injections into the main pulmonary artery only with single-projection angiography should be discouraged.

Venography

Clinical detection of deep venous thrombosis is unreliable; nearly 50% of patients with documented venous thrombosis have neither signs nor symptoms of disease (120). As a corollary, between 40% and 60% of patients with DVT can be shown to have silent PE (120). At present, several tests are available for assessing DVT. Those most widely used include positive contrast venography, color duplex sonography, and impedance plethysmography. Each has documented limitations. Positive contrast venography is the current standard for identification of venous thrombosis. Nonetheless, incomplete venous filling and other technical problems limit interpretation in up to 5% of cases, whereas in nearly 10%, interobserver disagreement occurs (121). Some evidence also indicates that contrast venography itself may induce venous thrombosis. Finally, contrast venography is less than accurate for assessing pelvic veins and the inferior vena cava.

In many institutions, color duplex sonography is now used in place of contrast venography as an initial means for assessing venous thrombosis (122). In addition to direct visualization of intraluminal clot, ancillary diagnostic criteria have been proposed, including assessing variations in vessels size after the Valsalva maneuver and, in particular, lack of compressibility (123). Although color-coded duplex sonography has been shown to have a sensitivity and specificity in the range of 95% for deep femoral and popliteal thrombi, it is less accurate for assessing calf and pelvic veins (121). Impedance plethysmography measures changes in the electrical impedance of a limb caused by altered venous flow resulting from venous obstruction. As such, it is nonspecific for acute DVT. Furthermore, optimal evaluation requires that if the initial study is normal, serial studies must be performed over a 2-week period.

Unfortunately, regardless of the type of examination, approximately 40% of patients with documented PE have no evidence of venous thrombi. Most often, this situation results from complete separation of clot from peripheral veins (124). Controversy exists concerning the significance of calf vein thrombi as compared with deep femoral venous thrombi. Although some investigators have argued that peripheral calf vein thrombi are clinically insignificant, others have noted that these ultimately lead to clot within more proximal veins (125).

CT Evaluation

To date, prospective studies have documented the utility of spiral–helical CT for assessing patients with suspected acute PE (49–54,62,65). Overall, these studies show that CT is an accurate method for detecting or excluding central PEs (Table 9-2).

At present, the greatest limitation of CT angiography has been in detecting emboli at the segmental and subsegmental

TABLE 9-2. *Prospective accuracy of CT for diagnosis of acute pulmonary emboli*

Study (reference)	Technique	Sensitivity (%)	Specificity (%)	Prevalence (%)
Remy-Jardin et al. (n = 42) (49)	5-mm sections; pitch, 1; RI, 3 mm	100	96	43
Teigen et al. (n = 60) (63)	Contiguous 6.75-mm sections (electron-beam CT)	75	98	38
Remy-Jardin et al. (n = 75) (52)	Both 5-mm sections; pitch, 1; RI, 3 mm; and 3-mm sections; pitch, 1.7; RI, 2 mm	91	78	52
Goodman et al. (n = 20) (51)	5-mm sections; pitch, 1; RI, NS	86 (central emboli); 63 (subsegmental)	92 (central emboli); 89 (subsegmental)	35
Van Rossum et al. (n = 77) (53)	5-mm sections; pitch, 1; RI, 4 mm	97	98	24
Mayo et al. (n = 142) (54)	3 mm; pitch, 1.8–2.0; RI, 1.5–3 mm	87	95	33
Garg et al. (n = 54[a]) (65)	3-mm sections; pitch, 2; RI, NS	67	100	25
Sostman et al. (n = 28[b]) (121)	5-mm sections; pitch, 1; RI, NS	Range, 62–92 (average, 75)	Range 73–100 (average, 89)	24

NS, not specified. RI, reconstruction interval.
[a] Sensitivity and specificity reported only for 26 patients with angiographic correlation.
[b] Sensitivity and specificity data reported independently for 5 readers.
Modified from ref. 103.

level. Using 5-mm sections, Goodman and associates (51) noted that whereas the sensitivity and specificity of CT for detecting central emboli were 86% and 92%, respectively, these numbers decreased to 63% and 89%, respectively, for subsegmental emboli. The failure to identify segmental and subsegmental arteries routinely using 5-mm sections is well documented. Ferretti and colleagues (62) found that of a total of 3,280 potentially analyzable segmental pulmonary arteries, 2,558 (78%) could be identified using 5-mm collimation (reconstruction interval, 2.5 mm). Overall, the mean number of segmental arteries identifiable per patient was 15.6 of 20 (62).

Assessment of segmental arteries is considerably enhanced with use of 3-mm collimation (Fig. 9-36); nonetheless, limitations remain. As documented by Remy-Jardin and colleagues (61), although CT allowed visualization of a mean of 17 (85%) of 20 potentially analyzable segmental pulmonary arteries, only a mean of 14. 8 (37%) of 40 potentially analyzable subsegmental arteries could be adequately assessed. The inability of helical CT to identify small peripheral emboli even when 3-mm collimation is used has been documented. As reported by Garg and associates (65) in a small series of 24 patients with angiographically documented PE, the prospective sensitivity of CT for detecting segmental or subsegmental PE was only 67%.

Both the incidence and, as important, the significance of subsegmental PEs are controversial. In a retrospective angiographic study, Oser and associates (126) identified PEs exclusively at the subsegmental level in 30% of cases. Similar data have been reported in prospective studies comparing CT with angiography (51,59). As documented in the more extensive PIOPED study, however, only 6% of patients with PE had thromboemboli limited to subsegmental arteries, and of these, fewer than 1% went on to develop recurrent PEs (111).

The significance of isolated subsegmental PEs is in doubt, especially in patients without underlying cardiopulmonary disease or evidence of associated DVT. Although investigators have frequently stated that the mortality rate in patients with untreated PEs is 30%, compared with 8% in treated patients, and the rate of recurrence is also higher in untreated patients (127), as reviewed by Egermayer and Town (109), few data, in fact, substantiate this claim. As documented by Hull and associates (112), among untreated patients without evidence of deep vein thrombosis, the recurrence rate was less than 2%. Similarly, Stein and coworkers (128), in a review of data from the PIOPED study, noted that when the 20 untreated patients, all with mild V/Q abnormalities, were compared with treated patients with similar V/Q abnormalities, no significant difference could be found either in mortality or morbidity. Based on these data, it would seem that missing isolated subsegmental PEs may only be of significance in patients with cardiovascular disease in whom even a small embolus may be clinically significant.

CT Venography

Investigators have proposed that routine contrast venography be replaced by CT venography. Baldt and associates (122) evaluated 52 consecutive patients with clinically suspected DVT by injecting a dorsal vein in each foot using dilute contrast media after which images were obtained from the ankles to the diaphragms. These authors noted a sensitivity of 100% and a specificity of 96% for CT venography: in two cases, thrombi within the inferior vena cava were identified only with CT venography. As noted by the authors of this study, potential advantages of CT venography include an 80% reduction in contrast load, increased sensitivity and specificity for evaluating pelvic and deep femoral veins, and less risk of phlebitis. Although CT venography remains to be established as a routine clinical tool, one modification suggested that is likely to gain widespread acceptance is the

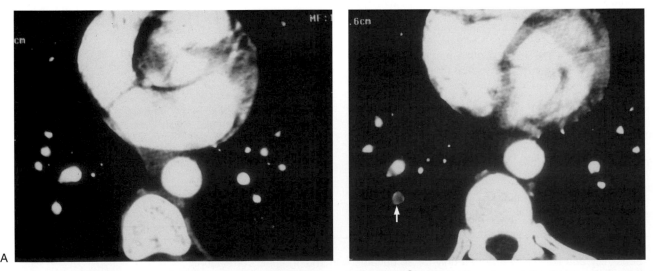

FIG. 9-36. Segmental pulmonary emboli: CT evaluation. **A, B:** Enlargments of sequential 3-mm sections through the right lower lobe show the presence of an isolated, discrete filling defect within the posterobasilar segmental artery (*arrow* in **B**).

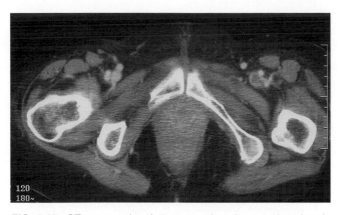

FIG. 9-37. CT venography. A 7-mm section shows a thrombus in the femoral vein in a patient with CT evidence of pulmonary emboli. Although acquisition of additional images through the abdomen, pelvis, and thigh after a routine pulmonary embolism study without administration of additional contrast media has been advocated by some investigators as an important component of CT evaluation of patients with clinically suspect pulmonary emboli, this remains to be verified.

idea of combined CT venography and pulmonary angiography. As first proposed by Loud and associates (55), instead of separate examinations, after routine CT pulmonary angiography, additional selected images are obtained every 5 cm from the diaphragms to the knees without additional contrast administration (Fig. 9-37). In an evaluation of 26 patients referred for CT angiography for suspected PE, DVT was detected in 8 patients, including 1 patient with inferior vena caval thombus; in distinction, PEs were documented in only 5 patients.

MR Evaluation

To date, several reports have addressed the accuracy of MR to diagnose PE, with conflicting results (80,91,129). In an early study using subsecond contrast-enhanced MRA, Loubeyre and associates (80) evaluted 23 consecutive patients with suspected PE and were able to identify all central PEs subsequently identified on pulmonary angiography. In distinction, MR was unable to identify emboli in peripheral arteries (see Fig. 9-23).

Similarly, Sostman and associates (129) compared contrast-enhanced helical CT with gradient-echo MR and found that among five readers of varying skill levels, the average sensitivity and specificity of CT were 75% and 89% ($n = 28$), respectively, whereas the average sensitivity and specificity of MR were 46% and 90%, respectively ($n = 25$). However, when data from experienced MR readers were evaluated, sensitivity and specificity improved to 71% and 97%, respectively. The low sensitivity of CT reported in this study is consistent with use of 5-mm collimation with a pitch of 1.

In comparison, Meaney and associates (91), in a study of 30 consecutive patients with suspected PE evaluated with both 3D gadolinium-enhanced, gradient-echo MR and angi-

ography reported that all 5 lobar and 16 of 17 segmental emboli identified by angiography were also identified by MR. Although these results are intriguing, determining the true clinical value of MR for assessing acute PE must await further validation.

Current Indications for CT Evaluation

Given the limitations of the various tests available for assessing patients with suspected venous thromboembolism, what should be the role of CT? Although definitive assessment remains to be established, the use of CT has certain compelling advantages. These include:

1. Direct visualization of PEs. The ability to identify PEs directly represents the single most important advantage of CT when compared with other imaging modalities. Furthermore, in the near future, improvements in scanner design clearly will allow contiguous 1- to 2-mm sections to be acquired in an even shorter period over considerably larger anatomic regions of interest than currently available. This capability ensures that CT will be both sensitive and specific for detecting even subsegmental PEs. These improvements should also have the additional beneficial effect of decreasing the number of inconclusive CT studies to less than the current estimate of 5% to 10%.

2. High interobserver agreement. As already noted, substantial interobserver disagreement has been documented, especially for interpreting indeterminate V/Q scans and identification of subsegmental PEs with pulmonary angiography. This finding has been further substantiated by preliminary data from a prospective multi-center European Pulmonary Embolism Trial (ESTIPEP) (113). Of 401 patients evaluated to date with V/Q scans, spiral CT and pulmonary angiography (performed in cases with intermediate- or low-probability V/Q scans as well as patients with discordant scintigraphic and CT results), interobserver agreement was significantly better for CT ($k = .71$) than for either V/Q scintigraphy ($k = .40$) or pulmonary angiography ($k = .35$). These data are comparable to similar findings reported by previous authors and represent an important advantage of CT angiography.

3. Added diagnostic accuracy resulting from simultaneous visualization of the entire thorax. As outlined previously, in a substantial percentage of cases, CT provides additional information, including otherwise unsuspected areas of pulmonary infarction, not identified by either routine chest radiographs or V/Q scans. In patients with either pleural or paranchymal abnormalities, CT still allows identification of central pulmonary emboli when other modalities would be more limited.

Given these advantages, we recommend the following guidelines for evaluating patients with suspected PE:

1. As suggested by Gefter and Palevsky (130), in patients without evidence of underlying cardiopulmonary disease

with a low clinical suspicion of PE, initial evaluation with V/Q scanning should remain the imaging procedure of choice. This recommendation is justified by the greater likelihood of a normal V/Q study combined with the high negative predictive value of this test result.

2. All other patients referred for diagnostic imaging with clinically suspected PE should be initially evaluated with CT. Given the advantages outlined earlier, little justification exists for first obtaining V/Q scans. Of particular concern is the well-documented finding that indeterminate V/Q scans are only intermittently followed by a more definitive imaging test. As emphasized by Rosenow (110), before therapy is instituted, a definitive diagnosis of venous thromboembolism must be established. Despite this recommendation, as documented by Khorasani and colleagues (118), all too often, clinical decisions are made based only on indeterminate V/Q scans. In this retrospective study of the medical records of 214 consecutive patients with clinically suspected PE and indeterminate V/Q scans, whereas treatment was instituted in 66 (331%), only 37% of these patients were treated on the basis of a definitive imaging test. Nearly identical results have been published by Murchison and associates (131). In their retrospective study of 94 patients with indeterminate V/Q studies identified over a 2-year period in Scotland for whom follow-up data were available, these authors showed that whereas 51 (55%) of these patients had no further workup, 19 (37%) were "unequivocally" diagnosed as having had PE, 18 of whom were treated with anticoagulant therapy.

3. CT studies should be complemented by an evaluation for venous thrombosis. Although an exact sequence has yet to be validated, a logical suggestion is that Doppler ultrasound or contrast venography should be performed first in patients with clinical signs or symptoms of venous thrombo-sis, whereas CT angiography should be performed first in patients with clinically suspect PE. This strategy has been shown to be cost-effective. Using a model created for analyzing the cost-effectiveness of available diagnostic algorithms for all realistic values of the pretest probability of PE using V/Q scans, ultrasound, D-dimer assay, conventional pulmonary angiography, and spiral CT (assuming a sensitivity of 88%), van Erkel and associates (132) showed that the single best strategy combined CT and ultrasound. Pending further validation, routine acquisition of combined CT angiography and venography may be anticipated to reduce the number of ultrasound examinations or contrast venograms performed.

4. Pulmonary angiography is reserved for those patients with limited cardiopulmonary reserve in whom the diagnosis of a subsegmental PE may be significant, or it may be used as a follow-up in patients with nondiagnostic CT examinations.

Chronic Pulmonary Embolism

In most cases, acute PEs resolve without sequelae. However, in approximately 5% of cases, lysis fails, with resultant incomplete resolution of clot. With organization, arteries become narrowed or occluded. Rarely this results in chronic pulmonary hypertension.

To date, several studies have described the range of CT findings in patients with chronic PE (133–136). As in patients with acute PE, these findings may be divided into two broad categories: vascular and parenchymal.

Vascular Changes

The hallmark of chronic PE is the demonstration of organized thrombi. Characteristically, these thrombi appear as either smooth or irregular eccentric mural defects (Fig. 9-

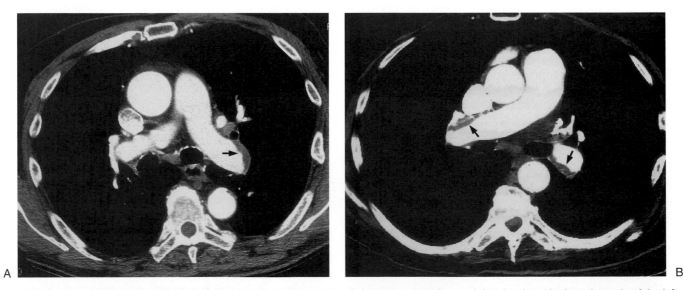

A   B

FIG. 9-38. Chronic pulmonary emboli. **A:** A 3-mm section shows a slightly irregular eccentric mural density along the lateral margin of the left interlobar pulmonary artery (*arrow*) characteristic of a chronic, organizing pulmonary embolus. **B:** A 3-mm section in a different patient from that in (**A**) and (**B**) shows the characteristic appearance of eccentric irregular mural densities involving both the right and left interlobar pulmonary arteries (*arrows*).

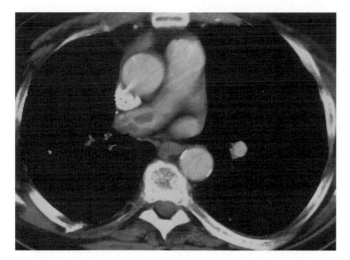

FIG. 9-39. Chronic pulmonary emboli. A 5-mm section shows several discrete filling defects within the right pulmonary artery. The pulmonary arteries in the right hilum are considerably smaller than those on the left side because of extensive stricturing. Disparity in the size of vessels is an important indication of chronic pulmonary thromboembolism.

38) (50). Frequently, they are associated with a marked disparity in the size of the central pulmonary arteries (Fig. 9-39). Indirect signs also may be present and include abrupt narrowing, webs and strictures, pouch defects (representing concave thrombi), and irregular vessel walls (Fig. 9-40) (134,136,137). In approximately 10% of cases, CT shows evidence of calcification (138). Ancillary vascular changes include identification of an enlarged right atrium as well as enlarged bronchial arteries in patients with CTEPH (138).

With the introduction of spiral CT, evaluation of temporal changes in patients with acute PE became possible. In a study of 62 patients with documented PEs in whom CT scans were obtained with a mean follow-up of 11 months, Remy-Jardin and colleagues (139) showed that complete resolution of central emboli occurred in only 48%; in the remaining cases, CT disclosed endovascular abnormalities including incomplete resolution of prior clot in 24 (39%) patients and the development of chronic PE in 8 (13%). More recently, Van Rossum and associates (140) obtained follow-up CT studies at 6 weeks in 19 patients with documented acute PE and found complete resolution in only 32% of cases (Fig. 9-41). Using a three-point grading system to assess severity of clot within central pulmonary arteries, these same authors documented that complete resolution was more likely to occur when initial CT scans show less extensive clot (140). Of the remainder, eccentric mural abnormalities could be identified in 22%, consistent with organization of acute emboli. These data have cast some doubt on the exact definition of acute versus chronic emboli. This is clinically important because differentiating chronic thrombi from acute recurrent PE is especially problematic with both V/Q imaging and pulmonary angiography.

Regardless of their precise age, compared with angiogra-

phy, CT has proved consistently more sensitive in detecting chronic central PE. Not only does CT allow visualization of arteries not opacified on pulmonary angiography, but also it is more sensitive in detecting smooth eccentric thrombi in central pulmonary arteries (Fig. 9-42) (83,136).

Parenchymal Changes

Distinct findings have been described in patients with chronic PE, especially those with chronic pulmonary hypertension. Most characteristic is the finding of mosaic perfusion, defined as well-defined geographic areas of ground glass attenuation often conforming to individual or groups of secondary pulmonary lobules, usually associated with marked disparity in size of segmental vessels (see Fig. 9-40; Fig. 9-43) (141,142). Additional less specific findings include parenchymal and linear densities, presumably the sequelae of prior pulmonary infarction. Unlike in acute PE, recognition of these lesions may play a crucial role in identifying patients with chronic PE, especially those with CTEPH. As pointed out by Bergin and associates (141), recognition of parenchymal changes is especially important because these patients usually present with nonspecific complaints and consequently are often first referred for noncontrast-enhanced high-resolution CT studies.

The value of mosaic perfusion as an indicator of chronic PE-related hypertension has been established. Sherrick and coworkers (142), in an evaluation of 64 patients with known pulmonary hypertension from a variety of causes, found that of 23 patients with pulmonary hypertension from vascular causes, mosaic attenuation could be identified in 17 (74%), compared with only 5% in patients with pulmonary hypertension due to underlying lung disease. Furthermore, of the 17 patients with pulmonary hypertension from vascular disease, 15 proved secondary to chronic PEs, and mosaic attenuation was present in 12 (80%). As noted by Bergin and associates (141), when the finding of mosaic perfusion is coupled with recognition of marked disparity in the size of segmental vessels within the lung, the combination is all but pathognomonic of chronic embolic pulmonary hypertension. In their study of 67 patients referred for high-resolution CT, including 28 patients with pulmonary hypertension, the sensitivity and specificity of these findings for distinguishing patients with chronic PE-related hypertension from other causes of pulmonary disease, including patients with nonthromboembolic pulmonary hypertension, exceeded 95% (141).

Chronic Thromboembolic Pulmonary Hypertension: Preoperative CT Evaluation

Although rare, identification of patients with CTEPH is important because, unlike other forms of primary (clinically occult) pulmonary hypertension, including plexigenic pulmonary arteriopathy and pulmonary venoocclusive disease, CTEPH may be reversed by pulmonary thromboendarterec-

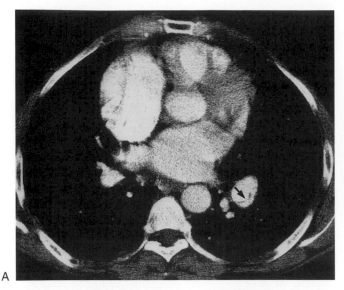
A

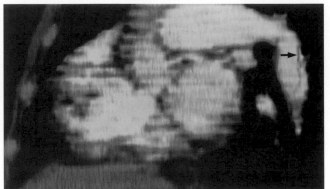
B

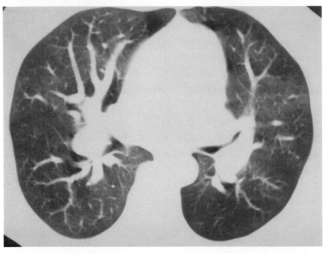
C

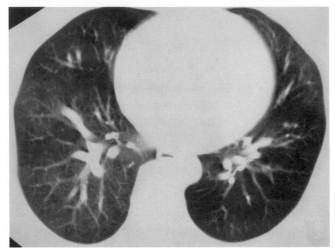
D

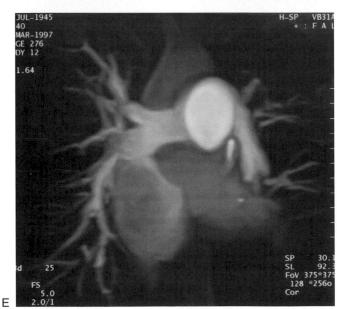
E

FIG. 9-40. Chronic pulmonary emboli: CT/MR correlation. **A:** A 5-mm section shows a curvilinear density within the left interlobar pulmonary artery (*arrow*) in this patient with chronic thromboembolic pulmonary artery hypertension. Note the marked enlargement of the right atrium. **B:** Multiplanar reconstruction shows to better advantage the appearance of a curvilinear line within a dilated left interlobar pulmonary artery (*arrows*). **C, D:** Sections through the middle and lower lung zones, imaged with wide windows, show the characteristic appearance of mosaic perfusion. Note the marked disparity in the size of lobar and segmental arteries, characteristic of chronic thromboembolic pulmonary hypertension. **E:** Coronal maximum intensity projection image from a breath-hold gadolinium-enhanced three dimensional MR angiogram shows markedly decreased perfusion with evidence of abruptly narrowed or strictured pulmonary arteries, especially to the left upper and lower lobes. These findings correlate with the appearance of the peripheral arterial bed shown in (**C**) and (**D**).

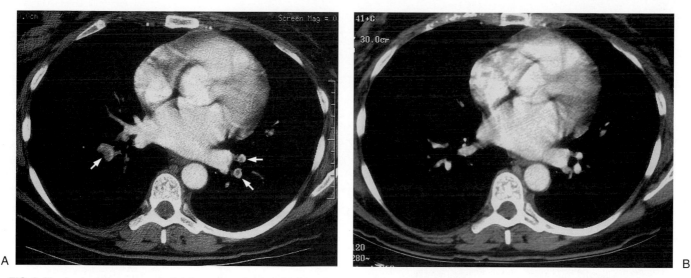

FIG. 9-41. Acute pulmonary emboli: follow-up evaluation. **A:** A 3-mm section shows pulmonary emboli in both right and left lower lobe pulmonary arteries (*arrows*). **B:** Follow-up study 2 months later shows complete resolution of previously identified filling defects (compare with **A**).

tomy. To date, several studies have assessed the accuracy of CT for predicting response to surgery with varying success (83,133,134,143). Schwickert and associates (133), for example, in a study of 74 patients with CTEPH using both conventional and spiral CT, found evidence of central pulmonary artery disease with a sensitivity of 77%, a specificity of 100%, and an accuracy of 80%.

As emphasized by Bergin and associates (83), preoperative evaluation of patients with suspected CTEPH represents a particularly difficult diagnostic challenge. This is because the presence of central pulmonary thrombi—defined as in-

volvement of all central arteries to the segmental level—is insufficient for determining response to therapy. Accurate preoperative assessment also requires determining the extent of surgically inaccessible disease produced by small vessel arteriopathy itself resulting from pulmonary hypertension.

The presence of central thromboembolism does not ensure a good response to surgery, especially in patients with severe cardiopulmonary compromise; as a corollary, the absence of central disease does not preclude a good surgical response. In their study correlating CT with surgical findings in 40 patients with documented CTEPH, Bergin and associates

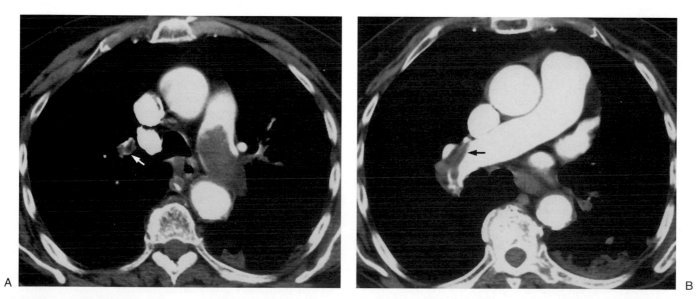

FIG. 9-42. A, B: Recurrent pulmonary emboli: 3-mm sections through the left main and right interlobar pulmonary arteries, respectively, in a patient with documented recurrent pulmonary emboli showing a large filling defect in the left main pulmonary artery (*arrow* in **A**) as well as a circular filling defect in the right upper lobe pulmonary artery (*arrow* in **A**). In addition, there is evidence of an eccentric mural filling defect along the lateral margin of the right interlobar pulmonary artery (*arrow* in **B**) and complete nonfilling in the lower lobe pulmonary arteries; these latter vessels are significantly smaller than normal. This case illustrates findings consistent with both acute and chronic pulmonary emboli.

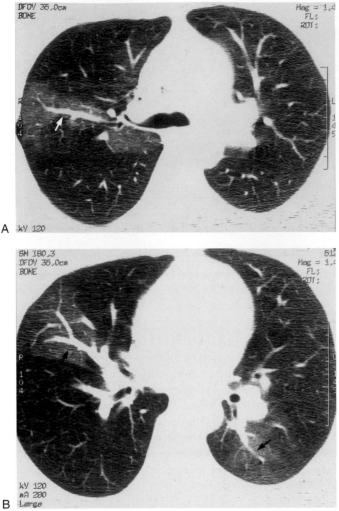

FIG. 9-43. Chronic pulmonary emboli: mosaic perfusion. **A, B:** These 3-mm sections through the right upper and middle lungs imaged with wide windows show evidence of mosaic perfusion in a patient with documented chronic thromboembolic pulmonary hypertension. Note discrete foci of ground glass attenuation within which markedly dilated lobar and segmental arteries can be defined (*arrows* in **A** and **B**), thus distinguishing this appearance from either diffuse infiltrative lung disease or air trapping.

(141) identified 3 patients without central pulmonary thrombi who nonetheless had good surgical responses with markedly decreased postoperative pulmonary vascular resistance.

Studies have documented that CT is more accurate than angiography for detecting central emboli. In the study reported by Bergin and colleagues (141), of 34 patients evaluated with both CT and angiography, CT proved significantly more sensitive (CT sensitivity ranging between 77% and 86% for 2 readers, versus angiographic sensitivity equal to 70%). This discrepancy was still greater when central arteries were assessed individually; of 20 surgically confirmed central arterial thrombi, CT detected between 16 and 20 (2 readers) compared with only 8 identified angiographically. The insensitivity of pulmonary angiography for identifying

well-epithelialized, smooth-contoured chronic central thrombi is well established. The value of CT is still further enhanced when direct evidence of segmental arterial abnormalities is coupled with evaluation of pulmonary parenchymal abnormalities, especially the finding of marked disparities in the size of segmental and subsegmental pulmonary arteries (141).

Nonetheless, angiography currently remains an important component of the diagnostic evaluation of patients with suspected CTEPH. As noted by Roberts and colleagues (134), angiography remains superior to CT for demonstrating webs, bands, and mural irregularities, especially in subsegmental arteries. Although a role for MR in evaluating these patients has yet to be established, in selected cases, MR may be of value as an ancillary imaging modality (see Fig. 9-40) (141).

PULMONARY ARTERY ANEURYSMS

The role of CT in the evaluation of pulmonary artery aneurysms has been well documented (Fig. 9-44). Although rare, pulmonary artery aneurysms are seen in a wide variety of conditions and have been associated with infection, with congenital heart disease, especially patent ductus arteriosus, atrial and ventricular septal defects, and congenital abnormalities of the pulmonary valve, with congenital and acquired primary vascular diseases, including both cystic medial necrosis and atherosclerosis, with congenital abnormalities, both isolated and associated with hereditary telangiectasia, and with penetrating and nonpenetrating trauma (Fig. 9-45) (144–146).

Pulmonary artery aneurysms also are associated with generalized vasculitis, including patients with Behçet's disease, Hughes-Stovin syndrome, and, less commonly, giant cell arteritis. In patients with Behçet's disease, pulmonary artery aneurysms are seen in association with a variety of vascular abnormalities, including venous occlusions and arterial aneurysms. These patients also develop aphthous stomatitis, genital ulcerations, and uveitis. In most cases, aneurysms are easily identified with either CT or MR (147–149).

Although the leading cause of pulmonary artery aneurysms is usually thought to be cystic medial necrosis, in association with both congenital and acquired cardiovascular diseases accompanied by pulmonary hypertension, investigators are increasingly aware of the problem of false aneurysms of the pulmonary artery developing as a consequence of Swan-Ganz catheterization. Ferretti and associates (150), in a review of seven false aneurysms in five patients identified over a 4-year period, noted that all these lesions occurred in either segmental or subsegmental arteries, in some cases as late as 19 days after removal of the catheter.

Radiologic diagnosis is frequently problematic (144). Although pulmonary artery aneurysms are generally visible, their appearance is rarely specific. Peripheral aneurysms may be mistaken for parenchymal nodules or metastases, unless accompanying vessels are identified; central lesions are easily confused with hilar adenopathy, masses, or even

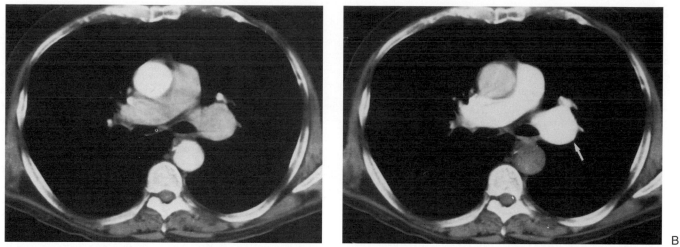

FIG. 9-44. Pulmonary artery aneurysm. **A, B:** Sequential sections from a dynamic-static contrast-enhanced sequence obtained at the level of the right main pulmonary artery in a patient with a left hilar mass identified on a routine chest radiograph (not shown). The interlobar pulmonary artery is aneurysmally dilated (*arrow* in **B**).

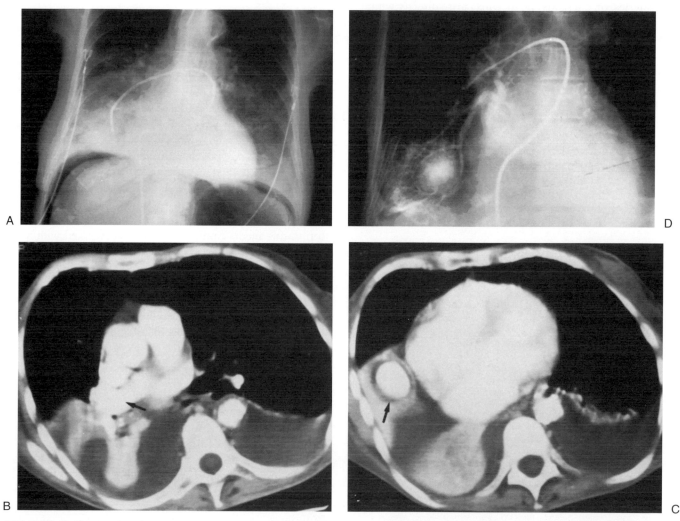

FIG. 9-45. Posttraumatic pulmonary artery aneurysm. **A:** PA radiograph shows the presence of a malpositioned Swan-Ganz catheter with its tip directed towards the base of the right lower lobe. Pneumoperitoneum is due to abdominal surgery. **B,C:** Sequential CT sections through the right main pulmonary artery (*arrow* in **B**) and the right lower lobe, respectively. A large pleural effusion is present, causing compression atelectasis of both the middle and right lower lobes. Within the collapsed middle lobe, marked contrast enhancement can be identified within an apparent vascular structure (*arrow*). **D:** Coned-down view from a selective right pulmonary artery arteriogram shows a peripheral pulmonary artery aneurysm corresponding in location to the tip of the Swan-Ganz catheter shown in **A**, and the large peripheral vascular structure identified within the middle lobe in **C**. (Case courtesy of Deborah Reede, M.D., Long Island College Hospital, NY.)

aortic aneurysms. As a consequence, definitive diagnosis traditionally has required pulmonary angiography. At present, both contrast-enhanced CT and MR have been shown to be reliable methods for diagnosis of both central and peripheral aneurysms, obviating more invasive studies in all cases save those for which therapeutic intervention is planned (151–154).

VASCULAR NEOPLASIA

In addition to PE, intravascular filling defects may also result from both primary and secondary (metastatic) tumors (see Figs. 9-32 and 9-33; Fig. 9-46). Although primary vascular tumors arising in the pulmonary arteries are rare, they are not unknown (Fig. 9-47) (104,105). Typically sarcomatous, these tumors may originate either within the right ventricle and extend through the valve into the main pulmonary arteries, or, alternatively, they may arise directly within the pulmonary arteries themselves. Histologically, pulmonary artery sarcomas are most frequently undifferentiated; specific subtypes include, most commonly, leiomyosarcomas and myxosarcomas, with rhabdomyosarcomas, fibrosarcomas, chondrosarcomas, and malignant mesenchymomas accounting for the remainder. Considerable overlap exists both in the CT and MR appearance of intravascular tumor and chronic organizing PE, in particular; in both cases, the result is often irregularly marginated filling defects. This problem may be solved, however, by noting contrast en-

hancement within tumor using either CT or gadolinium-enhanced MR (see Fig. 9-47) (106,107,155).

In addition to primary vascular tumors, tumor within pulmonary arteries may be caused by tumor arising either within the lung, hilum, or mediastinum. Although most cases are secondary to bronchogenic carcinoma, both extrathoracic metastases and primary intracardiac tumors may invade or cause obstruction of both pulmonary arteries and veins. Although rare, this type of tumor extension is easily identifiable with both contrast-enhanced CT and MR (Fig. 9-48) (156,157).

Encasement of the main pulmonary arteries is an absolute contraindication to resection in patients with bronchogenic carcinoma (Fig. 9-49). Although this condition is usually not problematic, overinterpretation should be avoided. Specifically, the finding of tumor adjacent to the main pulmonary arteries, regardless of extent, should not be interpreted as definitive evidence of unresectability.

Although tumor obstruction of hilar vessels is most often secondary to bronchogenic carcinoma, other lesions, both benign and malignant, have been reported to cause pulmonary artery obstruction (156,158,159). The CT appearance of pulmonary artery obstruction secondary to fibrosing mediastinitis, in particular, has been noted (Fig. 9-50) (160–162). This disorder causes a wide spectrum of clinical and radiographic changes, from incidental, asymptomatic disease to life-threatening hypertension. Usually the result histoplasmosis, a characteristic appearance of widespread mediastinal and hilar calcifications causing narrowing or obliteration of both pulmonary arteries and veins should suggest the diagnosis (see Fig. 9-50). Although alterations in the configuration of mediastinal and hilar vessels secondary to fibrosing mediastinitis have been documented with MR, the inability of MR to detect calcifications is a clear disadvantage (162).

Other causes of pulmonary artery compression include aneurysms of the ascending and descending aorta (163). Unfortunately, when the cause is other than vascular, accurate diagnosis usually necessitates histologic evaluation.

PULMONARY VENOUS DISEASE

Represented in this category are diverse entities for which evaluation of the pulmonary veins is important, including pulmonary vein varices, pulmonary venooocclusive disease, and tumor invasion of the pulmonary veins.

Both CT and MR are reliable, noninvasive methods for establishing the diagnosis of a pulmonary varix (164,165). Varices are easily identifiable as enlarged but otherwise normal pulmonary veins that directly drain into the left atrium, typically involving the right lower lobe and, less commonly, the left upper lobe and lingula (Fig. 9-51). Although commonly found in association with acquired heart disease, left atrial enlargement, and pulmonary venous hypertension, pulmonary varices also rarely occur as congenital local dilations of a segment of a pulmonary vein in otherwise normal

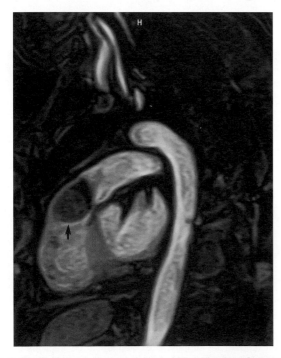

FIG. 9-46. Pulmonary artery neoplasm: MR evaluation. Oblique sagittal source image from breath-hold gadolinium-enhanced three dimensional MR angiogram (TR/TE 5/2 ms) demonstrates an enhancing mass within the pulmonary artery from metastatic melanoma (*arrow*).

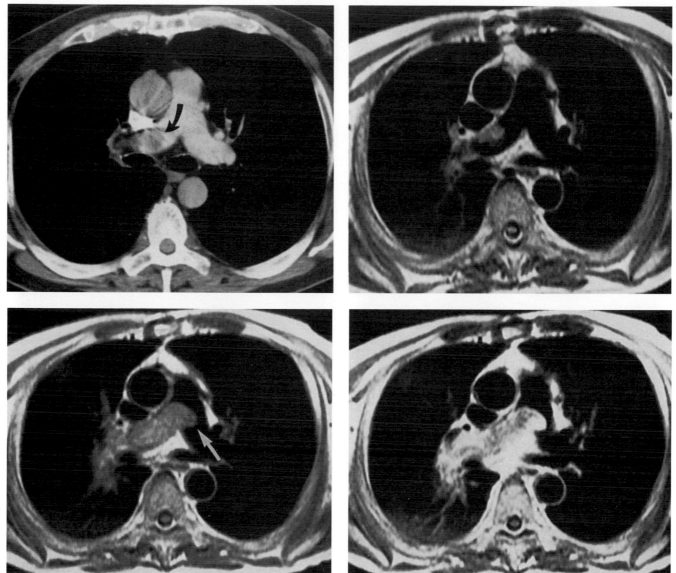

FIG. 9-47. A: CT scan at the level of the carina after a bolus injection of intravenous contrast medium shows a focal filling defect within the right main pulmonary artery (*arrow*). This appearance is nonspecific and may result from either tumor or thrombus. **B:** Every-beat gated, noncontrast-enhanced spin-echo MR section at the level of the carina shows an eccentric, slightly nodular intravascular filling defect within the right main pulmonary artery (compare with **A**). Additionally, one sees a subtle increase in signal intensity within the right lung as compared with the left lung, presumably reflecting vascular stasis and congestion. **C:** Every-beat gated, noncontrast-enhanced spin-echo MR image at the same level as **A** and **B**, 3 months later. A lobular mass of intermediate signal intensity is now clearly identifiable filling most of the lumen of the right main pulmonary artery, extending medially to partially obstruct the lumen of the left main pulmonary artery (*arrow*). A significant increase in the size of this lesion is apparent. **D:** Every-beat gated spin-echo MR image at the same level as shown in **C** obtained 1 minute after intravenous injection of gadolinium-diethylenetriaminepentaacetic acid (Gd-DTPA). Note the marked increase in the signal intensity of the intraluminal filling defect within the right main pulmonary artery as compared with the precontrast-enhanced image (compare with **C**). This finding is consistent with the presence of vascularized tissue as occurs within tumor, as distinct from a nonvascularized intraluminal thrombus. Again, note the presence of increased signal within the right lung, which also shows considerable signal enhancement after the intravenous injection of Gd-DTPA (compare with **A**). This lesion is a surgically verified pulmonary artery sarcoma. (From ref. 106, with permission.)

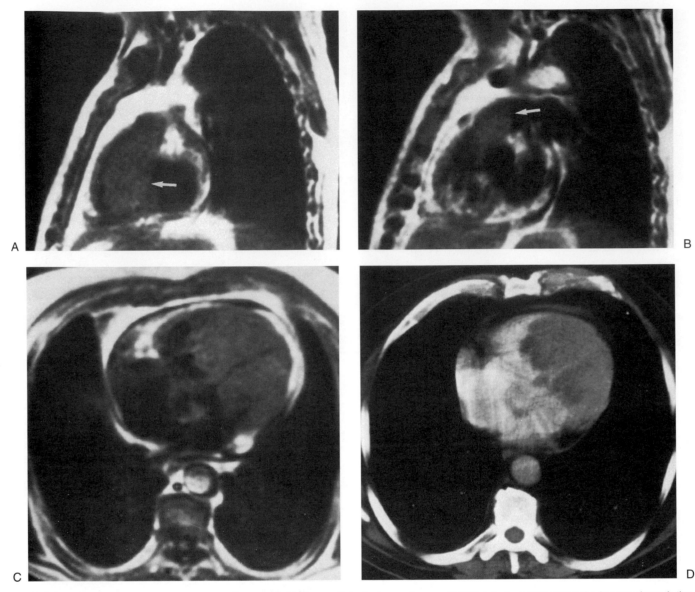

FIG. 9-48. Pulmonary artery metastases: melanoma. **A, B:** Sequential, electrocardiogram (ECG)-gated, sagittal spin-echo images through the right ventricular outflow tract and main pulmonary artery, respectively, show intermediate signal throughout the right ventricle (*arrow* in **A**) and within the proximal main pulmonary artery (*arrow* in **B**). **C, D:** ECG-gated axial spin-echo image and the corresponding contrast-enhanced axial CT section through the right and left ventricles confirm extensive intracardiac tumor. Biopsy confirmed metastatic melanoma.

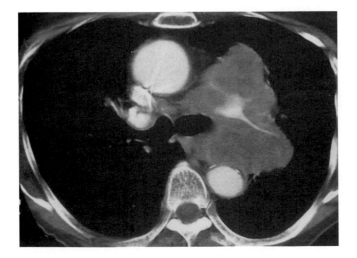

FIG. 9-49. Pulmonary artery obstruction resulting from bronchogenic carcinoma. A 3-mm contrast-enhanced section shows extensive tumor infiltration into the hilum and mediastinum resulting in encasement of the left pulmonary artery and obstruction of the left superior pulmonary vein.

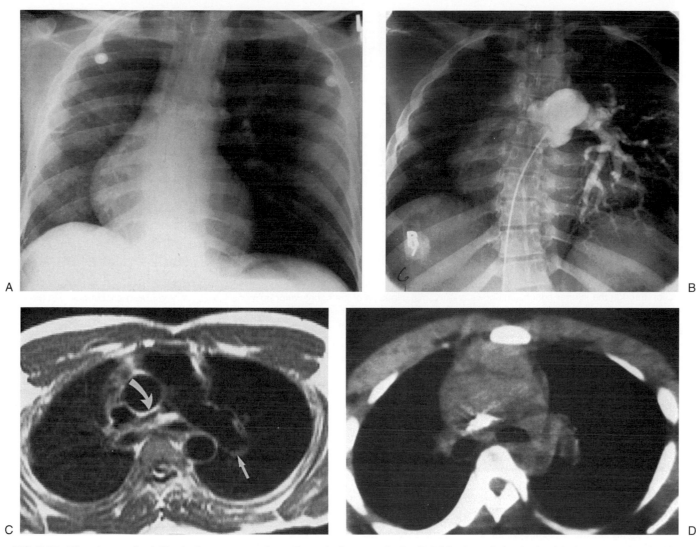

FIG. 9-50. Fibrosing mediastinitis. **A:** A posteroanterior radiograph shows markedly diminished ventilation in the right lung, associated with a shift of the heart and mediastinum to the right. Right hilar structures are difficult to identify. **B:** A pulmonary angiogram shows abrupt cutoff of the right main pulmonary artery, raising the possibility of obstruction secondary to tumor. **C:** Every-beat gated, axial spin-echo MR scan obtained just below the carina. The left pulmonary artery is slightly enlarged (*arrow*). The right main pulmonary artery is markedly attenuated (*curved arrow*). Although one sees a slight increase in the signal within the mediastinum adjacent to the right main pulmonary artery, the appearance is nonspecific. No obvious mediastinal mass is seen. **D:** Nonenhanced CT scan at the same level as (**C**), showing extensive mediastinal calcification in the region surrounding the right main pulmonary artery. Extensive mediastinal and hilar calcifications were present as well at numerous other levels (not shown). (Courtesy of Jerry Patt, M.D., Union Memorial Hospital, Baltimore, MD.)

patients. When a pulmonary varix masquerades either as a discrete pulmonary nodule or even as an arteriovenous malformation, bolus contrast administration is essential to show continuity between the varix and associated pulmonary veins. Characteristically, unlike typical arteriovenous malformations, isolated pulmonary varices enhance only during the phase of maximal venous opacification.

CT findings in patients with pulmonary venoocclusive disease have also been reported (Fig. 9-52) (166–170). In this rare entity, diffuse endothelial proliferation results in the occlusion of small pulmonary veins, resulting in severe pulmonary hypertension. Seen in association with several predisposing conditions, including viral infections, environ-

mental toxins, chemotherapy, radiation, and autoimmune diseases, this entity likely represents a nonspecific response to a wide variety of injuries (170). Because this disorder is typically fatal within a few years of onset, these patients should be considered candidates for lung transplantation. CT findings reflect a combination of parenchymal and hilar abnormalities. As reported by Swensen and associates (170) in their review of eight documented cases, the most common CT finding was the presence of smooth interlobular septal thickening associated with multifocal areas of ground glass attenuation; pathologically, these findings correlated with the presence of fibrosis and venous sclerosis. In 50% of cases, a mosaic pattern compatible with pulmonary hyper-

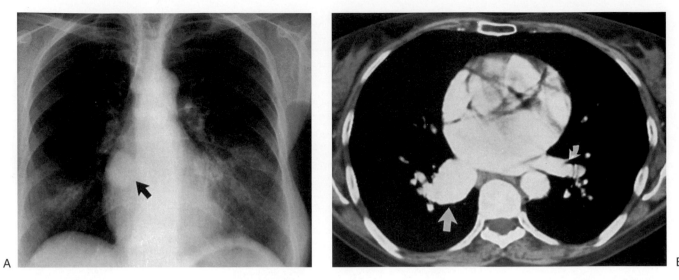

FIG. 9-51. Pulmonary varix. **A:** A posteroanterior radiograph shows a sharply defined right hilar mass (*arrow*). **B:** A contrast-enhanced CT section through the inferior right hilum shows aneurysmal dilatation of the right inferior pulmonary vein (*curved arrow*) contiguous with the left atrium. Compare with the appearance of normal left inferior pulmonary vein (*arrow*). This appearance is diagnostic of a pulmonary varix.

tension could be identified. When accompanied by enlarged pulmonary arteries with normal-sized pulmonary veins and left atrium, this constellation of parenchymal and vascular abnormalities strongly suggests pulmonary venoocclusive disease. Clinically, the diagnosis of venoocclusive disease should be suggested in patients with severe pulmonary hypertension, radiographic evidence of edema, and a normal pulmonary artery wedge pressure.

Involvement of the pulmonary veins with tumor also has been documented both with CT and MR (171). In patients with lung cancer, the finding of tumor within the pulmonary veins may signal the presence of intrapericardial extension, even without evidence of a filling defect within the left atrium (Fig. 9-53). Choe and associates (171), in a retrospec-

tive assessment of 19 patients with CT evidence of tumor extension into a pulmonary vein, found that 14 (73%) had intrapericardial extension at surgery. This was especially likely with involvement of the superior pulmonary veins. Although the presence of tumor within the pulmonary veins does not constitute evidence of unresectability, preoperative awareness of possible tumor extension into the left atrium is important. Although most often associated with direct extension of lung cancer, metastatic tumor also extends into the left atrium through the pulmonary veins (Fig. 9-54).

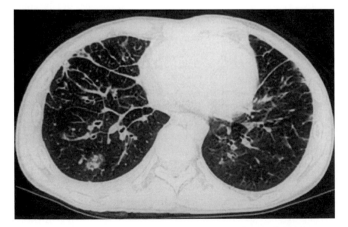

FIG. 9-52. Pulmonary venoocclusive disease. High-resolution CT section through the lower lobes shows smoothly thickened interlobar septa and bronchial wall thickening consistent with interstitial edema in a patient with documented pulmonary venoocclusive disease. (Courtesy of Stephen J. Swensen, M.D., Rochester, MN.)

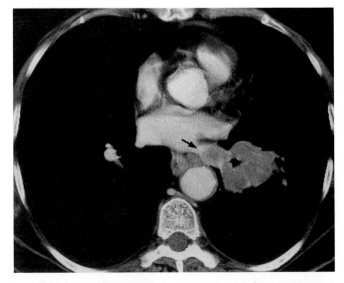

FIG. 9-53. Pulmonary vein obstruction: bronchogenic carcinoma. A 5-mm contrast-enhanced section shows tumor within the left hilum causing narrowing of the left lower lobe bronchi. Note the presence of a filling defect within the left inferior pulmonary vein resulting from tumor invasion and extension (*arrow*).

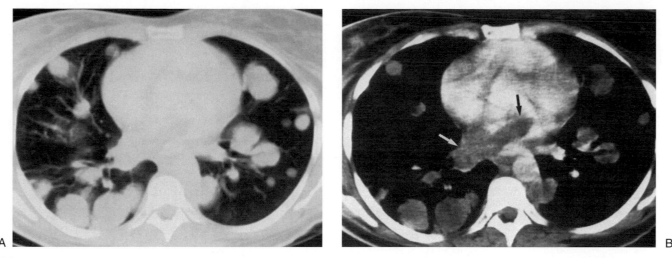

FIG. 9-54. Invasive (metastatic) uterine leiomyomatosis. **A, B:** CT section through the right inferior pulmonary vein, imaged with wide and narrow windows, respectively, after a bolus of intravenous contrast medium. Multiple nodules are present in both lungs of varying sizes, many clearly related to adjacent blood vessels (**A**). A large filling defect is also present within the left atrium and left inferior pulmonary vein, representing extension of tumor from the lungs into the left heart (*arrows* in **B**). (Courtesy of Ira Tyler, M.D., Albert Einstein Medical Center, Bronx, NY.)

REFERENCES

1. Guthaner DF, Wexler L, Harell G. CT demonstration of cardiac structures. *AJR Am J Roentgenol* 1979;133:75–81.
2. Kuriyama K, Gamsu G, Stern RG, Cann CE, et al. CT-determined pulmonary artery diameters in predicting pulmonary hypertension. *Invest Radiol* 1984;19:16.
3. Ackman Haimovici JB, Trotman-Dickenson B, Halpern EF, et al. Relationship between pulmonary artery diameter at computed tomography and pulmonary artery pressures at right-sided heart catheterization. *Acad Radiol* 1997;4:327–334.
4. Elliot FM, Reid L. Some new facts about the pulmonary artery and its branching pattern. *Clin Radiol* 1965;16:193.
5. Jefferson KE. The normal pulmonary angiogram and some changes seen in chronic nonspecific lung disease. I. The pulmonary vessels seen in the normal pulmonary angiogram. *Proc R Soc Med* 1965;58:677.
6. Webb WR. Radiologic imaging of the pulmonary hila. *Postgrad Radiol* 1986;6:145–168.
7. Murata K, Itoh H, Todo G, et al. Centrilobular lesions of the lung: demonstration by high-resolution CT and pathologic correlation. *Radiology* 1986;161:641–645.
8. Remy-Jardin M, Duyck P, Remy J, et al. Hilar lymph nodes: identification with spiral CT and histologic correlation. *Radiology* 1995;196:387–394.
9. Naidich DP, Khouri NF, Scott WJ, Wang KP, Siegelman SS. Computed tomography of the pulmonary hila. 1. Normal anatomy. *J Comput Assist Tomogr* 1981;5:459–467.
10. Naidich DP, Khouri NF, Stitik FP, McCauley DI, Siegelman SS. Computed tomography of the pulmonary hila. 2. Abnormal anatomy. *J Comput Assist Tomogr* 1981;5:468–475.
11. Webb WR, Glazer G, Gamsu G. Computed tomography of the normal pulmonary hilum. *J Comput Assist Tomogr* 1981;5:476–484.
12. Webb WR, Gamsu G, Glazer G. Computed tomography of the abnormal pulmonary hilum. *J Comput Assist Tomogr* 1981;5:485–490.
13. Naidich DP, Terry PB, Stitik FP, Siegelman SS. Computed tomography of the bronchi. 1. Normal anatomy. *J Comput Assist Tomogr* 1980;4:746–753.
14. Naidich DP, Stitik FP, Khouri NF, Terry PB, Siegelman SS. Computed tomography of the bronchi. 2. Pathology. *J Comput Assist Tomogr* 1980;4:754–762.
15. Webb WR, Gamsu G, Stark DD, Moore EH. Magnetic resonance imaging of the normal and abnormal pulmonary hila. *Radiology* 1984;152:89–94.
16. Furuse M, Saito K, Kunieda E, et al. Bronchial arteries: CT demonstration with arteriographic correlation. *Radiology* 1987;162:393–398.

17. Sherrick DW, DuShane JW. Agenesis of a main branch of the pulmonary artery. *AJR Am J Roentgenol* 1962;87:917–928.
18. Kieffer SA, Amplatz K, Anderson RC, Lillechei CW. Proximal interruption of a pulmonary artery. *AJR Am J Roentgenol* 1965;95:592–597.
19. Sotomora RF, Edwards JE. Anatomic identification of so-called absent pulmonary artery. *Circulation* 1978;57:624–633.
20. Sondheimer HM, Oliphant M, Schneider B, et al. Computerized axial tomography of the chest for visualization of "absent" pulmonary arteries. *Circulation* 1982;65:1020–1025.
21. Naidich DP, Rumancik WM, Ettenger NA, et al. Congenital anomalies of the lungs in adults: MR diagnosis. *AJR Am J Roentgenol* 1988;151:13–19.
22. Stone DN, Bein ME, Garris JB. Anomalous left pulmonary artery: two new adult cases. *AJR Am J Roentgenol* 1980;135:1259–1263.
23. Moncada R, Demos TC, Churchill R, Reyes C. Case report. Chronic stridor in a child: CT diagnosis of pulmonary vascular sling. *J Comput Assist Tomogr* 1983;7:713–715.
24. Berden WE, Baker DH, Wung JT. Complete cartilage-ring tracheal stenosis associated with anomalous left pulmonary artery: the ring-sling complex. *Radiology* 1984;152:57–64.
25. Hernandez RJ, Bank ER, Shaffeer EM, Snider AR, Rosenthal A. Comparative evaluation of the pulmonary arteries in patients with right ventricular outflow tract obstructive lesions. *AJR Am J Roentgenol* 1987;148:1189–1194.
26. Jacobstein MD, Fletcher BD, Nelson AD, Clampitt M, Alifid RJ. Magnetic resonance imaging: evaluation of palliative systemic-pulmonary artery shunts. *Circulation* 1984;70:650–656.
27. Park HS, Im JG, Jung JW, Yeon KM. Anomalous left pulmonary artery with complete cartilaginous ring. *J Comput Assist Tomogr* 1997;21:478–480.
28. Vogl TJ, Diebold T, Bergman C et al. MRI in pre- and postoperative assessment of tracheal stenosis due to pulmonary artery sling. *J Comput Assist Tomogr* 1993;17:878–886.
29. Dillon EH, Camputaro C. Partial anomalous pulmonary venous drainage of the left upper lobe vs duplication of the superior vena cava: distinction based on CT findings. *AJR Am J Roentgenol* 1993;160:375–379.
30. White CS, Baffa JM, Haney PJ, Campbell AB, NessAiver M. Anomalies of pulmonary veins: usefulness of spin-echo and gradient-echo MR images. *AJR Am J Roentgenol* 1998;170:1365–1368.
31. White CS, Baffa JM, Haney PJ, Pace ME, Campbell AB. Congenital anomalies of the thoracic veins: MR findings. *Radiographics* 1997;17:595–608.
32. Masui T, Seelos KC, Kersting-Sommerhoff BA, Higgins CB. Abnormalities of the pulmonary veins: evaluation with MR imaging and

comparison with cardiac angiography and echocardiography. *Radiology* 1991;181:645–649.

33. Choe YH, Lee HJ, Kim HS, et al. MRI of total anomalous pulmonary venous connections. *J Comput Assist Tomogr* 1994;18:243–249.

34. Baxter R, McFadden PM, Gradman M, Wright A. Scimitar syndrome: cine magnetic resonance imaging demonstration of anomalous pulmonary venous drainage. *Ann Thorac Surg* 1990;50:121–123.

35. Tisi GM, Friedman PJ, Peters RM, et al. Clinical staging of primary lung cancer. *Am Rev Respir Dis* 1983;127:659–664.

36. Engel S. *Lung structure.* Springfield, IL: Charles C Thomas, 1962.

37. Chang CH, Zinn TW. Roentgen recognition of enlarged hilar lymph nodes: an anatomic review. *Radiology* 1976;120:291–296.

38. Müller NL, Webb WR. Radiographic imaging of the pulmonary hila. *Invest Radiol* 1985;20:661–671.

39. Sone S, Higashihara T, Morimoto S, et al. CT anatomy of hilar lymphadenopathy. *AJR Am J Roentgenol* 1983;140:887–892.

40. Ashida C, Zerhouni EA, Fishman EK. CT demonstration of prominent right hilar soft tissue collections. *J Comput Assist Tomogr* 1987;11:57–59.

41. Nohl HC. An investigation of the anatomy of lymphatic drainage of the lungs: Hunterian lecture. *Ann R Coll Surg* 1972;51:157–176.

42. Gurney JW. No fooling around: direct visualization of pulmonary embolism. *Radiology* 1993;188:618–619.

43. Goodman LR, Lipchik RJ. Diagnosis of acute pulmonary embolism: time for a new approach. *Radiology* 1996;199:25–27.

44. Woodard PK. Pulmonary arteries must be seen before they can be assessed. *Radiology* 1997;204:11–12.

45. Hansell DM, Padley SPG. Continuous volume computed tomography in pulmonary embolism: the answer, or just another test? [Editorial] *Thorax* 1996;51:1–2.

46. Romano WM, Cascade PN, Korobkin MT, Quint LE, Francis IR. Implications of unsuspected pulmonary embolism detected by computed tomography. *Can Assoc Radiol J* 1995;46:363–367.

47. Winston CB, Wechsler RJ, Salazar AM, Kurtz AB, Spirn PW. Incidental pulmonary emboli detected at helical CT: effect on patient care. *Radiology* 1996;201:23–27.

48. Gosselin MV, Rubin GD, Leung AN, Rizk NW. Unsuspected pulmonary embolism: prospective detection on routine helical CT scans. *Radiology* 1998;208:209–215.

49. Remy-Jardin M, Remy J, Wattinne L, Giraud F. Central pulmonary thromboembolism: diagnosis with spiral volumetric CT with the single-breath-hold technique. Comparison with pulmonary angiography. *Radiology* 1992;185:381–387.

50. Teigen CL, Maus TP, Sheedy PF II, et al. Pulmonary embolism: diagnosis with electron-beam CT. *Radiology* 1993;188:839–845.

51. Goodman LR, Curtin JJ, Mewissen MW, et al. Detection of pulmonary embolism in patients with unresolved clinical and scintigraphic diagnosis: helical CT versus angiography. *AJR Am J Roentgenol* 1995;164:1369–1374.

52. Remy-Jardin M, Remy J, Deschildre F, et al. Diagnosis of pulmonary embolism with spiral CT: comparison with pulmonary angiography and scintigraphy. *Radiology* 1996;200:699–706.

53. Van Rossum AB, Treurniet FEE, Kieft GJ, Smith SJ, Schepersbok R. Role of spiral volumetric computed tomographic scanning in the assessment of patients with clinical suspicion of pulmonary embolism and an abnormal ventilation/perfusion lung scan. *Thorax* 1996;51:23–28.

54. Mayo JR, Remy-Jardin M, Müller NL, et al. Pulmonary embolism: prospective comparison of spiral CT with ventilation-perfusion scintigraphy. *Radiology* 1997;205:447–452.

55. Loud PA, Grossman ZD, Klippenstein DL, Katz DS, Shah R. Beyond CTPA: combined CT venography and pulmonary angiography to evaluate suspected thromboembolic disease (abstract). Society of Thoracic Radiology, 1998.

56. Costello P, Naidich DP. Protocols for helical CT of the chest. In: Silverman PM, ed. *Helical (spiral) computed tomography.* Philadelphia: Lippincott–Raven, 1998:65–101.

57. Remy-Jardin M, Remy J, Artaud D, Deschildre F, Fribourg M, Beregi JP. Spiral CT of pulmonary embolism: technical considerations and interpretive pitfalls. *J Thorac Imaging* 1997;12:103–117.

58. Kuzo RS, Goodman LR. CT evaluation of pulmonary embolism: technique and interpretation. *AJR Am J Roentgenol* 1997;169:959–965.

59. Van Rossum AB, Pattynama PMT, Tjin ER, et al. Pulmonary embolism: validation of spiral CT angiography in 149 patients. *Radiology* 1996;201:467–470.

60. Bankier AA, Janata K, Fleischmann D, et al. Severity assessment of acute pulmonary embolism with spiral CT: evaluation of two modified angiographic scores and comparison with clinical data. *J Thorac Imaging* 1997;12:150–158.

61. Remy-Jardin M, Remy J, Artaud D, Deschildre F, Duhamel A. Peripheral pulmonary arteries: optimization of the spiral CT acquisition protocol. *Radiology* 1997;204:157–163.

62. Ferretti GR, Bosson JL, Buffaz PD, et al. Acute pulmonary embolism: role of helical CT in 164 patients with intermediate probability at ventilation-perfusion scintigraphy and normal results at duplex US of the legs. *Radiology* 1997;205:453–458.

63. Teigen CL, Maus TP, Sheedy PF II, et al. Pulmonary embolism; diagnosis with contrast-enhanced electron-beam CT and comparison with pulmonary angiography. *Radiology* 1995;194:313–319.

64. Gosselin MV, Rubin GD. Altered intravascular contrast material flow dynamics: clues for refining thoracic CT diagnosis. *AJR Am J Roentgenol* 1997;169:1597–1603.

65. Garg K, Welsh CH, Feyerabend AJ, et al. Pulmonary embolism: diagnosis with spiral CT and ventilation-perfusion scanning. Correlation with pulmonary angiographic results or clinical outcome. *Radiology* 1998;208:201–208.

66. Costello P, Dupuy DE, Ecker CP, Tello R. Spiral CT of the thorax with reduced volume of contrast material: a comparative study. *Radiology* 1992;183:663–666.

67. Vanhoe L, Marchal G, Baert AL, Gryspeerdt S, Mertens L. Determination of scan delay time in spiral CT-angiography: utility of a test bolus injection. *J Comput Assist Tomogr* 1995;19:216–220.

68. Silverman P, Roberts S, Tiffl MC, Brown B, Fox SH. Helical CT of the liver: clinical application of a computer automated scanning technique—Smartprep—for obtaining images with optimal contrast enhancement. *AJR Am J Roentgenol* 1995;165:73–78.

69. Remy-Jardin M, Remy J, Cauvain O, et al. Diagnosis of central pulmonary embolism with helical CT: role of two-dimensional multiplanar reformations. *AJR Am J Roentgenol* 1995;165:1131–1138.

70. Brink JA, Woodard PK, Horesh L, et al. Depiction of pulmonary emboli with spiral CT: optimization of display window settings in a porcine model. *Radiology* 1997;204:703–708.

71. Posteraro RH, Sostman HD, Spritzer CE, Herfkens RJ. Cine-gradient-refocused MR imaging of central pulmonary emboli. *AJR Am J Roentgenol* 1989;152:465–468.

72. Erdman WA, Peshock RM, Redan HC, et al. Pulmonary embolism: comparison of MR images with radionuclide and angiographic studies. *Radiology* 1994;190:499–508.

73. Schiebler ML, Holland GA, Hatabu H, et al. Suspected pulmonary embolism: prospective evaluation with pulmonary MR angiography. *Radiology* 1993;189:125–131.

74. Gefter WB, Hatanabe H, Dinsmore BJ, et al. Pulmonary vascular cine MR imaging. *Radiology* 1990;176:761–770.

75. Hatabu H, Gefter WB, Kressel HY, et al. Pulmonary vasculature: high-resolution MR imaging. *Radiology* 1989;176:391–395.

76. MacFall J, Sostman H, Foo T. Thick-section, single breath-hold magnetic resonance pulmonary angiography. *Invest Radiol* 1992;27:318–322.

77. Grist TM, Sostman HD, MaFall JR, et al. Pulmonary angiography with MR imaging: preliminary clinical experience. *Radiology* 1993;189:523–530.

78. Wielopolski PA, Haacke EM, Adler LP. Three-dimensional MR imaging of the pulmonary vasculature: preliminary experience. *Radiology* 1992;183:465–472.

79. Wielopolski PA. Pulmonary arteriography. *Magn Reson Imaging Clin North Am* 1993;1:295–313.

80. Loubeyre P, Revel D, Douek P, et al. Dynamic contrast-enhanced MR angiography of pulmonary embolism: comparison with pulmonary angiography. *AJR Am J Roentgenol* 1994;162:1035–1039.

81. Revel D, Loubeyre P, Delignette A, et al. Contrast-enhanced magnetic resonance tomoangiography: a new imaging technique for studying thoracic great vessels. *Magn Reson Imaging* 1993;11:1101–1105.

82. Rubin GD, Herfkins RJ, Pelc NJ, et al. Single breath-hold pulmonary magnetic resonance angiography: optimization and comparison of three imaging strategies. *Invest Radiol* 1994;29:766–772.

83. Bergin CJ, Sirlin CB, Hauschildt JP, et al. Chronic thromboembolism: diagnosis with helical CT and MR imaging with angiographic and surgical correlation. *Radiology* 1997;204:695–702.

84. Laissy JP, Assayag P, Henryfeugeas MC, et al. Pulmonary time-of-

flight MR angiography at 1.0 T: comparison between 2D and 3D tone acquisitions. *Magn Reson Imaging* 1995;13:949–957.

85. Prince MR, Narasimham DL, Stanley JC, et al. Breath-hold gadolinium-enhanced MR angiography of abdominal aorta and its major branches. *Radiology* 1995;197:785–792.

86. Prince M, Grist TM, Debatin JF. *3D contrast MR angiography*. New York: Springer, 1997.

87. Gefter W, Hatabu H, Holland G, Osiason A. Pulmonary MR angiography. *Semin Ultrasound CT MR* 1996;17:316–323.

88. Isoda H, Ushimi T, Masui T, et al. Clinical evaluation of 3D time-of-flight MRA with breath holding using contrast media. *J Comput Assist Tomogr* 1995;19:911–919.

89. Leung DA, Mckinnon GC, Davis CP, et al. Breath-hold, contrast-enhanced, three-dimensional MR angiography. *Radiology* 1996;200:569–571.

90. Li KCP, Pelc LR, Napel SA, et al. MRI of pulmonary embolism using Gd-DTPA-polyethylene glycol polymer enhanced 3D fast gradient echo technique in a canine model. *Magn Reson Imaging* 1997;15:543–550.

91. Meaney JFM, Weg JG, Chenevert TL, et al. Diagnosis of pulmonary embolism with magnetic resonance angiography. *N Engl J Med* 1997;336:1422–1427.

92. Steiner P, McKinnon G, Romanowski B, et al. Contrast-enhanced, ultrafast 3D pulmonary MR angiography in a single breath-hold: initial assessment of imaging performance. *J Magn Reson Imaging* 1997;7:177–182.

93. Hatabu H, Gefter WB, Listerud J, et al. Pulmonary MR angiography utilizing phased-array surface coils. *J Comput Assist Tomogr* 1992;16:410–417.

94. Foo TKF, MacFall JR, Hayes CE, Sostman HD, Slayman BE. Pulmonary vasculature: single breath-hold MR imaging with phased-array coils. *Radiology* 1992;183:473–477.

95. Hatabu H. MR pulmonary angiography and perfusion imaging: recent advances. *Semin Ultrasound CT MRI* 1997;18:349–361.

96. Amundsen T, Kvaerness J, Jones RA, et al. Pulmonary embolism: detection with MR perfusion imaging of lung. A feasibility study. *Radiology* 1997;203:181–185.

97. Berthezene Y, Croisille P, Bertocchi M, et al. Lung perfusion demonstrated by contrast-enhanced dynamic magnetic resonance imaging: application to unilateral lung transplantation. *Invest Radiol* 1997;32:351–356.

98. Hennig J, Scheffler K, Laubenberger J, Strecker R. Time-resolved projection angiography after bolus injection of contrast agent. *Magn Reson Med* 1997;37:341–345.

99. Korosec F, Frayne R, Grist T, Mistretta C. Time-resolved contrast-enhanced 3D MR angiography. *Magn Reson Med* 1996;36:345–351.

100. Ladd ME, Gohde SC, Steiner P, et al. Virtual MR angioscopy of the pulmonary artery tree. *J Comput Assist Tomogr* 1996;20:782–785.

101. Greaves SM, Hart EM, Aberle DR. CT of pulmonary thromboembolism. *Semin Ultrasound CT MRI* 1997;18:323–337.

102. Coche EE, Müller NL, Kim K-I, Wiggs BR, Mayo JR. Acute pulmonary embolism: ancillary findings at spiral CT. *Radiology* 1998;207:753–758.

103. Remy-Jardin M, Remy J. Spiral CT of pulmonary embolism. In: Remy-Jardin M, Remy J, eds. *Spiral CT of the chest*. Berlin: Springer, 1996:201–230.

104. Anderson MB, Kriett JM, Kapelanski DP, Tarazi R, Jamieson SW. Primary pulmonary artery sarcoma: a report of six cases. *Ann Thorac Surg* 1995;59:1487–1490.

105. Cox JE, Chiles C, Aquino SL, Savage P, Oaks T. Pulmonary artery sarcomas: a review of clinical and radiologic features. *J Comput Assist Tomogr* 1997;21:750–755.

106. Weinreb JC, Davis SD, Berkman YM, Isom W, Naidich DP. Pulmonary artery sarcoma: evaluation using Gd-DTPA. *J Comput Assist Tomogr* 1990;14:647–649.

107. Kauczor H-U, Schwickert HC, Mayer E, et al. Pulmonary artery sarcoma mimicking chronic thromboembolic disease: computed tomography and magnetic resonance imaging. *Cardiovasc Intervent Radiol* 1994;17:185–189.

108. Matsumoto AH, Tegtmeyer CJ. Contemporary diagnostic approaches to acute pulmonary emboli. *Radiol Clin North Am* 1995;33:167–183.

109. Egermayer P, Town GI. The clinical significance of pulmonary embolism: uncertainties and implications for treatment. A debate. *J Intern Med* 1997;241:5–10.

110. Rosenow EC III. Venous and pulmonary thromboembolism: an algorithmic approach to diagnosis and management. *Mayo Clin Proc* 1995;70:45–49.

111. The Pioped Investigators. Value of the ventilation/perfusion scan in acute pulmonary embolism. Results of the prospective investigation of pulmonary embolism diagnosis (PIOPED). *JAMA* 1990;263:2753–2759.

112. Hull RD, Raskob GE, Pineo GF, Brant RF. The low-probability lung scan: a need for change in nomenclature. *Arch Intern Med* 1995;155:1847–1851.

113. Herold CJ, Remy-Jardin M, Grenier P, et al. Prospective evaluation of pulmonary embolism: initial results of the European multicenter trial (ESTIPEP). Annual Scientific Session of the Fleishner Society. Washington, DC, 1998.

114. Gottschalk A, Sostman HD, Juni JE, et al. Ventilation-perfusion scintigraphy in the PIOPED study. II. Evaluation of criteria and interpretations. *J Nucl Med* 1993;34:1119–1126.

115. Sostman HD, Coleman RE, DeLong DM, Newman GE, Paine S. Evaluation of revised criteria for ventilation-perfusion scintigraphy in patients with suspected pulmonary embolism. *Radiology* 1994;193:103–107.

116. Stein PD, Henry JW. Clinical characteristics of patients with acute pulmonary embolism stratified according to their presenting syndromes. *Chest* 1997;112:974–979.

117. Breslaw BH, Dorfman GS. Ventilation/perfusion scanning for prediction of the location of pulmonary emboli: correlation with pulmonary angiographic findings. *Radiology* 1992;185:180.

118. Khorasani R, Gudas TF, Nikpoor N, Polak JF. Treatment of patients with suspected pulmonary embolism and intermediate-probability lung scans: is diagnostic imaging underused? *AJR Am J Roentgenol* 1997;169:1355–1357.

119. Stein PD. Opinion response to acute pulmonary embolism: the role of computed tomographic imaging. *J Thorac Imaging* 1997;12:86–89.

120. Moser KM. Fatal pulmonary embolism: old pitfalls, new challenges. *Mayo Clin Proc* 1995;70:501–502.

121. Baldt MM, Zontsich T, Kainberger F, Fleischmann G, Mostbeck G. Spiral CT evaluation of deep venous thrombosis. *Semin Ultrasound CT MRI* 1997;18:369–375.

122. Baldt MM, Zontsich T, Stümpflen A, et al. Deep venous thrombosis of the lower extremity: efficacy of spiral CT venography compared with conventional venography in diagnosis. *Radiology* 1996;200:423–428.

123. Raghavendra BN, Horii SC, Hilton S, et al. Deep venous thrombosis: detection by probe compression of veins. *J Ultrasound Med* 1986;5:89–95.

124. Moser KM. Significance of silent pulmonary embolism in the specturm of thromboembolic disease. *Semin Respir Crit Care Med* 1996;17:17–21.

125. Kakkar VV, Flanc C, Howe CT, Nordyke RA. Natural history of postoperative deep venous thrombosis. *Lancet* 1969;2:230–235.

126. Oser RF, Zuckerman DA, Gutierrez FR, Brink JA. Anatomic distribution of pulmonary emboli at pulmonary angiography: implications for cross-sectional imaging. *Radiology* 1996;199:31–35.

127. Schauble JF, Anlyan WG, Deaton HL, et al. A study of recurrent pulmonary embolism. *Arch Surg* 1960;80:113–118.

128. Stein PD, Henry JW, Relyea B. Untreated patients with pulmonary embolism: outcome, clinical, and laboratory assessment. *Chest* 1995;107:931–935.

129. Sostman HD, Layish DT, Tapson VF, et al. Prospective comparison of helical CT and MR imaging in clinically suspected acute pulmonary embolism. *J Magn Reson Imaging* 1996;6:275–281.

130. Gefter WB, Palevsky HI. Opinion response to acute pulmonary embolism: The role of computed tomographic imaging. *J Thorac Imaging* 1997;12:97–100.

131. Murchison JT, Gavan DR, Reid JH. Clinical utilization of non-diagnostic lung scintigram. *Clin Radiol* 1997;52:295–298.

132. van Erkel AR, Vanrossum AB, Bloem JL, Klevit J, Pattynama PMT. Spiral CT angiography for suspected pulmonary embolism: a cost-effectiveness analysis. *Radiology* 1996;201:29–36.

133. Schwickert HC, Schweden F, Schild HH, et al. Pulmonary arteries and lung parenchyma in chronic pulmonary embolism: preoperative and postoperative CT findings. *Radiology* 1994;191:351–357.

134. Roberts HC, Kauczor HU, Schweden F, Thelen M. Spiral CT of pulmonary hypertension and chronic thromboembolism. *J Thorac Imaging* 1997;12:118–127.

135. King MA, Ysrael M, Bergin CJ. Pictorial essay. Chronic thromboembolic pulmonary hypertension: CT findings. *AJR Am J Roentgenol* 1998;170:955–960.

136. Tardivon AA, Musset D, Maitre S, et al. Role of CT in chronic pulmonary embolism: comparison with pulmonary angiography. *J Comput Assist Tomogr* 1993;17:345–351.

137. King MA, Bergin CJ, Yeung DWC, et al. Chronic pulmonary thromboembolism: detection of regional hypoperfusion with CT. *Radiology* 1994;191:359–363.

138. Kauczor H-U, Schwickert HC, Mayer E, et al. Spiral CT of bronchial arteries in chronic thromboembolism. *J Comput Assist Tomogr* 1994;18:855–861.

139. Remy-Jardin M, Louvegny S, Remy J, et al. Acute central thromboembolic disease: posttherapeutic follow-up with spiral CT angiography. *Radiology* 1997;203:173–180.

140. Van Rossum AB, Pattynama PMT, Ton ETA, Kieft GJ. Spiral CT appearance of resolving clots at 6 week follow-up after acute pulmonary embolism. *J Comput Assist Tomogr* 1998;22:413–417.

141. Bergin CJ, Rios G, King MA, et al. Accuracy of high-resolution CT in identifying chronic pulmonary thromboembolic disease. *AJR Am J Roentgenol* 1996;166:1371–1377.

142. Sherrick AD, Swensen SJ, Hartman TE. Mosaic pattern of lung attenuation on CT scans: frequency among patients with pulmonary artery hypertension of different causes. *AJR Am J Roentgenol* 1997;169:79–82.

143. Falaschi F, Palla A, Formichi B, et al. CT evaluation of chronic thromboembolic pulmonary hypertension. *J Comput Assist Tomogr* 1992;16:897–903.

144. Bartter T, Irwin RS, Nash G. Review: aneurysms of the pulmonary arteries. *Chest* 1988;94:1065–1079.

145. Butto F, Lucas RV, Edwards JE. Pulmonary arterial aneurysm: a pathologic study of five cases. *Chest* 1987;91:237–241.

146. SanDretto MA, Scanlon GT. Multiple mycotic pulmonary artery aneurysms secondary to intravenous drug use. *AJR Am J Roentgenol* 1984;143:89–90.

147. Tunaci A, Berkmen YM, Gokmen E. Thoracic involvement in Behçet's disease: pathologic, clinical and imaging features. *AJR Am J Roentgenol* 1995;164:51–56.

148. Numan F, Islak C, Berkmen T, Tuzun H, Cokyuksel O. Behçet disease: pulmonary arterial involvement in 15 cases. *Radiology* 1994;192:465–468.

149. Berkmen T. MR angiography of aneurysms in Behçet disease: a report of four cases. *J Comput Assist Tomogr* 1998;22:202–206.

150. Ferretti GR, Thony R, Link KM, et al. False aneurysm of the pulmonary artery induced by a Swan-Ganz catheter: clinical presentation and radiologic management. *AJR Am J Roentgenol* 1996;167:941–945.

151. Godwin JD, Webb WR. Dynamic computed tomography in the evaluation of vascular lung lesions. *Radiology* 1981;138:629–635.

152. Shin MS, Ceballos R, Bini RM, Ho KJ. Case report: CT diagnosis of false aneurysm of the pulmonary artery not demonstrated by angiography. *J Comput Assist Tomogr* 1983;7:524–526.

153. Daykin EL, Irwin GAL, Harrison DA. Case report: CT demonstration of a traumatic aneurysm of the pulmonary artery. *J Comput Assist Tomogr* 1986;10:323–324.

154. Jeang MK, Adyanthaya A, Kuo L, et al. Multiple pulmonary artery aneurysms: new use for magnetic resonance imaging. *Am J Med* 1986;81:1001–1004.

155. Winchester PA, Khilnani NM, Trost DW, et al. Technical note: endovascular catheter biopsy of a pulmonary artery sarcoma. *AJR Am J Roentgenol* 1996;167:657–659.

156. Shields JJ, Cho KJ, Geisinger KR. Pulmonary artery constriction by mediastinal lymphoma simulating pulmonary embolus. *AJR Am J Roentgenol* 1980;135:147–150.

157. Dore R, Alerci M, D'Andrea F, Giulio GD, Agostini AD, Volpato G. Intracardiac extension of lung cancer via pulmonary veins: CT diagnosis. *J Comput Assist Tomogr* 1988;12:565–568.

158. Marshall ME, Trump DL. Acquired extrinsic pulmonic stenosis caused by mediastinal tumors. *Cancer* 1982;49:1496–1499.

159. Hamper UM, Fishman EK, Khouri NF, Jogns CJ, Wang KP, Siegelman SS. Typical and atypical CT manifestations of pulmonary sarcoidosis. *J Comput Assist Tomogr* 1986;10:928–936.

160. Weinstein JB, Aronberg DJ, Sagel SS. CT of fibrosing mediastinitis: findings and their utility. *AJR Am J Roentgenol* 1983;141:247–251.

161. Berry DF, Buccigrossi D, Peabody J, Peterson KL, Moser KM. Review: pulmonary vascular occlusion and fibrosing mediastinitis. *Chest* 1986;89:296–301.

162. Farmer DW, Moore E, Amparo E, et al. Calcific fibrosing mediastinitis: demonstration of pulmonary vascular obstruction by magnetic resonance imaging. *AJR Am J Roentgenol* 1984;143:1189–1191.

163. Cramer M, Foley WD, Palmer TE. Compression of the right pulmonary artery by aortic aneurysms: CT demonstration. *J Comput Assist Tomogr* 1985;9:310–314.

164. Borokowski GP, O'Donovan PB, Troup BR. Pulmonary varix: CT findings. *J Comput Assist Tomogr* 1981;5:827–829.

165. Chaise LS, Soulen RL, Teplick S, Patrick H. Computed tomographic diagnosis of pulmonary varix. *J Comput Assist Tomogr* 1983;7:281–284.

166. Matsumoto AH, Parker LA, Delany D. CT demonstration of central pulmonary venous and arterial occlusive diseases. *J Comput Assist Tomogr* 1987;11:640–644.

167. Lombard CM, Churg A, Winokur S. Pulmonary veno-occlusive disease following therapy for malignant neoplasms. *Chest* 1982;92:871–876.

168. Maltby JD, Gouverne ML. CT findings in pulmonary venoocclusive disease. *J Comput Assist Tomogr* 1984;8:758–761.

169. Cassart M, Gevenois PA, Kramer M, et al. Pulmonary venoocclusive disease. *J Comput Assist Tomogr* 1993;160:759–760.

170. Swensen SJ, Tashjian JH, Myers JL, et al. Pulmonary venoocclusive disease: CT findings in eight patients. *AJR Am J Roentgenol* 1996;167:937–940.

171. Choe DH, Lee JH, Lee BH, et al. Obliteration of the pulmonary vein in lung cancer: significance in assessing local extent with CT. *J Comput Assist Tomogr* 1998;22:587–591.

172. Naidich DP. Volumetric CT in the evaluation of focal pulmonary disease. In: Remy-Jardin M, Remy J, eds. *Spiral CT of the chest*. Berlin: Springer, 1997:129–151.

173. Yamashita H. *Roentgenologic anatomy of the lung*. Tokyo: Igaku-Shoin, 1978.

CHAPTER 10

Pleura, Chest Wall, and Diaphragm

Very early in its development, the value of computed tomography (CT) was recognized in assessing pleural and chest wall diseases (1, 2). This reflects in part the wide range of pathology that affects these areas, as well as the accepted limitations of chest radiography, especially in the assessment of complex pleural and parenchymal disease. In this chapter, the value and limitations of CT in the assessment of diffuse and focal pleural disease, chest wall lesions, and the diaphragm will be discussed and illustrated. Potential applications of magnetic resonance (MR) also will be addressed.

THE PLEURA

There is no standardized technique for the evaluation of the pleura, chest wall, or diaphragm. Each case should be considered individually with regard to number of slices, section thickness, and use of intravenous contrast material. Posteroanterior (PA) and lateral radiographs are always obtained prior to the CT study. In most cases, standard 7- to 8-mm thick sections are sufficient to evaluate most pleural diseases. Although the use of high-resolution techniques is usually unnecessary, thin sections may be advantageous in detecting asbestos-related pleural plaques (3).

As will be extensively illustrated, the administration of intravenous contrast can play an indispensable role, especially in differentiating between pleural and parenchymal processes (4). In cases in which the major indication for CT is evaluation of complex pleuro-parenchymal disease, a bolus of intravenous (i.v.) contrast should be administered, with sections obtained helically, when available. This technique allows optimal visualization of parenchymal vasculature during the phase of maximum pulmonary artery and vein enhancement. In select cases, this initial sequence can be augmented by obtaining delayed images through regions of interest; sections obtained within minutes following the bolus administration of i.v. contrast may optimize visualization of the parenchyma, specifically when the lung is consolidated or collapsed. With helical acquisition it is also possible to generate multiplanar reconstructions. For this purpose, overlapping reconstructions are mandatory (see Chapter 1). Even if the disease process is localized, thorough examination of the entire chest is usually necessary to insure that other pertinent abnormalities are not missed.

CT Technique

CT is of greatest efficacy in (a) confirming the presence of a lesion; (b) determining its precise location and extent

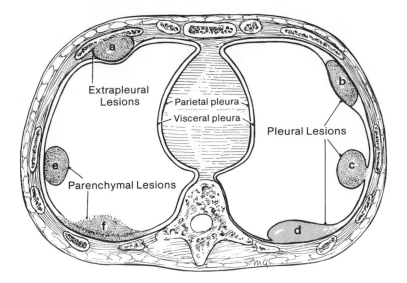

FIG. 10-1. Schematic drawing of the cross-sectional appearance, typical and atypical, of extrapleural, pleural, and peripheral parenchymal lesions. Extrapleural lesions displace the overlying parietal and visceral pleura (**A**), resulting in an obtuse angle between the lesion and the chest wall. Associated chest wall pathology (for example, rib erosion) helps define the lesion as extrapleural. Pleural lesions generally remain confined between the layers of the pleura and cause obtuse angles between the lesion and the chest wall (**B**). Pleural lesions, however, may be pedunculated (**C**), in which case they may prolapse into the pulmonary parenchyma, resulting in acute angles between the lesion and the chest wall. Additionally, pleural fibrosis may result in fusion of the parietal and visceral pleura (**D**), leading to abnormal configurations of pleural lesions and/or loculation of pleural fluid. Parenchymal lesions, if subpleural, abut the pleura (**E**), resulting in acute angulation with the chest wall. Clearly, while the mechanics vary, there is a considerable overlap in the cross-sectional appearance of extrapleural, pleural, and parenchymal lesions. In practical terms, all peripheral soft-tissue should be biopsied, regardless of site of origin.

as either primarily pulmonary or pleural; and (c) further characterizing the nature of the pathology by means of attenuation coefficients.

Localization

Peripheral lesions are generally classified as extrapleural, pleural, or parenchymal, and are usually characterized radiographically by the angle (either acute or obtuse) formed by the interface between the lesion and the adjacent pleura. Unfortunately, although CT is far superior to routine chest radiography in detecting the presence of pathology, there is considerable overlap in the cross-sectional appearance of these lesions, as shown in Figure 10-1.

Extrapleural lesions usually displace the overlying parietal and visceral pleura, resulting in an obtuse angle between the lesion and the chest wall (Fig. 10-2). Associated changes, such as rib destruction or muscle infiltration, help to confirm the site of origin as extrapleural, although these signs are often absent. Extrapleural lesions may prolapse into the adjacent lung, resulting in acute angulation between the lesion and the chest wall; however, this is uncommon.

Pleural lesions arising from the visceral or parietal pleura usually remain confined to the pleural space and have a configuration similar to that of extrapleural lesions. However, pedunculated pleural lesions, especially those arising from the visceral pleura, are an important exception (5,6). As shown in Figure 10-1, these may prolapse or invaginate into the adjacent pulmonary parenchyma. If the lesion is small, the appearance will mimic a peripheral, subpleural parenchy-

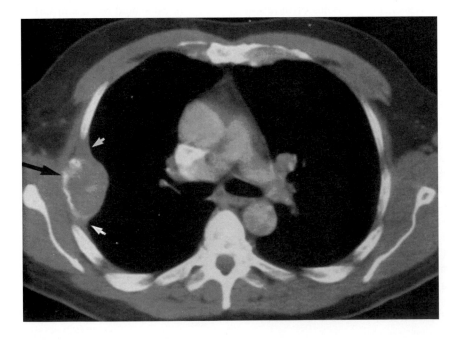

FIG. 10-2. Rib metastasis. CT section shows a lytic destructive rib lesion on the right side (*arrow*) associated with a large extraosseous soft-tissue component. Note obtuse angles between the lesion and the adjacent lung (*white arrows*).

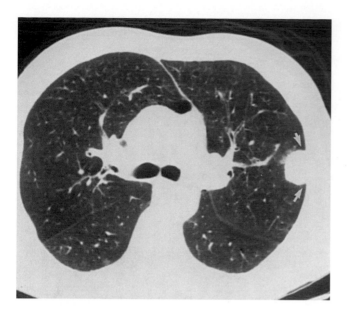

FIG. 10-3. Benign fibrous tumor of the pleura. Section through the left midlung shows a well-defined tumor mass on the left side, which at surgery proved to be a benign, pedunculated mesothelioma. Note acute angles between the lesion and adjacent lung, despite the pleural origin of this tumor (*arrows*).

mal nodule; if the lesion is larger and broad-based, the appearance of a pedunculated pleural lesion may mimic larger intraparenchymal subpleural lesions (Fig. 10-3).

The cross-sectional appearance of pleural pathology, especially loculated pleural fluid collections, will also be affected by pleural adhesions along the lesion margins. Pleurodesis restricts the mobility of the pleural layers; the result may be acute angulation between the pleural lesion and/or fluid, and the adjacent chest wall (see Fig. 10-1).

Pulmonary parenchymal lesions, when peripheral, may abut the pleura; this typically results in acute angulation between the lesion and the chest wall. However, if sufficiently large, parenchymal lesions may result in obtuse angles between the lesion and the chest wall, usually as the result of visceral and parietal pleural infiltration (see Fig. 10-1 and Fig. 10-4) (7). It cannot be overemphasized that evaluation of peripheral lung lesions that only abut pleural surfaces is extremely limited: The configuration of peripheral lung can-

cer in relation to the chest wall, for example, is of little use in determining whether or not there is histologic invasion of the pleura. As will be discussed in greater detail later, exclusion of tumor infiltration into the pleura or chest wall often requires biopsy.

Another potential pitfall in differentiating parenchymal from pleural disease is the presence of fluid within preexisting parenchymal cavities (8). As documented by Zinn and coworkers, fluid within bullae may precisely mimic the appearance of a loculated pleural fluid collection. In fact, in select cases, differentiation may be possible only by reference to previous chest radiographs documenting the presence of prior bullous lung disease (Fig. 10-5). Therefore, it is apparent that although the mechanics of pathology vary, the end result is that there may be considerable overlap in the cross-sectional appearance of extrapleural, pleural, and peripheral subpleural parenchymal lesions (see Fig. 10-1).

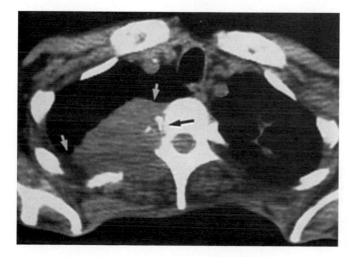

FIG. 10-4. Chest wall invasion: bronchogenic carcinoma. CT section through the lung apices shows a posterior lung mass on the right clearly invading both the chest wall and adjacent vertebral body (*straight arrow*). Note obtuse angles between the lesion and the adjacent lung (*white arrows*).

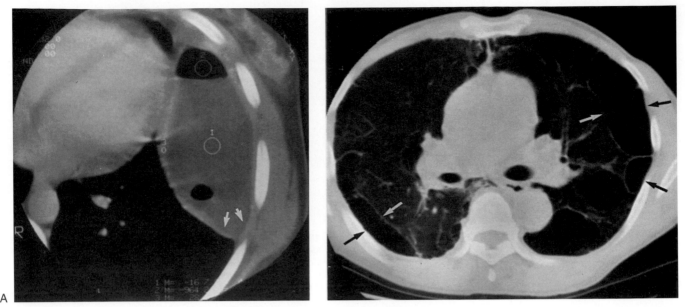

FIG. 10-5. A: Infected bulla. Enlargement of a CT section through the left midlung following a bolus of intravenous contrast media. A well-defined, smooth-walled, lenticular-shaped fluid collection (*arrows*) mimicking a split-pleura sign. Although this appearance suggests a loculated pleural fluid collection, at surgery this proved to be an infected bulla. **B:** CT section in a different patient showing characteristic appearance of numerous peripheral bullae (*arrows*). It is apparent that if any of these became fluid-filled, the appearance could precisely mimic that of loculated fluid within the pleural space (compare with **A**). (From ref. 8, with permission.)

Tissue Density Characteristics

As compared with routine chest radiographs, a major value of CT is its ability to provide improved contrast resolution. This has proven to be immensely valuable in assessing pleural pathology, especially in detecting the presence of pleural fluid (9–12). Less commonly, CT may help in differentiating a lipoma from a soft-tissue mass or cyst (Fig. 10-

6) (13). Unfortunately, although CT is extremely accurate in detecting the presence of pleural fluid, CT densitometry is of no value in differentiating among the various etiologies of pleural effusions. Specifically, CT numbers do not allow differentiation between transudative and exudative effusions, and cannot even be used reliably to detect chylous effusions (14–16). This is not to say that CT is of no value for differentiating between transudative and exudative effu-

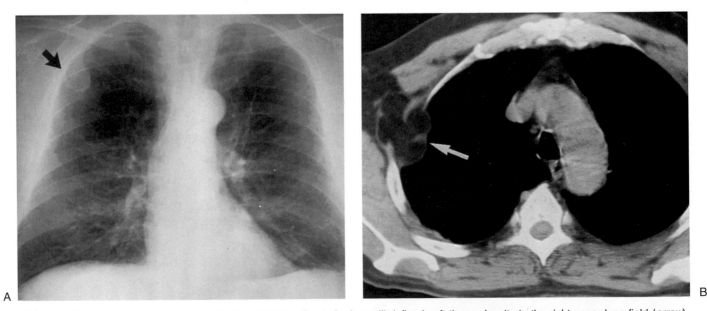

FIG. 10-6. Pleural/chest wall lipoma. **A:** Posteroanterior radiograph shows ill-defined soft-tissue density in the right upper lung field (*arrow*). Although suggestive of an extrapleural density, this appearance is nonspecific. **B:** CT section shows a lobular mass clearly composed of fat involving the chest wall and invaginating intrathoracically (*arrow*). This appearance is essentially pathognomonic of a lipoma.

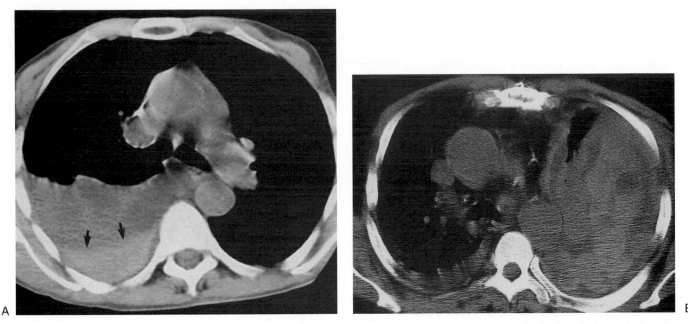

FIG. 10-7. Hemorrhagic effusions. **A:** Pleural hemorrhage. CT section shows a large right-sided pleural fluid collection within which there is a clear fluid-fluid level (*arrows*). The density within the dependent fluid collection measured within the range of acute hemorrhage, subsequently verified via thoracentesis. **B:** Noncontrast-enhanced CT section through a different patient than **A**, following trauma. There is a massive hemothorax present identifiable as inhomogrenous areas of high contrast. Note that in this case there is marked shift of the mediastinum and a small right pleural effusion.

sions: This distinction is possible in a significant percentage of cases based on the morphologic appearance of the pleural surfaces, as will be discussed in greater detail below.

In the setting of an acute bleed, CT may allow identification of hemorrhagic pleural effusions (Fig. 10-7). Rarely, CT also may be of value in detecting so-called milk of calcium effusions resulting from chronic inflammation (17).

Although CT easily detects the presence of even small pneumothoraces (Fig. 10-8) considerable limitations apply in the evaluation of soft-tissue masses, for which specific histologic diagnosis can be made only rarely. From a practi-

cal standpoint, any peripheral soft-tissue mass, regardless of its probable site of origin, should be biopsied.

Interlobar Fissures

The interlobar fissures represent invaginations of the visceral pleura, which, to a variable degree, separate the pulmonary lobes. A knowledge of fissural anatomy is essential in the localization and diagnosis of both pleural and parenchymal abnormalities. Interlobar fissures can be localized on CT in nearly all cases based on a knowledge of their anatomy

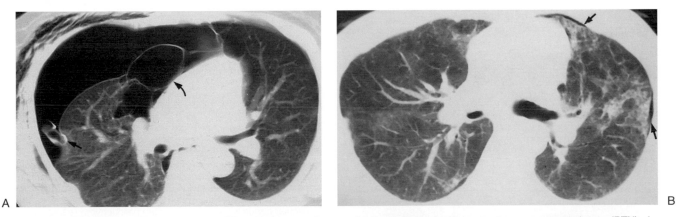

FIG. 10-8. Pneumothorax: CT evaluation. **A:** CT section in a patient previously diagnosed with a spontaneous pneumothorax (PTX) shows evidence of a residual large right pneumothorax despite the presence of a right-sided chest tube (*arrow*). In this case the persistent air leak was due to underlying bullous emphysema, identifiable as a cluster of cysts involving the medial aspect of the middle lobe (*curved arrow*). Not surprisingly, these were not initially identifiable on the admission radiograph. **B:** CT section in an AIDS patient shows ill defined areas of ground glass attenuation especially in the left upper lobe. Note the presence of a subtle, "occult" pneumothorax (*arrows*). These two cases point out the potential contribution of CT to both detect and characterize pneumothoraces.

(18,19), although their appearances vary depending on whether thick collimation (10 mm) or thin collimation (1 mm) is used. The normal CT appearances of the interlobar fissures have been described by a number of authors (3,18–24).

The Major (Oblique) Fissure

The major fissures serve to separate the lower lobe from the upper lobe on the left, and from the upper and middle lobes on the right. However, many patients have incomplete major fissures, with some contiguity between the parenchyma of adjacent lobes. In anatomic studies, the right major fissure is complete in only 30% of patients (9,25), although in an additional 30%, near compete separation is present. The right major fissure is more often complete inferiorly; complete separation of the right lower and middle lobes is present in about 53% of patients (25). On the left, the major fissure has been reported to be complete in 27% to 60% of

patients, although the extent of contiguity between lobes is often minimal (9,25).

The major fissures are oriented obliquely to the plane of scan. They originate along the anterior diaphragmatic pleural surface of each lung, angle posteriorly and superiorly, and terminate along the posterior pleural surfaces above the level of the aortic arch. The orientation of the major fissures varies at different levels. Within the lower thorax, the major fissures angle anterolaterally from the mediastinum, contacting the anterior third of the hemidiaphragms. In the upper thorax, the major fissures angle posterolaterally from the mediastinum.

Because of volume averaging, the appearance of a major (or oblique) fissure on CT obtained with 7 to 10 mm collimation is variable, and depends on the orientation of the fissure relative to the plane of cross-section. If the fissure is oriented perpendicular to the plane of scan, the fissure itself can be seen as a thin linear structure (Fig. 10-9); however, this is uncommon. In 60% to 84% of cases, the fissures are invisi-

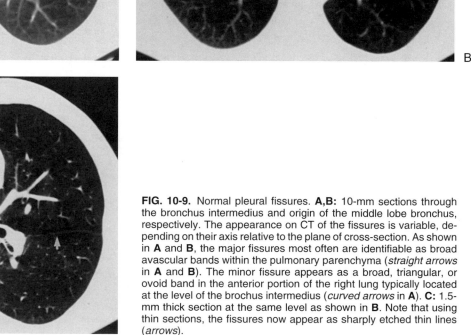

FIG. 10-9. Normal pleural fissures. **A,B:** 10-mm sections through the bronchus intermedius and origin of the middle lobe bronchus, respectively. The appearance on CT of the fissures is variable, depending on their axis relative to the plane of cross-section. As shown in **A** and **B**, the major fissures most often are identifiable as broad avascular bands within the pulmonary parenchyma (*straight arrows* in **A** and **B**). The minor fissure appears as a broad, triangular, or ovoid band in the anterior portion of the right lung typically located at the level of the brochus intermedius (*curved arrows* in **A**). **C:** 1.5-mm thick section at the same level as shown in **B**. Note that using thin sections, the fissures now appear as sharply etched thin lines (*arrows*).

ble, although their locations can be identified because of avascular bands, several cm in thickness, within the pulmonary parenchyma (see Fig. 10-9) (18,19,24). These bands appear "avascular" because of the small size of vessels located in the peripheral lung on either side of the fissure. In 4% to 21% of cases (18,24) the major fissures are localized by broad, ground-glass opacity bands, particularly when scans are obtained through the uppermost portions of the fissures. Presumably, this appearance is caused by volume averaging of the fissure with adjacent lung or congestion or hypoinflation of the dependent portions of the upper lobes, adjacent to the fissure. In support of the latter explanation, a dense band in the location of the fissure is more often seen on end-expiratory scans. Incompleteness of the fissure is difficult to diagnose on conventional CT because of these variations of its normal appearance. In nearly 20% of cases (26), a focal thickening of the fissure can be seen on CT, just above its point of contact with the diaphragm; this represents fat extending into the fissure.

On CT obtained using thin collimation or high-resolution technique, the major fissures usually appear as thin, well-defined lines, surrounded by a plane of avascular lung measuring about 1 cm in thickness. If the fissure is invisible on high resolution CT (HRCT), it may be incomplete. In some cases, cardiac motion during the scan results in a confusing artifact termed the "double-fissure" sign (27). When this artifact is present, the fissure is visible in two locations on the same scan.

The Minor (Horizontal) Fissure

The minor or horizontal fissure separates the superior aspect of the right middle lobe from the right upper lobe. Incompleteness of the minor fissure is common, occurring in 78% to 88% of patients. The minor fissure is most often incomplete laterally, with contiguity of the parenchyma of the upper and middle lobes (9,25).

On conventional CT obtained with 7 to 10 mm collimation, the minor fissure is rarely visible, as its position generally parallels the scan plane. Characteristically, however, the position of the minor fissure can be identified because of a broad avascular band in the anterior portion of the right lung, anterior to the major fissure, at the level of the bronchus intermedius (see Fig. 10-9). This avascular region represents peripheral lung on each side of the fissure, lying in or near the plane of scan. The avascular band is often triangular in shape, with one corner of the triangle at the pulmonary hilum, and the other two laterally, but considerable variation in the appearance of the minor fissure can be seen owing to variations in the orientation and curvature of the fissure. Less frequently, the avascular region of the minor fissure appears rectangular or round or elliptical in shape. Goodman and colleagues (22) labeled this avascular region the "right midlung window," and were able to identify this area of diminished vascularity in 92% of 50 patients.

Because the minor fissure often angles caudally, the lower lobe, middle lobe, and upper lobe can all be seen on a single scan (Figs 10-10–10-12). If this is the case, the major and minor fissures can have a similar appearance, with the major fissure being posterior and the minor fissure anterior; in this situation, the lower lobe is most posterior, the upper lobe is most anterior, and the middle lobe is in the middle. If the minor fissure is concave caudally, it can sometimes be seen in two locations or can appear ring-shaped, with the middle lobe between the fissure lines or in the center of the ring, and the upper lobe anterior to the most anterior part of the fissure (see Fig. 10-12).

The appearance of the minor fissure on scans obtained utilizing thin section or HRCT technique is quite variable (see Figs. 10-10 and 10-11) (20,28–30). Depending on its orientation and contour, the fissure may appear as (a) a thick or thin linear opacity, directed from anterior to posterior, and either medial or lateral in location (28,29) (see Figs. 10-10 and 10-11); (b) a thick or thin linear opacity, extending from medial to lateral, paralleling and anterior to the major fissure; (c) an ill-defined opacity resulting from the fissure lying in the plane of scan; (d) a circle or ring; or (e) a combination of these findings (see Figs. 10-10 and 10-11). However, in one study, the minor fissure appeared to be absent in 20% of cases and incomplete in 72% (28). Similar findings using 1.5-mm sections have been reported by Frija et al., who also found that the minor fissure was incomplete in 76% of cases (29).

Familiarity with the appearance of the minor fissure on thin section scans may help in differentiating middle lobe from right upper lobe lesions (28,30). In addition, as emphasized by Otsuji et al. (30), recognition of characteristic relationships between subsegmental bronchi and corresponding branches of the pulmonary artery can allow confident differentiation between adjacent lobes. Similar observations have been made by Berkman and colleagues, using visualization of the lowest tributary of the vein draining the anterior segment of the upper lobe. In these authors' experience, visualization of this vein allowed differentiation between the upper and middle lobe in 75% of their cases (28). Although they are of value in select cases, these distinctions require extremely detailed knowledge of subsegmental anatomy.

Accessory Fissures

Any segment of lung can be separated from adjacent segments by an accessory fissure; numerous accessory fissures have been identified (31–34). As many as 50% of lungs show some accessory fissure. Although these are not frequently of significance, a knowledge of their common appearances can be helpful.

An azygos fissure and azygos lobe are most common, occurring in less than 0.4% of subjects. The azygos fissure consists of 4 layers of pleura (2 parietal and 2 visceral), as the azygos vein originates in an extrapulmonary location. Altera-

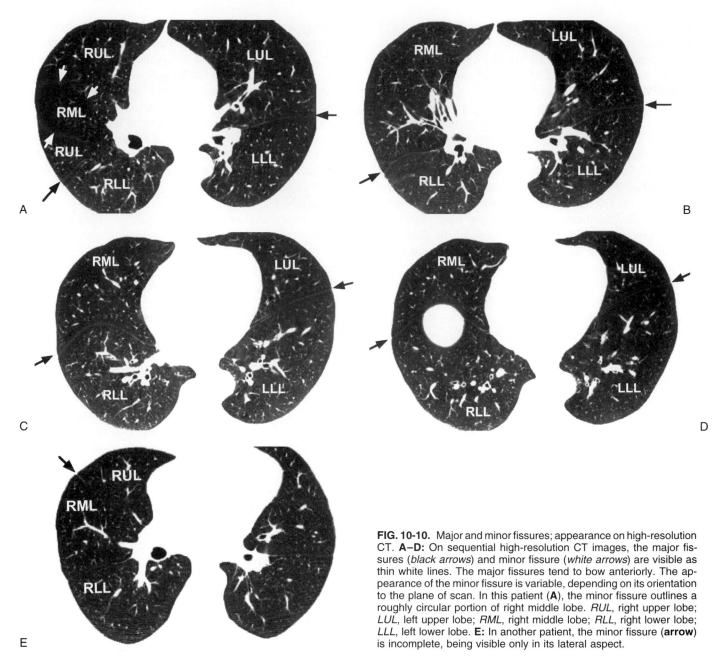

FIG. 10-10. Major and minor fissures; appearance on high-resolution CT. **A–D:** On sequential high-resolution CT images, the major fissures (*black arrows*) and minor fissure (*white arrows*) are visible as thin white lines. The major fissures tend to bow anteriorly. The appearance of the minor fissure is variable, depending on its orientation to the plane of scan. In this patient (**A**), the minor fissure outlines a roughly circular portion of right middle lobe. *RUL*, right upper lobe; *LUL*, left upper lobe; *RML*, right middle lobe; *RLL*, right lower lobe; *LLL*, left lower lobe. **E:** In another patient, the minor fissure (**arrow**) is incomplete, being visible only in its lateral aspect.

FIG. 10-12. Diagrammatic representation of the minor fissure, its orientation relative to the scan plane, and its appearance on high-resolution CT. If the minor fissure often angles caudally (**A**), the major and minor fissures can have a similar appearance, with the major fissure being posterior and the minor fissure anterior; in this situation, the lower lobe is most posterior, the upper lobe is most anterior, and the middle lobe is in the middle. If the minor fissure is concave caudally (**B**), the minor fissure can be seen in two locations or can appear ring-shaped or triangular, with the middle lobe between the fissure lines or in the center of the ring, and the upper lobe anterior to the most anterior part of the fissure.

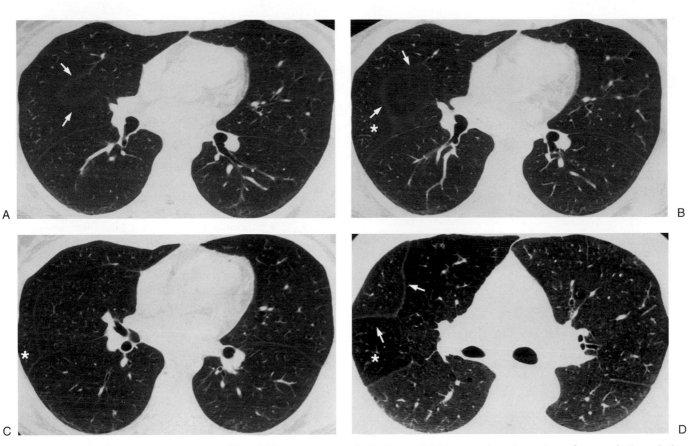

FIG. 10-11. Minor fissure of high-resolution CT-variable appearances. **A–C:** Sequential 1-mm sections from above downwards through the minor fissure. Note that in this case the apex of the middle lobe is rounded resulting in a circular appearance of the minor fissure in cross-section (*arrows* in **A** and **B**).Note that this results in a portion of the anterior segment of the right upper lobe extending lateral and posterior to the middle lobe (*asterisks* in **B** and **C**). **D:** High-resolution CT section in a different patient than **A–C**. In this case the highest point of the middle lobe is lateral: the result is a curvilinear appearance of the minor fissure (*arrows*). Note that in this case the right upper lobe (*asterisk*) extends directly behind the apex of the middle lobe. These appearances should not be misconstrued as abnormal. In select cases the ability to precisely identify the location of the minor fissure allows more precise localization of parenchymal disease.

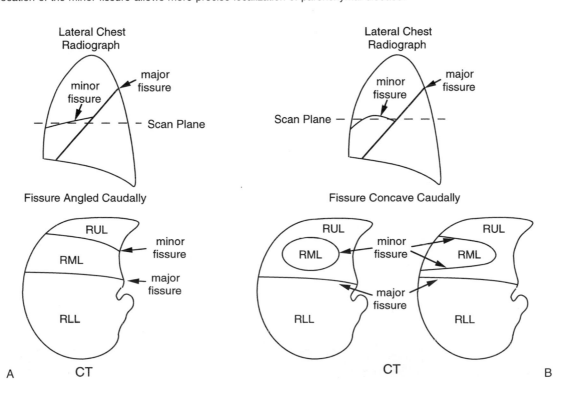

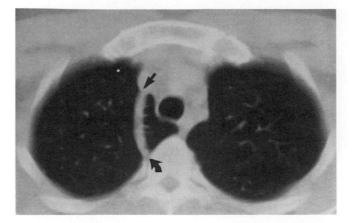

FIG. 10-13. Azygos lobe. 10-mm section through the upper lobes shows characteristic appearance of an azygos fissure and lobe. Note that the fissure extends from the lateral border of the right brachiocephalic vein anteriorly (*straight arrow*) to the right superior intercostal vein, posteriorly (*curved arrow*).

tions in the normal appearance of the lung and mediastinum produced by an azygos lobe have been well described (Fig. 10-13) (32). The azygos fissure limits the lateral margin of the azygos lobe, which frequently extends well behind the trachea and sometimes esophagus. The azygos fissure extends from the brachiocephalic vein, anteriorly, to a position adjacent to the right posterolateral aspect of the T4 or T5 vertebral body;

it is usually identifiable on CT as a thin, curved line. An azygos lobe represents parts of the apical or posterior segments of the right upper lobe. Although the bronchial supply of an azygos lobe is variable, an apical or anterior subsegmental branch of the apical segment is always present (35).

The inferior accessory fissure separates the medial basilar segment of either lower lobe from the remaining basal segments. It is present anatomically in 30% to 45% of lobes, although it is less commonly seen on CT (Fig. 10-14) (33). It extends laterally and anteriorly from the region of the inferior pulmonary ligament to join the major fissure.

Other accessory fissures that have been described include (a) the left minor fissure, anatomically present in approximately 15% of normal lungs, separating the anterior segment of the left upper lobe from the lingula (Fig. 10-15) (34); (b) a left "azygos" fissure, analogous to the more typical right azygos lobe, in which there is a malpositioned left superior intercostal vein (31); and (c) the superior accessory fissure, demarcating the superior segment from the remainder of the lower lobes (33). Identification of these accessory fissures rarely presents diagnostic difficulties; their recognition is of obvious benefit in identifying pathology related to the fissures (see Fig. 10-13), including loculated interfissural fluid collections. Although identification of benign processes involving both normal and accessory fissures is generally straightforward, it is unfortunate that identification of transfissural extension of tumor is more problematic.

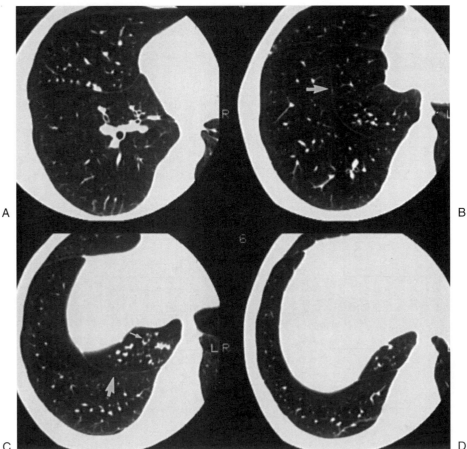

FIG. 10-14. Right inferior accessory fissure. **A–D:** Enlargements of sequential 1.5-mm sections through the right lung base show an accessory fissure identifiable as a thin curved line separating the medial basal segment of the right lower lobe from the remaining basilar segments (*arrows* in **B** and **C**). Note bronchiectasis limited only to the medial basal segment (*small arrow* in **C**).

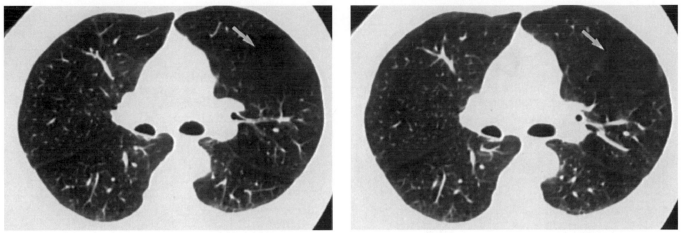

FIG. 10-15. Left minor fissure. **A,B:** Sequential sections through the left midlung show the presence of a left minor fissure, identifiable as a triangular area of decreased density (*arrows* in **A** and **B**), analogous to the appearance of the normal minor fissure in Figs. 10-9 and 10-10.

Inferior Pulmonary Ligaments and Phrenic Nerves

The inferior pulmonary ligaments (36–40) represent reflections of the parietal pleura that extend from just below the inferior margins of the pulmonary hila caudally and posteriorly to the diaphragm, and serve to anchor the lung to the mediastinum. The ligament can terminate before reaching the diaphragm, or extend over the medial diaphragmatic surface. The inferior pulmonary ligament is often contiguous with the intersublobar septum, dividing the medial from the posterior basal lung segments.

The CT appearance of these ligaments has been well described (36–40). In a review of 100 CT studies using 10-mm sections, Cooper and coworkers identified at least one of these ligaments in 42% of cases (37). Using 10-mm sections, Rost and Proto (40) could identify the left pulmonary ligament in 67% of cases, and the right inferior pulmonary ligament in 37% of cases. Both ligaments were seen in only 27% of cases (40). The inferior margins of these ligaments are variable; in their most caudal extension they may assume a triangular configuration as they reflect onto the diaphragm (Fig. 10-16).

It should be emphasized that the inferior pulmonary ligaments need to be distinguished from the phrenic nerves,

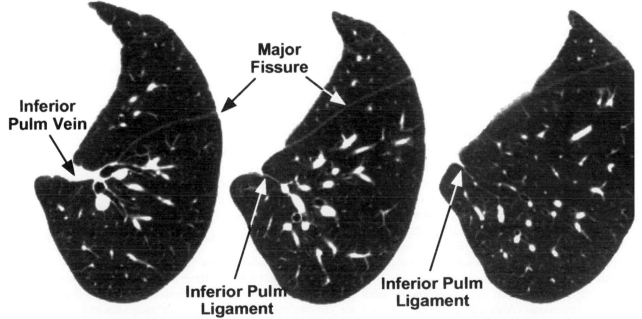

FIG. 10-16. A–C: High-resolution CT scans at 1-cm intervals showing the left inferior pulmonary ligament. **A:** The left inferior pulmonary vein and left major fissure are visible at the most cephalad level. **B,C:** The left inferior pulmonary ligament is visible as a triangular structure arising immediately caudal to the inferior pulmonary vein. This relationship is characteristic. A thin soft tissue septum within the adjacent lung represents the intersublobar septum.

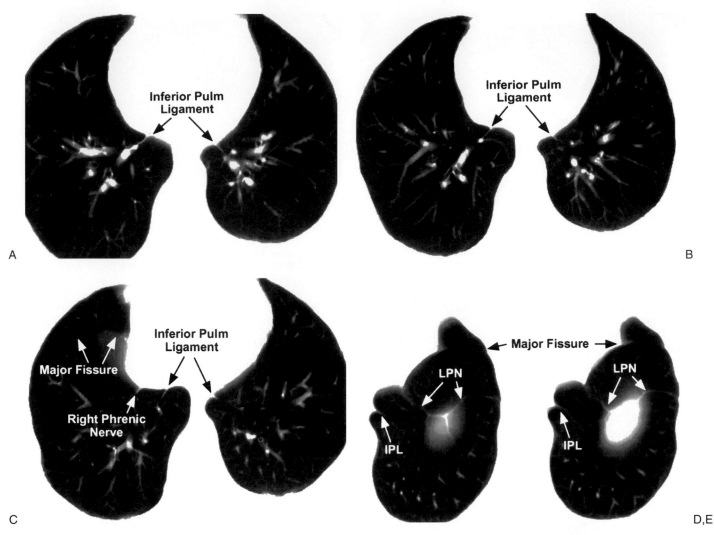

FIG. 10-17. Spiral CT in two patients showing the relationships between the inferior pulmonary ligaments, phrenic nerves, and major fissures. **A–C:** The inferior pulmonary ligaments arise below the level of the inferior pulmonary veins (**A**), and extend inferiorly (**B** and **C**), lying near the esophagus. The right phrenic nerve (**C**) results in a similar opacity anterior to the inferior pulmonary ligament, adjacent to the inferior vena cava. The right major fissure is visible more anteriorly. **D,E:** In another patient, two adjacent scans through the left lung show the location of the inferior pulmonary ligament (*IPL*), and the pleural reflections associated with the left phrenic nerve (*LPN*), just above the left hemidiaphragm. The major fissure is more anterior.

which may run nearby (see Fig. 10-16; Fig. 10-17). As documented by Taylor et al., the left phrenic nerve generally can be identified as a 1 to 3-mm rounded structure lying adjacent to the pericardium. In this study, identification of the right phrenic nerve proved more difficult (41). The relationship between the right inferior pulmonary ligament and right phrenic nerve has been examined in detail by Berkman et al. (36). Using anatomic specimens, these authors have shown that the right inferior pulmonary ligament appears as a thin, high-attenuation line frequently identifiable above or at the level of the diaphragm, usually extending from the region of the esophagus. Although previous reports have suggested that the right inferior pulmonary ligament can be identified on CT as a thin line extending from the lateral margin of the inferior vena cava, Berkman and coworkers have shown that in fact this line represents the right phrenic

nerve (see Fig. 10-17) (28). Accurate identification of the inferior pulmonary ligaments is important as alterations in the normal appearance of these ligaments typically are produced by pleural effusions, pneumothoraces, and lobar collapse (28,33,38).

The Pleural Surfaces and Adjacent Chest Wall

A number of structures, arranged in layers, surround the lung and line the inner aspect of the thoracic cavity (Fig. 10-18). Some can be identified on CT, and a knowledge of their anatomy is helpful in understanding normal CT findings and the appearances of pleural diseases.

The combined thickness of the layers of visceral and parietal pleura that surround the lung, and the fluid containing pleural space, is approximately 200 to 400 μm (0.2–0.4

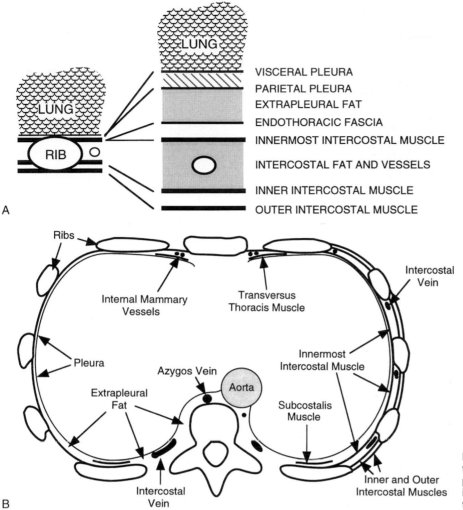

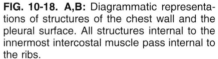

FIG. 10-18. A,B: Diagrammatic representations of structures of the chest wall and the pleural surface. All structures internal to the innermost intercostal muscle pass internal to the ribs.

mm). The parietal pleura consists of four layers and measures approximately 100 to 200 μm; the visceral pleura is anatomically similar to but somewhat thicker than the parietal pleura (42,43). The width of the pleural space, in studies of frozen thoraces, has been estimated to be 10 to 20 mm (44,45).

External to the parietal pleura is a layer of loose areolar connective tissue, which separates the parietal pleura from the endothoracic fascia. This fatty layer averages 250 μm in thickness in most locations (42,43), but can be markedly thickened over the lateral or posterolateral ribs, resulting in extrapleural fat pads several millimeters in thickness (46,47). The thoracic cavity is lined by the fibroelastic endothoracic fascia (approximately 250 μm in thickness) (42,43), which covers the surface of the intercostal muscles and intervening ribs, blends with the perichondrium and periosteum of the costal cartilages and sternum anteriorly, and posteriorly, is continuous with the prevertebral fascia, which covers the vertebral bodies and intervertebral discs.

External to the endothoracic fascia are a layer of fatty connective tissue and the three layers of the intercostal muscles. The innermost intercostal muscle (intercostales intimi)

passes between the internal surfaces of adjacent ribs and is relatively thin; it is separated from the inner and external intercostal muscles by the intercostal vessels and nerve. Although the innermost intercostal muscles are incomplete in the anterior and posterior thorax, other muscles (the transversus thoraces and subcostalis) can occupy the same relative plane, and are considered by some authors to be parts of the innermost intercostal muscles. Anteriorly, the transversus thoracis muscle consists of 4 or 5 slips, which arise from the xiphoid process or lower sternum, and pass superolaterally from the second to sixth costal cartilages. The internal mammary vessels lie external to the transversus thoracis. Posteriorly, the subcostal muscles are thin, variable muscles, which extend from the inner aspect of the angle of the lower ribs, crossing one or two ribs and intercostal spaces, to the inner aspect of a rib below.

CT Appearances

On HRCT in normals, a 1 to 2 mm thick soft-tissue density line is visible in the anterolateral and posterolateral intercostal spaces, at the point of contact between lung

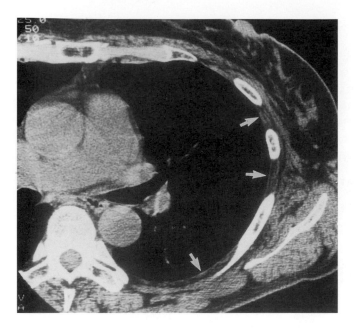

FIG. 10-19. Normal CT of the pleural surface and chest wall. On a high resolution CT scan, a thin line visible in the intercostal spaces (*arrows*) primarily represents the innermost intercostal muscle, but is also made up of the combined thicknesses of visceral and parietal pleura, the fluid-filled pleural space, endothoracic fascia, and fat layers. Although the pleurae, extrapleural fat, and endothoracic fascia pass internal to the ribs, they are not visible in this location on high resolution CT unless they are abnormally thickened.

and chest wall (Figs. 10-19 and 10-20). This line primarily represents the innermost intercostal muscle, but also reflects the combined thicknesses of visceral and parietal pleura, the fluid-filled pleural space, endothoracic fascia, and fat layers. Although the pleurae, extrapleural fat, and endothoracic fascia pass internal to the ribs, they are not visible in this location on HRCT unless they are abnormally thickened. Similarly, on conventional CT, a visible soft-tissue stripe, internal to a rib, is used to diagnose pleural thickening or effusion.

Normal extrapleural fat can be seen on HRCT internal to ribs in several locations, and can mimic pleural thickening

(Fig. 10-21) (3,46,47). The normal layer of extrapleural fat between the parietal pleura and the endothoracic fascia is notably thicker adjacent to the lateral ribs than in other sites (3,46,47). It is most abundant over the posterolateral fourth to eighth ribs and can result in fat pads several millimeters thick, which extend into the intercostal spaces. In normal subjects, these costal fat pads can be difficult to distinguish from pleural thickening or plaques when extended window settings (width 2,000 H) are used, but are very low in attenuation and difficult to see with soft-tissue window settings. In one study, extrapleural fat could be seen using extended windows in 12 of 15 normal subjects (3).

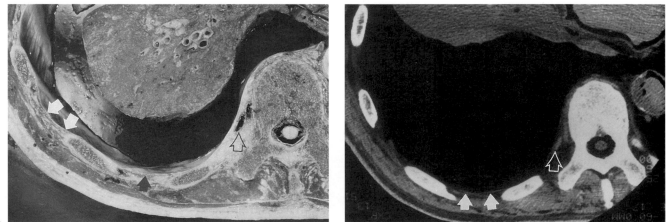

A B

FIG. 10-20. CT appearance of the normal pleura and chest wall. **A:** On a section of a cadaver, the parietal pleura and endothoracic fascia are visible as a white line (*white arrows*) at the internal surface of the chest wall. The innermost intercostal muscle (*black arrow*) lies external to these. Although the pleura and fascia pass internal to the ribs, they are not visible in this location on HRCT. In the paravertebral regions, the internal intercostal muscle is absent. Intercostal vessels (*open arrow*) lie within the paravertebral fat. **B:** High resoluion CT of the cadaver at the same level, photographed using a mediastinal window settings. A 1-mm to 2-mm line (*white arrows*) at the internal surface of the chest wall, in the intercostal spaces, represents the combined thicknesses of the parietal pleura, endothoracic fascia, and the innermost intercostal muscle. In a paravertebral location, the innermost intercostal muscle is absent and the combined parietal pleura and fascia are invisible or result in a very thin line. Intercostal vessels (*open arrows*) are visible within the fat external to the intercostal muscle or fascia.

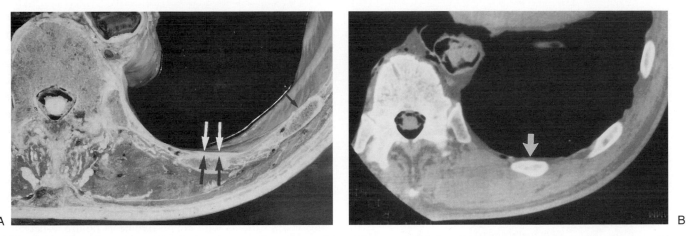

FIG. 10-21. Normal extrapleural fat. **A:** A cadaver section shows a fat pad (*large arrows*) internal to the posterior rib. More laterally, only a thin white stripe (*small arrow*) is seen internal to rib, representing the parietal pleura and endothoracic fascia. **B:** HRCT of the cadaver using a wide window width. The fat pad (*arrow*), internal to the most posterior rib segment is several mm thick. Note that fat pads are not visible internal to more lateral ribs.

The transversus thoracis and subcostalis muscles can also mimic pleural thickening in some patients. Anteriorly, at the level of the heart and adjacent to the lower sternum or xiphoid process, the transversus thoracis muscles are nearly always visible internal to the anterior ends of ribs or costal cartilages (Fig. 10-22) (3). Posteriorly, at the same level, a 1 to 2 mm thick line is sometimes seen internal to one or more ribs, representing the subcostalis muscle; this muscle is present in only a small percentage of patients (Fig. 10-23) (3). In contrast to pleural thickening, these muscles are smooth, uniform in thickness, and symmetric bilaterally.

Segments of intercostal veins are commonly visible in the paravertebral regions, and can mimic focal pleural thickening (see Fig. 10-23; Fig. 10-24). Continuity of these opacities with the azygos or hemiazygos veins can sometimes allow them to be correctly identified (3). Furthermore, when viewed using lung window settings, intercostal vein segments do not indent the lung surface; pleural plaques of the same thickness certainly would.

Because most segments of the ribs are obliquely oriented relative to the scan plane, each CT section typically traverses the upper edge, middle, and lower edge of most ribs. With either 1 cm collimation or HRCT, the normal 1 to 2 mm stripe of density, primarily representing the innermost intercostal muscle, can be seen internal to the tapering edges of the visible rib segments (i.e., internal to the upper and lower rib edges), mimicking pleural thickening (see Fig. 10-20B). This can be distinguished from pleural thickening in that the stripe is continuous with the normal innermost intercostal muscle in the adjacent interspaces. Also, this normal stripe will not usually be seen internal to the entire rib segment, but is visible only at its edges. However, when a rib segment is nearly horizontal, as is common posteriorly, the scan plane can traverse only a part of the upper or lower rib margin. In this case, the normal stripe can be seen internal to the entire length of the visible rib segment, mimicking pleural thickening. The visible rib segment will appear thinner than normal.

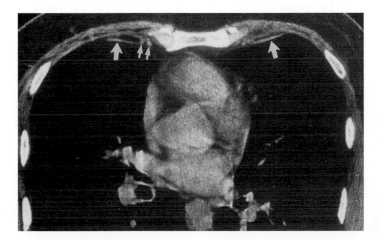

FIG. 10-22. High resolution CT in a normal subject shows the transversus thoraces muscles (*large arrows*). These lie internal to the innermost intercostal muscles and internal mammary vessels (*small arrows*).

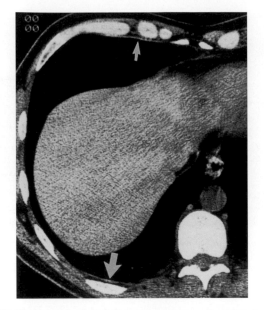

FIG. 10-23. Normal subcostalis and transversus thoraces muscles. High resolution CT in a normal subject at the level of the heart shows a well-defined linear opacity (*large arrow*), internal to the posterior rib, and separated from it by a fat pad. This represents the subcostalis muscle. Its location and appearance are characteristic. Anteriorly, (*small arrow*) the transversus thoracic muscle is visible passing internal to calcified costal cartilage. Paravertebral vein segments are also seen, joining azygos and hemiazygos veins.

Pleural Effusions: Clinical Characterization

Pleural effusions have traditionally been defined as either transudative or exudative. Transudative effusions result from systemic abnormalities that lead to an imbalance in hydrostatic and osmotic forces, resulting in the formation of protein-poor pleural fluid (Figs. 10-25 and 10-26). Common causes include congestive heart failure, cirrhosis, and nephrotic syndrome. In distinction, exudative effusions are usually associated with conditions that result either in increased permeability of abnormal pleural capillaries or lymphatic obstruction with resultant formation of protein-rich fluid (Fig. 10-27). Although the list of causes of an exudative effusion is quite long, most important are those caused by infection and malignancy. Traditionally, differentiation between transudative and exudative effusions has usually required thoracentesis. Using original criteria established by Light et al. (48), exudative effusions must meet one of the following criteria: (a) pleural fluid/serum total protein ratio of more than 0.5; (b) pleural fluid LDH/serum LDH ratio greater than 0.6; or (c) pleural fluid LDH greater than two-thirds the upper limit of normal for serum LDH. Transudative effusions are those that do not meet the above criteria. Using these criteria, despite somewhat lower specificity caused by decreased accuracy in identifying transudative effusions in patients with congestive heart failure, especially following diuresis, the sensitivity of these criteria for identifying exudates is generally greater than 95%. Although alternate measurements have been evaluated, including quantifying pleural fluid cholesterol and bilirubin and assessing the serum-pleural fluid albumin gradient, to date none has proved more accurate (49).

In addition to being classified as either transudative or exudative, effusions are also frequently defined as either parapneumonic or as an empyema (Fig. 10-28). Parapneumonic effusions are exudative effusions associated with an underlying parenchymal infection, most often pneumonia or a lung abscess, and are further subdivided as either simple or complicated. Complicated parapneumonic effusions are usually defined by one of the following criteria: (a) elevated pleural LDH greater than 1,000; (b) low pH (usually <7.1); or (c) low pleural glucose (<40 mg/dL). In distinction, effusions are considered empyemas only when cultures are positive.

The incidence of exudative parapneumonic effusions is dependent to some degree on the infecting organism, ranging from about 10% for pneumonias caused by *Streptococcus pneumoniae* to over 50% for those caused by *Staphylococcus pyogenes* (50). Regardless of the infecting organism, parapneumonic effusion have been noted to follow a natural his-

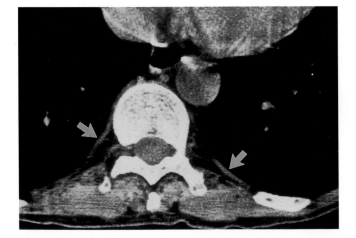

FIG. 10-24. Normal intercostal veins in a paravertebral location. High resolution CT shows normal intercostal veins (*arrows*) in a paravertebral location. The veins do not indent the pleura, and are typically seen only in segments.

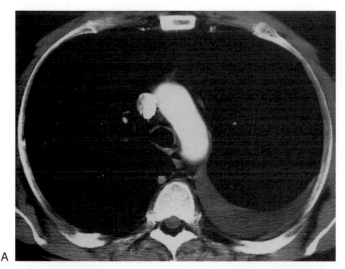

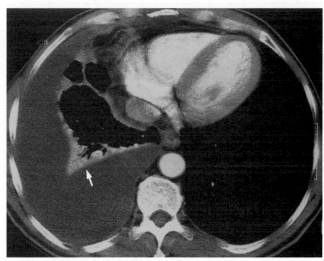

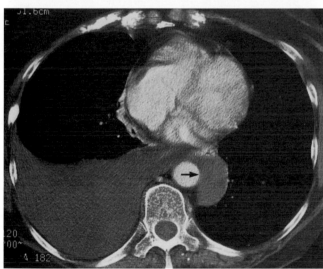

FIG. 10-25. Transudative effusions. **A:** Contrast-enhanced CT shows simple left sided transudative effusion. Note that neither the parietal or visceral pleura are thickened and that the effusion has a typically meniscoid configuration conforming to the shape of the posterior pleural space. **B:** Contrast-enhanced CT in a different patient than A shows a larger effusion this time causing marked compression atelectasis of the right lower lobe (*arrow*). Despite the large size of this effusion, again note lack of enhancement of the pleural surfaces, consistent with a transudative effusion. **C:** Contrast-enhanced CT section in a different patient than **A** or **B** again shows a large right sided effusion. In this case the effusion actually extends to the left hemithorax (*arrow*), presumably the result of fusion of pleural membranes with resultant direct communication between the right and left pleural spaces. Despite the large size of this effusion, there is no evidence of underlying compression atelectasis (compare with **B**). Again note lack of evidence of either visceral or parietal pleural thickening in this patient with a transudative effusion. Although an absence of pleural thickening is compatible with either a transudative or exudative effusion (including those associated with metastatic disease), this effectively eliminates an empyema.

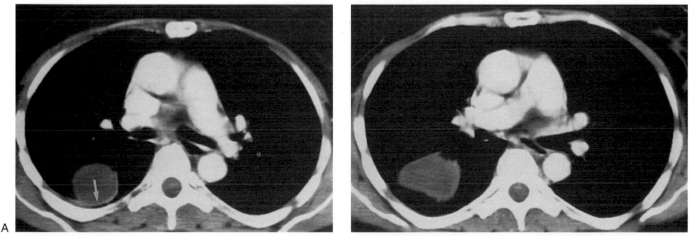

FIG. 10-26. Fissural pseudotumor: CT appearance. **A,B:** Sequential CT scans through the middle thorax show typical appearance of a loculated pseudotumor in the superior portion of the right major fissure. Characteristically, these conform to the expected position of the fissure, the posterior margin of which can be identified superiorly (*arrow* in **A**).

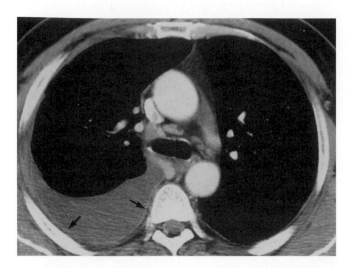

FIG. 10-27. Exudative effusion-metastatic breast cancer. Contrast-enhanced CT in a patient in a patient with known metastatic breast cancer. A right sided effusion is present associated with mild thickening and enhancement of the parietal pleura (*arrows;* compare with Fig. 10-25). Note presence of minimally enlarged mediastinal nodes. The finding of thickened parietal pleura is indicative of an exudative effusion and may be due to an empyema.

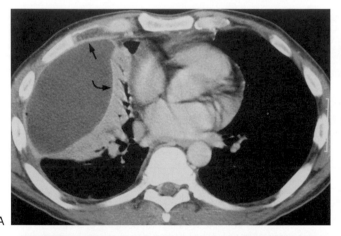

A

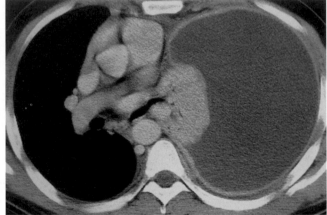

B

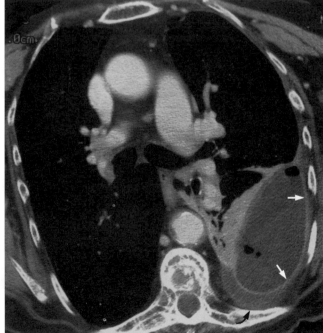

C

FIG. 10-28. Complicated parapneumonic effusions. **A:** Contrast-enhanced CT section shows loculated right effusion causing compression atelectasis of adjacent portions of the right middle and lower lobes. In this case there is smooth enhancement of both the parietal (*arrow*) and visceral (*curved arrow*) pleura giving rise to the so-called "split pleura" sign. Thoracentesis in this case confirmed that this was a complicated parapneumonic effusion requiring tube drainage. **B:** Contrast-enhanced CT in a different patient than **A** shows similar if more extensive changes as in **A**. There is a massive left sided effusion with evidence of uniformly thickened and enhancing parietal pleura. Although thoracentesis in this case was consistent with a simple parapneumnic effusion (pH = 7.32, protein = 5, glucose = 97, and LDH = 432), sputum cultures proved positive for *Mycobacterium avium*-intercellulare; subsequent pleural biopsy revealed noncaseating granulomas. **C:** Contrast-enhanced CT section in a different patient than **A** or **B** shows a large loculated effusion on the left side associated with compression atelectasis of the adjacent left lower lobe. There is moderate, smooth enhancement of the parietal pleura (*arrows*) in this case associated with considerable expansion of the extrapleural space within which apparent fluid density can be identified (*curved arrow*). Air within the pleural fluid is caused by prior thoracentesis, which confirmed the presence of a complicated parapneumonic effusion (see also Fig. 10-43).

tory. Three stages have been described, each of which is pathophysiologically and therapeutically distinct (51):

1. *Exudative or simple parapneumonic stage.* In this stage, an underlying pneumonic process causes inflammation of the visceral pleura, resulting in the accumulation of thin, uninfected pleural fluid, usually the result of increased capillary permeability, with resultant protein loss. A thoracentesis at this stage reveals a simple exudative parapneumonic effusion. Such uncomplicated or simple exudative parapneumonic effusions resolve without drainage, provided that the underlying cause of infection is adequately treated with appropriate antibiotics (52).

2. *Fibrinopurulent or complicated parapneumonic stage.* In this stage, large numbers of PMNs and bacteria accumulate in the pleural space, and sheets of fibrin are deposited over the visceral and parietal pleura. As a consequence, there is a progressive tendency toward fluid loculation as fluid resorption is impaired, presumably because of decreased lymphatic drainage (see Fig. 10-28). If the underlying infection is not adequately treated, the pleural fluid becomes infected. Furthermore, there is a tendency for progressive thickening of the extrapleural subcostal tissues to develop as well, presumably secondary to spread of infection and edema to the adjacent chest wall tissues (see Figs. 10-28 and 10-43). A thoracentesis performed at this stage reveals features characteristic of a complicated parapneumonic effusion as defined above. There is a tendency toward an increasing white blood cell count, decreasing glucose levels, and a decreased pH. Although controversial, in most centers complicated parapneumonic effusions are treated with immediate closed tube drainage.

3. *Organizing stage.* In this stage, there is an ingrowth of fibroblasts along the fibrin sheets lining the visceral and parietal pleura. The end result is pleural fibrosis, which acts as an inelastic membrane trapping the adjacent lung (50,52). Progression from the fibrinopurulent to the organizing stage may be quite rapid, occasionally occurring in the course of therapy with closed pleural tube drainage. In most cases, however, the organizing phase typically occurs within two to three weeks after initial pleural fluid formation. Eventually, especially if the infection is inadequately treated, the pleura may calcify, appearing initially as small, punctate foci involving both the visceral and parietal pleura, progressing to form a calcified rind of pleura (Fig. 10-29). Clinically, this most often occurs from tuberculous empyema, and was particularly common in the past following pneumothorax therapy. Whatever the etiology, with the formation of a fibrothorax there is contraction of the involved hemithorax and an expansion of the extrapleural fat. The underlying lung can no longer expand. Expansion of the extrapleural fat is especially characteristic, and may be accompanied by periosteal changes in the adjacent ribs (see Fig. 10-29A).

As documented by Schmitt et al., despite extensive pleural calcification, residual pleural fluid may be identified in a surprisingly high percentage of cases, especially when evaluated by CT (see Fig. 10-29; Fig. 10-30) (53). In their study of 140 patients with calcification of both the parietal and visceral pleura, these authors showed persistent pleural effusions in 22 (15%) of cases. This finding is especially important given the propensity for residual infection to result in either a bronchopleural fistula (Fig. 10-31) or a chest wall infection (empyema necessitatis) (Fig. 10-32) (54). Similar findings have been reported for tuberculous empyemas (55,56).

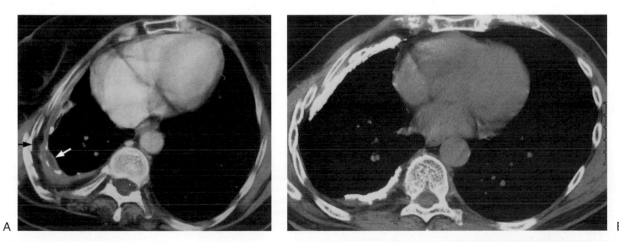

FIG. 10-29. Chronic tuberculous empyema. **A:** Contrast-enhanced section shows thickening and calcification of the pleura associated with marked expansion of the extrapleural space with fat (*black arrow*). There is also thickening of the cortex of the adjacent ribs and marked volume loss of the ipsilateral hemithorax. These findings are all characteristic of chronic pleural and periosteal inflammation, in this case caused by tuberculosis. Note that there is a small residual collection of fluid within the pleural space (*white arrow*). This represents a potential source of reactivation. **B:** Noncontrast enhanced section in a different patient than A shows more extensive pleural calcifications, again associated with pleural thickening and expansion of the extrapleural space with fat. This appearance is also consistent with chronic inflammation, in this case also caused by prior tuberculosis.

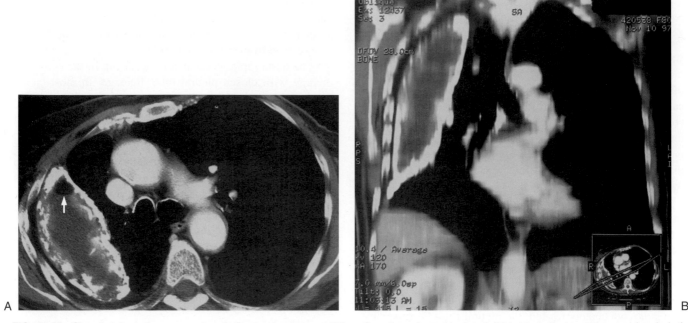

FIG. 10-30. Chronic tuberculous empyema. **A:** Contrast-enhanced CT section shows large loculated right sided effusion with extensive rind of calcification. A discrete fat-fluid level (*arrow*) can be identified within the pleural space, which can occasionally be identified in patients with long-standing chronic tuberulous empyemas. Note as well presence of expansion of the extrapleural fat and ipsilateral volume loss, all consistent with chronic inflammation. **B:** Coronal reformation showing to better advantage true extent of the loculated effusion.

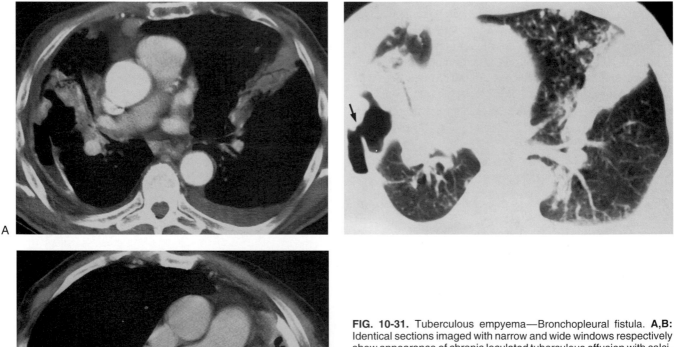

FIG. 10-31. Tuberculous empyema—Bronchopleural fistula. **A,B:** Identical sections imaged with narrow and wide windows respectively show appearance of chronic loculated tuberculous effusion with calcifications of the parietal and visceral pleural surfaces, expansion of the extrapleural fat, and ipsilateral volume loss. In this case there is an obvious bronchopleural fistula, best seen with wide windows (*arrow* in **B**), associated with extensive consolidation of both the middle lobe and left upper lobe. A small left effusion is also present. **C:** CT section in a different patient than **A** and **B** also shows evidence of a bronchopleural fistula (*curved arrow*) appearing in this patient with history of chronic tuberculous empyema. As shown in these cases, there is a propensity for chronic tuberculous empyemas to reactivate resulting in either a bronchopleural fistula or chest wall infection (empyema necessitatis; see Fig. 10-32).

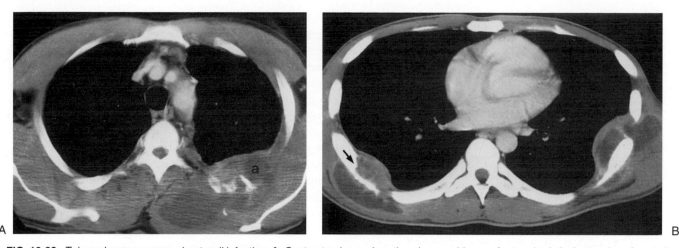

FIG. 10-32. Tuberculous empyema-chest wall infection. **A:** Contrast-enhanced section shows evidence of extensive lytic destruction of posterior ribs associated with a multiloculated chest wall abscess (*a*). **B:** Contrast-enhanced CT section in a different patient than **A** shows presence of bilateral chest wall abscesses again associated with lytic rib destruction on the right side (*arrow*). Both of these cases proved to have prior pleural disease with evidence of reactivation and extension into the chest wall (so-called empyema necessitans). In the case illustrated in **B**, presumably this was associated with hematogenous seeding resulting in tuberculous osteromyelitis on the right side.

CT Evaluation of Complex Pleuro-Parenchymal Disease

CT has been documented to be of considerable value in assessing all aspects of complex pleuro-parenchymal disease (57–62). In our experience, CT has been of greatest value in: (a) differentiation of pleural from parenchymal disease; (b) characterization of underlying parenchymal disease, including identification of necrotizing pneumonias, lung abscesses, and pulmonary infarcts; (c) characterization of pleural fluid as either free or loculated, as well as characterization of the appearance of the pleural membranes themselves; and (d) assessment and guidance of therapy.

It cannot be overemphasized that optimal evaluation of complex pleuro-parenchymal disease requires the use of a bolus of i.v. contrast media (Fig. 10-33). Besides allowing precise localization of fluid collections, i.v. contrast media may enhance both pleural membranes, especially when inflamed, and adjacent lung tissue. In most cases in which

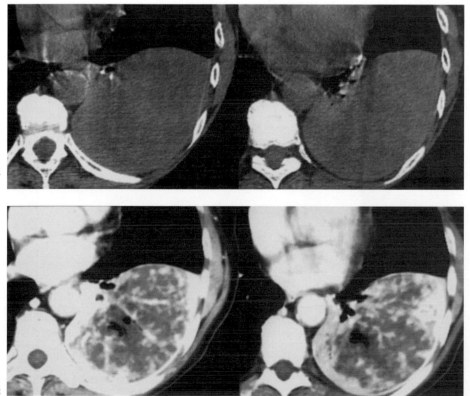

FIG. 10-33. Complex pleuro-parenchymal disease: role of intravenous contrast administration. **A,B:** Non-contrast-enhanced sections show apparent uniform soft-tissue density throughout the left lower lobe. **C,D:** Sections obtained at the same level as **A** and **B**, following a bolus of intravenous contrast media. There is evidence of extensive necrotizing pneumonitis throughout the left lower lobe. Contrast within intraparenchymal vessels is easily identified because of the uniform low density of the surrounding lung, a sign of extensive edema and or necrosis. This case clearly demonstrates the value of contrast enhancement for differentiating pleural from parenchymal disease, as well as a means for further characterizing parenchymal abnormalities when present.

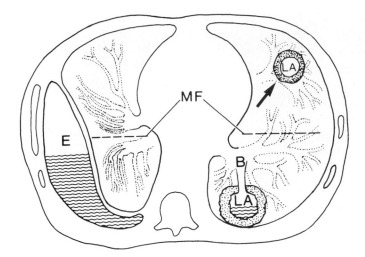

FIG. 10-34. CT differentiation between loculated pleural fluid collections/empyemas and lung abscess. Empyemas (*E*) typically appear lenticular in shape with a smooth wall, conform to the shape of the chest wall, and, if sufficiently large, cause compression of the adjacent lung with displacement of vessels and airways. Unlike infected bullae, empyemas may extend past the margins of the adjacent major fissure (*MF*). In distinction, lung abscesses (*LA*) lie within the substance of the lung. Initially, lung abscesses are smooth walled, and prior to communication either with an airway or the pleural space, contain no air (*arrow*). At this stage, administration of intravenous contrast may be invaluable, owing to marked enhancement of the abscess wall. Later, after communication with an adjacent bronchus (*B*), however, abscesses generally cause little displacement of surrounding structures within the lung. Although as drawn lung abscesses appear to form acute angles with the adjacent pleura and chest wall, in fact, in our experience, absence of this sign is unreliable.

there is suppurative lung disease, characteristic patterns of enhancement may be identified, allowing more precise determination of the nature and extent of underlying lung disease.

Differentiation of Pleural from Parenchymal Disease

The role of CT in differentiating pleural from parenchymal disease has been well established (57,58–61). Stark et al.

reported a retrospective review of 70 inflammatory thoracic lesions where CT alone was able to differentiate lung abscesses from empyemas in 100% of cases (60). In these authors' experience, lung abscesses characteristically appear spherical with an irregularly thick wall and cause little compression of the adjacent pulmonary parenchyma. By comparison, empyemas are usually lenticular with a smooth wall, conform to the shape of the chest wall, and, if sufficiently large, cause compression of the adjacent lung (Fig. 10-34). Unfortunately, not all cases fall into such easily classifiable subgroups. In our experience, in a small but significant percentage of cases, even using strict CT criteria, differentiation between lung abscesses and loculated pleural fluid collections/empyemas may be difficult (Fig. 10-35). In select cases, of course, both lung abscesses and empyemas may coexist, further complicating interpretation (Fig. 10-36). In fact, this differentiation may even prove difficult at surgery. In addition to occasional cases in which empyemas and lung abscesses appear to share similar characteristics, fluid within preexisting pulmonary cavities also may pose problems. As documented by Zinn et al., even the split-pleura sign may be misleading, as fluid within a bulla may have an identical appearance (see Fig. 10-5) (8). As noted previously, administration of a bolus of i.v. contrast medium may be of value in complicated cases (5,60).

It should also be noted that, rarely, tumor may also mimic the appearance of loculated pleural fluid (Fig. 10-37). The key to diagnosis in these cases is to note the presence of nodularity along the apparent pleural surfaces following contrast enhancement.

Characterization of Underlying Parenchymal Disease

In addition to differentiating pleural from parenchymal pathology, CT offers a unique opportunity to characterize lung disease. Given the spectrum of potential parenchymal causes of parapneumonic effusions, identification of the un-

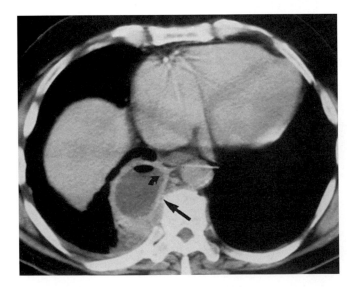

FIG. 10-35. Lung abscess vs. empyema: limitation in CT diagnosis. Contrast-enhanced CT section through the lower lobes shows a well-defined, smooth-walled fluid collection with a small air-fluid level within marginating the posterior mediastinum on the right (*arrow*). Despite the suggestion of a split-pleura sign (*curved arrow*) and the appearance of oblique angles along the margins of this lesion, at surgery this proved to be a thick-walled lung abscess associated with adjacent pleural thickening but without evidence of an empyema.

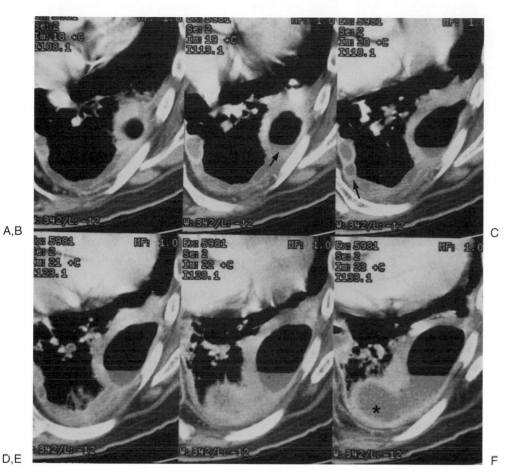

A,B
C
D,E
F

FIG. 10-36. CT differentiation: lung abscess vs. empyema. **A–F:** Sequential enlargements of views through the left lung base show findings suggestive of both a lung abscess and empyema. Superiorly there is a slightly irregular cavity with an air-fluid level within what appears to be the peripheral portion of the left lower lobe (*arrow* in **B**); more inferiorly, however, this cavity merges with what appears to be a loculated pleural effusion with an air-fluid level (*asterisk* in **F**). Note that medially, there are multiple small thick-walled fluid collections (*arrow* in **C**), which also have features suggestive of both lung abscesses and loculated effusions. In this case, a presumed lung abscess had ruptured into the pleural space resulting in a large bronchopleural fistula. Following therapy with a chest tube these findings resolved. This case illustrates that despite strict adherence to established criteria, differentiation between lung abscesses and empymas (especially those associated with a bronchopleural fistula) may be difficult if not impossible. In most of these cases, successful treatment requires that both abnormalities are assumed to be present.

derlying disease process may have both prognostic and therapeutic value.

In our experience, CT has been most useful in identifying lung abscesses. Lung abscesses are part of a spectrum of pulmonary suppurative processes characterized by necrosis and cavitation, most commonly associated with *Staphylococcus aureus*, *Pseudomonas aeruginosa*, *Klebsiella pneumoniae*, and anaerobes (63). The most common pathogenic mechanisms in their development are aspiration of oral flora, necrosis within an antecedent pneumonia, bronchial obstruction, septic emboli, and penetrating trauma. The necrosis and cavitation that frequently are associated with these infections tend to take several forms. Development of multiple small areas of necrosis, or cavitation within a larger area of necrosis, is generally termed necrotizing pneumonitis (63). By comparison, a lung abscess is characterized by a dominant focus of suppuration surrounded by a containing wall composed of well-vascularized fibrous and granulation tissue (see Fig. 10-34), supplied by hypertrophied bronchial arteries. This accounts for the association between lung abscesses and hemoptysis. Initially self-contained, communication is eventually established with nearby airways or with the adjacent pleural space into which the abscess contents are expelled. Rarely, these infections lead to pulmonary gangrene, characterized by still more extensive necrosis with resultant

sloughing of lung tissue. As previously discussed, all these manifestations of pulmonary suppuration are frequently accompanied by parapneumonic effusions or empyema.

Each of these forms of suppurative lung disease have characteristic CT appearances. Lung abscesses are easily recognized as homogeneous areas of low density surrounded by a markedly enhancing wall usually associated with a smooth inner contour (Fig. 10-38). Because of the presence of hypertrophied bronchial arteries, the wall of most lung abscesses tends to be extremely hypervascular (Fig. 10-39). This is especially the case in patients with superimposed fungal infections (Fig. 10-40). For this reason, optimal evaluation of lung abscesses is accomplished using a bolus injection of i.v. contrast, optimally timed to coincide with the early arterial phase of enhancement (see Fig. 10-40). Following communication with the pleural space or adjacent airways, lung abscesses cavitate; at this time their walls become thick and irregular (Fig. 10-41). In contrast, necrotizing pneumonitis is characterized by multiple, poorly defined foci of low density, unassociated with enhancing margins (see Fig. 10-33; Fig. 10-42). When extensive, this appearance merges with pulmonary gangrene. Although in typical cases differentiation between patients with lung abscesses and necrotizing pneumonitis is not associated with significant differences in therapy, this differentiation is of importance in those cases for

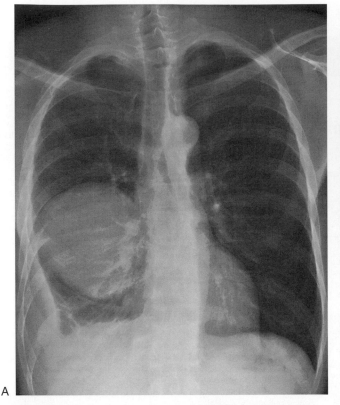

A

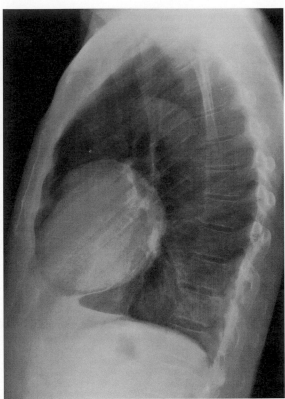

B

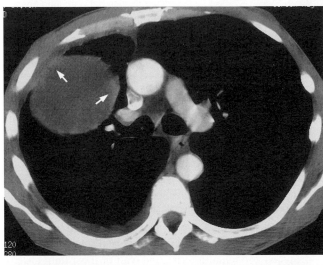

C

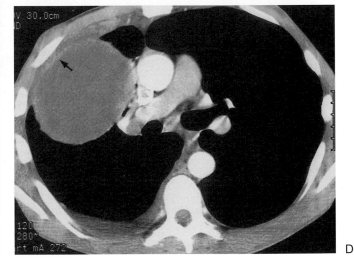

D

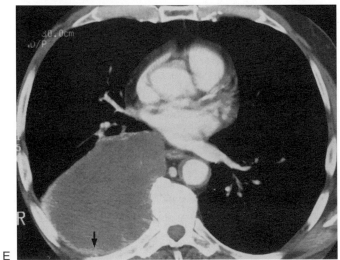

E

FIG. 10-37. Lung cancer mimicking loculated pleural fluid. **A,B:** Posteroanterior and lateral radiographs show well-defined mass on the right side thought to possibly represent loculated fluid within the minor fissure. **C,D:** Sequential sections show an apparently well defined fluid collection present anteriorly associated with a small quantity of both free pleural fluid posteriorly. This appearance mimics that of a fluid collection within the minor fissure. In retrospect, there is slight nodular thickening of the "pleural surfaces" (*arrow* in **C** and **D**). Following unsuccessful attempts at thoracentesis, this patient underwent an exploratory thoracotomy at which time this mass proved to be a necrotic nonsmall cell lung cancer. **E.** Contrast-enhanced CT section in a different patient than **A–D** also shows an apparent loculated pleural effusion on the right side. Note again, however, that there is subtle nodular thickening of the "pleura" (*arrow*). This also proved to be a necrotic nonsmall cell lung cancer.

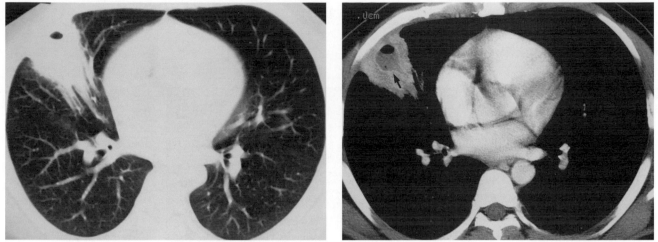

FIG. 10-38. Lung abscess. **A,B:** Identical sections imaged with wide and narrow windows, respectively, following a bolus of intravenous contrast media show characteristic appearance of a lung abscess within a focal area of parenchymal consolidation (*arrow* in **B**).

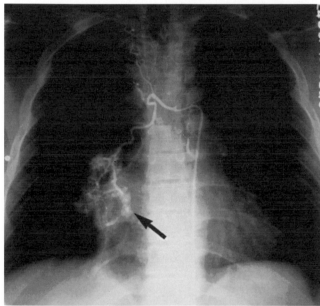

A

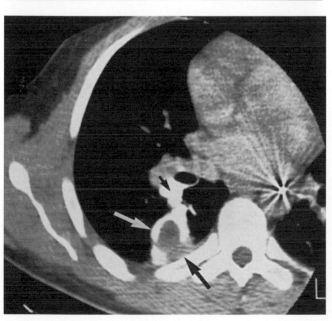

B

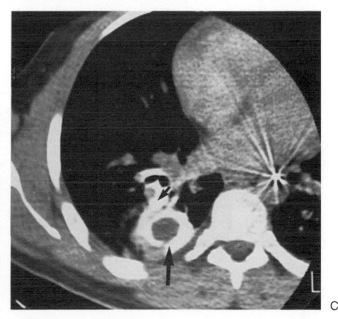

C

FIG. 10-39. Lung abscess: CT demonstration of hypertrophied bronchial arteries. **A:** Posteroanterior radiograph obtained following catheterization of the right bronchial artery. A focal area of hyperemia can be identified on the right, associated with considerable hypertrophy of the distal bronchial arteries (*arrow*). **B,C:** Enlargements of sequential sections through the right lower lobe in the same patient. In this case, CT scans were obtained with the catheter still in place within the right bronchial artery, using a slow drip infusion of intravenous contrast media. Hypertrophied bronchial arteries can be identified within the right hilum (*small arrows* in **B** and **C**) leading to a well-defined, smooth-walled fluid collection in the right lower lobe (*large arrow*). Note that the wall of this lesion is dramatically enhancing, consistent with a bronchial arterial blood supply. Surgically documented lung abscess.

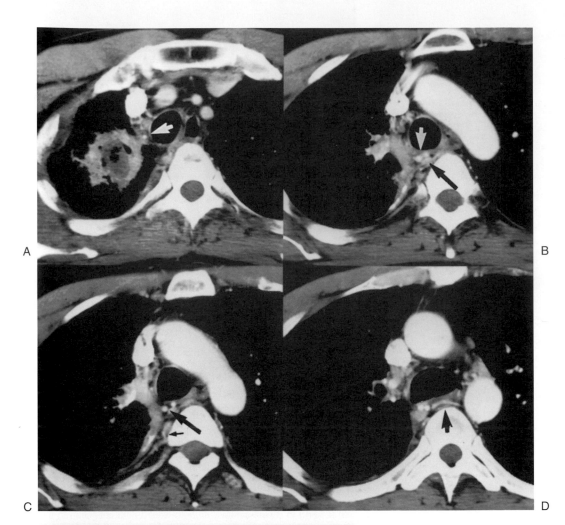

Fig. 10-40. Intracavitary aspergilloma: hypertrophied bronchial arteries **A–D:** Select 5-mm sections through the upper lobes from above down in a patient with a right upper lobe cavity presenting with hemoptysis. Following a bolus injection of 100 cc of 60% contrast material injected at a rate of 2 cc/second following a 20 second delay, note the presence of an enlarged right intercostal-bronchial trunk (*arrow* in **D**) within the posterior mediastinum behind the esophagus subsequently dividing into a right bronchial (*arrows* in *A–C*) and intercostal arteries (*small arrow* in **C**). Considerable enhancement of the wall of the abscess cavity is consistent with increased vascularity associated with chronic infection. **E:** Coned-down subtraction view from a select right bronchial artery injection confirms the presence of both an hypertrophied right bronchial artery extending into the right upper lobe as well as a prominent intercostal artery. Biopsy and culture confirmed fungal infection caused by *aspergillus*. (From Naidich DP. Volumetric CT in the evaluation of focal pulmonary disease. In: Remy-Jardin M, Remy J, eds. *Spiral CT of the chest*. Berlin: Springer, 1997:129–151, with permission.)

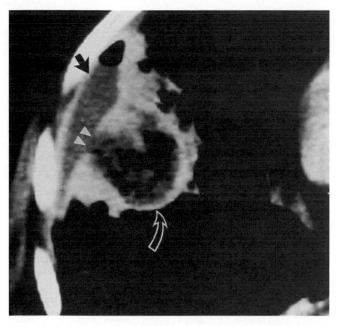

FIG. 10-41. Lung abscess: communication with the pleural space. Enlargement of a contrast-enhanced CT section through the right middle lung shows a typical lung abscess (*curved arrow*). In this case, the abscess is beginning to communicate with the adjacent pleural space (*arrowheads*), within which a small, loculated pleural fluid collection is beginning to form (*straight arrow*). Note the presence of air within both the pleural fluid collection and the abscess. (Case courtesy of Peter Nardi, M.D., Brooklyn, NY.)

which percutaneous drainage of lung abscesses may be considered (64). CT may also be valuable in detecting complications that may occur within abscesses, including the presence of intracavitary fungus balls (see Fig. 10-40). It should be noted that although cavitary lung neoplasms may mimic the

appearance of a lung abscess, in most cases there is only minimal enhancement of the tumor wall as compared with lung abscesses, especially in squamous cell carcinomas (65).

Pleural Effusions: CT Evaluation

Free Versus Loculated Effusions

Free pleural fluid has a characteristic appearance when seen in cross-section. Fluid typically looks "meniscoid," occupying the posterior pleural space in patients scanned in the supine position (see Fig. 10-25A). As effusions increase in size, they conform to the natural boundaries of the pleura. Laterally, these boundaries are formed by the lateral chest wall and the lateral aspect of the oblique fissures, into which fluid may track. Medially, these boundaries are formed by the inferior pulmonary ligaments. If sufficiently large, effusions usually result in compression atelectasis of the underlying lung (see Fig. 10-25B); this is not invariable, however, with large effusions often causing minimal if any change to the adjacent lung parenchyma (see Fig. 10-25C). Rarely, direct communication may be identified between the right and left pleural spaces, presumably the result of either congenital communications or following prior surgery (see Fig. 10-25C). In a surprising number of cases, small effusions may prove difficult to differentiate from pleural thickening and/or fibrosis. In these cases, scans obtained with the patient in the lateral decubitus position can be extremely helpful.

Fissural pseudotumors are also common and are usually secondary to congestive heart failure (66). Loculation of fluid within the fissures implies adherence of the pleural layers in the peripheral portions of the fissure, usually secondary to previous inflammatory disease. Identification of

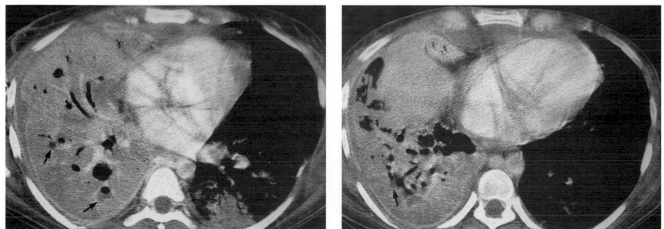

FIG. 10-42. Necrotizing pneumonia. **A,B:** Sequential contrast-enhanced sections show extensive consolidation throughout the entire right lung. Note that the right lung has heterogeneous low density with scattered small fluid collections easily identified (*arrows* in **A** and **B**) associated with small air-fluid collections. These findings are consistent with a necrotizing pneumonia associated with multiple small "microasbcesses." Vessels are easily identified traversing the right lung (so-called "positive angiogram" sign). Note that there is only a small quantity of pleural fluid left following drainage with a pleural tube. The pleural surfaces are clearly enhancing. Both blood cultures and pleural cultures were positive for Streptococcus pneumoniae. It cannot be overemphasized that this appearance is distinctly separate from that seen in patients with compressive atelectasis caused by an effusion in which there is no underlying infection. In these cases, following intravenous contrast enhancement there is uniform density throughout the collapsed lung (compare with Figs. 10-25B and 10-28).

interlobar fluid is significant because its appearance on CT may be confused with that of an intrapulmonary lesion. The typical radiographic appearance of loculated fissural fluid has been described by Baron (66).

Radiographically, fissural fluid usually is easily identified because: (a) the fluid collection lies in the expected region of the fissures; and (b) unless the fissure lies exactly perpendicular to the plane of the radiograph, the margins of the fluid collection appear hazy or poorly defined. These principles apply to the appearance of fluid within fissures on CT (see Fig. 10-26) (67). Fluid may collect in any portion of the fissures. If there is free communication between the lateral portion of the oblique fissure and the remainder of the pleural space, fluid will extend into the fissure and assume a characteristic triangular configuration with the apex pointing toward the hilum.

CT Characterization

Previous reports have examined the CT characteristics in patients with pleural effusions. In an early retrospective evaluation of 48 patients with pleural effusions who had a sonographically directed thoracentesis, Himmelman and Callen found a significant correlation between pleural fluid loculation and exudative pleural fluid chemistries. In addition, patients with loculated effusions tended to have larger effusions, longer hospitalizations, and more frequently required tube drainage (68). Seven of nine empyemas (78%) and 10 of 28 exudates (36%) were loculated. In 30% of cases,

pleural fluid loculation was identified, only by CT in 8%. None of these findings was noted in any patient with a transudative effusion.

More recently, Waite et al. reported evidence of pleural thickening following contrast enhancement on CT in nearly all patients with either empyemas or complicated parapneumonic effusions (69). Among 35 patients with documented thoracic empyema, 30 patients with malignant pleural effusions, and 20 patients with transudative effusions, Waite et al. found that enhancement of the parietal pleura was present in 96% of 25 patients with empyema who underwent contrast-enhanced CT scans. While 86% showed thickening of the parietal pleura, 60% showed thickening of the extrapleural subcostal tissues, and 35% showed increased attenuation of the extrapleural fat (Fig. 10-43; see Fig. 10-28) (69). Of 14 patients with complicated parapneumonic effusions, the thickness of the parietal pleura and extrapleural tissues averaged 3 mm and 3.5 mm, respectively, while in eight patients requiring decortication, the average thickness of these layers was 4 mm and 4.5 mm, respectively. In distinction, none of these findings were present in the 20 patients with transudative effusions (69).

In the most extensive study performed to date, Aquino et al. also evaluated CT findings in 80 consecutive patients (86 effusions) in whom correlative thoracenteses were performed (70). Specific CT signs evaluated included evidence of both parietal and visceral pleural thickening (further classified as either focal or diffuse, smooth or irregular), loculation, and evidence of expansion or edema of the extrapleural

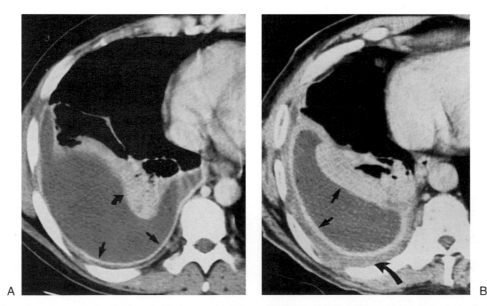

FIG. 10-43. Complicated parapneumonic effusion. **A:** Fibrinopurulent stage. Contrast-enhanced CT scan in a patient who had received antibiotics prior to admission. There is a moderate-sized right pleural effusion associated with volume loss and consolidation in the right lower lobe (*curved arrow*). The parietal pleura is slightly thickened and is clearly enhancing (*arrows*). Thoracentesis yielded clear pleural fluid without organisms. PH = 6.72; glucose = 22mg/dL; protein, = 5.4g/dL; LDH = 518 IU; WBC = 3,400/mm^3 with 70% polymorphonuclear leukocytes. This patient was subsequently successfully treated with closed-tube drainage. **B:** Fibrinopurulent stage. Contrast-enhanced CT scan in a different patient than shown in **A**. A loculated pleural effusion is present on the right side compressing the adjacent right lower lobe. There is marked thickening of both the visceral and parietal pleura (*arrows*). In addition, there is a considerable thickening of the extrapleural subcostal tissues, and increased attenuation of the extrapleural fat (*curved arrow*), presumably secondary to spread of infection or edema to the adjacent chest wall tissues.

space. Of 59 proved exudative effusions, 36 (61%) showed evidence of parietal pleural thickening. All cases of empyema ($n = 10$) and 56% of patients with exudative parapneumonic effusions, including all five patients with complicated parapneumonic effusions, had evidence of parietal pleural thickening. Overall, the specificity of this finding for exudative effusions proved to be 96% with a corresponding positive predictive value for 97% (70). Also of value was the finding of thickening and increased attenuation within the extrapleural fat, identifiable in 8 of 10 patients with empyemas. In distinction, the size or shape of effusions did not prove of diagnostic value. It should be noted that in the subset of patients with exudative malignant effusions, evidence of pleural thickening was present in only 11 (48%) of 23 cases.

Based on these data, Aquino et al., drew the following conclusions: (a) pleural thickening in association with an effusion in a patient with pneumonia indicates the presence of an exudative effusion; and (b) conversely, the absence of pleural thickening makes the likelihood of either a complicated parapneumonic effusion or empyema extremely unlikely.

It should be noted that although the thickness of the parietal pleura appears to correlate with the stage of parapneumonic effusions, there is little correlation between this appearance and the ability to predict which patients ultimately will require decortication. In a prospective study of serial CT scans in 10 patients following radiologic catheter drainage of empyemas, Neff et al. found that although the pleura was noticeably thickened four weeks following catheter removal in all patients, at 12 weeks the pleura was essentially normal in four patients, and showed only minimal or mild residual pleural thickening in the remainder (71).

Assessment and Guidance of Therapy

CT is of proven efficacy for assessing the response of patients to therapy. By identifying areas of loculated fluid, CT can be used to guide the appropriate placement of chest tubes. Although similar information may be obtained from a sinogram performed at the time of thoracentesis, sinograms do not provide any information concerning the nature of underlying parenchymal disease or associated chest wall pathology. Additionally, sinograms are of little value in disclosing the presence of multiple loculations, as frequently occurs in larger effusions. In patients with chest tubes, CT can be especially valuable by disclosing chest tubes inadvertently placed within the major fissures or within the lungs, as well as those inadequately positioned to ensure proper drainage (Fig. 10-44) (72,73). CT can help detect more serious complications of chest tube placement, including significant chest wall hemorrhage (Fig. 10-45). As documented by Stark et al., in a study of 26 patients with tube thoracostomies for treatment of empyema, malpositioned tubes were identi-

fied on frontal radiographs in only one of 21 patients while all were identified on CT (72). In addition to assessing the adequacy of chest tube placement, CT has also been proven effective in identifying residual changes caused by previous pleural tubes. CT may play an especially important role in the evaluation of patients who have undergone surgical therapy including thoracoplasties (Fig. 10-46), open drainage procedures including Eloesser window thoracostomies (Fig. 10-47), and even in patients who have been treated with oleothoraces or plombage (Fig. 10-48) (74–76).

Recently, considerable attention has been focused on radiologically guided percutaneous catheter drainage (PCD) of pleural fluid collections and pneumothoraces in both untreated and previously treated patients (77–82). Typically, these procedures are performed utilizing fluoroscopy, ultrasound, or CT, with comparable results (Fig. 10-49). Merriam et al., using a combination of imaging modalities, retrospectively reviewed the outcome of percutaneous catheter drainage of pleural fluid collections in 18 patients, including 16 patients with documented empyemas, nine of whom had previous unsuccessful surgical chest tube drainage (79). Twelve (80%) of 15 patients who had an adequate trial of guided drainage were cured. VanSonnenberg et al. reported similar results using both CT and ultrasound to drain 17 patients in whom previous conventional chest tube drainage had proven unsuccessful. In this study, 15 (88%) of patients were successfully drained, averting the need for open drainage (78). Using fluoroscopic guidance, Westcott successfully drained 11 of 12 patients with documented empyemas; in five of these patients, PCD was used as the sole means of drainage (77). Although most investigators advocate the use of closed pleural drainage in the initial management of complicated parapneumonic effusions, it should be noted that the use of closed drainage of empyemas is controversial (83–86). In a series of 70 patients with thoracic empyemas, closed tube thoracostomy was successful in only 35% of cases, while rib resection proved curative in 91% (84). Hood has argued that closed pleural drainage should be attempted only if the pleural process is less than three days duration; otherwise, patients should be treated with a rib resection with tube drainage (85).

In the absence of definitive data, it is apparent that the procedure of choice will remain a matter of individual physician's preference. This applies to the choice of imaging modality used to direct PCD as well. Ultrasonic guidance has the advantage of being relatively inexpensive and portable, allowing studies to be performed even in intensive care units. Unfortunately, ultrasound is far more operator-dependent than CT. Furthermore, despite claims to the contrary, CT is far more accurate in detecting underlying lung pathology, as well as in identifying multiple areas of loculation, especially when these are paramediastinal. Additionally, CT is not limited by bandages, drains, or tubes. Finally, it should be noted that in select cases, especially in those for whom there is a contraindication for the use of i.v. contrast media, MR may

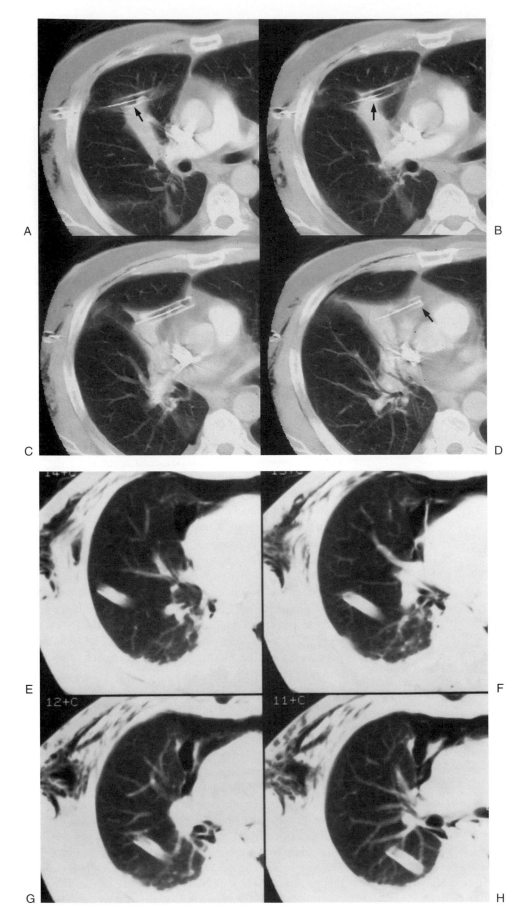

FIG. 10-44. Chest tube placement: CT evaluation. **A–D:** Enlargements of sequential images in a patient with atelectasis of the middle lobe shows a chest tube entering from the lateral chest wall traversing the right upper lobe to end with its distal tip seemingly within the mediastinum (*arrows* in **A**, **B**, and **D**). **E–H:** Enlargements of sequential images in a different patient than **A–D**, also shows a malpoisitioned chest tube traversing the right lower lobe. Note that in neither case is their evidence of apparent parenchymal laceration, or even a pneumothorax. In fact, the clinical significance of this type of malpositioning is largely a functional one related to incomplete drainage of preexisting pleural fluid or air.

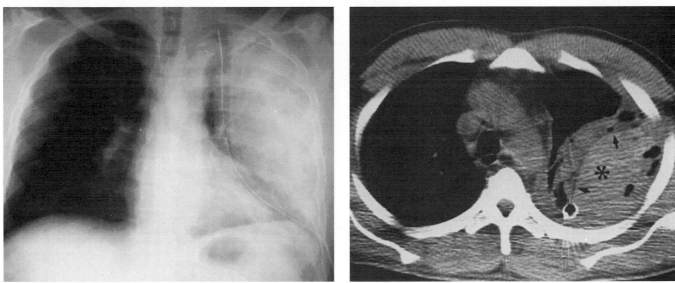

FIG. 10-45. Complication of closed chest tube placement: CT evaluation. **A:** Posteroanterior radiograph obtained shortly after placement of a left-sided chest tube shows nonspecific increased density on the left, suggestive of a loculated pleural collection. **B:** Noncontrast-enhanced CT section shows that the pleural tube is displaced medially by a large, high density, extrapleural fluid collection compressing and displacing the adjacent lung and pleura (*arrows*), consistent with extrapleural hemorrhage. At surgery these findings were confirmed to be secondary to traumatic injury to an intercostal artery that presumably occurred at the time of chest tube insertion.

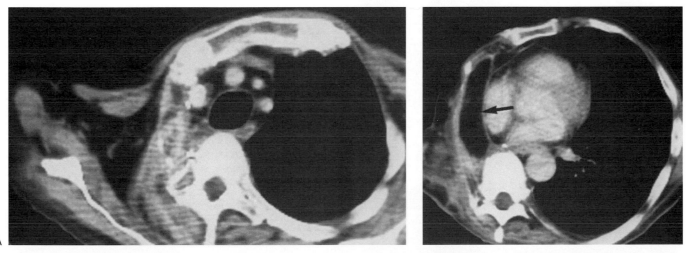

FIG. 10-46. Postsurgical assessment: thoracoplasty. **A,B:** Contrast-enhanced CT sections through the upper and lower chest, respectively, in a patient status-post a thoracoplasty for tuberculosis empyema. The entire right hemithorax is deformed, following surgical resection of numerous ribs and collapse of the ipsilateral hemithorax. Note that there has been a marked expansion of the extrapleural fat (*arrow* in **B**).

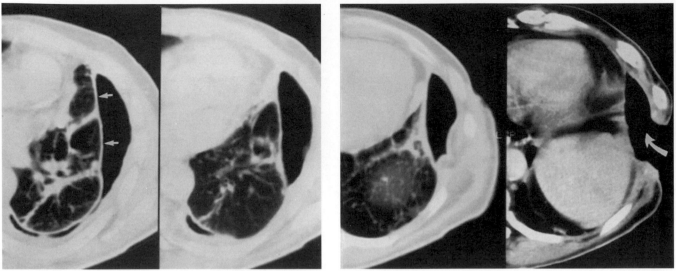

A,B   C,D

FIG. 10-47. Postsurgical assessment: Eloesser window thoracostomy. **A–C:** Sequential enlargements of sections through the lower right lung in a patient status postEloesser-window thoracostomy. The purpose of this procedure is to provide open drainage of chronic empyemas. Note that the visceral pleura is markedly thickened (*arrows* in **A**). Despite open communication through the chest wall, the left lung has not collapsed. **D:** Section obtained slightly more caudal than **C**, imaged with a narrow window confirming that there is an open communication with the pleural space (*curved arrow*).

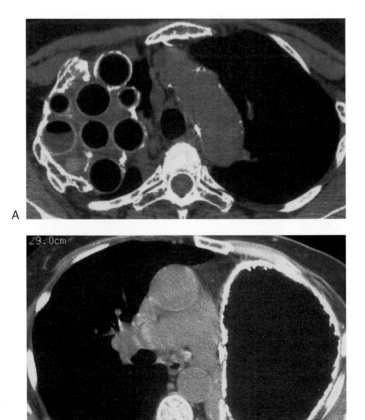

A

B

FIG. 10-48. Postoperative evaluation tuberculous empyemas. **A:**Noncontrast-enhanced CT section shows multiple rounded lucencies within the right hemithorax in a patient previously treated by plombage. Note the marked distortion of the ribs on the right side, consistent with prior thoracoplasty. **B:** Noncontrast-enhanced section through the middle lung in a different patient than **A**, shows that the entire left hemithorax is filled with uniform fat density, surrounded by a dense rim of calcification. This is the result of prior oleothorax. Similar to plombage, oleothorax used to be used in the therapy of TB and may occasionally still be identified in elderly patients.

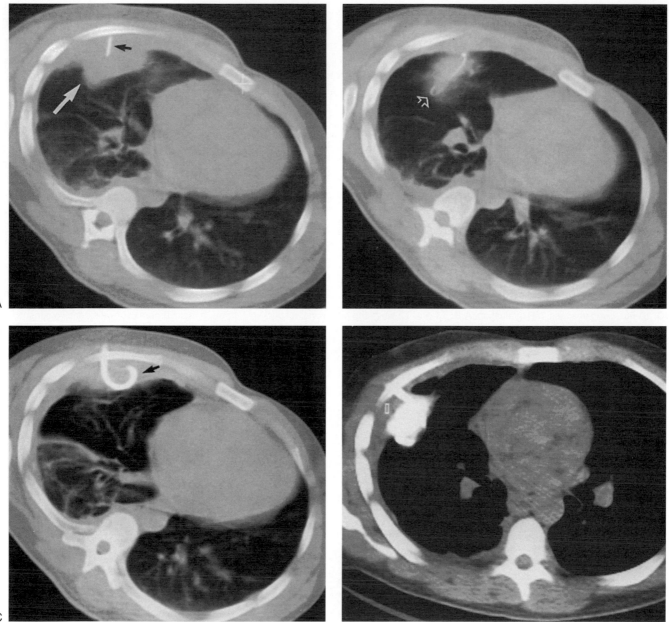

FIG. 10-49. CT-guided chest tube placement. **A:** CT section in a patient previously treated with a rib resection and open chest tube placement for an empyema. A moderate-sized, residual, loculated fluid collection is present within the lateral aspect of the minor fissure (*arrow*). Note that the patient has been placed in a slightly oblique position: the tip of a 22-gauge needle can be seen within the loculated fluid (*small arrow*). **B:** Section obtained at approximately the same level as **A**, following withdrawal of about 50 cc of pleural fluid. A guide-wire is now present within the minor fissure (*arrow*). **C:** Section at the same level as **A** and **B**, following placement of a catheter (*arrow*) within the minor fissure and withdrawal of the guidewire. **D:** Section at the same level as **A**, **B**, and **C**, following installation of approximately 10 cc of contrast material to confirm that the tube is in fact in the minor fissure.

be of value in differentiating pleural from parenchymal pathology, as well as detecting lung abscesses (Fig. 10-50).

Asbestos-Related Pleural Disease

Benign pleural manifestations of asbestos exposure include: (a) circumscribed pleural plaques; (b) benign exudative effusions; and (c) diffuse pleural fibrosis (87). Although these may be associated with underlying parenchymal abnor-

malities, they frequently occur independently (88). Of these, CT has proven most valuable in identifying pleural plaques and diffuse pleural thickening (89–97). The subject of CT findings in asbestosis is covered in detail in Chapter 6.

Circumscribed Pleural Plaques

Pleural plaques are the most common benign pleural manifestations of asbestos exposure (Figs. 10-51 and 10-52).

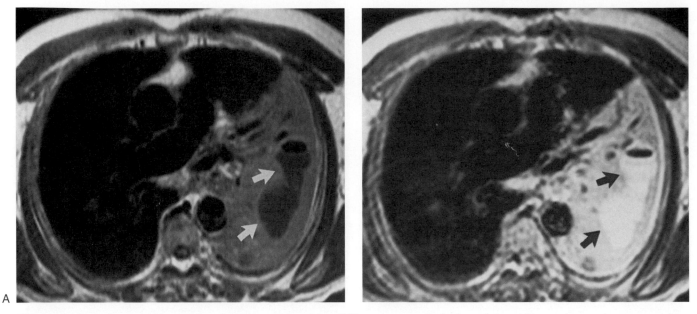

FIG. 10-50. Lung abscess: MR evaluation. **A,B:** T1-and T2-weighted MR scans, respectively, through the midthorax shows extensive consolidation throughout the entire left lung. A well-defined, smooth-walled, fluid-filled cavity can be identified within which there is a discrete air-fluid level (*arrows* in **A** and **B**). A central mass is also present, obliterating the left lower lobe bronchus and significantly narrowing the left upper lobe bronchus. In this case, MR clearly discloses the presence of a lung abscess developing distal to a central obstructing lesion.

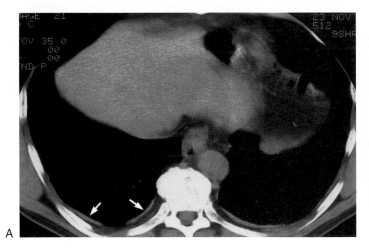

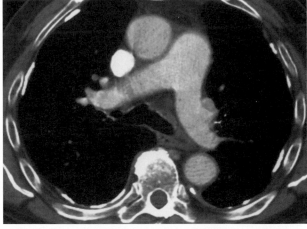

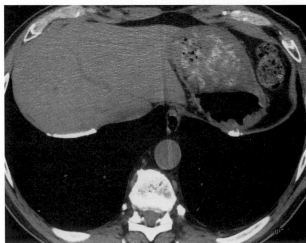

FIG. 10-51. Asbestos related pleural disease: calcified pleural plaques. **A:** Enlargement of a 10 mm section through the lung bases shows typical appearance of subtle noncalcified pleural plaques (arrows), identifiable as focal linear areas of pleural thickening. **B:** Contrast-enhanced section in a different patient than **A** shows typical appearance of bilateral calcified pleural plaques caused by prior asbestos exposure. **C:** Section through the lower lobes in a different patient than **A** or **B** show typical appearance of calcifications along the diaphragmatic pleura.

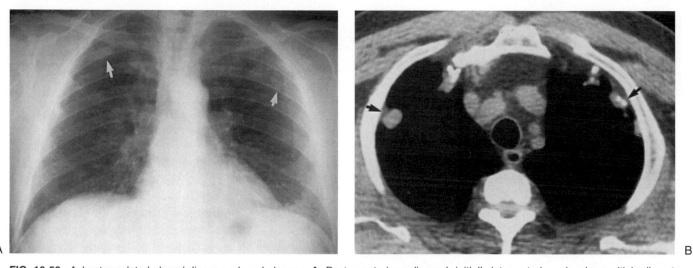

A   B

FIG. 10-52. Asbestos-related pleural disease: pleural plaques. **A:** Posteroanterior radiograph initially interpreted as showing multiple discrete pulmonary nodules, a common indication for obtaining CT (*arrows*). **B:** CT section through the great vessels shows calcified and noncalcified plaques bilaterally. In this case, many of these have a more nodular configuration than that shown in Fig. 10-51. Several appear to have prolapsed into the adjacent lung (*arrows*), accounting for the radiographic appearance of lung nodules.

They occur after a latency period of between 20 and 40 years, and generally are asymptomatic. Presumably the result of parietal pleural irritation caused by asbestos fibers protruding from the visceral pleural surface, it has also been hypothesized that fibers could pass from the lung via chest wall lymphatics to the parietal pleura (87). Typically, plaques appear as discrete, elevated, sharply defined foci of pleural thickening up to 15-mm thick (see Fig. 10-51) (94,98). Although usually found posterolaterally along the inferior costal margins as well as along the diaphragm, rarely plaques may involve the visceral pleura within fissures (99). Characteristically bilateral, some have observed a distinct unilateral, left-sided predominance (100). Calcifications occur in approximately 10% of plaques (96). These may appear punctate, linear, or occasionally "cake-like," especially when located along the diaphragmatic surfaces. Less commonly, calcified plaques may be pedunculated, in which case they may be mistaken for intraparenchymal nodules (see Fig. 10-52). Histologically, plaques are composed of predominantly acellular bundles of collagen usually described as having an undulated or "basketweave" configuration (88,101,102). Although plaques have been attributed to other causes including previous empyema and hemothorax, correlation between the presence of bilateral plaques and asbestos exposure is sufficiently high to warrant defining them as markers of previous dust exposure. A history of asbestos exposure can be elicited in >80% of individuals with pleural plaques (88,101,102). Pleural plaques are always benign.

Benign Exudative Effusions

Benign exudative effusions generally occur considerably earlier than other pleural manifestations of asbestos-related pleural disease, usually occurring within 10 to 20 years fol-

lowing exposure (87). They may be unilateral or bilateral, and recur in up to 30% of patients. As these effusions are usually nondescript and self-limited, their true incidence is difficult to determine. Epler et al. have reported identifying 35 cases (3.1%) of benign asbestos effusion among a survey group of 1,135 asbestos-exposed workers (103). Although the relationship between benign exudative effusions and the subsequent development of malignancy is unclear, it is unlikely that they represent a significant risk factor for mesothelioma (104). Nonetheless, as noted by Gefter et al., extra caution is probably warranted in those individuals with histories of asbestos exposure in whom a benign exudative effusion is identified (105).

Diffuse Pleural Thickening

In addition to pleural plaques and benign exudative effusions, diffuse pleural thickening may also result from asbestos exposure (Fig. 10-53) (87). Radiographic differentiation between these entities may be problematic. McLoud et al. have defined diffuse pleural thickening as a smooth, noninterrupted pleural density extending over at least one-fourth of the chest wall, with or without costophrenic angle obliteration (98). Unlike pleural plaques, diffuse pleural fibrosis presumably involves both the visceral and parietal pleural surfaces (see Fig. 10-53). The exact mechanism by which this occurs is controversial. It has been postulated that diffuse fibrosis results from an extension of underlying parenchymal disease to involve the adjacent visceral pleura (106). The frequency with which this occurs has been challenged, however. As documented by McLoud et al., in a study of 185 individuals with diffuse pleural thickening, this radiographic appearance proved to be the residue of a prior benign asbestos effusion in 31% of cases, and the result of confluent

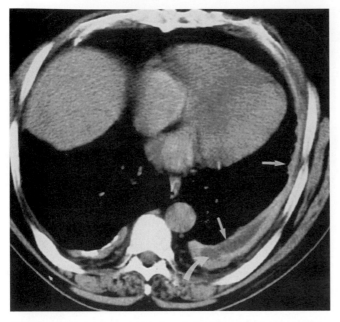

FIG. 10-53. Asbestos-related pleural disease: diffuse pleural fibrosis. Enlargement of a CT section through the left lung base shows a markedly thickened pleural rind, associated with marked expansion of the extrapleural fat (*arrows*). In addition, there is a small, residual pleural fluid collection identifiable as well (*curved arrow*). The presence of residual fluid suggests the possibility of a mesothelioma; however, pleural aspiration and biopsy showed only dense fibrosis and noninfected nonmalignant fluid. It is probable that with CT, small, residual pleural fluid collections will be recognized more commonly in patients with asbestos-related pleural fibrosis.

pleural plaques in 25%. In this study, only 10% of cases with diffuse pleural fibrosis proved to have underlying diffuse parenchymal fibrosis with extension to the visceral and parietal pleura (98). Differentiation between pleural plaques and diffuse pleural thickening is important, as the latter may be

associated with significant alterations in pulmonary function (87,98,107,108).

CT Evaluation of Benign Asbestos-Related Pleural Disease

As early as the late 1970s, Kreel and Katz showed CT to be significantly more sensitive than plain radiographs in the detection of asbestos-related pleural disease (2,89,90). In their series of 36 patients with known asbestos exposure, 27 (75%) individuals were found to have abnormal pleural thickening on CT, whereas 24 (66%) individuals had abnormalities detected on chest radiographs (90). In this same series, CT was 50% more sensitive in detecting pleural calcifications than were conventional radiographs.

It is apparent that there is a significant advantage to visualizing the pleural surfaces without superimposition of densities. Not only does CT allow a more precise assessment of the extent of pleural disease, but in a significant percentage of cases, CT can clarify otherwise indeterminate chest radiographic findings (91,94,109). As documented by Sargent et al., in a study of 30 patients with known asbestos exposure in whom radiographic interpretations were equivocal for the presence of pleural plaques, in 14 cases (48%), CT confirmed that the changes were caused by increased amounts of subpleural fat (Fig. 10-54) (46). Similar findings have been reported by Friedman et al. (95). In a study of 60 individuals with histories of occupational exposure to asbestos comparing the value of HRCT scans to routine radiographs for diagnosing pleural abnormalities, these authors showed the positive predictive value of chest radiographs to be 79%, compared with a positive predictive value of 100% for HRCT. Out of eight cases, false positive chest radiographs

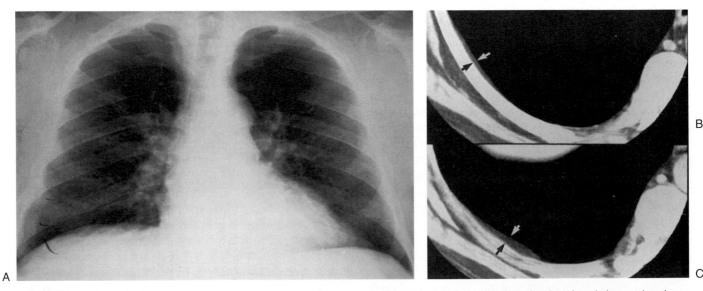

FIG. 10-54. Prominent extrapleural fat: CT evaluation. **A:** Posteroanterior radiograph initially interpreted as showing pleural plaques (*marks on right*) in a patient with documented exposure to asbestos. **B,C:** Enlargements of sequential CT scans obtained at the same level as in **A** shows the presence of prominent extrapleural fat pads (*arrows* in **B** and **C**), without evidence of pleural plaques or fibrosis.

proved to be secondary to extra subpleural fat in seven, and a prominent intercostal muscle in one.

The role of HRCT in the evaluation of benign asbestos-related pleural disease has also been evaluated by Aberle et al. In a study of 29 subjects with histories of occupational exposure to asbestos, these authors showed that pleural thickening was identified in 100% of cases using HRCT, compared with 93% using routine 10-mm thick CT sections (92). In addition to identifying pleural plaques, CT can be of value by disclosing diffuse pleural fibrosis. Gamsu et al. have suggested a useful CT definition of diffuse thickening: a continuous sheet of increased density at least 5-cm broad, 8-cm to 10-cm long, and more than 3-mm thick (96). It should be emphasized that care must be taken in assessing pleural thickness, especially when using HRCT. As shown by Im et al., in normal patients, identification of the usually pencil-thin line of the normal pleural surfaces may be obscured, especially in the paravertebral regions, because of a normal increase in the amount of extrapleural soft tissue caused by the incorporation of adjacent intercostal vessels (see Figs. 10-19–10-21 and 10-24) (3). As a consequence, the diagnosis with HRCT of diffuse pleural thickening requires that abnormalities be identified at several levels, preferably identifiable in other than just the paraspinal region.

The appearance of diffuse pleural thickening generally is easily differentiated from mesothelioma. Rabinowitz et al., however, have drawn attention to a variant of asbestos-related pleural fibrosis that closely mimics the appearance of malignant mesothelioma (110). In their series of 40 patients with known asbestos exposure, seven had a diffusely thickened, nodular pleura, indistinguishable from malignant mesotheliomas. None of these patients, however, had evidence of malignant transformation detected by multiple biopsies or by surgery. The significance of this type of fibrosis has yet to be established, as long-term follow-up studies of these patients was not undertaken (see Fig. 10-53).

Round Atelectasis

A variety of terms including folded lung, atelectatic pseudo-tumor, shrinking pleuritis with atelectasis, pleuroma, and rounded atelectasis, the most commonly used descriptive, refer to what is most often a manifestation of asbestos-related parenchymal and pleural disease (111). First described in this century, round atelectasis has been recognized with increasing frequency, especially with increasing use of CT to evaluate asbestos-exposed patients (94,96). Radiologically, round atelectasis usually presents as an incidental finding on routine chest radiographs (Figs. 10-55 and 10-56) (112,113). A distinct preponderance in men has been identified (114). Typically, conventional radiographs reveal a sharply defined pleural-based mass, ranging between 2 cm and 7 cm in size, usually located posteriorly in the lower lobes adjacent to an area of pleural thickening. Air-broncho-

grams may be present within. Characteristically, the mass is associated with vessels and bronchi that have a curvilinear appearance, coursing like a comet tail toward the hilum. These findings are associated with focal volume loss and often with hyperlucency of adjacent lung segments.

CT findings in round atelectasis have been extensively reviewed (94,96,115–120). The major CT sign is a rounded or wedge-shaped peripheral lung mass forming an acute angle with the adjacent pleura, which is almost invariably focally thickened. Additionally, vessels and bronchi can be identified curving toward the mass, creating a comet-tail appearance analogous to that seen on routine chest radiographs (see Figs. 10-55 and 10-56). Minor signs include focal emphysema, punctate areas of calcification, and uniform enhancement following administration of i.v. contrast media. Unfortunately, hypervascular lesions have been described in patients with asbestos-related pleural disease and lung cancers (121,122). Other tumors, albeit exceedingly rare, also have been described in association with asbestos-related disease (123,124).

Histologically, round atelectasis occurs adjacent to areas of both parietal and visceral pleural fibrosis (111). Round atelectasis probably results from at least one of two mechanisms. As hypothesized by Blesovsky, atelectasis probably results as a consequence of asbestos-induced pleural fibrosis (125). In support of this explanation, extensive fibrotic changes involving the adjacent visceral pleura have been verified pathologically (111,120). Alternatively, it is likely that in some cases round atelectasis results from compression of the lung caused by a pleural effusion causing infolding and distortion of the adjacent lung (126). Interestingly, parenchymal changes have been reported to resolve following decortication (111). Although generally associated with asbestos-related pleural disease, in fact, round atelectasis may result from any process that causes extensive focal pleural fibrosis (see Fig. 10-56). In an evaluation of 74 patients with rounded atelectasis evaluated by Hillerdal, 64 patients gave a prior history of asbestos exposure (114). Of the remaining 10 cases, two occurred following trauma and four occurred after a pleural exudate. Round atelectasis also has been described in association with histoplasmosis (127), as well as tuberculosis, including patients who have undergone therapeutic pneumothoraces (118).

In addition to the typical appearances described above, several variant forms of round atelectasis have been described. In patients with extensive pleural fibrosis, in particular, a pattern of single or multiple fibrous strands within the lung radiating toward a focal area of pleural thickening has been described in the absence of a definable parenchymal mass. These so-called ''crow's feet'' have been interpreted by some as the earliest manifestation of round atelectasis (Fig. 10-57) (128). As noted by Lynch et al, other benign lesions also occur in association with asbestos-exposure, including benign pleural-based masses, intrafissural pleural

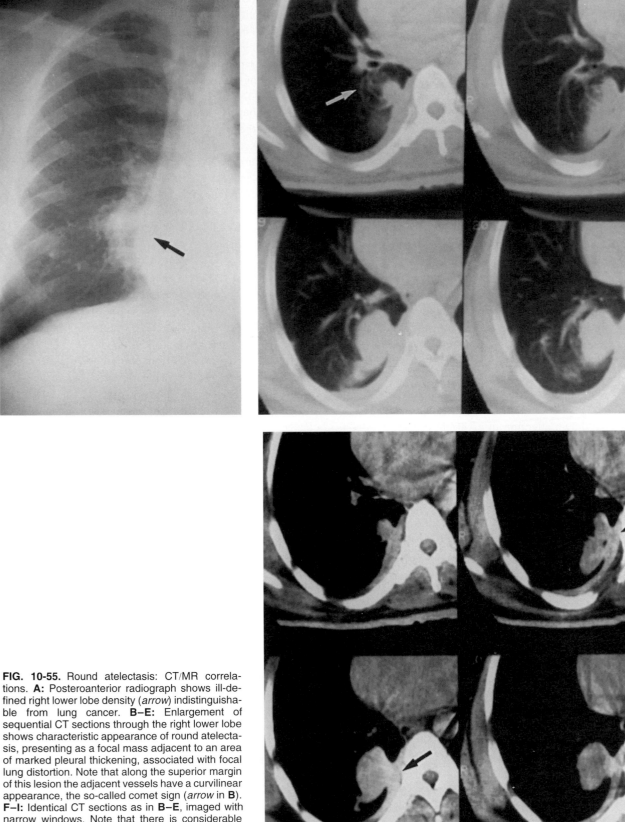

FIG. 10-55. Round atelectasis: CT/MR correlations. **A:** Posteroanterior radiograph shows ill-defined right lower lobe density (*arrow*) indistinguishable from lung cancer. **B–E:** Enlargement of sequential CT sections through the right lower lobe shows characteristic appearance of round atelectasis, presenting as a focal mass adjacent to an area of marked pleural thickening, associated with focal lung distortion. Note that along the superior margin of this lesion the adjacent vessels have a curvilinear appearance, the so-called comet sign (*arrow* in **B**). **F–I:** Identical CT sections as in **B–E**, imaged with narrow windows. Note that there is considerable pleural thickening, which is most prominent adjacent to the mass (*arrows* in **G** and **H**).

A

B,C

D,E

F,G

H,I

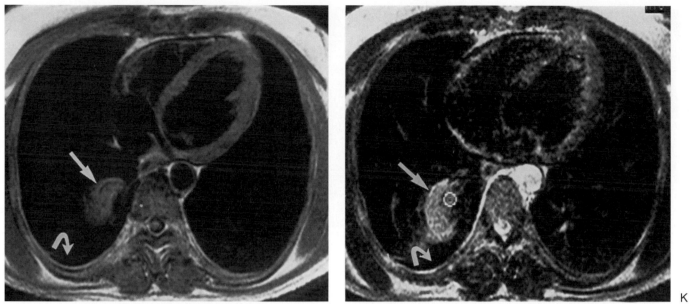

FIG. 10-55. *Continued.* **J,K:** T1- and T2-weighted images, respectively, both show a complex mass of intermediate signal intensity within the right lower lobe (*arrows*). Contrary to opinion, foci of round atelectasis do not represent areas of parenchymal fibrosis, but instead, infolded lung. It is therefore not surprising that considerable signal can be identified within these lesions, especially on T2-weighted scans. In distinction, note that the adjacent pleura, composed as it is of dense, mature fibrous tissue, generates no signal at all (*curved arrows* in **J** and **K**). Potentially, in equivocal cases, MR may be of value by confirming that the pleural thickening seen on CT does not represent tumor infiltration.

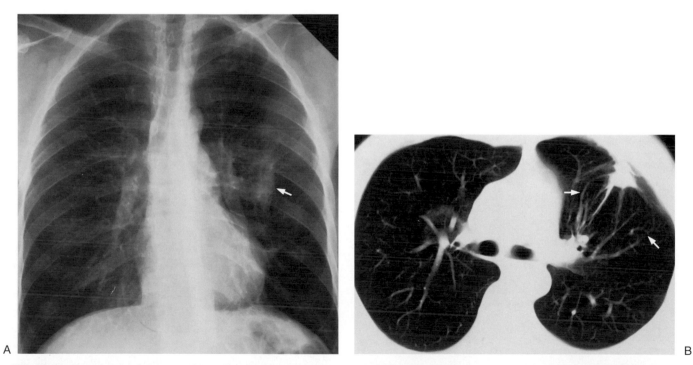

FIG. 10-56. Round atelectasis caused by prior tuberculosis. **A:** Posteroanterior chest radiograph shows ill defined nodular density in the left middle lung field (*arrow*). No other apparent pleural or parenchymal abnormality can be identified. **B,C:** Sequential images confirm focal, ill-defined density in the peripheral portion of the left upper lobe, extending to the pleural surface. Note the curvilinear configuration of the proximal left upper lobe vessels (*arrows* in **B** and **C**), the so-called "comet tail sign." **D:** Identical section as in **C**, imaged with narrow windows shows the presence of dense calcifications within the parenchymal mass; focal pleural thickening can be identified adjacent to this mass associated with a broad band of soft tissue leading from the calcifications to the pleural surface (*arrow*). Note that there are also bilateral hilar calcifications. In this case, round atelectasis has resulted from prior granulomatous infection with focal pleural and parenchymal scaring. (*continues*)

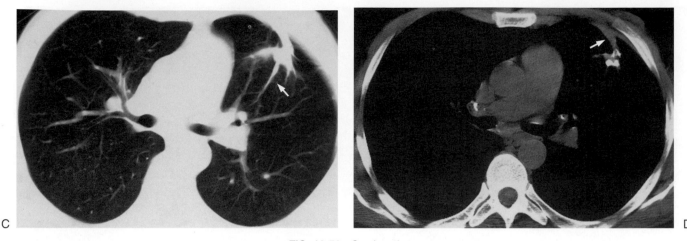

C   D

FIG. 10-56. *Continued.*

plaques, and masslike fibrotic sheets, especially adjacent to the hemidiaphragms (117). These authors have calculated that CT will detect asymptomatic benign masses in up to 10% of individuals with histories of significant exposure to asbestos.

In most cases, especially when there is a history of prior asbestos-exposure, the CT appearance of round atelectasis is sufficiently characteristic to obviate histologic verification, although careful follow-up surveillance is mandatory to insure an absence of growth. Alternatively, it has been suggested that suspicious lesions may also be evaluated with FDG-PET scans. As reported by McAdams et al, in their study of nine patients with 10 lesions, none proved positive, leading these authors to conclude that RA is not metabolically active on FDG imaging (129). These findings, while suggestive, clearly require further validation.

In our opinion, in those cases in which there is evidence of a change in size on follow-up CT studies, histologic evalu-

ation is indicated, even though it is well documented that areas of round atelectasis may continue to enlarge with time. It should also be noted that while rare, an association has been made between round atelectasis and malignant pleural mesothelioma (130). In particular, findings other than those described above as typically seen in patients with round atelectasis, such as diffuse pleural thickening or nodularity or pleural effusions, should suggest the possibility of coexistent malignancy.

Although MR has been used to evaluate round atelectasis, to date no consistent pattern of signal intensity within areas of rounded atelectasis has been found (118,131). However, MR may disclose the densely fibrotic nature of the adjacent visceral pleural thickening, eliminating possible confusion with tumor infiltration into the pleura (see Fig. 10-55).

Malignant Pleural Disease

Evaluation of patients with suspected pleural malignancy is an important practical use of CT. This is largely a reflection of the frequency of malignant pleural disease. Leff et al. have noted that approximately 25% of all pleural effusions in older patients in the general hospital setting are malignant in origin (132). In their series of 96 patients with carcinomatous involvement of the pleura, Chernow and Sahn showed that an effusion provided the basis for the first diagnosis of cancer in 44 of 96 patients (46%) (133).

Carcinoma of the lung is the most common cause of pleural malignancy, constituting between 35% and 50% of cases in most series. Breast cancer is also common, in some series equaling the incidence of lung cancer as a cause of malignant effusions. In approximately 7% of cases, the primary tumor site is unknown at the time of initial diagnosis; these frequently prove to be adenocarcinomas of "unknown origin" (50). Most unilateral malignant effusions are the result of pulmonary arterial tumor emboli seeding the visceral pleura with subsequent spread to the ipsilateral parietal

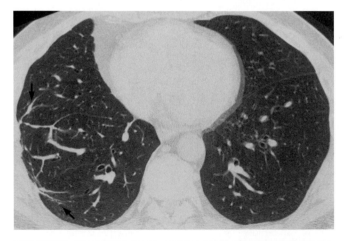

FIG. 10-57. Round atelectasis; early recognition by CT. High-resolution CT scan shows multiple curvilinear strands within the right lower lobe all oriented toward a slightly irregular and thickened pleural surface. These so-called "crow's feet" have been described as the earliest sign of developing round atelectasis (*arrows*).

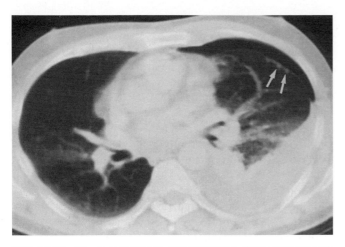

FIG. 10-58. Pleural metastases: CT correlation. CT section through the midthorax in a patient shows a moderate-sized left pleural effusion, following thoracentesis. A small anterior pneumothorax is present. Note that several small peripheral nodules can be identified involving the visceral pleural surface (*arrows*), which is particularly well seen owing to the pneumothorax. Most metastatic malignant effusions are the result of pulmonary arterial tumor emboli seeding the visceral pleura.

and talc, among others (50,138,139). As shown by Martini et al., in patients in whom initial tube thoracostomy is unsuccessful, pleurectomy may be effective; unfortunately, this procedure results in considerable morbidity and mortality (140).

Bronchogenic Carcinoma

As previously noted, bronchogenic carcinoma is the most frequent cause of a malignant pleural effusion, especially adenocarcinoma. As discussed in detail in Chapter 6, evidence of pleura involvement significantly alters the staging,

pleura (Fig. 10-58) (134). In distinction, bilateral malignant pleural effusions generally result from tumor spread to the liver, with subsequent hematogenous seeding. Pleural fluid may also accumulate in patients without direct pleural invasion. Mechanisms that have been proposed to account for paramalignant effusions include: (a) tumor obstruction of both central lymphatics and airways, with resultant pneumonia or atelectasis; (b) systemic effects of the disseminated tumor; and (c) results of radiation or drug therapy (50).

The definitive diagnosis of malignant pleural disease usually requires pleural fluid cytology, pleural biopsy, or even exploratory thoracotomy (135,136). In a review of recent literature, Sahn documented that the diagnostic yield from pleural fluid cytology was 66%, and from pleural biopsy was 46% (50). Combining procedures resulted in a 73% diagnostic yield. A diagnosis of pleural malignancy may be elusive. Ryan et al. emphasized that pleural effusions caused by malignancy may go undiagnosed even with careful examination of the pleura, lungs, and mediastinum at thoracotomy (137). In their retrospective study of the outcome of 51 patients with pleural effusions of indeterminate cause at thoracotomy, 25% were found later to have malignant pleural disease.

Malignant effusions usually imply a poor prognosis, although long-term survival has been reported, particularly in patients with metastatic breast carcinoma (50). In addition to radiation and chemotherapy, specific therapies that have been used to control malignant effusions include repeated thoracentesis, tube thoracostomy with or without the use of sclerosing agents, and pleurectomy (138). Although controversial in most centers, malignant effusions are initially treated by tube thoracostomy. Sclerosing agents that have been evaluated include tetracycline, bleomycin, quinacrine,

A
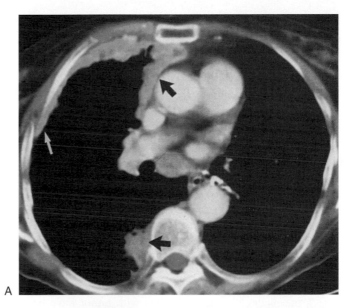

B
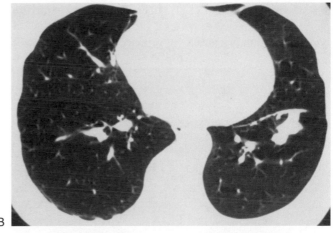

FIG. 10-59. A: Pleural seeding: CT evaluation. Contrast-enhanced CT section through the midthorax shows nodular thickened pleura in a patient with biopsy-proved adenocarcinoma of the lung. Note that pleural involvement is discontinuous, with foci of tumor infiltration (*arrows*) clearly separated by apparently normal intervening pleura. Enlarged subcarinal nodes are present as well. B: Section through the midlungs in a different patient than in A shows a lobulated mass in the anterobasilar segment of the left lower lobe subsequently verified as a nonsmall cell lung carcinoma on transthoracic needle biopsy. In this case, tumor directly extends to involve the major fissure (*arrow*), which is thickened and beaded in appearance (compare with normal right major fissure).

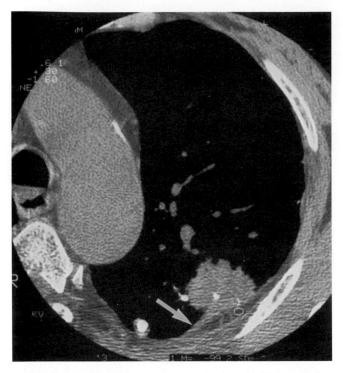

FIG. 10-60. Peripheral lung cancer: evaluation with high-resolution CT. Retrospective target reconstruction of the left lung in a patient with a peripheral lung cancer associated with apparent pleural thickening on posteroanterior and lateral chest radiographs (*not shown*). The mass clearly abuts the pleura, which is thickened (*arrow*). There is considerable expansion of the extrapleural fat adjacent to the mass, suggesting that there is no gross chest wall involvement. These findings were confirmed at surgery.

prognosis, and therapy of these tumors. The pathways by which the pleura becomes involved with tumor have been described by Heitzman et al. (141). Tumor may extend to the pleura secondary to reversal of the centripetal flow of lymph (commonly caused by primary central tumors), or

tumorous involvement of hilar nodes. Central venous obstruction also may be present. Alternatively, peripheral tumors may directly invade the adjacent pleura, either by tumor growth along peripheral perivascular-lymphatic sheaths, or by direct invasion of the adjacent pleura with subsequent pleural seeding (Fig. 10-59). Evidence of pleural seeding may be discovered in sites far removed from the primary tumor, including the mediastinal pleura (see Fig. 10-59A). Interestingly, not infrequently, tumor may involve the pleura without producing pleural fluid; these tumors may also involve the chest wall.

Unfortunately, assessment of pleural involvement is limited when tumors, both peripheral and central, abut the pleura but do not appear to directly invade either the chest wall or mediastinum (Fig. 10-60) (142–147). Even HRCT may offer little improvement; definitive evaluation usually still requires pleural biopsy (see Fig. 10-60). It has been suggested that this problem may be solved either with images obtained after therapeutic pneumothorax or using inspiration–expiration images. Although the presence of air within the pleural space helps to outline the pleural surfaces (see Fig. 10-58), adherence of lung to the pleural surfaces is nonspecific. This may result from either tumor infiltration of the parietal pleura and chest wall, or from previous adhesions. Similarly, some have suggested that the use of 3D surface reconstructions may be of value to identify pleural extension of tumor (see Fig. 4-6). To date, none of these applications has gained widespread clinical acceptance.

For similar reasons, CT is also limited in assessing patients with superior sulcus tumors because of problems related to cross-sectional imaging through the lung apices (Fig. 10-61). It should be noted, however, that CT is of value for assessing patients with asymmetric apical pleural thickening. Typically the result of prior tuberculous infection, "apical pleural thickening" in fact is a misnomer: In reality, it is the result of marked expansion of the apical extrapleural fat

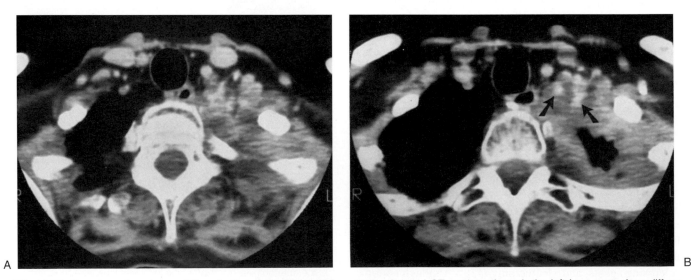

A   B

FIG. 10-61. Superior sulcus tumor: CT evaluation. **A,B:** Sequential contrast-enhanced CT sections through the left lung apex show diffuse infiltration of the pleura as well as the adjacent soft-tissue structures of the neck. Encasement of vessels by tumor is especially well visualized in **B** (*arrows*). Although in this case CT clearly depicts the extent of tumor, evaluation of apical tumors in general can be problematic with CT, which in most cases are most accurately assessed with MR.

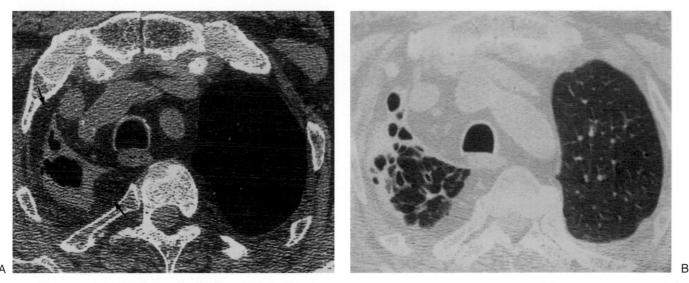

FIG. 10-62. Apical pleural thickening. **A:** High-resolution CT section through the right lung apex shows characteristic appearance of so-called "apical pleural thickening". In fact what appears radiologically to be thickened apical pleura in reality is due to marked expansion of apical extrapleural fat (*arrows*) usually in association with some element of volume loss and scaring in the adjacent lung parenchyma as is present in this case. This is exactly analogous to what occurs in patients with prior pleural infection (compare with Figs. 10-29 and 10-30), usually resulting from tuberculosis. **B:** High-resolution section obtained slightly below **A** shows typical cavitary and bronchiectatatic changes in the right apex caused by tuberculosis.

usually associated with some scarring and volume loss in the adjacent lung parenchyma (Fig. 10-62). The apical pleura itself is rarely sufficiently thickened to cause the radiographic changes to which it is typically attributed.

Another problem is encountered in evaluating patients with central endobronchial lesions with secondary obstruc-tive pneumonitis or apparent lobar collapse: Differentiation of infiltrate from tumor may be difficult. Similar to patients with Pancoast tumors (Fig. 10-63), MR is usually more accurate than CT in predicting parietal pleural and chest wall involvement in patients with underlying atelectasis (148–152).

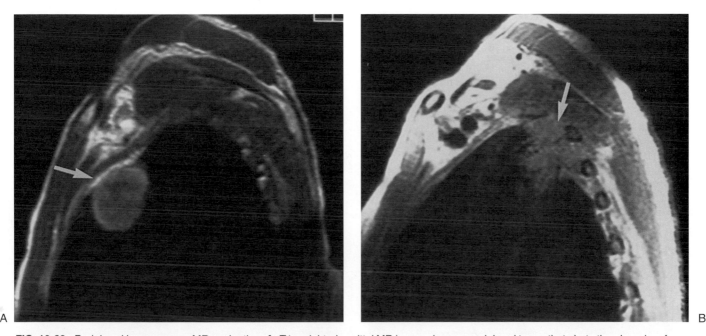

FIG. 10-63. Peripheral lung cancers: MR evaluation. **A:** T1-weighted sagittal MR image shows a peripheral tumor that abuts the pleural surface. Note that there is complete preservation of the extrapleural fat adjacent to the tumor (*arrow*), indicating that the chest wall is not grossly infiltrated by tumor. **B:** T1-weighted sagittal image in a different patient with a superior sulcus tumor. In this case, tumor has clearly invaded the adjacent chest wall, obliterating the normal extrapleural fat planes (*arrow*). Although CT is superior to MR in evaluating bony pathology, because of its greater contrast resolution, MR has proven more valuable than CT in detecting tumor infiltration into the soft tissues of the chest wall, especially infiltration into chest wall fat and adjacent muscles.

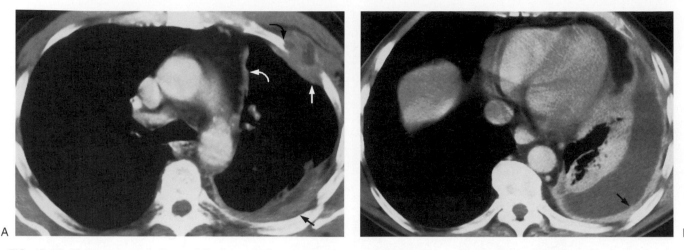

FIG. 10-64. Malignant mesothelioma. **A,B:** Sequential contrast-enhanced sections show nodular thickening involving both pleural surfaces (*arrows* in **A** and **B**) associated with loculated pleural fluid. The mediastinal pleura is subtly involved as well (*curved arrow* in **A**). Note presence of focal chest wall invasion anteriorly (*curved arrow* in **A**). There is considerable volume loss on the left typical of diffuse neoplastic involvement of the pleura.

Mesothelioma

Malignant pleural mesothelioma is a rare neoplasm representing less than 5% of pleural malignancies (50,153–155). The association between malignant mesotheliomas and asbestos exposure is well documented (50,155). Unlike the association between asbestos and bronchogenic carcinoma, the development of malignant mesotheliomas does not appear to be dose-related; tumors have been documented after only relatively trivial environmental or household exposure. It is probably for this reason that malignant mesotheliomas are frequently identified in patients without evidence of either pleural plaques or pleuropulmonary fibrosis (94). The risk of mesothelioma is related to the type of fiber to which patients are exposed. Crocidolite poses a far greater risk for development of a mesothelioma than either amosite or chrysolite (50,155). The latency period for the development of

malignant mesothelioma is long, generally between 20 and 30 years. Approximately 80% of mesotheliomas are pleural, while 20% are peritoneal (155).

The diagnosis of mesothelioma is often difficult to make. In particular, differentiating mesothelial neoplasia from mesothelial hyperplasia on one hand, and metastatic adenocarcinoma on the other may be problematic. As diagnosis typically requires extensive histopathologic examination, many have advocated the use of either thoracotomy or thoracoscopy to provide adequate tissue and provide more definitive staging (156). Recently, however, considerable success has been reported using closed needle biopsy under CT guidance (156). Relying on a combination of histochemical and immunohistochemical techniques, in particular the finding of positivity for keratin in 96.3% and negativity for CEA in 90%, Metintas et al. were able to prospectively diagnose 25 (83.3%) of 30 patients (156). As important, these authors

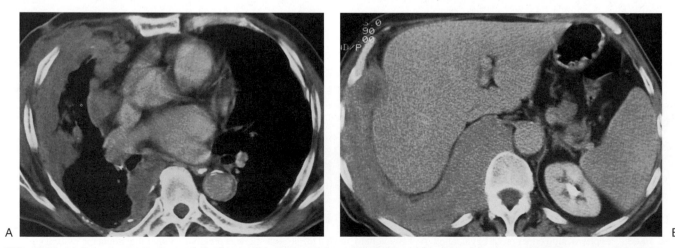

FIG. 10-65. Malignant mesothelioma. **A,B:** Sequential contrast-enhanced sections show extensive pleural thickening and nodularity more pronounced inferiorly affecting all pleural surfaces including the mediastinal pleura. In comparison to the case shown in Figure 10-64, there is only a small quantity of pleural fluid present. This is atypical, as most mesotheliomas are associated with large pleural effusions. Note that in this case there are contralateral calcified pleural plaques, consistent with prior exposure to asbestos. Extensive invasion of the chest wall and diaphragm in this case renders this tumor unresectable.

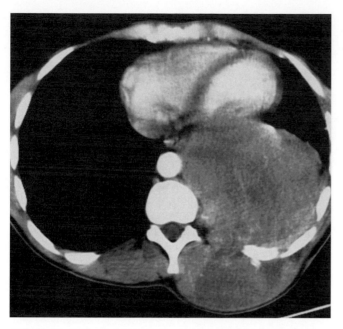

FIG. 10-66. Malignant mesothelioma: chest wall involvement. Contrast-enhanced CT scan shows extensive tumor involving the left lower lobe, ribs, and chest wall. This appearance is nonspecific, and initially suggested a primary lung cancer with secondary chest wall invasion. Malignant mesothelioma was biopsy-proved.

noted that local seeding occurred in only approximately 20% of cases, comparing favorably with both thoracoscopy and thoracotomy, both of which reportedly lead to seeding in up to 50% of cases.

Histologically, three forms of diffuse malignant mesothelioma have been recognized: epithelial, mixed, and sarcomatous (153). Characteristically, mesotheliomas grow by contiguous spread throughout the pleura, including the mediastinal pleural surfaces and the fissures (Figs. 10-

64–10-68). Not infrequently, spread occurs into the chest wall and the hemidiaphragms (see Figs. 10-64–10-68). Less frequently, mesotheliomas may metastasize hematogenously to mediastinal lymph nodes, as well as to the contralateral lung (50,155).

The appearance on CT of both "benign" and malignant mesotheliomas has been well described (94,96,110, 157–168). Characteristically, mesothelioma permeates the pleural space, causing the pleura to become markedly thickened, irregular, and nodular (see Figs. 10-64–10-68). The tumor often encircles the lung, which may then become entrapped (see Figs. 10-64 and 10-68). Effusions are present in up to 80% of cases. Ancillary findings include mediastinal and hilar lymphadenopathy and pulmonary nodules, which have been reported to be present in up to 60% of cases (96). Rarely, foci of calcification that have proved to represent areas of osteogenic sarcomatous degeneration may be identified (169).

In a review of 50 cases of documented diffuse malignant mesothelioma, Kawashima and Libshitz found 92% of cases had pleural thickening, 86% had thickening of the pleural surfaces of the interlobar fissures, and 74% had pleural effusions, but only 20% had evidence of pleural calcifications (165). Similarly, in a recent study of 84 patients with proved MPM, Sahin et al. also found that the most common findings included pleural thickening present in more than 90% of cases (168) with interfissural involvement, pleural effusions and ipsilateral volume loss noted in more than 70% of cases.

It should be emphasized that malignant mesotheliomas may rarely present as more localized masses, making CT distinction from benign fibrous tumors of the pleura extremely difficult (Fig. 10-69). It should also be noted that there are no CT-specific signs for mesothelioma; almost any malignancy involving the pleura can simulate the appearance of a mesothelioma (124,170).

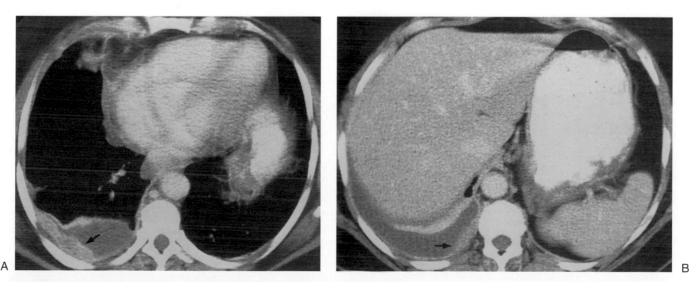

A   B

FIG. 10-67. Malignant mesothelioma. **A,B:** Sequential contrast-enhanced sections through the lung bases show atypical appearance of a relatively small loculated effusion associated with focal pleural thickening (*arrow* in **B**) and nodularity (*arrow* in **A**). Although these findings are more suggestive of pleural metastases, these findings proved to be caused by malignant mesothelioma.

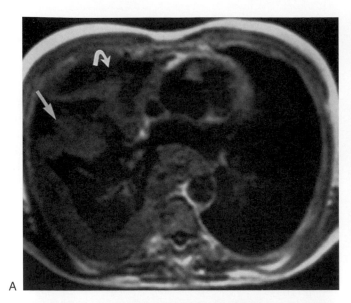

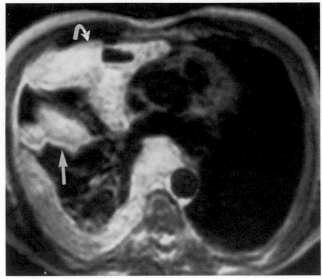

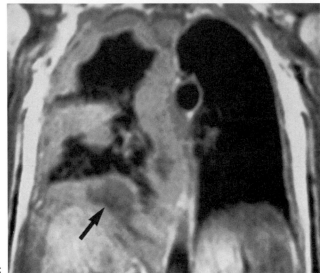

FIG. 10-68. Malignant mesothelioma: MR evaluation. **A,B:** T1- and T2- weighted images, respectively, through the lower chest in a patient with documented malignant mesothelioma. The pleura is circumferentially thickened and nodular, with evidence of tumor infiltration into the major fissure (*arrows* in **A** and **B**). **C:** Coronal T1-weighted image shows to better advantage of the full extent of tumor, from the lung apex to the diaphragms, including the fissures. Note the presence of another area of loculated fluid inferiorly (*arrow*). In this case, coronal images are of value by clearly delineating tumor extension into the diaphragm.

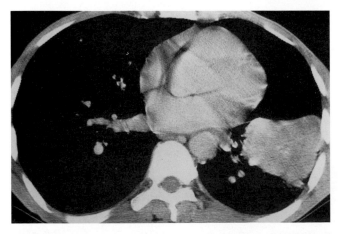

FIG. 10-69. Localized malignant mesothelioma. Contrast-enhanced section shows bulky nodular soft tissue mass apparently lying within or adjacent to the left major fissure. The remaining pleural surfaces are normal and there is no evidence of an effusion. Although this appearance suggested a possible diagnosis of a benign fibrous tumor of the pleura, histologically this proved to be a malignant mesothelioma.

Alexander et al. have shown that plain radiographs, compared with CT, frequently underestimate the disease extent (160). CT disclosed unexpected areas of involvement in each of their five cases. Extension into the contralateral chest was demonstrated in two cases, and extension into the abdomen and chest wall were each shown in one case. Similar findings have been reported by Sahin et al., who noted in a retrospective study of 84 patients with malignant pleural mesothelioma that of 17 (44%) patients in whom tumor was initially classified radiologically as stage 1, CT led to a reclassification to a higher stage (168).

Presently, the main value of CT has been to : (a) precisely delineate the intra- and extrathoracic extent of disease; (b) determine the best therapeutic approach; and (c) monitor the results of therapy. To date, a number of systems have been

TABLE 10-1. *Mesothelioma staging system: T designation*

Status	Region involved	Characteristics
T1a	Limited to ipsilateral parietal pleura, including mediastinal and diaphragmatic pleura	No involvement of visceral pleura
T1b	Ipsilateral parietal pleura, including mediastinal and diaphragmatic pleura	Scattered foci of tumor also involving visceral pleura
T2	Each ipsilateral pleural surface[a]	At least one of the following: • Involvement of diaphragmatic muscle • Confluent visceral pleural tumor (including fissures) or extension of tumor from visceral pleura into underlying pulmonary parenchyma
T3	Locally advanced but potentially resectable tumor; each ipsilateral pleural surface[a]	At least one of the following: • Involvement of endothoracic fascia • Extension into mediastinal fat • Solitary, completely resectable focus of tumor extending into soft tissues of chest wall • Nontransmural involvement of pericardium
T4	Locally advanced technically unresectable tumor; each ipsilateral pleural surface[a]	At least one of the following: • Diffuse extension or multifocal masses of tumor in chest wall, with or without associated rib destruction • Direct transdiaphragmatic extension of tumor to peritoneum • Direct extension of tumor to contralateral pleura • Direct extension of tumor to one or more mediastinal organs • Direct extension of tumor into spine • Tumor extending through to internal surface of pericardium with or without pericardial effusion, or tumor involving myocardium

[a] Parietal, mediastinal, diaphragmatic, and visceral pleura. See ref. 174.

proposed for staging malignant pleural mesotheliomas (MPM) (171). Reflecting recent advances in therapy, in particular the potential role of extrapleural pneumonectomy followed by radiation and chemotherapy to allow long term survival in a select population of patients (172,173), a new staging system has been proposed by the International Mesothelioma Interest Group (174). Using TNM descriptors, MPM has been grouped into four stages (Tables 10-1–10-3). Most important is the determination of T status. T1 describes early tumor confined to the ipsilateral hemithorax primarily involving the parietal pleura without evidence of pleural adhesions. In distinction, T2 designates tumor usually involving the diaphragmatic muscle that cannot be resected without removing the underlying lung. T3 tumors are those with evidence of locally advanced tumor extending into the endothoracic fascia, mediastinal fat or the surface of the pericardium that may nonetheless still be amenable to surgical resection. T4 lesions are those with locally advanced, surgically unresectable tumor caused by diffuse extension into the chest wall, direct extension through the diaphragm into the abdomen, or direct extension with encasement of mediastinal organs or the contralateral pleural space. Both N and M status are defined equivalent to their designation for staging nonsmall cell lung cancer (174). In addition to

TABLE 10-2. *Mesothelioma staging system: N and M designations*

Designation	Description
NX	Regional lymph nodes not assessable
N0	No regional lymph node metastases
N1	Metastases in ipsilateral bronchopulmonary or hilar lymph nodes
N2	Metastases in subcarinal or ipsilateral mediastinal lymph nodes, including ipsilateral internal mammary nodes
N3	Metastases in contralateral mediastinal, contralateral internal mammary, and ipsilateral or contralateral supraclavicular lymph nodes
MX	Distant metastases not assessable
M0	No distant metastases
M1	Distant metastases present

See ref. 174.

TABLE 10-3. *Mesothelioma: Staging*

Stage	Status	Lymph node	Metastases
Ia	T1a	N0	M0
Ib	T1b	N0	M0
II	T2	N0	M0
III	Any T3	Any N1 or N2	M0
IV	Any T4	Any N3	Any M1

See ref. 174.

stratifying patients into homogenous groupings to better assess the impact of prospective clinical trials, this staging system is designed to identify potentially resectable patients.

To date, attempts to accurately stage patients using either CT or MR have proved of limited value. As outlined by Patz et al., radiologic criteria for determining resectability include preservation of extrapleural fat planes, absence of an extrapleural soft tissue mass, smooth undersurface of the diaphragm, and normal CT attenuation values and MR signal characteristics of adjacent structures. By comparison, radiologic features indicative of unresectability include tumor encasing the diaphragm, invasion of extrapleural soft tissues or fat, or invasion, separation, or destruction of adjacent osseous structures (175). Using these criteria, these authors prospectively evaluated 41 consecutive patients with malignant pleural mesothelioma using both CT and MR, and found that while both CT and MR had >90% sensitivity for detecting signs of unresectability, corresponding specificity measured only between 25% and 50%. This remained true regardless of whether the location of the tumor evaluated was along the diaphragm, chest wall, or mediastinum (175). Although premature, these authors did note a potential benefit of MR as compared with CT because of improvements in visualization of the pleural surfaces owing to the ability to acquire images in multiple planes (see Fig. 10-68).

Metastatic Disease

Pleural metastases, apart from those caused by bronchogenic carcinoma, occur most frequently from primary neoplasms of the breast, gastrointestinal tract (including pancreas), kidneys, and ovaries (Figs. 10-70–10-73) (50,134, 136). Invasive thymoma also frequently involves the pleura, usually by contiguous invasion (Fig. 10-74). Malignant thymomas may also cause pleural seeding resulting in the development of discrete pleural masses often at a distance far removed from tumor within the anterior mediastinum (see Fig. 10-74; see also Chapter 2) (176,177).

In patients with metastatic disease, pleural effusions may develop for a variety of reasons. These include increased permeability of the capillaries supplying tumor implants, as well as increased capillary permeability caused by pleuritis associated with obstructive pneumonitis if present, direct tumor erosion of pleural blood and lymphatic vessels, and decreased removal of pleural fluid caused by mediastinal lymph node infiltration (50).

The same wide variation in the appearance on CT described for mesotheliomas may be seen with metastatic pleural disease (see Figs. 10-70–10-73). Pleural metastases may cause marked thickening and nodularity of the pleura associated with only a small quantity of pleural fluid. Alternatively, pleural metastases may cause large pleural effusions in which the foci of malignancy are difficult to identify. In a study of 86 patients evaluated with contrast-enhanced CT reported by O'Donovan and Eng (178), there was evidence of either smooth or irregular pleural thickening in 62% of cases. Although loculated fluid was present in 40%, focal soft tissue masses in association with fluid could be identified in only 10%.

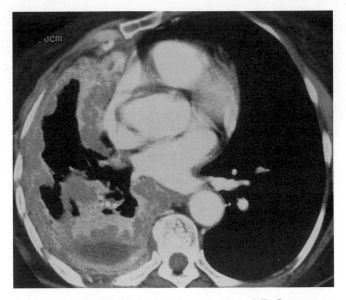

FIG. 10-70. Pleural metastases—breast cancer. **A,B:** Contrast-enhanced section shows pattern of diffuse nodular pleural thickening associated with loculated pleural fluid and marked ipsilateral volume loss—findings often associated with malignant mesothelioma. In fact, these findings are nonspecific; a pseudo-mesotheliomatous appearance is especially often seen in patients with metastatic adenocarcinoma (so-called adenocarcinoma of unknown primary). In this case, metastatic disease was secondary to breast carcinoma.

MR findings in patients with metastatic disease have been described (see Fig. 10-73) (179). In a study of 45 patients evaluated with both CT and MR, Falaschi et al. noted that while there was little difference between the morphologic appearance of tumors on both CT and MR, high-signal intensity was observed on T2-weighted images in all malignant lesions, but in only two benign lesions (sensitivity = 100%, specificity = 87%). It would appear that at least for a subset of lesions that are predominantly fibrous in nature, including pleural plaques, fibrothoraces and fibromas, MR may play a limited role as an ancillary method of evaluation.

Not infrequently, pleural biopsy will reveal adenocarcinoma of the pleura of unknown primary. Many of these are presumed to be secondary to primary adenocarcinomas of the lung, although the primary tumor may be obscured by the extensive pleural disease.

Pleural Lymphoma

It has been estimated that approximately 10% of malignant pleural effusions are the result of lymphoma (50). Pleural effusions are more likely to occur in non-Hodgkin's lymphomas (NHL) than with Hodgkin's disease (HD), and are more likely to occur in patients with extensive disease

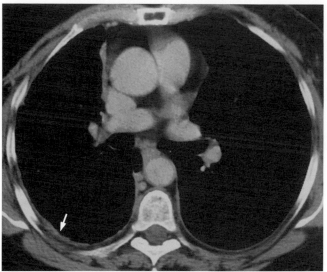

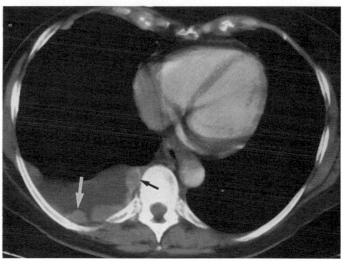

FIG. 10-71. Pleural metastases—breast cancer. **A:** Contrast-enhanced section shows subtle asymmetric thickening and nodularity along the posterior right pleural surface (*arrow*) and anterior mediastinal pleural surface in this patient with documented pleural metastases form breast cancer. **B,C:** Contrast-enhanced CT scans through the carina and the lower lobes in a patient status-post a right mastectomy. In addition to a moderate-sized right pleural effusion, enlarged internal mammary lymph nodes can be identified on the right (*small arrow*). The pleural surface is nodular and thickened superiorly (*large arrow* in **B**). Inferiorly, discrete pleural masses can be seen easily separable from the surrounding effusion (*arrows* in **C**). Metastatic breast cancer was biopsy-removed.

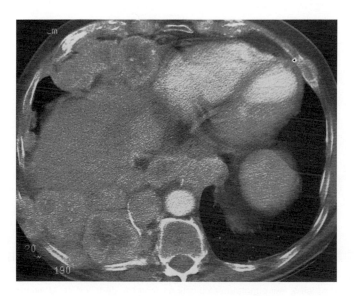

FIG. 10-72. Pleural metastases-melanoma. Contrast-enhanced section shows multiple nodular densities with a suggestion of rim enhancement infiltrating the pleural surfaces circumferentially. This unusual appearance is compatible with vascular neoplasms including metastatic renal cell carcinoma, among others. In this case, these findings proved secondary to metastatic melanoma.

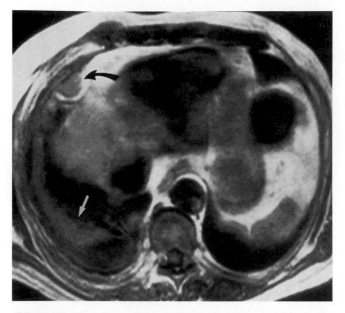

FIG. 10-73. Pleural metastases: MR evaluation. T1-weighted section in a patient with radiographic evidence of a nonspecific right-sided effusion (*not shown*). A pleural effusion is apparant on the right side compressing the adjacent right lower lobe (*arrow*). Additionally, there is an enlarged anterior mediastinal lymph node embedded in fat (*curved arrow*), strongly suggesting malignant disease. Adenocarcinoma of the pleura was documented.

of involvement of adjacent ribs with subsequent extension through the chest wall and pleura, or secondary to involvement of the adjacent lung (50,139).

As documented by Stolberg et al., lymphoma frequently causes subpleural deposits of tumor in the form of either nodules or plaques (Fig. 10-76) (183). Similar observations have been made by others (184). In a retrospective radiographic review of 112 nonselected patients with documented histiocytic lymphoma, Burgener and Hamlin showed that pleural involvement was present in 18% of cases, including four cases with localized pleural plaques (185). Shuman and Libshitz have documented a role for CT in detecting pleural involvement (186). In a series of 71 patients with both documented HD ($n = 47$) and NHL ($n = 24$) evaluated by CT, these authors showed solid pleural manifestations in 31%. Although this most probably does not represent a typical population of patients, as pointed out by the authors themselves, it is apparent that documentation of the presence of pleural disease can be of particular benefit in the development of appropriate treatment strategies, both following initial diagnosis and as a means for follow-up (187).

In select cases, the ability to identify chest wall involvement may also be important. In this regard, MR has recently been shown to be more accurate than CT for predicting the presence and assessing the extent of chest wall invasion (188,189). As recently reported by Carlsen et al., in a retrospective study comparing CT with MR in the evaluation of 57 patients, 22 of whom had chest wall or pleural involvement, chest wall disease was identified on MR in 20 patients compared with only seven with CT, while pleural involvement was detected on MR in 14 patients compared to only five with CT (188). Most important, three of 15 patients receiving radiation therapy in this study had their radiation ports changed on the basis of MR findings.

(Fig. 10-75) (180,181). Although distinctly uncommon at the time of initial diagnosis, up to 30% of patients with Hodgkin's disease may eventually develop effusions (182). In patients with lymphoma, pleural effusions result from a variety of causes including: impaired lymphatic drainage caused by obstruction of hilar and mediastinal lymph nodes, obstruction of the thoracic duct, frequently associated with a chylous effusion, and direct pleural infiltration as a result

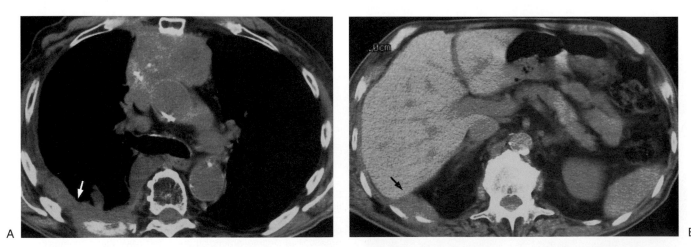

A   B

FIG. 10-74. Pleural metastases-invasive thymoma. **A,B:** Sequential noncontrast-enhanced sections show typical appearance of an invasive thymoma. A large homogenous anterior mediastinal mass is present within which a few punctate calcifications may be identified. In addition, there is marked pleural thickening noted especially along the posterior pleural surface (*arrow* in **A**). Note that there is also evidence of tumor involving the inferior pleural space in **B** (*arrow*): this is typical of "drop" metastases that often occur in patients with invasive thymoma, in particular (see Chapter 2).

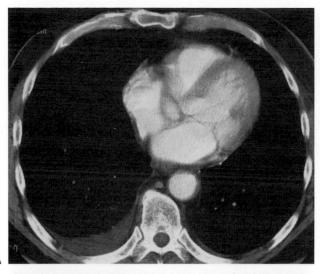

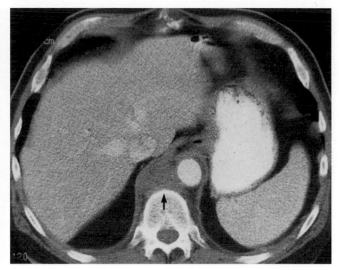

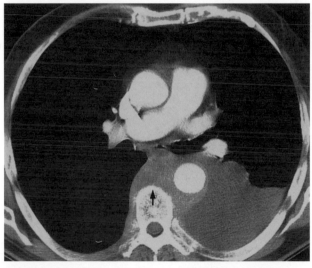

FIG. 10-75. Pleural lymphoma. **A:** Contrast-enhanced sections show nondescript right sided pleural effusion; note absence of pleural thickening or nodularity. **B:** Section at the level of the esophageal hiatus shows markedly enlarged retrocrural nodes (*arrow*). This combination of effusion with enlarged retrocrural and retroperitoneal nodes is especially suggestive of non-Hodgkin's lymphoma subsequently proved. **C:** Contrast-enhanced section in a different patient than shown in **A** and **B** shows extensive posterior adenopathy in a patient with known non-Hodgkin's lymphoma associated with an otherwise nondescript pleural effusion (*arrow*). This appearance is also characteristic and should suggest the correct diagnosis in most cases.

Postpneumonectomy Space

As described by Tsukada and Stark, complications are frequent following pneumonectomy, both in the immediate as well as the remote postsurgical period (190). Altogether, it has been estimated that pneumonectomy has a combined morbidity and mortality of approximately 30% (190).

As first shown by Biondetti et al., CT is especially efficacious in evaluating the postpneumonectomy space (see Fig. 5-32; Figs. 10-77–10-79) (191). As initially reported by these authors, in their series of 22 patients following pneumonectomy evaluated by CT, residual fluid was present in 13 (60%) of 22 cases, even years following surgery, while in nine (40%) of 22 cases, CT showed the postpneumonectomy space to be completely obliterated (191). Other findings identified were consequent to rotation and ipsilateral displacement of mediastinal and hilar structures, as well as hyperaeration of the contralateral lung.

To date, CT has proved most useful in the assessment of remote tumor recurrence (see Fig. 10-79). This can be identified in most cases as mediastinal or hilar masses or, less commonly, as discrete peripheral masses projecting into

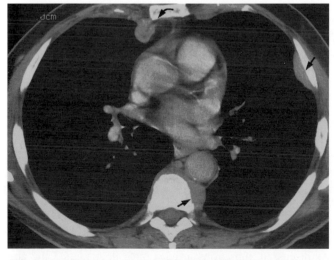

FIG. 10-76. Pleural lymphoma. Contrast-enhanced section shows separate discrete soft tissue masses (*arrows*) involving the left pleural space without evidence of an effusion at this level. Note also the presence of enlarged internal mammary nodes on the right (*curved arrow*). This appearance is compatible with involvement of the subpleural lymphatics in this patient with known non-Hodgkin's lymphoma.

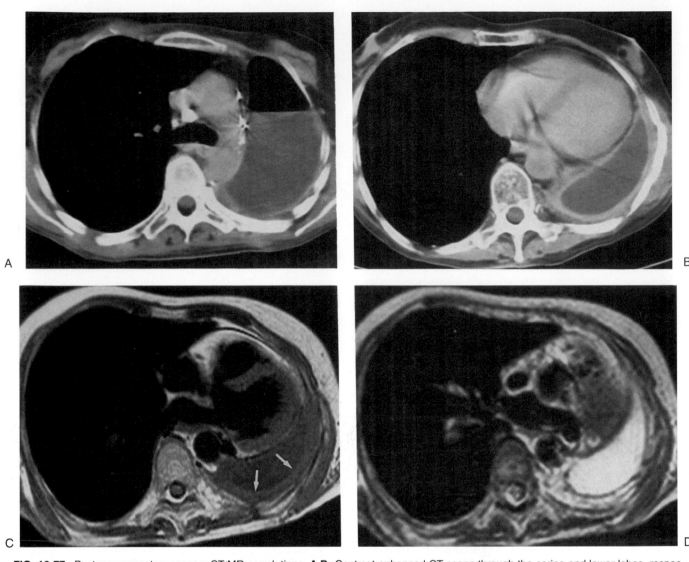

FIG. 10-77. Postpneumonectomy space: CT/MR correlations. **A,B:** Contrast-enhanced CT scans through the carina and lower lobes, respectively, show typical appearance following a recent pneumonectomy in a patient with lung cancer. A large air-fluid level can be seen in **A**. The pleural surfaces appear smooth, without evidence of focal masses or nodules. **C,D:** T1- and T2-weighted images, respectively, obtained at the same level through the lower chest in the same patient as shown in **A** and **B**, several months later. The pneumonectomy space is now entirely filled with fluid. The pleural surfaces are smooth without evidence of nodules or masses. Note that the pleural surfaces are most easily evaluated on the T1-weighted scans (*arrows* in **C**).

the lower-density fluid within the pneumonectomy space (192,193). Other complications for which CT may be of use include the development of a post-pneumonectomy empyema secondary to bronchopleural fistulae (see Fig. 10-78) (194). As shown by Shepard et al., CT also may also be valuable in diagnosing the so-called "right pneumonectomy syndrome" (195). In this condition, occurring sometimes years following surgery, patients develop symptoms of dyspnea and recurrent pulmonary infections in the left lung owing to compression of the distal trachea or left mainstem bronchus caused by the marked shift of the mediastinum to the right side.

Recently, MR has been used to evaluate the postpneumonectomy space (see Figs. 5-34 and 10-77) (196). Not surprisingly, the main advantage of MR is nonreliance on the use

of intravenous contrast administration to delineate hilar and mediastinal structures from recurrent tumor masses.

Malignant Pleural Disease Overview

Because of its unobstructed view of the pleural space, coupled with its ability to differentiate between fluid and soft-tissue densities, CT represents an important method for evaluating patients with suspected malignant pleural disease. As discussed, numerous articles have documented the appearance of pleural tumors, both benign and malignant. Specific CT signs that have been described for both primary and metastatic disease include circumferential thickening of the pleura and focal and/or diffuse nodularity of the pleura. Recently, Leung et al. in an evaluation of 74 patients with

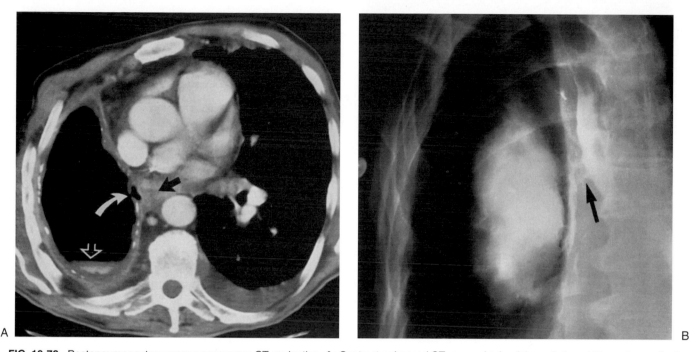

FIG. 10-78. Postpneumonectomy space empyema: CT evaluation. **A:** Contrast-enhanced CT scans obtained through the midthorax in a patient status post–right-sided pneumonectomy years prior for treatment of bronchiectasis. An air-fluid level is present within the pneumonectomy space, consistent with a fistula. Sections at the level of the carina and right mainstem bronchus show no evidence of airway pathology (*not shown*). Increased soft-tissue density is apparent in the region of the esophagus, which is difficult to identify (*straight arrow*). There is also a suggestion of a potential communication with the pneumonectomy space at this level (*curved arrow*). Note that the fluid level within the pneumonectomy space has extremely high density (*open arrow* in **B**). **B:** Coned-down view from an esophragm showing fistulous communication between the esophagus (*arrow*) and the pneumonectomy space.

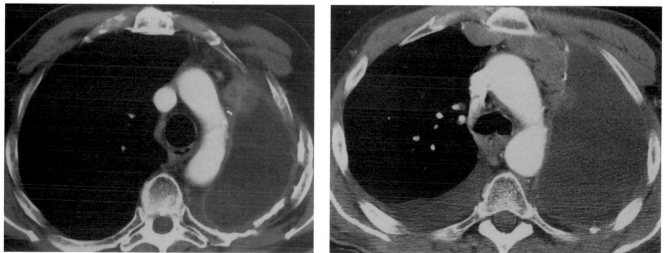

FIG. 10-79. Postoperative assessment—tumor recurrence. **A:** Contrast-enhanced section at the level of the aortic arch in a patient post–left-pneumonectomy for nonsmall cell lung cancer. There is evidence of an ill-defined soft tissue mass in the anterior mediastinum, consistent with tumor recurrence, subsequently proved by thoracentesis. **B:** Contrast-enhanced CT in a different patient than in **A**, following an extrapleural pneumonectomy for mesothelioma. Markedly enlarged anterior mediastinal nodes are apparent consistent with residual/recurrent tumor. The appearance of the left hemithorax following an extrapleural pneumonectomy is quite similar to that seen in patients at postpneumonectomy, as is the appearance of recurrent tumor.

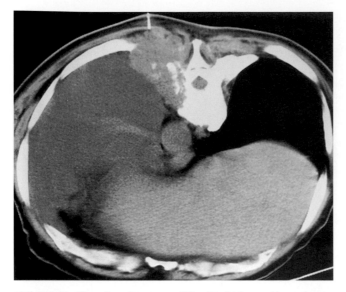

FIG. 10-80. Pleural malignancy—CT guided biopsy. Prone image obtained at the time of a transthoracic needle biopsy shows needle tip directed towards a large paraspinal mass causing erosion of the adjacent vertebral body. Previous thoracenteses and closed pleural biopsies had been nondiagnostic. Biopsy-proved metastatic adenocarcinoma.

proved diffuse pleural disease, including 39 cases of pleural malignancy, showed CT findings to be highly specific (197). Using the criteria of circumferential pleural thickening, nodular pleural thickening, parietal pleural thickening greater than 1 cm, and mediastinal pleural thickening alone or in combination, CT correctly diagnosed pleural malignancy in 28 of 39 cases (sensitivity = 72%; specificity = 83%). Significantly, in this series, circumferential pleural thickening proved to be 100% specific in predicting malignant pleural disease.

It is apparent that CT represents an important adjunct to routine chest radiography in the evaluation of patients with suspected malignant effusions. Although specific histologic diagnosis may be impossible, as documented by Leung et al., the appearance of malignant pleural disease is sufficiently characteristic to suggest the diagnosis, especially in those cases where establishing the diagnosis by conventional means, including pleuroscopy and thoracotomy, proves difficult (197). In these cases, CT may be of particular value by directing transthoracic needle biopsy of otherwise occult neoplasms (Fig. 10-80).

Benign Fibrous Tumors of the Pleura

Primary neoplasms of the pleura are rare tumors that are generally divided into two broad subgroups: localized, generally benign lesions, and diffuse, invariably malignant lesions (198). Variously referred to as localized pleural mesotheliomas or solid fibrous tumors of the pleura, these neoplasms represent only about 10% of primary pleural neoplasms (199). Unlike malignant mesotheliomas, there is no known association between localized pleural mesotheliomas and exposure either to asbestos or history of tobacco use. Usually presenting as incidental asymptomatic masses, these tumors have been associated with a number of extrathoracic abnormalities including pulmonary hypertrophic osteoarthropathy and digital clubbing, which have been reported to occur in as many as 20% of cases. Along with nonspecific joint pains, these findings have been noted to resolve following excision of these tumors. Other less common symptoms include those referable to large masses in the chest, including chest pain and hemoptysis. An association with hypoglycemia has also been noted (198).

Pathologically, these tumors are composed of a mixture of spindle-shaped fibroblastlike cells within a variable amount of collagenous stroma. Interestingly, the cell of origin of these tumors is not definitively known. In 30% to 50% of cases these tumors are pedunculated. Diagnosis usually requires surgical excision; transthoracic needle biopsy rarely provides sufficient tissue for definitive diagnosis.

CT findings have been described (157,199,200). These include well-defined, usually lobulated lesions ranging in size from solitary nodules to massive neoplasms occupying most of the pleural cavity (see Fig. 10-3; Fig. 10-81). Pleural effusions are conspicuously absent, given the large size of these lesions. Calcifications within these tumors are also rarely observed. Lee et al., in a series of nine cases, noted marked heterogeneous contrast enhancement in all eight evaluated following the administration of i.v. contrast (199). This they attributed to the presence of thin-walled venous sinusoids within tumors associated with thick-walled arteries and arterioles and dilated veins (199). In distinction, areas of low attenuation corresponded to foci of myxoid or hemorrhagic degeneration.

Although usually benign, localized malignant mesotheliomas do occur (see Fig. 10-69). Okike et al,, in a study of 60 patients with localized pleural mesotheliomas identified over a 25 year period, eight (13%) proved malignant (201). Similarly, Briselli et al., in a review of over 360 cases, found 12 percent to be malignant (202). Unfortunately, to date, no clinical or radiographic features allowing preoperative differentiation between malignant and benign localized fibrous tumors of the pleura have been reported. Although resection is usually definitive, in approximately 15% of cases, local recurrence will be observed.

THE CHEST WALL

The Sternum

The sternum and sternoclavicular joints are difficult to evaluate with plain radiographs, mainly because overlying structures are difficult to exclude from view on frontal and oblique projections. The sternoclavicular joints are angled obliquely, making their visualization particularly difficult. The potential role of CT to image the sternum has long been appreciated. Several reports have outlined in detail the nor-

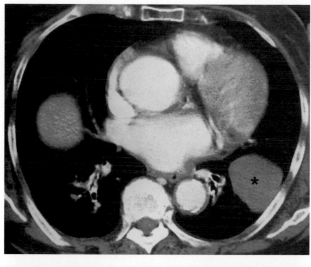

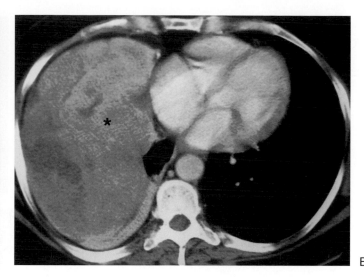

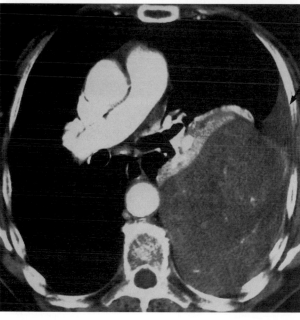

FIG. 10-81. Benign fibrous tumors of the pleura: CT spectrum. **A:** Contrast-enhanced section through the lower lobes shows a homogenous soft tissue mass in the region of the left major fissure (*asterisk*). **B:** Contrast-enhanced section in a different patient than A shows large, heterogeneous soft tissue mass occupying most of the inferior portion of the right hemithorax (*asterisk*) superficially mimicking the appearance of abnormal liver tissue. **C:** Contrast-enhanced section in a different patient than **A** or **B** also shows a markedly heterogeneous soft tissue mass occupying most of the inferior portion of the left hemithorax resulting in marked compression atelectasis of the left lower lobe. A small quantity of pleural fluid can be identified laterally anterior to the mass (*arrow*). Despite marked dissimilarities in the appearance of these tumors, they all represent biopsy proved benign fibrous tumors of the pleura.

mal appearance of the sternum and its articulations, including normal variants (Fig. 10-82) (203–208). With the patient's arms held above the head, the proximal portions of the clavicles have a steep obliquity and will appear in cross-section as elongated or oval structures. The sternal notch is easily defined between the clavicular heads. The manubrium is the widest part of the sternum and forms the anterior wall of the superior mediastinum. Superiorly, the middle part of the superior border of the manubrium is rounded; this portion is called the jugular notch. To each side of the jugular notch, posteriorly, an indentation in the manubrium can be identified; these are the clavicular notches, which represent the sternal part of the sternoclavicular joints. Sequential scans through the clavicular notches show close approximation of the sternum with the clavicular heads. Just below this, and somewhat more laterally, a rough projection in the contour of the manubrium can be defined, representing the point of

articulation between the sternum and the first costal cartilage.

The value of CT in assessing lesions of the sternoclavicular joints and sternum has been repeatedly documented (205,209–217). In their series of 17 patients with sternoclavicular abnormalities evaluated by CT, Destouet et al. demonstrated pathology better, or provided additional diagnostic information in the majority of cases (203). These included six cases of sternoclavicular joint dislocation, two cases of nonspecific synovitis and osteoarthritis, and two cases of osteomyelitis.

In our experience, CT has proven especially valuable: (a) in assessing the sternum following sternotomy, both to rule out postoperative infections and to evaluate the use of rotated pectoral flaps following sternal debridement (Figs. 10-83 and 10-84) (205–207,209–211); (b) to assess the sternum and sternoclavicular joints, especially in intravenous drug

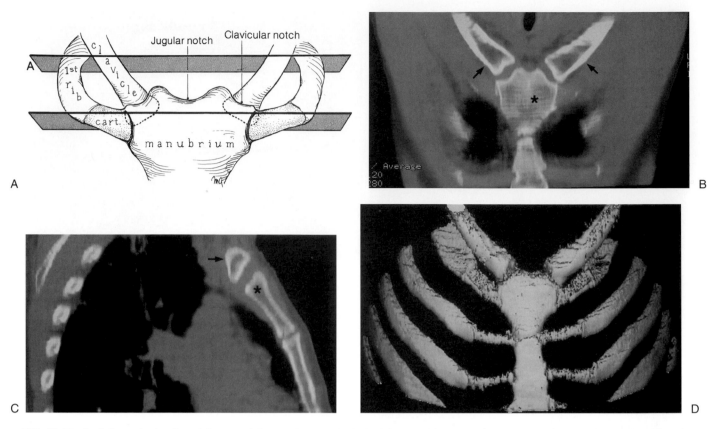

FIG. 10-82. A: Schematic drawing of the manubrium and sternoclavicular joints. A denotes a section through the distal clavicles above the level of the sternum. **B,C:** Coronal and parasagittal multiplanar reconstructions through the sternoclavicular joints generated from 3 mm helically acquired source images reconstructed every 2 mm provide good anatomic resolution of the manubrium (*asterisks* in **B** and **C**) as well as the distal clavicles (*arrows* in **B** and **C**). **D:** 3D surface reconstruction from the same case shown in **B** and **C** provides good anatomic delineation of the bony thorax.

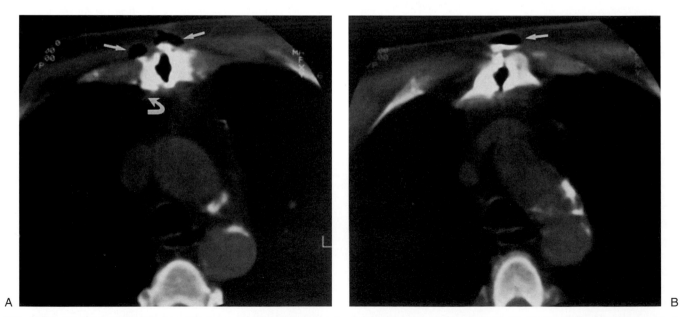

FIG. 10-83. Poststernotomy infection: CT sinogram. A,B: Enlargements of sequential CT sections through the sternum in a patient status-post sternotomy. This study was performed following injection of dilute contrast media into a catheter left in place following surgery. A space can be seen between the two halves of the sternum filled with contrast; additionally, pockets of air and contrast can be identified anteriorly in the chest wall (*arrows* in **A** and **B**) as well as posterirly, adjacent to the sternum (*curved arrow* in **A**). Note that there is no evidence of a significant fluid collection or contrast within the anterior mediastinum.

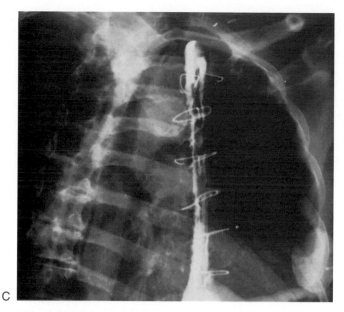

C

FIG. 10-83. *Continued.* **C:** Corresponding sinogram. Note that CT is far more precise in delineating the exact number and locations of fluid collections.

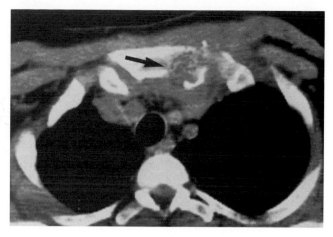

FIG. 10-85. Sternoclavicular osteomyelitis. CT section through the sternoclavicular joints shows lytic destruction of the lateral aspect of the sternum (*arrow*) as well as the distal clavicle, associated with considerable soft-tissue thickening in a known intravenous drug addict. Needle aspiration was positive for *Staphylococcal* infection.

users, to rule out infection, including associated mediastinitis (Fig. 10-85) (203,206,207,209,216–218); (c) to evaluate posttraumatic abnormalities (Fig. 10-86) (203,209,213,214); and (d) to evaluate patients in whom there is a clinical suspicion of a possible sternal lesion, especially in patients with

known breast cancer, as well as to evaluate sternal pathology following irradiation (203,207,209,212,219,220).

The Ribs

Although the ability of CT to assess rib pathology is somewhat limited by the oblique orientation of ribs relative to the CT scan plane, it is possible to accurately identify particular ribs, provided there is detailed knowledge of the CT appearances of their costovertebral and costotransverse articulations, as well as the relationship of the clavicle to the first rib (221). This anatomy is illustrated in Figures 10-87 and 10-88. Briefly, the heads of the first, tenth, eleventh, and

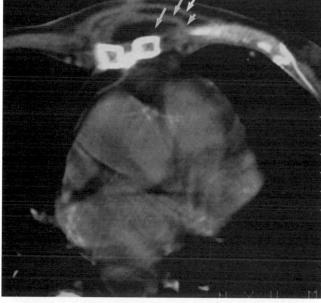

FIG. 10-84. Pectoral flaps: CT evaluation. Enlargement of a CT scan in a patient status-post sternotomy requiring bilateral pectoral flaps following sternal debridement. Concentric rings of alternating density (*short arrows*) and lucency (*long arrows*) can be identified anterior to the sternum, corresponding to attenuated muscle and fat, respectively. This appearance is pathognomonic and should not be confused with chest wall pathology. (From ref. 211, with permission.)

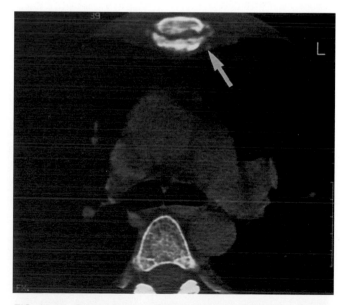

FIG. 10-86. Sternal fracture. Enlargement of a CT section through the sternum showing transverse fracture (*arrow*).

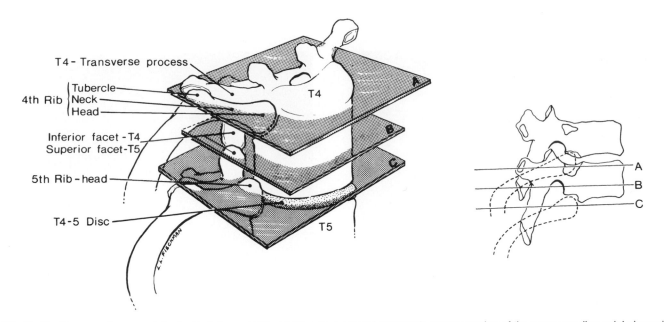

FIG. 10-87. Diagram of costovertebral articulations at T4 and T5, with a sagittal schematic representation of the corresponding axial planes in A, B, and C. (From ref. 211, with permission.)

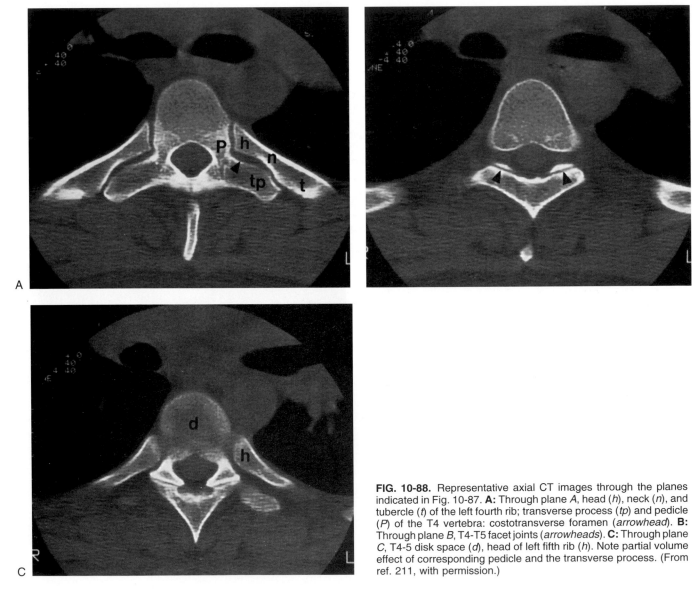

FIG. 10-88. Representative axial CT images through the planes indicated in Fig. 10-87. **A:** Through plane A, head (h), neck (n), and tubercle (t) of the left fourth rib; transverse process (tp) and pedicle (P) of the T4 vertebra: costotransverse foramen (arrowhead). **B:** Through plane B, T4-T5 facet joints (arrowheads). **C:** Through plane C, T4-5 disk space (d), head of left fifth rib (h). Note partial volume effect of corresponding pedicle and the transverse process. (From ref. 211, with permission.)

twelfth ribs articulate only with the body of the corresponding vertebra, while the heads of the second to ninth ribs articulate with the articular facet on the lateral aspect of the body of the corresponding vertebra, the intervening disc, and the demifacet on the vertebral body above. The first 10 ribs also articulate with their corresponding transverse processes. The intervening space between the neck of the rib and the transverse process is called the costotransverse foramen. Although only a short segment of each rib is visualized on an axial CT image because of the caudal slope of the ribs, the head and neck of a rib are usually in the same horizontal plane as the pedicle and the transverse process of the corresponding vertebra. Knowledge of these relationships allows individual ribs to be identified in most cases. As outlined by Bhalla et al. (221), this involves the following steps (Fig. 10-89):

1. Identify the first rib. The first rib is most easily identified on the axial image showing the middle third of the clavicle.
2. Identify the next two or three ribs on the same section by counting posteriorly along the rib cage. Each more posterior rib is numbered one higher than the rib anterior to it.
3. Proceed sequentially through the remaining images, concentrating on the costovertebral articulations. Each subsequent and numerically higher thoracic vertebra and the corresponding rib are enumerated.

4. Localize individual rib or pleural lesions by sequentially enumerating the ribs along the rib cage proceeding anteriorly from the spine. Each successive rib encountered represents the numerically preceeding rib.

In a retrospective review of 12 cases with documented rib pathology, Bhalla et al. (221) successfully localized 21 lesions, including 17 costal and five thoracic spine lesions, using this approach.

Axilla and Chest Wall

Detailed evaluation of the soft tissue structures of the chest wall requires thorough familiarity with normal cross-sectional anatomy. Anatomic relationships in the region of the axilla are especially important given the significance of this area for identifying chest wall neoplasia, especially manifestations of breast cancer and lymphoma, as well as identifying lesions that affect the brachial plexus. Sequential cross-sectional anatomic illustrations of the axilla are shown in detail in Figures 10-90–10-92. As described by Fishman et al., the axilla is a pyramidal-shaped space between the upper arm and the chest wall, with the apex directed superiorly and the base directed downward (222). The boundaries of the axilla include: (a) an anterior wall formed by the pectoralis major and minor muscles, subclavius muscles, clavipectoral facia, and the suspensory ligament of the axilla; (b) a posterior

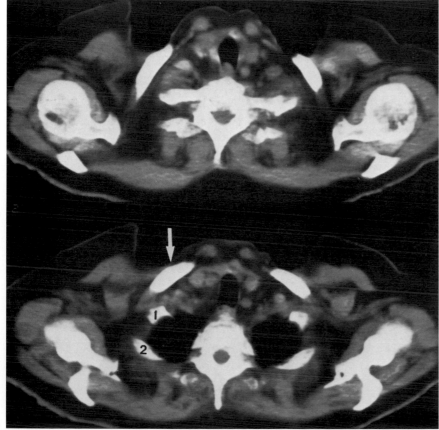

FIG. 10-89. Counting ribs: CT technique. **A–J:** 10 sequential CT images. The ribs (labeled 1 through 7) are most easily counted as follows: First identify the first rib by recognizing the characteristic relationships between the anterior portion of the first rib and the axillary vessels and clavicle (*arrow* in **B**). Then, at this same level, identify the second and third ribs by counting posteriorly along the rib cage. Finally, proceed sequentially through the remaining images, concentrating on the costovertebral articulations. In this case, a lytic lesion can be identified in the sixth rib on the right (*arrow* in **J**).

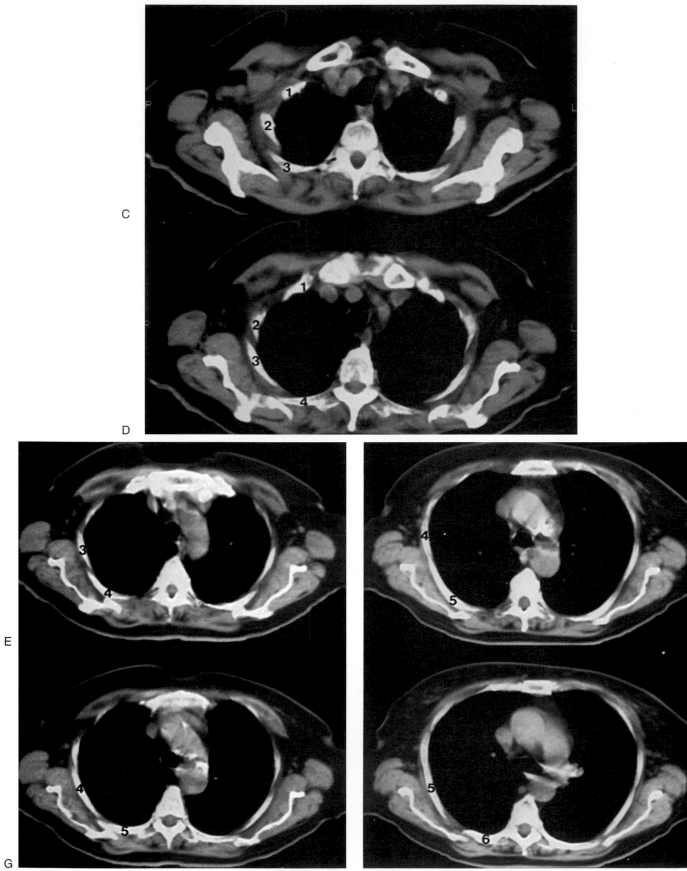

FIG. 10-89. *Continued.*

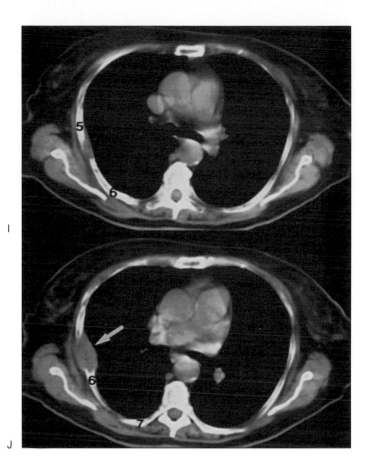

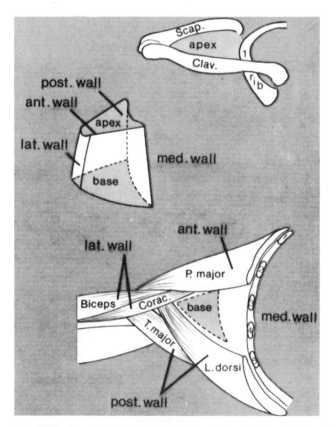

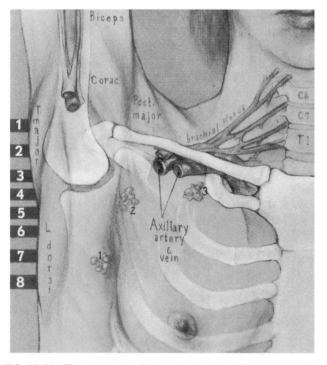

FIG. 10-89. *Continued.*

FIG. 10-90. The boundaries of the axilla. *Lat wall*, lateral wall; *ant wall*, anterior wall; *P major*, pectoralis major; *med wall*, medial wall; *L dorsi*, latissimus dorsi; *post wall*, posterior wall; *T major*, teres major; *Cora c*, coracobrachialis. (From ref. 222, with permission.)

FIG. 10-91. The structures of the normal axilla, with corresponding characteristic transaxial segments labeled 1 to 8. *Corac*, coracobrachialis; *Pect major*, pectoralis major; *L dorsi*, latissimus dorsi; *T major*, teres major. (From ref. 222, with permission.)

717

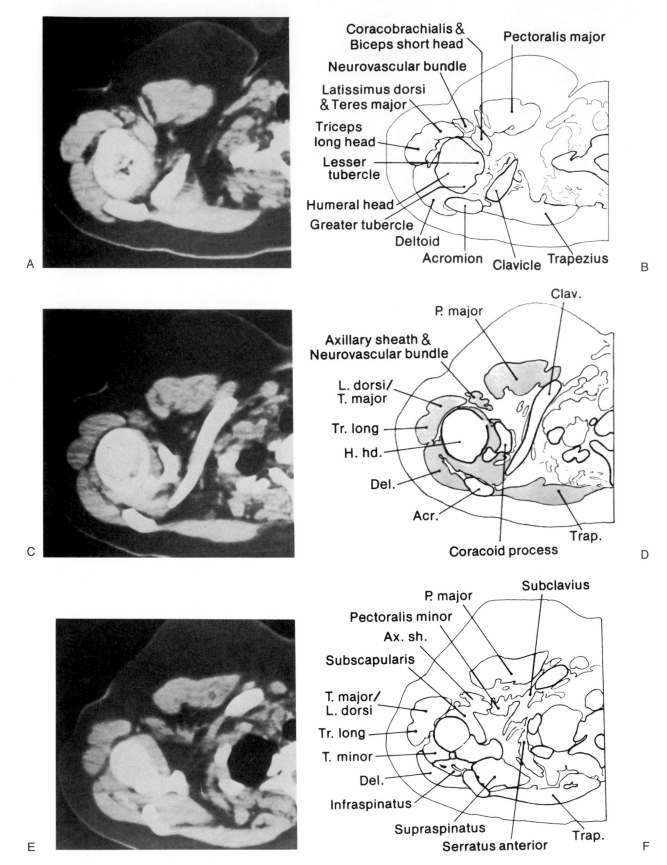

FIG. 10-92. CT anatomy of the axilla. Sequential CT images and corresponding line through the axilla, from above-downward, corresponding to the 8 planes identified in Fig. 10-91. **A,B:** Correspond to level 1, Fig. 10-19. **C,D:** Correspond to level 2, Fig. 10-91. **E,F:** Correspond to level 3, Fig. 10-91.

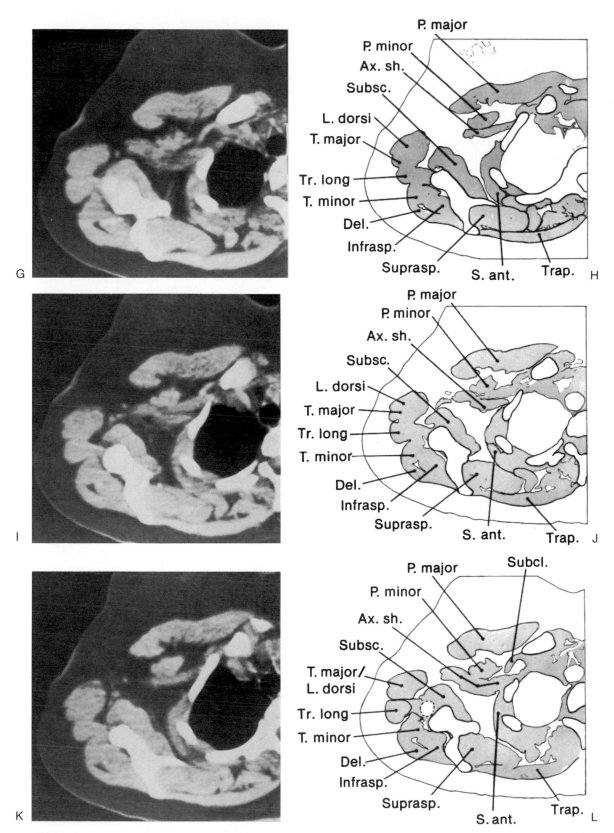

FIG. 10-92. *Continued.* **G,H:** Correspond to level 4, Fig. 10-91. **I,J:** Correspond to level 5, Fig. 10-91. **K,L:** Correspond to level 6, Fig. 10-91.

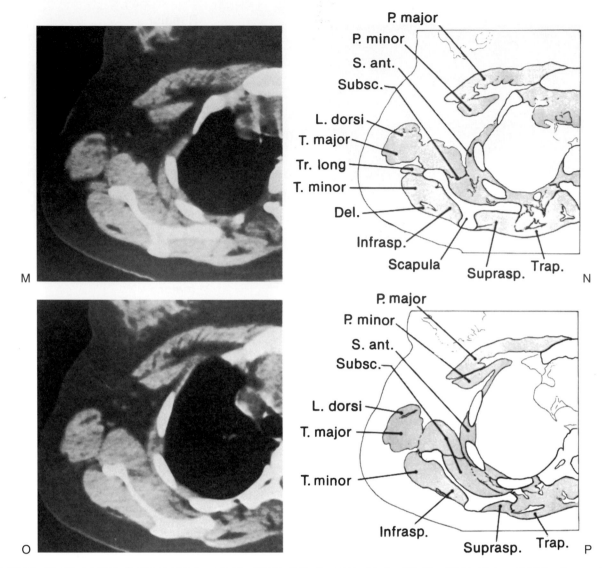

FIG. 10-92. *Continued.* **M,N:** Correspond to level 7, Fig. 10-91. **O,P:** Correspond to level 8, Fig. 10-91. (From ref. 222, with permission.)

wall, formed by the subscapularis, latissimus dorsi, and teres major muscles; (c) a medial wall, formed by the first through the fifth ribs, their intercostal spaces, and the serratus anterior muscle; (d) a lateral wall, formed by the humerus and the coracobrachial and biceps brachii muscles; (e) an apex formed by the clavicle and upper border of the scapula and outer border of the first rib; and finally, (f) a base formed by the anterior and posterior axillary folds, the serratus anterior muscle, and the chest wall. In the CT assessment of axillary structures it must be kept in mind that when patients are scanned with their arms up, the axilla is open laterally.

Important landmarks within the axilla include the axillary artery and vein and the cords of the brachial plexus, all of which are enclosed in a connective tissue sheath, the axillary sheath. Of these only the artery and vein can be identified as discrete structures on CT. The axillary vein courses cephalad and lies successively on the anterior, medial, and inferior sides of the axillary artery. With the arm raised, characteristi-

cally the vein tends to lie anterior to the artery throughout its course. In addition to these structures, numerous lymph node chains are also present within the axilla. Although variably described, these usually include: (a) nodes located between the inferolateral margin of the pectoralis minor muscle and the latissimus dorsi muscle; (b) nodes located behind the pectoralis muscle in the axilla; and (c) nodes located between the superomedial margin of the pectoralis muscle and the thoracic inlet (222,223). Additional nodes identifiable by CT include interpectoral lymph nodes, normally seen only as small dots in the interpectoral fat (224).

Knowledge of the axilla and remaining chest wall anatomy has proven clinically useful in assessing patients with breast cancer, especially following radiation and/or surgery (Figs. 10-93 and 10-94) (220,225–229). The appearance of the normal postoperative chest wall after mastectomy as well as the CT appearance of tumor recurrence have been well described by Shea et al. (227,228). As shown by these au-

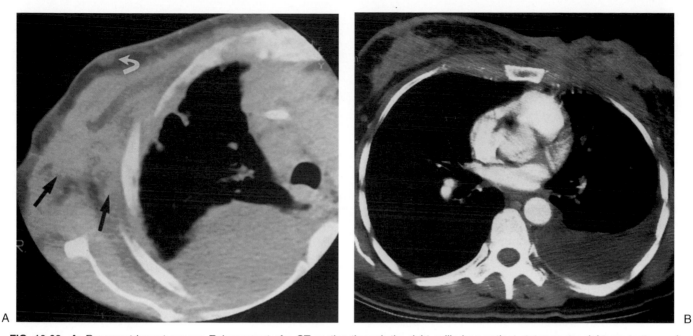

FIG. 10-93. A: Recurrent breast cancer. Enlargement of a CT section through the right axilla in a patient status-post a right mastectomy. A poorly marginated soft-tissue mass can be identified within the axilla (*arrows*) associated with subcutaneous nodules (*curved arrow*). In addition, nodular tumor implants can be associated with a large pleural effusion; mediastinal lymphadenopathy is present as well. **B:** Contrast-enhanced section in a different patient than **A** shows extensive soft tissue infiltration of the anterior chest wall. Predominantly involving the left breast, tumor can be seen to infiltrate the anterior chest wall muscles on the left, as well as the extending into the subcutaneous tissues of the right breast. Right sided effusion proved to be caused by metastatic disease.

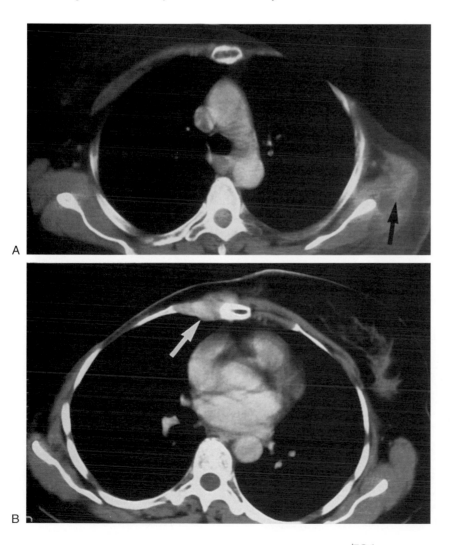

FIG. 10-94. Recurrent breast cancer: chest wall evaluation. **A:** CT scan in a patient status-post left mastectomy shows an ill-defined soft-tissue mass anterior to the scapula (*arrow*). Recurrent breast cancer was biopsy-proved. **B:** CT scan in another patient following a left mastectomy. A poorly defined soft-tissue mass can be identified just to the right of the sternum (*arrow*). Recurrent breast cancer was biopsy-proved.

thors, in a study of 19 patients suspected of tumor recurrence following mastectomy, CT allowed identification of tumor recurrence in all 15 cases in which recurrence was biopsy-proved. Similar results have been previously reported by Gouliamos et al. (220). In an evaluation of 64 patients following mastectomies for breast cancer, these authors found that 21 of these patients had axillary adenopathy, 11 of whom had metastatic disease subsequently verified histologically, while nine showed internal mammary node enlargement, and six had local chest wall recurrence. As shown by Lindfors et al., CT can detect foci of tumor recurrence unsuspected on physical examination (229). In their study of 42 patients with local and/or regional recurrence of breast cancer, of 33 patients with clinical evidence of chest wall recurrence, 16 patients (49%) had areas of disease identified by CT that were clinically unsuspected. Despite these reports in our experience, in the absence of unequivocal tumor mass or extensive adenopathy, differentiation between postoperative changes and tumor recurrence can be problematic. In these cases we advise either follow-up CT scans or biopsy, depending on the specific clinical setting.

In addition to breast cancer, a wide variety of diseases, both benign and neoplastic, may result in the development of axillary or chest wall adenopathy or masses (209,220,230–238). These generally are nonspecific and frequently require biopsy (Figs. 10-95–10-101). In exceptional cases, CT can provide specific tissue diagnoses. In patients with chest wall lipomas, for example, CT may play an invaluable role by excluding more significant pathology, especially in patients with previously documented malignancies (see Fig. 10-6) (13,234–236). As illustrated in Figure 10-97, however, care must be taken to insure that no solid or soft-tissue elements are present. In the face of these or evidence of growth, these lesions should be biopsied.

CT can also be of specific value in identifying patients with chest wall abscesses, especially those associated with

tuberculosis (see Fig. 10-32) (54–56,230,239). CT also has proven to be of diagnostic aid in detecting chest wall infiltration in patients with actinomycosis (see Fig. 10-99) (209,240–242). In select cases, MR may also be of value to precisely delineate the extent of chest wall involvement (Fig. 10-100).

As previously discussed, considerable interest has focused on the role of CT in detecting neoplastic infiltration of the chest wall, especially in patients with lung cancer (see Figs. 10-4 and 10-61) (142–146). The value of CT in detecting other infiltrating lesions, including mesothelioma (see Figs. 10-63–10-65) (160–166,243) and lymphoma (52,180,184, 186,187) have also been described. In general, CT is only effective in patients with relatively extensive tumor, as has been emphasized previously; CT is considerably less accurate in assessing patients with only minimal or subtle chest wall infiltration (Fig. 10-101).

In distinction, CT is especially sensitive in detecting chest wall collaterals that may develop in patients with central tumors causing superior vena caval obstruction (244–247). In general, these are easily distinguished from transient thoracic venous collaterals that may be seen normally in occasional patients following the bolus administration of i.v. contrast (248). It should be emphasized that as noted by Engel et al., identification of venous obstruction is contingent on recognizing both decreased opacification of central veins and enlarged collaterals: neither, in itself is sufficient for diagnosis of venous obstruction as collateral veins are frequently identifiable owing to flow dynamics in patients receiving rapid infusions of contrast media (249). As shown by Gosselin and Rubin, in select cases, CT angiography may augment conventional CT evaluation of venous obstruction by allowing identification of abnormal temporal relationships following contrast enhancement (250).

Finally, CT may play an important role in assessing patients with trauma, including iatrogenic causes such as in-

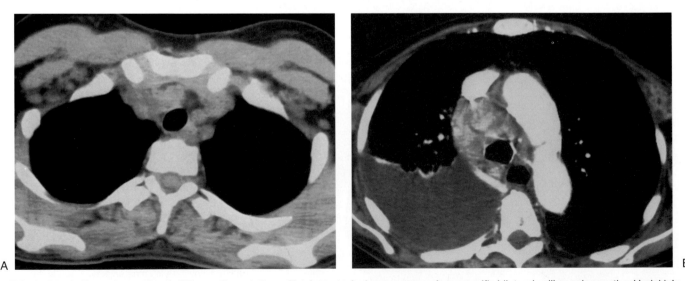

FIG. 10-95. Axillary adenopathy. **A:** CT scan through the axilla shows typical appearance of nonspecific bilateral axillary adenopathy. Hodgkin's disease was biospy-proved. **B:** Contrast-enhanced section in a different patient than **A** shows extensive mediastinal and left axillary nodes with evidence of marked heterogeneous contrast enhancement. This case proved to be due to non-Hodgkin's lymphoma.

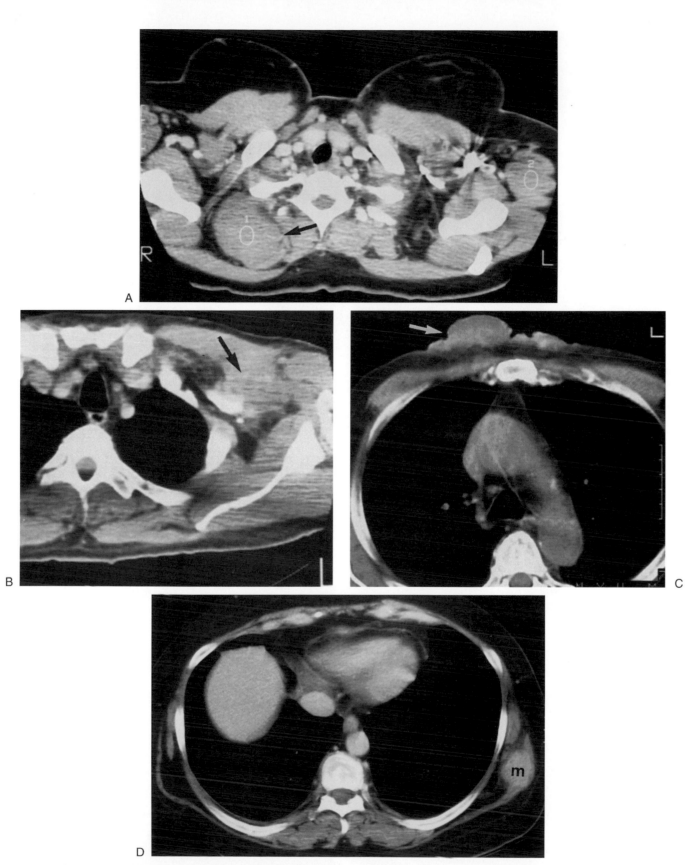

FIG. 10-96. Soft-tissue masses in the chest wall and axilla: CT appearances. **A:** CT scan at the level of the thoracic inlet shows a well-defined soft-tissue mass posteriorly (*arrow*). Benign desmoid tumor was biopsy-proved. **B:** CT scan through the left axilla shows enlarged axillary lymph nodes or masses associated with a loss of the normal facial planes within the axilla. Melanoma was biopsy-proved. **C:** Enlargement of a CT scan through the anterior midthorax shows a lobular exophytic soft-tissue mass involving the skin, sparing the immediate subcutaneous fat (*arrow*). Basal cell carcinoma was biopsy-proved. These cases have in common the presence of nonspecific soft tissue masses in either the chest wall or axilla. Although CT allows precise localization of these tumors in most cases, CT rarely obviates biopsy. **D:** Contrast-enhanced CT through the lung bases shows focal soft tissue mass in the left chest wall (*m*). Biopsy proved metastatic nonsmall cell lung cancer.

723

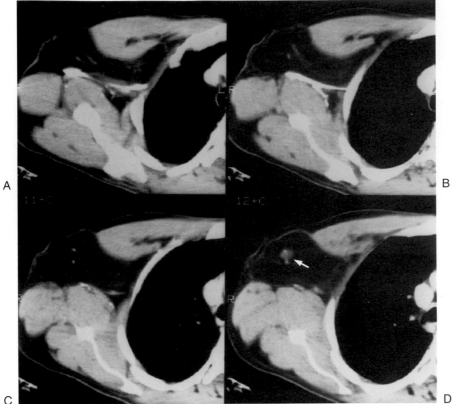

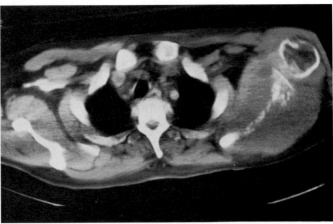

FIG. 10-97. Liposarcoma. **A–D:** Enlargements of sections through the right axilla and chest wall show a fat density mass causing separation of the chest wall muscles. Although most of this mass appears composed of well-differentiated fat, at least one soft tissue nodule can be identified within this lesion (*arrow* in **D**; compare with Fig. 10-6). Despite the benign appearance of this lesion, growth led to excisional biopsy, which documented well-differentiated liposarcoma.

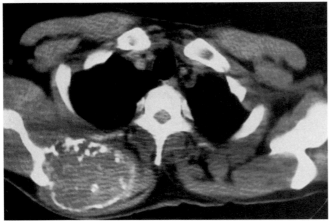

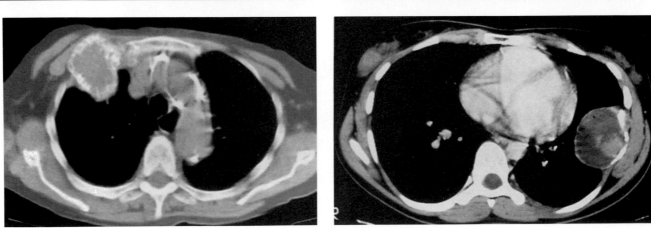

FIG. 10-98. Bony lesions of the thorax: CT scans in four different patient showing a variety of bony chest wall lesions. As with soft-tissue masses, the CT appearance of these lesions is rarely specific. **A:** Chondrosarcoma of the right scapula. **B:** Ewings sarcoma of the left scapula. **C:** Hemangioma arising within a rib. **D:** Aneurysmal bone cyst within a rib.

724

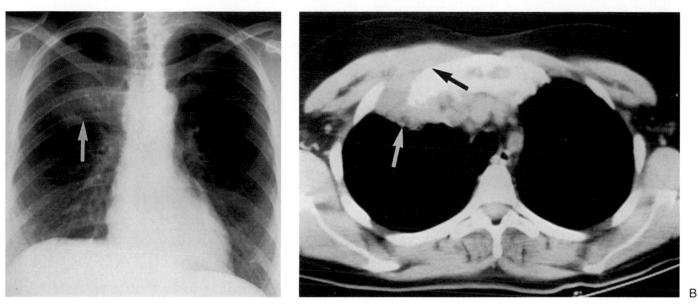

FIG. 10-99. Actinomycosis. **A:** Posteroanterior radiograph shows a poorly defined, nonspecific area of increased density on the right (*arrow*). **B:** CT scan through the sternum increased soft-tissue density (*arrows*) involving the chest wall, corresponding to the ill-defined density seen on the PA radiograph. Actinomycosis was biopsy-proved. (Case courtesy of Robert Maissel, M.D., Queens, NY.)

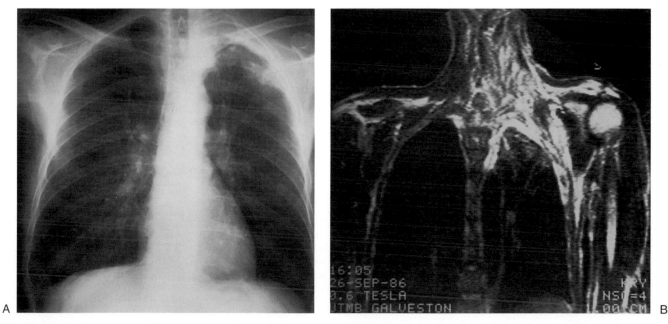

FIG. 10-100. Actinomycosis—MR evaluation. **A:** Posteroanterior chest radiograph shows evidence of asymmetric increased density in the left apex. **B:** Coronal T2-weighted image shows diffuse increased signal intensity within the chest wall and lower neck. Changes caused by documented actinomycosis. (Case courtesy of Sanford A. Rubin, M.D., Galveston, Texas.)

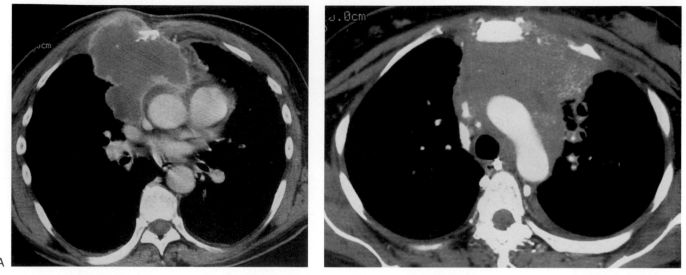

FIG. 10-101. Chest wall invasion—lymphoma. **A:** Contrast-enhanced section shows bulky necrotic anterior mediastinal mass with invasion of both the anterior chest wall and sternum. **B:** Contrast-enhanced section at the level of the aortic arch in a different patient than in **A,** shows homogeneous soft tissue mass in the anterior mediastinum. There is slight loss of fascial planes on the left side consistent with tumor infiltration. Although usually obvious, chest wall invasion caused by lymphoma may be exceedingly subtle. In these cases, MR may be of value owing to superior contrast resolution.

dwelling chest wall catheters, chest tubes, and pacemakers, as well as postsurgical changes (245,251–261). CT may detect unsuspected small pneumothoraces (see Fig. 10-8B) or hemothoraces, especially following rib fractures or abdominal trauma (262), and also allows identification of sternoclavicular dislocation and sternal fractures (see Fig. 10-86), including retrosternal hematomas, injuries involving the thoracic spine, scapular injuries, and pulmonary lacerations and contusions (Fig. 10-102) (259). As documented by Tocino et al., CT frequently detects small, incidental pneumothoraces following head trauma, a finding that can be important in patients requiring mechanical ventilation (253). Similar findings have been reported following abdominal trauma (252,262). As documented by Mirvis et al., CT may also be

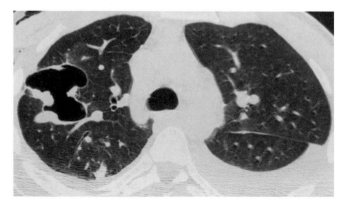

FIG. 10-102. Pulmonary contusion. Section through the upper lobes in a patient following a motor vehicle accident with extensive subcutaneous emphysema on the right. There is an unusual shaped airspace in the right lung extending to the pleural surface consistent with pulmonary laceration caused by accompanying rib fractures (*not shown*). Note the presence of bilateral effusions, larger on the left side, without evidence of a pneumothorax.

of value in assessing patients with multisystem trauma to identify possible thoracic sources of infection, including both lung abscesses and empyemas (257). CT also can play a role in evaluating late sequelae of trauma, including the finding of post-traumatic lung herniation (Fig. 10-103) (261,263).

MR Evaluation of the Pleura and Chest Wall

Compared with other usages, little has been written concerning the use of MR to evaluate pleural disease. Although some correlations have been found in both in vitro and in vivo between MR signal intensities and pleural fluid composition, MR has not yet proven to be a reliable means for differentiating among various etiologies of pleural effusions (15,264–267). In a study of 22 patients with pleural effusions from a variety of etiologies evaluated by MR, Davis et al. have shown apparently consistent quantitative and qualitative relationships between the MR signal characteristics of transudative versus exudative effusions (266). Using a triple spin-echo multislice sequence, these authors found that as indicated by relative signal intensity ratios, effective T2 relaxation times, and/or qualitative visual assessment, complex exudates (infected or malignant) were always brighter than simple exudates, which in turn were always brighter than transudates, regardless of which echo was evaluated (266). Furthermore, MR proved of additional value by clearly differentiating between free and loculated effusions, as well as identifying coexistent underlying lung disease. Despite these findings, however, no clear clinical role for the use of MR in evaluating pleural fluid collections has yet emerged. MR has also been used to evaluate patients with malignant mesotheliomas of both the pleura and pericardium

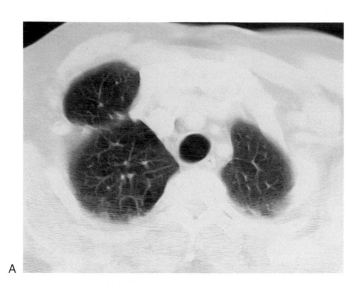

FIG. 10-103. Traumatic lung hernia **A:** Section through the right lung apex shows large anterior lung hernia. **B,C:** Corresponding sagittal and coronal views showing to better advantage the true extent of lung herniation.

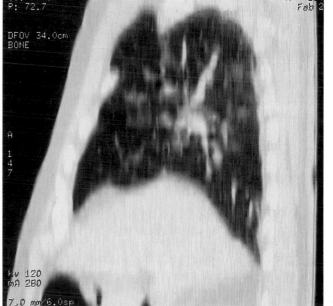

(see Fig. 10-68). Although MR clearly delineates the extent of tumor, and also allows differentiation between pleural tumor and fluid, the role for MR in assessing malignant effusions has yet to be firmly established (267,268).

If the role of MR is limited in the evaluation of pleural disease, a considerably more convincing argument can be made for the use of MR in the evaluation of chest wall pathology (see Figs. 10-63 and 10-100). The main advantages of MR for evaluating the chest wall are multiplanar imaging and increased contrast resolution. This may have implications for those patients for whom surgery is planned, in order to better delineate the disease extent.

To date, the most important application of MR has been in evaluating chest wall invasion in patients with lung cancer (see Fig. 10-63). As previously discussed, CT is of only limited use in assessing parietal pleural and chest wall invasion. By comparison, MR has proven significantly more ac-

curate in assessing tumor infiltration, especially in patients with superior sulcus tumors (148–152,269). In a study of 31 patients evaluated with both thin-section CT scans and MR. Heelan et al. showed that MR was 94% accurate in detecting tumor invasion into the chest wall as compared with 63% accuracy for CT (149). In these authors' opinion, the improved accuracy of MR appeared to be related primarily to improved visualization of anatomy obtained with coronal and sagittal images. In a study of 10 patients with superior sulcus tumors evaluated with MR. McLoud et al. also showed MR to be of value in detecting chest wall and mediastinal invasion. MR proved to be particularly sensitive for detecting tumor infiltration into the soft tissues of the chest wall caused by marked differences in the signal intensity of tumor as compared to both fat and muscle on T2-weighted sequences in particular. Unfortunately, in this same series, MR failed to identify subsequently confirmed rib destruction in five patients because of poor visualization of cortical bone (150). Recently, MR has also been proven more sensitive than CT in detecting chest wall involvement by malignant lymphoma (188,189). In a study of 28 patients examined with both CT and MR, Bergin et al. showed that while CT detected chest wall invasion in seven sites in four patients, MR showed chest wall lesions in 14 cites in seven patients (52).

MR has also been used to evaluate a variety of other chest wall masses, both benign and malignant, including lipomatous lesions and soft-tissue hemangiomas and even abnormalities involving the sternum and clavicles (270). Although MR has been shown to help identify chest wall infections, MR is less accurate in detecting osteomyelitis compared with CT (271).

Finally, a number of reports have confirmed that MR may be useful in the evaluation of both the brachial plexus and the supraclavicular region (272–274). The advantages of multiplanar imaging for these regions is apparent, especially as compared with CT. As shown by Rapoport et al., in an evaluation of 32 patients with symptoms referable to the brachial plexus, in six of the 12 cases of neoplasia in which CT scans were also obtained, MR showed more extensive disease in all (273). In the remaining six cases, findings were sufficiently characteristic on MR to obviate the need for additional imaging studies altogether. Additionally, MR provided definitive diagnoses in three cases of trauma. Similar findings have been reported by Castagno and Shuman (274).

THE DIAPHRAGM

Anatomy

The diaphragm is a musculotendinous layer, which in addition to its function in respiration, serves to separate the thorax and abdomen. It consists of a fibrous central tendon, divided, into middle, right, and left leaflets (Fig. 10-104), and muscle fibers, which inset into the central tendon, and arise from all parts of the inner aspect of the body wall (275). Based on the origin of its muscle fibers, the diaphragm is considered to consist of an anterior or sternocostal part and a posterior or lumbar part, which may be functionally distinct (276).

The sternocostal or anterior part of the diaphragm arises from the inner aspect of the sternum and xiphoid process and the seventh through twelfth ribs and costal cartilages, and inserts into the anterior portions of the middle, right, and left leaflets (Fig. 10-105). The xiphoid process and costal cartilages form an inverted V- or U-shaped arch when viewed from the front, and the anterior diaphragm assumes a similar shape (277–279).

The posterior diaphragm is more properly referred to as the lumbar part of the diaphragm (280,281). It is made up of the right and left diaphragmatic crura (see Fig. 10-104), and fibers arising from the right and left medial and lateral arcuate ligaments (282). The crura originate from the anterolateral surfaces of the bodies of the first three lumbar vertebrae on the right, and the first two lumbar vertebrae on the left. The medial and lateral arcuate ligaments represent thickenings of the thoracolumbar fascia overlying the anterior surfaces of the psoas and quadratus lumborum muscles (280,281). The medial arcuate ligament arises from the lateral margin of the L1 vertebral body and inserts on the transverse process of L1. The lateral arcuate ligament arises from the transverse process of the L1 vertebral body and inserts on the 12th rib (see Fig. 10-104; Fig. 10-106). Muscle fibers arising from both the crura and arcuate ligaments arch forward to insert into the posterior aspects of the middle, right, and left leaflets.

CT Appearances

Near its dome, the diaphragm lies in or near the plane of scan and is impossible to identify as a specific structure

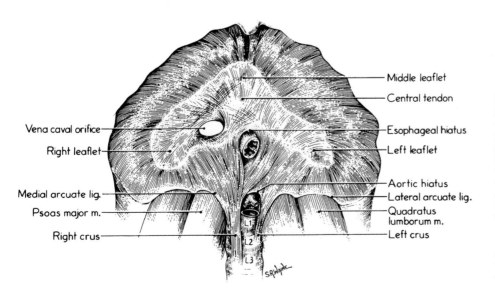

FIG. 10-104. Schematic diagram of the lumbar portion of the diaphragm, as viewed from below. This portion is composed of the crura, which arise from the anterolateral surfaces of the first three lumbar vertebrae on the right and the first two lumbar vertebrae on the left, respectively, and fibers that arise from the medial and lateral arcuate ligaments. These ligaments represent thickenings of the thoracolumbar fascia overlying the anterior surface of the psoas and quadratus muscles. Note that as drawn, no clear line of demarcation separates the crura from the remainder of the posterior portions of the diaphragm.

Labels in figure:
Middle leaflet
Central tendon
Vena caval orifice
Right leaflet
Esophageal hiatus
Left leaflet
Medial arcuate lig.
Psoas major m.
Right crus
Aortic hiatus
Lateral arcuate lig.
Quadratus lumborum m.
Left crus

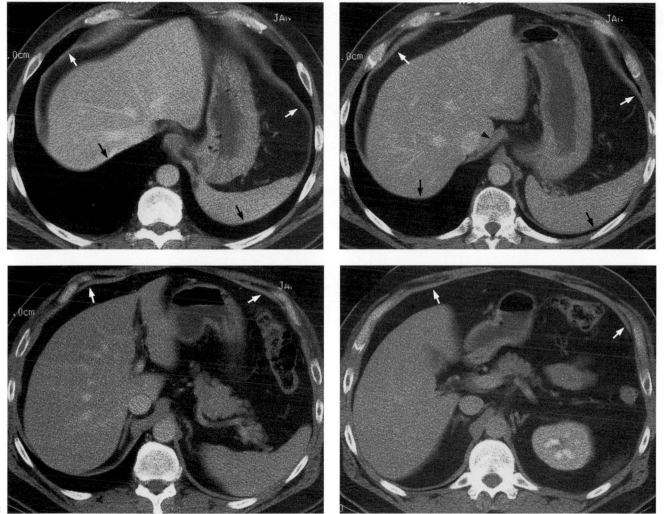

FIG. 10-105. Normal anatomy. **A–D:** Sequential 7 mm sections through the diaphragm beginning at the level of the esophageal hiatus and proceeding downwards. The hemidiaphragms can be visualized as separate structures only when marginated centrally by peritoneal or retroperitoneal fat (*white arrows* in **A–D**), or peripherally by air within the lungs, or by extraperitoneal fat . Visualization is lost when the diaphragms abut a structure of similar density (for example, the liver or spleen) (*Straight black arrows* in **A** and **B**). The position of the diaphragm can still be inferred, however, from knowledge of characteristic anatomic relationships. At all levels, the lung and pleura lie adjacent and peripheral to the diaphragm; abdominal viscera, fat, and retroperitoneal structures lie adjacent and central to the hemidiaphragms. Note posteriorly the appearance of a normal esophageal hiatus defined by the medial margins of the crura, bilaterally (*arrowheads* in **B**).

because of volume averaging (see Fig. 10-105). Furthermore, visualization of the normal diaphragm, measuring only a few millimeters in thickness, is difficult when the diaphragm abuts structures of similar density, such as the liver and spleen. The diaphragm can be visualized as a separate structure only when it is imaged at an angle to its surface, its outer aspect is marginated by air in the lungs or extraperitoneal fat, and its inner aspect is marginated by intraperitoneal or retroperitoneal fat or when there is an alteration in the density of adjacent viscera, as may occur in patients with marked fatty infiltration of the liver (Fig. 10-107).

Anterior Diaphragm

The anterior diaphragm is visible in 87% of patients (279) with the left side being seen more often than the right. In a study of 102 normal adults, Patterson and Teates could identify portions of the left anterior diaphragm in 82 individuals, while the right anterior diaphragm was visible in only 13 (277). The anterior diaphragm is variable in appearance, but characteristically assumes one of three appearances, depending on the cephalocaudal relationship between the xiphoid and the central tendon of the diaphragm (279). In those individuals in whom the middle leaflet lies superior to the xiphoid, the anterior diaphragm appears as a smooth or slightly undulating line that is continuous across the midline with the lateral diaphragmatic attachments (Fig. 10-108). This appearance is present in nearly 50% of individuals. In distinction, if the apex of the middle leaflet of the central tendon lies inferior to the xiphoid, the anterior muscle fibers will be oriented opposite to muscle fibers in the lateral portion of the diaphragm; this results in apparent discontinuity of the

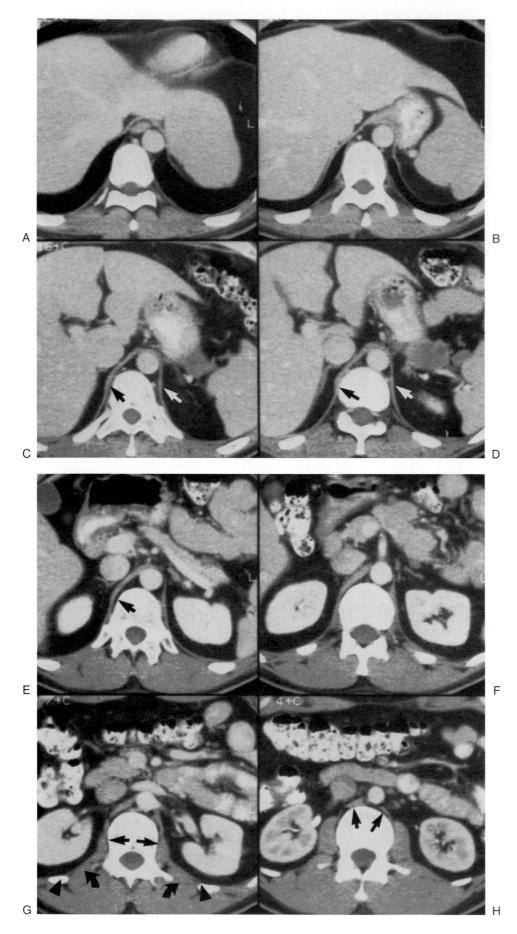

FIG. 10-106. Normal anatomy. **A–H:** Sequential 10-mm thick sections from the level of the esophageal hiatus to the inferior portions of the crura. The medial and lateral aruate ligaments lie anterior to the uppermost portions of the psoas (*arrows* in **G**) and quadratus muscles (*curved arrows* in **G**). The lateral arcuate ligaments insert into the 12th rib (*arrowheads* in **G**). Note that the crura at all levels bilaterally merge imperceptibly with the remainder of the posterior portions of the diaphragms (*arrows* in **C–E**), and that the crura themselves are thin, smooth structures. In its inferiormost extent, the crura are all that remain of the diaphragm, and should not be mistaken for adenopathy (*arrows* in **H**).

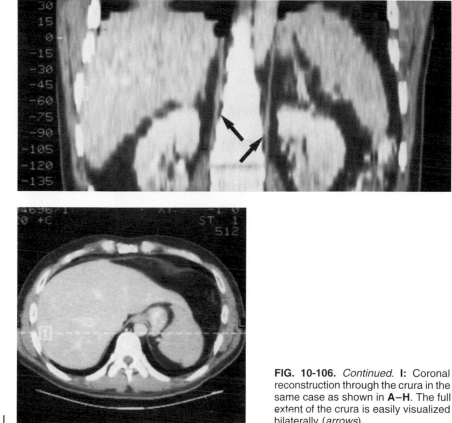

FIG. 10-106. *Continued.* I: Coronal reconstruction through the crura in the same case as shown in **A−H**. The full extent of the crura is easily visualized bilaterally (*arrows*).

costal diaphragm, with the lateral portion of the diaphragm diverging and opening anteriorly toward the sternum. This appearance occurs in approximately 30% of individuals. Lastly, if the dome of the central tendon and the xiphoid are at the same level, the anterior muscle fibers lie almost en-

tirely within the scan plane; as a consequence, these appear as broad, poorly defined bands.

Lateral and Posterior Diaphragm

Lateral and posterior to its dome, the position of the diaphragm can usually be inferred from a knowledge of characteristic anatomic relationships between the diaphragm and surrounding structures. Specifically, below the level of the dome of the diaphragm, the lungs and pleura lie peripheral to the diaphragm whereas the abdominal viscera, retroperitoneal spaces, and fat lie central to the diaphragm. However, as pointed out in Figure 10-104, only those portions of the hemidiaphragms outlined centrally by fat will be identifiable as discrete lines. When the diaphragm abuts structures of similar density, such as the liver or spleen, the line of the diaphragm is invisible.

Segments of the posteromedial diaphragm on either side are often outlined by abdominal fat, allowing them to be demonstrated as discrete structures. On the right, fat outlining the medial hemidiaphragm defines the most cephalad extent of the posterior pararenal space. Naidich and colleagues (280) identified fat in this region in 62 (82%) of 75 cases. On the left, the visibility of this fat layer is less consistent, probably owing to variations in the size and shape of the spleen. Retroperitoneal fat along the posterior border of the right lobe of the liver serves as a marker identifying the

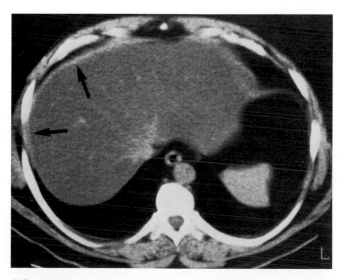

FIG. 10-107. Normal anatomy. CT section through the base of the lungs shows that the right hemidiaphragm can be visualized almost along its entire course owing to marked fatty infiltration of the liver (*arrows*).

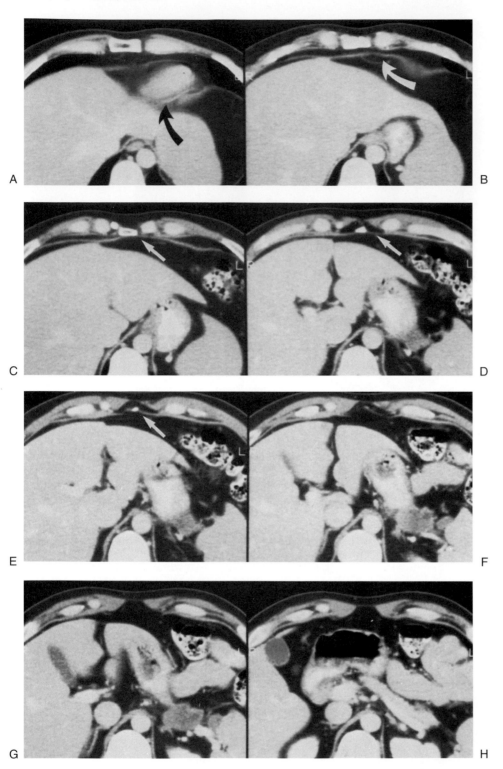

FIG. 10-108. The costal diaphragm: normal anatomy. **A–H:** Enlargements of sequential 10-mm thick sections through the costal diaphragm. This portion of the diaphragm arises from the posterior surfaces of the lower six costal cartilages and inserts into the anterolateral border of the central tendon. Additionally, fibers attach the middle leaflet to the xiphoid (*arrows* in **C–E**). Note the close association between the inferior portion of the pericardium and the central tendon (*curved arrow* in **A**). Most commonly, the costal portion of the diaphragm appears as a continuous, slightly undulating line that is continuous across the midline with the lateral diaphragmatic attachments (*curved arrow* in **B**). This results when the middle leaflet lies superior to the xiphoid.

right coronary ligament. As will be discussed, identification of the right coronary ligament may be of particular value when attempting to differentiate intraperitoneal from pleural fluid.

On the left side, the anatomy appears less constant, particularly at the level of the esophageal hiatus. This is probably caused by variability in the shape and position of the spleen.

Analogous to what is seen on the right, retroperitoneal fat within the posterior pararenal space typically marginates the anteromedial aspect of the left hemidiaphragm (see Figs. 10-105 and 10-107). Fat in this same space marginates the spleen, accounting for the so-called "bare area" of the spleen (see Fig. 10-105) (283), Inferiorly, as on the right, a clear distinction between fat in the left perirenal space and the left posterior pararenal space generally is not possible. As will be discussed later, differentiation between retroperitoneal fat and peritoneal fat around the spleen is also difficult unless fluid is present in one or the other space.

The amount of intraabdominal and retroperitoneal fat that is present varies from patient to patient. In some cases, an unusual quantity of fat may be present anteriorly, under the diaphragm, allowing the diaphragm to be clearly defined.

Diaphragmatic Crura

The crura ascend anterior to the spine, on each side of the aorta, and pass medially and anteriorly, joining the muscular diaphragm anterior to the aorta to form the aortic hiatus (see Fig. 10-106). The right crus, which is larger and longer than the left, arises from the first three lumbar vertebrae; the left crus arises from the first two lumbar segments (281,284). The aortic hiatus and the anterior crura are invariably demonstrated by CT (275,280,281,284). CT scans at caudal levels show the individual crura as discrete oval or round structures positioned posterolateral to the aorta and anterior to the vertebral column. The larger and longer right crus has a greater cross-sectional diameter than the left and is visible at lower levels (see Fig. 10-106). Variations in the cross-sectional appearance of the crura have been described (275,280, 281,284).

The diaphragmatic crura can be mistaken for enlarged lymph nodes or masses because of their rounded appearance; paraaortic lymph nodes can indeed be seen in a similar position. However, on contiguous CT scans, the crura merge gradually with the diaphragm at more cephalad levels, allowing them to be correctly identified. The diameter of the crura vary with lung volume, increasing in thickness at full inspiration, as compared with expiration (285–287).

Although the crura can be identified as discrete structures anterior to the aorta, laterally they merge with fibers from the medial arcuate ligaments. A smooth transition between the crura and the remainder of the lumbar portion of the diaphragm (that is, fibers arising from the medial arcuate ligaments) is seen in as many as 90% of individuals (280) (see Figs. 10-104 and 10-106). Less commonly, there is an abrupt transition, and on occasion, actual separation between the various components of the lumbar diaphragms can be seen.

The most cephalad section at which the crura can be identified is at the level of the esophageal hiatus (see Figs. 10-105 and 10-106). Typically, at this level the anteromedial margin of the right crus can be identified because of retroperitoneal fat within the posterior pararenal space (see Fig. 10-105). Fat within this space has been identified in approximately 80% of normal subjects (280). More inferiorly, the right adrenal gland can be recognized within the perirenal space (see Fig. 10-105). At this level, differentiation between perirenal fat and posterior pararenal fat can rarely be made.

Inferiorly, the lumbar portion of the diaphragm extends to the arcuate ligament. As previously noted, the arcuate

ligaments represent thickenings of the thoracolumbar fascia overlying the anterior surfaces of the psoas major and quadratus lumborum muscles. In cross-section, these muscles will lie just posterior and medial to the arcuate ligaments. Characteristically, the crura are the only portions of the diaphragm visible below the level of the arcuate ligaments (Fig. 10-4). The psoas and quadratus muscles can also be defined, but they are no longer in contact with the diaphragm.

Normal Variants

A number of normal variants have been described (280,285–289). The significance of these lies primarily in their not being confused with significant pathology.

Nodularity

In some patients, and in some locations, the diaphragm may assume a nodular configuration, mimicking the appearance of a tumor (Fig. 10-109). Presumably, this appearance is caused by infoldings or invaginations of contracted and foreshortened muscle bundles. In a series of 150 consecutive scans, a nodular appearance could be identified on the left in nearly 25% of cases, involving the crura in approximately 30% of cases, and on the right were identified in only 5% of cases (289). The lower frequency of a nodular appearance on the right is presumably caused by pressure exerted on the diaphragm by the adjacent liver (289). Importantly, these changes appear to be related to the patients' age; as noted by Rosen et al. (289), diaphragmatic pseudotumors were visible in 60% of patients older than 70 years, in 27% of patients between 50 and 69 years of age, and in only 5% of those under 50 years.

Caskey et al. have also studied age-related changes in the appearance of the hemidiaphragms (288). In a study of 120 individuals evaluated by CT, these authors failed to note any appreciable change in the thickness of the diaphragm with age, even when the appearance was correlated with other indicators of physical condition, including skeletal muscle status, obesity, pulmonary emphysema, and the presence of an esophageal hiatal hernia. In agreement with Rosen et al. (289), however, these authors also noted a generalized increase in nodularity and irregularity, especially of the left hemidiaphragm, in older patients.

Silverman et al., have noted nodular areas abutting the lateral diaphragmatic surfaces in as many as 5% of routine abdominal CT studies and have attributed these to inferolateral extensions of the lateral arcuate ligaments reflecting over the quatrus lumborum muscles to fuse with the diaphragm (282).

Changes with Respiration

As first described by Rosen et al., variations in the degree of inspiration may have a profound effect on the cross-sectional appearance of the diaphragm (289). Specifically on

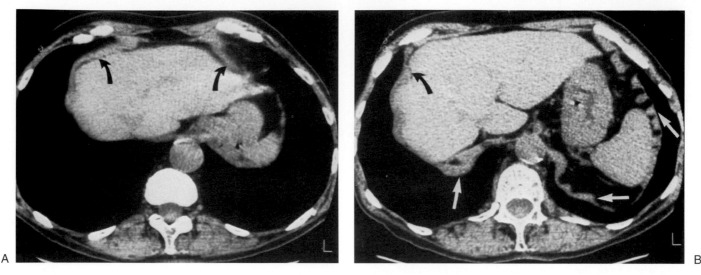

FIG. 10-109. Diaphragmatic pseudotumors. **A,B:** Ten-mm thick CT sections through the costal and lumbar portions of the diaphragm, respectively. Note the marked lobularity of the diaphragmatic surfaces both anteriorly (*curved arrows* in **A** and **B**), and posterolaterally (*arrows* in **B**). This appearance is caused by infoldings of contracted and foreshortened muscle fibers resulting from a deep inspiratory effort. This phenomenon appears at least in part to be age-related.

scans obtained in deep inspiration, nodularity of the diaphragm is accentuated (see Fig. 10-109) (285–287,289) these changes are reversible when expiratory scans are obtained. The diameter of the crura also vary with lung volume, increasing at full inspiration. Also, nodularity is accentuated on the left side when scans are obtained with patients in the right lateral decubitus position.

Retrocrural Air

Occasionally, air within the most medial and inferior portions of the lower lobes, in apparent isolation from the remainder of the lung, can be seen on CT. This normal variant

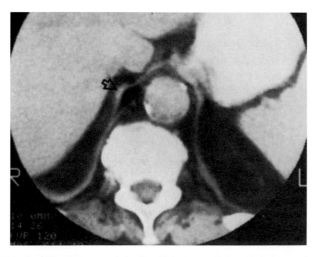

FIG. 10-110. Retrocrural air. Air within the medial and inferior portion of the right lower lobe can be identified; it is marginated anteriorly by the medial portion of the right hemidiaphragm (*arrow*) and posteriorly by visceral and parietal pleura.

has been described by Silverman et al. as "retrocrural air" (290). As shown in Figure 10-110, this represents air within lung posterior to the medial aspect of the right hemidiaphragm, marginated posteriorly by visceral and parietal pleura. This finding is visible in approximately 1% of normal subjects. The only significance of this is that it is a normal variant not to be confused with true retrocrural (i.e., retroperitoneal and/or posterior mediastinal) air.

Diaphragmatic Defects

The most common pathways that allow communication between the abdomen and thorax are the aortic and esophageal hiatuses (see Figs. 2-85 and 2-105–2-107). Another potential pathway for spread of disease between the abdomen and thorax is focal defects in the hemidiaphragms. Posteriorly, the most common of these defects is caused by persistence of the embryonic pleuroperitoneal canal (so-called Bochdalek's hernia) (Fig. 10-111). Although it has been reported that these defects occur in up to 90% of cases on the left side, it has, in fact, been shown that right-sided defects are also common (see Fig. 10-111) (291). In an evaluation of 940 patients studied with CT, Gale identified 60 Bochdalek's hernias in 52 patients for a surprisingly high prevalence of 6% (292). As surprising, left-sided hernias proved only twice as common as right-sided hernias. Herniation of abdominal structures through this defect may occur, and may simulate intrathoracic masses (291–294). Herniation is presumably facilitated by lower intrathoracic pressure, as opposed to intraabdominal pressure on the undersurface of the diaphragms, forcing them up into the thorax.

Recently, the precise nature of these posterior defects has been questioned. In an attempt to correlate the appearance

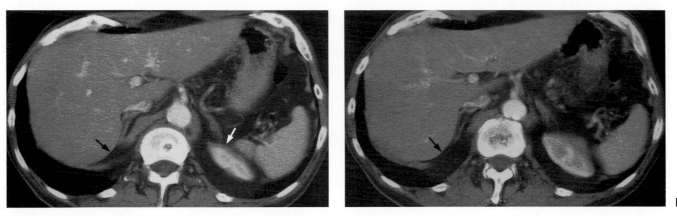

FIG. 10-111. Bochdalek hernia. **A,B:** Sequential contrast-enhanced sections show typical appearance of intrathoracic herniation of the left kidney through a defect in the left hemidiaphragm, a Bochdalek hernia. Note that a similar defect is present on the right side as well through which some retroperitoneal fat has herniated (*arrows* in **A** and **B**). Bilateral posterior diaphragmatic defects are not unusual incidental findings on CT.

of the diaphragms with age, Caskey et al., described three types of diaphragmatic defects: type 1, in which a localized defect can be identified in the thickness of the diaphragm without loss of diaphragmatic continuity; type 2, in which an apparent defect can be identified where muscle fibers appear to separate into layers parallel to the diaphragmatic contour; and type 3, any defect in which a portion of the diaphragm appears absent, typically associated with protrusion of omental fat (288). As shown by these authors, the appearance of diaphragmatic defects appears related to both age and the presence of pulmonary emphysema. In a review of 120 scans, these authors found that none of their patients in their 20s or 30s demonstrated defects of any type, whereas 56% of patients in their 60s and 70s proved to have defects. A significant association between diaphragmatic defects and pulmonary emphysema was also noted, especially in men. Based on these findings, these authors have suggested that many of the diaphragmatic defects identified, especially posteriorly in older patients, represent acquired defects occurring in areas of structural weakness, perhaps themselves embryologic in origin.

Regardless of their origin, congenital diaphragmatic defects are easily identified with CT (see Fig. 10-111) (291–294). Commonly identified on plain chest radiographs as areas of eventration, these defects characteristically are associated with protrusion of omental or even retroperitoneal fat. Care must be taken not to confuse these focal protrusions of intraperitoneal fat with intrapulmonary masses, especially when images are viewed sequentially through the lower thorax .

Herniation of intraabdominal fat and/or viscera may also occur in the anterior portions (costal portions) of the diaphragms, resulting in a paracardiac mass (so-called Morgagni's hernia) (see Fig. 2-85) (295). CT is efficacious, first, in defining such masses as fatty, and second, in demonstrating continuity between this fat and abdominal fat. The actual

point of the diaphragmatic defect may be definable using parasagittal reconstructions.

Diaphragmatic Rupture

In addition to congenital abnormalities, defects in the diaphragm may also be the result of both blunt and penetrating trauma. Diaphragmatic rupture usually occurs on the left side (in up to 95% of patients) and may go undiagnosed for years following both blunt and penetrating injuries (296–298). As pointed out by Heiberg et al., radiologic diagnosis of diaphragmatic rupture may be difficult (299) as this entity is frequently misdiagnosed as an elevated hemidiaphragm, left lower lobe atelectasis, left pleural effusion, or left subphrenic fluid collection and/or abscess. As documented by Lee et al., in a study of 50 patients with acute diaphragmatic rupture caused by blunt injury, nearly all had evidence of other associated thoracic, abdominal and/or pelvic injuries (300). Unfortunately, despite the long time interval, chronic traumatic diaphragmatic rupture may eventuate in patients presenting with symptoms of acute intestinal obstruction secondary to infarction and/or strangulation of herniated bowel or viscera (301,302).

CT findings in patients with diaphragmatic rupture have been extensively reported (see Fig. 10-111; Figs. 10-112–10-115) (299,303–310). CT can identify discontinuities in the course of the diaphragm, especially along the posterolateral aspect, an appearance, which, when sufficiently severe, may aptly be described as the "absent diaphragm sign" (see Fig. 10-113). Superiorly, near the dome of the diaphragm, CT identification of diaphragmatic discontinuity is considerably more difficult. In these cases, recognition of diaphragmatic rupture usually necessitates identification of intrathoracic herniation of fat or abdominal contents. As noted by Shakelton et al., identification in these cases is

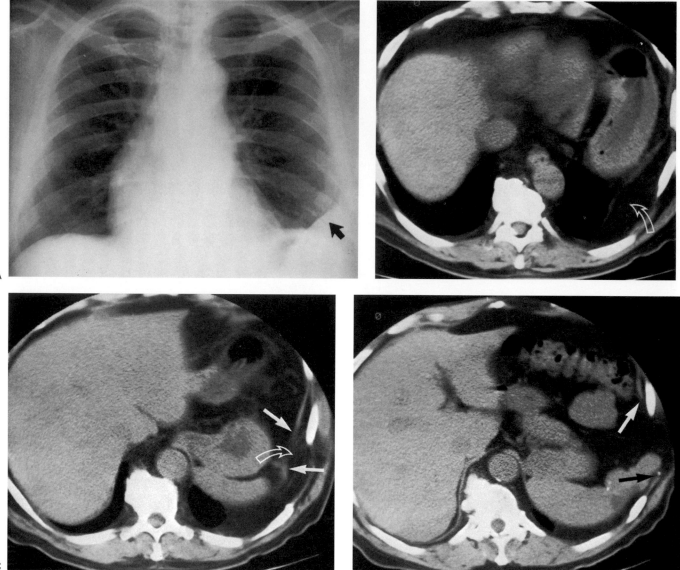

FIG. 10-112. Traumatic diaphragmatic rupture. **A:** Posteroanterior radiograph shows ill-defined density at the left costophrenic angle (*arrow*). **B–D:** Sequential 10-mm thick CT sections through the left hemidiaphragm. The left hemidiaphragm is discontinuous: there is wide separation of the diaphragmatic margins (*arrows* in **C** and **D**) through which considerable intraabdominal fat has herniated (*curved arrows* in **B** and **C**).

simplified when herniated organs manifest a "waist" or collar sign (310). Rarely, diaphragmatic rupture will be accompanied by rupture of the adjacent pericardium resulting in herniation of abdominal contents into the pericardial sac (see Fig. 10-115).

Unfortunately, it is well established that CT is of only limited use in the diagnosis of diaphragmatic rupture. As reported by Shapiro et al., in an evaluation of 12 patients with traumatic diaphragmatic rupture, only five (42%) CT studies were positive (306). Similar findings have been reported by Murray et al. who demonstrated a sensitivity of only 61% and a specificity of 87% for the CT diagnosis of diaphragmatic rupture (309). Reliance on axial imaging is the major limitation of CT; in our experience, the use of

multiplanar reconstructions around the diaphragm have proved of a only marginal value, likely caused by poor spatial resolution and the presence of frequent artifacts that themselves may mimic diaphragmatic disruption. Some have suggested that better results would be obtained using MR (311) in select cases, however, to date this application has not received widespread clinical acceptance.

Peridiaphragmatic Fluid Collections

Accurate localization of peridiaphragmatic fluid requires detailed knowledge of normal cross-sectional anatomy through the lung bases and upper abdomen. The key to accurate localization of peridiaphragmatic fluid is identification

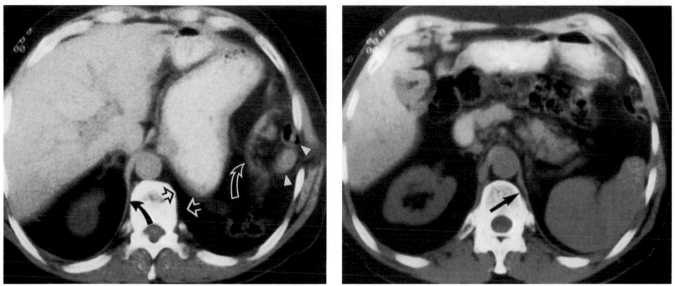

A   B

FIG. 10-113. Traumatic diaphragmatic rupture: the absent diaphragm sign. **A,B:** Ten-mm thick CT sections from above-downward through the left hemidiaphragm. Note that in **A**, in the location in which the left hemidiaphragm is usually seen, no distinct line is identifiable (*arrows* in **A**) as compared to the normal appearance of the right hemidiaphragm (*black curved arrow* in **A**). A portion of the left hemidiaphragm at this level is identifiable more medially (*open curved arrow* in **A**). There has been some herniation of both fat and a portion of colon into the lower left hemithorax (*arrowheads*). Note that inferiorly, the left hemidiaphragm is easily recognized in its usual position (*arrow* in **B**). This apparent loss of the diaphragm has proven to be an especially valuable sign for diagnosing traumatic diaphragmatic rupture.

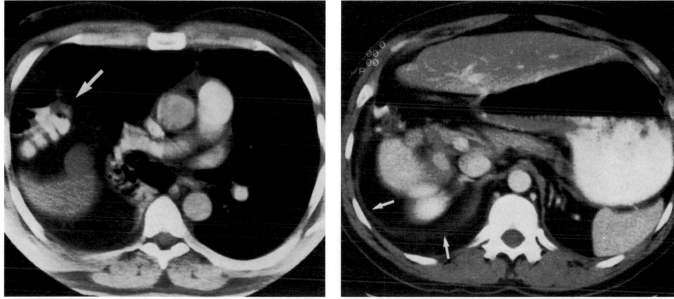

A   B

FIG. 10-114. Right-sided traumatic diaphragmatic rupture. **A–C:** 10-mm thick CT sections through the right upper quadrant from above-downward show characteristic appearance of herniation of bowel and fat into the right hemithorax (*arrow* in **A**) secondary to traumatic rupture of the right hemidiaphragm. The right hemidiaphragm itself can be identified in **B** (*arrows*), appearing somewhat thickened and displaced medially. Diaphragmatic discontinuity can be identified in **C** (*arrows*). (*continues*)

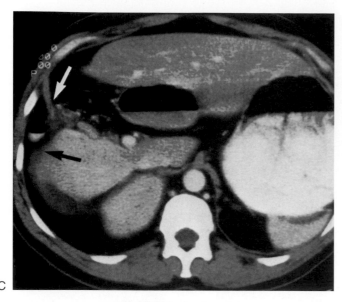

C

FIG. 10-114. *Continued.*

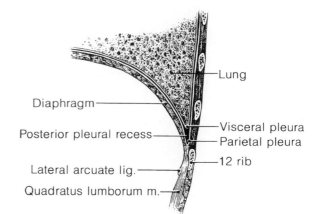

FIG. 10-116. Schematic diagram of a sagittal section through the lateral arcuate ligament. The lung is invested with visceral pleura. Below the inferior edge of the lung there is a potential space, the posterior pleural recess, which is defined anteriorly and posteriorly by layers of parietal pleura. The diaphragm always lies central to the lung and pleura when seen in cross-section.

of the hemidiaphragms, because these represent the interface between the thorax and the abdomen (312). In principle, at all levels the lungs and pleura lie adjacent and peripheral to the diaphragm while the abdominal viscera, fat, and intraperitoneal spaces lie adjacent and central to the diaphragm. Precise anatomic localization of the diaphragm depends on awareness of these anatomic relationships.

As shown in Figure 10-116, a schematic drawing of a sagittal section through the diaphragm at the level of the lateral arcuate ligament and upper portion of the quadratus muscle, the lungs and pleura always lie peripheral to the diaphragm. The lung is invested with visceral pleura. Just below the most inferior portion of the lung there is a

space—generally a potential space—referred to as the posterior pleural recess. This space is defined anteriorly and posteriorly by layers of parietal pleura. Fibers of the lumbar portion of the diaphragm extend below the posterior pleural recess, ending at the lateral arcuate ligament at the level of the 12th rib.

Identification of the posterior pleural recesses is critical when evaluating peridiaphragmatic fluid collections, as this space represents the most inferior, dependent recess of the pleural space: it is this space that will be filled first by free pleural fluid (312). Although the posterior pleural recess is usually a potential space, on occasion it can be identified with CT in normal individuals (Fig. 10-117).

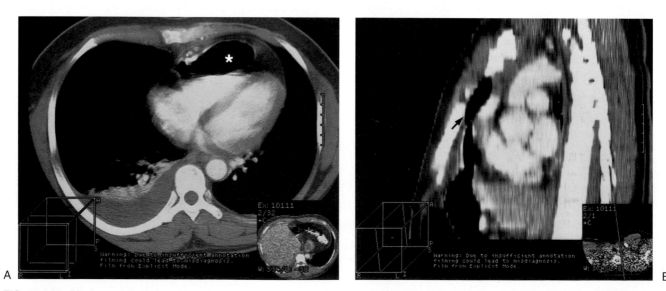

A   B

FIG. 10-115. Diaphragmatic and pericardial rupture. **A:** Contrast-enhanced section shows apparent air collection in front of the right ventricle (*asterisk*). Note presence of moderate right effusion as well. **B:** Sagittal reconstruction shows that the air in front of the ventricle in fact represents bowel that has herniated through both the diaphragm and pericardium (*arrow*).

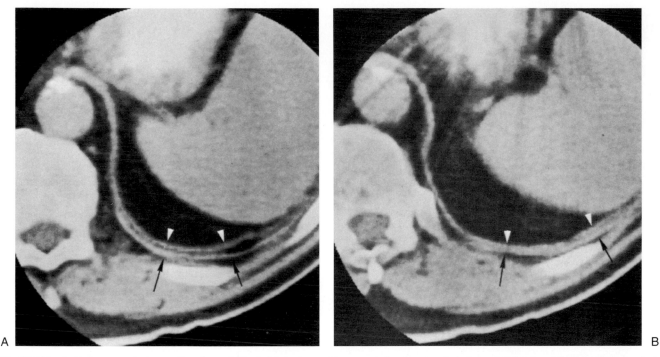

FIG. 10-117. A: Enlargement of a section through the left lung base. The lung is bordered anteriorly by the left hemidiaphragm and anterior parietal and visceral pleura (*arrowheads*). Posteriorly, the lung is bordered by posterior visceral and parietal pleura (*arrows*). **B:** Magnification of a section through the posterior pleural recess, 5 mm below **A**. Visceral pleura is no longer present at this level. This space is bordered anteriorly by the left hemidiaphragm and anterior parietal pleura, which are indistinguishable (*arrowheads*). Posteriorly, this space is defined by the posterior parietal pleura (*arrows*).

As illustrated in Figure 10-118, peridiaphragmatic fluid can be localized to one of four potential spaces: the pleural cavity, the lung, the peritoneum, or the retroperitoneum.

Four main criteria have been proposed to differentiate pleural from peritoneal fluid (312–315):

1. The "diaphragm sign." As already discussed, direct visualization of the diaphragm itself allows accurate localization of peridiaphragmatic fluid collections, as fluid peripheral to the diaphragm is intrathoracic while fluid central to the diaphragm is intraabdominal (Fig. 10-119).
2. The "displaced crura sign" results from the interposition

of pleural fluid between the crus and adjacent vertebra, with resultant anterior displacement of the crus.

3. The "interface sign," first described by Teplick et al., is based on the nature of the interface between the liver and adjacent fluid (314). This interface is hazy in the case of pleural fluid, but distinct in the case of ascites.

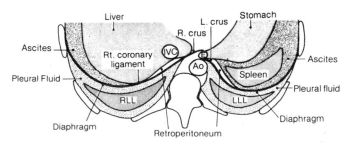

FIG. 10-118. Schematic drawing of the potential spaces in which peridiaphragmatic fluid may collect. Accurate identification of the diaphragm is critical. Fluid within the pleural spaces or lung lies peripheral to the hemidiaphragms; intraperitoneal or retroperitoneal fluid lies central to the hemidiaphragms. On the right side intraperitoneal fluid is restricted medially at the level of the right coronary ligament. *Ao*, aorta; *E*, esophagus; *IVC*, inferior vena cava; *LLL*, left lower lobe; *RLL*, right lower lobe.

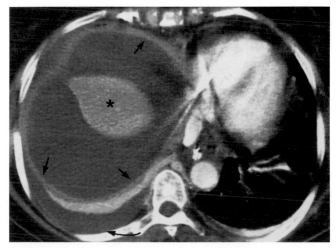

FIG. 10-119. Peridiaphragmatic fluid localization. Contrast-enhanced section through the dome of the liver (*asterisk*) shows evidence of both ascites and right pleural effusion. In this case ascites clearly lies central to the diaphragm (*arrows*) whereas the effusion and associated linear band of atelectatic lung lie peripheral and posterior to the diaphragm (*curved arrow*).

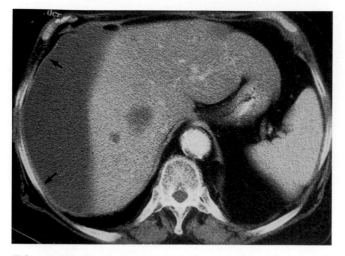

FIG. 10-120. Peridiaphragmatic fluid localization. Contrast-enhanced section through the liver in a patient with ascites shows fluid marginating the right lobe of the liver, clearly lying central to the diaphragm (*arrows*). Note that the fluid does not extend to cover the bare area of the liver.

4. The "bare area sign" is based on recognition that identification of the bare area of the liver indicates fluid within the peritoneum (Fig. 10-120).

As documented by Halvorsen et al., familiarity with each of these signs usually allows accurate localization of peridiaphragmatic fluid collections (103,316,317). Applying the above-mentioned four criteria to 52 cases with ascites (*n* = 13), right pleural effusions (*n* = 25), or both ascites and right pleural effusions (n = 14), retrospectively, these authors found that although none of the four criteria proved entirely reliable by itself, together these signs allowed accurate localization of peridiaphragmatic fluid collections in all cases (103). For differentiating between ascites and pleural effusions, the diaphragm sign proved to have the highest sensitivity (97%) but was frequently indeterminate, while the bare area sign proved most accurate (92%) but was of little value in patients with pleural effusions. The displaced crura sign, while relatively specific, is contingent on pleural

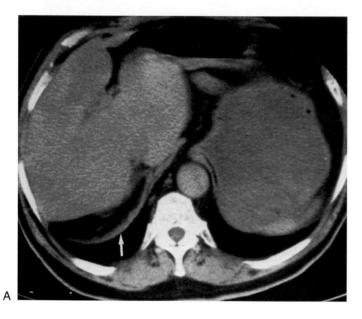

A

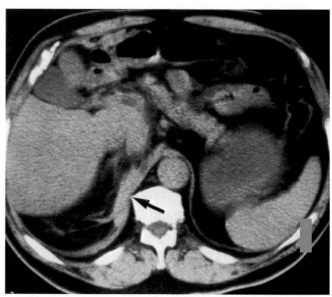

B

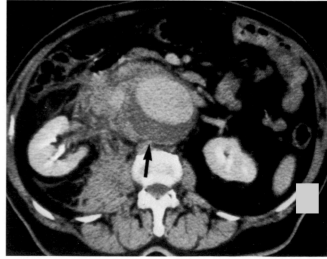

C

FIG. 10-121. Retroperitoneal fluid localization. **A–C:** Ten-mm thick CT sections from above-downward show apparent thickening of the right hemediaphragm superiorly (*arrow* in **A**). Inferiorly, a high-density retroperitoneal fluid collection can be identified (*arrow* in **B**), the result of hemorrhage into the retroperitoneum from a leaking abdominal aortic aneurysm (*arrow* in **C**).

fluid extending medially and was therefore inaccurate in patients with loculated effusions, proving to be indeterminate in almost 25% of cases. In cases in which both ascites and pleural fluid were present, the interface sign proved most valuable, although its accuracy was only 75% (103).

Additional CT findings have been described as potential pitfalls in differentiating pleural from peritoneal fluid. Silverman et al. have noted that a combination of atelectasis and subpulmonic pleural fluid in particular may be misleading because subsegmental atelectasis may result in a curvilinear band at the lung base that superficially may simulate the hemidiaphragm (290). Similar findings have been reported by Federle et al. (12). In these cases, variability in the appearance of pleural fluid at the lung base probably reflects differences in the anatomy of the pulmonary ligaments (4,36). If there are incomplete attachments of these ligaments, the lower lobes are free to float on pleural fluid provided the lung is not stiffened by disease and there are no adhesions between the lung and the adjacent pleura. In distinction, when these attachments are complete, the base of the lung may become tethered inferiorly, despite the presence of even sizable pleural effusions; the result may be the appearance of a ''pseudodiaphragm sign.''

Potential difficulty may also be encountered in identifying basilar lung consolidation and/or atelectasis with or without associated pleural fluid (312). Superficially, areas of dense parenchymal consolidation may mimic an effusion, especially when small.

Underneath the diaphragm, both peritoneal and retroperitoneal fluid may abut the diaphragm (318–320). Retroperitoneal fluid will conform to the anatomic space and/or structures involved, e.g., posterior pararenal versus perirenal spaces. The psoas muscles are also retroperitoneal, and, as discussed above, are intimately related to the arcuate ligaments. Generally, differentiation between retroperitoneal and intraperitoneal fluid is not difficult. This is especially true in cases where retroperitoneal fluid accumulates secondary to a leaking abdominal aortic aneurysm (Fig. 10-121) (321,322).

In distinction, intraperitoneal fluid will collect in the peritoneal spaces and will therefore be restricted by the peritoneal reflections. These are best visualized following intraperitoneal injection of dilute contrast media (Fig. 10-122). On the right side, peritoneal fluid is restricted posteromedially by the right coronary ligament. This results in a characteristic medial tapering of intraperitoneal fluid (the ''bare area sign'') (see Figs. 10-120 and 10-122). It should be remembered, however, that superiorly, ascites, when massive, may collect under the domes of the diaphragm on both the left and right sides (i.e., above the level of the coronary ligaments), thereby limiting considerably the value of the bare-area sign. On the left side, intraabdominal (intraperitoneal) fluid is easy to identify because it will characteristically be central to the left hemidiaphragm and, additionally, will surround the

spleen. As noted previously, identification of intraperitoneal fluid around the spleen is facilitated by recognition of a bare area, analogous to that of the liver (283).

As already discussed, the medial aspect of the left hemidiaphragm is generally outlined by retroperitoneal fat in the upper portion of the left posterior pararenal space. Unlike the right side, the configuration of this portion of the posterior pararenal space and its relationship to the diaphragm may be variable. This variability should not cause confusion since in both cases, intraabdominal fluid can be localized central to the left hemidiaphragm.

Anterior subdiaphragmatic fluid collections also are characteristic in appearance. As shown by Halvorsen et al., fluid may become confined to the anterior left subphrenic space (316). This space is defined on the right side by the falciform ligament and on the left by the left coronary ligament, which extends from the dorsal aspect of the liver posteriorly to the diaphragm (Fig. 10-123).

The anterior subphrenic space extends superiorly to the dome of the diaphragm. Importantly, this fluid lies central to the anterior aspect of the left hemidiaphragm; additionally, fluid in this space will lie adjacent to the left lobe of the liver in a manner analogous to that of free intraperitoneal fluid, which surrounds the spleen posteriorly.

Despite clarification of normal cross-sectional anatomy of the pleural, peritoneal, and retroperitoneal spaces, certain cases remain difficult to evaluate. This is especially true when pleural fluid is sufficiently massive to cause inversion of the hemidiaphragms, since pleural fluid may then simulate the appearance of intraabdominal fluid (323,324). In these cases and others, multiplanar reconstructions may prove helpful by further delineating anatomic relationships (Fig. 10-124).

The Diaphragm as Pathway for the Spread of Disease

The diaphragm usually serves to localize disease in either the thorax or abdomen. However, extension through the diaphragm can occur via several pathways. Direct contiguous spread most commonly occurs through the preexisting normal channels of communication, that is, the aortic and esophageal hiatuses.

The esophageal hiatus is an elliptical opening just to the left of the midline and is formed by the decussation of muscle fibers originating from the diaphragm around the lower esophagus. The margins of the hiatus are formed by the medial portions of the diaphragmatic crura (279,280,284, 325). As the esophagus passes through the upper margin of the hiatus, it assumes an oblique orientation; the gastroesophageal junction itself lies just below the diaphragm. On cross-section, the abdominal or submerged portion of the esophagus typically appears cone-shaped with its base at the junction of the gastric fundus (326).

Sliding hiatal hernias typically are manifest as widening

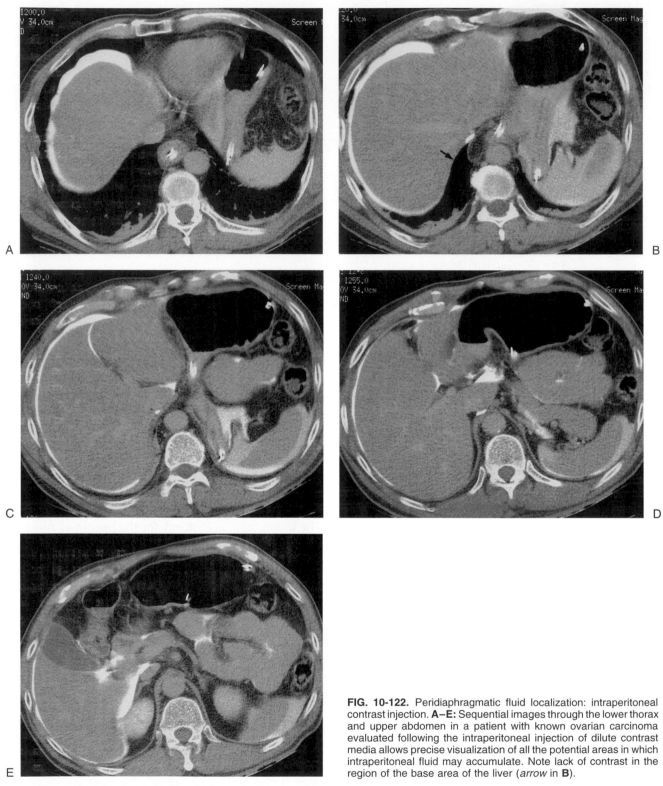

FIG. 10-122. Peridiaphragmatic fluid localization: intraperitoneal contrast injection. **A–E:** Sequential images through the lower thorax and upper abdomen in a patient with known ovarian carcinoma evaluated following the intraperitoneal injection of dilute contrast media allows precise visualization of all the potential areas in which intraperitoneal fluid may accumulate. Note lack of contrast in the region of the base area of the liver (*arrow* in **B**).

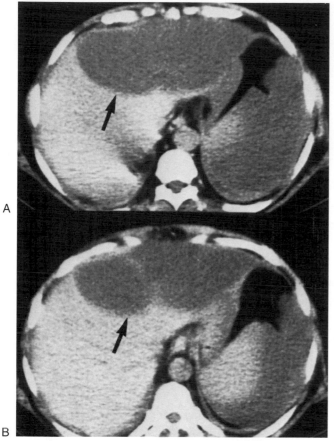

FIG. 10-123. Anterior subphrenic fluid. **A,B:** Sequential 10-mm thick CT sedtions through the upper abdomen show characteristic appearance of intraperitoneal fluid in the anterior subphrenic space, defined on the right by the falciform ligament and superiorly by the anterior aspect of the left hemidiaphragm. In addition, fluid in this space lies adjacent to the left lobe of the liver (*arrows* in **A** and **B**).

of the esophageal hiatus on cross-section (see Figs. 2-105 and 2-107). Measurements of the standard width of the esophageal hiatus, defined as the distance between the medial margins of the crura, have been reported (288,327). As documented by Caskey et al., the width of the esophageal hiatus clearly enlarges with age, especially in men (288). Measuring an average 1.25 cm in individuals in their 20s, the esophageal hiatus progressively widens each decade, measuring greater than 3 cm on average in individuals in their 70s. Hiatal hernias typically present little difficulty in diagnosis. They are frequently associated with an apparent increase in mediastinal fat surrounding the distal esophagus, secondary to herniation of omentum through the phrenicoesophageal ligament. Fluid within herniated peritoneum anterior to the contrast-filled stomach may occasionally be identified as well (328).

In addition to hiatal hernias, the esophageal hiatus serves as a passage for the spread of malignancy, especially that arising in the esophagus and stomach (see Fig. 2-98). Esophageal varices also may traverse the esophageal hiatus (329,330); in these cases, CT is especially valuable in detecting paraesophageal varices (see Fig. 2-105). Frequently these present as nonspecific mediastinal soft-tissue masses, necessitating differentiation from enlarged periesophageal lymph nodes or other posterior mediastinal masses. Despite the accuracy of endoscopy and esophagography to detect esophageal varices, paraesophageal varices have previously required angiography for definite diagnosis.

CT has proven particularly valuable in diagnosing esophageal perforation (see Figs. 2-111 and 2-112). This potentially lethal condition frequently results in peridiaphragmatic fluid collections both above and below the diaphragm. Unfortunately, as documented by Han et al., chest radiographs may be normal in up to 12% of patients (331). In select cases, CT may prove invaluable by delineating the extent of associated mediastinal, pleural, parenchymal disease, and subdiaphragmatic disease (332,333).

More rarely, the esophageal hiatus serves as the pathway for the spread of pancreatic fluid collections (Fig. 10-125). The key to evaluating these fluid collections is analysis of contiguous sections from the lung bases to the upper abdomen. It should be noted that fluid in the lesser sac may appear to extend past the crural margins, occasionally even mimicking the appearance of thrombosis of the inferior vena cava (334). This appearance should not be confused with true mediastinal extension of disease.

The aortic hiatus is another important path for the spread of disease. As shown by Zerhouni et al. (176), malignant thoracic neoplasms, especially those involving the pleura, can extend into the retroperitoneum by this route. The propensity for tumor spread through the aortic hiatus is related to two anatomic features. First, the phrenicoesophageal membrane affixes the esophagus to the crura in most individuals. This may preferentially direct tumor spread through the aortic hiatus. Second, the thoracic duct traverses the aortic hiatus providing a direct lymphatic pathway between the thorax and abdomen. These facts explain the frequent finding of retrocrural adenopathy as a clue to the simultaneous presence of intrathorax and abdominal malignancy. Less frequently, the aortic hiatus serves as the pathway for fluid spread between the thorax and abdomen (see Fig. 2-20).

Although disease usually spreads between the abdomen and thorax by means of a diaphragmatic defect—either congenital or acquired—the diaphragm itself, on occasion, may actually serve as a pathway for disease, both inflammatory and malignant (55,177,186). This is most typically encountered in patients with diffuse malignant pleural disease, especially mesotheliomas (Fig. 10-65).

In this setting, the diaphragm may become involved by tumor; the result is that tumor tracks along the diaphragm

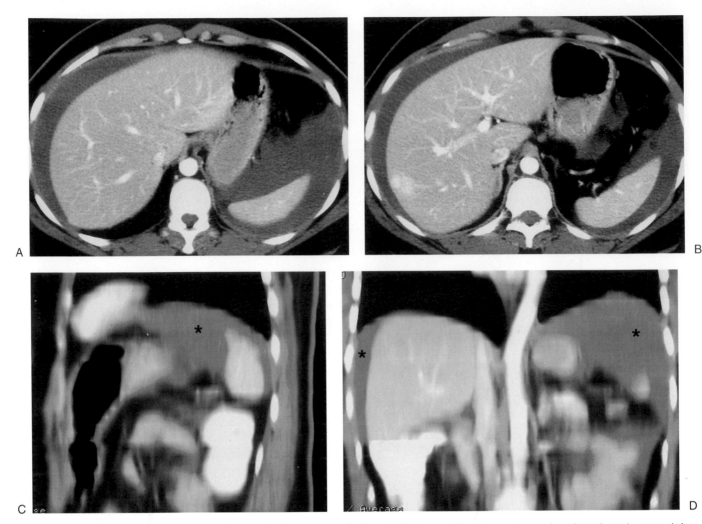

FIG. 10-124. Peridiaphragmatic fluid collections- multiplanar reconstructions. **A,B:** Sequential contrast-enhanced sections through upper abdomen show evidence of extensive ascites surrounding both the liver and spleen. **C,D:** Coronal and sagittal reconstructions help to further localize the precise location of intraperitoneal fluid (*asterisks* in **C** and **D**) owing to sharp margin of the diaphragm.

to gain entry into the abdomen. A similar appearance has been described in patients with invasive thymomas and lymphomas, and may be expected to be seen in any tumor that originates in viscera adjacent to the diaphragms (see Fig. 10-73; Fig. 10-126) (177,186).

Analogous to the spread of tumor, the diaphragm may also serve as a means of extension of infection. In our experience, this is most frequently secondary to tuberculosis, although a similar appearance may be seen with other infections including actinomycosis. Infections may also occur following abdominal surgery (Fig. 10-127).

Finally tumors may arise within the diaphragm (335). This is exceptionally rare, and frequently presents diagnostic dilemmas. An example of a surgically confirmed hemangiopericytoma arising in the diaphragm is shown in Figure 10-128. The intimate relationship between the tumor and the diaphragm is obvious, but the appearance should not be con-

sidered characteristic. Such cases invariably require surgery to actually confirm the precise origin of the lesion.

MR Evaluation of the Diaphragm

To date, the role of MR in evaluating disease in and around the diaphragm has been quite limited. Although isolated reports have shown the efficacy of MR in evaluating thoracic and abdominal wall infections, diaphragmatic rupture, Morgagni hernias, mediastinal pseudocysts, and even diaphragmatic endometriosis, no large series has ever been reported comparing MR with CT in the evaluation of peri-diaphragmatic fluid collections (271,311,336–338). Given the superior contrast resolution of MR and advantages that accrue from coronal and sagittal imaging, it may be anticipated that at least in select cases, MR may ultimately prove of value in the assessment of peridiaphragmatic disease (Figs. 10-129–10-131).

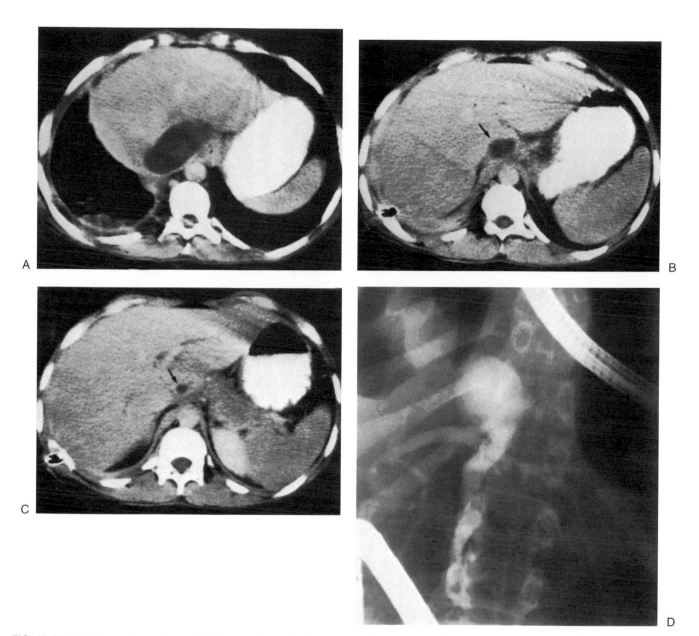

FIG. 10-125. Mediastinal pseudocyst. In this case, the key to the diagnosis is evaluation of sequential images through the thoraco-abdominal junction. **A:** Section shows a large fluid collection in the posterior mediastinum, adjacent to the esophagus. **B:** Section just above the esophageal hiatus. The fluid collection seen in A is still present, although smaller in size, lying anterior to the crura and lateral to the distal esophagus (*arrow*). **C:** Section at the level of the pancreas. A small fluid collection can be identified in the region of the head of the pancreas (*arrow*). In this case fluid has tracked from the retroperitoneum, through the esophageal hiatus, to localize in the posterior mediastinum. Communication of these fluid collections could be established by reviewing sequential images (not all are shown). **D:** Oblique view from an endoscopic retrograde cholangiopancreatogram confirming the diagnosis.

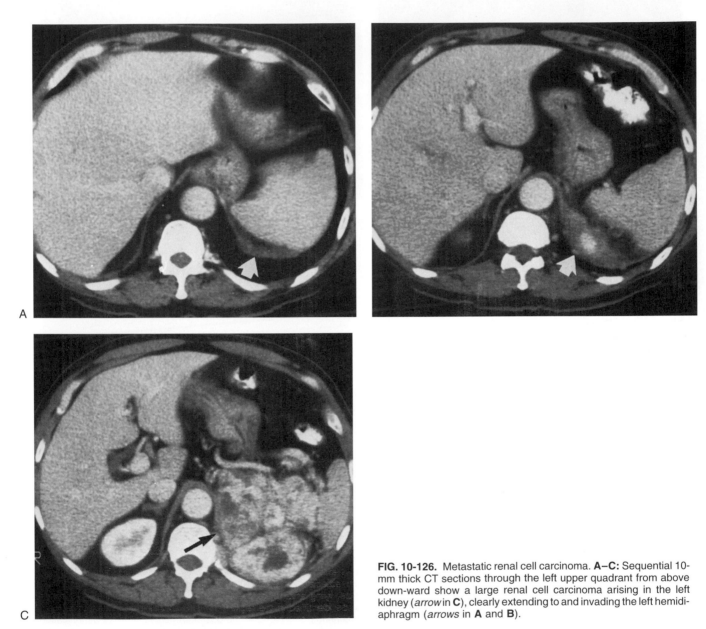

FIG. 10-126. Metastatic renal cell carcinoma. **A–C:** Sequential 10-mm thick CT sections through the left upper quadrant from above down-ward show a large renal cell carcinoma arising in the left kidney (*arrow* in **C**), clearly extending to and invading the left hemidi-aphragm (*arrows* in **A** and **B**).

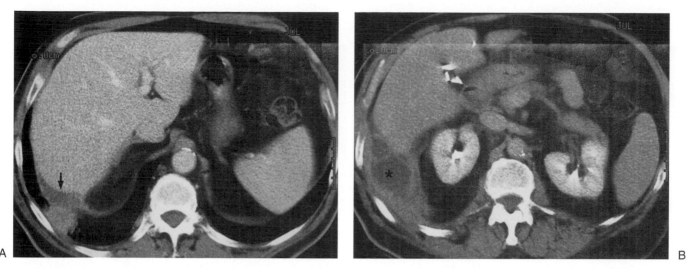

FIG. 10-127. Diaphragm as pathway for spread of infection. **A,B:** Sequential contrast-enhanced sections through the upper abdomen in a patient following recent cholecysectomy with spiking fevers. There is an ill-defined fluid collection in the right upper quadrant (*asterisk* in **B**) that extends superiorly to the diaphragm, which is thickened (*arrow* in **A**). A focal area of consolidation is also apparent in the right lower lobe. CT guided transabdominal aspiration confirmed the presence of pus.

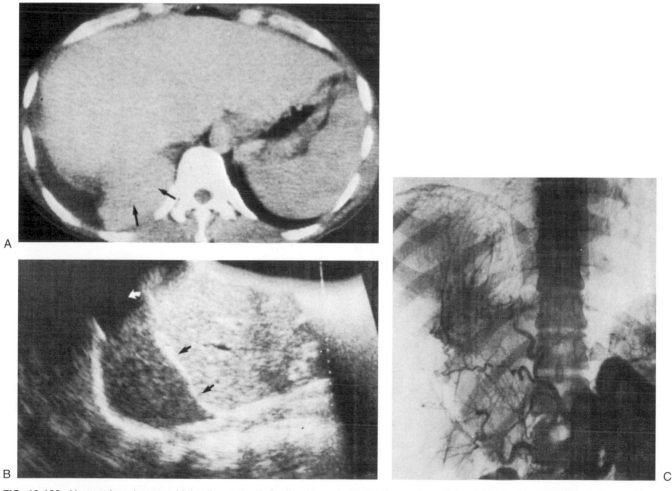

FIG. 10-128. Hemangiopericytoma (right diagram). **A:** Section through the inferior portion of the right pleural space. There is considerable pleural fluid, as well as a large oval soft-tissue mass, clearly peripheral to the hemidiaphragm (*arrows*). **B:** Longitudinal sonogram through the liver. The diaphragm is well-defined (*arrows*). Superior and adjacent to the diaphragm is an echogenic mass, above which pleural fluid can be identified (*white arrow*). **C:** Coned-down view from a celiac angiogram shows a markedly hypervascular mass being fed by a hypertrophied phrenic artery. Biopsy proven hemangiopericytoma arising in the right diaphragm.

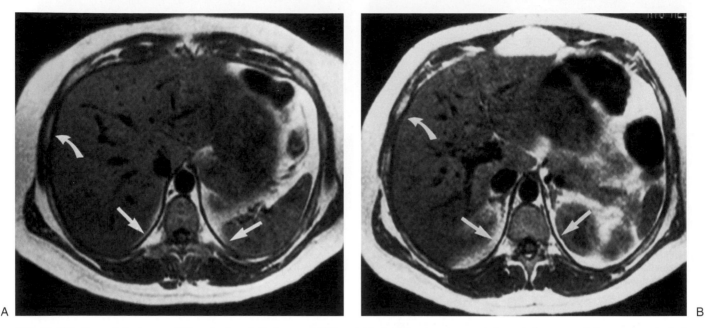

A   B

FIG. 10-129. Normal diaphragm: MR evaluation. **A,B:** Sequential T1-weighted axial spin-echo scans through the upper abdomen show typical appearance of the diaphragms, recognizable as a distinctly low signal intensity line, marginated centrally and peripherally by high signal intensity fat (*arrows* in **A** and **B**). Note that, because of increased contrast resolution, the line of the diaphragm can also be appreciated marginating the lateral aspect of the liver (*curved arrows* in **A** and **B**; compare with Fig. 10-105).

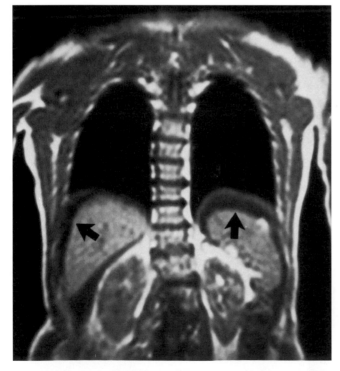

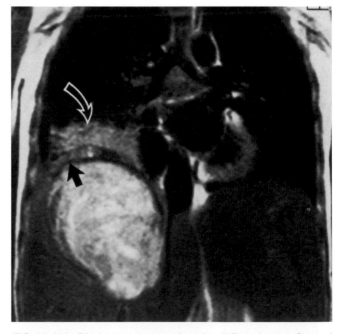

FIG. 10-130. Peridiaphragmatic fluid localization-ascites: evaluation with MR. Coronal T1-weighted MR scan clearly shows the presence of ascites surrounding both the liver and spleen (*arrows*), recognizable as a low signal intensity fluid collection.

FIG. 10-131. Diaphragmatic tumor invasion: MR evaluation. Coronal T1-weighted scan through the liver shows a large, necrotic tumor mass in the liver extending superiorly to involve the diaphragm (*arrow*). Note the presence of basilar consolidation, as well, in the right lower lobe (*curved arrow*). Given the inherent advantages of multiplanar imaging and superior contrast resolution, MR should be of benefit in difficult cases for defining the true extent of peridiaphragmatic tumor.

REFERENCES

1. Pugatch RD, Faling IJ, Robbins AH, Snider GL. Differentiation of pleural and pulmonary lesions using computed tomography. *J Comput Assist Tomogr* 1978;2:601–606.
2. Kreel L. Computed tomography of the lungs and pleura. *Semin Roentgenol* 1978;13:213–225.
3. Im JG, Webb WR, Rosen A, Gamsu G. Costal pleura: appearances at high-resolution CT. *Radiology* 1989;171:125–131.
4. Bressler EL, Francis IR, Glazer GM, Gross BH. Bolus contrast medium enhancement for distinguishing pleural from parenchymal lung disease: CT features. *J Comput Assist Tomogr* 1987;11:436–440.
5. Berne AS, Heitzman ER. The roentgenographic signs of pedunculated pleural tumors. *AJR Am J Roentgenol* 1962;87:892–895.
6. Lewis MI, Horak DA, Yellin A, et al. The case of the moving intrathoracic mass. *Chest* 1985;88:897,898.
7. Williford ME, Hidalgo H, Putman CE, Korobkin M, Ram PC. Computed tomography of pleural disease. *AJR Am J Roentgenol* 1983;140:909–914.
8. Zinn WL, Naidich DP, Whelan CA, et al. Fluid within preexisting pulmonary air-spaces: a potential pitfall in the CT differentiation of pleural from parenchymal disease. *J Comput Assist Tomogr* 1987;11:441–448.
9. Raasch BN, Carsky EW, Lane EJ, et al. Radiographic anatomy of the interlobar fissures: a study of 100 specimens. *AJR Am J Roentgenol* 1982;138:1043.
10. Maffessanti M, Tommasi M, Pelegrini P. Computed tomography of free pleural effusions. *Eur J Radiol* 1987;7:87–90.
11. Griffin DJ, Gross BH, McCracken S, Glazer GM. Observations on CT differentiation of pleural and peritoneal fluid. *J Comput Assist Tomogr* 1984;8:24–28.
12. Federle MP, Mark AS, Guillaumin ES. CT of subpulmonic pleural effusions and atelectasis: criteria for differentiation from subphrenic fluid. *AJR Am J Roentgenol* 1986;146:685–689.
13. Epler GR, McLoud TC, Munn CS, Colby TV. Pleural lipoma. Diagnosis by computed tomography. *Chest* 1986;90:265–268.
14. Levi C, Gray JE, McCullough E, Hattery RR. The unreliability of CT numbers as absolute values. *AJR Am J Roentgenol* 1982;139:443–447.
15. Vock P, Effman EL, Hedlund LW, Lischko MM, Putman CE. Analysis of the density of pleural fluid analogs by computed tomography. *Invest Radiol* 1984;19:10–15.
16. Rawkin RN, Raval B, Finley R. Case report. Primary chylopericardium: combined lyhmphoangiographic and CT diagnosis. *J Comput Assist Tomogr* 1980;4:869–870.
17. Im J-G, Chung JW, Han MC. Milk of calcium pleural collections: CT findings. *J Comput Assist Tomogr* 1993;17:613–616.
18. Marks BW, Kuhns IR. Identification of the pleural fissures with computed tomography. *Radiology* 1982;143:139–141.
19. Friga J, Schmit P, Katz M, Vadrot D, Laval-Jeantet M. Computed tomography of the pleural fissures: normal anatomy. *J Comput Assist Tomogr* 1982;6:1069–1074.
20. Chasen MH, McCarthy MJ, Gilliland JD, Floyd JL. Concepts in computed tomography of the thorax. *RadioGraphics* 1986;6:793–832.
21. Genereux GP. The posterior pleural reflections. *AJR Am J Roentgenol* 1983;141:141–149.
22. Goodman LR, Golkow RS, Steiner RM, et al. The right mid-lung window. *Radiology* 1982;143:135–138.
23. Proto AV, Ball JB. Computed tomography of the major and minor fissures. *AJR Am J Roentgenol* 1983;140:439–448.
24. Proto AV, Ball JB. The superolateral major fissures. *AJR Am J Roentgenol* 1983;140:431–437.
25. Yamashita H. *Roentgenologic anatomy of the lung.* Stuttgart: Thieme, 1978.
26. Gale ME, Grief WF. Intrafissural fat: CT correlation with chest radiography. *Radiology* 1986;160:333–336.
27. Mayo JR, Müller NL, Henkelman RM. The double-fissure sign: a motion artifact on thin-section CT scans. *Radiology* 1987;165:580–581.
28. Berkman YM, Auh YH, Davis SD, Kazam E. Anatomy of the minor fissure: evaluation with thin-section CT. *Radiology* 1989;170:647–651.
29. Frija J, Yana C, Laval-Jeantet M. Letter to the editor. Anatomy of the minor fissure: evaluation with thin-section CT. *Radiology* 1989;173:571–572.
30. Otsuji H, Hatakeyama M, Kitamura I, et al. Right upper lobe versus right middle lobe: differentiation with thin-section high-resolution CT. *Radiology* 1989;172:653–656.
31. Takasugi JE, Godwin JD. Left azygos lobe. *Radiology* 1989;171:133–134.
32. Speckman JM, Gamsu G, Webb WR. Alterations in CT mediastinal anatomy produced by an azygos lobe. *AJR Am J Roentgenol* 1981;137:47–50.
33. Godwin JD, Tarver RD. Accessory fissures of the lung. *AJR Am J Roentgenol* 1985;144:39–47.
34. Austin JHM. The left minor fissure. *Radiology* 1986;161:433–436.
35. Boyden EA. The distribution of bronchi in gross anomalies of the right upper lobe, particularly lobes subdivided by the azygos vein and those containing pre-eparterial bronchi. *Radiology* 1952;58:797.
36. Berkmen YM, Davis SD, Kazam E, et al. Right phrenic nerve: anatomy, CT appearance, and differentiation from the pulmonary ligament. *Radiology* 1989;173:43–46.
37. Cooper C, Moss AA, Buy JN, Stark DD. CT appearance of the normal inferior pulmonary ligament. *AJR Am J Roentgenol* 1983;141:237–240.
38. Godwin JD, Vock P, Osborne DR. CT of the pulmonary ligament. *AJR Am J Roentgenol* 1983;141:231–236.
39. Rabinowitz JG, Cohen BA, Mendelson DS. The pulmonary ligament. *Radiol Clin North Am* 1984;22:659–672.
40. Rost RC Jr, Proto AV. Inferior pulmonary ligament: computed tomographic appearance. *Radiology* 1983;148:479–483.
41. Taylor GA, Fishman EK, Kramer SS, Siegelman SS. CT demonstration of the phrenic nerve. *J Comput Assist Tomogr* 1983;7:411–414.
42. Bernaudin J-F, Fleury J. Anatomy of the blood and lymphatic circulation of the pleural serosa. In: Chrétien J, Bignon J, Hirsch A, eds. *The pleura in health and disease.* New York: Marcel Dekker, 1985:101–124.
43. Policard A, Galy P. *La Plevre.* Paris: Masson, 1942.
44. Agostoni E, Miserocchi G, Bonanni MV. Thickness and pressure of the pleural liquid in some mammals. *Respir Phys* 1969;6:245–256.
45. Staub NC, Wiener-Kronish JP, Albertine KH. Pleural liquid and solute exchange. In: Chrétien J, Bignon J, Hirsch A, eds. *The pleura in health and disease.* New York: Marcel Dekker, 1985:170.
46. Sargent EN, Boswell WD, Ralls PW, Markovitz A. Subpleural fat pads in patients exposed to asbestos: distinction from non-calcified pleural plaques. *Radiology* 1984;152:273–277.
47. Vix VA. Extrapleural costal fat. *Radiology* 1974;112:563–565.
48. Light RW, Macgrefor I, Luchsinger PCea. Pleural effusions: the diagnostic separation of transudates from exudates. *Ann Int Med* 1972;77:507–513.
49. Bartter T, Akers SM, Pratter MR. The evaluation of pleural effusion. *Chest* 1994;106:1209–1214.
50. Sahn SA. The Pleura. *Amer Rev Resp Dis* 1988;138:184–234.
51. Management of non-tuberculous empyema. *Am Rev Resp Dis* 1962;85:935.
52. Light RW. Management of parapneumonic effusions. *Chest* 1976;70:3–4.
53. Schmitt WGH, Hubener KH, Rucker HC. Pleural calcification with persistent effusion. *Radiology* 1983;149:633–638.
54. Bhatt GM. Case report. CT demonstration of empyema necessitatis. *J Comput Assist Tomogr* 1985;1985:1108–1109.
55. Peterson MW, Austin JHM, Yip AC, McManus RP, Jaretzki A. Case report. CT findings in transdiaphragmatic empyema necessitatis due to tuberculosis. *J Comput Assist Tomogr* 1987;1987:704–706.
56. Hulnick DH, Naidich DP, McCauley DI. CT of pleural tuberculosis. *Radiology* 1983;149:759–765.
57. Baber CEJ, Hedlund LW, Oddson TA, Putman CE. Differentiating empyemas and peripheral pulmonary abscesses. The value of computed tomography. *Radiology* 1980;1980:755–758.
58. Shin M, Ho, K. J. Computed tomographic characteristics of pleural empyema. *J Comput Tomogr* 1983;7:179–182.
59. Williford ME, Godwin JD. Computed tomography of lung abscess and empyema. *Radiol Clin North Am* 1983;21:575–583.
60. Stark DD, Federle MP, Goodman PC, Podrasky AE, Webb WR. Differentiating lung abscess and empyema: radiography and computed tomography. *AJR Am J Roentgenol* 1983;141:163–167.
61. Peters ME, Gould HR, McCarthy TM. Identification of a bronchopleural fistula by computerized tomography. *Comput Tomogr* 1983;7:267–270.

62. Naidich DP. Radiologic evaluation of pleural disease. In: Hood RM, ed. *Surgical diseases of the pleura and chest wall.* Philadelphia: WB Saunders, 1986:95.

63. Bartlett JG. Anaerobic bacterial pneumonitis. *Am Rev Respir Dis* 1979;119:19–23.

64. Robinson BR. The treatment of lung abscess. *Current Concepts* 1985; 87:709–710.

65. Viamonte MJ, Parks RE, Smoak WM. Guided catheterization of the bronchial arteries. Part 2. Pulmonary and mediastical neoplasms. *Radiology* 1965;1965:205–230.

66. Baron MG. Radiologic notes in cardiology: interlobar effusion. *Circulation* 1971;44:475–483.

67. Pecorari A, Weisbrod GL. Computed tomography of pseudotumoral pleural fluid collections in the azygoesophageal recess. *J Comput Assist Tomogr* 1989;13:803–805.

68. Himmelman RB, Callen PW. The prognostic value of loculations in parpneumonic pleural effusions. *Chest* 1986;90:852–856.

69. Waite RJ, Carbonneau RJ, Balikian JP, et al. Parietal pleural changes in empyema: appearances at CT. *Radiology* 1990;175:145–150.

70. Aquino SL, Webb WR, Gushiken BJ. Pleural exudates and transudates: diagnosis with contrast-enhanced CT. *Radiology* 1994;192: 803–808.

71. Neff CC, vanSonnenberg E, Lawson DW, Patton AS. CT follow-up of empyemas: pleural peels resolve after percutaneous catheter drainage. *Radiology* 1990;176:195–197.

72. Stark DD, Federle MP, Goodman PC. CT and radiographic assessment of tube thoracostomy. *AJR Am J Roentgenol* 1983;141:253–258.

73. Webb WR, LaBerge JM. Radiographic recognition of chest tube malposition in the major fissure. *Chest* 1984;85:81–83.

74. Panicek DM, Randall PA, Witanowski LS, Raasch BN, Heitzman ER. Chest tube tracks. *Radiographics* 1987;7:321–342.

75. Shapiro MP, Gale ME, Daly BD. Eloesser window thoracostomy for treatment of empyema; radiographic appearance. *AJR Am J Roentgenol* 1988;150:549–552.

76. Mullin DM, Rodan BA, Bean WJ, Gocke TM, Feng TS. Computed tomography of oleothorax. *CT* 1987;10:197–199.

77. Westcott J. Percutanaeous catheter drainage of pleural effusion and empyema. *AJR Am J Roentgenol* 1985;144:1189–1193.

78. vanSonnenberg E, Nakamoto SK, Mueller PR, et al. CT and ultrasound-guided catheter drainage of empyemas after chest-tube failure. *Radiology* 1984;151:349–353.

79. Merriam MA, Cronan JJ, Dorfman GS, Lambiase RE, Haasa RA. Radiographically guided percutaneous catheter drainage of pleural fluid collections. *AJR Am J Roentgenol* 1988;151:1113–1116.

80. Moulton JS, Moore PT, Mencici RA. Treatment of loculated pleural effusions with transcatheter intracavitary urokinase. *AJR Am J Roentgenol* 1989;153:941–945.

81. Hunnam GR, Flower CDR. Radiologically guided percutaneous catheter drainage of empyemas. *Clin Radiol* 1988;39:121–126.

82. Reinhold C, Illescase FF, Atri M, Bret PM. Treatment of pleural effusions and pneumothorax with catheters placed percutaneously under imaging guidance. *AJR Am J Roentgenol* 1989;152:1189–1191.

83. Berger HA, Morganroth ML. Immediate drainage is not required for all patients with complicated parapneumonic effusions. *Chest* 1990; 97:731–735.

84. Orringer MB. Thoracic empyema; back to basics. *Chest* 1988;93: 901–902.

85. Hood RM. *Surgical diseases of the pleura and chest wall.* Philadelphia: WB Saunders, 1987.

86. Hoover EL, Hsu H-K, Ross MJ, et al. Reappraisal of empyema thoracis. Surgical intervention when the duration of illness is unknown. *Chest* 1986;90:511–515.

87. Rudd RM. New developments in asbestos-related pleural disease. *Thorax* 1996;51:210–216.

88. Sison RF, Hruban RH, Moore GW, et al. Pulmonary disease associated with pleural "asbestos" plaques. *Chest* 1989;95:831–835.

89. Kreel L. Computer tomography in the evaluation of pulmonary asbestosis: preliminary experiences with the EMI general purpose scanner. *Acta Radiodl [Diagn] (Stockh)* 1976;17:405–412.

90. Katz D, Kreel L. Computed tomography in pulmonary asbestosis. *Clin Radiol* 1979;30:207–213.

91. Gefter WB, Epstein DM, Miller WT. Radiographic evaluation of asbestos-related chest disorders. *CRC Crit Rev Diagn Imaging* 1984; 21:133–181.

92. Aberle DR, Gamsu G, Ray CS, Feurstein IM. Asbestos-related pleural and parenchymal fibrosis: detection with high-resolution CT. *Radiology* 1988;166:729–734.

93. Aberle DR, Hamsu G, Ray CS. High-resolution CT of benign asbestos-related diseases: clinical and radiologic correlation. *AJR Am J Roentgenol* 1988;151:883–891.

94. Aberle DR, Balmes JR. Computed tomography of asbestos-related pulmonary and pleural diseases. *Clin Chest Med* 1991;12:115–131.

95. Friedman AC, Fiel SB, Fisher MS, et al. Asbestos-related pleural disease and asbestosis: a comparison of CT and chest radiography. *AJR Am J Roentgenol* 1988;150:269–275.

96. Gamsu G, Aberle DR, Lynch D. Computed tomography in the diagnosis of asbestos-related thoracic disease. *J Thorac Imag* 1989;4:61–67.

97. Al Jarad N, Poulakis N, C. PM, Rubens MB, Rudd RM. Assessment of asbestos induced pleural disease by computed tomography-correlation with chest radiograph and lung function. *Resp Med* 1991;85:203–208.

98. McLoud TC, Woods BO, Carrington CB, Epler GR, Gaensler EA. Diffuse pleural thickening in an asbestos-exposed population: prevalence and causes. *AJR Am J Roentgenol* 1985;144:9–18.

99. Rupp SB, Jolles H. Calcified plaque in the superior portion of the major fissure. An unusual manifestation of asbestos exposure. *Chest* 1989;96:1436–1437.

100. Withers BF, Ducatman AM, Yang WN. Roentgenographic evidence for predominant left-sided location of unilateral pleueral plaques. *Chest* 1984;95:262–264.

101. Craighead JE, Abraham JL, Churg A. et al. The pathology of asbestos-associated diseases of the lungs and pleural cavities: diagnostic criteria and proposed grading schema. *Arch Pathol Lab Med* 1982;106: 544–596.

102. Churg A. Asbestos fibers and pleural plaques in a general autopsy population. *Am J Pathol* 1982;109:88–96.

103. Epler GR, McLoud TC, Gaensler EA. Prevalence and incidence of benign asbestos pleural effusion in a working population. 1982;247: 617–622.

104. Halvorsen RA, Fedyshin PJ, Korobkin M, Thompson WM. CT differentiation of pleural effusion from ascites. An evaluation of four signs using blinded analysis of 52 cases. *Invest Radiol* 1986;21:391–395.

105. Gefter WB, Conant EF. Issues and controversies in the plain-film diagnosis of asbestos-related disorders in the chest. *J Thorac Imag* 1988;3:11–28.

106. Becklake MR. State of the art: asbestos-related disease of the lung and other organs; their epidemiology and implications for clinical practice. *Am Rev Respir Dis* 1976;114:187–227.

107. Jones RN, McLoud T, Rockoff SD. The radiographic pleural abnormalities in asbestos exposure; relationship to physiologic abnormalities. *J Thorac Imag* 1988;3:57–66.

108. Schwartz DA, Fuortes LJ, Galvin JR, et al. Asbestos-induced pleural fibrosis and impaired lung function. *Am Rev Respir Dis* 1990;141: 321–326.

109. Bégin R, Boctor M, Bergeron D, et al. Radiographic assessment of pleuropulmonary disease in asbestos workers: posteroanterior, four view films, and computed tomograms of the thorax. *Br J Ind Med* 1984;41:373–383.

110. Rabinowitz JG, Elfremidis SC, Cohen B, et al. A comparative study of mesothelioma and asbestosis using computed tomographpy and conventional chest radiography. *Radiology* 1982;144:453–460.

111. Menzies R, Fraser R. Round atelectasis. Pathologic and pathogenetic features. *Am J Surg Pathol* 1987;11:674–681.

112. Schneider H, Felson B, Gonzalez L. Rounded atelctasis. *AJR Am J Roentgenol* 1980;134:225–232.

113. Mintzer RA, Gore RM, Vogelzang RL, Holz S. Rounded atelctasis and its association with asbestos-induced pleural disease. *Radiology* 1981;139:567–570.

114. Hillerdal G. Rounded atelectasis: clinical experience with 74 patients. *Chest* 1989;95:836–941.

115. Doyle TC, Lawler GA. CT features of rounded atelectasis of the lung. *AJR Am J Roentgenol* 1984;143:225–228.

116. McHugh K, Blaquiere RM. CT features of rounded atelectasis. *AJR Am J Roentgenol* 1989;153:257–260.

117. Lynch DA. Asbestos-related focal lung masses: manifestations on conventional and high-resolution CT scans. *Radidology* 1988;169: 603–607.

118. Batra P, Brown K, Hayashi K, Mori M. Rounded atelectasis. *J Thorac Imag* 1996;11:187–197.

119. Ren H, Hruban RH, Kuhlman JE, et al. Computed tomography of rounded atelectasis. *J Comput Assist Tomogr* 1988;12:1031–1034.

120. Ren H, Hruban RH, Kuhlman JE, et al. Case report. Computed tomography of rounded atelectasis. *J Comput Assist Tomogr* 1989;12:1031–1034.

121. Taylor PM. Dynamic contrast enhancement of asbestos-related pulmonary pseudotumors. *Br J Radiol* 1988;61:1070–1072.

122. Coleman BG, Eplstein DM, Arger PH, Miller WT. Case report. CT features of an unusual hypervascular lung carcinoma complicating chronic asbestos related pleural disease. *J Comput Assist Tomogr* 1985;9:554–557.

123. Sinner WWN. Pleuroma—a cancer mimicking atelectatic pseudotumor of the lung. *Fortschr Geb Rontgenst Nuklarmed Erganzungsband* 1980;133:578–585.

124. Reifsnyder AC, Smith HJ, Mullhollan TJ, Lee EL. Case Report. Malignant fibrous histiocytoma of the lung in a patient with a history of asbestos exposure. *AJR Am J Roentgenol* 1990;154:65–66.

125. Blesovsky A. The folded lung. *Br J Dis Chest* 1966;60:19–22.

126. Hanke R, Kretzschmar R. Rounded atelectasis. *Semin Roentgenol* 1980;15:174–182.

127. Stancato-Pasik A, Mendelson DS, Marom Z. Case Report. Rounded atelecctasis caused by histoplasmosis. *AJR Am J Roentgenol* 1990;155:275,276.

128. Hillerdal G. Asbestos-related pleural disease. *Semin Respir Med* 1987;9:65–74.

129. McAdams HP, Erasmus JJ, Patz EF, Goodman PC, Coleman RE. Evaluation of patients with round atelectasis using 2-(18F)fluoro-2-deoxy-D-glucose PET. *J Comput Assist Tomogr* 1998;22:601–604.

130. Munden RF, Libshitz HI. Rounded atelectasis and mesothelioma. *AJR Am J Roentgenol* 1998;170:1519–1522.

131. Verschakelen JA, Demaerel P, Coolen J, et al. Rounded atelectasis of the lung: MR appearance. *AJR Am J Roentgenol* 1989;152:965–966.

132. Leff A, Hopewell PC, Costello J. Pleural effusion from malignancy. *Ann Intern Med* 1978;88:532–537.

133. Chernow B, Sahn SA. Carcinomatous involvement of the pleura: an analysis of 96 patients. *Am J Med* 1977;63:695–702.

134. Meyer PC. Metastatic carcinoma of the pleura. *Thorax* 1966;21:437–443.

135. Scerbo J, Keltz H, Stone DJ. A prospective study of closed pleural biopsies. *JAMA* 1971;218:377–380.

136. Salyer WR, Eggleston JC, Erozan YS. Efficacy of pleural needle biopsy and pleural fluid cytology in the diagnosis of malignant neoplasm involving the pleura. *Chest* 1975;67:536–539.

137. Ryan CJ, Rodgers RF, Unni KK, Hepper NGG. The outcome of patients with pleural effusions of indeterminate cause at thoracotomy. *Mayo Clin Proc* 1981;56:145–149.

138. Tattersall MHN, Boyer MJ. Management of malignant effusions. *Thorax* 1990;45:81–82.

139. Miller KS, Sahn S. Chest tubes. Indications, technique, management and complications. *Chest* 1987;1987:258–264.

140. Martini N, Beatatie, E. J. Indications for pleurectomy in malignant effusion. *Cancer* 1875;35:734–738.

141. Heitzman ER, Markarian B, Raasch ON, et al. Annual oration. Pathways of tumor spread through the lung: radiologic correlations with anatomy and pathology. *Radiology* 1982;144:3–14.

142. Webb WR, Jeffrey RB, Godwin JD. Thoracic computed tomography in superior sulcus tumors. *J Comput Assist Tomogr* 1981;5:361–365.

143. Glazer HS, Duncan MJ, Aronberg DJ, et al. Pleural and chest wall invasion in bronchogenic carcinoma: CT evaluation. *Radiology* 1985;157:191–194.

144. Pennes DR, Glazer GM, Wimbish KJ, et al. Chest wall invasion by lung cancer: limitations of CT evaluation. *AJR Am J Roentgenol* 1985;144:507–511.

145. Shin MS, Anderson SD, Myers J, Ho KJ. Case report. Pitfalls in CT evaluation of chest wall invasion by lung chest. *J Comput Assist Tomogr* 1986;10:136–138.

146. Pearlberg JL, Sandler MA, Beute GH, Lewis JWJ, Madrazo BL. Limitations of CT in evaluation of neoplasms involving chest wall. *J Comput Assist Tomogr* 1987;11:290–293.

147. Glazer HS, Kaiser LR, Anderson DJ, et al. Indeterminate mediastinal invasion in bronchogenic carcinoma: CT evaluation. *Radiology* 1989;173:37–42.

148. Grenier P, Dubray B, Carettte MF, et al. Preoperative thoracic staging of lung cancer: CT and MR evaluation. *Diagn Inter Radiol* 1989;173(P):69.

149. Heelan RT, Demas BE, Caravelli JF, et al. Superior sulcus tumors. *Radiology* 1989;170:637–641.

150. McLoud TC, Filion RB, Edelman RR, Shepard JO. MR imaging of superior sulcus carcinoma. *J Comput Assist Tomogr* 1989;13:233–239.

151. Webb WR, Jensen BJ, Sollito R, et al. Bronchogenic carcinoma: staging with MR compared with staging with CT surgery. *Radiology* 1985;156:117–124.

152. Haggar AM, Pearlberg JL, Froelich JW, et al. Chest-wall invasion by carcinoma of the lung: detection by MR imaging. *AJR Am J Roentgenol* 1987;148:1075–1078.

153. Adams VI, Unni KK, Muhm JR, Jett JR, Ilstrup DM, Bernatz PE. Diffuse malignant mesosthelioma of pleura. Diagnosis and survival in 92 cases. *Cancer* 1986;58:1540–1551.

154. Martini N, McCormack PM, Bains MS, et al. Current review. Pleural mesotheliona. *Ann Thorac Surg* 1987;43:113–120.

155. Dunn MM. Asbestos and the lung. *Chest* 1989;95:1304–1308.

156. Metintas M, Ozdemir N, Isiksoy S, et al. CT-guided pleural needle biopsy in the diagnosis of malignant mesothelioma. *J Comput Assist Tomogr* 1995;19:370–374.

157. Dedrick CG, McLoud TC, Shepard JO, Shipley RT. Computed tomography of localized pleural mesothelioma. *AJR Am J Roentgenol* 1985;144:275–280.

158. Spizarny DL, Gross BH, Shepard J-A O. CT findings in localized fibrous mesothelioma of the pleural fissure. *J Comput Assist Tomogr* 1986;10:942–944.

159. Kreel L. Computed tomography in mesothelioma. *Semin Oncol* 1981;8:302–312.

160. Alexander E, Clark RA, Colley DP, Mitchell SE. CT of malignant pleural mesothelioma. *AJR Am J Roentgenol* 1981;137:287–291.

161. Grant DC, Seltzer SE, Antman KH, Finberg HJ, Koster K. Computed tomograqphy of malignant pleural mesothelioma. *J Comput Assist Tomogr* 1983;7:626–632.

162. Mirvis S, Dutcher JP, Haney PJ, Whitley NO, Aisner J. CT of malignant pleural mesothelioma. *AJR Am J Roentgenol* 1983;140:665–670.

163. Salonen O, Kivissarikjold-Nordenstam C-G, Somer K, Mattson K, Tammilehto L. Computed tomography of pleural lesions with special reference to the mediastinal pleura. *Acta Radiol Diagn (Stokh)* 1986;27:527–531.

164. Rusch VW, Godwin JD, Shuman WP. The role of computed tomography scanning in the initial assessment and the follow-up of malignant pleural mesothelioma. *J Thoracic Cardiovasc Surg* 1988;96:171–177.

165. Kawashima A, Libshitz HI. Malignant pleural mesothelioma: CT manifestations in 50 cases. *AJR Am J Roentgenol* 1990;155:965–969.

166. Shin MS, Berland LL, Ho K-J. Case report. Postoperative malignant seroma: CT demonstration of its formation mechanisms. *Comput Assist Tomogr* 1984;8:1001–1004.

167. Uri AJ, Schulman ES, Scott RD, Rose LJ. Diffuse contralateral pulmonary metastases in malignant mesothelioma. An unusual radiographic presentation. *Chest* 1988;93:433–434.

168. Sahin AA, Coplü L, Selçuk ZT, et al. Malignant pleural mesothelioma caused by environmental exposure to asbestos or erionite in rural Turkey: CT findings in 84 patients. *AJR Am J Roentgenol* 1993;161:533–537.

169. Raizon A, Schwartz A, Hix W, Rockoff SD. Calcification as a sign of sarcomatous degeneration of malignant pleural mesotheliomas: A new CT finding. *J Comput Assist Tomogr* 1996;20:42–44.

170. Taylor DR, Page W, Hughes D, Vargese G. Metastatic renal cell carcinoma mimicking pleural mesothelioma. *Thorax* 1987;42:901–902.

171. Patz EF, Rusch VW, Heelan R. The proposed new international TNM staging system for malignant pleural mesothelioma: Application to imaging. *Am J Roentgenol* 1996;166:323–327.

172. Sugarbaker DJ, Jaklitsch MT, Liptay MJ. Mesothelioma and radical multimodality therapy: Who benefits? *Chest* 1995;107:S345–S350.

173. Sugarbaker DJ, Garcia JP, Richards WG, et al. Extrapleural pneumonectomy in the multimodality therapy of malignant pleural mesothelioma—Results in 120 consecutive patients. *Ann Surg* 1996;224:288–294.

174. Rusch VW. A proposed new international TNM staging system for malignant pleural mesothelioma from the international mesothelioma interest group. *Lung Cancer J Iaslc* 1996;14:1–12.

175. Patz EF, Shaffer K, Piwnica-Worms DR, et al. Malignant pleural mesothelioma: value of CT and MR imaging in predicting resectability. *AJR Am J Roentgenol* 1992;159:961–966.

176. Zerhouni EA, Scott WW, Baker RR, Wharam MO, Siegelman SS.

Invasive thmyomas: diagnosis and evaluation by computed tomography. *J Comput Assist Tomogr* 1982;6:92–100.

177. Scatariage JC, Fishman EK, Zerhouni EA, Siegelman SS. Transdiaphragmatic extension of invasive thymoma. *AJR Am J Roentgenol* 1985;144:31–35.

178. O'Donovan PB, Eng P. Pleural changes in malignant pleural effusions: appearance on computed tomography. *Cleveland Clin J Med* 1994; 61:127–131.

179. Falaschi F, Battolla L, Mascalchi M, et al. Usefulness of MR signal intensity in distinguishing benign from malignant pleural disease. *Am J Roentgenol* 1996;166:963–968.

180. Blank N, Casttellino RA. The intrathoracic manifestations of the malignant lyumphomas and leukemia. *Semin Roentgenol* 1980;15: 227–245.

181. Xaubet A, Diumenjo MC, Marin A, et al. Characteristics and prognostic value of pleural effusions in non-Hodgkin's lymphomas. *Eur J Respir Dis* 1985;66:135–140.

182. Fisher AMH, Kendall B, Van Leuven BD. Hodgkin's disease: a radiologic survey. *Clin Radiol* 1962;13:115–127.

183. Stolberg HO, Patt NL, MacEwan KF, Warwick OH, Brown TC. Hodgkin's disease of the lung: radiologic-pathologic correlation. *AJR Am J Roentgenol* 1964;192:96–115.

184. Ellert J, Kreel L. The role of computed tomography in the initial staging and subsequent management of the lymphomas. *J Comput Assist Tomogr* 1980;4:368–391.

185. Burgener FH, Hamlin DJ. Intrathoracic histiocytic lymphoma. *AJR Am J Roentgenol* 1981;136:499–504.

186. Shuman LS, Libshitz HI. Pictorial essay. Solid pleural manifestations of lymphoma. *AJR Am J Roentgenol* 1984;142:269–273.

187. Bernadreschi P, Bonechi I, Urbano U. Recurrent pleural effusion as manifesting feature of primary chest wall Hodgkin's disease. *Chest* 1988;94:424–426.

188. Carlson SE, Bergin CJ, Hoppe RT. MR imaging to detect chest wall and pleural involvemnt in patients with lyhmphoma: effect on radiation therapy planning. *AJR Am J Roentgenol* 1993;160:1191–1195.

189. Bergin CJ, Healy MJ, Zincone GE, Castellino RA. MR evaluation of chest wall involvement in malignant lymphoma. *J Comput Assist Tomogr* 1990;14:928–933.

190. Tsukada G, Stark P. Pictorial essay. Postpneumonectomy complications. *AJR Am J Roentgenol* 1997;169:1363–1370.

191. Biondetti PR, Fiore D, Sartori F, Colognato A, Ravaseni S. Evaluation of the post-pneumonectomy space by computed tomography. *J Comput Assist Tomogr* 1982;6:238–242.

192. Glazer HS, Aronberg DJ, Sagel SS, Bahman E. Utility of CT in detecting postpneumonectomy carcinoma recurrence. *AJR Am J Roentgenol* 1984;142:487–494.

193. Peters JC, Desai KK. CT demonstration of postpneumonectomy tumor recurrence. *AJR Am J Roentgenol* 1983;141:259–262.

194. Heater K, Revzani L, Rubin JM. CT evaluation of empyema in the postpneumonectomy space. *AJR Am J Roentgenol* 1985;145:39–40.

195. Shepard J-AO, Grillo HC, McLoud TC, Dedrick CG, Spirzarny DL. Right-pneumonectomy syndrome: radiologic findings and CT correlation. *Radiology* 1986;161:661–664.

196. Laissy J-P, Rebibo G, Iba-Zizen M-T, Cabanis EA, Benozio M. MR appearance of the normal chest after pneumonectomy. *J Comput Assist Tomogr* 1989;13:248–252.

197. Leung AN, Müller NL, Miller RR. CT in differential diagnosis of diffuse pleural disease. *AJR Am J Roentgenol* 1990;154:487–492.

198. Robinson LA, Reilly RB. Localized pleural mesothelioma. The clinical spectrum. *Chest* 1994;106:1611–1615.

199. Lee KS, Im JG, Choe KO, Kim CJ, Lee BH. CT findings in benign fibrous mesothelioma of the pleura: pathologic correlation in nine patients. *AJR Am J Roentgenol* 1992;158:983–986.

200. Mendelson DS, Meary E, Buy JN, Pigeau I, Kirshner PA. Localized fibrous pleural mesothelioma; CT findings. *Clin Imaging* 1991;15: 105–108.

201. Okike N, Bernatz PE, Woolner LB. Localized mesothelioma of the pleura. *J Thorac Cardiovasc Surg* 1978;75:363–372.

202. Briselli M, Mark EJ, Dickersin GR. Solitary fibrous tumors of the pleura: eight new cases and review of 60 cases in the literature. *Cancer* 1981;47:2678–2689.

203. Destouet JM, Gilula LA, Murphy WA, Sagel SS. Computed tomography of the sternoclavicular joint and sternum. *Radiology* 1981;138: 123–128.

204. Goodman LR, Teplick SK, Kay H. Computed tomography of the normal sternum. *AJR Am J Roentgenol* 1983;141:219–223.

205. Goodman LR, Kay HR, Teplick SK, Mundth ED. Complications of median sternotomy: computed tomographic evaluation. *AJR Am J Roentgenol* 1983;141:225–230.

206. Hatfield MK, Gross BH, Glazer GM, Martel W. Computed tomography of the sternum and its articulations. *Skeletal Radiol* 1984;11: 197–203.

207. Stark P, Jaramillo D. Pictorial essay. CT of the sternum. *AJR Am J Roentgenol* 1986;147:72–77.

208. Stark P, Watkins GE, Hildebrandt-Stark HE, Dunbar RD. Episternal ossicles. *Radiology* 1987;165:143–144.

209. Jafri SZ, Roberts JL, Bree RL, Tubor HD. Computed tomography of chest wall masses. *RadioGraphics* 1989;9:51–68.

210. Carter AR, Sostman HD, Curtis AM, Swett HA. Thoracic alterations after cardiac surgery. *AJR Am J Roentgenol* 1983;140:475–481.

211. Leitman BS, Naidich DP, McCauley SI. Computed tomography of pectoral flaps. *J Comput Assist Tomogr* 1988;12:392–393.

212. Aoki J, Mosser RP, Kransdork MJ. Chondrosarcoma of the sternum: CT features. *J Comput Assist Tomogr* 1989;13:806–810.

213. Levinsohn EM, Bunnell WP, Wuan HA. Computed tomography in the diagnosis of dislocations of the sternoclavicular joint. *Clin Orthop* 1979;140:12–16.

214. Burnstein MI, Pozniak A. Case report: Computed tomography with stress maneuver to demonstrate sternoclavicular joint dislocation. *J Comput Assist Tomogr* 1990;14:159–160.

215. Sartoris DJ, Schreiman JS, Kerr R, Resnick CS, Resnick D. Sternoclavicular hyperostosis; a review and report of 11 cases. *Radiology* 1986; 158:125–128.

216. Rafii M, Firooznia H, Golimbu C. Computed tomography of septic joints. *CT* 1985;9:51–60.

217. Alexander PW, Shin MS. CT manifestations of sternoclavicular pyarthrosis in patients with intravenous drug abuse. *J Comput Assist Tomogr* 1990;14:104–106.

218. Pollack MS. Staphylococcal mediastinitis due to sternoclavicular pyarthrosis: CT appearance. *J Comput Assist Tomogr* 1990;14:924–928.

219. Gautard R, Dusssault RG, Chahlaoui J, Duranceau A, Sylvestsre J. Contribution of CT in thoracic bony lesions. *J Can Assoc Radiol* 1981; 32:39–41.

220. Gouliamos AD, Carter BL, Emami B. Computed tomography of the chest wall. *Radiology* 1980;134:433–436.

221. Bhalla M, McCauley DI, Golimbu C, Leitman BS, Naidich DP. Counting ribs on chest CT. *J Comput Assist Tomogr* 1990;14:590–594.

222. Fishman EK, Zinreich ES, Jacobs CG, Rostock REA, Siegelman SS. CT of the axilla: normal anatomy and pathology. *RadioGraphics* 1986;6:475–502.

223. Goldberg RP, Austin RM. Computed tomography of axillary and supraclavicular adenopathy. *Clin Radiol* 1985;36:593–596.

224. Holbert BL, Holbert JM, Libshitz HI. CT of interpectoral lymph nodes. *AJR Am J Roentgenol* 1987;149:687–688.

225. Scatarige JC, Boxen I, Smathers RL. Interal mammary lymphadenopathy: imaging of a vital lymphatic pathway in breast cancer. *RadioGraphics* 1990;10:857–870.

226. Scatarige JC, Fishman EK, Zinreich ES, Brem RF, Almaraz R. Internal mammary lymphadenopathy in breast cancinoma: CT appraisal of anatomic distribution. *Radiology* 1988;167:89–91.

227. Shea WJ, de Geer G, Webb WR. Chest wall after mastectomy. Part 1. CT appearance of normal postoperative anatomy, postirradiation changes and optimal scanning techniques. *Radiology* 1987;162: 157–161.

228. Shea WJ, de Geer G, Webb WR. Chest wall after mastectomy. Part 2. CT appearance of tumor recurrence. *Radiology* 1987;162:162–164.

229. Lindfors KK, Meyer JE, Busse PM, Kopans DB, Munzenrider JE, Sawicka JM. Evaluation of local and regional breast cancer recurrence. *AJR Am J Roentgenol* 1985;145:833–837.

230. Leitman BS, Firooznia H, McCauley DI, et al. The use of computed tomography in the evaluation of chest wall pathology. *J Comput Tomogr* 1983;7:399–405.

231. Hudson TM, Vandergriend RA, Springfield DS, et al. Aggressive fibromatosis: evaluation by computed tomography and angiography. *Radiology* 1984;150:495–501.

232. Berthoty DP, Shulman HS, Miller HAB. Elasatofibroma: chest wall pseudotumor. *Radiology* 1986;1986:341–342.

233. Marin ML, Austin JHM, Markowitz AM. Elastofibroma dorsi: CT demonstration. *J Comput Assist Tomogr* 1987;11:675–677.

234. Faer MJ, Burnam RE, Beck CL. Transmural thoracic lipoma: demonstration by computed tomography. *AJR Am J Roentgenol* 1978;130:161–163.

235. Sullivan WT. Extrapleural fat prolapse mimicking recurrent bronchogenic carcinoma. *CT* 1986;10:277–279.

236. Buxton RC, Tan CS, Khine NM, et al. Atypical transmural thoracic lipoma: CT diagnosis. *J Comput Assist Tomogr* 1988;12:196–198.

237. Biondetti PR, Fiore D, Perin B, Ravasini R. Infiltrative angiolipoma of the thoracoabdominal wall. *J Comput Assist Tomogr* 1982;6:847.

238. Wilinsky J, Costello P, Clouse ME. Liposarcoma involving the scapula. *CT* 1984;8:341–343.

239. Whalen MA, Naidich DP, Post JD, Chase NE. Computed tomography of spinal tuberculosis. *J Computed Assist Tomogr* 1983;7:25–30.

240. Webb WR, Sagel SS. Actinomycosis involving the chest wall: CT findings. *AJR Am J Roentgenol* 1982;139:1007–1009.

241. Allen H, A., Scatarige JC, Kim MH. Actinomycosis: CT findings in six patients. *AJR Am J Roentgenol* 1987;149:1255–1258.

242. James R, Heneghan MA, Lipansky V. Thoracic actinomycosis. *Chest* 1985;87:536–637.

243. Rabinowitz JG, Efremidis SC, Cohen B, et al. A comparative study of mesothelioma and asbestosis using computed tomograpy and conventional chest radiography. *Radiology* 1982;144:453–460.

244. Trigaux J-P, Beers BV. Thoracic collateral venous channels: normal and pathologic CT findings. *J Comput Assist Tomogr* 1990;14:769–773.

245. Yedlicka JW, Schultz K, Moncada R, Flisak M. CT findings in superior vena cava obstruction. *Semin Roentgenol* 1989;24:84–90.

246. Moncada R, Cardella R, Demos TC, et al. Evaluation of superior vena cava syndrome by axial CT and CT phlebography. *AJR Am J Roentgenol* 1984;143:731–736.

247. Bechtold RE, Wolfman NT, Karstaedt N, Choplin RH. Superior vena cava obstruction: detection using CT. *Radiology* 1985;157:485–487.

248. Gerard PS, Lefkovitz Z, Golbey SH, Bryk D. Transient thoracic venous collaterals: an incidental CT finding. *J Comput Assist Tomogr* 1986;10:75–77.

249. Engel IA, Auh YH, Rubenstien WA, Sniderman K, Whalen JP, Kazam E. CT diagnosis of mediastinal and thoracic inlet venous obstruction. *AJR Am J Roentgenol* 1983;141:521–526.

250. Gosselin MV, Rubin GD. Altered intravascular contrast material flow dynamics: clues for refining thoracic CT diagnosis. *Am J Roentgenol* 1997;169:1597–1603.

251. Toombs BD, Sandler LM, Lester RG. Computed tomography of chest trauma. *Radiology* 1981;140:733–738.

252. Wall SD, Federle MP, Jeffrey RB, Brett CM. CT diagnosis of unsuspected pneumothorax after blunt abdominal trauma. *AJR Am J Roentgenol* 1983;141:919–921.

253. Tocino IM, Miller WH, Freerick PR, Bahr AL, Thomas F. CT detection of occult pneumothorax in head trauma. *AJR Am J Roentgenol* 1984;143:987–990.

254. Murphy FB, Small WC, Wichman RD, Chalif M, Bernardino ME. CT and chest radiography are equally sensitive in the detection of pneumothorax after CT-guided pulmonary interventional procedures. *AJR Am J Roentgenol* 1990;154:45–46.

255. Vargas FC, Vas W, Carlin B, Morris L, Salimi Z. Case report. Radiographic and CT demonstration of mammary emphysema. *J Comput Assist Tomogr* 1985;9:560–562.

256. Wagner RB, Crawford WO Jr, Schimpf PP. Classification of parenchymal injuries of the lung. *Radiology* 1988;167:77–82.

257. Mirvis SE, Rodriguez A, Whitley NO, Tarr RJ. CT evaluation of thoracic infections after major trauma. *AJR Am J Roentgenol* 1985;144:1183–1187.

258. Sivit CJ, Taylor GA, Eichelberger MR. Chest injury in children with blunt abdominal trauma; evaluation with CT. *Radiology* 1989;171:815–818.

259. Kerns SB, Gay SB. Pictorial essay. CT of blunt chest trauma. *AJR Am J Roentgenol* 1990;154:55–60.

260. Nguyen TH, Hoang T-A, Dash N, et al. Latissimus dorsi cardiomyoplasty: radiographic findings. *AJR Am J Roentgenol* 1988;150:545–547.

261. Seibel DG, Hopper KD, Ghaed N. Case report. Mammographic and CT detection of extrathoracic lung herniation. *J Comput Assist Tomogr* 1987;11:537–538.

262. Wolfman NT, Gilpin JW, Bechtold RE, Meredith JW, Ditesheim JA. Occult pneumothorax in patients with abdominal trauma: CT studies. *J Comput Assist Tomogr* 1993;17:56–59.

263. Bhalla M, Leitman BS, Forcade C, et al. Lung hernia: radiographic features. *AJR Am J Roentgenol* 1990;154:51–53.

264. Brown JJ, van Sonnenberg E, Gerber KH, Strich G, Wittich GR, Slutsky RA. Magnetic resonance relaxation times of percutaneously obtained normal and abnormal body fluids. *Radiology* 1985;727–731.

265. Terrier F, Revel D, Pajannen H, et al. MR imaging of body fluid collections. *J Comput Assist Tomogr* 1986;10:953–962.

266. Davis SD, Henschke CI, Yankelevitz DF, Cahill PT, Yi Y. MR imaging of pleural effusions. *J Comput Assist Tomogr* 1990;14:192–198.

267. Lorigan JG, Libshitz HI. MR imaging of malignant pleural mesothelioma. *J Comput Assist Tomogr* 1989;13:617–620.

268. Vogel HJP, Wondergem JHM, Falke THM. Mesothelioma of the pericardium; CT and MR findings. *J Compu Assist Tomogr* 1989;13:543–546.

269. Webb RW, Gatsonois C, Zerhouni EA, et al. CT and MR in staging non-small cell bronchogenic carcinoma: Report of the Radiological Diagnostic Oncology Group. *Radiology* 1989;173(P):69.

270. Dooms GC, Hricak H, Solitto RA, Higgins CB. Lipomatous tumors and tumors with fatty component: MR imaging potential and comparison of MR and CT results. *Radiology* 1985;157:479–483.

271. Sharif HS, Clark DC, Aabed MY, et al. MR imaging of thoracic and abdominal wall infections: comparison with other imaging procedures. *AJR Am J Roentgenol* 1990;154:989–995.

272. Blari DN, Rapoport S, Sostman HD, Blair OC. Normal brachial plexus: MR imaging. *Radiology* 1987;165:763–767.

273. Rapoport S, Blair DN, McCarthy SM, et al. Brachial plexus: correlation of MR imaging with CT and pathologic findings. *Radiology* 1988;167:161–165.

274. Castagno AA, Shuman WP. MR imaging in clinically suspected brachial plexus tumors. *AJR Am J Roentgenol* 1987;149:1219–1222.

275. Panicek DM, Benson CB, Gottlieb RH, Heitzman ER. The diaphragm: anatomic, pathologic, and radiologic considerations. *RadioGraphics* 1988;8:385–425.

276. De Troyer A, Sampson M, Sigrist S, et al. The diaphragm: two muscles. *Science* 1981;213:237–238.

277. Patterson NW, Teates CD. CT measurements of the anterior portions of the diaphragm with illustrative abnormal cases. *Comput Radiol* 1985;9:61–65.

278. Kleinman PK, Raptopoulos V. The anterior diaphragmatic attachments: an anatomic and radiologic study with clinical correlates. *Radiology* 1985;155:289–293.

279. Gale EM. Anterior diaphragm: variations in the CT appearance. *Radiology* 1986;161:635–639.

280. Naidich DP, Megibow AJ, Ross CR, Beranbaum ER, Siegelman SS. Computed tomography of the diaphragm: normal anatomy and variants. *J Comput Assist Tomogr* 1983;7:633–640.

281. Shin MS, Berland LL. Computed tomography of retrocrural spaces: normal, anatomic variants, and pathologic conditions. *AJR Am J Roentgenol* 1985;145:81–86.

282. Silverman PM, Cooper C, Zeman RK. Lateral arcuate ligaments of the diaphragm: anatomic variations at abdominal CT. *Radiology* 1992;185:105–108.

283. Vibhakar SD, Bellon EM. The bare area of the spleen: a constant CT feature of the ascitic abdomen. *AJR Am J Roentgenol* 1984;141:953–955.

284. Callen PWQ, Filly RA, Korobkin M. Computed tomographic evaluation of the diaphragmatic crura. *Radiology* 1978;126:413–416.

285. Williamson BR, Gouse JC, Rohrer DG, Teates CD. Variation in the thickness of the diaphragmatic crura with respiration. *Radiology* 1987;163:683–684.

286. Nightingale RC, Dixon AK. Crural change with respiration: a potential mimic of disease. *Br J Radiol* 1984;57:101–102.

287. Anda S, Roysland P, Fougner R, Stovring J. CT appearance of the diaphragm varying with respiratory phase and muscular tension. *J Comput Assist Tomogr* 1986;10:744–745.

288. Caskey CI, Zerhouni EA, Fishman EK, Rahmouni AD. Aging of the diaphragm: a CT study. *Radiology* 1989;171:385–389.

289. Rosen A, Auh YH, Rubenstein WA, et al. CT appearance of diaphragmatic pseudotumors. *J Comput Assist Tomogr* 1983;7:995–999.

290. Silverman PM, Baker ME, Mahoney BS. Atelectasis and subpulmonic fluid: a CT pitfall in distinguishing pleural from peritoneal fluid. *J Comput Assist Tomogr* 1985;9:763–766.

291. Demartini WJ, House AJS. Partial Bochdalek's herniation: computerized tomographic evaluation. *Chest* 1980;77:702–704.

292. Gale ME. Bochdalek hernia: prevalence and CT characteristics. *Radiology* 1985;156:449–452.

293. Curley FJ, Hubmayr RD, Raptopoulos V. Bilateral diaphragmatic densities in a 72 year old woman. *Chest* 1984;86:915–917.

294. Weinshelbaum AM, Weinshelbaum EI. Incarcerated adult Bochdalek hernia with splenic infarction. *Gastrointest Radiol* 1982;7:287–289.

295. Fagelman D, Caridi JG. CT diagnosis of hernia of Morgagni. *Gastroinest Radiol* 1984;9:153–155.

296. Wiencek RG, Wilson RF, Steiger Z. Acute injuries of the diaphragm. An analysis of 165 cases. *J Thorac Cardiovasc Surg* 92;92:989–993.

297. Hegarty MM, Bryer JV, Angorn IB, Baker LW. Delayed presentation of traumatic diaphragmatic hernia. *Ann Surg* 1978;188:229–233.

298. Degiannis E, Levy RD, Sofianos C, et al. Diaphragmatic herniation after penetrating trauma. *Br J Surg* 1996;83:88–91.

299. Heiberg E, Wolverson MK, Hurd RN, B. J-L, Sundaram M. Case report: CT recognition of traumatic rupture of the diaphragm. *AJR Am J Roentgenol* 1980;1980:369–392.

300. Lee WC, Chen RJ, Fang JF, et al. Rupture of the diaphragm after blunt trauma. *Eur J Surg* 1994;160:479–483.

301. Aronchick JM, Epstein DM, Gefter WB, Miller WT. Chronic traumatic diaphragmatic hernia: the significance of pleural effusion. *Radiology* 1988;168:675–678.

302. Radin DR, Ray MJ, Halls JM. Strangulated diaphragmatic hernia with pneumothorax. *AJR Am J Roentgenol* 1986;146:321–322.

303. Demos TC, Solomon C, Posniak HV, Flisak MJ. Computed tomography in traumatic defects of the diaphragm. *Clin Imag* 1989;13:62–67.

304. Leekam RN, Ilves R, Shankar L. Case report. Inversion of gall-bladder secondary to traumatic herniation of liver: CT findings. *J Comput Assist Tomogr* 1987;11:163–164.

305. Gurney J, Harrison WL, Anderson JC. Omental fat simulating pleural fluid in traumatic diaphragmatic hernia: CT characteristics. *J Comput Assist Tomogr* 1985;9:1112–1114.

306. Shapiro MJ, Heiberg E, Durham RM, Luchtfeld W, Mazuski JE. The unreliability of CT scans and initial chest radiogrpahs in evaluating blunt trauma induced diaphragmatic rupture. *Clin Radiol* 1995;51:27–30.

307. Shah R, Sabanathan S, Mearns AJ, Choudhury AK. Traumatic rupture of diaphragm. *Ann Thorac Surg* 1995;60:1444–1449.

308. Worthy SA, Kang EY, Hartman TE, Kwong JS, Mayo JR, Müller NL. Diaphragmatic rupture: CT findings in 11 patients. *Radiology* 1995;194:885–888.

309. Murray JG, Caoili E, Gruden JF, Evans SJJ, Halvorsen RA, Mackersie RC. Acute rupture of the diaphragm due to blunt trauma: Diagnostic sensitivity and specificity of CT. *Am J Roentgenol* 1996;166:1035–1039.

310. Shackleton KL, Stewart ET, Tahylor AJ. Traumatic diaphragmatic injuries: spectrum of radiographic findings. *Radiographics* 1998;18:49–59.

311. Mirvis SE, Keramati B, Buckman R, Rodriguez A. Case report. MR imaging of traumatic diaphragmatic rupture. *J Comput Assist Tomogr* 1988;12:147–149.

312. Naidich DP, Megibow AJ, Hilton S, Hulnick DH, Siegelman SS. Computed tomography of the diaphragm: peridiaphragmatic fluid localization. *J Comput Assist Tomogr* 1983;7:641–649.

313. Dwyer A. The displaced crus: a sign for distinguishing between pleural fluid and ascites on computed tomography. *J Comput Assist Tomogr* 1978;2:598–599.

314. Teplick JG, Teplick SK, Goodman L, Haskin ME. The interface sign: a computed tomographic sign for distinguishing pleural and intraabdominal fluid. *Radiology* 1982;144:359–362.

315. Alexander ES, Proto AU, Clark RA. CT differentiation of subphrenic abscess and pleural effusion. *AJR Am J Roentgenol* 1983;140:47–51.

316. Halvorsen RA, Jones MA, Rice RP, Thompson WM. Anterior left subphrenic abscess: characteristic plain film and CT appearance. *AJR Am J Roentgenol* 1982;139:283–289.

317. Halvorsen RA, Fedyshin PJ, Korobkin M, Foster WL, Thompson WM. Ascites or pleural effusion? CT differentiation: four useful criteria. *RadioGraphics* 1986;6:135–149.

318. Meyers MA. *Dynamic radiology of the abdomen: normal and pathologic anatomy.* 2nd ed. New York: Springer-Verlag, 1982.

319. Rubenstein WA, Auh YH, Whalen JP, Kazam E. The perihepatic spaces: computed tomographic and ultrasound imaging. *Radiology* 1985;149:231–239.

320. Dodds WJ, Foley WD, Lawson TL, Stewart ET, Taylor A. Anatomy and imaging of the lesser peritoneal sac. *AJR Am J Roentgenol* 1985;14:567–575.

321. Rosen A, Korobkin M, Silverman P, Moore AJ, Jr., Dunnick NR. CT diagnosis of ruptured abdominal aortic aneurysms. *AJR Am J Roentgenol* 1984;143:262–268.

322. Hopper KD, Sherman JL, Ghaed N. Aortic rupture into retroperitoneum (letter). *AJR Am J Roentgenol* 1985;145:435–437.

323. Katzen BT, Choi WS, Friedman MH, Green IJ, Hindle WV, Zellis A. Pseudo-mass of the liver due to pleural effusion and inversion of the diaphragm. *AJR Am J Roentgenol* 1978;131:1077–1078.

324. Dallemand S, Twersky J, Gordon DH. Pseudomass of the left upper quadrant from inversion of the left hemidiaphragm: CT diagnosis. *Gastrointest Radiol* 1982;7:57–59.

325. Thompson WM, Halvorsen RA, Williford ME, Foster WL, Korobkin M. Computed tomography of the gastroesophageal junction. *RadioGraphics* 1982;2:179–193.

326. Govoni AF, Whalen JP, Kazam E. Hiatal hernia: a relook. *RadioGraphics* 1983;3:612–644.

327. Ginalski JM, Schnyder P, Moss AA. Incidence and significance of a widened esophageal hiatus at CT scan. *J Clin Gastroenterol* 1984;6:467–470.

328. Godwin JD, MacGregor JM. Case report: Extension of ascites into the chest with hiatal hernia: visualization on CT. *AJR Am J Roentgenol* 1987;148:31–32.

329. Clark KE, Foley WD, Lawson TL, Berland LL, Maddison FE. CT evaluation of esophageal and upper abdominal varices. *J Compu Assist Tomogr* 1980;4:510–515.

330. Balthazar EJ, Naidich DP, Megibow AJ, Lefleur RS. CT evaluation of esophageal varices. *AJR Am J Roentgenol* 1987;148:131–135.

331. Han SY, McElvein RB, Aldrete JS. Perforation of the esophagus: correlation of site and cause with plain film findings. *AJR Am J Roentgenol* 1985;145:537–540.

332. Glenny RW, Fulkerson WJ, Ravin CE. Occult spontaneous esophageal peforation. Unusual clinical and radiographic presentation. *Chest* 1987;92:562–565.

333. Pezzulli FA, Aronson D, Goldberg N. Case report. Computed tomography of mediastinal hematoma secondary to unusual esophageal laceration: a Boerhaave variant. *J Comput Assist Tomogr* 1989;13:129–131.

334. Raval B, Hall JT, Jackson H. Case report. CT diagnosis of fluid in the lesser sac mimicking thrombosis of inferior vena cava. *J Comput Assist Tomogr* 1985;9:956–958.

335. Müller NL. Case report. CT features of cystic teratoma of the diaphragm. *J Comput Assist Tomogr* 1986;10:325–326.

336. Yeager BA, Guglielmi GE, Schiebler ML, Gefter WB, Kressler HY. Magnetic resonance imaging of Morgagnai hernia. *Gastrointest Radiol* 1987;12:296–298.

337. Winsett MZ, Amparo EG, Fagan CJ, Bedi DG, Gallagher P, Nealon WH. Case report. MR imaging of mediastinal pseudocyst. *J Comput Assist Tomogr* 1988;12:320–322.

338. Posniak HV, Keshavarzian A, Jabamoni R. Diaphragmatic endometriosis: CT and MR findings. *Gastrointest Radiol* 1990;15:349–351.

Subject Index

halo sign in, 298–299, 299f
MR evaluation of, 299, 300f
in non-AIDS immunocompromised
patient, 445–446, 445f, 446f
pulmonary embolism vs., 634f
pulmonary nodules in, 400, 401f
Aspiration
transbronchial. *See* Transbronchial
needle aspiration/biopsy
transthoracic, of solitary pulmonary
nodule, 332–334, 333f, 336
Atelectasis
adhesive, 247, 247f, 250
causes of, 228
cicatrization, 237–242, 242f–245f
compression (passive), 242–247, 245f,
246f, 673f, 683
CT evaluation of, 228–247
left upper lobe
cicatrization, 243f
compression, 246f
CT-MR correlation in, 248f
obstructive, 232–236, 232f, 236f,
237f, 240f
lingular
compression, 246f
obstructive, 236
lower lobe
compression, 245f, 246f
MR evaluation of, 249f
obstructive, 232f, 237, 239f, 240f
middle lobe
cicatrization, 244f
compression, 246f
obstructive, 232f, 234f–235f,
236–237, 238f–239f
MR evaluation of, 247–250, 248f, 249f
nonobstructive, 237–247
causes of, 241t
on MRI, 32f, 33, 34t
obstructive (resorption), 228–237
CT appearance of, 230–237,
231f–241f, 232t
mechanisms and causes of, 228–230,
229t
MRI appearance of, 33, 33f, 34t
nonobstructive vs., MR
differentiation of, 455
right upper lobe
cicatrization, 242f, 245f
obstructive, 230–232, 232f–235f
round, 693–696, 694f–696f
superior segment, obstructive, 237,
240f
Atelectatic pseudotumor (round
atelectasis), 693–696, 694f–696f
Atheromas, aortic, 565–567, 567f
Atherosclerosis
aortic aneurysm with, 539–541, 541f,
543, 546f, 548f
penetrating aortic ulcer in, 554–556,
556f–559f, 561f
Attenuation
decreased
in bronchiolar disease, 272t,
278–280, 278f, 279f
in diffuse lung disease, 403–406,
406f

ground-glass. *See* Ground-glass
attenuation
of lung, 395
in mediastinal mass differential
diagnosis, 54–57
mosaic. *See* Mosaic perfusion
Autolobectomy, due to cicatrization, 241
Autopneumonectomy
due to cicatrization, 241
CT of, curved reconstruction of,
167f–168f
Axilla, 715–722, 717f–723f
boundaries of, 715–720, 717f
CT anatomy of, 717f–720f, 720
Axillary artery, 720
Axillary lymph nodes, 720
Axillary vein, 720
Azygoesophageal recess, 51–53, 52f, 203,
203f
masses involving, 57t
Azygos arch, 50f, 51, 581, 581f, 583f,
586f
Azygos continuation, 586f, 587, 587f
Azygos fissure, 663–666, 666f
Azygos lobe, 663–666, 666f
Azygos lymph node, 90
Azygos vein, 51f, 52f, 53, 581, 581f,
583f–585f
prominent, bronchial wall thickening
vs., 202

B
Bacillary angiomatosis, in AIDS,
488–489
Bacterial infections. *See also specific
infections*
in AIDS, 469–472, 470f–473f
CD4 lymphocyte level and, 466
Pneumocystis pneumonia vs.,
467–468, 467f
Balloon angioplasty, for coarctation of the
aorta, 533
Bare area sign, in peridiaphragmatic fluid
localization, 739, 740, 740f, 741
Bartonella henselae infection, in AIDS,
488–489
Basal cell carcinoma, of chest wall, 723f
Basilar zone of chest, 161, 163f
Bayesian analysis, in assessing CT
characteristics of solitary
pulmonary nodules, 331–332
Behçet's disease, pulmonary artery
aneurysm in, 646
Biopsy
in diffuse lung disease, 451–454, 452f
percutaneous needle, CT planning and
guidance of, 16–18
pleural, CT-guided, 17, 18, 710f
for malignant mesothelioma
diagnosis, 700–701
in solitary pulmonary nodule
assessment, 332–334, 333f, 335f,
336
transbronchial. *See* Transbronchial
needle aspiration/biopsy
Bird breeder's lung. *See* Hypersensitivity
pneumonitis

Black blood imaging, in MR angiography,
28, 512–513
Bleomycin, pulmonary fibrosis due to,
438
Bochdalek's hernia, 124, 734–735, 735f
Boerhaave's syndrome, 142f, 143
Bone marrow transplantation
obliterative bronchiolitis after, 278,
279f
pulmonary complications of, 443f,
444–445, 446f, 453
BOOP. *See* Bronchiolitis obliterans, with
organizing pneumonia
Brachial plexus, MR evaluation of, 728
Brachiocephalic artery, 519
Brachiocephalic veins, 43, 46f–47f, 581,
582f–584f
MRI of, 591–594
obstruction of, 584f
Brain metastases, from lung cancer, MR
evaluation of, 371–372
Breast cancer
lymph node involvement in, 90f, 116
pleural involvement in, 674f, 696, 704f,
705f
pulmonary nodule due to, 295f
recurrent, axilla and chest wall
assessment in, 720–722, 721f
thymic involvement in, 76
Bronchial arteries, 615
Bronchial dilatation, in bronchiectasis,
252–256, 256t
Bronchial stricture
lobar atelectasis due to, 229
after transplantation, 181
CT display of, 169f, 174
Bronchial tapering, lack of, in
bronchiectasis, 253f, 254–256,
256f, 257f
Bronchial tumor. *See* Endobronchial
tumor
Bronchial wall thickening, in
bronchiectasis, 256, 256t, 258f
Bronchiectasis, 250–270
in allergic bronchopulmonary
aspergillosis, 267–270, 268f, 269f
in atypical mycobacterial infection,
266–267, 266f
bronchial dilatation in, 252–256, 256t
bronchial wall thickening in, 256, 256t,
258f
bronchographic findings in, 251
causes of, 250–251, 250t, 266–270
central, allergic bronchopulmonary
aspergillosis and, 268, 268f
classification of, 251, 253f
CT technique in, 254f–255f, 257f,
262–263
cylindric, 253f
cystic, 253f
in cystic fibrosis, 267
diagnostic criteria for, on CT,
251–259, 256t
expiratory scanning in, 254f, 263
hemoptysis and, 281–282, 282t
lack of bronchial tapering in, 253f,
254–256, 256f, 257f